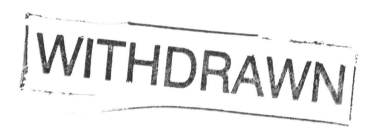

SIDE EFFECTS OF DRUGS ANNUAL

VOLUME 39

SIDE EFFECTS OF DRUGS ANNUAL

VOLUME 39

A Worldwide Yearly Survey of New Data
in Adverse Drug Reactions

Editor

SIDHARTHA D. RAY, PHD., FACN

Manchester University College of Pharmacy, Natural and Health Sciences, USA

ELSEVIER

Elsevier
Radarweg 29, PO Box 211, 1000 AE Amsterdam, Netherlands
The Boulevard, Langford Lane, Kidlington, Oxford OX5 1GB, United Kingdom
50 Hampshire Street, 5th Floor, Cambridge, MA 02139, United States

First edition 2017

Notices
Knowledge and best practice in this field are constantly changing. As new research and experience broaden our understanding, changes in research methods, professional practices, or medical treatment may become necessary.

Practitioners and researchers must always rely on their own experience and knowledge in evaluating and using any information, methods, compounds, or experiments described herein. In using such information or methods they should be mindful of their own safety and the safety of others, including parties for whom they have a professional responsibility.

To the fullest extent of the law, neither the Publisher nor the authors, contributors, or editors, assume any liability for any injury and/or damage to persons or property as a matter of products liability, negligence or otherwise, or from any use or operation of any methods, products, instructions, or ideas contained in the material herein.

ISBN: 978-0-444-63948-6
ISSN: 0378-6080

For information on all Elsevier publications visit our
website at https://www.elsevier.com/books-and-journals

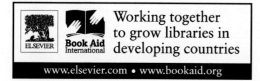

Working together
to grow libraries in
developing countries

www.elsevier.com • www.bookaid.org

Publisher: Zoe Kruze
Acquisition Editor: Zoe Kruze
Editorial Project Manager: Shellie Bryant
Production Project Manager: Surya Narayanan Jayachandran
Cover Designer: Victoria Pearson

Typeset by SPi Global, India

Contributors

Sara Al-Dahir   College of Pharmacy, Xavier University of Louisiana, New Orleans, LA, United States

Asima N. Ali   Campbell University College of Pharmacy and Health Sciences, Buies Creek; Wake Forest Baptist Health, Internal Medicine Clinic, Winston-Salem, NC, United States

Jennifer L. Babin   University of Utah College of Pharmacy, Salt Lake City, UT, United States

Mario V. Beccari   School of Pharmacy and Pharmaceutical Sciences, State University of New York at Buffalo, Buffalo, NY, United States

Tina C. Beck   University of the Incarnate Word Feik School of Pharmacy, San Antonio, TX, United States

Robert D. Beckett   Manchester University College of Pharmacy, Natural and Health Sciences, Fort Wayne, IN, United States

Renee A. Bellanger   Feik School of Pharmacy, University of the Incarnate Word, San Antonio, TX, United States

Nicholas T. Bello   School of Environmental and Biological Sciences, Rutgers, The State University of New Jersey, New Brunswick, NJ, United States

Matthew Bessesen   Manchester University College of Pharmacy, Natural and Health Sciences, Fort Wayne, IN, United States

Adrienne T. Black   3E Company, Warrenton, VA, United States

Alison Brophy   Overlook Medical Center, Summit, NJ, United States

Kezia Brown   University of Utah College of Pharmacy, Salt Lake City, UT, United States

Rebecca A. Buckler   Jefferson Health—Methodist Hospital Division, Philadelphia, PA, United States

Maria Cardinale   Ernest Mario School of Pharmacy, Rutgers, The State University of New Jersey, Piscataway; Saint Peter's University Hospital, New Brunswick, NJ, United States

Pierre S. Chue   Canadian Consortium for Early Intervention in Psychosis, University of Alberta, Edmonton, AB, Canada

Joy Creaser-Thomas   Institute of Life Science 1, Swansea University, Swansea, United Kingdom

Medhane G. Cumbay   Marian University College of Osteopathic Medicine, Indianapolis, IN, United States

Kendra M. Damer   Butler University College of Pharmacy and Health Sciences, Indianapolis, IN, United States

Gwyneth A. Davies   School of Medicine, Swansea University, Swansea, United Kingdom

Jon F. Davis   Washington State University, Pullman, WA, United States

Rahul Deshmukh   College of Pharmacy, Rosalind Franklin University of Medicine and Science, North Chicago, IL, United States

Sujana Dontukurthy   New York Presbyterian—Brooklyn Methodist Hospital, Brooklyn, NY, United States

Shadi Doroudgar   Touro University California College of Pharmacy, Vallejo, CA, United States

Tyler S. Dougherty   South College School of Pharmacy, Knoxville, TN, United States

Haley Ethredge   PCOM School of Pharmacy, Suwanee, GA, United States

Kirk Evoy   College of Pharmacy, University of Texas at Austin, Austin, TX, United States

Jingyang Fan   SIUE School of Pharmacy, Edwardsville, IL, United States

Joanna Fawkner-Corbett   Royal Liverpool Hospital, Liverpool, Merseyside, United Kingdom

Rozette Fawzy   Manchester University College of Pharmacy, Natural and Health Sciences, Fort Wayne, IN, United States

Hannah R. Fudin   University of Utah College of Pharmacy, Salt Lake City, UT, United States

Jason C. Gallagher   Temple University, Philadelphia, PA, United States

Jason A. Garcia-Trevino   University of the Incarnate Word Feik School of Pharmacy, San Antonio, TX, United States

Nathan T. Goad   Wake Forest Baptist Health, Internal Medicine Clinic, Winston-Salem, NC, United States

Tatsya Gomi   Ohashi Medical Center, Toho University, Tokyo, Japan

David L. Gordon   Flinders Medical Centre, Adelaide, South Australia, Australia

Joshua P. Gray   United States Coast Guard Academy, New London, CT, United States

Holly Gurgle   University of Utah College of Pharmacy, Salt Lake City, UT, United States

Alison Hall   Royal Liverpool Hospital, Liverpool, Merseyside, United Kingdom

Alisyn L. Hansen University of Utah College of Pharmacy, Salt Lake City, UT, United States

Makoto Hasegawa Ohashi Medical Center, Toho University, Tokyo, Japan

Sandra Hrometz College of Pharmacy, Natural and Health Sciences, Manchester University, Fort Wayne, IN, United States

Jason Isch Graduate Medical Education, Saint Joseph Health System, Mishawaka, IN, United States

Carrie M. Jung Butler University College of Pharmacy and Health Sciences; Butler University, Eskenazi Health, Indianapolis, IN, United States

Allison Kalstein New York Presbyterian—Brooklyn Methodist Hospital, Brooklyn, NY, United States

Justin B. Kaplan Rutgers, The State University of New Jersey, Piscataway; Hackensack University Medical Center, Hackensack, NJ, United States

Jennifer J. Kim Greensboro Area Health Education Center, Greensboro; University of North Carolina Eshelman School of Pharmacy, Chapel Hill, NC, United States

Nora Klemke Lutheran Health Network, Fort Wayne, IN, United States

Justin G. Kullgren The Ohio State University Wexner Medical Center, Columbus, OH, United States

Dirk W. Lachenmeier Chemisches und Veterinäruntersuchungsamt (CVUA) Karlsruhe, Karlsruhe, Germany

Dustin Linn Manchester University College of Pharmacy, Natural, and Heath Sciences, Fort Wayne, IN, United States

Carrie M. Maffeo Butler University College of Pharmacy and Health Sciences, Indianapolis, IN, United States

Tamara Malm Yale-New Haven Hospital, New Haven; University of Saint Joseph School of Pharmacy, University of Saint Joseph, West Hartford, CT, United States

Arduino A. Mangoni School of Medicine, Flinders University and Flinders Medical Centre, Bedford Park, SA, Australia

Dianne May University of Georgia College of Pharmacy, Augusta, GA, United States

Cassandra Maynard SIUE School of Pharmacy, Edwardsville, IL, United States

Renee McCafferty Manchester University College of Pharmacy, Natural and Health Sciences, Fort Wayne, IN, United States

Dayna S. McManus Yale-New Haven Hospital, Yale University, New Haven, CT, United States

Calvin J. Meaney School of Pharmacy and Pharmaceutical Sciences, State University of New York at Buffalo, Buffalo, NY, United States

Philip B. Mitchell Black Dog Institute, Sydney, NSW, Australia

Vicky Mody PCOM School of Pharmacy, Suwanee, GA, United States

Irandokht K. Najafabadi PCOM School of Pharmacy, Suwanee, GA, United States

Toshio Nakaki Teikyo University School of Medicine, Tokyo, Japan

John D. Noti National Institute for Occupational Safety and Health, Centers for Disease Control and Prevention, Morgantown, WV, United States

Igho J. Onakpoya University of Oxford, Oxford, United Kingdom

Michael G. O'Neil South College School of Pharmacy, Knoxville, TN, United States

Sreekumar Othumpangat National Institute for Occupational Safety and Health, Centers for Disease Control and Prevention, Morgantown, WV, United States

Kent Owusu Yale-New Haven Hospital, New Haven, CT, United States

Michelle M. Peahota Thomas Jefferson University Hospital, Philadelphia, PA, United States

Mary E. Pisano Novant Health, Winston Salem, NC, United States

Jasmine M. Pittman Parkwest Medical Center, Knoxville, TN, United States

Sarah Quick Manchester University College of Pharmacy, Natural, and Heath Sciences; Lutheran Hospital of Indiana, Fort Wayne, IN, United States

Hanna Raber College of Pharmacy, University of Utah, Salt Lake City, UT, United States

Vignaresh Rajasundaram Abertawe Bro Morgannwg University Health board, Singleton Hospital, Swansea, United Kingdom

Meenakshi R. Ramanathan The University of North Texas Health Science Center System College of Pharmacy, Fort Worth, TX, United States

Brittney A. Ramirez University of the Incarnate Word Feik School of Pharmacy, San Antonio, TX, United States

Sidhartha D. Ray Manchester University College of Pharmacy, Natural and Health Sciences, Fort Wayne, IN, United States

David Reeves College of Pharmacy and Health Sciences, Butler University; St. Vincent Indianapolis Hospital, Indianapolis, IN, United States

Matthew B. Roberts Flinders Medical Centre, Adelaide, South Australia, Australia

James M. Sanders The University of North Texas Health Science Center System College of Pharmacy; JPS Health Network, Fort Worth, TX, United States

Shaun P. Say College of Pharmacy, Natural and Health Sciences, Manchester University, Fort Wayne, IN, United States

Laura A. Schalliol South College School of Pharmacy, Knoxville, TN, United States

Christina M. Seeger Feik School of Pharmacy, University of the Incarnate Word, San Antonio, TX, United States

Ajay Singh South University School of Pharmacy, Savannah, GA, United States

Arno G. Siraki University of Alberta, Edmonton, AB, Canada

Sunil Sirohi Laboratory of Endocrine and Neuropsychiatric Disorders, College of Pharmacy, Xavier University of Louisiana, New Orleans, LA, United States

Anna Smith Laboratory of Endocrine and Neuropsychiatric Disorders, College of Pharmacy, Xavier University of Louisiana, New Orleans, LA, United States

Helen E. Smith Feik School of Pharmacy, University of the Incarnate Word, San Antonio, TX, United States

Jonathan Smithson School of Psychiatry, University of New South Wales, Sydney, NSW, Australia

Lisa V. Stottlemyer Pennsylvania College of Optometry, Elkins Park, PA; Wilmington VA Medical Center, Wilmington, DE, United States

Natalia Suhali-Amacher Manchester University College of Pharmacy, Fort Wayne, IN, United States

Kelan L. Thomas Touro University California College of Pharmacy, Vallejo, CA, United States

Katie Traylor University of Utah College of Pharmacy, Salt Lake City, UT, United States

Emily C. Tucker Flinders Medical Centre, Adelaide, South Australia, Australia

Kyle Turner University of Utah College of Pharmacy, Salt Lake City, UT, United States

Nisha Vithlani Laboratory of Endocrine and Neuropsychiatric Disorders, College of Pharmacy, Xavier University of Louisiana, New Orleans, LA, United States

Kirby Welston University of Georgia College of Pharmacy, Athens, GA, United States

Anna Woods University of Utah College of Pharmacy, Salt Lake City, UT, United States

Joel Yarmush New York Presbyterian—Brooklyn Methodist Hospital, Brooklyn, NY, United States

Matthew R. Zahner East Tennessee State University, Johnson City, TN, United States

Deborah Zeitlin Butler University College of Pharmacy and Health Sciences; Indiana University Health, Indianapolis, IN, United States

Contents

ROBERT D. BECKETT, NORA KLEMKE, MATTHEW BESSESEN, AND SIDHARTHA D. RAY

MICHAEL G. O'NEIL, AND JUSTIN G. KULLGREN

Preface

Side Effects of Drugs: Annual (SEDA) is a yearly publication focused on existing, new and evolving side effects of drugs encountered by a broad range of healthcare professionals including physicians, pharmacists, nurse practitioners and advisors of poison control centres. This 39th edition of SEDA includes analyses of the side effects of drugs using both clinical trials and case-based principles which include encounters identified during bedside clinical practice over the 12–14 months since the previous edition. SEDA seeks to summarize the entire body of relevant medical literature into a single volume with dual goals of being comprehensive and of identifying emerging trends and themes in medicine as related to side effects and adverse drug effects (ADEs).

With a broad range of topics authored by practicing clinicians and scientists, SEDA is a comprehensive and reliable reference to be used in clinical practice. The majority of the chapters include relevant case studies that are not only peer-reviewed, but also have a forward-looking, learning-based focus suitable for practitioners as well as students in training. The nationally known contributors believe this educational resource can be used to stimulate an active learning environment in a variety of settings. Each chapter in this volume has been reviewed by the editor, experienced clinical educators, actively practicing clinicians and scientists to ensure the accuracy and timeliness of the information. The overall objective is to provide a framework for further understanding the intellectual approaches in analysing the implications of the case-studies and their appropriateness when dispensing medications, as well as interpreting adverse drug reactions (ADRs), toxicity and outcomes resulting from medication errors.

This volume of SEDA has included new perspectives from pharmacogenomics/pharmacogenetics and personalized medicine and USFDA's advisories. Due to the advances in science, the genetic profiles of patients must be considered in the aetiology of side effects, especially for medications provided to very large populations. This marks the first phase of genome-based personalized medicine, in which side effects of common medications are linked to polymorphisms in one or more genes. A focus on personalized medicine should lead to major advances for patient care and awareness among clinicians to deliver the most effective medication for the patient. This modality should considerably improve 'appropriate medication use' and enable the clinicians to pre-determine 'good versus bad responders' and help reduce ADRs. Overall, clinicians will have a better control on 'predictability and preventability' of ADEs induced by certain medications. Over time, it is anticipated that pharmacogenetics and personalized medicine will become an integral part of the practice sciences. SEDA will continue to highlight the genetic basis of side effects in future editions.

The collective wisdom, expertise and experience of the editor, authors and reviewers were vital in the creation of a volume of this breadth. Reviewing the appropriateness, timeliness and organization of this edition consumed an enormous amount of energy by the authors, reviewers and the editor, which we hope will facilitate the flow of information both inter-professionally among health practitioners, professionals in training and students, and will ultimately improve patient care. Scanning for accuracy, rebuilding and reorganizing information between editions is not an easy task; therefore, the editor had the difficult task of accepting or rejecting information. The editor will consider this undertaking worthwhile if this publication helps to provide better patient care; fulfils the needs of the healthcare professionals in sorting out side effects of medications, medication errors or adverse drug reactions; and stimulates interest among those working and studying medicine, pharmacy, nursing, physical therapy, chiropractic, and those working in the basic therapeutic arms of pharmacology, toxicology, medicinal chemistry and pathophysiology.

Editor of this volume gratefully acknowledges the leadership provided by the former editor Prof. J. K. Aronson and will continue to maintain the legacy of this publication by building on their hard work. The editor would also like to extend special thanks for the excellent support and assistance provided by Ms. Zoe Kruze (Publisher, serials and series) and Ms. Shellie Bryant (Editorial Project Manager) during the compilation of this work.

Sidhartha D. Ray
Editor

Special Reviews in SEDA 39

Table of Essays, Annuals 1–38

Abbreviations

The following abbreviations are used throughout the SEDA series.

2,4-DMA	2,4-Dimethoxyamfetamine
3,4-DMA	3,4-Dimethoxyamfetamine
3TC	Lamivudine (dideoxythiacytidine)
ADHD	Attention deficit hyperactivity disorder
ADP	Adenosine diphosphate
ANA	Antinuclear antibody
ANCA	Antineutrophil cytoplasmic antibody
aP	Acellular pertussis
APACHE	Acute physiology and chronic health evaluation (score)
aPTT	Activated partial thromboplastin time
ASA	American Society of Anesthesiologists
ASCA	*Anti-Saccharomyces cerevisiae* antibody
AUC	The area under the concentration versus time curve from zero to infinity
AUC$_{0 \to x}$	The area under the concentration versus time curve from zero to time x
AUC$_{0 \to t}$	The area under the concentration versus time curve from zero to the time of the last sample
AUC$_\tau$	The area under the concentration versus time curve during a dosage interval
AVA	Anthrax vaccine adsorbed
AZT	Zidovudine (azidothymidine)
BCG	Bacillus Calmette Guérin
bd	Twice a day (bis in die)
BIS	Bispectral index
BMI	Body mass index
CAPD	Continuous ambulatory peritoneal dialysis
CD [4, 8, etc]	Cluster of differentiation (describing various glycoproteins that are expressed on the surfaces of T cells, B cells and other cells, with varying functions)
CI	Confidence interval
C$_{max}$	Maximum (peak) concentration after a dose
C$_{ss.max}$	Maximum (peak) concentration after a dose at steady state
C$_{ss.min}$	Minimum (trough) concentration after a dose at steady state
COX-1 and COX-2	Cyclo-oxygenase enzyme isoforms 1 and 2
CT	Computed tomography
CYP (e.g. CYP2D6, CYP3A4)	Cytochrome P450 isoenzymes
D4T	Stavudine (didehydrodideoxythmidine)
DDC	Zalcitabine (dideoxycytidine)
DDI	Didanosine (dideoxyinosine)
DMA	Dimethoxyamfetamine; *see also* 2,4-DMA, 3,4-DMA
DMMDA	2,5-Dimethoxy-3,4-methylenedioxyamfetamine
DMMDA-2	2,3-Dimethoxy-4,5-methylenedioxyamfetamine
DTaP	Diphtheria + tetanus toxoids + acellular pertussis
DTaP-Hib-IPV-HB	Diphtheria + tetanus toxoids + acellular pertussis + IPV + Hib + hepatitis B (hexavalent vaccine)
DT-IPV	Diphtheria + tetanus toxoids + inactivated polio vaccine
DTP	Diphtheria + tetanus toxoids + pertussis vaccine
DTwP	Diphtheria + tetanus toxoids + whole cell pertussis
eGFR	Estimated glomerular filtration rate
ESR	Erythrocyte sedimentation rate
FDA	(US) Food and Drug Administration
FEV$_1$	Forced expiratory volume in 1 s
FTC	Emtricitabine
FVC	Forced vital capacity
G6PD	Glucose-6-phosphate dehydrogenase
GSH	Glutathione
GST	Glutathione S-transferase
HAV	Hepatitis A virus
HbA$_{1c}$	Hemoglobin A$_{1c}$
HbOC	Conjugated Hib vaccine (Hib capsular antigen polyribosylphosphate covalently linked to the nontoxic diphtheria toxin variant CRM197)
HBV	Hepatitis B virus

HDL, LDL, VLDL	High-density lipoprotein, low-density lipoprotein, and very low density lipoprotein (cholesterol)
Hib	*Haemophilus influenzae* type b
HIV	Human immunodeficiency virus
hplc	High-performance liquid chromatography
HPV	Human papilloma virus
HR	Hazard ratio
HZV	Herpes zoster virus vaccine
ICER	Incremental cost-effectiveness ratio
Ig (IgA, IgE, IgM)	Immunoglobulin (A, E, M)
IGF	Insulin-like growth factor
INN	International Nonproprietary Name (rINN = recommended; pINN = provisional)
INR	International normalized ratio
IPV	Inactivated polio vaccine
IQ [range], IQR	Interquartile [range]
JE	Japanese encephalitis vaccine
LABA	Long-acting beta-adrenoceptor agonist
MAC	Minimum alveolar concentration
MCV4	4-valent (Serogroups A, C, W, Y) meningococcal Conjugate vaccine
MDA	3,4-Methylenedioxyamfetamine
MDI	Metered-dose inhaler
MDMA	3,4-Methylenedioxymetamfetamine
MenB	Monovalent serogroup B meningoccocal vaccine
MenC	Monovalent serogroup C meningoccocal conjugate vaccine
MIC	Minimum inhibitory concentration
MIM	Mendelian Inheritance in Man (see http://www.ncbi.nlm.nih.gov/omim/607686)
MMDA	3-Methoxy-4,5-methylenedioxyamfetamine
MMDA-2	2-Methoxy-4,5-methylendioxyamfetamine
MMDA-3a	2-Methoxy-3,4-methylendioxyamfetamine
MMR	Measles + mumps + rubella
MMRV	Measles + mumps + rubella + varicella
MPSV4	4-Valent (serogroups A, C, W, Y) meningococcal polysaccharide vaccine
MR	Measles + rubella vaccine
MRI	Magnetic resonance imaging
NMS	Neuroleptic malignant syndrome
NNRTI	Non-nucleoside analogue reverse transcriptase inhibitor
NNT, NNT_B, NNT_H	Number needed to treat (for benefit, for harm)
NRTI	Nucleoside analogue reverse transcriptase inhibitor
NSAIDs	Nonsteroidal anti-inflammatory drugs
od	Once a day (omne die)
OMIM	Online Mendelian Inheritance in Man (see http://www.ncbi.nlm.nih.gov/omim/607686)
OPV	Oral polio vaccine
OR	Odds ratio
OROS	Osmotic-release oral system
PCR	Polymerase chain reaction
PMA	Paramethoxyamfetamine
PMMA	Paramethoxymetamfetamine
PPAR	Peroxisome proliferator-activated receptor
ppb	Parts per billion
PPD	Purified protein derivative
ppm	Parts per million
PRP-CRM	*See* HbOC
PRP-D-Hib	Conjugated Hib vaccine(Hib capsular antigen polyribosylphosphate covalently Linked to a mutant polypeptide of diphtheria toxin)
PT	Prothrombin time
PTT	Partial thromboplastin time
QALY	Quality-adjusted life year
qds	Four times a day (quater die summendum)
ROC curve	Receiver-operator characteristic curve
RR	Risk ratio or relative risk
RT-PCR	Reverse transcriptase polymerase chain reaction
SABA	Short-acting beta-adrenoceptor agonist
SMR	Standardized mortality rate
SNP	Single nucleotide polymorphism
SNRI	Serotonin and noradrenaline reuptake inhibitor
SSRI	Selective serotonin reuptake inhibitor

SV40	Simian virus 40
Td	Diphtheria + tetanus toxoids (adult formulation)
Tdap:	Tetanus toxoid + reduced diphtheria toxoid + acellular pertussis
tds	Three times a day (ter die summendum)
TeMA	2,3,4,5-Tetramethoxyamfetamine
TMA	3,4,5-Trimethoxyamfetamine
TMA-2	2,4,5-Trimethoxyamfetamine
t_{max}	The time at which C_{max} is reached
TMC125	Etravirine
TMC 278	Rilpivirine
V_{max}	Maximum velocity (of a reaction)
wP	Whole cell pertussis
VZV	*Varicella zoster* vaccine
YF	Yellow fever
YFV	Yellow fever virus

ADRs, ADEs and SEDs: A Bird's Eye View

Sidhartha D. Ray*,1, Adrienne T. Black†

*Manchester University College of Pharmacy, Fort Wayne, IN, United States
†3E Services, 3E Company, Warrenton, VA, United States
1Corresponding author: sdray@manchester.edu

INTRODUCTION

Adverse drug events (ADEs), drug-induced toxicity and side effects are a significant concern. ADEs are known to pose significant morbidity, mortality, and cost burden to society; however, there is a lack of strong evidence to determine their precise impact. The landmark Institute of Medicine (IOM) report *To Err is Human* implicated adverse drug events in 7000 annual deaths at an estimated cost of $2 billion [1]. However, the US Department of Health and Human Services estimates 770 000 people are injured or die each year in hospitals from ADEs, which costs up to $5.6 million each year per hospital excluding the other accessory costs (e.g., hospital admissions due to ADEs, malpractice and litigation costs, or the costs of injuries). Nationally, hospitals spend $1.56–5.6 billion each year, to treat patients who suffer ADEs during hospitalization [2]. A second landmark study suggests that approximately 28% of ADEs are preventable, through optimization of medication safety and distribution systems, provision and dissemination of timely patient and medication information, and staffing assignments [3]. Subsequent recent investigations suggest these numbers might be conservative estimates of the morbidity and mortality impact of ADEs [4].

Analysis of ADEs, ADRs, Side Effects and Toxicity

A recent report suggested that ADEs and/or side effects of drugs occur in approximately 30% of hospitalized patients [5]. The American Society of Health-System Pharmacists (ASHP) defines medication mishap as unexpected, undesirable, iatrogenic hazards or events where a medication was implicated [6]. These events can be broadly divided into two categories: (i) medication errors (i.e., preventable events that may cause or contain inappropriate use) and (ii) adverse drug events (i.e., any injury, whether minor or significant, caused by a medication or lack thereof). Another significant ADE-generating category that can be added to the list is: lack of incorporation of pre-existing condition(s) or pharmacogenetic factors. This work focuses on adverse drug events; however, it should be noted that adverse drug events may or may not occur secondary to a medication error.

The lack of more up-to-date epidemiological data regarding the impact of ADEs is largely due to challenges with low adverse drug event reporting. ASHP recommends that health systems implement adverse drug reaction (ADR) monitoring programs in order to (i) mitigate ADR risks for specific patients and expedite reporting to clinicians involved in care of patients who do experience ADRs and (ii) gather pharmacovigilance information that can be reported to pharmaceutical companies and regulatory bodies [7]. Factors that may increase the risk for ADEs include polypharmacy, multiple concomitant disease states, pediatric or geriatric status, female sex, genetic variance, and drug factors, such as class and route of administration. The Institute for Safe Medication Practices (ISMP) defines high-alert medications as those with high risk for harmful events, especially when used in error [8]. Examples of high-alert medications include antithrombotic agents, cancer chemotherapy, insulin, opioids, and neuromuscular blockers.

Terminology

ADEs may be further classified based on expected severity into adverse drug reactions (ADRs) or adverse effects (also known as side effects). ASHP defines ADRs as an "unexpected, unintended, undesired, or excessive response to a drug" resulting in death, disability, or harm [7]. The World Health Organization (WHO) has traditionally defined an ADR as a "response to a drug which is noxious and unintended, and which occurs at doses normally used"; however, another proposed definition, intended to highlight the seriousness of ADRs is "an appreciably harmful or unpleasant reaction, resulting from an intervention related to the use of a medicinal product, which predicts hazard from future administration and warrants prevention or specific treatment, or alteration of the dosage regimen, or withdrawal of the product" [9]. Under all definitions, ADRs are distinguished from side effects in that they generally necessitate some type of modification to the patient's therapeutic regimen. Such modifications could include discontinuing treatment, changing medications, significantly altering the dose, elevating or prolonging care received by the patient, or changing diagnosis or prognosis. ADRs include drug allergies, immunologic hypersensitivities, and idiosyncratic reactions. In contrast, side effects, or adverse effects, are defined as "expected, well-known reaction resulting in little or no change in patient management" [7]. Side effects occur at predictable frequency and are often dose related, whereas ADRs are less foreseeable [9,10].

Two additional types of adverse drug events are drug-induced diseases and toxicity. Drug-induced diseases are defined as an "unintended effect of a drug that results in mortality or morbidity with symptoms sufficient to prompt a patient to seek medical attention, require hospitalization, or both" [11]. In other words, a drug-induced disease has elements of an ADR (i.e., significant severity, elevated levels of patient care) and adverse effects (i.e., predictability, consistent symptoms). Toxicity is a less precisely defined term referring to the ability of a substance "to cause injury to living organisms as a result of physicochemical interaction" [12]. This term is applied to both medication and non-medication types of substances, while "ADRs," "side effects," and "drug-induced diseases" typically only refer to medications. When applied to medication use, toxicity typically refers to use at higher than normal dosing or accumulated supratherapeutic exposure over time, while ADRs, side effects, and drug-induced diseases are associated with normal therapeutic use.

Although the title of this monograph is "Side Effects of Drugs," this work provides emerging information for all adverse drug events including ADRs, side effects, drug-induced diseases, toxicity, and other situations less clearly classifiable into a particular category, such as effects subsequent to drug interactions with other drugs, foods, and cosmetics. Pharmacogenetic considerations have been incorporated in several chapters as appropriate and subject to availability of literature.

Adverse drug reactions are described in SEDA using two complementary systems, EIDOS and DOTS [13–15]. These two systems are illustrated in Figs. 1 and 2 and general templates for describing reactions in this way are shown in Figs. 3–5. Examples of their use have been discussed elsewhere [16–20]. As the clinicians are becoming more cognizant about different types of ADRs, reports in this arena are growing faster than one can imagine; few recent articles are listed for reference [21–27].

EIDOS

The EIDOS mechanistic description of adverse drug reactions [15] has five elements:

- the Extrinsic species that initiates the reaction (Table 1);
- the Intrinsic species that it affects;
- the Distribution of these species in the body;
- the (physiological or pathological) Outcome (Table 2), which is the adverse effect;
- the Sequela, which is the adverse reaction.

- *Extrinsic species:* This can be the parent compound, an excipient, a contaminant or adulterant, a degradation product, or a derivative of any of these (e.g. a metabolite) (for examples see Table 1).
- *Intrinsic species:* This is usually the endogenous molecule with which the extrinsic species interacts; this can be a nucleic acid, an enzyme, a receptor, an ion channel or transporter, or some other protein.
- *Distribution:* A drug will not produce an adverse effect if it is not distributed to the same site as the target species that mediates the adverse effect. Thus, the pharmacokinetics of the extrinsic species can affect the occurrence of adverse reactions.
- *Outcome:* Interactions between extrinsic and intrinsic species in the production of an adverse effect can result in physiological or pathological changes (for examples see Table 2). Physiological changes can involve either increased actions (e.g. clotting due to tranexamic acid) or decreased actions (e.g. bradycardia due to β(beta)-adrenoceptor antagonists). Pathological changes can involve cellular adaptations (atrophy, hypertrophy, hyperplasia, metaplasia and neoplasia), altered cell function (e.g. mast cell degranulation in IgE-mediated anaphylactic reactions) or cell damage (e.g. cell lysis, necrosis or apoptosis).
- *Sequela:* The sequela of the changes induced by a drug describes the clinically recognizable adverse drug reaction, of which there may be more than one. Sequelae can be classified using the DoTS system.

DoTS

In the DoTS system (SEDA-28, xxvii–xxxiii), 1,2) adverse drug reactions are described according to the Dose at which they usually occur, the Time-course over which they occur, and the Susceptibility factors that make them more likely, as follows:

- *Relation to dose*
  - Toxic reactions (reactions that occur at supratherapeutic doses)
  - Collateral reactions (reactions that occur at standard therapeutic doses)

- ○ Hypersusceptibility reactions (reactions that occur at subtherapeutic doses in susceptible individuals)
- *Time course*
  - ○ Time-independent reactions (reactions that occur at any time during a course of therapy)
- *Time-dependent reactions*
  - ○ Immediate or rapid reactions (reactions that occur only when drug administration is too rapid)
  - ○ First-dose reactions (reactions that occur after the first dose of a course of treatment and not necessarily thereafter)
  - ○ Early tolerant and early persistent reactions (reactions that occur early in treatment then either abate with continuing treatment, owing to tolerance, or persist)
  - ○ Intermediate reactions (reactions that occur after some delay but with less risk during longer term therapy, owing to the 'healthy survivor' effect)
  - ○ Late reactions (reactions the risk of which increases with continued or repeated exposure)
  - ○ Withdrawal reactions (reactions that occur when, after prolonged treatment, a drug is withdrawn or its effective dose is reduced)
  - ○ Delayed reactions (reactions that occur at some time after exposure, even if the drug is withdrawn before the reaction appears)
- *Susceptibility factors*
  - ○ Genetic (Ex. Variations in expression of certain drug-metabolizing enzymes)
  - ○ Age (newborn, pediatric, young adult, adult and old age)
  - ○ Sex (gender differences—hormonal variations)
  - ○ Physiological variation (e.g. weight, pregnancy)
  - ○ Exogenous factors (for example the effects of other drugs, devices, surgical procedures, food,

phytochemicals & nutraceuticals, alcoholic beverages, smoking etc.)
  - ○ Diseases (ongoing but latent with no clinical signs, pre-existing and obvious)
  - ○ Environmental factors (drinking water containing trace chemicals; breathing polluted air)

WHO Classification

Although not systematically used in Side Effects of Drugs Annual, the WHO classification, used at the Uppsala Monitoring Center, is a useful schematic to consider in assessing ADRs and adverse effects. Possible classifications include:

- Type A (dose-related, "augmented"): more common events that tend to be related to the pharmacology of the drug, have a mechanistic basis, and result in lower mortality
- Type B (non-dose-related, "bizarre"): less common, unpredictable events that are not related to the pharmacology of the drug
- Type C (dose-related and time-related, "chronic"): events that are related to cumulative dose received over time
- Type D (time-related, "delayed"): events that are usually dose-related but do not become apparent until significant time has elapsed since exposure to the drug
- Type E (withdrawal, "end of use"): events that occur soon after the use of the drug
- Type F (unexpected lack of efficacy, "failure"): common, dose-related events where the drug effectiveness is lacking, often due to drug interactions

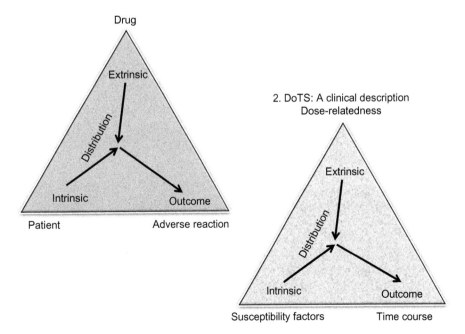

FIG. 1 Describing adverse drug reactions using two complementary systems. Note that the triad of drug–patient–adverse reaction appears outside the triangle in EIDOS and inside the triangle in DoTS, which leads to Fig. 2.

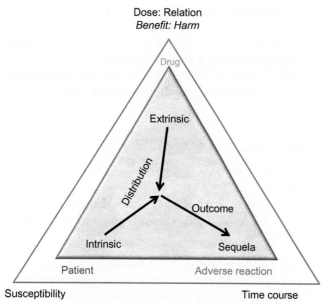

Dose: Relation
Benefit: Harm

FIG. 2 How the EIDOS and DoTS systems relate to each other. Here the two triangles in Fig. 1 are superimposed, to show the relation between the two systems. An adverse reaction occurs when a drug is given to a patient. Adverse reactions can be classified mechanistically (EIDOS) by noting that when the Extrinsic (drug) species and an Intrinsic (patient) species, are co-Distributed, a pharmacological or other effect (the Outcome) results in the adverse reaction (the Sequela). The adverse reaction can be further classified (DoTS) by considering its three main features—its Dose-relatedness, its Time-course, and individual Susceptibility.

REFERENCES ON ADVERSE DRUG REACTIONS

[1] Kohn, LT, Corrigan JM, Donaldson MS, editors. *To Err is Human: Building a Safer Health System.* Washington, DC National Academy Press; 1999: 1–8.
[2] US Department of Health & Human Services Report: http://archive.ahrq.gov/research/findings/factsheets/errors-safety/aderia/ade.html.
[3] Leape LL, Bates DW, Cullen DJ, et al. Systems analysis of adverse drug events. JAMA. 1995; 274 (1):35–43.
[4] James JT. A new, evidence-based estimate of patient harms associated with hospital care. J Patient Saf. 2013; 9(3):122–128.
[5] Wang G, Jung K, Winnenburg R, Shah NH. A method for systematic discovery of adverse drug events from clinical notes. J Am Med Inform Assoc. 2015 Jul 31. pii: ocv102. doi: 10.1093/jamia/ocv102.
[6] Society of Health-Systems Pharmacists. Positions. Medication Misadventures. http://www.ashp.org/DocLibrary/BestPractices/MedMisPositions.aspx.
[7] American Society of Health-Systems Pharmacists. Guidelines. ASHP Guidelines on adverse drug reaction monitoring and reporting. http://www.ashp.org/DocLibrary/BestPractices/MedMisGdlADR.aspx.
[8] Institute for Safe Medication Practices. ISMP list of high-alert medications in acute care settings. http://www.ismp.org/Tools/institutionalhighAlert.asp.

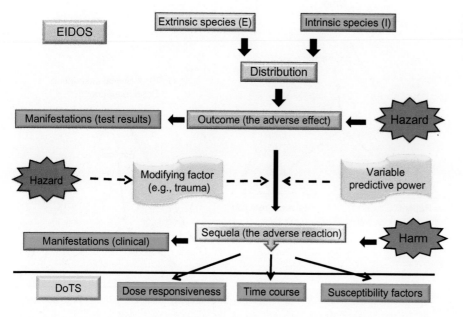

FIG. 3 A general form of the EIDOS and DoTS template for describing an adverse effect or an adverse reaction.

FIG. 4 A general form of the EIDOS and DoTS template for describing two mechanisms of an adverse reaction or (illustrated here) the balance of benefit to harm, each mediated by a different mechanism.

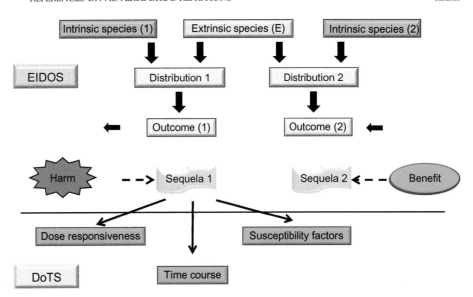

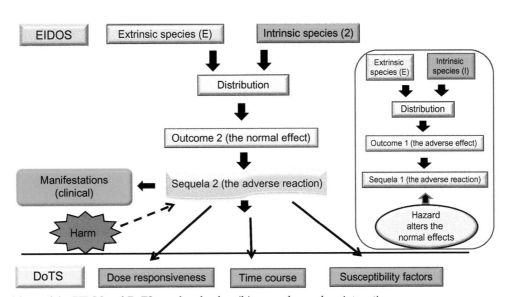

FIG. 5 A general form of the EIDOS and DoTS template for describing an adverse drug interaction.

[9] Edwards IR, Aronson JK. Adverse drug reactions: Definitions, diagnosis, and management. Lancet. 2000; 356:1255–59.

[10] Cochrane ZR, Hein D, Gregory PJ. Medication misadventures I: adverse drug reactions. In: Malone PM, Kier KL, Stanovich JE, Malone MJ, editors. Drug Information: A Guide for Pharmacists, 5th edition. New York, NY: McGraw-Hill; 2013.

[11] Tisdale JE, Miller DA, editors. Drug-Induced Diseases: Prevention, Detection, and Management. 2nd edition. Bethesda, MD: American Society of Health-System Pharmacists; 2010.

[12] Wexler P, Abdollahi M, Peyster AD, et al., editors. Encyclopedia of Toxicology. 3rd edition. Burlington, MA: Academic Press, Elsevier; 2014.

[13] Aronson JK, Ferner RE. Joining the DoTS. New approach to classifying adverse drug reactions. BMJ. 2003; 327:1222–1225.

[14] Aronson JK, Ferner RE. Clarification of terminology in drug safety. Drug Saf. 2005; 28(10):851–870.

[15] Ferner RE, Aronson JK. EIDOS: a mechanistic classification of adverse drug effects. Drug Saf. 2010; 33(1):13–23.

[16] Callréus T. Use of the dose, time, susceptibility (DoTS) classification scheme for adverse drug reactions in pharmacovigilance planning. Drug Saf. 2006; 29(7):557–566.

[17] Aronson JK, Price D, Ferner R.E. A strategy for regulatory action when new adverse effects of a licensed product emerge. Drug Saf. 2009; 32(2):91–98.

TABLE 1 The DIDOS Mechanistic Description of Adverse Drug Effects and Reactions

Feature	Varieties	Examples
E. Extrinsic species	1. The parent compound	Insulin
	2. An excipient	Polyoxyl 35 castor oil
	3. A contaminant	1,1-Ethylidenebis [l-tryptophan]
	4. An adulterant	Lead in herbal medicines
	5. A degradation product formed before the drug enters the body	Outdated tetracycline
	6. A derivative of any of these (e.g. a metabolite)	Acrolein (from cyclophosphamide)
I. The intrinsic species and the nature of its interaction with the extrinsic species		
(a) Molecular	1. Nucleic acids	
	(a) DNA	Melphalan
	(b) RNA	Mitoxantrone
	2. Enzymes	
	(a) Reversible effect	Edrophonium
	(b) Irreversible effect	Malathion
	3. Receptors	
	(a) Reversible effect	Prazosin
	(b) Irreversible effect	Phenoxybenzamine
	4. Ion channels/transporters	Calcium channel blockers; digoxin and Na^+–K^+–ATPase
	5. Other proteins	
	(a) Immunological proteins	Penicilloyl residue hapten
	(b) Tissue proteins	N-acetyl-p-benzoquinone-imine (paracetamol [acetaminophen])
(b) Extracellular	1. Water	Dextrose 5%
	2. Hydrogen ions (pH)	Sodium bicarbonate
	3. Other ions	Sodium ticarcillin
(c) Physical or physicochemical	1. Direct tissue damage	Intrathecal vincristine
	2. Altered physicochemical nature of the extrinsic species	Sulindac precipitation
D. Distribution	1. Where in the body the extrinsic and intrinsic species occur (affected by pharmacokinetics)	Antihistamines cause drowsiness only if they affect histamine H_1 receptors in the brain
O. Outcome (physiological or pathological change)	The adverse effect (see Table 2)	
S. Sequela	The adverse reaction (use the Dose, Time, Susceptibility [DoTS] descriptive system)	

TABLE 2 Examples of Physiological and Pathological Changes in Adverse Drug Effects (Some Categories Can Be Broken Down Further)

Type of change	Examples
1. Physiological changes	
(a) Increased actions	Hypertension (monoamine oxidase inhibitors); clotting (tranexamic acid)
(b) Decreased actions	Bradycardia (beta-adrenoceptor antagonists); QT interval prolongation (antiarrhythmic drugs)
2. Cellular adaptations	
(a) Atrophy	Lipoatrophy (subcutaneous insulin); glucocorticosteroid-induced myopathy
(b) Hypertrophy	Gynecomastia (spironolactone)
(c) Hyperplasia	Pulmonary fibrosis (busulfan); retroperitoneal fibrosis (methysergide)
(d) Metaplasia	Lacrimal canalicular squamous metaplasia (fluorouracil)
(e) Neoplasia	
– Benign	Hepatoma (anabolic steroids)
– Malignant	
– Hormonal	Vaginal adenocarcinoma (diethylstilbestrol)
– Genotoxic	Transitional cell carcinoma of bladder (cyclophosphamide)
– Immune suppression	Lymphoproliferative tumors (cyclosporin)
3. Altered cell function	IgE-mediated mast cell degranulation (class I immunological reactions)
4. Cell damage	
(a) Acute reversible damage	
– Chemical damage	Periodontitis (local application of methylenedioxymetamfetamine [MDMA, 'ecstasy'])
– Immunological reactions	Class III immunological reactions
(b) Irreversible injury	
– Cell lysis	Class II immunological reactions
– Necrosis	Class IV immunological reactions; hepatotoxicity (paracetamol, after apoptosis)
– Apoptosis	Liver damage (troglitazone)
5. Intracellular accumulations	
(a) Calcification	Milk-alkali syndrome
(b) Drug deposition	Crystal-storing histiocytosis (clofazimine) Skin pigmentation (amiodarone)

[18] Calderón-Ospina C, Bustamante-Rojas C. The DoTS classification is a useful way to classify adverse drug reactions: a preliminary study in hospitalized patients. Int J Pharm Pract. 2010; 18(4):230–235.

[19] Ferner RE, Aronson JK. Preventability of drug-related harms. Part 1: A systematic review. Drug Saf. 2010; 33(11):985–994.

[20] Aronson JK, Ferner RE. Preventability of drug-related harms. Part 2: Proposed criteria, based on frameworks that classify adverse drug reactions. Drug Saf. 2010; 33(11):995–1002.

[21] Saini VK, Sewal RK, Ahmad Y, Medhi B. Prospective Observational Study of Adverse Drug Reactions of Anticancer Drugs Used in Cancer Treatment in a Tertiary Care Hospital. Indian J Pharm Sci., 2015; 77(6):687–93.

[22] White RS; Thomson Reuters Accelus. Pharmaceutical and Medical Devices: FDA Oversight. Issue Brief Health Policy Track Serv. 2015; 28:1–97.

[23] Davies EA, O'Mahony MS. Adverse drug reactions in special populations—the elderly. Br J Clin Pharmacol., 2015; 80(4):796–807.

[24] Mouton JP, Mehta U, Parrish AG, et al. Mortality from adverse drug reactions in adult medical inpatients at four hospitals in South Africa: a cross-sectional survey. Br J Clin Pharmacol., 2015; 80(4):818–26.

[25] Bouvy JC, De Bruin ML, Koopmanschap MA. Epidemiology of adverse drug reactions in Europe: a review of recent observational studies. Drug Saf., 2015; 38(5):437–53.

[26] Bénard-Laribière A, Miremont-Salamé G, Pérault-Pochat MC, et al. Incidence of hospital admissions due to adverse drug reactions in France: the EMIR study. (EMIR Study Group on behalf of the French network of pharmacovigilance centres). Fundam Clin Pharmacol., 2015; 29(1):106–11.

[27] Coleman JJ, Pontefract SK. Adverse drug reactions. Clin Med (Lond). 2016; 16(5):481–485. Review. https://www.ncbi.nlm.nih.gov/pubmed/27697815.

PHARMACOGENOMICS CONSIDERATIONS

It has long been known that individuals respond differentially to the same medication regardless of dose and that these differences may result in adverse drug reactions. These differences may be explained using pharmacogenomics (also known as pharmacogenetics), the study of how genes affect the individual responses to drugs. A primary goal of this field is to characterize the relationship between genetic variations and drug responses and, with advances in genetic knowledge and technology, the role of pharmacogenomics has been recognized as a primary factor in the development of adverse drug reactions. Greater use of pharmacogenomics may replace, in part or in full, the "one-size-fits-all" approach to drug prescription in favor of a more tailored pharmacological approach for each individual that may increase efficacy of the medication while reducing the risk of adverse drug reactions. This is the promise of individualized or personalized medicine.

The genetic variations between individuals may be described by polymorphisms in their genetic code, also known as genetic variants. These variations may be caused by the presence or absence of an entire gene or, more typically, are the result of single-nucleotide polymorphisms (SNPs). The SNPs create genetic variants that are similar but different to the wild-type gene present in the majority of the population. The impact of SNPs is profound in affecting how genes and their products (proteins that comprise enzymes, transporters, membrane and intracellular receptors, membrane channels, to name a few) may be regulated or expressed. Such changes are associated with drug pharmacokinetics or pharmacodynamics, affecting both the efficacy and development of adverse drug reactions. Of particular interest in the field of pharmacogenetics is the role of polymorphisms in drug-metabolizing enzymes, ion transporters and human leukocyte antigens (HLA).

Enzymes and Transporters

It has been reported that polymorphisms in one gene superfamily, the cytochrome P450s (CYP) are associated with up to 60% of drug-induced toxicity. Other drug-metabolizing enzymes with variation-inducing toxicity include N-acetyl transferase type 2 (NAT2), thiopurine methyltransferases (TPMT), dihydropyrimidine dehydrogenase (DPD), uridine diphosphateglucuronosyl transferases (UGT) and organic anion transporters (OAT). As an illustration of the importance of pharmacogenetics in this area, genomic analysis has recently confirmed the association of long QT syndrome (LQTS) induced by a number of drugs including antibiotics, antipsychotics, chemotherapeutics, antiemetics, opioid analgesics and antiarrhythmics with KCNH2 and SCN5A mutations. Examples of the genetic variants with the primary gene and the associated drug with adverse effects are shown in Table 3.

Human Leukocyte Antigens (HLA)

The HLA family comprises over 200 genes, forming the human major histocompatibility complex (MHC). Associated adverse drug reactions may occur through

TABLE 3 Genetic Polymorphisms and Drug-Induced Adverse Reactions

Gene	Variant/ polymorphism	Drug	Adverse effects
CYP2D6	CYP2D6*4	Atorvastatin	Myopathy
CYP3A4	CYP3A4*20	Paclitaxel	Neuropathy
	CYP3A4*25		
CYP3A5	CYP3A5*3	Atorvastatin	Myopathy
CYP2C9	CYP2C9*2	Warfarin	Bleeding, thrombosis
	CYP2C9*3	Phenytoin	Severe cutaneous adverse reactions
CYP2C19	CYP2C19*2	Clopidogrel	Cardiovascular events
NAT 2		Isoniazid	Hepatotoxicity, neuropathy
TPMT		Thiopurines	Myelosupression
DPD	rs3918290 rs67376798 rs1801158 rs55886062	5-Fluorouracil	Neutropenia
UGT	rs34815109	Irinotecan	Neutropenia, myelosuppression
SLCO1B1 (OAT)	rs2306283 rs4149056	Statins	Myopathy
ACYP2	rs1872328	Cisplatin	Ototoxicity

TABLE 4 Examples of HLA Allele Variants and Associated Drug-Induced Adverse Reactions

Reaction	Drug	HLA variant(s)
Hypersensitivity	Abacavir	HLA-B*5701, HLA-DR7 ,HLA-DQ3
Stevens–Johnson syndrome (SJS)/toxic epidermal necrolysis (TEN) and Severe cutaneous adverse reactions	Allopurinol	HLA-B*5801
Hypersensitivity and SJS/TEN	Carbamazepine	HLA-B*1502, HLA-A3101
Hepatoxicity	Co-Amoxiclav	HLA-DRB1*15:01, HLA-A*0201, HLA-B*1801
Hepatotoxicity	Flucloxacillin	HLA-B*5701
Systemic lupus erythematosus	Hydralazine	HLA-DR4
SJS/TEN	Lamotrigine	HLA-B*3801
Hepatoxicity	Lumiracoxib	HLA-DRB*1501, HLA-DQA*0102
Systemic lupus erythematosus	Minocycline	HLA-DQB1
SJS/TEN	Nevirapine	HLA-B*3505, HLA-C0401
SJS/TEN	Phenytoin	HLA-B*1502
Hepatoxicity	Ticlopidine	HLA-A*3303
Hepatoxicity	Ximelagatran	HLA-DRB1*0701

direct or indirect interaction of the drug with a specific HLA allele, thereby initiating an immune response and causing an adverse effect. These HLA-mediated reactions are typically hypersensitivity reactions but they also include drug-induced injury to such organs and the liver, kidney, skin, muscle, heart, to name a few. As these reactions are dependent upon the presence of specific HLA alleles, the phenotype or ethnicity of an individual is of particular interest in determining if a medication may cause unwanted effects.

Due to the risk of adverse drug reactions, HLA genotyping is commonly done prior to prescribing many medications. In the case of abacavir, screening for the presence of *HLA-B*5701* is required by American and European regulatory authorities prior to the initiation of treatment. Similarly, genetic screening for *HLA-B*1502* and *HLA-B*5801* before administration of carbamazepine or allopurinol has become commonplace in several Asian countries. A number of drug-induced reactions have been associated with specific variants in the HLA genes and several examples are shown in Table 4. The HLA Adverse Drug Reaction Database also provides an up-to-date listing of HLA alleles and the associated adverse drug reactions (http://www.allelefrequencies.net/hla-adr/default.asp).

Genetic Testing Technology

The ability to conduct genetic testing may be limited by cost and/or computing power. In addition, it is critical to know how the drug is metabolized, transported, etc. and what key enzymes or molecules are involved in these processes. It must also be noted that even strong associations from genomic studies are not the equivalent of clinical relevancy as degree of relevancy is dependent upon the relative frequency of the genetic variation in the affected population, the disease phenotype and the severity of the outcome/reaction.

The following section describes the general categories of genomic testing.

1. Linkage mapping: This analysis is a tracking method to identify patterns of DNA phenotypes or markers within families (i.e., hemophilia, brown eye color, etc.). Linkage mapping is generally not a useful tool for the detection of a genetic basis for the occurrence of an adverse drug reaction although identification of an individual with a suspect phenotype may lead to more focused genetic testing.

2. **Genome-wide association (GWA) studies:** GWA studies analyze data from large cohorts to detect genetic variations via high-throughput analysis of SNPs in each individual's genome. Although genotyping of SNPs was initially used as a means to better understand human disease, this method has increasingly been used to study the genetic basis for adverse drug reactions. It is likely that as costs and application limitations decrease, whole genomic analysis will become the preferred method.

3. **Next-generation sequencing methods:** While whole genome sequencing is currently possible and may be preferential, the processing power for analysis of the data is prohibitive for the majority of users. As a result, a subset of the genome, the exome or all exons (protein coding regions), is typically analyzed in whole exome sequencing (WES). This technique allows identification of any variations within this section of the genome; a major drawback, however, is that any variations in other areas of the genome such as in introns (regulatory coding regions) is not included.

The US FDA has provided a "Table of Pharmacogenomic Biomarkers in Drug Labeling" with current labeling information for numerous drugs that includes pharmacogenetics information (genetic variations, polymorphisms, etc.) for each medication. This table also provides a recommendation on genetic testing and/or screening to be conducted prior to prescription (https://www.fda.gov/downloads/Drugs/ScienceResearch/ResearchAreas/Pharmacogenetics/UCM545881.pdf). An additional resource, "Actionable Pharmacogenetics in FDA Labeling", succinctly describes the recommended actions to be taken for each medication based on the FDA information (http://www.wolterskluwercdi.com/blog/actionable-pharmacogenetics-fda-labeling/). The FDA has also issued a guidance document for recommended pharmacogenetic and genetic tests intended for drug sponsors and FDA reviewers involved in preparing and reviewing premarket approval applications (PMA) and premarket notification (510(k)) submissions (https://www.fda.gov/RegulatoryInformation/Guidances/ucm077862.htm).

CONCLUSION

The availability of genetic testing technology and increasing knowledge about genetic variation-associated adverse drug reactions has elevated the role of pharmacogenomics in designing the drug regimen tailored to the individual patient (individualized or personalized medicine). An individual's genetic profile would, therefore, determine what medication would be most appropriate along with the most effective dosing regimen to increase the drug effectiveness and reduce the probability of adverse drug reactions. To this goal, the Clinical Pharmacogenetics Implementation Consortium (CPIC) has issued genetic testing and dosing guidelines for over 200 drugs (https://cpicpgx.org/genes-drugs).

Although pharmacogenetic testing is becoming more widespread in application, it is not expected that this approach will completely eliminate standard therapeutic monitoring or measurement of other phenotype variables. It is known that adverse reactions may be affected by other factors such as drug–drug interactions, age, sex, ethnicity and comorbities. In the future, it is likely that there will be a blending of the different methods to provide the most appropriate therapeutic approach.

REFERENCES

[1] Ray SD, Thomas, K and Kisor DF. **ADRs, ADEs and SEDs: A Bird's Eye View** Editorial Article—In: Ray SD, Editor. Side Effects of Drugs: Annual: A worldwide yearly survey of new data in adverse drug reactions, Vol. 38: pp. xxvii–xli, 2016. [R]. http://www.sciencedirect.com/science/article/pii/S0378608016300605.

[2] Ray SD, Beckett RD, Kisor DF, Gray JP and Kiersma ME. **ADRs, ADEs and SEDs: A Bird's Eye View** In: Ray SD, Editor. Side Effects of Drugs: Annual: A worldwide yearly survey of new data in adverse drug reactions, Vol. 37, pp. XXVII–XXXIX, Elsevier; 2015. [R]. http://www.sciencedirect.com/science/article/pii/S0378608015000616.

[3] Kullak-Ublick GA, Andrade RJ, Merz M, et al. Drug-induced liver injury: Recent advances in diagnosis and risk assessment. 2017. Gut. 66(6): 1154–1164. [3R]

[4] Lauschke VM, Ingelman-Sundberg M. The importance of patient-specific factors for hepatic drug response and toxicity. 2016. Int. J. Mol. Sci. 17(10): 1714–1741. [R]

[5] Maggo SD, Savage RL, Kennedy MA. Impact of new genomic technologies on understanding adverse drug reactions. 2016. Clin. Pharmacokinet. 55(4): 419–436. [R]

[6] Maagdenberg H, Vijverberg SJ, Bierings MB, et al. Pharmacogenomics in pediatric patients: towards personalized medicine. 2016. Paediatr. Drugs. 18(4): 251–260. [R]

[7] O'Donnell PH, Danahey K, Ratain MJ. The outlier in all of us: why implementing pharmacogenomics could matter for everyone. 2016. Clin. Pharmacol. Ther. 99(4): 401–404. [R]

[8] Su SC, Hung SI, Fan WL, et al. Severe cutaneous adverse reactions: the pharmacogenomics from research to clinical implementation. 2016. Int. J. Mol. Sci. 17(11): 1890–1990. [R]

IMMUNOLOGICAL REACTIONS

The immunological reactions are diverse and varied but considered specific. Nearly five decades ago, Karl Landsteiner's ground-breaking work "The Specificity of Serological Reactions" set the standard in experimental immunology. Several new discoveries in immunology in the 20th century, such as, 'CD' receptors (cluster of differentiation), recognition of 'self' versus 'non-self', a large family of cytokines and antigenic specificity became instrumental in describing immunological reactions. The most widely accepted classification divides immunological reactions (drug allergies or otherwise) into four pathophysiological types:

A. Type I hypersensitivity: (naphylaxis, immediate type)
B. Type II hypersensitivity: (antibody-mediated cytotoxic reactions, cytotoxic type) or
C. Type III hypersensitivity: (immune complex-mediated reactions, toxic-complex syndrome)
D. Type IV hypersensitivity: (cell-mediated immunity, delayed-type hypersensitivity)

Although this classification was proposed more than 30 years ago, it is still widely used today [1–3].

Type I Reactions (IgE-Mediated Anaphylaxis; Immediate Hypersensitivity)

In type I reactions, the drug or its metabolite interacts with immunoglobulin (IG) IgE molecules bound to specific type of cells (mast cells and basophils). This triggers a process that leads to the release of pharmacological mediators (histamine, 5-hydroxytryptamine, kinins, and arachidonic acid derivatives) which cause the allergic response. The development of such a reaction depends exclusively upon exposure to the same assaulting agent (antigen, allergen or metabolite) for the second time and the severity depends on the level of exposure. The clinical effects [2] are due to smooth muscle contraction, vasodilatation, and increased capillary permeability. The symptoms include faintness, light-headedness, pruritus, nausea, vomiting, abdominal pain, and a feeling of impending doom (angor animi). The signs include urticaria, conjunctivitis, rhinitis, laryngeal edema, bronchial asthma, pulmonary edema, angioedema, and anaphylactic shock. In addition, takotsubo cardiomyopathy can occur as well as Kounis syndrome (an acute coronary episode associated with an allergic reaction). Not all type I reactions are IgE-dependent; however, adverse reactions that are mediated by direct histamine release have conventionally been called anaphylactoid reactions but are better classified as non-IgE-mediated anaphylactic reactions. Cytokines, such as, inteleukin (IL)-4, IL-5, IL-6 and IL-13 either mediate or influence this class of hypersensitivity reaction. Representative agents that are known to induce such reactions include: gelatin, gentamicin, kanamycin, neomycin, penicillins, polymyxin B, streptomycin and thiomersal [1–3].

Type II Reactions (Cytotoxic Reactions)

Type II reactions involve circulating immunoglobulins G (IgG) or M (IgM) (or rarely IgA) binding with cell surface antigens (membrane constituent or protein) and interacting with an antigen formed by a hapten (drug or metabolite) and subsequently fixing complement. Complement is then activated leading to cytolysis. Type II reactions often involve antibody-mediated cytotoxicity directed to the membranes of erythrocytes, leukocytes, platelets, and probably hematopoietic precursor cells in the bone marrow. Drugs that are typically involved are methyldopa (hemolytic anemia), aminopyrine (leukopenia), and heparin (thrombocytopenia) with mostly hematological consequences, including thrombocytopenia, neutropenia, and hemolytic anemia [1–3].

Type III Reactions (Immune Complex Reactions)

In type III reactions, formation of an immune complex and its deposition on tissue surface serve as primary initiators. Occasionally, immune complexes bind to endothelial cells and lead to immune complex deposition with subsequent complement activation in the linings of blood vessels. Circumstances that govern immune formation or immune complex disease remain unclear to date, and it usually occurs without symptoms. The clinical symptoms of a type III reaction include serum sickness (β-lactams), drug-induced lupus erythematosus (quinidine), and vasculitis (minocycline). Type III reactions can result in acute interstitial nephritis or serum sickness (fever, arthritis, enlarged lymph nodes, urticaria, and maculopapular rashes) [1–3].

Type IV Reactions (Cell-Mediated or Delayed Hypersensitivity Reactions)

Type IV reactions are initiated when a hapten–protein antigenic complex sensitizes T lymphocytes (T cells). Upon re-exposure to the immunogen, the activity of the sensitized T-cells usually results in severe inflammation in the affected areas. Type IV reactions are exemplified by contact dermatitis while pseudoallergic reactions may resemble allergic reactions clinically but are not immunologically mediated. Examples of Type IV reactions include asthma and rashes caused by aspirin and maculopapular erythematous rashes due to ampicillin or amoxicillin in the absence of penicillin hypersensitivity. This reaction may also be caused by sulfonamides, anticonvulsants (phenytoin, carbamazepine, and phenobarbital), NSAIDs (aspirin, naproxen, nabumetone, and ketoprofen), antiretroviral agents and cephalosporins [1–4].

Other Types of Reactions

Several types of adverse drug reactions do not easily fit into the general classification scheme. These include most cutaneous hypersensitivity reactions (such as toxic epidermal necrolysis), 'immune-allergic' hepatitis and hypersensitivity pneumonitis. Another difficulty is that allergic drug reactions can occur via more than one mechanism; picryl chloride in mice induces both type I and type IV responses. Several articles are included in this review to serve as a pointer to this field [4–12].

REFERENCES

[1] Coombs RRA, Gell PGH. Classification of allergic reactions responsible for clinical hypersensitivity and disease. In: Gell PGH, Coombs RRA, Lachmann PJ, editors. Clinical Aspects of Immunology. London: Blackwell Scientific Publications; 1975. pp. 761–81.

[2] Schnyder B, Pichler W. Mechanisms of Drug-Induced Allergy. Mayo Clin Proc. Mar 2009; 84(3): 268–272.

[3] Boyman O, Comte D, Spertini F. Adverse reactions to biologic agents and their medical management. Nat Rev Rheumatol., 2014 Aug 12. doi: 10.1038/nrrheum.2014.123. [Epub ahead of print].

[4] Brown SGA. Clinical features and severity grading of anaphylaxis. J Allergy Clin Immunol 2004; 114(2): 371–6.

[5] Johansson SGO, Hourihane JO, Bousquet J, Bruijnzeel-Koomen C, Dreborg S, Haahtela T, Kowalski ML, Mygind N, Ring J, van Cauwenberge P, van Hage-Hamsten M, Wüthrich B. A revised nomenclature for allergy. An EAACI position statement from the EAACI nomenclature task force. Allergy 2001; 56(9): 813–24.

[6] Uzzaman A, Cho SH. Chapter 28: Classification of hypersensitivity reactions. Allergy Asthma Proc. 2012 May–Jun; 33 Suppl 1:S96–9.

[7] Descotes J, Choquet-Kastylevsky G. Toxicology, 2001; 158(1–2):43–9. Gell and Coombs's classification: is it still valid?

[8] Corominas M, Andrés-López B, Lleonart R. Severe adverse drug reactions induced by hydrochlorothiazide: A persistent old problem. Ann Allergy Asthma Immunol., 2016; 117 (3):334–5.

[9] Velickovic J, Palibrk I, Miljković B, et al. Self-reported drug allergies in surgical population in serbia. Acta Clin Croat. 2015; 54(4):492–9.

[10] Yip VL, Alfirevic A, Pirmohamed M. Genetics of immune-mediated adverse drug reactions: a comprehensive and clinical review. Clin Rev Allergy Immunol., 2015; 48(2–3):165–75.

[11] Agúndez JA, Mayorga C, García-Martin E. Drug metabolism and hypersensitivity reactions to drugs. Curr Opin Allergy Clin Immunol. 2015; 15(4):277–84.

[12] Wheatley LM, Plaut M, Schwaninger JM. et al. Report from the National Institute of Allergy and Infectious Diseases workshop on drug allergy. J Allergy Clin Immunol., 2015; 136(2):262-71.e2.

ANALYSIS OF TOXICOLOGICAL REACTIONS

Potentiation Reactions

This type of reaction occurs when either one non-toxic chemical interacts with another non-toxic chemical or one non-toxic chemical interacts with another toxic chemical at low doses (subtoxic, acutely toxic) results in a greater level of toxicity. An alternate interpretation could be when two drugs are taken together and one of them intensifies the action of the other. In such scenarios, if the final result is high toxicity, then the final outcome is called potentiation (increasing the toxic effect of 'Y' by 'X'). Results usually lead to unanticipated level of cell death in the form of apoptosis, necrosis, autophagy and apocrosis (or necraptosis, aponecrosis). Theoretically, it can be expressed as: $x + y = M$ $(1 + 0 = 4)$.

Examples:

(i) When chronic or regular alcohol drinkers consume therapeutic doses of acetaminophen, it can lead to alcohol-potentiated acetaminophen-induced hepatoxicity (cause: ethanol-induced massive CYP2E1 induction in the liver)

(ii) Administration of iron supplements in patients on doxorubicin therapy may cause potentiation of doxorubicin-induced cardiotoxicity (cause: hydroxyl radical formation and redox cycling of doxorubicin)

(iii) Phenergan®, an antihistamine, when given with a painkilling narcotic such as Demerol® can intensify the narcotic effect; reducing the dose of the narcotic is advised

(iv) Ethanol potentiation of CCl4-induced hepatotoxicity

(v) Use of phenytoin and calcium-channel blockers combination should be used with caution.

Synergistic Effect

Synergism is somewhat similar to potentiation. When two drugs are taken together that are similar in action, such as barbiturates and alcohol, which are both depressants, an effect exaggerated out of proportion to that of each drug taken separately at the given dose may occur (mathematically: $1 + 1 = 4$). Normally, taken alone, neither substance would cause serious harm, but if taken together, the combination could cause coma or death. Another example is when smokers get exposed to asbestos, resulting in the development of lung cancer.

Additive Effect

Additive effect is defined as a consequence which follows exposure to two or more agents which act jointly but do not interact, the total effect is the simple sum of the effects of separate exposure to the agents under the same conditions. This could be represented by $1 + 1 = 2$:

Examples:
(i) a barbiturate and a tranquilizer given together before surgery to relax the patient
(ii) the toxic effect on bone marrow resulting after AZT + ganciclovir or AZT + clotrimazole administration.

Antagonistic Effects

Antagonistic effects are when two drugs/chemicals are administered simultaneously or one closely followed by the other with the net effect of the final outcome of the reaction being negligible or zero. This could be expressed by $1 + 1 = 0$. An example might be the use of a tranquilizer to stop the action of LSD.

Examples:
(i) When ethanol is administered to methanol-poisoned patient
(ii) NSAIDs administered to diuretics (hydrochlorothiazide/furosemide): Reduce diuretics effectivness
(iii) Certain β-blockers (INDERAL®) taken to control high blood pressure and heart disease, counteract β-adrenergic stimulants, such as Albuterol®.

REFERENCES

[1] Ray SD, Mehendale HM. Potentiation of CCl4 and CHCl3 hepatotoxicity and lethality by various alcohols. Fundam Appl Toxicol. 1990; 15(3):429–40.

[2] Gammella, E., Maccarinelli, F., Buratti, P., et al. The role of iron in anthracycline cardiotoxicity. Front Pharmacol. 2014; 5:25. doi: 10.3389/fphar.2014.00025. eCollection 2014.

[3] NLM's Toxlearn tutorials: http://toxlearn.nlm.nih.gov/Module1.htm.

[4] NLM's Toxtutor (visit interactions): http://sis.nlm.nih.gov/enviro/toxtutor/Tox1/a42.htm.

[5] Smith MA, Reynolds CP, Kang MH, et al. Synergistic activity of PARP inhibition by talazoparib (BMN 673) with temozolomide in pediatric cancer models in the pediatric preclinical testing program. Clin Cancer Res., 2015; 21(4):819–32.

[6] Niu F, Zhao S, Xu CY, et al. Potentiation of the antitumor activity of adriamycin against osteosarcoma by cannabinoid WIN-55,212-2. Oncol Lett. 2015; 10(4):2415–2421.

[7] Calderon-Aparicio A, Strasberg-Rieber M, Rieber M. Disulfiram anti-cancer efficacy without copper overload is enhanced by extracellular H2O2 generation: antagonism by tetrathiomolybdate. Oncotarget. 2015; 6(30):29771–81.

[8] Zajac J, Kostrhunova H, Novohradsky V, et al. Potentiation of mitochondrial dysfunction in tumor cells by conjugates of metabolic modulator dichloroacetate with a Pt(IV) derivative of oxaliplatin. J Inorg Biochem. 2016; 156:89–97.

[9] Nurcahyanti AD, Wink M. Cytotoxic potentiation of vinblastine and paclitaxel by L-canavanine in human cervical cancer and hepatocellular carcinoma cells. Phytomedicine. 2015; 22(14):1232–7.

[10] Lu CF, Yuan XY, Li LZ, et al. Combined exposure to nano-silica and lead-induced potentiation of oxidative stress and DNA damage in human lung epithelial cells. Ecotoxicol Environ Saf. 2015; 122:537–44.

[11] Kuchárová B, Mikeš J, Jendželovský R, et al. Potentiation of hypericin-mediated photodynamic therapy cytotoxicity by MK-886: focus on ABC transporters, GDF-15 and redox status. Photodiagnosis Photodyn Ther. 2015; 12(3):490–503.

[12] Djillani A, Doignon I, Luyten T, et al. Potentiation of the store-operated calcium entry (SOCE) induces phytohemagglutinin-activated Jurkat T cell apoptosis. Cell Calcium. 2015; 58(2):171–85.

[13] Yoon E, Babar A, Choudhary M. et al. Acetaminophen-Induced Hepatotoxicity: a Comprehensive Update. J Clin Transl Hepatol. 2016; 4(2): 131–142.

[15] Ray SD, Corcoran, G.B. "Apoptosis and Cell Death", 3rd Edition, Vol. I, Chapter-11, Pp. 247-312, in Ballantyne, Marrs and Syversen Eds., 'General and Applied Toxicology'; Wylie Publishing, UK, 2009. http://onlinelibrary.wiley.com/doi/10.1002/9780470744307.gat015/abstract.

[14] Betharia S, Farris FF, Corcoran GB, Ray SD. 'Mechanisms of Toxicity' In: Wexler, P. (Ed.),

Encyclopedia of Toxicology, 3rd edition vol 3. Elsevier Inc., Academic Press, pp. 165–175, 2014. http://www.sciencedirect.com/science/article/pii/B9780123864543003298.

GRADES OF ADVERSE DRUG REACTIONS

Drugs and chemicals may exhibit adverse drug reactions (ADRs or adverse drug effects) that may include unwanted (side effects), uncomfortable (system dysfunction), or dangerous effects (toxic). ADRs are a form of manifestation of toxicity which may occur after overexposure or high-level exposure or, in some circumstances. ADRs may also occur after exposure to therapeutic doses but often an underlying cause (pre-existing condition) is present. In contrast, 'Side effect' is an imprecise term often used to refer to a drug's unintended effects that occur within the therapeutic range [1]. Risk–benefit analysis provides a window into the decision-making process prior to prescribing a medication. Patient characteristics such as age, gender, ethnic background, pre-existing conditions, nutritional status, genetic pre-disposition or geographic factors, as well as drug factors (e.g., type of drug, administration route, treatment duration, dosage, and bioavailability) may profoundly influence ADR outcomes. Drug-induced adverse events can be categorized as unexpected, serious or life-threatening.

Adverse drug reactions are graded according to intensity, using a scheme that was originally introduced by the US National Cancer Institute to describe the intensity of reactions to drugs used in cancer chemotherapy [2]. This scheme is now widely used to grade the intensity of other types of adverse reactions, although it does not always apply so clearly to them. The scheme assigns grades as follows:

- Grade 1 ≡ mild;
- Grade 2 ≡ moderate;
- Grade 3 ≡ severe;
- Grade 4 ≡ life-threatening or disabling;
- Grade 5 ≡ death.

Then, instead of providing general definitions of the terms "mild", "moderate", "severe", and "life-threatening or disabling", the system describes what they mean operationally in terms of each adverse reaction, in each case the intensity being described in narrative terms. For example, hemolysis is graded as follows:

- Grade 1: Laboratory evidence of hemolysis only (e.g. direct antiglobulin test; presence of schistocytes).
- Grade 2: Evidence of red cell destruction and ≥2 g/dL decrease in hemoglobin, no transfusion.
- Grade 3: Transfusion or medical intervention (for example, steroids) indicated.

- Grade 4: Catastrophic consequences (for example, renal failure, hypotension, bronchospasm, emergency splenectomy).
- Grade 5: Death.

Not all adverse reactions are assigned all grades. For example, serum sickness is classified as being of grade 3 or grade 5 only; i.e. it is always either severe or fatal.

The system is less good at classifying subjective reactions. For example, fatigue is graded as follows:

- Grade 1: Mild fatigue over baseline.
- Grade 2: Moderate or causing difficulty performing some activities of daily living.
- Grade 3: Severe fatigue interfering with activities of daily living.
- Grade 4: Disabling.

Attribution categories can be defined as follows:

(i) Definite: The adverse event is clearly related to the investigational agent(s).
(ii) Probable: The adverse event is likely related to the investigational agent(s).
(iii) Possible: The adverse event may be related to the investigational agent(s).
(iv) Unlikely: The adverse event is doubtfully related to the investigational agent(s).
(v) Unrelated: The adverse event is clearly NOT related to the investigational agent(s).

REFERENCES

[1] Merck Manuals: http://www.merckmanuals.com/professional/clinical_pharmacology/adverse_drug_reactions/adverse_drug_reactions.html.
[2] National Cancer Institute. Common Terminology Criteria for Adverse Events v3.0 (CTCAE). 9 August, 2006. http://ctep.cancer.gov/protocolDevelopment/electronic_applications/docs/ctcaev3.pdf.

FDA PREGNANCY CATEGORIES/CLASSIFICATION OF TERATOGENICITY

The FDA has established five categories to indicate the potential of a drug to cause birth defects if used during pregnancy. The categories are determined by the reliability of documentation and the risk to benefit ratio. They do not take into account any risks from pharmaceutical agents or their metabolites in breast milk. The pregnancy categories are:

Category A: Adequate and well-controlled studies have failed to demonstrate a risk to the fetus in the first trimester of pregnancy and there is no evidence of risk in later trimesters.

Example drugs or substances: levothyroxine, folic acid, magnesium sulfate, liothyronine.

Category B: Animal reproduction studies have failed to demonstrate a risk to the fetus and there are no adequate and well-controlled studies in pregnant women.

Example drugs: metformin, hydrochlorothiazide, cyclobenzaprine, amoxicillin, pantoprazole.

Category C: Animal reproduction studies have shown an adverse effect on the fetus and there are no adequate and well-controlled studies in humans, but potential benefits may warrant use of the drug in pregnant women despite potential risks.

Example drugs: tramadol, gabapentin, amlodipine, trazodone, prednisone.

Category D: There is positive evidence of human fetal risk based on adverse reaction data from investigational or marketing experience or studies in humans, but potential benefits may warrant use of the drug in pregnant women despite potential risks.

Example drugs: lisinopril, alprazolam, losartan, clonazepam, lorazepam.

Category X: Studies in animals or humans have demonstrated fetal abnormalities and/or there is positive evidence of human fetal risk based on adverse reaction data from investigational or marketing experience, and the risks involved in use of the drug in pregnant women clearly outweigh potential benefits.

Example drugs: atorvastatin, simvastatin, warfarin, methotrexate, finasteride.

Category N: FDA has not classified the drug.

Example drugs: aspirin, oxycodone, hydroxyzine, acetaminophen, diazepam.

Examples of drugs approved since June 30th, 2015 showing various new pregnancy and lactation subsections in their labels [3]:

- Addyi (flibanserin)—indicated for generalized hypoactive sexual desire disorder (HSDD) in premenopausal women.
- Descovy (emtricitabine and tenofovir alafenamide fumarate)—indicated for HIV-1 infection.
- Entresto (sacubitril and valsartan)—indicated for heart failure.
- Harvoni (ledipasvir and sofosbuvir)—indicated for chronic viral hepatitis C infection (HCV).
- Praluent (alirocumab)—indicated for heterozygous familial hypercholesterolemia, or patients with atherosclerotic heart disease who require additional lowering of LDL-cholesterol.
- Vosevi (sofosbuvir, velpatasvir and voxilaprevir)—indicated for chronic hepatitis C infection (HCV).

- Nerlynx (neratinib)—indicated for early stage HER2-overexpressed breast cancer, , following adjuvant trastuzumab-based therapy.
- Rituxan Hycela (rituximab and hyaluronidase human)—indicated for follicular lymphoma, diffuse large B-cell lymphoma (DLBCL), and chronic lymphocytic leukemia (CLL).
- Mydayis (amphetamine mixed salts)—indicated for attention deficit hyperactivity disorder (ADHD). Kevzara (sarilumab)—indicated for rheumatoid arthritis.
- Radicava (edaravone)—indicated for amyotrophic lateral sclerosis (AML).
- Imfinzi (durvalumab)—indicated for urothelial carcinoma

On December 3, 2014, the FDA issued a final rule for the labeling of drugs during pregnancy and lactation, titled "Content and Format of Labeling for Human Prescription Drug and Biological Products; Requirements for Pregnancy and Lactation Labeling"; this rule is also informally known as the "Pregnancy and Lactation Labeling Rule (PLLR)".

The rule changes the content and format for drug labeling information and the new labeling requirements include:

- *Elimination the pregnancy letter categories (A, B, C, D and X)*
  - *Text provides specific information in each section to assist with making benefit– risk decisions when medication is needed*
- *Labeling sections are changed*
  - *Old: Pregnancy, Labor and Delivery, Nursing Mothers*
  - *New: Pregnancy (includes L&D), Lactation (includes nursing mothers), Females and Males of Reproductive Potential*
- *Requirement that the label is updated as new information becomes available*

The PLLR changes are effective as of June 30, 2015. Prescription medications and biologics approved after this date will use the new format while older material will have a 3-year phase-in for the new labeling. These changes are not applicable to over-the-counter (OTC) products.

REFERENCES

[1] Doering PL, Boothby LA, Cheok M. Review of pregnancy labeling of prescription drugs: is the current system adequate to inform of risks? Am J Obstet Gynecol 2002; 187(2): 333–9.

[2] Ramoz LL, Patel-Shori NM. Recent changes in pregnancy and lactation labeling: retirement of risk categories. Pharmacotherapy, 2014; 34(4):389–95. doi: 10.1002/phar.

[3] Drugs.com: http://www.drugs.com/pregnancy-categories.html.

[4] FDA. Pregnancy and Lactation Labeling (Drugs) Final Rule. https://www.fda.gov/downloads/drugs/guidancecomplianceregulatoryinformation/guidances/ucm450636.pdf; https://www.fda.gov/Drugs/DevelopmentApprovalProcess/DevelopmentResources/Labeling/ucm093307.htm.

Clinicians are suggested to be aware of the information contained in the following literature originating from regulatory agencies:

[5] FDA/CDER SBIA Chronicles. Drugs in Pregnancy and Lactation: Improved Benefit-Risk Information. January 22, 2015. URL: http://www.fda.gov/downloads/Drugs/DevelopmentApprovalProcess/SmallBusinessAssistance/UCM431132.pdf.

[6] FDA Consumer Articles. Pregnant? Breastfeeding? Better Drug Information Is Coming. Updated: December 17, 2014. URL: https://www.drugs.com/fda-consumer/pregnant-breastfeeding-better-drug-information-is-coming-334.html.

[7] FDA News Release. FDA issues final rule on changes to pregnancy and lactation labeling information for prescription drug and biological products. December 3, 2014. URL: http://www.fda.gov/NewsEvents/Newsroom/Press Announcements/ucm425317.htm.

[8] Mospan C. New Prescription Labeling Requirements for the Use of Medications in Pregnancy and Lactation. CE for Pharmacists. Alaska Pharmacists Association. April 15, 2016. URL: http://www.alaskapharmacy.org/files/CE_Activities/0416_State_CE_Lesson.pdf.

[9] Australian classification: https://www.tga.gov.au/australian-categorisation-system-prescribing-medicines-pregnancy#.U038WfmSx8E.

CONCLUSION

Adverse drug events, including ADRs, side effects, drug-induced diseases, toxicity, pharmacogenetics and immunologic reactions, represent a significant burden to patients, health care systems, and society. It is the goal of *Side Effects of Drugs Annual* to summarize and evaluate important new evidence-based information in order to guide clinicians in the prevention, monitoring, and assessment of adverse drug events in their patients. The work provides not only a summary of this essential new data, but suggestions for how it may be interpreted and implications for practice.

1

Central Nervous System Stimulants and Drugs That Suppress Appetite

Nicholas T. Bello*,1, Matthew R. Zahner†

*School of Environmental and Biological Sciences, Rutgers, The State University of New Jersey, New Brunswick, NJ, United States
†East Tennessee State University, Johnson City, TN, United States
1Corresponding author: ntbello@rutgers.edu

Abbreviations

ADHD	attention deficit hyperactive disorder
LDX	lisdexamfetamine dimesylate
MA	methamphetamine
MAP	methamphetamine-induced psychosis
MAS	mixed amphetamine salts
MDA	3,4-methylenedioxyamphetamine
MDMA	3,4-methylenedioxymetamphetamine
RCT	randomized-controlled trial
STEMI	ST segment elevation myocardial infarction

AMPHETAMINE AND AMPHETAMINE DERIVATES [SEDA-34, 1; SEDA-35, 1; SEDA-36, 1; SEDA-37, 1; SEDA-38, 1]

In two phase III randomized clinical trials of lisdex-amfetamine dimesylate (LDX) for binge eating disorder (BED), LDX (50 or 70 mg/day; $n=192$ for study 1; $n=181$ for study 2) was compared with placebo ($n=187$ for study 1; $n=185$ for study 2) for 12 weeks. All subjects had moderate to severe BED. In both studies >50% of subjects reported mild or moderate treatment emergent adverse events (TEAEs). The most common LDX-induced TEAEs were dry mouth (39.6% for study 1; 33.1% for study 2), insomnia (17.7% for study 1; 10.5% for study 2) or headache (13.5% for study; 17.7% for study 2). No placebo TEAEs was >10%. There was an increase at 12 weeks for hemodynamic measurements for both studies. LDX caused a 4.41–6.31 bpm increase for pulse rate, 0.2–1.45 mm Hg increase in systolic pressure, and 1.06–1.83 mm Hg increase diastolic blood pressure [1C].

Organs and Systems

Cardiovascular

A 39-year-old African American female without a history of coronary artery disease became unresponsive shortly after being admitted to the hospital. She was in ventricular-fibrillation cardiac arrest with a 99% thrombotic occlusion of the mid-distal left anterior descending coronary artery. She had a positive toxicological screen for amphetamines, but only admitted to using a natural weight loss dietary supplement. Thrombus was suspected to be secondary to catecholamine-induced platelet aggregation [2A].

A 35-year-old male with a 15 year history of methamphetamine abuse presented with dyspnea and chest pain. Symptoms had persisted for 2 weeks prior to seeking medical attention. Multiple thrombi were found in both ventricles of the heart. Following cessation of methamphetamine no additional thrombi were noted at 3 month follow-up [3A].

A 31-year-old male with no past medical history developed progressive cardiogenic shock following a 48 hours treatment for dyspnea, prolonged orthopnea, peripheral edema, and lethargy. This incident emerged during 2 months of abstinence of methamphetamine after being a heavy user for 8 years. Cardiogenic shock was suspected to result from the methamphetamine-induced cardiomyopathy. The patient had normal left ventricular function following a 12-month period of drug abstinence and treatment with perindopril (uptitrated to 10 mg/QD) and carvedilol (uptitrated to 12.5 mg/BID) [4A].

A 55-year-old male arrived at the emergency department after swallowing an egg-sized amount of methamphetamine. Patient presented with progressive sympathomimetic intoxication and autonomic instability. Because methamphetamine is lipophilic, an intravenous bolus (100 mL) of Intralipid (20%) was administered. Within 20 min, his pulse, respiratory rate, and temperature began to normalize. After a 5-day hospital stay in a telemetry unit, he was discharged. Rapid recovery from methamphetamine toxicity was attributed to the trial of lipid emulsion therapy [5A].

Psychiatric

Methamphetamine-induced psychosis (MAP) is often times clinically indistinguishable from paranoid schizophrenia (SZ). The set of psychiatric symptoms were characterized in MAP ($n = 33$; 76% male) and SZ ($n = 69$; 58% male) adult subjects. For a MAP diagnosis, onset of symptoms had to be within 1 month of intoxication or withdrawal. Duration of symptoms had to be ≥ 4 weeks. MAP subjects displayed more voice conversing and auditory hallucinations than SZ subjects (48.5% vs 20.3%, $P = 0.003$ for both symptoms). After adjusting for age, there was an association for thought broadcasting in the SZ subjects (adjusted OR = 3.02; 95% CI 1.12–8.15, $P = 0.028$) [6c]. In another study, MAP subjects ($n = 53$) had more visual hallucinations (30.2% vs 11.3%, $P = 0.017$) and somatic or tactile hallucinations (20.8% vs 3.8%, $P = 0.008$) than SZ subjects ($n = 50$). The SZ subjects had higher scores of conceptual disorganization ($P = 0.002$), mannerism/posturing ($P = 0.011$), blunted affect ($P = 0.005$), emotional withdrawal ($P = 0.016$), motor retardation ($P = 0.007$), and the summation of negative symptoms ($P = 0.029$) compared with MAP subjects. Notably, MAP subjects in this study had continued with symptoms, even 1 month after methamphetamine discontinuation [7c].

In an examination of MAP patients ($n = 152$) in a hospital in northern Iran, it was revealed that 146 patients (96.1%) had delusions or hallucinations and 115 (75.6%) has at least one form of violent behavior in the past month. The most common type of delusions were persecutory (85.5%), reference (38.8%), grandiosity (32.9%), and infidelity (30.2%), whereas most hallucinations were auditory (51.3%). Of those MAP patients that were married, most violent behavior was intimate partner violence (61.2%) [8C].

In a prospective study of MAP patients ($n = 50$), 50% remained abstinent of methamphetamine at a 3-month time point. Most clinical symptoms, except for depressive symptoms, improved with methamphetamine abstinence in this patient population. A higher negative score at initial admission to treatment hospital was associated with a greater risk of methamphetamine relapse ($P = 0.028$) [9c].

Two cases of mixed amphetamine salts (MAS)-induced somnambulism in pediatric patients were reported. The first case was a 13-year-old female diagnosed with ADHD that had been on methylphenidate for 7 years. Before her diagnosis of ADHD, at age 5 years old she had 2 episodes of somnambulism, but no other episodes since that time. She also had a family history of sleepwalking. One week after her medication was switched to MAS extended release (10 mg daily), she had 2 episodes of sleepwalking. The second case was an 8-year-old male that began MAS extended release (uptitrated to 10 mg). His mother reported several episodes of somnambulism after the first month of starting treatment. The boy's medication was switched to a delayed release formulation of methylphenidate and no further incidences of sleep walking were noted [10A].

Drug–Drug Interactions

A 32-year-old female was taking MAS-extended release formulation (30 mg/day) to treat ADHD symptoms for >10 years had co-morbidity of alcohol use disorder for 5 years. As part of her alcohol cessation program she was administered disulfiram for 1 month. She was admitted into an inpatient psychiatric unit after a 1-day onset of paranoid delusions. Cessation of both drugs completely resolved the psychotic symptoms after 4 days. The authors speculate that disulfiram inhibits dopamine beta-hydroxylase to augment the amphetamine-induced frontostriatal dopamine transmission and decreases brain levels of norepinephrine to produce acute psychosis [11A].

Genotype–Drug Interactions

Polymorphisms of the catechol-O-methyltransferase (COMT) were studied in the post-mortem blood and cerebrospinal fluid of fatal methamphetamine abusers ($n = 28$) and fatal psychotropic drug intoxication ($n = 22$). Those fatal methamphetamine abusers that carried the rs4633 T allele and rs4680 A allele had significantly higher CSF dopamine concentrations than the methamphetamine abusers with the CC genotype of rs4633 and GG genotype of rs4680, ($P = 0.004$, $P = 017$, respectively). There were no such genotype interactions with fatal psychotropic drug cases [12c].

Ecstasy (3,4-Methylenedioxy-N-Methylamphetamine; MDMA)

In order to determine the long-term impact of MDMA during pregnancy, the development of the offspring of MDMA users were followed up to the age of 2-years old. A total of 93 children were assessed as infants, 4-, 12-, 18- and 24-months, of age. Children of pregnant women that were heavy users of MDMA (averaged 1.7 ± 1.8 tablets/week) had persistent motor delays evident from 4-month to 24-months of age (OR = 2.19, 95% CI = 1.02–4.70, $P < 0.045$) [13c].

Organs and Systems

Death

A 29-year-old male was brought to a tertiary care center unresponsive. He had a history of MDMA use. The chemical analysis report was positive for ethanol and MDMA in the blood, urine and visceral tissue. The cause of death was respiratory failure due to disseminated intravascular coagulation (DIC) as a consequence of MDMA and ethanol consumption [14A].

METHYLPHENIDATE [SEDA-34, 5; SEDA-35, 1; SEDA-36, 1; SEDA 37, 1; SEDA-38, 1]

An open-label trial of methylphenidate was initiated in advance pancreatic cancer patients ($n = 71$) to combat associated fatigue. Methylphenidate (titrated from 5 mg to 10 mg after 2 weeks) was initiated for 4 weeks (treatment duration ranged from 4 to 24 weeks) and self-reported fatigue was assessed throughout. A total of 9 patients (13%) dropped out of the study due to the treatment-emergent adverse effects. The most common adverse events attributed to methylphenidate were weight loss (6%), decreased appetite (4%), insomnia (3%), rapid pulse rate (3%), tremor (1%), nervousness (1%), xerostomia (1%), and anorexia (1%). 4% of the methylphenidate-treated patients experienced nausea, but nausea could also be attributed to the chemotherapeutic agents used to treat the advance pancreatic cancer [15c].

Methylphenidate (2–30 mg) was compared alone or in combination with risperidone (0.25–2 mg) for the treatment of ADHD single blind randomized control trial in preschool children (mean age 4.5 years old; $n = 42$). Study length was 6 weeks and children were assessed at 3 weeks and 6 weeks for improvement of ADHD symptoms. Three children were discontinued treatment with methylphenidate for decreased appetite, increased agitation, and increased nervousness and aggression. In contrast, two children in the methylphenidate and risperidone were discontinued for severe increase in appetite and sleepiness. The most common reported adverse effects with methylphenidate were insomnia (33.3%), anorexia (25%), agitation (8.3%), and nervousness (4.2%). Anorexia (21.7%), sedation (17.4%), enuresis (13%), phobia (8.7%), and nervousness (8.7%) were reported in the methylphenidate and risperidone treated group [16c].

Organs and Systems

Cardiovascular

A 45-year-old male developed thoracic palpations a few days after beginning methylphenidate treatment for ADHD. After 2 months, he sought medical attention for the condition. His dose of methylphenidate at the time of evaluation was 36 mg (for each working day). An electrocardiogram revealed 3 ventricular extrasystoles a minute and a Holter monitor showed 3249 ventricular extrasystoles in 24 hours. Normal electrocardiograms with no extrasystoles were obtained 7 months after cessation of methylphenidate [17A].

A 21-year-old male presented to the emergency department with acute chest pains that developed overnight and continued until the morning. From his electrocardiogram and elevated troponin levels, he was diagnosed with ST elevation myocardial infarction (STEMI). It was revealed that patient had begun methylphenidate for the ADHD symptoms 3 days prior to admission into the emergency department. Based on coronary angiogram, it was suggested that STEMI a methylphenidate-induced coronary vasospasm. Methylphenidate was stopped and 1 week later the patient was asymptomatic [18A].

Reproductive Systems

A 14-year-old male with ADHD symptom began methylphenidate osmotic-controlled release oral delivery system (OROS; 27 mg). Because at age 6-years old the patient previously had surgery to correct undescended testis, testosterone levels were routinely monitored. After 13 days of beginning the methylphenidate OROS treatment, blood testosterone levels dropped. Blood testosterone levels return to normal levels 2 weeks following cessation of methylphenidate. The mechanisms for this interaction are unknown [19A].

Skin

An 11-year-old male with ADHD and social and generalized anxiety had several episodes of itching and mild skin eruptions on his arm and chest. He had no known allergies and his skin reactions were attributed to a psychological origin. He had been intermittently taking sertraline (uptitrated to 50 mg) for 4 months and started developing attention problems in school. He was restarted on sertraline (50 mg) and methylphenidate (27 mg) was added to his treatment. After 4 months he showed improvement, so the dose of methylphenidate was increased to 57 mg. After 1 week of the increased dose of methylphenidate, he developed a wide spread nonpruritic maculopapular skin rash. His rash resolved 10 days following discontinuation of methylphenidate and sertraline. The authors noted other reports of skin eruptions associated with methylphenidate [20A].

Drug–Drug Interaction

A 13-year-old male with a history of schizophrenia, bipolar disorder, autism, and ADHD was receiving risperidone (1.5 mg BID), oxcarbazepine, and methylphenidate. The patient developed weight gain, which was thought to be secondary to risperidone. When the dose of risperidone was tapered (to 0.5 mg BID), he developed severe painful cervical dystonia and upper extremity dyskinesia with agitation and restlessness. The extrapyramidal symptoms were thought to be precipitated by the interaction between the lower risperidone dose and methylphenidate [21A].

METHYLXANTHINES

Caffeine [SEDA-32, 14; SEDA-33, 11; SEDA-34, 6; SEDA-36, 1; SEDA-37, 1; SEDA-38, 1]

A case crossover design in which pregnant women diagnosed with preeclampsia ($n = 286$) were assessed for potential triggers. The data were retrospectively collected in 7 day blocks (a total of 2 weeks) in the time before preeclampsia. The experiment window was day 1–7, whereas the control window was day 8–14 before the preeclampsia event. Caffeine intake (OR 0.26, 95% CI: 0.17–0.39) was inversely associated with onset of preeclampsia [22C].

In a prospective study of neonates ($n = 313$) the frequency and characteristics of adverse drug reactions (ADR) were examined. Of the 2166 prescriptions, caffeine citrate had the highest number of ADR. Caffeine was prescribed 282 and was associated with 19 ADR. The ADR were cardiovascular (6 tachycardia and 3 hypertension events), gastrointestinal (1 hemorrhaging and 2 vomiting), central nervous system disorders (6 stimulation events, such as irritability, restlessness, and jitteriness), and 1 ADR was high bilirubin blood levels (>7.1 mg/dL) [23C].

Organs and Systems

Cardiovascular

Caffeine is often used to treat apnea in premature neonates. Two cases of arrhythmia developed in neonates within 24 hours following an eye examination. The first case was a 22 day infant that developed bradycardia that persisted for 48 hours following an eye examination with phenylephrine 1%–cyclopentolate 0.2% eyedrops. A similar incident occurred 16 days later following a second eye examination. On both days, the infant was receiving caffeine for apnea. The second case was in a 9-week-old infant that developed acute atrial tachycardia approximately 12 hours after an eye examination with phenylephrine 2.5%–cyclopentolate 0.5% eye drops. The infant was receiving domperidone, omeprazole, and caffeine citrate. Caffeine was discontinued for at least 72 hours. No further cardiac issues were noted when caffeine was reintroduced [24A].

SELECTIVE NOREPINEPHRINE REUPTAKE INHIBITORS ATOMOXETINE [SEDA-34, 4; SEDA-36, 1; SEDA-37, 1; SEDA-38, 1]

In a systematic review of the available literature from 2001 to 2014, the safety of atomoxetine was examined. The safety topics include suicidality (15 studies), aggression/hostility (3 studies), psychosis/mania (7 studies), hepatotoxicity (7 studies), cardiovascular effects (29 studies), and growth and development (28 studies). Atomoxetine treatment did not result in an increased risk for suicidality, aggression/hostility behaviors, or seizures frequency. Liver damage associated with atomoxetine treatment were reported rare and were noted as severe in some of the reviewed literature. Cardiovascular changes, in particular the risk for prolonged QT segments, were also commonly reported, but there was no severe or serious cardiovascular risks noted with atomoxetine. Decreases in growth (height and weight) were noted in the first month of atomoxetine treatment, but this decline appears to normalize with more prolonged atomoxetine treatment (>2 years) [25M].

Organ and Systems

Drug–Drug Interactions

A 26-year-old female receiving fluoxetine (40 mg, QD) for affect dysregulation was also prescribed atomoxetine for underlining ADHD-related issues. She received atomoxetine at 40 mg QD, which was increased to 40 mg BID. After 4 days of the uptitration, the patient developed acute chest pain and dyspnea. The electrocardiogram revealed an acute anteroseptal STEMI and echocardiogram revealed apical akinesis and hyperkinesis. Following some additional tests, the patient was diagnosed with Takotsubo cardiomyopathy. After 5 weeks atomoxetine (uptitrated to 65 mg QD; 40 and 25 mg doses) was reintroduced. The patient was without incident after a 16 weeks follow-up. Therefore, clinicians should be aware of the possibility of fluoxetine inhibiting CYP2D6 to increase the levels of atomoxetine to cause a norepinephrine-induced cardiotoxicity [26A].

A 17-year male diagnosed with ADHD combined subtype was receiving atomoxetine (uptitrated to 60 mg/day). The patient became more irritable with each incremental dose of atomoxetine, so atomoxetine was discontinued and he was switched to aripiprazole (5 mg/kg/day). After the second dose of aripiprazole, which was 36 hours after the last dose of atomoxetine, the patient developed abrupt and painful contractions in the neck. Patient was administered biperiden (5 mg) and his aripiprazole-induced acute dystonia was resolved within minutes. Aripiprazole was discontinued and the patient's neurological examination was normal 2 days later [27A].

A 13-year female diagnosed with ADHD and mild intellectual disability was receiving atomoxetine (80 mg/day). She complained of hypomanic symptoms (e.g., increased sexual desire, excessive talking, and poor sleep patterns) and atomoxetine was discontinued and began same day treatment with aripiprazole (5 mg/day). Approximately 5 hours after initiation of aripiprazole treatment she developed difficulties in swallowing and contraction of mouth muscles. She was treated with biperiden (5 mg) and her aripiprazole-induced dystonia was resolved within minutes. She was prescribed risperidone without further cardiac symptoms [27A].

VIGILANCE PROMOTING DRUGS

Modafinil and Armodafinil [SEDA-34, 6; SEDA-36, 1; SEDA-37, 1; SEDA-38, 1]

In a meta-analysis of 16 randomized-controlled trials (RCT) involving patients receiving modafinil ($n=723$) or armodafinil ($n=1009$) for the treatment of obstructive sleep apnea several mild or moderate TEAEs were noted. Discontinuation from the RCT was <12% for both medications. Headache was the most common TEAE with a risk ratio of 1.78 (95% CI: 1.20–2.65) and 2.04 (95% CI: 1.36–3.05) for modafinil and armodafinil, respectively. Anxiety/nervousness had a risk ratio of 3.89 (95% CI: 1.48–10.23) and 5.01 (95% CI: 1.83–13.70) for modafinil and armodafinil, respectively. Nausea had a risk ratio of 3.13 (95% CI: 1.29–7.61) and 1.85 (95% CI: 1.02–3.36) for modafinil and armodafinil, respectively. Insomnia was reported for modafinil with a risk ratio of 5.30 (95% CI: 1.54–18.18) [28M].

An 8-week RCT for the use modafinil (200 mg/day) as an adjunctive treatment to haloperidol in schizophrenic patients ($n=50$) reported several TEAEs. These mild TEAEs included headache ($n=4$), nausea ($n=3$), and anxiety ($n=3$). These TEAEs, however, did not result in an increase in dropout rate [29c].

A 4-week open-label trial of armodafinil (uptitrated to 150 mg/day) was examined in women ($n=20$) experiencing menopause-related fatigue. No serious TEAEs were reported. Only 3 women (12%) dropped out from the study because of jitteriness, headache, and hypertension. Hypertension was a pre-existing condition in the patient reporting the TEAE of hypertension [30c].

A 6-month open-label multicenter trial of armodafinil (uptitrated to 200 mg/day) was performed in patients with bipolar I depression. Patients that had initially completed an 8-week RCT of armodafinil were allowed to enroll a 6-month open trial. In all of the enrolled patients ($n=867$; 8-week RCT and 6 month open-label), at least 1 AE was reported by 423 (49%) patients. The most common TEAEs were headache (11%), insomnia (6%), and anxiety (5%). A total of 26 patients (3%) had severe TEAEs and only headache ($n=3$), insomnia ($n=3$), and nausea ($n=2$) occurred in >1 patient. The study was discontinued by 57 patients (7%) because of TEAEs. The reported the discontinued TEAEs were mania ($n=11$), anxiety ($n=7$), depression ($n=5$), nausea ($n=5$), insomnia ($n=5$), and suicidal ideation ($n=2$). During the open-labeled phase, specifically, a total of 27 (3%) had ≥ 1 serious TEAEs. Serious TEAEs included mania ($n=5$), bipolar I disorder ($n=3$), and suicidal ideation ($n=3$). A total of 19 (2%) of patients in the 6-month phase reported TEAE that required expedite reporting, these included skin reactions ($n=8$), hypersensitivity reaction ($n-2$), suicidal ideation ($n=7$), suicide attempt ($n=1$), acute psychosis ($n=1$) [31MC].

Organs and Systems

Psychiatric

A 54-year-old male with a history of drug abuse arrived at the emergency department complaining of anxiety and demanding benzodiazepines. Besides benzodiazepines, he was taking high doses of armodafinil (1200 mg/daily) intermittent for 2 years. Although he had a prescription for armodafinil (250 mg/daily), he supplemented this prescription with armodafinil purchased on the internet. He described the feeling of taking excessive doses of armodafinil as "like you are smoking crack cocaine". He also reported paranoid delusions and after a 5-day inpatient drug detoxification protocol he was transferred to overnight inpatient psychiatric facility. He was discharged with gabapentin 300 mg (every 8 hours), thiamine 100 mg (TID), folic acid 1 mg (daily), and nicotine patch 14 mg [32A].

A 35-year-old male with bipolar affective disorder for over 7 years had 4 episodes of depression and 2 episodes of mania. He was referred to a psychiatric unit because of his reported excessive sexual desires and his exceeding high daily dose of modafinil. His daily modafinil dose had been 400–600 mg/daily for 3 years. A few weeks prior to his examination, he had increased his daily dose of modafinil to 800–1000 mg and had begun to develop the hypersexual behaviors. He underwent a gradual and slow reduction of modafinil at a rate of 100 mg every 2 days. He was also administered clonazepam (2 mg/day) to mitigate the withdrawal symptoms.

This was completed over a 3-week period. He was placed a structures relapse program prior to discharge that included lithium (600 mg/day), lamotrigine (200 mg/day), and venlafaxine (150 mg/day) [33A].

DRUGS THAT SUPPRESS APPETITE [SEDA-34, 8; SEDA-36, 1; SEDA-37, 1; SEDA-38, 1]

A meta-analysis of 28 RCT ($n = 29\,018$), which include all FDA-approved weight loss medications (orlistat, lorcaserin, naltrexone–bupropion, phentermine–topiramate, and liraglutide) was conducted. Lorcaserin [SEDA-37, 1; SEDA-38, 1] had the lowest odds of being discontinued due to adverse events (OR 1.34; 95% CI: 1.05–1.76). In contrast, the highest odds of being discontinued were liraglutide (OR 2.95; 95% CI: 2.11–0.23) and naltrexone sustained-release/bupropion sustained-release [SEDA-37, 1] (OR 2.64; 95% CI: 2.10–3.35) [34M].

PHENTERMINE [SEDA-34, 8; SEDA-36, 1, SEDA-37, 1; SEDA-38, 1]

Organs and Systems

Gastrointestinal

A 36-year-old obese female was admitted into the emergency department with an acute onset of severe abdominal pain as her primary symptom. She was constipation for 2 weeks prior with rectal bleeding. A colonoscopy revealed an extensive segment of inflammation, edema, and necrotic membrane in the descending colon. Biopsies confirmed ischemic colitis. No other causes were evident; however, the patient revealed she was taking phentermine (37.5 mg/day) for 2 years. Phentermine is only FDA-approved for the short-term weight loss and only prescribed for 8 weeks. The authors speculate that ischemic colitis was caused by prolonged phentermine-induced adrenergic mesenteric vasoconstriction [35A].

PARASYMPATHOMIMETICS [SEDA-34, 9, SEDA-36, 1; SEDA-37, 1; SEDA-38, 1]

A systematic review and meta-analysis of 21 RCT ($n = 9509$) of acetylcholinesterase inhibitors, donepezil, galantamine [SEDA-37, 1; SEDA-38, 1], and rivastigmine (patch and oral formulation) for the treatment of mild-to-moderate Alzheimer's disease were performed. All medications, except donepezil, had a higher rate of discontinuation due to TEAEs than placebo. The most common TEAEs were nausea, vomiting, diarrhea, and dizziness. The risk for diarrhea associated with galantamine and the risk for dizziness associated with rivastigmine (patch) were not significant compared with placebo [36M].

In a review of the California state-wide pediatric (>19-years old) poison control cases ($n = 189$) exposed to anti-dementia drugs, only 1 case was intentional ingestion (rivastigmine in a suicide attempt). A majority of the accidental ingestions were of donepezil ($n = 108$) followed by memantine ($n = 57$). Symptoms were reported in 38 cases with the most common symptoms were gastrointestinal ($n = 21$). These symptoms were nausea, vomiting, diarrhea. CNS depression was another set of symptoms commonly reported ($n = 15$) [37C].

DONEPEZIL [SEDA-34, 10; SEDA-36, 1; SEDA-37, 1; SEDA-38, 1]

Organ and Systems

Psychiatric

A 72-year-old female with probable Alzheimer's disease was receiving donepezil (10 mg/daily) for 1 month. She was also receiving duloxetine (30 mg/daily) for fibromyalgia for 8 years. Within 1 week of increasing the dosage of donepezil from 5 mg to 10 mg/daily, the patient developed increased cognitive and behavioral disorganization, hyperreligiosity, hypersexuality, delusions, insomnia, agitation, and violent behaviors. Discontinuation of donepezil and duloxetine and initiation of risperidone (uptitrated to 1.5 mg/daily) for 2 weeks returned her mental status to normal. Donepezil-induced mania caused by elevated brain acetylcholine and drug–drug interactions with duloxetine are speculated as possible mechanisms of action [38A].

A 79-year-old female receiving tianeptine (12.5 mg; BID) was initiated on donepezil (uptitrated to 10 mg/daily) for 2 month after experiencing memory loss and poor performance on Mini-Mental State Examination. After 2 weeks of increasing the daily dose of donepezil from 5 mg to 10 mg, the patient reported a dramatic increase in sexual desire and insomnia. Her libido was still elevated when the daily dose of donepezil was reduced back to 5 mg. Discontinuation of donepezil restored her normal libido levels. She received galantamine (8 mg/daily) and had no libido issues for 6 years. Patient remained on the tianeptine throughout the entire period. The difference in the mechanism of action galantamine and donepezil are discussed. The action of donepezil as an allosteric modulator of cholinergic receptors is noted [39A].

MEMANTINE [SEDA-34, 1]

Organ and Systems

Cardiovascular

A 70-year-old male with Alzheimer's disease was admitted to the hospital for diabetes mellitus. Upon examination, it was noted that he had complete right bundle branch block (CRBBB). The patient received haloperidol (1.5 mg/daily), lorazepam (3 mg/daily), oxypertine (20 mg/daily) and memantine (uptitrated to 20 mg/daily) during his hospitalization. After 54 days, patient developed a prolonged QTc (504 ms) on his electrocardiogram. Discontinuation of haloperidol, oxypertine, and memantine reduced his QTc to 474 ms. With the reintroduction of haloperidol and memantine a similar prolonged QTc developed. After a 3 week discontinuation of memantine only, QTc returned to basal levels (450 ms). The mechanism of memantine-induced prolonged QTc is unknown [40A].

RIVASTIGMINE [SEDA-34, 10; SEDA-36, 1; SEDA-37, 1; SEDA-38, 1]

In a randomized double-blind Phase II trial in patients with Parkinson disease, rivastigmine ($n = 65$) was compared with placebo for gait stability. During the 32-week study period 2184 adverse events occurred. A majority of these reported adverse events were report as falls ($n = 1875$ with 678 falls in rivastigmine-treated and 1197 in placebo-treated subjects). A total of 27 adverse events were characterized as serious ($n = 14$ in rivastigmine group with 2 listed as probable/definitely related to treatment). The most common TEAEs associated with rivastigmine were nausea (31%, $n = 20$) and vomiting (17%, $n = 11$). No adverse effects were considered to be related to rivastigmine at the 52 week follow-up period [41c].

Rivastigmine transdermal (9.5 mg/daily) was compared with rivastigmine oral formulation (12 mg/day) in randomized double-blind 24-week study in patients with probable Alzheimer's disease ($n = 501$). The 56.7% of patients receiving the patch and 62.5% of patients receiving oral capsules reported mild or moderate TEAEs. Gastrointestinal adverse events, nausea, vomiting, and diarrhea, were reported less in the patch group (15.8%) compared with oral capsule group (28.7%). Application site pruritus was more prevalent in the patch group (10.9%) compared with oral capsule group (2.8%). Application site pruritus was the cause of discontinuation in 4.9% of the patients receiving the patch, compared with 0.8% of the oral capsule group [42C].

Organ and Systems

Skin

An 80-year-male patient with chronic pulmonary obstructive pulmonary disease and Alzheimer's disease was being treated with rivastigmine (3 mg/BID) for 1 month developed hypertrichosis. Increased pigmentation and hair growth was confined to dorsal side of forearms with symmetrical distribution. No other symptoms were noted. Considering the cognitive benefit of rivastigmine, medication was continued and the patient was monitored. There was no extension of the hypertrichosis at the 1-year follow-up. Acetylcholinesterase inhibitors have been noted to induced hair growth and dermatitis [43A].

References

[1] McElroy SL, Hudson J, Ferreira-Cornwell MC, et al. Lisdexamfetamine dimesylate for adults with moderate to severe binge eating disorder: results of two pivotal phase 3 randomized controlled trials. Neuropsychopharmacology. 2016;41:1251–60 [C].

[2] Perez-Downes J, Hritani A, Baldeo C, et al. Amphetamine containing dietary supplements and acute myocardial infarction. Case Rep Cardiol. 2016;2016:6404856 [A].

[3] Janardhanan R, Kannan A. Methamphetamine cardiotoxicity: unique presentation with multiple Bi-ventricular thrombi. Am J Med. 2016;129:e3–4 [A].

[4] Stokes MB, Fernando H, Taylor AJ. Cardiogenic shock secondary to methamphetamine induced cardiomyopathy requiring veno-arterial extra-corporeal membrane oxygenation. Int J Cardiol. 2016;207:134–5 [A].

[5] Tse J, Ferguson K, Whitlow KS, et al. The use of intravenous lipid emulsion therapy in acute methamphetamine toxicity. Am J Emerg Med. 1732;2016(34):e3–4 [A].

[6] Shelly J, Uhlmann A, Sinclair H, et al. First-rank symptoms in methamphetamine psychosis and schizophrenia. Psychopathology. 2016;49:429–35 [c].

[7] Wang LJ, Lin SK, Chen YC, et al. Differences in clinical features of methamphetamine users with persistent psychosis and patients with schizophrenia. Psychopathology. 2016;49:108–15 [c].

[8] Zarrabi H, Khalkhali M, Hamidi A, et al. Clinical features, course and treatment of methamphetamine-induced psychosis in psychiatric inpatients. BMC Psychiatry. 2016;16:44 [C].

[9] Javadian S, Shabani A, Shariat SV. Clinical course of methamphetamine-induced psychotic disorder in a 3-month follow-up. Prim Care Companion CNS Disord. 2016;18:6 [c].

[10] Pinnaka S, Gosai K, Czekierdowski C, et al. Somnambulism during monotherapy with mixed amphetamine salts. J Clin Psychopharmacol. 2016;36:187–9 [A].

[11] Spiegel DR, McCroskey A, Puaa K, et al. A case of disulfiram-induced psychosis in a previously asymptomatic patient maintained on mixed amphetamine salts: a review of the literature and possible pathophysiological explanations. Clin Neuropharmacol. 2016;39:272–5 [A].

[12] Matsusue A, Ishikawa T, Michiue T, et al. Association between cerebrospinal fluid dopamine concentrations and catechol-O-methyltransferase gene polymorphisms in forensic autopsy cases of methamphetamine abusers. Forensic Sci Int. 2017;270:159–64 [c].

[13] Singer LT, Moore DG, Min MO, et al. Motor delays in MDMA (ecstasy) exposed infants persist to 2 years. Neurotoxicol Teratol. 2016;54:22–8 [c].

[14] Chandra YG, Shetty AR, Jayanth SH, et al. A death due to ecstasy—a case report. Med Leg J. 2016;84:46–8 [A].

[15] Jiang Z, Butler-Bowen H, Rodriguez T, et al. Role of methylphenidate in the treatment of fatigue in advanced pancreatic cancer population. Ann Gastroenterol. 2016;29:536–43 [c].

[16] Safavi P, Dehkordi AH, Ghasemi N. Comparison of the effects of methylphenidate and the combination of methylphenidate and risperidone in preschool children with attention-deficit hyperactivity disorder. J Adv Pharm Technol Res. 2016;7:144–8 [c].

[17] Montastruc F, Montastruc G, Montastruc JL, et al. Cardiovascular safety of methylphenidate should also be considered in adults. BMJ. 2016;353:i3418 [A].

[18] Baumeister TB, Wickenbrock I, Perings CA. STEMI secondary to coronary vasospasm: possible adverse event of methylphenidate in a 21-year-old man with ADHD. Drug Saf Case Rep. 2016;3:10 [A].

[19] Akaltun I. Report of a 14-year-old boy whose testosterone level decreased after starting on methylphenidate. J Child Adolesc Psychopharmacol. 2016;26:181 [A].

[20] Kaya I, Coskun M. Diffuse maculopapular rash with increasing dosage of methylphenidate. J Clin Psychopharmacol. 2016;36:106–7 [A].

[21] Perez CA, Garcia SS, Yu RD. Extrapyramidal symptoms as a result of risperidone discontinuation during combination therapy with methylphenidate in a pediatric patient. J Child Adolesc Psychopharmacol. 2016;26:182 [A].

[22] Ford JB, Schemann K, Patterson JA, et al. Triggers for preeclampsia onset: a case-crossover study. Paediatr Perinat Epidemiol. 2016;30:555–62 [C].

[23] Belen Rivas A, Arruza L, Pacheco E, et al. Adverse drug reactions in neonates: a prospective study. Arch Dis Child. 2016;101:371–6 [C].

[24] Ahmad A, Mondal T, Klein B. Atrial arrhythmia after newborn eye exam, to caffeine or not to caffeine? J Neonatal Perinatal Med. 2016;9:427–31 [A].

[25] Reed VA, Buitelaar JK, Anand E, et al. The safety of atomoxetine for the treatment of children and adolescents with attention-deficit/ hyperactivity disorder: a comprehensive review of over a decade of research. CNS Drugs. 2016;30:603–28 [M].

[26] Naguy A, Al-Mutairi H, Al-Tajali A. Atomoxetine-related takotsubo cardiomyopathy. J Psychiatr Pract. 2016;22:232–3 [A].

[27] Basay O, Basay BK, Ozturk O, et al. Acute dystonia following a switch in treatment from atomoxetine to low-dose aripiprazole. Clin Psychopharmacol Neurosci. 2016;14:221–5 [A].

[28] Kuan YC, Wu D, Huang KW, et al. Effects of modafinil and armodafinil in patients with obstructive sleep apnea: a meta-analysis of randomized controlled trials. Clin Ther. 2016;38:874–88 [M].

[29] Shoja Shafti S, Akbari S. Intractability of deficit syndrome of schizophrenia against adjunctive modafinil. J Clin Psychopharmacol. 2016;36:45–9 [c].

[30] Meyer F, Freeman MP, Petrillo L, et al. Armodafinil for fatigue associated with menopause: an open-label trial. Menopause. 2016;23:209–14 [c].

[31] Ketter TA, Amchin J, Frye MA, et al. Long-term safety and efficacy of armodafinil in bipolar depression: a 6-month open-label extension study. J Affect Disord. 2016;197:51–7 [MC].

[32] Jerry JM, Shirvani N, Dale R. Addiction to armodafinil and modafinil presenting with paranoia. J Clin Psychopharmacol. 2016;36:98–100 [A].

[33] Swapnajeet S, Bn S, Gourav G. Modafinil dependence and hypersexuality: a case report and review of the evidence. Clin Psychopharmacol Neurosci. 2016;14:402–4 [A].

[34] Khera R, Murad MH, Chandar AK, et al. Association of pharmacological treatments for obesity with weight loss and adverse events: a systematic review and meta-analysis. JAMA. 2016;315:2424–34 [M].

[35] Sharma P, Krishnamoorthy P. Colon ischemia after weight-loss medication in a 36-year-old woman. Conn Med. 2016;80:213–5 [A].

[36] Kobayashi H, Ohnishi T, Nakagawa R, et al. The comparative efficacy and safety of cholinesterase inhibitors in patients with mild-to-moderate Alzheimer's disease: a Bayesian network meta-analysis. Int J Geriatr Psychiatry. 2016;31:892–904 [M].

[37] Thornton SL, Pchelnikova JL, Cantrell FL. Characteristics of pediatric exposures to antidementia drugs reported to a poison control system. J Pediatr. 2016;172:147–50 [C].

[38] Hategan A, Bourgeois JA. Donepezil-associated manic episode with psychotic features: a case report and review of the literature. Gen Hosp Psychiatry. 2016;38. 115.e1–4 [A].

[39] Segrec N, Zaman R, Pregelj P. Increased libido associated with donepezil treatment: a case report. Psychogeriatrics. 2016;16:70–2 [A].

[40] Kajitani K, Yanagimoto K, Monji A, et al. Memantine exacerbates corrected QT interval prolongation in Alzheimer's disease: a case report from an unintentional rechallenge. J Am Geriatr Soc. 2016;64:232–3 [A].

[41] Henderson EJ, Lord SR, Brodie MA, et al. Rivastigmine for gait stability in patients with Parkinson's disease (ReSPonD): a randomised, double-blind, placebo-controlled, phase 2 trial. Lancet Neurol. 2016;15:249–58 [c].

[42] Zhang ZX, Hong Z, Wang YP, et al. Rivastigmine patch in Chinese patients with probable Alzheimer's disease: a 24-week, randomized, double-blind parallel-group study comparing rivastigmine patch (9.5 mg/24 h) with capsule (6 mg Twice Daily). CNS Neurosci Ther. 2016;22:488–96 [C].

[43] Imbernon-Moya A, Podlipnik S, Burgos F, et al. Acquired localized hypertrichosis induced by rivastigmine. Case Rep Dermatol Med. 2016;2016:7296572 [A].

2

Antidepressants

Jonathan Smithson*, Philip B. Mitchell†,1

*School of Psychiatry, University of New South Wales, Sydney, NSW, Australia
†Black Dog Institute, Sydney, NSW, Australia
1Corresponding author: phil.mitchell@unsw.edu.au

GENERAL

Cardiovascular

Vascular Outcomes

Studying 238 963 patients with a first diagnosis of depression, Coupland et al. examined for associations between a range of newly commenced antidepressants and three vascular outcomes (myocardial infarction [MI], stroke or transient ischemic attack, and arrhythmia) over a 5-year period [1MC]. They found that 772 patients had a MI, 1106 a stroke or transient ischemic attack, and 1452 an arrhythmia. While there were no significant associations between antidepressants as a broad class and these vascular outcomes, there were some significant associations with specific agents. A reduced risk of MI (aHR 0.58, 95% CI; 0.42–0.79) was found in the first year for SSRIs compared to no antidepressants. However, when specific antidepressants were considered, fluoxetine was associated with reduced risk (aHR 0.44, 95% CI; 0.27–0.72) of MI, while the tricyclic antidepressant (TCA) lofepramine was linked with increased risk (aHR 3.07, 95% CI; 1.50–6.26). Risk of arrhythmias was increased during the first 28 days of treatment with tricyclic and related antidepressants (aHR 1.99, 95% CI; 1.27–3.13), while a reduced risk was found with fluoxetine over the full 5 years (aHR 0.74, 95% CI; 0.59–0.92). Intriguingly, in light of previous concerns about torsades de pointes (see SEDA-36, 14), there was no association between citalopram and arrhythmias, even at doses in excess of 40 mg.

In view of a prior inconsistent literature, Noordam et al. specifically examined risk of myocardial infarction (MI) with antidepressants [2C]. 744 subjects in their cohort of 9499 developed MI during follow-up. After adjustment for cardiovascular risk factors and depression, they found that antidepressants were associated with a lower risk of MI (OR 0.71; 95% CI 0.51–0.98) compared with no antidepressants. There were no significant differences in risk to MI between SSRIs and other antidepressants.

Valvular Heart Disease

Drug-induced valvular heart disease (VHD) generally presents as cardiac-valvular regurgitation.

Using a National Health Insurance Research database, a nested case–control study examined for association between antidepressants and VHD in an ethnically Chinese population. The authors found that antidepressants were associated with an increased risk of new onset VHD, with specific risk varying with different agents [3M]. Current use of antidepressants was associated with a 1.4-fold increase in risk (adjusted odds ratio [aOR] 1.44; 95% confidence interval [CI] 1.17–1.77), with a dose–response association observed between cumulative duration of VHD and cumulative antidepressant dose. Increased risk of VHD was more likely with antidepressants in those with underlying congestive heart failure (aOR 4.04; 95% CI [3.14–5.19]), MI (aOR 2.10; 95% CI [1.73–2.55]), chronic kidney disease (aOR 2.14; 95% CI [1.58–2.89]), hypertension (aOR 1.77; 95% CI [1.46–2.14]), and chronic obstructive pulmonary disease (aOR 1.62; 95% CI [1.23–2.14]). TCAs were associated with a significantly higher risk of VHD (aOR 1.40 [1.05–1.87]) compared to other antidepressants.

Arrhythmia/Torsades de Pointes

There has been controversy over the relationship between antidepressants and prolonged QT interval/torsades de pointes (TdP), particularly with the related FDA black box warning for citalopram (SEDA-36, 14; SEDA-37, 24). Danielsson et al. performed a large nationwide case–control study of 286 092 patients aged ≥65 years who died outside hospital over a 6-year period and 1 430 460 matched controls [4C]. They found that antidepressants which had been previously classified as having "known" or "possible" TdP risk were associated with a higher adjusted risk for mortality (OR 1.53, 95% CI; 1.51–1.56 and OR 1.63, 95% CI; 1.61–1.67, respectively) compared with antidepressants classified as having "conditional" risk (i.e. drugs which are associated with TdP but only under certain circumstances of their use) (OR 1.25, 95% CI; 1.22–1.28). The risk ranking for commonly used antidepressants was: mirtazapine > citalopram > sertraline >amitriptyline. Interestingly, the adjusted hazard ratios for citalopram and mirtazapine were almost identical to those previously described by Coupland et al. [5C].

Nervous System

Stroke

Studies examining the association between antidepressants and stroke have yielded inconsistent findings. More recent studies have suggested that SSRIs may be linked with increased risk of ischemic [6C] or hemorrhagic stroke [7C], or both [8C,9C]. This association has been linked to the strength of inhibition of serotonin reuptake. There have been two relevant recent meta-analyses.

First, Hackam and Mrkobrada found SSRIs to be associated with an increased risk of hemorrhagic stroke (both intracerebral and intracranial) hemorrhage, but noted absolute risks to be very low [10M]. Using an estimated global incidence of such strokes of 24.6 per 100 000 person-years, they estimated one additional intracerebral bleeding episode per 10 000 persons treated for 1 year [11M]. Second, Shin et al.'s meta-analysis of 13 studies found SSRIs to be associated with an increased risk of all types of stroke [(aOR), 1.40; 95% (CI), 1.09–1.80], ischemic stroke (aOR 1.48; 95% CI 1.08–2.02) and hemorrhagic stroke (aOR 1.32; 95% CI 1.02–1.71), although the authors cautioned that any confounding of depression could not be excluded [12M]. Second, Renoux et al., in a 19.5-year population-based cohort study of 1 363 990 incident users of antidepressants, assessed the risk for intracranial hemorrhage (ICH) associated with SSRIs compared with TCAs among new users of antidepressants [13C]. They found that SSRIs were associated with an increased risk of ICH compared to TCAs (RR, 1.17; 95% CI, 1.02–1.35) with this risk being highest during the first 30 days of use (RR, 1.44; 95% CI, 1.04–1.99). They also found that the risk was greater with stronger serotonin reuptake inhibitors (RR, 1.25; 95% CI, 1.01–1.54).

Other studies have examined the association between antidepressants and subclinical cerebrovascular events. Several years ago (SEDA-37, 18), Aarts et al., using a cross-sectional design, reported that antidepressants with a high serotonin affinity did not cause subclinical microbleeds on brain magnetic resonance imaging (MRI) [14C]. Recently, the first prospective study of this association found antidepressants to be associated with an increased risk of incident first-ever microbleeds after 4 years of follow-up, irrespective of antidepressant class, with this statistical relationship persisting after accounting for depressive symptoms and cardiovascular risk [15C]. The prevalence of intracranial microbleeds in this study was much higher than that for stroke; the authors interpreting this as indicating that symptomatic hemorrhages are "just the tip of the iceberg". Further, Akoudad et al. [15C] examined 2559 participants aged 45 years or older who had no prior history of microbleeds. After a mean of 3.9 years, the overall incidence of cerebral microbleeds was 3.7%, with antidepressants significantly associated with increased risk (OR, 2.22; 95% CI, 1.31–3.76) compared with non-use. While there was no difference in risk between antidepressant classes, antidepressants with intermediate serotonin affinity were associated with the highest risk for microbleeds (OR, 3.07; 95% CI, 1.53–6.17) compared with non-use. Antidepressants with high serotonin affinity were associated with incidence of microbleeds, although results did not reach statistical significance (odds ratio, 2.18; 95% CI, 0.90–5.29), perhaps due to insufficient statistical power. Interpreting their findings, the authors emphasized the possibility of a "reverse causality" whereby the microbleeds themselves may lead to antidepressant prescription, as it is possible that microbleeds may contribute to the progression of depression.

Seizures

SSRIs are known to lower seizure threshold [16R], though most evidence for this is derived from clinical trials not specifically designed to investigate this relationship. Bloechliger et al. assessed the risk of a first seizure in depressed patients, without other risk factors for seizures, treated with antidepressant medications in an observational retrospective follow-up study with a nested case–control analysis using a national database [17C]. Compared with no antidepressants, risk of seizures was increased with SSRIs (aOR 1.98, 95% CI; 1.48–2.66) and SNRIs (aOR 1.99, 95% CI; 1.20–3.29), but not TCAs. Considering specific antidepressants, citalopram (aOR 1.69 [95% CI; 1.25–2.28]), sertraline (aOR 2.53 [95% CI; 1.49–4.30]), fluoxetine (aOR 1.51 [95% CI; 1.06–2.16]), and venlafaxine (aOR 2.52 [95% CI; 1.44–4.42]) were all associated with significantly increased risk.

Dementia/Cognitive Impairment

The nature of the association between depression, dementia and antidepressant treatment is complex

[18R]. Antidepressant drugs have been variously shown to either increase or decrease risk of dementia. A recent meta-analysis and a national register study have addressed this relationship.

Moraros et al. conducted a meta-analysis of English-language studies over the last decade examining the association between antidepressants and cognitive impairment or dementia [19M]. All but one of the five studies were population-based, with the meta-analysis including 1477626 participants. Antidepressant usage was associated with a twofold increase in the odds of dementia/cognitive impairment (OR=2.17; 95% CI: 1.41–3.33; $I^2=84.9\%$). The finding appeared to be unrelated to age, with significantly increased odds ratios in studies with an average age ≥ 65 years (OR=1.65 95% CI: 1.18–2.31; $I^2=35.2\%$) and those with all subjects ≤ 65 years (OR=3.25 95% CI: 3.19–3.32; $I^2=0\%$). The authors concluded that individuals with cognitive impairment or AD/dementia were more likely to have been prescribed an antidepressant drug, with this association stronger if the antidepressant drug was commenced before the age of 65.

Lee et al. investigated the relationship between antidepressants and the later risk of developing dementia in a population-based retrospective case–control study utilizing a national health insurance database [20C]. They identified two clinical groups older than 40 years of age: 5394 cases with major depression that were diagnosed with dementia over the following 6 years, and 5232 controls that had major depression but no history of dementia. The investigators found that the risk of later onset of dementia differed with the various antidepressants classes. The risk was reduced with tricyclic antidepressants (TCAs) (OR=0.24; 95% CI, 0.22–0.27), but increased with SSRIs (OR=2.48; 95% CI, 2.27–2.71), MAOIs (OR=1.86; 95% CI, 1.47–2.36), heterocyclic antidepressants (OR=1.44; 95% CI, 1.32–1.57) and other antidepressants (OR=2.05; 95% CI, 1.85–2.27). The apparent "protective" effect of TCAs was dose related as the cumulative dose of TCAs increased, whereas with the SSRIs, MAOIs, and heterocyclic antidepressants, increases in cumulative dose were associated with increased risk of dementia. This apparent reduction in risk of dementia with TCAs has been reported elsewhere [21C].

In summary, the nature of the interrelationships between depression, dementia and antidepressant treatment remains unclear.

Hematological

Bleeding Risk

SSRIs have been consistently reported to lead to increased risk of bleeding (SEDA-36, p11; SEDA-37, p16; SEDA-38, p11). Laporte et al. have conducted a meta-analysis of case–control and cohort studies investigating bleeding risk with SSRIs to quantify this risk [22R]. Overall, their series of meta-analyses found an increased risk of bleeding with SSRIs of about 40%: (i) 42 observational studies [OR 1.41 (95% CI 1.27–1.57), $P<0.0001$]; (ii) 31 case–control studies involving 1255073 patients [OR 1.41 (95% CI 1.25–1.60)]; and (iii) 11 cohort studies involving 187956 patients [OR 1.36 (95% CI 1.12–1.64)].

Reproductive System (Pregnancy, Development and Infancy)

Pregnancy

Up to 5% of pregnant women receive a diagnosis of depression [23C,24C] and up to 10% of pregnant women receive an antidepressant during pregnancy in developed countries [25C,26C,27C]. The use of SSRIs during pregnancy has been repeatedly associated with complications for both mother and infant (SEDA-36, p13; SEDA-37, p18; SEDA-38, p12), including intrauterine growth retardation, preterm birth [28M], low birth weight, prematurity, post-partum haemorrhage (PPH) [29C,30MC,31M], miscarriage, poor neonatal adaptation (PNA) [32M], persistent pulmonary hypertension of the newborn (PPHN) [33M], neonatal complications, birth defects, neurodevelopmental disorders and autism [34M]. It has been difficult to ascribe causality in this research field, with adverse fetal effects potentially being due to either the mother's antidepressant use or her depression, or the multiplicity of other factors known to affect the health of mother and infant [35R]. The number of women exposed to antidepressants during pregnancy appears to be increasing, with some surveys suggesting that up to 7.5 percent of pregnant women take antidepressants while pregnant [36C].

Fetal Malformations

Previous meta-analyses [37M,38M,39M], and pooled national registry studies [40MC] have indicated an association between SSRI exposure and congenital heart defects (CHD), although there is as yet no firm consensus as to the strength of such risk (SEDA-36, p13; SEDA-37, p18; SEDA-38, p12).

To clarify this issue, Bérard et al. recently reported on a meta-analysis of the risk of cardiac malformations associated with gestational exposure to paroxetine, while taking into account indication, study design and reference category [41M]. First, when they included studies where the comparison group of women unexposed to paroxetine included those using other antidepressants, they found that first trimester use of paroxetine led to an increased risk of any major congenital malformation (pooled OR 1.23, 95% CI 1.10–1.38). Second, when the reference group was restricted to those not taking any antidepressants, the increase in risk was similar. When the authors focused on major cardiac malformations in particular, risk with paroxetine, compared with non-paroxetine exposure (comparison subjects could on other antidepressants) was significantly increased (pooled OR 1.28, 95% CI 1.11–1.47; $n = 18$ studies), particularly risk of bulbus cordis and cardiac septal closure anomalies (pooled OR 1.42, 95% CI 1.07–1.89; $n = 8$ studies). Further, risks to atrial septal defects (pooled OR 2.38, 95% CI 1.14–4.97; $n = 4$ studies) and right ventricular outflow track defects (pooled OR 2.29, 95% CI 1.06–4.93; $n = 4$ studies) were significantly elevated.

Jordan et al. investigated the teratogenicity SSRIs in the 3 months before and after the first day of last menstrual period (LMP). Using three national population-based congenital anomaly registries linked to healthcare databases which contained prospectively collected prescription information, they included 519117 deliveries [42C]. They found that SSRIs 3 months either side of the LMP were associated with a greater likelihood of severe congenital heart defects (CHD) (OR 1.50, 95% CI 1.06–2.11) and the composite adverse outcome of 'anomaly or stillbirth' (OR 1.13, 1.03–1.24). There was a strong trend towards an increased prevalence of 'all major anomalies' with SSRIs, though this did not reach formal statistical significance (OR 1.09, 0.99–1.21). Further, there was a significant dose–response relationship between SSRI dose and risk of severe CHD (meta-regression OR 1.49, 1.12–1.97). The investigators noted that the additional absolute risk of teratogenesis associated with SSRIs was small but opined that the high prevalence of SSRI use in general, and in pregnancy in particular, emphasizes the public health importance of the association, justifying modifications to preconception care.

Preeclampsia

The relationship between use of antidepressants in pregnancy and gestational hypertension (GH) or pre-eclampsia (PE) remains unclear, with contradictory findings [43C,44C] (SEDA-36, p13). DeOcampo et al., in a small prospective cohort study over 10 years, examined the association between the discontinued and continued use of antidepressants and risk for GH and PE [45c]. Women who discontinued antidepressants before 20 weeks of gestation (discontinuers) and those who continued antidepressant use at or after 20 weeks of gestation (continuers) were compared with non-users for risk of GH and PE. 3471 women met the inclusion criteria for the study, with 129 developing GH without PE and 141 PE. The investigators found that "continuers" were at significantly greater risk of GH (aOR 1.83; 95% CI; 1.05–3.21). Focusing on specific antidepressant classes, and after adjusting for potential confounding factors, SNRI (but not SSRI) continuation was associated with increased risk of GH (aOR 4.96; 95%CI 1.33–18.56) but

not PE. Continuers using two or more antidepressant drug classes had increased risk for PE.

Preterm Birth and Size

Any potential relationship between antidepressants and preterm birth (PTB) needs to consider the potential impact of depression per se. A number of studies have associated maternal depression during pregnancy with an increased risk of intrauterine growth restriction (IUGR) [46C], preterm birth (PTB) [47C,48C], and low birth weight (LBW) [49C,50C], while other studies have reported no such association [51C,52C]. A recent meta-analysis suggests that depression during pregnancy is itself associated with an elevated risk of IUGR, PTB and LBW [53M], although the nature of the association is not uncertain. The complexity of these issues is highlighted by recent studies from China and Sweden which have also reported paternal depression to be associated with LBW, perhaps highlighting the role and impact of psychosocial factors in these outcomes [54C,55C].

The risk of confounding by indication (i.e. depression) generally, and in low birth weight specifically, is perhaps highlighted by the results of Venkatesh et al.'s study of women screened for depression before delivery, which found that those with depressive symptoms had an increased likelihood of preterm and 'very preterm' delivery as well as having a small for gestational age (SGA) neonate, but that this risk was not apparent among women treated with an antidepressant [56R]. This report comprised an observational cohort study of 7267 women, 11% of whom were identified as depressed. Adjusting for multiple potential confounding factors, they found that depressed women had an increased risk of preterm birth ([aOR] 1.27, 95% CI 1.04–1.55) and very preterm birth (aOR 1.82, 95% CI 1.09–3.02) as well as of having a SGA neonate (aOR 1.28, 95% CI 1.04–1.58). In secondary analyses they found for the women who were treated with an antidepressant during pregnancy, depressive symptoms were not significantly associated with increased risk of preterm/very preterm birth or an SGA neonate.

However, the risk of PTB in women using SSRIs during pregnancy remains controversial. Given the known association between maternal depression and PTB and LBW, as well as the obvious impact of psychosocial factors, it is therefore critical to control for these factors when examining any association between antidepressant use in pregnancy and these complications.

Eke et al. evaluated the risk of PTB in cases of maternal exposure to SSRIs during pregnancy [57M]. They identified eight relevant studies which had a comparison group of unexposed pregnant women. These studies included a total of 1237669 women; 93982 were in the exposure group and 1143687 in the control group. The incidence of PTB was significantly higher in women treated with

SSRIs compared against controls (aOR 1.24, 95% CI 1.09–1.41). When women with depression but without exposure to SSRIs during pregnancy (i.e. depressed women treated with psychotherapy alone) were compared to the SSRI group, those taking SSRIs were found to have an increased risk of PTB (OR 1.17, 95% CI 1.10–1.25), which corresponded to an absolute risk of 6.8% vs 5.8%. The authors concluded that pregnant women who received SSRIs during pregnancy had a significantly higher risk of developing PTB compared with controls, and that this risk remained significant when compared with depressed women who did not receive SSRIs.

In a population-based study, Cantarutti et al. examined the effect of antidepressants on risk of PTB and LBW [58C]. The investigators found that those mothers who continued to use antidepressants during pregnancy had a 20% increased prevalence of both PTB and LBW compared to those who had never used antidepressants. Interestingly, however, when compared to women who had stopped antidepressants during pregnancy, those who continued antidepressants during pregnancy were not at increased risk of PTB and LBW.

Using national register data, Nezvalová-Henriksen et al. addressed shared genetic and family level confounding in a sibling-controlled prospective cohort study investigating the effects of prenatal SSRI exposure and maternal depression on birthweight and gestational age [59C]. They found that SSRI exposure during two or more trimesters was associated with a significant decrease in birthweight of 205 g and a decrease in gestational length of 4.9 days.

Viktorin et al. investigated the association between SSRIs in pregnancy and offspring size using a national register population-based cohort of 392 029 children, of whom 6572 (1.7%) were exposed to SSRIs during pregnancy, and 1625 (0.4%) who were exposed to a mother with depression but not treated with an SSRI. Children not exposed to depression or SSRI were used as the reference group [60C]. Compared to depressed mothers who did not use an antidepressant, mothers who used SSRIs gave birth to children with lower birth length and smaller birth head circumference, and who were a shorter gestational age at birth and a more likely to be preterm. To account for unmeasured parental genetic and environmental confounders, a within-family design was also undertaken, using women who gave birth to more than one child with the same father, and for whom the children were discordant for SSRI exposure. Using that within-family analysis, the only significant association was between SSRI exposure and reduced gestational age [-2.27 days; 95% CI −3.79 to −0.75; P = 0.004). To address the effect of depression per se, the investigators compared children of depressed mothers without SSRI exposure with children of mothers with no depression or SSRIs. The children of depressed mothers without SSRI

exposure also had lower gestational age (-1.69; 95% CI −2.51 to −0.86; P < 0.001) and a higher probability of preterm birth (OR 1.31; 95% CI 1.07–1.60; P = 0.009). Overall, the study could not exclude the possibility that the relationship between SSRIs and offspring size may be due to depression itself.

Persistent Pulmonary Hypertension of the Newborn

A decade ago, a large case–control study reported a sixfold increase in the risk of PPHN among infants whose mothers were exposed to an SSRI in late pregnancy [61C], leading to the FDA issuing a public health advisory warning on the potential increased risk of PPHN [62S]. However, after subsequent inconsistent studies, the US advisory was revised in 2011, stating that "there have been conflicting findings from new studies evaluating this potential risk, making it unclear whether use of SSRIs during pregnancy can cause PPHN" [63S].

A recent retrospective cohort study of 143 281 pregnancies has examined the association between infants exposed to SSRI, SNRI, and other antidepressant use during pregnancy, and risk of PPHN [64C]. After adjustment for maternal depression, the authors found that SSRIs during the second half of pregnancy was associated with an increased risk of PPHN compared to no antidepressants (aOR 4.29, 95% CI; 1.34–13.77); SNRIs were not associated with increased risk, although the authors cautioned that this may have been due to a lack of statistical power.

A retrospective national register study of 741 040 singleton births estimated the rate of admissions to NICUs, as well as neonatal morbidity, following exposure to antidepressant drugs in utero [65C]. The investigators found that following maternal use of an SSRI, 13.7% of the infants were admitted to the NICU compared with 8.2% in the non-exposed population (aOR: 1.5 [95% CI: 1.4–1.5]). SSRI treatment during late pregnancy was associated with an increased risk of admission to NICU (16.5%) when compared with treatment during early pregnancy for which the risk was 10.8% (aOR: 1.6 [95% CI: 1.5–1.8]). Maternal use of an SSRI was associated with an increased frequency of respiratory and central nervous system disorders and hypoglycemia. This study also found an increased rate of PPHN in infants exposed to SSRIs in late pregnancy compared with early pregnancy, with a number needed to harm (NNTH) of 285.

Postpartum Hemorrhage (PPH)

Perhaps the strongest evidence to date for an association between antidepressant use close to delivery and increased risk of PPH has been that of Palmsten et al. [66MC] who found a 1.47-fold increased risk. Several studies have been directed at this issue over the last year. Grzeskowiak et al. [67C], in a retrospective cohort study, investigated the association between antidepressant use in late pregnancy and risk of primary PPH. Using hospital data, 30 198 pregnancies from 24 266 women were identified and pharmacy dispensing records used to determine antidepressant use during pregnancy. Compared with unexposed controls, women exposed to antidepressants had an increased risk of PPH (aRR 1.53; 95% CI 1.25–1.86). Antidepressant use in late gestation was associated with a risk of both severe PPH (aRR 1.84; 95% CI 1.39–2.44), and postpartum anemia (aRR 1.80; 95% CI 1.46–2.22). Late gestation antidepressant exposure was associated with an adjusted excess risk of 5.8% for any PPH, with a NNH of 17; the adjusted excess risk for severe PPH was 3.9% (95% CI 1.5%–6.1%), with a corresponding NNH of 26.

A further larger retrospective population-based cohort study also examined the association between SSRIs and SNRIs and PPH, using data from a 10-year period involving 225 973 women with 322 224 pregnancies [68M]. After adjustment for potential confounders, the authors found an increased risk of PPH in the 1390 patients who were exposed to a SNRIs in the final month of pregnancy (aOR 1.76, 95% CI, 1.47–2.11), corresponding to 4.1 additional cases per 100 treated. No relationship was observed between SSRI use in the final month of pregnancy and postpartum hemorrhage. Mid-pregnancy exposure was not associated with an increased risk.

Jiang et al. conducted a meta-analysis of all observational studies to estimate the risk of PPH among those taking antidepressants during pregnancy. They identified eight studies involving more than 40 000 instances of PPH [69M]. They found that the risk of developing PPH was 1.32-fold higher (RR 1.32; 95% CI; 1.17–1.48) in mothers receiving antidepressants, with all classes being associated with greater risk. Furthermore, the authors noted that the closer to delivery antidepressants were prescribed, the greater the risk of PPH.

Autism

The association between prenatal exposure to SSRIs and childhood autism spectrum disorder (ASD) remains controversial. Three new meta-analyses have recently been published. First, Boukhris et al. undertook a cohort study of 145 456 singleton live births over a 12-year period [70C]. After adjustment for potential confounding variables, the use of an antidepressant during the second and/or third trimester was associated with a significantly increased risk of autism spectrum disorder, even after accounting for a maternal history of depression (aHR, 1.75; 95% CI; 1.03–2.97). Second, Kaplan et al. [71R] reported on a meta-analysis of case–control studies which demonstrated a significantly increased risk of ASD in the offspring of children who were prenatally exposed to SSRIs during different exposure time windows (except third trimester for which there was no significant association). In their interpretation of their own findings, Kaplan et al. remained concerned that they could not

exclude maternal depression as a cause of this observed association. Third, Kobayashi et al. performed a meta-analysis using of five case–control and three cohort studies to quantify risk of ASD in offspring exposed to SSRIs in utero. They found that the SSRI group had a significantly higher risk of ASD than the SSRI non-exposed group (pooled OR 1.45, 95% CI 1.15–1.82). However, when they confined their analysis to the offspring of women with psychiatric disorders, the SSRI group did not show an increased ASD risk compared to non-exposed subjects (pooled OR 0.96, 95% CI 0.57–1.63). In other words, similar to Kaplan et al., Kobayashi et al. could not exclude maternal psychiatric illness as a potential major confounding factor.

Neurodevelopmental Disorders

The impact of prenatal SSRI exposure on vulnerability to adverse neurodevelopmental outcomes is confounded by many factors, including maternal and paternal mental illness [72R]. Data on the association between prenatal SSRI exposure and long-term neurodevelopment are limited, and the evidence inconclusive [73R]. Recent research has suggested that gestational SSRI exposure might adversely impact motor development in the offspring [74c,75c,76c], although the findings have been inconsistent and potentially complicated by the effects of maternal mood disorder. It has been suggested that untreated depression before and after delivery may have adverse developmental effects on the offspring [77R].

Brown et al. examined the relationship between gestational SSRI exposure and speech/language, scholastic, and motor disorders in offspring up to early adolescence in a large prospective birth cohort study of 845 345 pregnant women and their singleton offspring [78C]. Using registry data on maternal use of antidepressants and depression-related psychiatric disorders during pregnancy three exposure groups of offspring were identified: 15 596 in the SSRI-exposed group, 9537 in the unmedicated maternally depressed group, and 31 207 in the unexposed group, whose mothers had no psychiatric illness and no SSRIs. The investigators found that the offspring of mothers using SSRIs at least twice during pregnancy had a 37% increased risk of speech/language disorders compared with offspring of the unmedicated group, after accounting for maternal depression (hazard ratio, 1.37; 95% CI, 1.11–1.70; P = 0.004).

Handal et al. examined the association between prenatal exposure to SSRIs and motor development in children whilst also taking into account the effect of maternal symptoms of anxiety and depression in a population-based prospective pregnancy cohort study [79C]. 51 404 singleton pregnancies were identified from a national register, with use of SSRIs for the 6 months before pregnancy and during pregnancy recorded. The investigators found that, compared with no SSRI exposure, and after adjusting for symptoms of anxiety and depression before and during pregnancy, prolonged SSRI exposure was associated with a delay in fine motor development (odds ratio 1.42, 95% CI; 1.07–1.87), with the severity of maternal depression only partially explaining the association. When subjects were stratified according to depression after pregnancy, no impact on the estimated effect of SSRIs was observed. The authors concluded that long-term prenatal SSRI exposure was weakly associated with delayed motor development independent of depression.

Malm et al. investigated the impact of gestational exposure to SSRIs on offspring neurodevelopment [80C] in a national register study over a 15-year period, including 845 345 singleton live births. Abnormal neurodevelopment was defined by the cumulative incidence of depression, anxiety, ASD and ADHD up to the age of 14 years. The cumulative incidence of depression among those exposed prenatally to SSRIs was higher than those whose mothers had a psychiatric disorder but were not on antidepressants (adjusted HR = 1.78; 95% CI = 1.12–2.82; $P = 0.02$). There were, however, no differences in the rates of anxiety disorders, ASD and ADHD diagnoses in offspring. Comparing SSRI exposed to unexposed individuals, the hazard ratios were significantly elevated for each outcome.

Falls and Fractures

There is evidence that depression is associated with a significant reduction in lumbar and hip mineral density in older adults and that depression is an independent risk factor for falling [81M]. Additionally, there is now a consistent literature linking antidepressants, including SSRIs, with increased risk of falls and fractures. This has been recently replicated in a study of primary care patients older than 65 years, in whom SSRIs were associated with a significant increase in fall risk compared with nonusers of antidepressants (aHR 1.66; 95% CI: 1.58–1.73) [82C]. In a further study of an older population, Carrière et al. [83C] examined the association between the use of SSRIs and falls or fractures in a three-city population-based 4-year prospective study of 6599 community dwelling subjects aged ≥ 65 years. After adjusting for depression and other potential confounders, compared to those taking no antidepressants, the use of SSRIs at study entry (baseline) was significantly associated with a higher risk of falls (HR, 95% CI = 1.58, 1.23–2.03) and fractures (HR, 95% CI = 1.61, 1.16–2.24). Citalopram was associated with the highest risk of falls (multi adjusted HR, 95% CI = 2.31, 1.35–3.96) and fluoxetine with a twofold increase in risk of fractures (multi-adjusted HR, 95% CI = 2.07, 1.28–3.32).

When considering those who had taken SSRIs throughout the 4-year period, compared to those who had never used an SSRI, an increased risk of fracture was observed (HR, 95% CI = 1.78, 1.15–2.78). The risk of falls was similarly increased in those who continued treatment with an SSRI over the entire 4-year period, with the risk of falls at 4 years for the "continuing" group 88% higher than those who had never taken an SSRI (aHR 1.88, 95% CI 1.36–2.61). The authors noted that their results indicated an increase of about 60% in the 4-year risk of falls and fractures for those taking SSRIs at baseline and an even greater increase (around 80%) in chronic users, with this increased risk being independent of residual depressive symptoms.

Wang et al. conducted a large nested case–control study using a Taiwanese National Health Insurance Research Database. Current users of serotonergic antidepressants had an increased risk of fracture ((aOR) 1.16 [95% CI 1.07–1.25]) with the risk of fracture comparable between SSRI and SNRI users. A higher risk of fractures was also found in patients with osteoporosis (aOR 3.05 [2.73–3.42]) or a history of falling (aOR 6.13 [3.41–11.0]) [84C].

Sensory Systems

Acute Angle-Closure Glaucoma

Medications may precipitate acute angle-closure glaucoma (AACG) via either adrenergic- or anticholinergic-induced dilation of the pupil, resulting in physical obstruction of outflow of intraocular fluid. AACG may lead to eye pain, visual disturbance, ocular swelling and redness; if not recognized and treated rapidly, this may lead to permanent blindness. There have been consistent reports linking SSRIs and AACG (SEDA-37, 9 and 10).

To clarify details of this relationship, Chen et al. conducted a case–control study using a national healthcare insurance database over an 11-year period [85C]. The authors found a 5.8-fold increased risk of AACG associated with "immediate use" (within 7 days of treatment initiation) of SSRIs (OR 5.8, 95% CI 1.89–17.9), but no increased risk with "non-immediate use" (within 8–30 days). Among the "immediate" SSRI users, the risk of AACG was greatest in the high dose group (OR 8.53, 1.65–44.0).

SELECTIVE SEROTONIN RE-UPTAKE INHIBITORS (SSRIs) [SED-15, 3109; SEDA-31, 18; SEDA-32, 33; SEDA-33, 26; SEDA-34, 17; SEDA-35, 30; SEDA-36, 14; SEDA-37, 23; SEDA-38, 16]

Escitalopram

Telangiectasia

Iatrogenic telangiectasia is a poorly understood dermatological effect of several drugs, including venlafaxine

[86A] and may be triggered by photo-exposure. Huang et al. suggested that serotonin released around skin appendages is involved in the regulation of inflammation and immune reactions, and that serotonin receptors mediate cutaneous vasoconstriction and stimulate cytokine release from keratinocytes and lymphocytes [87R]. Although escitalopram has been associated with mucocutaneous undesired effects, few cases of photosensitivity have been reported in controlled trials and postmarketing surveillance, and none involved telangiectasia. A case of photo-distributed telangiectasia following use of escitalopram has been reported [88A]:

A previously healthy 81-year-old woman was referred with 4 days history of telangiectatic skin lesions: visible small linear red blood vessels (broken capillaries). She had commenced escitalopram (10 mg daily) 11 days previously for depression. She was on no other medications, and had no history of photosensitivity, rosacea or application of topical steroids. Physical examination showed several asymptomatic telangiectasias and angiomatous-like macules and papules, widely distributed on face, forearms and dorsum of both hands. Laboratory tests, including liver function tests, ANA, ENA, Scl-70 antibody and ANCA were within normal values. Histological examination revealed a normal epidermis; but blood vessels in the superficial dermis were prominent and focally dilated. A mild lymphocytic infiltrate with rare eosinophils was present. Since distribution in photoexposed areas suggested a light-induced adverse reaction, photo testing was performed. Patch tests were performed with standard photoallergens and 5% and 10% escitalopram in petrolatum, and were negative; photo-patch test with the same substances and a single suberythematous dose of 30 J/cm2 UVA on her upper back resulted in the appearance of telangiectatic lesions after 28 hours with escitalopram only (at both 5% and 10% strengths), providing evidence of a photo-induced drug reaction. Due to the relationship between administration and onset of telangiectasia, and the confirmation by phototesting, the escitalopram was ceased and the patient treated with oral methylprednisolone (16 mg/day with progressive reduction) and oral nicotinamide (500 mg/day) which led to a progressive and complete resolution of lesions after 1 month. Re-challenge was refused by the patient.

Fluoxetine

Henoch–Schonlein Purpura

There have been a small number of case reports of adult patients with urticarial and eukocytoclastic vasculitis related to SSRIs, particularly paroxetine and fluoxetine, generally within weeks of initiation of treatment [89A,90A]. There have been no reports of vasculitis in children or adolescents in association with SSRI treatment. A case has been reported of a 15-year-old boy who developed Henoch–Schonlein Purpura (HSP) during fluoxetine treatment [91A]:

A 15-year-old boy, with a 1-week history of treatment with fluoxetine, presented to the ER with a widely spread skin rash on his lower legs and pain in his ankles and knees. As the lesions were raised and purpuric, vasculitis was considered. There was no medical of psychiatric history of note, and he had become depressed in the context of the recent death of his father.

Investigations were normal, including complete blood count, blood chemistry, liver function tests, total serum immunoglobulin E, immunoglobin M, immunoglobulin A, and coagulation tests (the activated partial thromboplastin time and prothrombin time). Urinalysis showed slight proteinuria. D-dimer level was 3468 µg/L (<550), and fibrinogen level was 332.02, consistent with vasculitis. The diagnosis of HSP was made, and fluoxetine ceased. Treatment with methylprednisolone 40 mg qid and ranitidine 100 mg qid was commenced after which vasculitic symptoms resolved in 2 months.

In this case, vasculitis emerged after 1 week of fluoxetine treatment and, in addition to the characteristic rash, the patient had evidence suggestive of renal involvement and arthritis. There were no abnormal standard laboratory results or past history consistent with other possible causes of HSP. Accordingly, fluoxetine was the only possible causative factor related to vasculitis in this patient and on application of the Naranjo scale scored was 6 revealing "probable causative association" [92R].

Sertraline

Drug-Induced Liver Injury With Vanishing Bile Duct Syndrome

Vanishing bile duct syndrome (VBDS) is an acquired progressive destruction and disappearance of interlobular bile ducts causing chronic cholestasis. It may be associated with infections, drugs, toxins, oncologic, and immunologic processes [93R]. A case of bile duct paucity in a healthy teenager with resolution of symptoms following cessation of sertraline has been reported [94A]. Although sertraline is a well-recognized cause of drug-induced liver injury (DILI), it has not previously been implicated in VBDS.

A 15-year-old boy with depression had been treated with sertraline 75 mg daily for 6 months. He presented with a 1-month history of jaundice, pruritus, nausea, anorexia and pale stools. He reported no rashes, fevers, hospitalizations or other medical problems. Family history was negative for liver disease and he denied the use of alcohol, illicit drugs or supplements. There were no other medication exposures in the months prior to onset of symptoms. Two weeks after onset, laboratory investigations revealed elevated total bilirubin, direct bilirubin, aspartate aminotransferase (AST), and alanine aminotransferase (ALT), and normal international normalized ratio. White cell count was 6.4 × 103 µL and his infectious work up negative, including hepatitis A IgM, hepatitis B surface antigen, and

Hep C polymerase chain reaction. Abdominal ultrasound revealed a 16 cm liver span, enlarged for age, multiple gallstones without obstruction, and mildly enlarged spleen. Because of worsening nausea, pruritus, and rising bilirubin in the absence of ductal obstruction, liver biopsy was performed. Pathology revealed preserved lobular architecture with 14–16 portal tracts notable for rare bile duct profiles, minimal lymphocytic infiltration, and marked hepatocellular and canalicular cholestasis. Further investigations were performed, specifically, evaluation for rare causes of ductopenia, including an echocardiogram, absence of butterfly vertebrae detected by radiograph, and an unremarkable ophthalmologic examination. Screening was performed for the most common heritable causes of cholestatic liver disease in children, and was negative. Urine bile acids were not consistent with a bile acid synthesis defect. Markers for autoimmune hepatitis including antinuclear antibody and smooth muscle antibody were negative. Magnetic resonance cholangiopancreatogram was normal. Despite initiation of ursodiol to dissolve gallstones, the patient's cholestasis and fatigue progressed over 1 month. Total bilirubin peaked at 33.7 mg/dL with direct bilirubin 29.2 mg/dL. As the patient had rising bilirubin levels without any etiology for ductopenia being established, sertraline was discontinued because of concern for moderate to severe DILI evidenced by elevated alanine aminotransferase and total bilirubin and need for hospitalization. Within 4 weeks of discontinuation, his total bilirubin had decreased. Four months after medication cessation, his laboratory tests were within normal limits. Antidepressant therapy was later recommended with fluoxetine and hepatic tests remained normal 9 months later.

SEROTONIN AND NORADRENALINE RE-UPTAKE INHIBITORS (SNRIs)

Venlafaxine and Desvenlafaxine [SED-15, 3614; SEDA-31, 22; SEDA-32, 35; SEDA-33, 32; SEDA-34, 20; SEDA-35, 32; SEDA-36, 19; SEDA-37, 25; SEDA-38, 17]

Venlafaxine

BRUISING

Although many studies examine SSRI-induced bleeding, relatively few address the risk of SNRI-induced bleeding. Five case reports documenting venlafaxine-associated bleeding have been made [95A,96A,97A,98A,99A]. A further case of venlafaxine-induced bruising has been reported [100A]:

A 34-year-old woman with a history of depression, posttraumatic stress disorder, and Graves' disease, reported significant bruising for 10 days after starting the SNRI venlafaxine. She noticed small bruises mostly on her lower extremities reporting that the bruising began after commencing venlafaxine and worsening after the dose was titrated to 75 mg daily. The bruises appeared after playing with her children and old bruises did not resolve. She was also taking zolpidem, lorazepam, levothyroxine, and an over-the-counter iron supplement daily. She denied the use of nonsteroidal anti-inflammatory drugs or antiplatelet agents, or any medical or family history of blood dyscrasias or platelet disorders. All laboratory results were within normal range except for her measured sodium level of 133 mmol/L, mean platelet volume of 11.2 fL, and mean corpuscular hemoglobin concentration of 32.7%. Platelet, iron, thyroid, and liver abnormalities were excluded. A trial of bupropion was started, and venlafaxine was tapered over a 7-day period. At review 4 weeks after discontinuing venlafaxine, the bruising had resolved, but Ms A reported troubling side effects with bupropion, including palpitations and insomnia. She ceased bupropion and requested to restart a trial of venlafaxine despite the previous symptoms of bruising.

POOR NEONATAL ADAPTATION WITH FAILURE TO THRIVE

A case of poor neonatal adaptation with poor feeding and failure to thrive—possibly secondary to maternal venlafaxine use—has been reported [101A]:

A 1-month-old girl presented with poor weight gain and feeding interrupted by apparent distress and easy fatigability. The infant was born at term with her mother's pregnancy significant for an exacerbation of pre-existing depression and anxiety at 15 weeks followed by the use of venlafaxine, olanzapine, quetiapine and temazepam. Venlafaxine was continued as monotherapy from 20 weeks gestation for the remainder of the pregnancy and in early breastfeeding. The maternal dose of venlafaxine was high at 300 mg. At delivery her birth weight was 4309 g (>97th centile) and weight on admission 4326 g. On the third day of life, the infant demonstrated extensor posturing and cycling of the limbs which was assessed as possibly seizure related. Neurological examination was normal, although the infant's suck was noted to be un-coordinated and easily fatigued. EEG and MRI were normal. Phenobarbitone was initiated but subsequently ceased due to excessive sedation.

Venlafaxine and its major metabolite (O-desmethylvenlafaxine) are concentrated in breast milk (milk:plasma ratio of 3–4:1), a high infant proportion/dose when compared with other antidepressants. In this case, due to concerns about the effect of a high dose of venlafaxine upon the infant, and its concentration in breast milk, breast feeding was suspended which resulted in an improvement in alertness and a weight gain of 314 g over 7 days. Exposure to antidepressant medications in utero may precipitate the onset of a range of symptoms such as tremors, jitteriness, irritability, muscle tone regulation disorders, excessive crying, sleep disturbance, tachypnea and feeding problems after delivery. These symptoms describe the "poor neonatal adaptation syndrome" (PNA) and have been considered suggestive of a withdrawal syndrome, due to similar clinical features to SSRI discontinuation syndrome in adults. The authors noted that it may be difficult clinically to distinguish PNA occurring as part of a withdrawal syndrome from direct SSRI and SNRI toxicity causing overstimulation of the serotonergic system [102R]. They noted that symptoms of toxicity may occur 8–48 hours after birth, but withdrawal symptoms generally present directly after birth. Complicating the clinical picture further, toxicity and withdrawal symptoms may coexist [103R]. Depending upon the presentation and maternal dose of antidepressant, it may be appropriate to suspend or continue breast feeding.

Milnacipran

Piloerection

In 2007, the first case of piloerection in a patient receiving milnacipran hydrochloride was reported [104A]. Interestingly, in a recent case report, that patient's biological sister has also presented with piloerection occurring frequently all over her body, which also began shortly after initiation of milnacipran hydrochloride (50 mg/day) and which increased with dose escalation, disappearing after several months without change to her medication regime [105A].

Piloerection is induced by contraction of the arrector pili muscles following the activation of α1-adrenoceptor [106A]. Although there are few reports of piloerection following treatment with tricyclic antidepressants, these are ostensibly related not to the stimulation of α1-adrenoceptors, but their inhibition. Milnacipran, however, has a low potential for α1-adrenoceptor inhibition, instead inhibiting the reuptake of endogenous norepinephrine into nerve terminals, increasing the endogenous concentration of norepinephrine in the synaptic cleft, leading to piloerection.

Mirtazapine [SED-15, 2536; SEDA-32, 36; SEDA-33, 33; SEDA-34, 22; SEDA-35, 34; SEDA-36, 21; SEDA-37, 28]

Although edema is described in the product information, only five cases of mirtazapine-associated peripheral edema have been reported [107A,108A,109A,110A,111A]. Two further cases of mirtazapine-associated peripheral edema, from the same institution, have been recently reported, both in elderly patients [112A].

A 74-year-old woman was admitted due with psychotic depression with catatonic features. Her medications on admission included lorazepam, clonazepam, venlafaxine and thyroxine. She had comorbid diagnoses of breast cancer in remission and hypothyroidism. Benzodiazepines were ceased in preparation for electroconvulsive therapy and mirtazapine commenced 7 days later increased to 60 mg over the next 2 weeks. Aripiprazole was commenced on day 15 and increased to 10 mg by day 20. She was noted to have bilateral pitting edema of the lower limbs 4 weeks after admission. Clinical examination and pathology investigations, including sonography, chest X-ray and trans-thoracic echocardiogram were normal. Aripiprazole was ceased due to extra-pyramidal side effects. Frusemide 80 mg twice-daily did not improve the peripheral edema. Seven days after mirtazapine was changed to sertraline edema completely resolved.

A 70-year-old woman was admitted with deterioration in her mood and development of melancholic features. Her medical history included controlled hypertension and fibromyalgia. She had been on duloxetine, diazepam, aspirin, valsartan, hydrochlorothiazide, tramadol and oxycodone. Mirtazapine was commenced and increased to 30 mg within 5 days of admission which was followed by the development of peripheral edema of the lower limbs and mouth ulcers. Clinical examination and pathology investigations, including sonography, chest X-ray and trans-thoracic echocardiogram were normal. Mirtazapine was decreased and agomelatine commenced which was followed by the complete resolution of edema and mouth ulcerations. After exclusion of more common etiologies, a diagnosis of mirtazapine-associated peripheral edema was made.

A full resolution of edema following cessation of mirtazapine and a Naranjo score of 6 in both cases suggest a 'probable' adverse drug reaction. The authors noted that all reported cases of mirtazapine-associated peripheral edema have occurred at a dosage of 30 mg/day or greater.

References

[1] Coupland C, et al. Antidepressant use and risk of cardiovascular outcomes in people aged 20 to 64: cohort study using primary care database. BMJ. 2016;352:i1350 [MC].

[2] Noordam R, et al. Use of antidepressants and the risk of myocardial infarction in middle-aged and older adults: a matched case-control study. Eur J Clin Pharmacol. 2016;72(2):211–8 [C].

[3] Lin CH, et al. Antidepressants and valvular heart disease: a nested case-control study in Taiwan. Medicine (Baltimore). 2016;95(14):e3172 [M].

[4] Danielsson B, et al. Antidepressants and antipsychotics classified with torsades de pointes arrhythmia risk and mortality in older adults—a Swedish nationwide study. Br J Clin Pharmacol. 2016;81(4):773–83 [C].

[5] Coupland C, et al. Antidepressant use and risk of adverse outcomes in older people: population based cohort study. BMJ. 2011;343:d4551 [C].

[6] Chen Y, et al. Risk of cerebrovascular events associated with antidepressant use in patients with depression: a population-based, nested case-control study. Ann Pharmacother. 2008;42:177–84 [C].

[7] Smoller JW, et al. Antidepressant use and risk of incident cardiovascular morbidity and mortality among postmenopausal women in the Women's Health Initiative study. Arch Intern Med. 2009;169:2128–21391 [C].

[8] Hung CC, et al. The association of selective serotonin reuptake inhibitors use and stroke in geriatric population. Am J Geriatr Psychiatry. 2013;21:811–5 [C].

[9] Wu CS, et al. Association of cerebrovascular events with antidepressant use: a case-crossover study. Am J Psychiatry. 2011;168:511–21 [C].

[10] Hackam DG, Mrkobrada M. Selective serotonin reuptake inhibitors and brain hemorrhage. A meta-analysis. Neurology. 2012;79(18):1862–5 [M].

[11] van Asch CJ, et al. Incidence, case fatality, and functional outcome of intracerebral haemorrhage over time, according to age, sex, and ethnic origin: a systematic review and metaanalysis. Lancet Neurol. 2010;9:167–76 [M].

[12] Shin D, et al. Use of selective serotonin reuptake inhibitors and risk of stroke: a systematic review and meta-analysis. J Neurol. 2014;261(4):686–95 [M].

[13] Renoux C, et al. Association of selective serotonin reuptake inhibitors with the risk for spontaneous intracranial hemorrhage. JAMA Neurol. 2017;74(2):173–80 [C].

[14] Aarts N, et al. Inhibition of serotonin reuptake by antidepressants and cerebral microbleeds in the general population. Stroke. 2014;45:1951–7 [C].

[15] Akoudad S, et al. Antidepressant use is associated with an increased risk of developing microbleeds. Stroke. 2016;47(1):251–4 [C].

[16] Pisani F, et al. Effects of psychotropic drugs on seizure threshold. Drug Saf. 2002;25(2):91–110 [R].

[17] Bloechliger M, et al. Risk of seizures associated with antidepressant use in patients with depressive disorder: follow-up study with a nested case–control analysis using the clinical practice research datalink. Drug Saf. 2016;39(4):307–21 [C].

[18] Kessing LV. Depression and the risk for dementia. Curr Opin Psychiatry. 2012;25(6):457–61 [R].

[19] Moraros J, et al. The association of antidepressant drug usage with cognitive impairment or dementia, including Alzheimer disease: a systematic review and meta-analysis. Depress Anxiety. 2017;34 (3):217–26. http://dx.doi.org/10.1002/da.22584 [Epub ahead of print] [M].

[20] Lee CW, et al. Antidepressant treatment and risk of dementia: a population-based, retrospective case-control study. J Clin Psychiatry. 2016;77(1):117–22 [C].

[21] Kessing LV, Forman JL, Andersen PK. Do continued antidepressants protect against dementia in patients with severe depressive disorder? Int Clin Psychopharmacol. 2011;26(6): 316–322 [C].

[22] Laporte S, et al. Bleeding risk under selective serotonin reuptake inhibitor (SSRI) antidepressants: a meta-analysis of observational studies. Pharmacol Res. 2017;118:19–32 [R].

[23] Nordeng H, et al. Pregnancy outcome after exposure to antidepressants and the role of maternal depression: results from the Norwegian Mother and Child Cohort Study. J Clin Psychopharmacol. 2012;32:186–94 [C].

[24] Sandanger I, et al. Prevalence, incidence and age at onset of psychiatric disorders in Norway. Soc Psychiatry Psychiatr Epidemiol. 1999;34:570–9 [C].

[25] Meunier MR, Bennett IM, Coco AS. Use of antidepressant medication in the United States during pregnancy, 2002–2010. Psychiatr Serv. 2013;64:1157–60 [C].

[26] Hanley GE, Mintzes B. Patterns of psychotropic medicine use in pregnancy in the United States from 2006 to 2011 among women with private insurance. BMC Pregnancy Childbirth. 2014;14:242 [C].

[27] Charlton R, et al. Selective serotonin reuptake inhibitor prescribing before, during and after pregnancy: a population-based study in six European regions. BJOG. 2015;122:1010–20 [C].

[28] Huybrechts KF, et al. Preterm birth and antidepressant medication use during pregnancy: a systematic review and meta-analysis. PLoS One. 2014;9(3):e92778 [M].

[29] Salkeld E, Ferris LE, Juurlink DN. The risk of postpartum hemorrhage with selective serotonin reuptake inhibitors and other antidepressants. J Clin Psychopharmacol. 2008;28(2):230–4 [C].

[30] Palmsten K, et al. Use of antidepressants near delivery and risk of postpartum hemorrhage: cohort study of low income women in the United States. BMJ. 2013;347:f4877 [MC].

[31] Grigoriadis S, et al. Prenatal exposure to antidepressants and persistent pulmonary hypertension of the newborn: systematic review and meta-analysis. BMJ. 2014;348:f6932 [M].

[32] Kieviet N, et al. Serotonin and poor neonatal adaptation after antidepressant exposure in utero. Acta Neuropsychiatr. 2017;29(1): 43–53 [M].

[33] Grigoriadis S, et al. Prenatal exposure to antidepressants and persistent pulmonary hypertension of the newborn: systematic review and meta-analysis. BMJ. 2014;348:f6932 [M].

[34] Ross LE, et al. Selected pregnancy and delivery outcomes after exposure to antidepressant medication: a systematic review and meta-analysis outcomes after antidepressant use in pregnancy. JAMA Psychiat. 2013;70:436–43 [M].

[35] Alwan S, Friedman JM, Chambers C. Safety of selective serotonin reuptake inhibitors in pregnancy: a review of current evidence. CNS Drugs. 2016;2:1–7 [R].

[36] Andrade SE, et al. Use of antidepressant medications during pregnancy: a multisite study. Am J Obstet Gynecol. 2008;198:194. e191–5 [C].

[37] Nikfar S, et al. Increasing the risk of spontaneous abortion and major malformations in newborns following use of serotonin reuptake inhibitors during pregnancy: a systematic review and updated meta-analysis. Daru. 2012;20(1):75 [M].

[38] Myles N, et al. Systematic meta-analysis of individual selective serotonin reuptake inhibitor medications and congenital malformations. Aust N Z J Psychiatry. 2013;47(11):1002–12 [M].

[39] Grigoriadis S, et al. Antidepressant exposure during pregnancy and congenital malformations: is there an association? A systematic review and meta-analysis of the best evidence. J Clin Psychiatry. 2013;74(4):e293–308 [M].

[40] Wemakor A, et al. Selective serotonin reuptake inhibitor antidepressant use in first trimester pregnancy and risk of specific congenital anomalies: a European register-based study. Eur J Epidemiol. 2015;30(11):1187–98 [MC].

[41] Bérard A, et al. The risk of major cardiac malformations associated with paroxetine use during the first trimester of pregnancy: a systematic review and meta-analysis. Br J Clin Pharmacol. 2016;81(4):589–604 [M].

[42] Jordan S, et al. Selective serotonin reuptake inhibitor (SSRI) antidepressants in pregnancy and congenital anomalies: analysis of linked databases in Wales, Norway and Funen Denmark. PLoS One. 2016;11(12)e0165122 [C].

[43] Palmsten K, et al. Antidepressant use and risk for preeclampsia. Epidemiology. 2013;24(5):682 [C].

[44] Avalos LA, Chen H, Li DK. Antidepressant medication use, depression, and the risk of preeclampsia. CNS Spectr. 2015;20(01): 39–47 [C].

[45] DeOcampo M, et al. Risk of gestational hypertension and preeclampsia in women who discontinued or continued antidepressant medication use during pregnancy. Am J Obstet Gynecol. 2016;214(1):S366 [c].

[46] Steer RA, et al. Self-reported depression and negative pregnancy outcomes. J Clin Epidemiol. 1992;45(10):1093–9 [C].

[47] Dayan J, et al. Prenatal depression, prenatal anxiety, and spontaneous preterm birth: a prospective cohort study among women with early and regular care. Psychosom Med. 2006;68(6):938–46 [C].

[48] Orr ST, James SA, Blackmore Prince C. Maternal prenatal depressive symptoms and spontaneous preterm births among

African-American women in Baltimore Maryland. Am J Epidemiol. 2002;156(9):797–802 [C].

[49] Neggers Y, Goldenberg R, Cliver S, et al. The relationship between psychosocial profile, health practices, and pregnancy outcomes. Acta Obstet Gynecol Scand. 2006;85(3):277–85 [C].

[50] Rahman A, et al. Impact of maternal depression on infant nutritional status and illness: a cohort study. Arch Gen Psychiatry. 2004;61(9):946–52 [C].

[51] Copper RL, et al. National Institute of Child Health and Human Development Maternal-Fetal Medicine Units Network. The preterm prediction study: maternal stress is associated with spontaneous preterm birth at less than thirty-five weeks' gestation. Am J Obstet Gynecol. 1996;175(5):1286–92 [C].

[52] Andersson L, et al. Neonatal outcome following maternal antenatal depression and anxiety: a population-based study. Am J Epidemiol. 2004;159(9):872–81 [C].

[53] Grote NK, et al. A meta-analysis of depression during pregnancy and the risk of preterm birth, low birth weight, and intrauterine growth restriction. Arch Gen Psychiatry. 2010;67(10):1012–24 [M].

[54] Liu C, et al. Prenatal parental depression and preterm birth: a national cohort study. BJOG. 2016;123(12):1973–82 [C].

[55] Fan C, et al. Paternal factors to the offspring birth weight: the 829 birth cohort study. Int J Clin Exp Med. 2015;8(7):11370 [C].

[56] Venkatesh KK, et al. Association of antenatal depression symptoms and antidepressant treatment with preterm birth. Obstet Gynecol. 2016;127(5):926–33 [R].

[57] Eke A, Saccone G, Berghella V. Selective serotonin reuptake inhibitor (SSRI) use during pregnancy and risk of preterm birth: a systematic review and meta-analysis. BJOG. 2016;123(12):1900–7 [M].

[58] Cantarutti A, et al. Is the risk of preterm birth and low birth weight affected by the use of antidepressant agents during pregnancy? A population-based investigation. PLoS One. 2016;11(12):e0168115 [C].

[59] Nezvalová-Henriksen K, et al. Effect of prenatal selective serotonin reuptake inhibitor (SSRI) exposure on birthweight and gestational age: a sibling-controlled cohort study. Int J Epidemiol. 2016;45(6):2018–29 [C].

[60] Viktorin A, et al. Selective serotonin re-uptake inhibitor use during pregnancy: association with offspring birth size and gestational age. Int J Epidemiol. 2016;45(1):170–7 [C].

[61] Chambers CD, et al. Selective serotonin-reuptake inhibitors and risk of persistent pulmonary hypertension of the newborn. N Engl J Med. 2006;354(6):579–87 [C].

[62] US Food and Drug Administration. Public health advisory: treatment challenges of depression in pregnancy and the possibility of persistent pulmonary hypertension in newborns. 7/19/2006;2006, http://www.fda.gov/Drugs/DrugSafety/PostmarketDrugSafetyInformationforPatientsandProviders/ucm124348.htm [S].

[63] US Food and Drug Administration. FDA drug safety communication: selective serotonin reuptake inhibitor (SSRI) antidepressant use during pregnancy and reports of a rare heart and lung condition in newborn babies, 2012, Available from URL: [Accessed 2017 Jan 11]. http://www.fda.gov/Drugs/DrugSafety/ucm283375.htm [S].

[64] Bérard A, et al. SSRI and SNRI use during pregnancy and the risk of persistent pulmonary hypertension of the newborn. Br J Clin Pharmacol. 2017;83(5):1126–33 [C].

[65] Nörby U, et al. Neonatal morbidity after maternal use of antidepressant drugs during pregnancy. Pediatrics. 2016;138(5) e20160181 [C].

[66] Palmsten K, et al. Use of antidepressants near delivery and risk of postpartum hemorrhage: cohort study of low income women in the United States. BMJ. 2013;347:f4877 [MC].

[67] Grzeskowiak LE, et al. Antidepressant use in late gestation and risk of postpartum haemorrhage: a retrospective cohort study. BJOG. 2016;123(12):1929–36 [C].

[68] Hanley GE, et al. Postpartum hemorrhage and use of serotonin reuptake inhibitor antidepressants in pregnancy. Obstet Gynecol. 2016;127(3):553–61 [M].

[69] Jiang HY, et al. Antidepressant use during pregnancy and risk of postpartum hemorrhage: a systematic review and meta-analysis. J Psychiatr Res. 2016;83:160–7 [M].

[70] Boukhris T, et al. Antidepressant use during pregnancy and the risk of autism spectrum disorder in children. JAMA Pediatr. 2016;170(2):117–24 [C].

[71] Kaplan YC, et al. Prenatal selective serotonin reuptake inhibitor use and risk of autism spectrum disorder in the children: a systematic review and meta-analysis. Reprod Toxicol. 2016;60:174 [R].

[72] El Marroun H, et al. Maternal use of antidepressant or anxiolytic medication during pregnancy and childhood neurodevelopmental outcomes: a systematic review. Eur Child Adolesc Psychiatry. 2014;23:973–92 [R].

[73] Oyebode F, et al. Psychotropics in pregnancy: safety and other considerations. Pharmacol Ther. 2012;135(1):71–7 [R].

[74] Pedersen LH, Henriksen TB, Olsen J. Fetal exposure to antidepressants and normal milestone development at 6 and 19 months of age. Pediatrics. 2010;125:e600–8 [c].

[75] Casper RC, et al. Length of prenatal exposure to selective serotonin reuptake inhibitor (SSRI) antidepressants: effects on neonatal adaptation and psychomotor development. Psychopharmacology (Berl). 2011;217:211–9 [c].

[76] Galbally M, Lewis AJ, Buist A. Developmental outcomes of children exposed to antidepressants in pregnancy. Aust N Z J Psychiatry. 2011;45:393–9 [c].

[77] Kingston D, Tough S, Whitfield H. Prenatal and postpartum maternal psychological distress and infant development: a systematic review. Child Psychiatry Hum Dev. 2012;43(5):683–714 [R].

[78] Brown AS, et al. Association of selective serotonin reuptake inhibitor exposure during pregnancy with speech, scholastic, and motor disorders in offspring. JAMA Psychiat. 2016;73(11):1163–70 [C].

[79] Handal M, et al. Motor development in children prenatally exposed to selective serotonin reuptake inhibitors: a large population-based pregnancy cohort study. BJOG. 2016;123(12):1908–17 [C].

[80] Malm H, et al. Gestational exposure to selective serotonin reuptake inhibitors and offspring psychiatric disorders: a national register-based study. J Am Acad Child Adolesc Psychiatry. 2016;55(5):359–66 [C].

[81] Stubbs B, et al. Depression and reduced bone mineral density at the hip and lumbar spine: a comparative metaanalysis of studies in adults 60 years and older. Psychosom Med. 2016;78:492–500 [M].

[82] Coupland C, et al. Antidepressant use and risk of adverse outcomes in older people: population based cohort study. BMJ. 2011;343:d4551 [C].

[83] Carrière I, et al. Patterns of selective serotonin reuptake inhibitor use and risk of falls and fractures in community-dwelling elderly people: the Three-City cohort. Osteoporos Int. 2016;27(11):3187–95 [C].

[84] Wang CY, et al. Serotonergic antidepressant use and the risk of fracture: a population-based nested case–control study. Osteoporos Int. 2016;27(1):57–63 [C].

[85] Chen HY, et al. Association of selective serotonin reuptake inhibitor use and acute angle-closure glaucoma. J Clin Psychiatry. 2016;77(6):692–6 [C].

[86] Vaccaro M, et al. Photodistributed eruptive telangiectasia: an uncommon adverse drug reaction to venlafaxine. Br J Dermatol. 2007;157(4):822–4 [A].

[87] Huang J, et al. Immunohistochemical study of serotonin in lesions of chronic eczema. Int J Dermatol. 2004;43(10):723–6 [R].

[88] Vaccaro M, et al. Photodistributed telangiectasia following use of escitalopram. Allergol Int. 2016;65(3):336–7 [A].

[89] Margolese HC, et al. Cutaneous vasculitis induced by paroxetine. Am J Psychiatry. 2001;158(3):497 [A].

[90] Welsh JP, Cusack CA, Ko C. Urticarial vasculitis secondary to paroxetine. J Drugs Dermatol. 2005;5(10):1012–4 [A].

[91] Süleyman A, et al. Henoch–Schönlein Purpura during treatment with fluoxetine. J Child Adolesc Psychopharmacol. 2016;26(7):651 [A].

[92] Naranjo CA, et al. Naranjo ADR probability scale. Clin Pharmacol Ther. 1981;30:239–45 [R].

[93] Reau NS, Jensen DM. Vanishing bile duct syndrome. Clin Liver Dis. 2008;12(1):203–17 [R].

[94] Conrad MA, Cui J, Lin HC. Sertraline-associated cholestasis and ductopenia consistent with vanishing bile duct syndrome. J Pediatr. 2016;169:313–5 [A].

[95] Tham CJ, Trew M, Brager N. Abnormal clotting and production of factor VIII inhibitor in a patient treated with venlafaxine. Can J Psychiatry. 1999;44(9):923–4 [A].

[96] Linnebur SA, Saseen JJ, Pace WD. Venlafaxine-associated vaginal bleeding. Pharmacotherapy. 2002;22(5):652–5 [A].

[97] Benazzi F. Hemorrhages during escitalopram-venlafaxine-mirtazapine combination treatment of depression. Can J Psychiatry. 2005;50(13):877 [A].

[98] Sarma A, Horne MK. Venlafaxine-induced ecchymoses and impaired platelet aggregation. Eur J Haematol. 2006;77(6):533–7 [A].

[99] Ghio L, Puppo S, Presta A. Venlafaxine and risk of upper gastrointestinal bleeding in elderly depression. Curr Drug Saf. 2012;7(5):389–90 [A].

[100] Carpenter JE, et al. Venlafaxine-induced bruising: a case report. Prim Care Companion CNS Disord. 2016;18(3). http://dx.doi.org/10.4088/PCC.15l01886 [A].

[101] Tran MM, Fancourt N, Ging JM, et al. Failure to thrive potentially secondary to maternal venlafaxine use. Australas Psychiatry. 2016;24(1):98–9 [A].

[102] Sie SD, et al. Maternal use of SSRIs, SNRIs and NaSSAs: practical recommendations during pregnancy and lactation. Arch Dis Child Fetal Neonatal Ed. 2012;97(6):F472–6 [R].

[103] Kieviet N, Dolman KM, Honig A. The use of psychotropic medication during pregnancy: how about the newborn. Neuropsychiatr Dis Treat. 2013;9:1257–66 [R].

[104] Hori S, et al. Piloerection induced by replacing fluvoxamine with milnacipran. Br J Clin Pharmacol. 2007;63(6):665–71 [A].

[105] Matsuo N, et al. Sisters who developed piloerection after administration of milnacipran. Int J Clin Pharmacol Ther. 2016;54(3):208–11 [A].

[106] Stephens MDB. Drug-induced piloerection in man: an alpha 1-adrenoceptor agonist effect? Hum Toxicol. 1986;5:319–24 [A].

[107] Kutscher EC, Lund BC, Hartman BA. Peripheral edema associated with mirtazapine. Ann Pharmacother. 2001;35(11):1494–5 [A].

[108] Lin CE, Chen CL. Repeated angioedema following administration of venlafaxine and mirtazapine. Gen Hosp Psychiatry. 2010;32:e1–2 [A].

[109] Sarısoy G. Peripheral edema associated with olanzapine-mirtazapine combination: a case report. Bull Clin Psychopharmacol. 2011;21(3):249–52 [A].

[110] Çam B, Kurt H. Peripheral edema associated with mirtazapine: a case report. Anatolian J Psychiatry. 2013;14(1):84–6 [A].

[111] Saddichha S. Mirtazapine associated tender pitting pedal oedema. Aust N Z J Psychiatry. 2013;48:487 [A].

[112] Lai FY, Shankar K, Ritz S. Mirtazapine-associated peripheral oedema. Aust N Z J Psychiatry. 2016;50(11):1108 [A].

3

Lithium

Kelan L. Thomas[1], *Shadi Doroudgar*

Touro University California College of Pharmacy, Vallejo, CA, United States

[1]Corresponding author: kelan.thomas@tu.edu

INTRODUCTION

Lithium is widely accepted as the gold standard treatment for bipolar disorder according to psychiatry practice guidelines [1S,2R,3R,4R]. A recent population-based cohort study ($N=5089$), using UK health records from 1995 to 2013, confirmed this superior efficacy by demonstrating that lithium was a more successful maintenance treatment monotherapy than olanzapine, valproate or quetiapine, based on its longer duration to treatment failure (for 75% of subjects): 2.05 years [95% CI 1.63–2.51] vs 1.13 [95% CI 0.64–0.84], 0.98 [95% CI 0.84–1.18] and 0.76 years [95% CI 0.64–0.84], respectively [5MC]. These researchers also analyzed a population-based cohort study ($N=6671$), using UK health records from 1995 to 2013, comparing lithium to the same medications (olanzapine, valproate, quetiapine) and found that lithium use was associated with the highest rates of chronic kidney disease (all P-values <0.001) and new onset hypercalcemia (all P-values ≤ 0.013), but lowest rate of weight gain (all P-values <0.001) [6MC]. They also demonstrated that lithium had a higher rate of thyroid disease than olanzapine and valproate (both P-values ≤ 0.012), but lower rates of hypertension than olanzapine ($P=0.017$) [6MC].

A recent review suggested that an estimated 67%–90% of patients treated with lithium experience at least one side effect, and also proposed strategies for managing lithium side effects like polyuria, polydipsia, tremor, weight gain, cognitive impairment, sexual dysfunction and dermatological disorders [7R].

Organs and Systems

Cardiovascular

Lithium's potential cardiovascular adverse effects, including heart rate and rhythm changes, have been well documented in adults. However, there is little information about cardiotoxicity in pediatric populations. A recent case report from Singh and colleagues has illustrated the possible cardiac manifestations of lithium poisoning in a child taking lithium 750 mg/day for 3 months, whose symptoms of muffled speech, poor muscle tone and shuffling gait worsened after switching from methylphenidate to amantadine. The 5-year-old boy with ADHD and bipolar disorder presented in an obtunded state, appearing disoriented, agitated and combative, along with notable signs of dysarthria, truncal ataxia and hand tremors. His serum lithium was significantly elevated at 5.4 mEq/L, while an ECG showed a QRS interval of 128 ms, QTc interval 590 ms, ST segment depression 1–2 mm with T-wave inversions, heart rate around 100 bpm, and his atrial rate was less than the ventricular rate, which authors suggested was consistent with sinus node depression and a junctional escape rhythm. The patient was treated with hemodialysis over 48 hours, which steadily decreased lithium levels. The QRS and QTc intervals decreased proportionally with decreasing lithium levels, demonstrating correlation coefficients of $R^2=0.98$ and $R^2=0.95$, respectively. The authors suggest that it was difficult to be certain exactly which ECG changes were attributable to lithium alone or electrolyte abnormalities, but concluded the two were probably related. They also caution that children's families should be aware of lithium toxicity warning signs, particularly muffled speech, shuffling gait and poor muscle tone, which were early clinical manifestations in this case [8A].

Nervous System

COGNITIVE DYSFUNCTION

A recent review of lithium and cognition, in patients with bipolar disorder, suggested that lithium may cause reversible psychomotor retardation, but appears to have no impact on attention. The authors also suggested that any impact on processing speed, executive functioning, intellectual ability or memory remains unclear due to contradictory evidence available in the literature [9R].

Sabater and colleagues conducted a cross-sectional study ($N=98$), comparing lithium monotherapy, anticonvulsants only, lithium plus anticonvulsants, and healthy controls, to determine the effect of lithium and anticonvulsants on neurocognition in stable patients with bipolar disorder. The group with lithium monotherapy ($N=29$) had preserved long-term memory (measured by Wechsler Memory Scale-Revised Delayed Auditory Memory, Delayed Visual Memory, Auditory Recognition Delayed, and Delayed Memory tests), short-term auditory memory (measured by Wechsler Memory Scale-Revised Immediate Auditory Memory), and attention (measured by Trail Making Test-A) when compared to healthy controls, while the other comparison groups did not, which was consistent with the above review [9R] finding that lithium had no impact on attention. The authors concluded that lithium may have less cognitive impairment than anticonvulsants and therefore suggested that lithium may be a more appropriate long-term treatment option for stable patients with bipolar disorder [10c].

Neuromuscular Functioning

TREMOR

Neuromuscular side effects, such as tremor and acute cerebellar toxicity, have been associated with lithium therapy, but the mechanism for these adverse reactions during therapy remains uncertain. Lei and colleagues conducted a retrospective neuroimaging analysis study ($n=20$) to evaluate if low-dose lithium (450 mg/day) treatment over 3 months had the potential to increase nigral iron levels in subjects meeting criteria for ultrahigh risk of psychosis, determined by using the Comprehensive Assessment of the At Risk Mental State (CAARMS). In animal models, nigral iron elevation has been linked to parkinsonian features (such as hand tremor), cognitive loss and neurodegeneration. The MRI analysis found that subjects treated with lithium for 3 months had significant reductions in substantia nigra average T2 relaxation time compared with baseline scans (-5%, $P=0.007$) and treatment as usual control scans (-7%, $P<0.001$), which they suggested was consistent with iron accumulation. In animal models, lithium (3.6 mg/kg daily) administered for 3 weeks was shown to lower brain levels of tau protein, while increasing nigral iron levels, so they also demonstrated that tau-knockout mice were protected from lithium-induced iron elevation and neurotoxicity. Therefore, the authors suggested that the MRI neuroimaging findings might potentially explain lithium's neuromuscular side effects, particularly hand tremor [11c,E].

Irreversible neurological sequelae are rare with lithium, but have been reported and diagnosed as Syndrome of Irreversible Lithium-Effectuated Neurotoxicity (SILENT) when neurological dysfunction persists for 2 months after lithium cessation in the absence of prior neurological illness. Banwari and colleagues describe two such cases of persistent cerebellar dysfunction after acute lithium toxicity and subsequent cessation. The first case was a 35-year-old male with bipolar disorder, who was stable taking lithium 1200 mg/day for several years. He presented to the emergency room with vomiting, ataxia, coarse hand tremors, dysarthria, dysdiadochokinesia, finger–nose dysmetria and gaze-evoked nystagmus on examination. He reported taking extra doses to induce sleep (2000 mg/day) for the previous 2 days and he had the following abnormally elevated labs: serum lithium 4.42 mEq/L, creatinine 2.3 mg/dL, blood urea 68 g/dL, and TSH 10.52 mIU/mL. The patient was treated with six sessions of hemodialysis, and on day 12 his elevated labs had all substantially decreased: serum lithium 0.9 mEq/L, creatinine 1.2 mg/dL, blood urea 52 mg/dL, and TSH 4.51 mIU/mL. Upon discharge he was only prescribed lorazepam 2 mg orally as needed for insomnia, but was still dysarthric, finger–nose dysmetric and unable to walk without support. At 6 months follow-up, he had disarticulate speech, hand tremors, dysrhythmokinesia, saccadic dysmetria and an unsteady gait, but his serum lithium was undetectable at <0.2 mEq/L and all other labs were normal.

The second case reported was a 55-year-old man with a 20-year history of bipolar disorder, who was stable taking lithium 900 mg and olanzapine 10 mg daily for many years. Prior to hospitalization for his current manic episode, he had been poorly adherent with his medication and subsequently decompensated. On day 3 of the psychiatric admission, he developed a fever and cough with expectoration, along with an elevated leukocyte count (14 100/cumm), and was treated for an upper respiratory tract infection with cefadroxil 500 mg twice daily. On day 5, he rapidly developed lethargy, nausea, abdominal pain, diarrhea, disorientation and unsteadiness. He still had an elevated leukocyte count (15 200/cumm), but his serum lithium was also elevated 2.52 mEq/L, while all other labs were normal. Lithium was immediately discontinued, but on day 10 he had prominent intention tremors, finger–nose and knee–heel dysmetria, rebound nystagmus and truncal instability with a tendency to fall. Upon discharge his lithium was 0.3 mEq/L and he was prescribed olanzapine 10 mg and lorazepam 1 mg daily. After 12 months of follow-up, he had scanning dysarthria, limb incoordination and a clumsy ataxic gait. The authors propose that acute lithium overdose in the first case and fever in the setting of infection for the second case were contributory since these are both known risk factors predisposing patients to SILENT [12A].

DOWNBEAT NYSTAGMUS

Nystagmus is known to occur with acute lithium intoxication but may also occur at normal blood levels. Jørgenson and colleagues described a 62-year-old woman with bipolar disorder who was being treated with 600 mg/day of lithium for the past 4 weeks, in addition to her previous regimen of valproate 1500 mg/day, lamotrigine 75 mg/day and venlafaxine 375 mg/day. She presented with extremity tremor, generalized weakness and recurrent falls. Upon neurological examination, she was found to have normal mental status, saccadic eye movements, gross extremity tremor and unsteady gait. While working up other potential causes, MRI, CSF, EEG findings were all normal and paraneoplastic autoantibodies were negative. Lab results included a serum lithium 0.78 mmol/L, magnesium 0.87 mmol/L and vitamin B12 688 pmol/L. During the following 3 weeks of hospitalization, the patient experienced cognitive impairment, tremor, ataxia, and complained of diplopia. At this time, further exam revealed downbeat nystagmus, upward gaze deviation and horizontal gaze palsy. No voluntary pursuit movements or horizontal saccades could be elicited and a doll's head maneuver to activate vestibulo-ocular reflexes did not overcome the gaze palsies. Lithium intoxication was suspected and since the serum lithium had increased to 1.0 mmol/L, the medication was discontinued. Within 1 week, serum lithium decreased to 0.2 mmol/L and her symptoms significantly improved. Seven weeks after initial presentation, tremor, cognitive function, vertical and horizontal eye movements had all normalized, although there were still some residual low-amplitude nystagmus and oscillopsia on down gaze and some degree of retrograde amnesia. Therefore, after ruling out alternative causes of nystagmus and considering the temporal relationship for symptomatic improvement, the authors concluded that the downbeat gaze nystagmus and horizontal gaze palsy were caused by lithium intoxication [13A].

NEUROLEPTIC MALIGNANT SYNDROME

Another rare, but serious neuromuscular side effect that has been reported for lithium is neuroleptic malignant syndrome (NMS). Patil and colleagues reported a 74-year-old female with a 30-year history of bipolar disorder and hypothyroidism, who was taking lithium 400 mg, valproate 500 mg and levothyroxine 100 μg daily for 2 years with no dosage changes. She presented to the emergency department complaining of high fever and generalized weakness over the previous 10 days, but her family also noticed decreased oral intake during the week and altered consciousness over the previous 4 days. During examination she was disoriented, confused, afebrile and had generalized rigidity with BP 150/70 mm Hg. She also had the following abnormal labs: serum lithium 2.5 mEq/L, WBC $21.5 \times 10^3/\mu$L, CK 637 IU/L and sodium 107 mEq/L. A diagnosis of NMS was made based on presence of elevated CK, muscle rigidity and previous fevers, along with several supplementary symptoms such as abnormal blood pressure, altered consciousness and leukocytosis. After discontinuation of psychotropics, IV fluids, and supportive management, her symptoms abated over 2 weeks and there was minimal rigidity at the time of discharge. The authors suggested a plausible mechanism for lithium-induced NMS: lithium may reduce the effects of dopamine by preventing intracellular cAMP accumulation and this dopamine hypoactivity could lead to the development of NMS [14A].

Sensory Systems

DYSGEUSIA AND HYPOSMIA

Metallic taste is an acute reversible side effect of lithium therapy in up to 20% of patients, but persistent dysgeusia and hyposmia after discontinuing lithium is rare. De Coo and Haan report a 55-year-old man who was prescribed lithium for chronic cluster headache prophylaxis and developed an unpleasantly strange taste, along with diminished smell, about a week after initiation. The patient had already been taking verapamil 480 mg/day and sodium valproate 2000 mg/day, but due to a high frequency of cluster headaches, the lithium 800 mg/day was added. He reported a metallic taste after 1 week, complaining that his taste was altered for coffee and chocolate and that he could taste creamy, spicy, sweet, salty, and sour foods only minimally. He also reported a diminished sense of smell, complaining that he could no longer detect gas or perfume odors and he noticed a chemical smell perception for foods like fried meat and onions. Serum lithium level was only 0.35 mmol/L 13 days after starting lithium 800 mg/day, but he decided to discontinue the medication after about 3 weeks of therapy due to these taste and smell disturbances. He reported that the metallic taste quickly disappeared after discontinuation, but the impaired sense of taste and smell actually increased for several weeks before stabilizing. In a follow-up visit 9 months later, his dysgeusia and hyposmia had still not improved. This is the first case report of long-term smell and taste disturbances after discontinuing lithium according to authors, since all previous cases reported a return to normal taste and smell within days following lithium discontinuation [15A].

Endocrine

THYROID

Lithium prescribing information has specific warnings about hypothyroidism and hypercalcemia with or without hyperparathyroidism. Lambert and colleagues conducted a retrospective cohort study of medical claims for patients with bipolar disorder ($n = 27\,574$) to compare hypothyroidism risk among nine medications commonly prescribed to treat bipolar disorder: lithium, lamotrigine, valproate, carbamazepine, oxcarbazepine, quetiapine, aripiprazole, risperidone and olanzapine. The subjects had at least 1 year of no prior hypothyroidism or bipolar disorder drug treatment, but had subsequently started bipolar drug monotherapy and then had at least one thyroid test. After adjusting for age, sex, physician visits and thyroid tests covariates, the mean 4-year cumulative risks were: lithium 8.8%, quetiapine 8.3%, lamotrigine 7.1%, valproate 7.0%, aripiprazole 7.0%, carbamazepine 6.7%, risperidone 6.5%, olanzapine 6.4% and oxcarbazepine 6.3%. While lithium had a higher risk of hypothyroidism when compared to all other treatments combined as one group, the risk was not different when lithium was compared to each agent individually. A linear fit estimated that patients taking lithium were also administered thyroid tests roughly 2–3 times more often than patients taking the other medications. Despite lithium's slightly higher risk of hypothyroidism, the authors concluded that thyroid abnormalities occur somewhat frequently in patients with bipolar disorder regardless of drug treatment. As a result, thyroid tests should be regularly checked in patients with bipolar disorder [16MC].

Harari and colleagues conducted an analysis ($N=178$), with a mother–child cohort in Argentina, to determine the effect of lithium levels in drinking water on calcium homeostasis during pregnancy. Multivariable-adjusted mixed-effects logistic regression modeling, adjusted for gestational age, season of sampling, maternal age, urinary arsenic and serum boron, demonstrated that every $25 \mu L/L$ increase in blood lithium concentration was associated with a 3.46 higher odds [95% CI 1.04–11.5] of having vitamin D_3 concentrations <50 nmol/L and 4.64 higher odds [95% CI 1.11–19.3] of having vitamin $D_3 < 30$ nmol/L. In a multivariable-adjusted mixed-effects linear regression model, adjusted for the same covariates, every $25 \mu L/L$ increase in blood lithium concentration was inversely associated with vitamin D_3 concentrations (-6.1 nmol/L [95% CI -9.5 to -2.6]), urinary calcium (-29 mg/L [95% CI -51 to -7.2]), and urine magnesium (-8.9 mg/L [95% CI -16 to -2.1]). These findings suggest that drinking water with elevated lithium levels may impair calcium homeostasis in pregnant women, particularly vitamin D_3 concentration, which could have potential negative effects on maternal and fetal health, including infectious diseases, preeclampsia, developmental programming and fetal skeletal development [17C].

PARATHYROID

The prevalence of hyperparathyroidism has been reported to reach 6.3% after 19 years of treatment with lithium. As lithium is a calcium-sensing receptor (CaSR) antagonist, blocking this receptor could lead to lower calcium sensitivity by parathyroid cells and subsequent decrease of negative feedback inhibition on parathyroid hormone (PTH) secretion. Ruiz Pardo and colleagues report three cases of female patients (Case 1: 63 years old, Case 2: 29 years old, and Case 3: 74 years old) treated with lithium 1200 mg/day for bipolar disorder who developed hyperparathyroidism. The duration of lithium treatment was 15, 10 and 19 years, respectively. Laboratory results showed elevated PTH (656 pg/mL, 93 mg/dL, 96 mg/dL) and elevated calcium (16.3, 10.8, 11 mg/dL) in all cases, respectively. Case 1 had symptoms of neurological impairment (coma), whereas Case 2 and 3 were asymptomatic. All three cases had indications for surgical intervention due to persistent hypercalcemia after lithium withdrawal. The surgeons decided to treat all cases with bilateral cervical exploration and excision (without intraoperative PTH measurement) and found this procedure be a safe and effective treatment strategy since none of these cases had persistence or recurrence [18A].

Metabolism

Ricken and colleagues suggest lithium augmentation is a well-established treatment strategy for patients with major depressive disorder (MDD) who have an insufficient antidepressant response. However, weight gain associated with lithium augmentation is a potential side effect that may cause patients to discontinue therapy. Although the mechanism of lithium-induced weight gain is not well understood, leptin is thought to play a role. Leptin is a hormone involved in the regulation of food intake and energy expenditure, as well as neuroendocrine and immune functions. Leptin and leptin receptor resistance have been previously associated with weight gain from other psychiatric medications. This association prompted the authors to investigate the relationship between leptin and body mass index (BMI) in a cohort of German patients using lithium augmentation for MDD. Adult patients (>18 years) with MDD who had an indication for lithium augmentation and a Hamilton Depression Rating Scale (HDSR-17) score ≥ 12 were included ($n=89$). Leptin serum concentrations were measured at baseline and 4 weeks after starting lithium augmentation and analyzed using linear mixed-effects models. The model estimated a BMI-increase of 0.24 kg/m^2 from baseline to endpoint, where the following variables demonstrated a significant positive effect on BMI: time ($P=0.016$), leptin ($P=0.0003$), male gender ($P=0.027$) and adiposity (BMI ≥ 30) at baseline ($P<0.0001$). The authors concluded that leptin signaling may be involved with lithium-induced weight gain, but suggest further research is warranted since this is only the first study to test this association [19c].

Salivary Glands

Lithium is known to cause dry mouth, due its inhibition of adenylyl cyclase, but only a few cases of hypersalivation have been reported. Bou Khalil and colleagues report a 50-year-old female with bipolar disorder who started lithium 800 mg/day 3 days before a psychiatric hospitalization and was also taking diazepam, olanzapine, levothyroxine, and valsartan during the admission. The patient reported hypersalivation, polyuria and a constant salty taste upon admission with a serum lithium concentration of 0.9 mEq/L. The physical and laboratory examination findings were normal and patient reported also having hypersalivation the last time she was prescribed lithium a year prior. Her case scored a 6 on the Naranjo Adverse Drug Reaction Probability Scale, indicating a probable adverse drug reaction to lithium. The authors point out that valsartan is an angiotensin-receptor blocker, which could increase lithium accumulation in the intracellular compartment and in her saliva. They suggest this drug interaction could be a possible explanation for the symptoms in this patient, despite her therapeutic lithium levels (0.7–0.9 mEq/L) [20A].

Urinary Tract

KIDNEYS

It is well known that lithium use has been limited by adverse effects on the kidneys with 2–3 times increased risk of chronic kidney disease (CKD). Risk factors for lithium-induced renal dysfunction include supratherapeutic doses or concomitant administration with drugs known to increase lithium exposure, such as non-steroidal anti-inflammatory drugs, angiotensin-converting enzyme inhibitors or angiotensin receptor blockers. However, cases of CKD are still reported when lithium concentrations are maintained within the therapeutic window.

A recent systematic review of the literature published through 2015 by Rej and colleagues investigated the effects of lithium on the development of nephrogenic diabetes insipidus (NDI) and chronic kidney disease (CKD) using molecular markers. They evaluated molecular alterations in 3510 records from 71 pre-clinical studies and two clinical studies. Molecular changes were reported in calcium signaling, sodium/solute transport, vasopressin/aquaporin, extracelluar-regulated pathway signaling, nitric oxide, inositol monophosphate, prostaglandin, G protein-coupled receptors, and inflammation-related pathways in lithium-associated renal disease. The authors suggest these changes may lead to a lower vasopressin response, which can reduce urea transporter and aquaporin expression causing NDI, and potentially progress to CKD via inflammation and oxidative stress [21R].

In addition to increased risk of CKD, the risk of lithium-induced renal neoplasia has also been recently investigated as lithium-induced inhibition of Glycogen Synthase Kinase 3 beta (GSK-3β) is thought to increase the risk of inflammation and cancer in the kidneys. A case–control study by Pottegard and colleagues identified 9444 cases of Upper Urinary Tract Cancers (UUTC) from 2000 to 2012 in Denmark residents prescribed lithium for at least 5 years. After exclusions, the remaining 6477 cases were matched by age and sex to 259 080 cancer-free controls. After adjusting for confounders, including education, diseases or use of drugs that could affect risk of UUTC or renal function, logistic regression modeling demonstrated no significant change in estimated risk for overall UUTC [OR 1.3; 95% CI 0.8–2.2], localized disease [OR 1.6; 95% CI 0.8–3.0] or renal pelvis/ureter cancers [OR 1.7, 95% CI 0.5–5.4]. Therefore, the authors concluded that lithium was unlikely to increase the risk of UUTC [22MC].

Second-Generation Effects

Pregnancy

Pregnancy may increase the risk of depressive symptoms in bipolar disorder, but since lithium is teratogenic it is important to carefully weigh the risk and benefits of lithium, although it remains one of the most effective medications for bipolar depression. A review by Hogan and Freeman summarized the evidence regarding lithium use during pregnancy. It is well known that first trimester exposure to lithium can increase the risk of Ebstein's anomaly, a malformation of the tricuspid valve that may eventually require surgery. The estimated incidence of Ebstein's anomaly is roughly 1/1000 live births in those with first trimester lithium exposure and only 1/20 000 live births in the general population. Therefore, a level II ultrasound and fetal echocardiography at 16–20 weeks gestation is recommended to assess for the malformation in pregnant women treated with lithium during the first trimester.

Late antenatal lithium use has been associated with neonatal adverse effects such as lethargy, hypotonia and respiratory distress. Other neonatal complications like arrhythmias, nephrotoxicity, hepatic dysfunction, hypothyroidism, and diabetes insipidus may be mitigated by discontinuation of lithium 24 to 48 hours prior to planned delivery or at labor onset during spontaneous deliveries.

Lithium levels and the patient's mood should be carefully monitored during pregnancy since physiologic changes, including alterations in vascular volume and the glomerular filtration rate, as well as preeclampsia and hyperemesis, can lead to changes in serum lithium concentration. The authors explain that standard guidelines recommend weekly serum levels, along with thyroid and renal function labs, during the month before the expected delivery date, but only monthly monitoring starting at 20 weeks gestation [23R].

Lactation

The postpartum period is also associated with a higher risk of psychiatric symptoms in patients with bipolar disorder. Therefore, some mothers may require treatment of symptoms with lithium and it is important to weigh the risks for breastfed infants against the potential benefits for the mother. Uguz and Sharma conducted a systematic review of literature published from 1995 to 2015 and identified two studies and three case reports of patients treated with lithium doses between 600 and 1350 mg/day during lactation ($n=26$). Infant ages at the time of assessment ranged from 5 days to 15 months. The reports suggested that a considerable amount of lithium is excreted in breast milk with one study demonstrating a mean milk-to-plasma (M/P) ratio of 0.53 (range 0.34–0.7). Mild hypotonia and elevations in serum and creatinine, TSH and urea nitrogen, were also reported. The infants' serum lithium concentrations ranged from undetectable to 0.47 mEq/L, while the infant/maternal ratio of serum drug concentration (IS/MS) ratio ranged from 0.10 to 0.58. One study also reported mean relative infant dose (RID), which was 12.2% (range 0%–30%), which represented the weight-adjusted infant dose relative to the weight-adjusted maternal dose. The authors concluded that, although lithium is excreted in breast milk, the adverse effect frequency for infants exposed through breast milk is relatively low. The authors suggested that while lithium is not contraindicated during lactation, it should be considered only when there is a lack of alternative options since lithium does have a relatively high exposure in infants and limited data on potential effects [24R].

Susceptibility Factors

R A retrospective case–control study using electronic health records from a large New England health system was conducted by Castro and colleagues to determine risk factors for lithium-induced renal insufficiency. The study included adult patients (≥18 years) who had been prescribed lithium between 2006 and 2013. Patients with documented "renal failure" ICD-9 code or GFR < 60 mL/min were categorized as cases ($n=1445$) and were matched 1:3 to controls without renal insufficiency using risk set sampling ($n=4306$). Multivariate logistic regression models in the training set, adjusted for baseline clinical and demographic features, demonstrated that female sex [OR 1.75; 95% CI 1.49–2.08], white race [OR 1.53; 95% CI 1.21–1.94], older age [OR 1.55; 95% CI 1.44–1.65], history of hypertension [OR 2.62; 95% CI 2.18–3.16], history of smoking [OR 1.27; 95% CI 1.06–1.53], a diagnosis of schizophrenia or schizoaffective disorder [OR 1.63; 95% CI 1.31–2.03], and overall medical comorbidity burden measured by Charlson index [OR 1.46; 95% CI 1.31–1.64] were associated with renal insufficiency. Once-daily lithium dosing [OR 0.79; 95% CI 0.69–0.93] and concomitant antidepressants [OR 0.67; 95% CI 0.58–0.80] were associated with a lower risk of renal failure in the full cohort analysis. Mean lithium levels were also examined in fully adjusted models, which demonstrated that incrementally higher therapeutic levels were associated with a higher risk of renal failure than subtherapeutic levels < 0.6 mEq/L: 0.6–0.8 mEq/L [OR 1.42; 95% CI 1.14–1.77], 0.8–1.0 mEq/L [OR 2.03; 95% CI 1.56–2.65], and >1.0 mEq/L [OR 2.20; 95% CI 1.43–3.38] [25MC].

In addition to predicting risk with regression models containing demographic and clinical variables, using pharmacogenetics to predict who may be susceptible to lithium-induced renal toxicity could provide another novel strategy to minimize treatment risks. Tsermpini and colleagues genotyped 70 patients from an Italian lithium clinic for 45 tag single-nucleotide polymorphisms (SNPs) previously shown to be associated with kidney function or lithium's mechanism of action. Only one SNP, rs378448, demonstrated a significant effect on estimated glomerular filtration rate (eGFR) in a multiple regression analysis ($P=0.011$). The regression model also included covariates known to affect eGFR, such as years of lithium exposure, gender, age and smoking status. They also found a significant interaction term, rs378448*years of lithium exposure ($P=0.033$), which suggested that this SNP from the first intron of the Acid Sensing Ion Channel neuronal-1 (ACCN1) gene. This gene encodes the ASIC2 sodium channel protein and may modulate the effect of lithium exposure-years on eGFR. In addition, the lowest eGFR values were found for carriers of the rs378448 CC genotype [26c].

Interactions

Drug–Drug Interactions

Lithium has a narrow therapeutic index and small changes in dose or serum concentration may lead to clinically significant adverse drug reactions. Finley provided an updated review of drug interactions with lithium, primarily focused on the pharmacokinetic evidence generated over the last two decades.

The pharmacokinetics of lithium is essential to understanding the possible drug–drug interactions with other agents. It is estimated that brain concentrations are 50% lower than peripheral concentrations once steady state is achieved. However, lithium's terminal half-life in the brain is 6–12 hours longer than in the periphery, accounting for prolonged pharmacodynamic effects even when plasma concentrations have decreased. A number of medication classes have a risk of drug–drug interactions with lithium, primarily due to alterations in lithium's renal elimination. The non-steroidal anti-inflammatory drugs, ACE inhibitors, ARBs, thiazide and loop diuretics can increase lithium serum concentrations up to 40%, while potassium sparing diuretics appear to have no effect on lithium concentration. In contrast, osmotic diuretics (mannitol and urea) and methyl xanthines (e.g. theophylline, aminophylline and caffeine) can enhance the clearance of lithium from the body and decrease lithium concentrations by 40%–60%. Antipsychotics, the antiepileptic drug carbamazepine, and calcium channel blockers typically have no effect on lithium concentrations, but do have some reports of increased neurotoxicity when co-administered with lithium. Often, the clinical significance of drug interactions with lithium may be unpredictable, but careful monitoring is especially important in patients with dehydration, electrolyte abnormalities and renal insufficiency [27R].

Mood stabilizers may be prescribed in combination with atypical antipsychotics for patients with bipolar disorder or schizoaffective disorder, but there have been several case reports of neurotoxicity with lithium and antipsychotics. Hsu and colleagues report a 55-year-old male with a diagnosis of schizoaffective disorder who had been taking lithium and olanzapine for 2 years was hospitalized for acute treatment of a manic episode. Upon admission, he was prescribed lithium 600 mg/day and olanzapine 10 mg/day, which were then titrated up to lithium 900 mg/day and olanzapine 20 mg/day over a week. Due to poor blood glucose control during the first 2 weeks, olanzapine was discontinued and risperidone 25 mg intramuscular injection was administered, with subsequent oral dosing of risperidone 4.5 mg/day initiated a week later. A few days later the patient developed delirium, muscle rigidity, slurred speech, and his urine output decreased. His labs revealed an elevated serum lithium 1.2 mEq/L, creatinine 1.33 mg/dL, BUN 24 mg/dL and CK 975 U/L. The patient fully recovered 2 days after discontinuation of this combination and his labs returned to baseline: serum lithium 0.82 mEq/L, creatinine 0.82 mg/dL and BUN 12 mg/dL. Upon rechallenge with this combination at decreased doses (lithium 600 mg/day and risperidone 3 mg/day), he once again exhibited signs of delirium, elevated serum lithium 1.54 mEq/L and creatinine 1.36 mg/dL 3 days later. Upon discontinuation, the symptoms and labs once again resolved with serum lithium 1.06 mEq/L, and creatinine 0.88 mg/dL a day later. Finally, he was restarted on risperidone 2 mg/day monotherapy and was stable for the following 2 years on risperidone 2–3 mg/day without any recurrence of neurotoxicity or nephrotoxicity. These adverse reactions of delirium and acute kidney injury were considered to be due to the lithium–risperidone interaction based on a Naranjo Adverse Drug Reaction Probability Scale score of 10, which suggests a "definite" drug adverse reaction.

Hsu and colleagues also summarized case reports from the literature and found seven other similar cases with lithium doses between 450 and 1500 mg/day and risperidone doses between 2 and 6 mg/day. Neurotoxicity was reported in all cases, including four delirium cases and four NMS cases, which usually occurred during the first 3 weeks of concomitant therapy. The authors suggested two hypotheses for neurotoxicity, either by direct lithium intoxication or an excessive reduction in dopamine activity due to risperidone's postsynaptic dopamine receptor antagonism and lithium's inhibition of presynaptic dopamine release. Based on their case report and literature review, the authors concluded that the combination of lithium and risperidone should be closely monitored for neurological signs during the first 3 weeks [28A].

References

[1] National Institute for Health and Care Excellence (NICE). Bipolar disorder: the assessment and management of bipolar disorder in adults, children and young people in primary and secondary care (CG185). Available from https://www.nice.org.uk/guidance/CG185/; 2017. Published September 2014. Last updated February 2016. Accessed January 11, 2017. [S].

[2] Yatham LN, Kennedy SH, Parikh SV, et al. Canadian Network for Mood and Anxiety Treatments (CANMAT) and International Society for Bipolar Disorders (ISBD) collaborative update of CANMAT guidelines for the management of patients with bipolar disorder: update 2013. Bipolar Disord. 2013;15: 1–44 [R].

[3] Grunze H, Vieta E, Goodwin GM, et al. The World Federation of Societies of biological psychiatry (WFSBP) guidelines for the biological treatment of bipolar disorders: update 2012 on the long-term treatment of bipolar disorder. World J Biol Psychiatry. 2013;14(3):154–219 [R].

[4] American Psychiatric Association. Practice guideline for the treatment of patients with bipolar disorder (revision). Am J Psychiatry. 2002;159(Suppl 4):1–50 [R].

[5] Hayes JF, Marston L, Walters K, et al. Lithium vs. valproate vs. olanzapine vs. quetiapine as maintenance monotherapy for bipolar disorder: a population-based UK cohort study using electronic health records. World Psychiatry. 2016;15(1):53–8 [MC].

[6] Hayes JF, Marston L, Walters K, et al. Adverse renal, endocrine, hepatic, and metabolic events during maintenance mood stabilizer treatment for bipolar disorder: a population-based cohort study. PLoS Med. 2016;13(8). e1002058 [MC].

[7] Gitlin M. Lithium side effects and toxicity: prevalence and management strategies. Int J Bipolar Disord. 2016;4(1):27 [R].

[8] Singh D, Akingbola A, Ross-ascuitto N, et al. Electrocardiac effects associated with lithium toxicity in children: an illustrative case and review of the pathophysiology. Cardiol Young. 2016;26(2): 221–9 [A].

[9] Paterson A, Parker G. Lithium and cognition in those with bipolar disorder. Int Clin Psychopharmacol. 2017;32(2):57–62 [R].

[10] Sabater A, García-blanco AC, Verdet HM, et al. Comparative neurocognitive effects of lithium and anticonvulsants in long-term stable bipolar patients. J Affect Disord. 2016;190:34–40 [c].

[11] Lei P, Ayton S, Appukuttan AT, et al. Lithium suppression of tau induces brain iron accumulation and neurodegeneration. Mol Psychiatry. 2016;22:396–406. Epub ahead of print. [c,E].

[12] Banwari G, Chaudhary P, Panchmatia A, et al. Persistent cerebellar dysfunction following acute lithium toxicity: a report of two cases. Indian J Pharmacol. 2016;48(3):331–3 [A].

[13] Jørgensen JS, Landschoff Lassen L, et al. Lithium-induced downbeat nystagmus and horizontal gaze palsy. Open Ophthalmol J. 2016;10:126–8 [A].

[14] Patil V, Gupta R, Verma R, et al. Neuroleptic malignant syndrome associated with lithium toxicity. Oman Med J. 2016;31(4): 309–11 [A].

[15] De Coo IF, Haan J. Long lasting impairment of taste and smell as side effect of lithium carbonate in a cluster headache patient. Headache. 2016;56(7):1201–3 [A].

[16] Lambert CG, Mazurie AJ, Lauve NR, et al. Hypothyroidism risk compared among nine common bipolar disorder therapies in a large US cohort. Bipolar Disord. 2016;18(3):247–60 [MC].

[17] Harari F, Åkesson A, Casimiro E, et al. Exposure to lithium through drinking water and calcium homeostasis during pregnancy: a longitudinal study. Environ Res. 2016;147:1–7 [C].

[18] Ruiz Pardo J, Ríos Zambudio A, Rodríguez González JM, et al. Lithium-associated hyperparathyroidism. Med Clin (Barc). 2016;146(8):e43–4 [A].

[19] Ricken R, Bopp S, Schlattmann P, et al. Leptin serum concentrations are associated with weight gain during lithium augmentation. Psychoneuroendocrinology. 2016;71:31–5 [c].

[20] Bou Khalil R, Souaiby L, Ghossan R, et al. Hypersalivation as an adverse drug reaction related to lithium carbonate: a case report. J Clin Psychopharmacol. 2016;36(6):739–40 [A].

[21] Rej S, Pira S, Marshe V, et al. Molecular mechanisms in lithium-associated renal disease: a systematic review. Int Urol Nephrol. 2016;48(11):1843–53 [R].

[22] Pottegård A, Hallas J, Jensen BL, et al. Long-term lithium use and risk of renal and upper urinary tract cancers. J Am Soc Nephrol. 2016;27(1):249–55 [MC].

[23] Hogan CS, Freeman MP. Adverse effects in the pharmacologic management of bipolar disorder during pregnancy. Psychiatr Clin North Am. 2016;39(3):465–75 [R].

[24] Uguz F, Sharma V. Mood stabilizers during breastfeeding: a systematic review of the recent literature. Bipolar Disord. 2016;18(4):325–33 [R].

[25] Castro VM, Roberson AM, Mccoy TH, et al. Stratifying risk for renal insufficiency among lithium-treated patients: an electronic health record study. Neuropsychopharmacology. 2016;41(4):1138–43 [MC].

[26] Tsermpini EE, Zhang Y, Niola P, et al. Pharmacogenetics of lithium effects on glomerular function in bipolar disorder patients under chronic lithium treatment: a pilot study. Neurosci Lett. 2017;638:1–4 [c].

[27] Finley PR. Drug interactions with lithium: an update. Clin Pharmacokinet. 2016;55(8):925–41 [R].

[28] Hsu CW, Lee Y, Lee CY, et al. Neurotoxicity and nephrotoxicity caused by combined use of lithium and risperidone: a case report and literature review. BMC Pharmacol Toxicol. 2016;17(1):59 [A].

4

Drugs of Abuse

Hannah R. Fudin*,¹, Jennifer L. Babin*, Alisyn L. Hansen*,
Sidhartha D. Ray†

*University of Utah College of Pharmacy, Salt Lake City, UT, United States
†Manchester University College of Pharmacy, Natural and Health Sciences, Fort Wayne, IN, United States
¹Corresponding author: hannah.fudin@pharm.utah.edu

INTRODUCTION

Drug use and abuse continues to be a significant problem affecting the population worldwide. Among 15–64 year-olds, there are about 207 400 drug-related deaths each year or about 43.5 deaths per million (2014). These deaths have remained stable, but they are preventable and unacceptable. One-third to one-half of drug-related deaths are caused by overdose, with the majority attributed to opioids. Worldwide about 1 in 20 adults (250 million people), aged 15–64 misused or abused at least one drug in 2014. An estimated >29 million people suffer from drug use disorders, of those 12 million inject drugs. Now that this problem has been identified worldwide, policies should be set in place that are aimed at the overall social, economic and environmental community development to prevent and treat drug misuse and abuse based on scientific evidence which will result in decreased unnecessary adverse effects (AE), toxicity, and mortality [1S].

CANNABINOIDS: SYNTHETIC

Synthetic cannabinoid use was first reported in Europe in the early 2000s, and in the United States (U.S.) in 2008 [2r]. Synthetic cannabinoids are two to 100 times more potent than Δ9-tetrahydrocannabinol (THC), with higher cannabinoid receptor binding affinities [3S]. Altogether there are >50 individual compounds marketed with various names including "K2" and "Spice." Synthetic cannabinoids are often dissolved in a solvent, then applied to dry plant material and smoked. Users cite using synthetic cannabinoids because they provide a more intense psychoactive effect than marijuana and are usually undetectable on routine drug screening [4c,A]. From January to May 2015 there were 3572 calls to poison control centers in the U.S. related to synthetic cannabinoid use. Most commonly reported adverse effects (AE) included agitation ($n = 1262$ [35%]), tachycardia (1035 [29%]), drowsiness or lethargy (939 [26%]), and vomiting (585 [16%]) [5c].

Cardiovascular

A 39-year-old (YO) Caucasian male with a history of depression, deep vein thrombosis, and tobacco use was brought to the emergency department (ED) after cardiac arrest. Before arrival the patient was found to have ventricular fibrillation and required four direct current shocks. An electrocardiogram (ECG) demonstrated ST-elevation and the serum troponin-T level was 4398ng/L. Coronary angiography showed a left anterior descending arterial occlusion, so the patient underwent thrombectomy and stent placement. An acquaintance reported that he smoked "Black Mamba," a synthetic cannabinoid, within three hours of his presentation. Urine toxicology confirmed synthetic adamantyl-group cannabinoids but no other drugs of abuse. The authors note that ECG changes after synthetic cannabinoid use could be related to tachycardia, hypertension, and hypokalemia. This case is unusual since most previous reports of acute myocardial infarction have been associated with the synthetic cannabinoid class JWH [6A].

Another case involved a 16 year-old-male (YOM) with exercise-induced asthma and tobacco use who presented with 24 hours of continuous non-radiating substernal chest pressure associated with dyspnea, nausea, and vomiting (N/V). Two hours prior to symptom onset he used a synthetic cannabinoid. His initial troponin level was 1.47 ng/mL peaking at 8.29 ng/mL, and an ECG showed ST-segment elevation in the inferolateral leads. The patient was started on a nitroglycerin infusion, and on hospital day three verapamil was added. By day four, nitroglycerin was stopped, but an ECG continued to show ST-elevations. The patient underwent cardiac catheterization, which revealed no abnormalities [7A].

Respiratory

A case series examined four males aged 18–24 presenting with pulmonary symptoms, abnormal lung exams, and decreased oxygen levels on room air (79%–84%). Two patients confirmed synthetic cannabinoid use, but the others were unsure if they smoked natural marijuana or a synthetic cannabinoid. On initial chest radiography all patients had diffuse miliary-micronodular patterns and on chest computerized tomography (CT) all patients had diffuse tiny centrilobular nodules and tree-in-bud-pattern. Video-assisted thoracoscopic surgical biopsy was performed on three patients, which demonstrated organizing pneumonia with plugs of loose organizing granulation tissue or intra-alveolar fibrin in the distal bronchioles, patchy bronchiolocentric fibrosis, and scattered eosinophilia. An infectious pneumonia source was ruled out in all patients. One patient had mild residual symptoms at follow-up and moderate airflow limitation on pulmonary function testing. Two patients had chronic dyspnea, cough and moderate to severe airway obstruction, and the fourth patient died due to respiratory failure prior to discharge. The authors note that this is the first report of chest radiograph and CT descriptions of organizing pneumonia secondary to synthetic cannabinoid use [8A].

A 29-YOM with schizoaffective disorder presented with severe agitation after smoking a synthetic cannabinoid. Significant vitals included a mild fever of 37.9°C, heart rate (HR) of 109 beats/minute, and labs demonstrated leukocytosis (18.5 K/μL) with predominant neutrophilia (83.4%). Chest imaging revealed diffuse reticular-nodular and interstitial infiltrates. The patient was treated with sedatives, antibiotics, and intravenous fluids. Twenty-four hours after admission he was afebrile and his chest radiograph showed pulmonary infiltrate resolution. The authors diagnosed the patient with inhalation fever caused by synthetic cannabinoid [9A].

Nervous System

An observational case series identified 35 patients presenting to the ED at a single hospital with reported synthetic cannabinoid use. The median patient age was 34.6 years (range 14–58 years), and 31 were male.

Symptoms included altered mental status (AMS) ($n=24$ [61%]), tachycardia ($n=16$ [46%]), seizures ($n=14$ [40%]), hypertension ($n=6$ [17%]), and hallucinations ($n=2$ [6%]). Twenty-five patients (71.4%) were discharged from the ED, but seven (20%) required care in the intensive care unit (ICU), and five (14%) were intubated. All patients recovered after drug use. Routine urine and blood samples were tested for synthetic cannabinoids in 26 patients. Samples from 15 patients were positive for N-[(1S)-1-(aminocarbonyl)-2-methylpropyl]-1-(cyclohexylmethyl)-1H-indazole-3-carboxamide (AB-CHMINACA). An additional five patients had suspected AB-CHMINACA exposure based on metabolite presence. Concomitant substance use included ethanol ($n=7$) and cocaine ($n=6$) [10c].

Schwartz et al. describe seven patients (ages 16–30) simultaneously presenting to the hospital with anxiety and agitation after smoking synthetic cannabinoid at a party. Three exhibited combative and aggressive behavior. A couple weeks later, a 24-YOM presented with disorientation and delayed-onset seizures several days after smoking the same synthetic cannabinoid. During the same period, a U.S. official was evaluated in the ED for lethargy, forgetfulness, anxiety, difficulty sleeping, N/V, and chest discomfort. He reported that two days prior to admission he was manipulating packaged synthetic cannabinoid as part of his job duties with Latex gloves but no respiratory protection. Blood samples for all except one of the patients were collected and were positive for N-(1-amino-3,3-dimethyl-1-oxobutan-2-yl)-1-pentyl-1H-indazole-3-carboxamide (ADB-PINACA), which is found in the product "Crazy Clown" [4c,A].

Six hours after smoking synthetic cannabinoid, a 23-YOM and daily synthetic cannabinoid user developed generalized tonic–clonic seizure activity with urinary incontinence and tongue lacerations, witnessed by his wife. The patient smoked the substance again three hours later, and four hours after the second dose he experienced a second seizure. The patient denied any seizure history, other illicit drug use or medications, and a urine drug screen (UDS) was negative for THC and ethanol. Five synthetic cannabinoid variations were found in his blood samples: BB-22, AM2233, PB-22, 5F-PB-22, and JWH-122 [11A].

Urinary Tract

Case series have previously reported renal impairment associated with synthetic cannabinoids. Gudsoorkar and Perez provide an additional patient case who developed acute kidney injury (AKI) after synthetic cannabinoid use. A 26-YOM presented after having seizure-like activity followed by altered consciousness. He had been smoking synthetic cannabinoids for the past two days, and his last inhalation was the night prior to his presentation.

Laboratory studies revealed serum creatinine (SCr) 2.3 mg/dL, blood urea nitrogen (BUN) 25 mg/dL, and creatinine phosphokinase (CPK) 2337 units/L. His fractional excretion of sodium (5.09) was consistent with intrinsic renal failure, and a renal ultrasound showed no abnormalities. On hospital day four, the patient's SCr peaked at 8.1 mg/dL and his BUN was 53 mg/dL. He required one hemodialysis session for volume overload, and at discharge his SCr was 2 mg/dL. The authors note that while AKI associated with synthetic cannabinoid use may be reversible with supportive treatment, the long-term effect on the kidneys is still unknown [12A].

Thermoregulation

A 27-YO African-American male with schizophrenia experienced extreme agitation and disruptive behavior after a witnesses saw him smoking synthetic cannabinoids. His initial temperature was 106.1°F, and his HR was 173 beats/minute. Abnormal labs at admission included SCr 2.2, lactate 4.1, and CPK 1341. Within an hour his temperature decreased to 101.7°F with cooling measures. His CPK level peaked at 57050 on hospital day two, and aspartate transaminase (426), alanine transaminase (193), and international normalized ratio (2.2) were also elevated. After their initial peaks, the CPK and liver enzymes trended down, and the patient was discharged after 10 days. The authors believe this is the first publication that shows an association between synthetic cannabinoid use and hyperthermia [13A].

Death

Labay et al. identified 25 deaths involving ≥1 synthetic cannabinoid detected through toxicology testing. The cases included 19 males and six females aged 15–61. Eight synthetic cannabinoid variations were detected, most commonly AM-2201, XLR-11, and various JWH compounds. Synthetic cannabinoid blood concentrations ranged from 0.11 to 105 ng/mL. Sixteen cases were positive for only one synthetic cannabinoid, and nine had concomitant use of other illicit drugs. Based on the data, the authors concluded that patients with excited delirium, trauma or other accidents, overconsumption of other drugs, and pre-existing cardiopulmonary disease are at greater mortality risk when using synthetic cannabinoids [14c].

A 25-YOM with a history of alcohol and psychoactive substance abuse obtained three brands of synthetic cannabinoids at 11:00. He smoked one of the products (Czeszący grzebień) in a pipe while drinking a beer. Around 14:00–15:00 the patient was sleepy and had slurred speech and difficulty communicating. At 16:50 the patient used another product, "Mocarz," and within minutes collapsed with wheezing and vomiting. Around 17:30, after being found pulseless, he was initially successfully resuscitated but died after cardiac arrest on hospitalization day four. Significant symptoms prior to death included body temperature 33.0–37.3°C, severe upper body erythema, chest muscle contraction, diarrhea, and bleeding from injection sites. Before death, (methyl 2-{[1-(cyclohexylmethyl)-1H–indol-3-yl]formamido}-3,3-dimethylbutanoate) (MDMB-CHMICA) was found in his blood at 5.6 ng/mL, drawn eight hours after the patient's initial synthetic cannabinoid use. After death, varying amounts of MDMB-CHMICA were found in the blood, bile, brain, stomach, liver, and kidney [15A]. Another case involved a 22-YO with asystole after smoking a synthetic cannabinoid. Emergency medical services (EMS) was able to initially reestablish spontaneous circulation, but the next day the patient was declared dead due to brain hypoxia. On autopsy anoxic brain damage and pneumonia were found. Two hours after the patient was found lifeless, serum samples were collected and revealed MDMB-CHMICA (1.4 ng/mL), subtherapeutic mirtazapine, THC (1.5 ng/mL), and cetirizine. The authors concluded that death was most likely caused by MDMB-CHMICA [16A]. Another author notes that MDMB-CHMICA intoxication severity cannot be directly correlated with serum concentrations. During forensic case work, the authors detected MDMB-CHMICA in 140 serum samples, ranging from 0.10 to 91 ng/mL (median 0.67 ng/mL, mean 3.5 ng/mL). Several cases had concentrations similar to the patient presented by Westin et al., but they did not show signs of severe toxicity [17r].

Shanks and Behonick report the case of a 34-YOM who died after using a synthetic cannabinoid. Autopsy screening for drugs and ethanol was negative except for synthetic cannabinoid (S)-methyl-2-(1-(5-fluoropentyl)-1H-indazole-3-carboxa-mido)-3-methylbutanoate (5F-AMB). Previously reported deaths in patients using this drug involved other substances, making this the first case in which 5F-AMB was the sole substance contributing to death [18A].

Genotoxicity

Genotoxicity studies were conducted using four synthetic cannabinoids: (1-(5-fluoropentyl)-1H-indol-3-yl)(naphthalen-1-yl)methanone (AM-2201), (1-pentyl-1H-indol-3yl)(2,2,3,3-tetramethylcyclopropyl)methanone (UR-144), 1-(5-fluoropentyl)-N-(tricyclo[3.3.1.13,7yl)-1H-indazole-3-carboxamide (5F-AKB-48), and 1-(5-fluor-pentyl)-N-(naphtalen-1-yl)-1H-indazole-3-carboxamide (AM-2201-IC)]. Based on the study results, researchers concluded that these compounds cause damage to DNA at the chromosomal level but do not cause gene mutations [19E].

Age

A study conducted in Turkey retrospectively analyzed 16 pediatric patients (15 males; average age 15.4 ± 1.7 years) diagnosed with synthetic cannabinoid intoxication. Four patients had concomitant alcohol exposure and one had ecstasy co-administration. Psychoactive effects observed were agitation ($n=10/16$ [62.5%]), anxiety (10/16 [62.5%]), perceptual changes (7/13 [53.8%]), hallucinations (4/13 [30.8%]), panic attack (4/13 [30.8%]), numbness (2/13 [15.4%]), and euphoria (2/16 [12.5%]). Physical symptoms that occurred in $\geq 30\%$ of patients included eye redness, N/V, altered consciousness, sweating, mydriasis, slurred speech, hypotension, tachycardia, bradycardia, and syncope [20c].

A case of unintentional pediatric exposure in a 10-month-old female found chewing on a synthetic cannabinoid cigarette was recently published. She was brought to the ED within 30 minutes, and her initial physical exam (PE) was unconcerning. However, within 90 minutes the child required intubation. Routine imaging and laboratory studies were unremarkable except for positive influenza A. Her serum was analyzed for synthetic cannabinoids, and AB-PINACA (42 ng/mL) was detected. After 36 hours, the child was extubated and fully recovered [21A].

Recent studies have demonstrated potential for synthetic cannabinoids treatment in various diagnosis [22C]. Most studies reported mild to moderate AE that were Gastrointestinal (GI) or Central Nervous System (CNS) related. In patients treated for seizure common (>10% reported) AE events ($n=128$ [79%]) included somnolence ($n=41$ [25%]), decreased appetite ($n=31$ [19%]), diarrhea ($n=31$ [19%]), fatigue ($n=21$ [13%]), and convulsion ($n=18$ [11%]) [21C]. Patients taking >15 mg/kg/day (vs less) cannabidiol were significantly more likely to report diarrhea or related side effects (e.g., weight loss) [22C]. Additional reported AE (cannabidiol plus valproate treatment) included mild to moderate thrombocytopenia ($n=5$ [3%]), mildly elevated liver function tests ($n=11$ [7%]) and hyperammonaemia ($n=1$ [1%]) [22C]. Ball et al. evaluated cannabidiol (oromucosal spray [Sativex®]) for Multiple Sclerosis (MS) treatment ($n=68$). Total all-causality AE were reported by (41 [13.1%]) in the safety population ($n=320$). The most common AEs ($\geq 1\%$ incidence) were all mild to moderate and including dizziness ($n=18$ [5.6%]), confusion ($n=8$ [2.5%]), somnolence ($n=4$ [1.25%]) and nausea ($n=4$ [1.25%]) [23C]. Patients treated with THC (0.125 mg/kg IV) or placebo [24c] for postoperative nausea and vomiting (PONV) prevention were evaluated ($n=40$) [23c]. Most reported AEs included sedation and confusion but HR did not differ significantly between groups. Significantly more THC (vs placebo) patients were too sedated to perform initial psychotropic AE evaluation and significantly more THC patients were confused after one hour. Randomized controlled trials ($n=23$) were reviewed in chemotherapy-induced nausea and vomiting (CINV) cases for cannabinoid treatment to evaluate effectiveness and tolerability in adults with a various cancer types. Results demonstrated that compared to placebo patients receiving cannabinoids reported fewer AE for N/V but more AE overall [25M]. Efficacy and safety were studied for dementia-related neuropsychiatric symptoms (NPS) in patients receiving treatment with THC ($n=24$) 1.5 mg or placebo ($n=26$) thrice daily for three weeks. Mild or moderate AEs were similar, and no vital signs (VS), weight, or episodic memory effects or serious AEs were observed [26c].

Few AEs ($n=20$ [12%]) were reported for the above trials including status epilepticus, diarrhea, pneumonia, and weight loss, possibly related to cannabidiol use [23C,27C]. MS patients ($n=493$) reported ≥ 1 serious AE (35% and 28%) for THC (median dose = 14 mg/day) and placebo therapy, respectively [27C], and fewer serious AE ($n=2$) were reported including mental impairment and suicidal ideation [23C]. Pronounced AEs ($n=4$) reported for PONV treatment included extreme and sustained mood swings or anxiety and one patient fighting and screaming when awakening [24C]. Cannabinoids were discontinued in multiple studies due to AEs including nervous system-related serious AE ($n=3$) including psychiatric ($n=2$) and GI ($n=1$) [23C], and 'feeling high', dizziness, sedation and dysphoria [25M]. Treatment was discontinued for PONV due to inefficiency and clinically unacceptable side effects for this setting [24C].

CANNABINOIDS: NON-SYNTHETIC

Marijuana is becoming more available with continuous legalization throughout the U.S. [28MC]. More potent marijuana formulations including edibles, wax, oils, and dabs have been directly linked to toxicity and death [28MC,29A].

Hancock-Allen et al. report edible marijuana use leading to mortality in a 19-YOM. He purchased marijuana cookies and followed instructions to eat one-sixth portion. After 30–60 minutes without feeling affects the descendent consumed the entire cookie. Over the following two hours he displayed erratic speech and hostile behaviors, followed by jumping off the fourth-floor balcony, resulting in death from trauma. Toxicology results found 10 times (49 ng/mL) the serum concentration compared to the legal driving limit (5 ng/mL in Colorado). This is the first reported case attributing death to marijuana consumption without polysubstance use since Colorado approved recreational cannabis use in 2012 [29A].

Pierre et al. reports two cases associated with emergent psychosis resulting from concentrated THC extract use, cannabis 'wax', 'oil', or 'dabs' [30A]. Concerns are being raised about physicians recommending these products for medical purposes especially considering increased reported psychosis cases. The first reported case presented was a 17-YOM with no previous psychiatric history besides recreational cannabis use one to two times per week for two years. Patient then began using cannabis wax 'a few times.' Over the next three weeks he developed paranoid concerns including checking locks and fear of sleeping alone. He progressed to full delusions about being 'possessed by Satan' and getting 'caught in the middle of a war between the Free Masons and the Illuminati.' Patient presented to the ED with symptoms including confusion, disorganization and agitation with mild fever, tachycardia, hypertension, diaphoresis and photophobia. After revealing an unremarkable UDS, he was admitted to psychiatry and treated with risperidone 3 mg/day for one week. His VSs and psychotic symptoms normalized to baseline, and he was discharged on day 12. Risperidone was gradually tapered over six months then discontinued without psychosis recurrence and continued cannabinoid abstinence [30A]. The second case was similar but the patient (28-YOM) was self-treating by inhaling wax products ("Fire OG" and "Mystery") with a vaporizer and water pipe for 18 months before developing paranoid concerns that he was "being 'targeted' by Mexican gangs and that he could 'see the future.'" Patient displayed significant disorganization, thought blocking, and paranoia. He was treated with olanzapine 20 mg/day but switched to risperidone 2 mg/day on day two, prior to discontinuing anti-psychotic medications for suspicion of drug-induced psychosis. Day seven-to-eight, patient presented with two catatonic episodes displaying mutism, catalepsy, and waxy flexibility and treated with lorazepam 2 mg thrice daily which resolved catatonia. Psychotic symptoms diminished with risperidone re-initiation and up-titration over the following week. Patient was discharged on day 17, treated with risperidone outpatient and then slowly down-titrated for two months. Patient remained psychosis free without psychosis treatment, while maintaining cannabis abstinence [30A].

Hall reviewed literature for AE from cannabis use over 20 years. Results demonstrated increased car accident risk and cannabinoid dependence, poor psychosocial outcomes and mental health in adulthood associated with regular adolescent cannabis use. Acute AEs identified for cannabis use included modest fetal birth-weight reduction (pregnancy use) and risk-doubling for car crashes while intoxicated, with risk increasing substantially with alcohol co-administration. Psychosocial-related adverse outcomes with chronic use occur in 1:10 adulthood-and 1:6 adolescent-aged initiation. Similarly, cannabis-use initiated in adolescence increases risk two-fold for developing psychotic symptoms and is associated with increased cognitive impairment, lower educational attainment, illicit drug use, schizophrenia or a two-fold increase for developing psychotic diagnosis in adulthood. Physical health-related adverse outcomes for chronic cannabis use included increased risk for developing chronic bronchitis (regular smokers) [31r].

The first known case using dexmedetomidine treatment to support cannabis toxicity was reported in a 19-month-old male presenting to the ED hemodynamically stable with somnolence, periodic agitation, spontaneous breathing on room air (SPO$_2$ 96%), and apneic periods. He was responsive to painful stimulus with jarring cry, and isocoric and isocyclic midpoint pupils. Patient's mother reported that somnolence developed 12 hours prior, after the child consumed something on the park grounds. The UDS, immunochemical result was THC positive. Patient started having sudden-onset agitation and violent behavioral outbursts between calm periods so non-pharmacological methods were used first including quiet ambience, toys, colors, etc., but at a later stage, the patient was given bolus midazolam 1 mg to control agitation. Following the bolus, the patient had obstructive apneic periods, at which time the provider chose to use dexmedetomidine continuous infusion 0.4 μg/kg/hour and increase the rate to 0.7 μg/kg/hour to curb agitation. After 24 hours, dexmedetomidine was progressively reduced and patient returned to full consciousness. Dexmedetomide seemed the appropriate therapeutic choice allowing for "cooperative" sedation with decreased respiratory depression (RD) risk compared to benzodiazepines [32A]. Furthermore, Haney et al. demonstrate effective therapy for non-treatment seeking, chronic cannabinoid users. Researchers conducted a double-blind, placebo-controlled human laboratory study where naltrexone 50 mg ($n = 23$) maintenance treatment was used for the reinforcing, subjective, psychomotor and cardiovascular effects associated with active and inactive cannabinoid use. Compared to placebo ($n = 28$), naltrexone significantly reduced both active cannabis self-administration and its positive subjective effects (good effects). Placebo participants were 7.6 times (95%; CI: 1.1–51.8) more likely to self-administer active cannabis compared to naltrexone participants. Additionally, naltrexone had intrinsic effects including decreased ratings for friendliness, food intake, and systolic blood pressure (SBP) while increasing spontaneous reports of stomach upset and headache. This has been the first reported study to demonstrate naltrexone maintenance treatment effectively decreasing cannabis self-administration and 'good effect' rating for non-treatment-seeking daily cannabis smokers [33c].

ALCOHOL

According to the World Health Organization, the average daily pure alcohol consumption for people ≥15 years was 13.5 g in 2010. Many people occasionally drink more than average, with 16% of people worldwide participating in heavy episodic drinking. Although low-risk alcohol use patterns have reported benefits for some disease states, alcohol consumption is also associated with >200 diseases and injury conditions, including alcohol dependence, liver cirrhosis, cancer, infectious diseases and death [34S].

Nervous System

Previous studies demonstrated that alcohol intoxication is associated with disinhibition. Therefore, Claus and Hendershot sought to determine if differences in baseline working memory capacity influence disinhibition level. Fourteen males aged 21–35 were tested to determine their baseline working memory, then they consumed alcohol to attain a breath alcohol concentration (BAC) ≥ 0.06 g%. Study results suggested that individuals with low working memory capacity are more affected by alcohol intoxication, which authors concluded may make them more likely to perform risky behaviors under alcohol influence. However, this was a small study and the authors noted that unequal drinking duration and marijuana use between the groups may have influenced the results [35c].

Sensory Systems

Brasil et al. compared 24 participants aged 18–29 who, on average, had routinely been consuming alcohol for five years at 5.6 times/month and 138 g/day to control subjects of the same age with no alcohol consumption. An ophthalmologist determined that all enrolled subjects had a normal exam. Non-invasive tests used to detect subclinical visual alterations were administered to each participant. Based on the results, the authors concluded that regular alcohol consumption in young adults causes subclinical color vision impairment compared to young adults who do not consume alcohol [36c].

Immunologic

Aliphatic alcohols, alcohols that contain more than two carbon atoms, are produced by alcoholic fermentation and have been detected in non-regulated and regulated alcoholic beverages. Aliphatic alcohols are associated with greater hepatotoxicity than ethanol and may also produce additional toxicities, including immune system impairment. Pal et al. collected blood from 15 healthy volunteers, separated the monocytes, and treated the cells with aliphatic alcohol solutions. The authors found that monocyte phagocytosis was inhibited in a concentration-dependent manner by aliphatic alcohols. It should be noted that aliphatic alcohol concentration varies based on product, and even large-volume consumption of some beverages would not produce sufficient blood aliphatic alcohol concentrations to inhibit phagocytosis. It is possible that consumption of other alcoholic beverages with higher aliphatic alcohol concentrations could lead to impaired immunity, but this effect has not been shown in vivo [37E].

Genetic Factors

After alcohol consumption, ethanol is initially metabolized to acetaldehyde, a carcinogen. In individuals with active aldehyde dehydrogenase (ALDH2) enzymes, acetaldehyde is further metabolized rapidly to non-toxic acetate and is undetectable in the blood. However, some people, especially individuals of Eastern Asian descent, have impaired or absent ALDH2 enzyme activity. Enzyme-deficient individuals who drink alcohol have been shown to have increased head, neck, and esophageal cancer risk compared to those with normal ALDH2 enzymes [38c,39R]. Maejima et al. sought to determine how ALDH2 deficiency affects acetaldehyde concentration in gastric juice after ethanol 0.5 g/kg administration via nasogastric tube in 19 healthy Japanese males who were non-smokers and normal social drinkers. In subjects with functioning ALDH2 enzymes, the intragastric alcohol infusion caused only a small increase in gastric juice acetaldehyde concentration, but in ALDH2-deficient participants, there was a comparative mean 5.6-fold increase in the area under the curve ($P < 0.0001$), and acetaldehyde levels remained elevated throughout the 120-minute study period. The authors suggested that gastric mucosa exposure to acetaldehyde may be a mechanism of gastric cancer development in individuals with ALDH2 deficiency who consume alcohol [38c].

Recently, differences in the mu-opioid receptor gene OPRM1 among individuals have been associated with individual variation in alcohol response. To provide further evidence for the gene involvement, Hendershot et al. studied 40 heavy alcohol drinkers aged 19–21. Study participants self-administered intravenous alcohol over 120-minutes by pushing a button until they achieved a pleasurable intoxication level without AE. The authors found that subjects with the 118G variant of OPRM1 had more alcohol requests and a subsequently higher peak breath alcohol concentration compared to participants with the 118A variant (94.90 mg% vs 74.46 mg%) [40c].

Long et al. studied the GRM8 gene, which is involved in glutamate modulation. The authors determined that two single-nucleotide gene polymorphisms, rs886003 and rs17862325, were associated with alcohol dependence symptoms in a European American adult sample. The trend was also seen in African-American participants but was not statistically significant, possibly due to a lack of power [41c].

Drug–Drug Interactions

The US Food and Drug Administration (FDA) issued a warning in 2015 concerning the interaction between alcohol and varenicline, a prescription smoking cessation medication. According to reports submitted to the FDA, some patients who consume alcohol while taking varenicline experience increased alcohol intoxication, unusual or aggressive behavior, or amnesia. Patients did not experience these effects when drinking similar alcohol amounts prior to starting varenicline [42S].

BENZODIAZEPINES

Benzodiazepine (BZD) abuse is increasing and is widely implicated in drug overdose deaths. Falling just behind opioid analgesics, BZDs are one of the most common drugs associated with ED visits due to nonmedical use of prescription drugs [43C,44C]. Prescribing patterns within the US Veteran's Administration demonstrate that up to 27% of patients who received a prescription for an opioid medication, also received a prescription for a BZD. Furthermore, receipt of BZD while taking opioid analgesics led to an increase of death from drug overdose (2.33, 95% CI 2.05–2.64) [45c].

Over recent years a rise of abuse of BZD analogs has been noted [46r]. Designer BZDs have been described to cause dangerous situations in case reports [47r,48r]. Phenazepam, described as a new long-acting synthetic BZD has been documented to induce delirium in a case report of a 19-YO patient [48r]. Another new, and life-threatening, BZD, flubromazolam, has been described to cause severe intoxication in a young adult patient [47r].

Pancreas

Liaw et al. described the risk of acute pancreatitis associated with BZD poisoning in a population-based cohort study. This study found a significant association between BZD poisoning and acute pancreatitis, noting that BZD poisoning had a 5.33-fold increased risk of acute pancreatitis compared to those without BZD poisoning (HR 5.33, 95% CI 2.26–12.60) [49c].

Nervous System

A fatal BZD overdose was described by Aljarallah and Al-Hussain noting acute fatal posthypoxic leukoencephalopathy. The group was not able to identify underlying pathophysiology or recommended treatment for this scenario [50A].

While effects of BZD therapy on cognition are widely known, this concern has been expanded to patients seemingly recovered after only light sedation with midazolam.

Investigators Hsu et al. determined that patients who received midazolam for light sedation for endoscopy had significant impairment of psychomotor speed, memory, learning, working memory, and sustained attention for up to 2 hours following the procedure in some patients. This study highlights additional risk for patients of advanced age [51C]. A similar study evaluating midazolam sedation in pediatric dentistry noted no significant side effects but demonstrated that paradoxical reactions were the most common minor AE ($n = 11$, 6.5%) [52c].

Clobazam use, specifically in patients with Lennox–Gastaut syndrome, has been demonstrated to lead to increased risk of aggression-related adverse events in pediatric patients both with and without a personal history of aggressive behavior [53C].

Fluid Balance

Clobazam, primarily used for the treatment of epilepsy and seizure disorders, has been implicated as causing pedal edema in four patients within one-to-three months of therapy initiation. The edema completely subsided within six weeks of therapy discontinuation. Of note, the patients described no benefit to diuretic therapy and additional edema workup was unremarkable [54c].

Pharmacogenetics

It has recently been discovered that pharmacogenetics may alter one's risk for falls associated with BZD use. Ham et al. evaluated 11 485 community-dwelling individuals based on their CYP2C9 variants and BZD use. When compared to nonusers, current BZD users carrying a CYP2C9*2 or *3 allele had a 45% increased fall risk (HR, 1.45, 95% CI 1.21–1.73) suggesting that reduced CYP2C9 enzyme activity may indeed increase the risk of falls in patients taking BZD medication [55C].

Special Populations

It is well known that BZDs are potentially inappropriate medications in older adults [56R]. Lorazepam has been considered the BZD of choice in older adults [57c]. A study by Pomara et al. evaluated lorazepam in 37 cognitively intact elderly individuals demonstrated that patients exhibit significantly poorer recall and slowed psychomotor performance following acute lorazepam administration [57c]. Another study observed 387 elderly patients admitted due to pure BZD poisoning. When compared to younger patients, elderly had significantly higher rates of coma, respiratory failure, and pneumonia [58C]. Another study by Maeda et al. detail the increased risks associated with triazolam use. This study documents 40% increased pneumonia risk, 30% risk of trauma, and 30% increased risk of pressure ulcer in regular triazolam users when compared to matched nonusers [59C].

Additionally, Scheifes et al. noted that of 103 adults with intellectual disability and challenging behavior had significant adverse event rates when exposed to psychotropic drugs including BZDs [60C].

Flumazenil

Flumazenil, a short acting benzodiazepine antagonist, is typically not recommend in BZD overdose situations due to concern for seizures and arrhythmias. An ED observational study of 23 patients found that 15% of patients had clinically significant mental status improvement and no patients experienced seizures with the use of flumazenil [61c]. However, a recently published meta-analysis confirms that routine use of flumazenil should be avoided due to the risk of serious AE. This meta-analysis found that serious AEs (convulsions and arrhythmia) were significantly increased in the flumazenil group when compared to placebo (3.81, 95% CI 1.28–11.39, $P=0.02$) [62C].

SYMPATHOMIMETICS: METHAMPHETAMINE

Methamphetamine has many associated negative consequences. Many chronic abusers exhibit significant symptoms related to mood and sleep disturbances. Three published studies have discussed advances in the mechanisms underlying neurotoxicity and new methamphetamine toxicities: pseudovasculitis and rhabdomyolysis [63r,64r,65C]. A case study of a young female demonstrates a strong case suggestive of vasculitis, however, further determined to be drug-induced pseudovasculitis [63r]. O'Connor et al. evaluated data to assess prevalence of rhabdomyolysis in sympathomimetic toxicity. Patients taking methamphetamine accounted for 40% of the cohort. Methamphetamine use was considered to be less risk for rhabdomyolysis when compared to cathinones [65C].

OPIOIDS: HEROIN

Heroin is a semisynthetic product produced by morphine acetylation that may be smoked, snorted, or injected. Like non-illicit opioids, heroin produces analgesia, along with drowsiness, euphoria, and a sense of detachment. Negative side effects include RD, N/V, and constipation. With repeated heroin use, tolerance and physical dependence occur, and users may develop abscesses, endocarditis, pneumonia, liver disease, or kidney impairment. In 2015 around 2% of people ≥12 YO in the U.S. reported heroin use during their lifetime [66S,67S].

Cardiovascular

Patients with Brugada phenocopy show a Brugada-like ECG pattern without true congenital Brugada syndrome. Rambod et al. present a 44-YOM with heroin use and Brugada phenocopy. His urine UDS was positive for opiates, and his serum alcohol level was 267 mg/dL. His initial ECG showed a Brugada type 1 pattern, with resolution on subsequent ECGs. ECG changes, mainly QTc prolongation and bradyarrhythmia, have previously been reported in patients who use heroin. The authors concluded that Brugada phenocopy may be another ECG abnormality associated with heroin use but acknowledged that it is difficult to attribute this case solely to heroin since the patient had also consumed alcohol [68A].

Respiratory

A 49-YOM presented with sudden-onset dyspnea and severe hypoxia. His respiratory rate (RR) was 32 breaths/minute, oxygen saturation (O_2 sat) on room air <80%. He had diffuse fine crackles on pulmonary auscultation, and chest CT revealed large ground-glass infiltration of the lungs associated with parenchymal reticulations and centrolobular emphysema. Bronchial aspiration lavage and blood cultures were negative. The patient reported tobacco use and sniffing heroin the previous day as well as seven months earlier. Within 48 hours the patient had clinically improved with only supportive care. A repeat CT scan 10 days later revealed resolution of the ground-glass infiltration but emphysema persisted, which was corroborated by pulmonary function studies. The authors diagnosed the patient with acute interstitial pneumonia related to heroin inhalation. They also noted that the patient's presentation was similar to interstitial pneumonia reports following intravenous heroin use [69A].

Nervous System

Bui et al. describe a 25-YO female with a two-year history of heroin inhalation and bipolar disorder who was found unconscious shortly after heroin use. Her Glasgow Coma Scale (GCS) score was 6, HR was elevated (109 beats/minute), and blood pressure (BP) was 168/44 mmHg. She had intact corneal, cough, and gag reflexes, bilateral Babinski signs, and both pupils measured 4 mm and were reactive. Brain imaging showed enlarged ventricles, communicating ventriculomegaly, and cerebellar enhancement, so an external ventricular drain was placed emergently. The patient then became responsive but developed a resting tremor and cogwheeling. After 13 days she received a ventriculoperitoneal shunt, and at discharge her GCS score was 15, but she was bedridden and required constant nursing attention. After three months she was significantly improved but had some residual deficits. The authors hypothesized that her refractory hydrocephalus with a communicating element was a complication of heroin inhalation [70A].

In response to the previously described case, Dastur et al. reported a 28-YOM who developed progressive parkinsonism > four weeks after heroin inhalation and eventual unresponsiveness. On exam, he had sluggish pupils, downward ocular deviation, and intermittent tonic spasms. Brain imaging revealed symmetric white matter lesions, ventriculomegaly with sulcal effacement, and tonsillar herniation. The fourth ventricle was obliterated by cerebellar swelling, so the patient underwent emergency ventriculostomy placement and dexamethasone was started. After initial improvement, the patient deteriorated seven days later, and his family requested comfort care. Two months later the patient died. The authors suggested that the delayed hydrocephalus following heroin inhalation in this case may be due to a prolonged blood–brain barrier permeability caused by heroin. They also questioned whether the heroin-use duration, recent abuse frequency, possible heroin impurity, and genetic factors played a role in the patient's presentation [71r].

Heroin use has also been associated with spongiform leukoencephalopathy. According to Pirompanich et al., most cases have occurred in patients who inhaled heroin. These authors report a less common spongiform leukoencephalopathy case associated with intravenous heroin injection. A 41-YOM was hospitalized and intubated four hours after intravenous heroin injection (unknown amount). Brain imaging showed diffuse brain swelling and electroencephalography (EEG) demonstrated a pattern consistent with toxic or metabolic encephalopathy. The patient was discharged after 12 days with only mild cognitive improvement, but five days later he exhibited increased confusion with no additional heroin use, and one week later he was readmitted to the hospital with confusion, akinetic mutism, spasticity, and hyperreflexia of all extremities. A lumbar puncture and most labs were within normal limits, but magnetic resonance imaging (MRI) results were abnormal. Based on the patient's clinical presentation and repeat imaging results, spongiform leukoencephalopathy was diagnosed. He was discharged from the hospital 19 days after admission with minimal improvement. When he followed up three months later, he had improvement in spasticity, could follow one-step commands, and showed improvement on imaging, but EEG still demonstrated severe diffuse encephalopathy. At a six-month follow-up appointment, his spasticity and dysarthria were both very mild, and EEG showed mild diffuse encephalopathy. The authors suggest four potential heroin-associated mechanisms of spongiform leukoencephalopathy: direct toxicity from heroin or additives, mitochondrial dysfunction, hypoxia, and genetic predisposition, such as cytochrome 450 2D6 gene polymorphism. All previously reported intravenous heroin-associated spongiform leukoencephalopathy cases have involved males aged 30–46. The disease onset occurred around three weeks after heroin use for most patients, and many experienced unconsciousness, akinetic mutism, and spastic quadriplegia. Of the reported case outcomes, only one patient died [72A].

Genetic Factors

As with alcohol, variations in the mu-opioid receptor gene *OPRM1* also influence response to heroin. A recent study found that a sample of Caucasian males with the 118G allele who were chronic, regular heroin users reported more negative consequences of heroin use, more failed quit attempts, and were more likely to seek treatment for heroin use compared to individuals with the 118AA variant [73c].

OPIOIDS: SYNTHETIC

In 2015, 20.5 million Americans ≥12 years had a substance use disorder. Of those, 2 million disorders involved prescription pain relievers, and 591000 involved heroin [74MC]. The leading cause for accidental death in the U.S. is drug overdose ($n = 52404$ [2015]). The main force driving this epidemic is opioid addiction, indicated by 20101 overdose deaths related to prescription pain relievers, and 12990 related to heroin in 2015 [75MC]. Nordic countries have seen similar patterns demonstrating fatal poisonings in drug addicts. Opioids were the main intoxicants (2012) for fatal poisonings in drug addicts represented by Denmark (87%), Norway (85%), Sweden (82%) and Finland (62%). Buprenorphine is the major intoxicant in Finland for opioid-related deaths, with cases increasing 19%–54% (2002−2012) and deaths in Sweden, with cases accounting for 14% (2012). Heroin/Morphine is the main intoxicant in Norway, accounting for the most (44%) fatal overdose cases. Oxycodone related death increased in all Nordic countries except Denmark and fentanyl poisonings nearly doubled in Finland and Sweden with other countries having either none or few cases. Only few tramadol- and oxycodone-positive cases were reported in Nordic countries overall, but tramadol-positive cases increased in Finland [75MC].

Multiple studies about intoxication have separated patients based upon identification for opioid misuse or abuse in patients with a valid and/or non-valid prescription [76C,77C,78c,79MC,80c,81MC,82R,83MC,84A].

Ries et al. compared demographics, clinical and survival characteristics for primary care patients using illicit drugs in the past 90-days and were further characterized by past 30-day use with no opioids ($n=472$) or any opioids ($n=396$) [76C]. Any opioid use further classified as non-prescribed ($n=228$) or as prescribed ($n=168$). As a group, opioid users (vs non-opioid users) were significantly less physically and psychiatrically healthy and were a larger burden to medical services. They were significantly more likely (2.61 times) to die one-to-five years after study enrollment, and die from accidental poisoning. Compared to appropriate opiate users, opiate misusers were more likely to have "serious drug problems" (IVDU, greater risk of HIV). Patients using non-prescribed opioids (vs prescribed) were significantly less likely to use marijuana, more likely to use alcohol, more likely to be homeless, and be admitted for chemical dependence treatment both before and after the study [76C].

Novel Illicit Drugs/Analogs

Novel illicit drugs and analogs are emerging worldwide, specifically new fentanyl analogs [85r]. To circumvent drug abuse legislation, new psychoactive substance (NPS) products claim to contain compounds that are legal to sell, possess, and use, often labeled as "not for human consumption." The European Union warning system operated by European Monitoring Centre for Drugs and Drug Addiction identified 236 NPS (May 2005–Dec. 2012) [85r].

Peterson et al. reported increased fentanyl deaths (2013–2015) from an investigation by University of Florida and Ohio Department of Health, in collaboration with the CDC [86MC]. Fentanyl deaths (2013–2014) increased in Florida (115%) and in Ohio (526%). In Florida (Jan.–Jun. 2015) fentanyl analogs use resulted in 49 fatal drug overdoses including acetyl fentanyl ($n=26$), butyryl-fentanyl ($n=5$), and beta-hydroxythiofentanyl ($n=18$). Toxicological panels could not distinguish illicit manufactured fentanyl (IMF) from pharmaceutical fentanyl (PF), but findings supported fentanyl death upsurge in Florida and Ohio (2013–2015) correlating closely to increased IMF supply, as opposed to diverted PF [86MC].

Illicit Substances: Nervous System

Vo et al. report poisoning overdoses related to ingestion of fentanyl-contaminated counterfeit Norco in three California Bay Area counties [87A]. Two patients admitted to ED for N/V, CNS and RD 30 min after ingesting (what appeared to be) Norco (hydrocodone/APAP) which was purchased a few days earlier. California poison control centers identified an additional five cases. All cases contained promethazine which has not previously been reported as an additive in adulterated fentanyl-containing products. Chronic opioid users have more recently been using promethazine to "potentiate the high" from opioids [88C].

1-Cyclohexyl-4-(1,2-diphenylethyl)piperazine (MT-45) is a synthetically substituted piperazine and a novel opioid-like psychoactive substance available over the Internet [89r]. MT-45 has availability via the internet originating from sources in China, Canada, Germany, India and Sweden. The effects from MT-45, desired and unwanted, are similar to other opioids. Reported withdrawal symptoms after use included restlessness, dehydration, "feeling hungover". MT-45 also has a desirably long half-life, up to 12 hours. Only one user stated the reason for co-using MT-45 with cannabis was "to accentuate the high from cannabis because MT-45 was not sufficient on its own." Two deaths in the U.S. (from acute intoxication) and twenty-one in Sweden resulted from MT-45 use, with eight reporting MT-45 as the primary cause [89r].

Respiratory

Rhode Island (RI) overdose deaths caused by illicit drugs increased (2011–2013), overtaking pharmaceutical overdose rates [90S] and fentanyl-related overdose deaths (2009–2015) by increasing 15-fold [91S]. Fentanyl has greater than 200 chemical derivatives and is 80–100 times more potent than morphine [92A,93E]. Furthermore, RI State Health Laboratory associated frequent opioid-related deaths (Mar.–May 2013) to acetyl fentanyl [94c]. Acetyl fentanyl (N-phenyl-N-[1-(2-phenylethyl)-4-piperidinyl]-acetamide, monohydrochloride) is four- to five-fold more potent than heroin, about threefold less potent than fentanyl and about 15-fold more potent than morphine [95A]. Acetyl fentanyl is considered an illicit synthetic opioid substance, not approved by the FDA nor commercially available. RI office of State Medical Examiners describe the first instance acetyl fentanyl was identified in the U.S. for drug overdose deaths. This research helped to develop an acetyl fentanyl chemical standard which is now commercially available through the national reference laboratory [95A]. A recently described acetyl fentanyl overdose death case was reported. A 24-YOM with past medical history (PMH) only significant for heroin abuse was declared dead at the scene. Upon completed autopsy, significant findings demonstrated three recent punctures in his forearm and the antecubital fossa. Lungs were edematous and congested. Earlier cases reported fentanyl fatalities which included additional drugs, whereas this is the first case reporting no other drugs detected [96A]. In a separate study, McIntyre et al. describe the first fatal overdose case containing acetyl- and butyr-fentanyl. Butyr-fentanyl (or butyr-fentanyl; desmethyl-fentanyl) [N-(1-phenylethyl)-4-piperidinyl)-N-phenylbutyramide] is about tenfold less potent than fentanyl, not currently scheduled in the U.S. and illegal in the United Kingdom (U.K.). The case describes a 44-YOM with PMH of heroin abuse. At the scene a syringe was found only containing butyr-fentanyl, but gastric contents contained substantial butyr-fentanyl levels (lesser extent acetyl fentanyl) describing intoxication from oral and intravenous routes. Remarkable findings for edematous and congested lungs were also described [96A].

Cole et al. describe the first butyr-fentanyl, non-fatal overdose, resulting in clinically significant hemoptysis, acute lung injury, hypoxic respiratory failure, and diffuse alveolar hemorrhage [96A]. A previously healthy 18-YOM with PMH of heroin abuse, snorted (what he believed to be) acetyl fentanyl purchased from the internet. He presented to the ED tachypnic, with blood in his nares, coughing up blood, increased work of breathing and coarse rales. Chest X-ray revealed bilateral "batwing"-shaped perihilar, predominant airspace opacities containing diffuse increased interstitial markings. The patient experienced pulmonary edema, acute lung injury and diffuse alveolar hemorrhage (rare for opioid overdose). UDS was positive for fentanyl and opiates but further analysis revealed fentanyl as a false-positive. High-performance gas chromatography and mass spectrometry (GC/MS) revealed butyr-fentanyl demonstrating cross-reactivity with the fentanyl immunoassay [97A]. Also concerning, was the incorrect product labeling shown from two cases where butyr-fentanyl was sold and labelled as such but contained about 10 times more potent fentanyl. Results from two butyr-fentanyl-labelled products (one white powder and one nasal spray) for two different patients demonstrated negative butyr-fentanyl and positive for fentanyl. Further analysis identified that fentanyl was the major active ingredient, accounting for the elevated potency [98A].

Additionally, for the first time, fentanyl analogs, 4-flurobutyrfentanyl (4F-butyrfentanyl) [98A] and 4-methoxybutyrfentanyl were described in overdose cases [99A]. Analysis for the 4F-butyrfentanyl nasal spray (test-purchase) showed no other NPS. Patient obtained the drug from the internet and reported consuming "one pill." Patient displayed similar symptoms to opioid overdose including disorientation, unsteadiness, slurred speech, hypotension (90/60 mmHg), miotic pupils [98A].

Nervous System: Fentanyl Analogs

Helander et al. describe 14 analytically confirmed fentanyl-analog cases (Apr.–Nov. 2015) involving two novel substances, 4-methoxybutyrfentanyl [4-MeO-butyrfentanyl] ($n=3$), furanylfentanyl ($n=1$), and 4-MeO-butyrfentanyl plus furanylfentanyl ($n=1$) [99A]. One furanylfentanyl (Nov. 2015) and zero 4-MeO-butyrfentanyl-related cases had been previously reported. The furanylfentanyl-positive patient brought a nasal spray in an unlabeled blue bottle that contained mainly furanylfentanyl and 5% 4-MeO-butyrfentanyl. Furanylfentanyl ($n=2$) and 4-MeO-butyrfentanyl ($n=4$)-positive patients displayed unconsciousness and RD, clinical similar to opioid overdose [99A]. ICU treatment (one-month duration) was necessary in one acetyl fentanyl case and in another acetyl fentanyl case, the patient died from cerebral hemorrhage [90A]. Increased novel, potent fentanyl-analog use with products obtained via the internet continues to result in deadly intoxications by causing life-threatening pulmonary toxicity, RD and sedation.

Nervous System: Drug–Drug Interactions

The first opioid cases resulting in serotonin syndrome without the co-administration of other serotonergic agents were recently described [100A,101A]. One case involved fentanyl [101A], and the other, fentanyl plus methadone [100A]. Seven YOM presented with frontal intracerebral hemorrhage, but before surgery was completed, patient experienced a tremor episode in his lower limbs [101A]. Four hours post-surgery patient had several shivering and tremor episodes. Mild fever was detected but infection was ruled out, and tremors progressed, associated with tachycardia. Brain CT revealed adequate hematoma evacuation. Midazolam and fentanyl doses were doubled and at 48-hour post-operative, patient experienced episodes of generalized hypertonia, tremors, fever, tachycardia, and arterial hypertension lasting three-to-four minutes. EEG was negative for epileptic discharges. Bilateral mydriasis was then observed identifying neurological deterioration. Generalized hypertonia, severe deep-tendon hyperreflexia and spontaneous-inducible clonus on legs were observed, accompanied by tachycardia and hypertension. CT scan was negative for intracranial abnormality. Fentanyl was immediately withdrawn and symptoms dramatically improved within one hour. These cases should raise awareness for clinicians when assessing patients taking one or multiple serotonergic narcotics with regards to precipitating serotonin syndrome [101A].

Reisner et al. report a two YO female who suffered accidental opioid overdose also resulting in CNS and cardio-pulmonary symptoms [84A]. She presented with AMS requiring cardiorespiratory support and required emergency posterior fossa decompression, partial cerebellectomy and CSF drainage due to cerebellar edema. This was the first report where surgical decompression was used to treat cerebellar edema associated with opioid overdose in a child. Neurosurgeons should know the clinical and neuroimaging findings for opioid-induced acute leukoencephalopathy because cerebellitis in children, leading to acute obstructive hydrocephalus needs prompt diagnosis and surgical interventions [84A].

Auditory

A reproducible acute subjective bilateral temporary hearing loss occurring after oxymorphone inhalation is described [102A]. This ADR was reported in one of 2011 patients receiving oxymorphone ER in phase II and III trials with mild outcomes and unknown causality. The patient crushed and snorted oxymorphone ER and presented with subjective bilateral temporary hearing loss. Hearing loss began to improve three hours after presenting to ED and completely resolved by the next day. He also reported a previous oxymorphone ER inhalation where he obtained similar hearing loss symptoms [102A]. Providers should be aware that opioids can be associated with hearing loss which is rare and could be underreported.

Endocrine

Recently new hypoglycemia cases have been associated with opioid use in adults [103C,104MC] and pediatrics [105A], specifically involving methadone and tramadol. An evaluation was completed for hypoglycemic incidence with inpatients receiving methadone compared to fentanyl, hydromorphone, and morphine. This is the first human study observing blood glucose changes for methadone compared to other opioids. Multivariable logistic regression showed significant associations between methadone and hypoglycemia (oral equivalent dose >40 mg/day or patient-controlled analgesia). When using doses >8 mg/day, a dose–response relationship was observed, but increased hypoglycemia risk was not evidenced for other opioids [102C].

Dermatologic

Doris et al. describe a fentanyl case where the transdermal patch was applied to eczematous skin [106A]. A 19-YOM with eczema history was found by paramedics. He was unresponsive with poor respiratory effort and a widespread erythematous rash. Paramedics observed constricted pupils and administered naloxone treatment. Patient's father disclosed that he gave his own fentanyl patches to alleviate patient's distressful eczema symptoms. The patient had removed the patch prior to collapsing but suffered life-threatening opioid toxicity through eczematous skin. This was the first opioid toxicity case with fentanyl patches resulting from a chronic skin condition where the natural skin barrier mechanism is impaired, increasing permeability and drug absorption [106A].

Cardiac

Loperamide abuse in large doses (50–300 mg) for euphoric effects and opioid withdrawal treatment is resulting in increased AEs including cardiotoxicity and CNS depression [107C,108A,109A,110A]. Eggleston et al. identified 22 loperamide abuse cases reported to New York poison control centers. Multiple cases reported opioid abuse ($n=15$), withdrawal symptoms after loperamide cessation ($n=15$), and ECG abnormalities including QTc-prolongation ($n=15$ [68%]), QRS-prolongation ($n=9$ [41%]) and ventricular dysrhythmia ($n=8$ [36%]). The average reported dose was 358 mg/day, and serum loperamide levels were 25–875 times the therapeutic range. The National Poison Database System identified 179 cases with irregular cardiac conduction ($n=24$ [13%]), ventricular tachycardia (VT) or fibrillation ($n=16$ [9%]), other dysrhythmias ($n=10$ [6%]), other ECG changes ($n=5$[3%]), and reported deaths ($n=4$) [107C].

Spinner et al. [108A] describe a loperamide misuse case in a previously healthy female with significant history for cholecystectomy, eight years earlier. Since then she self-treated chronic diarrhea with loperamide, increasing from 2 mg capsules to an entire bottle (144 mg/day for 20 years). Patient developed cardiac pauses, non-sustained VT, and eventually sustained VT with hemodynamic instability. She required cardiopulmonary resuscitation (CPR), multiple cardioversions, and pacemaker placement. Lasoff et al. report ventricular dysrhythmias from loperamide abuse [109C]. 24-YOM presented with generalized weakness and found in VT. He was taking loperamide 400 mg daily plus cimetidine (recommended from online forum to maximize effect). Similarly, the second ever case with intentional loperamide abuse for opioid effects was reported in a 19-YOM with known drug abuse history. Autopsy revealed distended bladder and bloody oral purge with non-toxic UDS levels for alprazolam, fluoxetine and marijuana. The cause of death was loperamide abuse [110A].

Opioid Use Treatment: Death/Toxicity

In Australia, investigation proved that polysubstance-use type, nature or amount could explain the increased non-fatal overdose risk among people with severe psychological distress who inject drugs ($n=2673$) [111MC]. Subutex, suboxone, and methadone were negatively associated with non-fatal overdose in those without psychological distress but not with psychological distress. The only profile associated with non-fatal overdose without psychological distress was polysubstance use with morphine and oxycodone. Furthermore, Jones et al. demonstrated significant positive correlation (2002–2006) between methadone distribution and overdose death rates ($r=0.89$) and methadone diversion ($r=0.95$) [112C].

Fatal and non-fatal incidences are increasing in children and adults with increased methadone use for detoxification [77C,78c,113A,114C]. A six YOM brought to the ED for suspected asthma exacerbation, presented unresponsive with diffusely diminished breath sounds bilaterally, wheezing, pinpoint pupils and UDS positive for methadone. Increased methadone utilization for opioid withdrawal treatment and chronic pain requires clinician awareness. Two cases report toddlers who drank their "father's drug" [80c]. In one case deliberate methadone administration to their child was suspected more than once. In four adolescent cases aged 16, 22, 29, and 38, methadone was consumed while partying, and they were found dead the next morning by casual acquaintances [80c].

Methadone-related poisonings have been increasing over the past few years in the U.S., Denmark and Italy [83C,86c,113A,114C,115A]. For adults, fatal methadone poisonings have been associated more so with patients enrolled in a methadone treatment program as opposed to obtaining methadone illegally without a prescription [115A,80c]. Additionally, patients with psychiatric disorders have increased risk for methadone related deaths compared to their counterparts [114C].

In addition to methadone, buprenorphine [81MC, 83MC,115A,116A,117A], used for substitution therapy, has also shown elevated risk for opioid-related deaths [83MC]. In England and Wales, poisoning with methadone or buprenorphine for use in opioid substitution therapy has been reported [81MC]. Drug-related mortality data was drawn for methadone and buprenorphine (2007–2012) which demonstrated 2366 methadone-related and 52 buprenorphine-related deaths corresponding to 17 333 163 methadone and 2 602 374 buprenorphine issued prescriptions. Patient deaths included those who consumed opioids legally and illegally (not prescribed). Pooled overdose death rates from methadone (0.137/1000 prescriptions) was compared to buprenorphine (0.22/1000 prescriptions) which generated a relative risk ratio (6.23; 95% CI 4.79–8.10) demonstrating that buprenorphine is sixfold safer than methadone among the general population [81MC].

Opioid Black Box Warnings (BBW)

The FDA issued a new BBW (Mar. 2016) mandating a class-wide for all immediate-release opioids warning, "serious risks of misuse abuse, addiction, overdose and death associated with these medications" and "they are only for patients with severe enough pain to justify opioids and for which other treatments were not sufficient or tolerated." The FDA clarified dosing (instructions, initial, and dose changes) warning [...] cessation in addicted patients. Th[...] additional safety labeling for all [...] "chronic maternal use of opioids [...] result in neonatal opioid withdr[...] may be life-threatening if not r[...] using protocols developed by [...] Additional labeling information [...] the endocrine system, including "a rare but serious disorder of the adrenal glands and decreased sex hormone levels" [118S]. Supplemental BBW issued by the FDA (8/31/16) indicates required labeling for patients taking opioids and benzodiazepines to include details that co-administration can be fatal [119C] (Table 1).

ELECTRONIC CIGARETTES

Electronic cigarettes (EC) are small battery-powered electronic devices, heating liquid to produce vapor and typically contain nicotine and flavors. ECs are highly advertised through the media, as "healthy substitutes" to conventional cigarettes (CC) to aid smoking cessation or circumventing smoking ban in public places [127MC]. The CDC and FDA analyzed data from National Youth Tobacco Surveys (NYTS) to determine prevalence and trends for current tobacco use among 6th–8th and 9th–12th graders (2011–2015). Among sixth–twelfth graders, ECs are the most used tobacco product (5.3%) and current tobacco-users preferred ECs (3 million) compared to other tobacco products. About 4.7 million (2015) sixth–twelfth graders are current tobacco users. Over 2.3 million use ≥ 2 tobacco products and among ninth-twelfth graders, ECs (16%) were the most common tobacco source. Current EC-use increased significantly for sixth–eighth but not ninth–twelfth graders. Current EC-use among sixth–twelfth significantly increased non-linearly (1.5–16%) [128MC]. Bunnell et al. analyzed data from NYTS (2011–2013) identifying youth intention to smoke. The quantity of ever-smoking youths who used ECs increased threefold, from 79 000 to >263 000. Intention to smoke conventional cigarettes varied between ever EC-users (43.9%) and never-users (21.5%). Ever EC-users exposure to pro-tobacco advertisement had higher reported odds for having smoking intentions compared to never-users [129MC].

Cho and Paik investigated the association between EC-use and asthma diagnosis (<12 months) for South Korean high-school students ($n=35 904$). Asthma prevalence was associated with "current EC" ($n=98$ [3.9%]), "former EC" ($n=46$ [2.2%]) "never EC" ($n=530$ [1.7%]), respectively. Overall, when compared to the reference population and adjusting for CC-use, EC-users had both increased association with asthma and higher absence likelihood due to severe asthmatic symptoms

TABLE 1 Opioid Pharmacogenetics [120C,121c,122C,123c,124R,125E,126A]

Objectives	Gene/Allele	Population	Clinical Affect	Practical Implications
1. To analyze opioid-positive UDS for patients with opioid dependence (methadone and buprenorphine). 2. To analyze five common haplotypes contained by MOR-1 in a ~13kb 3′ untranslated region on the OPRM1 gene [120C]	OPMR-1 rs10485058	European Americans ($n = 582$)	– In silico analysis: predicts miR-95-3p would interact with the G, but not the A allele for rs10485058 – Luciferase assays: miR-95-3p decreased reporter activity for constructs with G allele of rs10485058 but not A – Some methadone patients (A/A genotype at rs10485058) were less likely to have methadone-positive UDS compared to combined genotype-group A/G and G/G ($P = 0.0064$) – Note: Method was done by immunoassay testing and will vary based on the assigned laboratory cut-off – Rs10485058 predicted self-reported relapse rates for an independent Australian patient population with European descent [$n = 1215$]) receiving opioid substitution therapy ($P = 0.003$)	Medication treatment for opioid dependence could improve outcomes if selected based on rs10485058
To determine CYP2B6*6, influence and other allelic variants encountered, on methadone concentrations, clearance, and metabolism [121c]	CYP2B6*1/*1; $n = 21$ CYP2B6*1/*6; $n = 20$ CYP2B6*6/*6; $n = 17$ CYP2B6*1/*4; $n = 1$ CYP2B6*4/*6; $n = 3$ CYP2B6*5/*5; $n = 2$	Healthy volunteers in genotype cohorts	Oral dosing: – S-methadone apparent clearance in CYP2B6*1/*6 and CYP2B6*6/*6 subjects (1.6 ± 0.5 and 1.2 ± 0.6) was significantly less than in CYP2B6*1 homozygotes (2.3 ± 1.5) – R-methadone apparent oral clearance was significantly less in CYP2B6*6 than CYP2B6*1 homozygotes 1.6 ± 0.7 vs 2.4 ± 1.2, respectively – R- and S-methadone apparent oral clearance was three- and fourfold greater in CYP2B6*4 carriers IV dosing: – S-methadone systemic clearance in CYP2B6*1/*6 and CYP2B6*6/*6 was significantly less than in CYP2B6*1 homozygotes – Hepatic clearance (mL/kg/minute) was significantly less in CYP2B6*6/*6 compared with CYP2B6*1/*1 subjects for S-methadone (0.8 ± 0.4 and 1.3 ± 0.3) but not R-methadone (1.0 ± 0.3 and 1.3 ± 0.3) Both: – Intravenous and oral R- and S-methadone metabolism were significantly lower in CYP2B6*6 carriers compared with CYP2B6*1 homozygotes, and greater in CYP2B6*4 carriers – Methadone metabolism and clearance were lower in African-Americans due to the CYP2B6*6 genetic polymorphism	S-enantiomer accumulation is known to widen Qtc interval. CYP 2B6 accumulation is dependent on decreased S-enantiomer metabolism and elevated risk of ventricular tachycardia due to torsade de pointes. Individual patients can be identified by CYP2D6 genetics, to decrease risk for methadone toxicity and drug interactions based on metabolism and clearance

Objective	Gene/SNP	Participants	Findings	Clinical significance
To identify genetic determinants and characterize genetic mechanisms for the methadone (R- and S-enantiomers) plasma concentrations, in a genome-wide pharmacogenetics study [122C]	SNP: rs17180299 Genes: SPON1, GSG1L, and CYP450	– 360 Heroin-dependent patients undergoing MMT (>3 months). – Resided in Taiwan and were Han Chinese – >18 YO – Diagnosed with heroin dependence	– A significant single nucleotide polymorphism (SNP), rs17180299 (raw $P = 2.24*10-8$), was identified, accounting for 9.541% variation in the methadone R-enantiomer plasma concentration – Associated with methadone S-enantiomer plasma concentration, 17 haplotypes were identified on SPON1, GSG1L, and CYP450 genes – Haplotypes accounted for ~25% variation in overall S-methadone plasma concentration – The association between the S-methadone plasma concentration and CYP2B6, SPON1, and GSG1L were replicated in another independent study and gene expression experiment revealed that CYP2B6, SPON1, and GSG1L can be activated concomitantly through a constitutive and rostane receptor activation pathway	S-enantiomer accumulation is known to widen Qtc interval. CYP 2B6 accumulation is dependent on decreased metabolism of the S-enantiomer and elevated risk of ventricular tachycardia due to torsade de pointes. Results can be applied to patients on methadone maintenance therapy to predict treatment responses and methadone-related deaths
To evaluate the association between ABCC3 gene variants and respiratory depression (RD) [123c]	ATP binding cassette gene ABCC3 Allele A at rs4148412 and allele G at rs729923	Children ($n=316$) and adolescents ($n=67$) with post-operative RD	Hepatic morphine efflux and morphine metabolite clearance significantly increasing prolonged RD	– 3-glucuronide metabolite accumulation increases neurotoxicity risk – 6-glucurine metabolite accumulation causes increased opioid agonist effects such as analgesia, euphoria, diminished GI motility, and RD
1. To quantify hydrocodone (HC) and hydromorphone (HM) metabolite pharmacokinetics (PK) with pharmacogenetics (PGen) phenotypes in CYP2D6: – Ultra-rapid metabolizer (UM) – Extensive metabolizer (EM) – Poor metabolizer (PM) 2. To develop an HC phenotype-specific dosing strategy for HC that accounts for HM production using clinical PK integrated with PGen for patient safety [124R]	2D6 polymorphism	Healthy white men and women without comorbidities or history of opioid use, or any other drug use or nutraceutical use, age 26.3 ± 5.7 years (range, 19–36 years) and weight 71.9 ± 16.8 kg (range, 50–108 kg) Participants: 5 CYP2D6 EM and 6 CYP2D6 PM phenotypes	– Clearance was reduced by nearly 60% and the T½ was increased by about 68% compared with EMs – HC elimination reduced by 70% in PM – HC clearance was UM>EM>PM – HC's apparent volume of distribution was not significantly different among UMs, EMs, and PM – For the CYP2D6 phenotypes, the mean predicted HM levels were within HM's therapeutic range, indicating HC has significant phenotype-dependent pro-drug effects	Ultra-rapidly CYP2D6 metabolizers will rapidly convert hydrocodone to hydromorphone, the latter of which is more potent. This can lead to an elevated risk for opioid overdose

Continued

TABLE 1 Opioid Pharmacogenetics [120C,121c,122C,123c,124R,125E,126A]—cont'd

Objectives	Gene/Allele	Population	Clinical Affect	Practical Implications
To detect allelic variants described as non-functional to explain some circumstances of death post-mortem tramadol cases [125E]	2D6 polymorphism	Both methodologies were successfully applied to 100 post-mortem blood samples and evaluated the relation between toxicological and genetic results	The developed methodology is important to enhance genetic tool application to forensic toxicology and pathology. A Sanger sequencing methodology was developed detecting genetic variants causing absent or reduced CYP2D6 activity (alleles: *3,*4,*6,*8,*10 and *12) This methodology and GC/MS for detecting and quantifying tramadol and its main metabolites in blood samples was fully validated according to international guidelines	Ultra-rapid CYP2D6 metabolizers will rapidly convert Tramadol to O-desmethyl tramadol, the latter of which has more potent opioid agonist properties and higher bonding affinity to the mu receptor. This can lead to an elevated risk for opioid overdose
To assess whether post-mortem methadone findings in breastfed infants are clinically and/or toxicologically significant [126A]	CYP2B6*6 Haplotype Single nucleotide polymorphism ABCB1 gene	Two cases of deceased breast-fed infants of mothers on methadone maintenance programs	Case 1: The infant was found to be homozygous for the CYP2B6*6 haplotype, associated with methadone-related adult mortality due to impaired ability to metabolize methadone. This infant was also heterozygous for SNPs in the ABCB1 gene associated with partially impaired efflux activity Case 2: This infant was also heterozygous for the three SNPs in ABCB1 associated with decreased P-glycoprotein (pGP) activity. This efflux transporter is expressed in the blood–brain barrier (BBB) luminal membrane and when impaired it is associated with increased methadone amount reaching the brain	pGP is responsible for pulling methadone back into the gut and diminishing oral methadone absorption. Similarly, pGP controls the amount of methadone that passes through the BBB. If pGP activity is reduced, more methadone is absorbed orally and more passes into the CNS resulting in toxicity

[130MC]. In Mexico where ECs are banned, middle-school students ($n = 10\,146$) were assessed regarding their EC-use. EC-triers were compared to students who tried CC-only, EC plus CC, and neither type (never-triers) [131MC]. More students (51%) had heard about ECs and believed (19%) they were less harmful than CCs but less (10%) had actually tried ECs. Exclusive EC-triers (4%) had significantly higher technophilia (media use), and internet tobacco advertising exposure compared to CC-triers (19%) and never-triers (71%), but not compared to dual-triers (6%). Similar trends were reported in New Zealand, amongst 14–15 YO "EC-triers" demonstrating tripled prevalence from (7% [2012]–20% [2014]) [132MC]. Recent prevalence estimates for EC trials particularly were elevated European youths 12–19 YO including Finnish (17%) (2013) [133MC], North West England (2013) (19%) [134MC], Polish (2010 – 2011) (24%) [135MC], Irish (2014) [136C] and 19-24 YO Romanians (25%) (2013) [137C,138C]. Additionally, Polish University students, medical ($n = 545$) and non-medical ($n = 523$) were polled. More non-medical University students (195 [31.46%]) were EC-ever-users compared to medical (141 [25.87%]) students. Some respondents viewed ECs as safer ($n = 456$ [42.70%]) than CCs but most ($n = 912$ [85.39%]) viewed ECs as generally unhealthy [127MC].

EC-use is becoming more popular among adolescents [128MC,131MC,132MC,134MC,135MC,136C,137C], which has been driven by electronic media advertising resulting in changed intentions [138C] and perceptions [127MC] associated with EC-use. Leventhal et al. sought to gain insight about psychiatric comorbidities associated with adolescent EC-use and dual-use (EC plus CC). Researchers identified ninth-graders in Los Angeles with a self-report, measuring CC- or EC-use, emotional disorders, substance use, and transdiagnostic psychiatric phenotypes consistent with the NIMH-Research Domain Criteria Initiative. Students identified use as non-users ($n = 2557$ [77.3%]), EC-only ($n = 412$ [12.4%]), CC-only ($n = 152$ [4.6%]), or EC plus CC ($n = 189$ [5.6%]). EC-only use was significantly more common than CC-only (4.6%) and dual (5.7%), but dual-use was significantly more common than CC-use only. Adolescents using CC-only reported lower internalizing syndromes (depression, generalized anxiety, panic, social phobia, and obsessive–compulsive disorder) and transdiagnostic phenotypes (i.e., distress intolerance, anxiety sensitivity, rash action during negative affect) compared to EC-users only. For EC-users only, depression, panic disorder, and anhedonia were more prominent than non-users. A pattern was recognized for externalizing outcomes (mania, rash action during positive affect, alcohol drug use/abuse) and anhedonia, indicating lowest comorbidity amongst non-users, moderate in single-product-users and highest in dual-users [138C].

Conversely, from a survey completed by 146 million working U.S. adults, about 5.5 million (3.8%) were current EC-users which was significantly associated with a higher prevalence among males (4.5%), non-Hispanic whites (4.5%), and ages 18–24 years (5.1%), annual family income <$35\,000$ (5.1%), no health insurance (5.9%), residing in the Midwest region (4.5%), and fair or poor health (5.7%). EC-use was also significantly higher among current CC-users (16.2%) and non-combustible tobacco use [139MC]. A New South Wales survey (2014) identified current EC-user prevalence (1.3%) and EC-ever-triers (8.4%). The authors estimated about 78\,000 people were current EC-users in NSW which was considered relatively low compared with other countries (U.S. and U.K.) [140MC].

Rogers et al. report a case where a 36-YOM used propylene glycol (PG) EC, filled with acetyl fentanyl for additional relaxation. He purchased "what he called 'synthetic opium'" online, which he used to fill the EC and inhale vapors. Since the product was purchased online, it seemed 'legal' to the patient. He started using ECs more frequently while on medical leave for a planned patent foramen ovale closure, discovered three months prior when admitted for a TIA. Family found the patient with AMS and activated 9-1-1. Patient presented aroused by painful stimuli, with RD, pinpoint pupils, hypoxemia (O_2 sat: 85%), and GCS = 6. His mental and respiratory status improved when receiving intravenous naloxone. Afterward, patient also admitted to adding "synthetic opium" to alcoholic beverages [141A].

Chen et al. describe a case with intentionally ingested e-liquid nicotine (up to 3000 mg) in a 24-year-old-female (YOF). She was found with a suicide note, partially ingested whiskey bottle and two empty 15-mL nicotine vials (100 mg/mL). She had pulseless electrical activity, which returned to spontaneous circulation after undergoing CPR for 10 minutes (BP:74/53 mmHg HR:106 beats/minute, RR:14 breaths/minute via mechanical ventilation). The PE reported pupils fixed and dilated 5 mm, pale and clammy skin, urine and stool incontinence, without wheezes or rales. Shortly after, patient presented with myoclonic jerks in her neck progressing to whole body myoclonus. ECG demonstrated sinus tachycardia, QRS 96 ms, QTC 483 ms and UDS was notable for plasma nicotine and cotinine levels each >1000 ng/mL. GC/MS revealed nicotine, cotinine and patient home medications (trazodone, fluoxetine, and olanzapine). Patient continued having uncontrollable limb myoclonus, despite intravenous lorazepam (6 mg), phenytoin (1800 mg) and levetiracetam (1000 mg). Results from the MRI indicated multiple acute infarcts, consistent with severe anoxic brain injury. Due to her poor prognosis, she was transitioned to comfort care and died three days post-ingestion [142A].

EC ingestion can be deadly and has also been seen with unintentional toxicity especially in young children. Center for Tobacco Products voluntary reports exposures and included four child-related reports with one infant death caused from choking on an EC-cartridge, one due to burns following EC explosion, and two due to passive exposures including breathing problems, and "raspy voice" after passive aerosol exposure [143c]. Similarly, Texas poison control network (TPCN) (Jan. 2009–Feb. 2014) evaluated EC exposures reported with cases more than doubling each year (2009–2014). The majority ($n=119/225$ [53%]) occurred among individuals aged <5 YO and >20 YO (93/225 [41%]). The most common exposure route was ingestion (78%), but other routes include inhalation, dermal, ocular, and multiple routes. The majority were unintentional and mild or moderate. Clinically related AEs most reported (>5%) were vomiting (20%), nausea, headache, ocular irritation, dizziness. During the same period 2888 tobacco/nicotine product exposure was reported to TPCN, and ECs (7%) were responsible for a minimal product exposures [144C]. TPCN separately analyzed children (Jan. 2010–Jun. 2014) and reported increasing EC toxic exposures ($n=203$) for ages zero–five. Most exposures were children ages one (32%) and two (42%) and exposed via ingestion (93%). Most common clinical AEs were GI-related (vomiting (24%) and less common AEs were neurologic (drowsiness/lethargy), and respiratory (cough/choke). Serious exposures (11%) included cardiovascular (HTN, tachycardia) and respiratory (cyanosis, hyperventilation/tachypnea, respiratory arrest) [145C]. EC exposure continues to increase with use but the exposed majority are young children through ingestion and often non-serious outcomes.

Although EC toxicity continues to rise [143c,144C, 145C], ECs are perceived as lower risk compared to CCs [127MC,146MC,147c]. Tan et al. examined associations between self-reported EC exposure to advertising, media coverage, interpersonal discussion and second hand vapor (SHV) and perceived harms ($n=1449$). This is the first study investigating public perceptions about SHV harms in a national sample (U.S. adults) associated with information exposure. Results demonstrated significantly less perceived health risk with SHV and lower comparative harm between SHV and second hand smoke (SHS). Negative ad exposure perceptions and interpersonal discussion were significantly associated with higher perceived harm to their health for SHV and SHS. While negative media coverage perception was significantly associated with higher concern about breathing SHV and health impact, positive perception resulted from interpersonal discussion [146MC]. Practical observations have been identified by providers, patients and community members about EC perceptions [147c]. Providers identified that EC-use was most commonly seen among daily smokers rather than occasional or light smokers. One smokeless tobacco-user likened EC-use to smokeless tobacco pre-packaged in single serving pouches. EC-users also identify lower cost, flavor variety and long-lasting nature as benefits to EC-compared to CC-products. Providers and community

leaders voice concern about tobacco screening practices within primary care settings which fail to detect or address ECs with screening questions. One EC-user commented, "They're like, 'Well, you know, I only smoke 3 cigarettes a day', and I asked them, 'Well, do you smoke any e-cigarettes?' 'Yeah, but that's not a cigarette'" [147c].

Although perceptions about ECs, active and passive exposures are more collectively positive, toxicity and AE continue. The U.S. FDA, Center for Tobacco Products (CTP) reviewed voluntary reports from consumers, healthcare professionals and public members about tobacco-associated AEs from passive exposure (1/2012–12/2014). Reports involved non-users (40/136) with 35 related to passive aerosol exposure. The most common symptoms reported were respiratory ($n=26$) including asthma exacerbations, bronchitis, cough, difficulty breathing and pneumonia. Additional symptoms included eye irritation ($n=8$), headache ($n=8$), nausea ($n=6$), sore throat/irritation ($n=6$), dizziness ($n=5$), and racing/irregular HR ($n=5$). Reports ($n=11$) were associated with recurrent, repeated exposure, AE ($n=6$) in multiple individuals, seeking medical attention ($n=6$). Reports with pre-existing conditions ($n=27$) included respiratory or allergic ($n=11$), while others included burns ($n=3$) and lip cheilitis ($n=1$). Although AEs are only reported in small numbers here, reporting is voluntary and is therefore most likely underestimated [143c]. Multiple studies [148E,149c] have identified harmful chemicals released in the vapor from ECs including volatile organic compounds, PG, formaldehyde, acetaldehyde, glycerol, and carbonyls. Even though the levels are detectable, all have been within indoor air quality guideline limits.

Multiple studies have compared ECs to CCs and have demonstrated similarities among the comparisons. There has been some discrepancies as to whether ECs should be used for smoking cessation. In a Cochrane review of 24 completed studies, investigators found higher abstinence rates (9%) from using ECs after six months compared to placebo (4%) in 662 participants [150M]. They also found one study comparing ECs to nicotine patches which did not show a significant difference in abstinence rates (584 participants). Authors concluded that although the evidence seems positive, the review lacks many large RCTs accounting for low grade evidence. Conversely Kalkhoran et al. reviewed 20 studies evaluating differences between EC- and CC-smoking cessation irrespective to motivation for use. Researchers found that the odds for cigarette cessation was 28% lower for ECs compared to CCs and recommended that ECs should not be used for smoking cessation aids until evidence can support their use [150R,151R].

A positive AE profile has been associated with EC-use [143c,145C], specifically Hartmann-Boyce et al. did not identify any studies with reported serious AE related to EC-use in their review. The most reported AEs were mouth and throat irritation, resolving with time. One RCT provided data on the participant proportion experiencing any AEs which was similar throughout the study arms comparing ECs vs placebo (298 participants) and ECs vs patch (456 participants). Additionally, Cravo et al. sought to evaluate the safety profile when switching from CCs to ECs (nicotine = 2%) for 12 weeks in a randomized, parallel group clinical study. They demonstrated a positive AE profile for EC-use. No clinically significant product-related findings were observed during the study in terms of VSs, ECG, lung function tests and standard clinical laboratory parameters. The commonly reported AEs ($n = 495/1515$) were identified as being related to nicotine withdrawal symptoms including headache (47.4%), sore throat, desire to smoke, cough, increased appetite, nasopharyngitis and irritability reported by subjects but only a minimal amount (6%) were identified to probably or definitely be related to ECs. Laboratory markers were decreased for EC subjects including nicotine in urine and three toxicant biomarkers known to be present in CCs including benzene, acrolein and 4-[methylnitrosamino]-1-[3-pyridyl]-1-butanone [152MC]. Additionally, Walele et al. evaluated EC safety by comparing ECs (nicotine concentration 0%, 0.4%, 0.9%, 2%) to CCs (0.6 mg) and a licensed nicotine inhalator (Nicorette®, 15 mg) in 12 participants [153c]. Only mild and moderate AEs were reported, and there were no differences between groups. CC-users showed increased exhaled CO levels, similar to other studies [155c]. All products similarly decreased smoking urges and nicotine withdrawal symptoms. Furthermore, Yan designed a clinical study to characterize EC-users' exposure to nicotine and acute effect on blood pressure and HR compared to CCs [154c]. Five different ECs and one CC (Marlboro) were randomized in 23 participants for 10 days. HR, SBP and diastolic BP (DBP) were significantly elevated in CC- vs EC-users. EC-use had no impact on exhaled CO levels vs CCs (CO exhalation >eight times baseline). All products significantly increased HR and DBP compared to baseline but CCs demonstrated a most significant HR increase and ECs (Menthol (2.4% Nic, Gly) had significantly lower DBP increase than CCs. A significant correlation resulted from the data trend between nicotine plasma levels and increased HR [154c]. Another advantage to switching from CCs to ECs was described for the first time evaluating long-term body weight changes for CC-users [155C]. Participants were invited to quit or reduce smoking by switching to ECs in a prospective, randomized controlled trial, measuring CC consumption and body weight in Italy (Jun. 2010–Feb. 2011). Significant differences were seen among continuous smoking phenotypes, for quitters at week-12 and -24, gaining 2.4 (±4.3Kg) and 2.9 (±4.4Kg), respectively but at 52-weeks weight gain was not significant 1.5 (±5kg) compared to failures and reducers. Failure

to reduce or quit smoking demonstrated significantly decreased to weight gain compared to successfully quitting at week-12 and -24 [155C]. Overall, EC-use showed some positive benefits for CC abstinence and AE profile, including reported mild AE and protective mechanism to weight gain, but when motivation for EC-users is taken into account, the results show decreased abstinence rates in EC-users compared to CC-users. The evidence is mixed and more large controlled trials should be conducted before determining the place for ECs in smoking cessation therapy.

EC-use compared to CC-use continues to demonstrate a more favorable safety profile. Hecht et al. evaluated 28 EC smokers who had not smoked CCs for at least two months but were using ECs to compare toxicants and carcinogenic metabolites [156c]. Results demonstrated significantly lower 1-HOP, total NNAL, 3-HPMA, 2-HPMA, HMPMA, and SPMA in urine for EC- compared to CC-user [156c]. Conversely, Kosmider et al. demonstrated much greater carcinogenic concentration with formaldehyde and acetaldehyde when high voltage devices were used, although still lower concentration than CCs [157E]. Inhaling these carcinogens increases the risk for oral and lung cancer and in preclinical experimental models. EC vapor was also associated with increased inflammation, oxidative stress, and disruption of endothelial barrier function [157E].

Two products have been developed to decrease the health risks associated with ECs and both studies evaluated the same primary outcomes to compare biomarkers between groups compared to non-smoker levels [158E,159C]. Shepperd et al. investigated whether exposure to reduced-toxicant-prototype cigarette (RTP), could reduce harmful exposure to smoke constituents. They evaluated changes in Biomarkers of Exposure (BoE), Effective Dose (BoED) and Biological Effect (BoBE) in Hamburg, Germany. Participants were switched to either control (same cigarette) or RTP [159C]. Authors demonstrated increased BoE for controls over the study period, but most BoE and all BoED significantly decreased for RTP smokers. BoBE was similar across groups but also very variable within individuals [159C]. Similarly, Haziza et al. developed a Tobacco Heating System (THS) 2.2, Modified Risk Tobacco Product, designed to heat tobacco without burning it. The study design was a five-day exposure, controlled, parallel-group, open-label clinical study with 160 healthy subjects who smoked, randomized into three groups. BoBE was similar across groups and/or too variable within individuals to detect any changes. Authors demonstrated significantly reduced biomarkers in the THS group, compared to the CC-group and approached smoking abstinence. THS was well tolerated and had increased consumption and total puff volume but had nicotine exposure similar to CCs. Relative to CCs on day five, the THS group had significantly reduced biomarkers for COHb (77%), 3-HPMA (58%), MHBMA (92%), and S-PMA (94%). Furthermore, reductions were seen in total NNAL (56%), Total NNN (76%), Total 1-OHP (56%), 4-ABP (85%), 1-NA (96%), 2-NA (88%), o-toluidine (58%), CEMA (87%), HEMA (68%), 3-HMPMA (77%), and total-3-OHeB[a]P (72%) for the THS- relative to the CC-group [160C].

Studies have demonstrated that EC sales lack appropriate drug content and safety labeling which could cause some toxicities and AEs. Morris et al. assessed U.S. internet EC retailers (Jun. 2013) to identify consumer protection to accidental poisonings. From 21 retailers, the most common e-liquid volumes were 10- and 30-mL (36 mg/mL), but four sites sold ≥500-mL bottles. Multiple concentrations were offered ranging from 0% to 3.6% nicotine (36 mg/mL) but two sites sold 75 mg/mL concentrated, and one offered 100 mg/mL. Warnings for nicotine were found on 13 sites (59%) but only six (29%) were posted on the homepage and seven (33%) were available in downloadable versions or frequently asked questions. Conversely, no sites included poisoning hazards to children or pets on their home page, only three sites (14%) stated all bottles had child-resistant caps, and one offered optional child-resistant packaging [161c]. Similarly, Buettner-Schmidt found some (35%) child-resistant containers from 94 sampled containers [162E] and Salt Lake County (SLCo) found e-liquids (28%) lacked child-resistant containers [162E]. Furthermore, not only do concentrations vary between retailers, but also the nicotine concentration labeling has variable accuracy. Buettner-Schmidt et al. sought to determine labeling accuracy observed at 16 unlicensed vape stores selling ECs in North Dakota. Seventy e-liquid samples were collected claiming to contain nicotine content, demonstrating e-liquid quantity variation (by ≥10%) less than labelled (34%) and one sample contained >172% labeled quantity. In samples ($n = 23$) claiming 0 mg/mL, 10 (43%) contained nicotine. Four stores also provided opportunity to add more nicotine to e-liquids [162E]. Equivalently, SLCo Health Department (2014) in Utah demonstrated multiple discrepancies (≥10%) to advertised nicotine content in e-liquids; 61% e-liquids (not listing zero concentration), ranging from <88% to >840% advertised. Additionally, 28% listed nicotine concentration on containers without child-resistant caps [163E].

On a larger scale, Goniewicz et al. sought to compare differences in e-liquid discrepancies for ECs worldwide by measuring e-liquid concentrations (2013–2014) in the U.S. ($n = 32$), South Korea ($n = 29$), Poland ($n = 30$), respectively [164E]. Overall the labelled nicotine concentration in these countries significantly varied (19%) among discrepancies (>20%) compared to their labelled nicotine concentrations. The U.S. e-liquid nicotine concentrations varied (±20%; range 0–36.6 mg/mL) from labelled content (28%) and nicotine traces were found in three "nicotine-free" labelled containers [164E]. Multiple discrepancies were found for South Korean products, including non-detectable nicotine levels ($n = 19$ [66%]) but other products varied from 6.4 ± 0.7 to 150.3 ± 7.9 mg/mL (labelled as "pure nicotine"). Five (28%) demonstrated >20% difference in content compared to the label [164E]. In Poland, nicotine concentrations varied from 0 (five cases) to 24.7 ± 0.1 mg/mL but only three (10%) demonstrated significant discrepancies (>20%) for labelled nicotine concentrations compared to analyzed e-liquids. Nicotine was not detected in any products labeled "nicotine-free" and only three products (10%) showed differences between labelled and detected nicotine concentrations >20% [164E]. Despite Poland demonstrating the most accurate analyzed e-liquids, the European Commission implemented (May 2016) new regulations taking effect after the above study. Of the 10 key changes for tobacco product sales in the European Union, three were specific to EC products including safety and quality requirements, packaging and labelling rules, monitoring and required reporting related to ECs every five years [165S].

CONCLUSION

Drug misuse and abuse has become a worldwide epidemic. One factor that has eliminated boundaries and thus attributed to drug availability is increased access via the internet for any age, race, sex, economic class, or education level. Increased awareness and novel science including pharmacogenomics, allows for enhanced and individualized treatment to progress, benefiting the patients and potentially decreasing AE, drug–drug interactions, toxicities and mortality resulting from this growing epidemic.

References

[1] United Nations Office on Drugs and Crime, World Drug Report 2016 (United Nations publication, Sales No. E.16.XI.7) [S]..
[2] Cooper ZD. Adverse effects of synthetic cannabinoids: management of acute toxicity and withdrawal. Curr Psychiatry Rep. 2016;18(5):52 [r].
[3] Riederer AM, Campleman SL, Carlson RG, et al. Acute poisonings from synthetic cannabinoids—50 U.S. toxicology investigators consortium registry sites, 2010–2015. MMWR Morb Mortal Wkly Rep. 2016;65(27):692–5 [S].
[4] Schwartz MD, Trecki J, Edison LA, et al. A common source outbreak of severe delirium associated with exposure to the novel synthetic cannabinoid ADB-PINACA. J Emerg Med. 2015;48(5):573–80 [c,A].
[5] Law R, Schier J, Martin C, et al. Notes from the field: increase in reported adverse health effects related to synthetic cannabinoid use—United States, January–May 2015. MMWR Morb Mortal Wkly Rep. 2015;64(22):618–9 [c].

[6] McIlroy G, Ford L, Khan JM. Acute myocardial infarction, associated with the use of a synthetic adamantyl-cannabinoid: a case report. BMC Pharmacol Toxicol. 2016;17:2 [A].

[7] McKeever RG, Vearrier D, Jacobs D, et al. K2—not the spice of life; synthetic cannabinoids and ST elevation myocardial infarction: a case report. J Med Toxicol. 2015;11(1):129–31 [A].

[8] Berkowitz EA, Henry TS, Veeraraghavan S, et al. Pulmonary effects of synthetic marijuana: chest radiography and CT findings. AJR Am J Roentgenol. 2015;204(4):750–7 [c].

[9] Chinnadurai T, Shrestha S, Ayinla R. A curious case of inhalation fever caused by synthetic cannabinoid. Am J Case Rep. 2016;17:379–83 [A].

[10] Tyndall JA, Gerona R, De Portu G, et al. An outbreak of acute delirium from exposure to the synthetic cannabinoid AB-CHMINACA. Clin Toxicol (Phila). 2015;53(10):950–6 [c].

[11] Schep LJ, Slaughter RJ, Hudson S, et al. Delayed seizure-like activity following analytically confirmed use of previously unreported synthetic cannabinoid analogues. Hum Exp Toxicol. 2015;34(5):557–60 [A].

[12] Gudsoorkar VS, Perez Jr. JA. A new differential diagnosis: synthetic cannabinoids-associated acute renal failure. Methodist Debakey Cardiovasc J. 2015;11(3):189–91 [A].

[13] Sweeney B, Talebi S, Toro D, et al. Hyperthermia and severe rhabdomyolysis from synthetic cannabinoids. Am J Emerg Med. 2016;34(1):121. e1-2 [A].

[14] Labay LM, Caruso JL, Gilson TP, et al. Synthetic cannabinoid drug use as a cause or contributory cause of death. Forensic Sci Int. 2016;260:31–9 [c].

[15] Adamowicz P. Fatal intoxication with synthetic cannabinoid MDMB-CHMICA. Forensic Sci Int. 2016;261:e5–10 [A].

[16] Westin AA, Frost J, Brede WR, et al. Sudden cardiac death following use of the synthetic cannabinoid MDMB-CHMICA. J Anal Toxicol. 2016;40(1):86–7 [A].

[17] Angerer V, Franz F, Schwarze B, et al. Reply to 'Sudden cardiac death following use of the synthetic cannabinoid MDMB-CHMICA. J Anal Toxicol. 2016;40(3):240–2 [r].

[18] Shanks K, Behonick G. Death after use of the synthetic cannabinoid 5F-AMB. Forensic Sci Int. 2016;262:e21–4 [A].

[19] Koller VJ, Ferk F, Al-Serori H, et al. Genotoxic properties of representatives of alkylindazoles and aminoalkyl-indoles which are consumed as synthetic cannabinoids. Food Chem Toxicol. 2015;80:130–6 [E].

[20] Besli GE, Ikiz MA, Yildirim S, et al. Synthetic cannabinoid abuse in adolescents: a case series. J Emerg Med. 2015;49(5):644–50 [c].

[21] Thornton SL, Akpunonu P, Glauner K, et al. Unintentional pediatric exposure to a synthetic cannabinoid (AB-PINACA) resulting in coma and intubation. Ann Emerg Med. 2015;66(3):343–4 [A].

[22] Devinsky O, Marsh E, Friedman D, et al. Cannabidiol in patients with treatment-resistant epilepsy: an open-label interventional trial. Lancet Neurol. 2016;15(3):270–8 [C].

[23] Ball S, Vickery J, Hobart J, et al. The cannabinoid use in progressive inflammatory brain disease (CUPID) trial: a randomised double-blind placebo-controlled parallel-group multicentre trial and economic evaluation of cannabinoids to slow progression in multiple sclerosis. Health Technol Assess. 2015;19(12):1–187. vii-viii, xxv-xxxi. [C].

[24] Kleine-Brueggeney M, Greif R, Brenneisen R, et al. Intravenous delta-9-tetrahydrocannabinol to prevent postoperative nausea and vomiting: a randomized controlled trial. Anesth Analg. 2015;121(5):1157–64 [c].

[25] Smith LA, Azariah F, Lavender VT, et al. Cannabinoids for nausea and vomiting in adults with cancer receiving chemotherapy. Cochrane Database Syst Rev. 2015;11:CD009464 [M].

[26] van den Elsen GA, Ahmed AI, Verkes RJ, et al. Tetrahydrocannabinol for neuropsychiatric symptoms in dementia: a randomized controlled trial. Neurology. 2015;84(22):2338–46 [c].

[27] Trojano M, Vila C. Effectiveness and tolerability of THC/CBD oromucosal spray for multiple sclerosis spasticity in Italy: first data from a large observational study. Eur Neurol. 2015;74(3–4):178–85 [C].

[28] Azofeifa A, Mattson ME, Schauer G, et al. National estimates of marijuana use and related indicators—national survey on drug use and health, United States, 2002–2014. MMWR Surveill Summ. 2016;65(11):1–28 [MC].

[29] Hancock-Allen JB, Barker L, VanDyke M, et al. Notes from the field: death following ingestion of an edible marijuana product—Colorado, March 2014. MMWR Morb Mortal Wkly Rep. 2015;64(28):771–2 [A].

[30] Pierre JM, Gandal M, Son M. Cannabis-induced psychosis associated with high potency "wax dabs" Schizophr Res. 2016;172(1–3):211–2 [A].

[31] Hall W. What has research over the past two decades revealed about the adverse health effects of recreational cannabis use? Addiction. 2015;110(1):19–35 [r].

[32] Cipriani F, Mancino A, Pulitano SM, et al. A cannabinoid-intoxicated child treated with dexmedetomidine: a case report. J Med Case Reports. 2015;9:152 [A].

[33] Haney M, Ramesh D, Glass A, et al. Naltrexone maintenance decreases cannabis self-administration and subjective effects in daily cannabis smokers. Neuropsychopharmacology. 2015;40(11):2489–98 [c].

[34] World Health Organization. Global status report on alcohol and health 2014. Geneva: WHO Press; 2014 [S].

[35] Claus ED, Hendershot CS. Moderating effect of working memory capacity on acute alcohol effects on BOLD response during inhibition and error monitoring in male heavy drinkers. Psychopharmacology (Berl). 2015;232(4):765–76 [c].

[36] Brasil A, Castro AJ, Martins IC, et al. Colour vision impairment in young alcohol consumers. PLoS One. 2015;10(10)e0140169 [c].

[37] Pal L, Arnyas EM, Bujdoso O, et al. Aliphatic alcohols in spirits inhibit phagocytosis by human monocytes. Immunopharmacol Immunotoxicol. 2015;37(2):193–201 [E].

[38] Maejima R, Iijima K, Kaihovaara P, et al. Effects of ALDH2 genotype, PPI treatment and L-cysteine on carcinogenic acetaldehyde in gastric juice and saliva after intragastric alcohol administration. PLoS One. 2015;10(4)e0120397 [c].

[39] Chang JS, Hsiao JR, Chen CH. ALDH2 polymorphism and alcohol-related cancers in Asians: a public health perspective. J Biomed Sci. 2017;24(1):19 [R].

[40] Hendershot CS, Claus ED, Ramchandani VA. Associations of OPRM1 A118G and alcohol sensitivity with intravenous alcohol self-administration in young adults. Addict Biol. 2016;21(1):125–35 [c].

[41] Long EC, Aliev F, Wang JC, et al. Further analyses of genetic association between GRM8 and alcohol dependence symptoms among young adults. J Stud Alcohol Drugs. 2015;76(3):414–8 [c].

[42] fda.gov [Internet]. Silver Spring, MD: U.S. Food and Drug Administration; 2017. [cited 2017 March 22]. Available from, http://www.fda.gov [S].

[43] Bachhuber MA, Maughan BC, Mitra N, et al. Prescription monitoring programs and emergency department visits involving benzodiazepine misuse: early evidence from 11 United States metropolitan areas. Int J Drug Policy. 2016;28:120–3 [C].

[44] Jones CM, McAninch JK. Emergency department visits and overdose deaths from combined use of opioids and benzodiazepines. Am J Prev Med. 2015;49(4):493–501 [C].

[45] Park TW, Saitz R, Ganoczy D, et al. Benzodiazepine prescribing patterns and deaths from drug overdose among US veterans receiving opioid analgesics: case-cohort study. BMJ. 2015;350: h2698 [c].

[46] O'Connell CW, Sadler CA, Tolia VM, et al. Overdose of etizolam: the abuse and rise of a benzodiazepine analog. Ann Emerg Med. 2015;65(4):465–6 [r].

[47] Lukasik-Glebocka M, Sommerfeld K, Tezyk A, et al. Flubromazolam—a new life-threatening designer benzodiazepine. Clin Toxicol (Phila). 2016;54(1):66–8 [r].

[48] Ali A, Jerry JM, Khawam EA. Delirium induced by a new synthetic legal intoxicating drug: phenazepam. Psychosomatics. 2015;56(4):414–8 [r].

[49] Liaw GW, Hung DZ, Chen WK, et al. Relationship between acute benzodiazepine poisoning and acute pancreatitis risk: a population-based cohort study. Medicine (Baltimore). 2015;94(52) e2376 [c].

[50] Aljarallah S, Al-Hussain F. Acute fatal posthypoxic leukoencephalopathy following benzodiazepine overdose: a case report and review of the literature. BMC Neurol. 2015;15:69 [A].

[51] Hsu YH, Lin FS, Yang CC, et al. Evident cognitive impairments in seemingly recovered patients after midazolam-based light sedation during diagnostic endoscopy. J Formos Med Assoc. 2015;114(6):489–97 [C].

[52] Papineni McIntosh A, Ashley PF, Lourenco-Matharu L. Reported side effects of intravenous midazolam sedation when used in paediatric dentistry: a review. Int J Paediatr Dent. 2015;25(3):153–64 [c].

[53] Paolicchi JM, Ross G, Lee D, et al. Clobazam and aggression-related adverse events in pediatric patients with Lennox-Gastaut syndrome. Pediatr Neurol. 2015;53(4):338–42 [C].

[54] Mathew T, D'Souza D, Nadimpally US, et al. Clobazam-induced pedal edema: an unrecognized side effect of a common antiepileptic drug. Epilepsia. 2016;57(3):524–5 [c].

[55] Ham AC, Ziere G, Broer L, et al. CYP2C9 genotypes modify benzodiazepine-related fall risk: original results from three studies with meta-analysis. J Am Med Dir Assoc. 2017;18(1). 88.e81–88.e15 [C].

[56] By the American Geriatrics Society 2015 Beers Criteria Update Expert Panel. American Geriatrics society 2015 updated beers criteria for potentially inappropriate medication use in older adults. J Am Geriatr Soc. 2015;63(11):2227–46 [R].

[57] Pomara N, Lee SH, Bruno D, et al. Adverse performance effects of acute lorazepam administration in elderly long-term users: pharmacokinetic and clinical predictors. Prog Neuropsychopharmacol Biol Psychiatry. 2015;56:129–35 [c].

[58] Vukcevic NP, Ercegovic GV, Segrt Z, et al. Benzodiazepine poisoning in elderly. Vojnosanit Pregl. 2016;73(3):234–8 [C].

[59] Maeda T, Babazono A, Nishi T, et al. Quantification of adverse effects of regular use of triazolam on clinical outcomes for older people with insomnia: a retrospective cohort study. Int J Geriatr Psychiatry. 2016;31(2):186–94 [C].

[60] Scheifes A, Walraven S, Stolker JJ, et al. Adverse events and the relation with quality of life in adults with intellectual disability and challenging behaviour using psychotropic drugs. Res Dev Disabil. 2016;49–50:13–21 [C].

[61] Nguyen TT, Troendle M, Cumpston C, et al. Lack of adverse effects from flumazenil administration: an ED observational study. Am J Emerg Med. 2015;33(11):1677–9 [c].

[62] Penninga ER, Graudal N, Ladekarl MB, et al. Adverse events associated with flumazenil treatment for the management of suspected benzodiazepine intoxication—a systematic review with meta-analyses of randomised trials. Basic Clin Pharmacol Toxicol. 2016;118(1):37–44 [C].

[63] Fowler AH, Majithia V. Ultimate mimicry: methamphetamine-induced pseudovasculitis. Am J Med. 2015;128(4):364–6 [r].

[64] Yu S, Zhu L, Shen Q, et al. Recent advances in methamphetamine neurotoxicity mechanisms and its molecular pathophysiology. Behav Neurol. 2015;2015:103969 [r].

[65] O'Connor AD, Padilla-Jones A, Gerkin RD, et al. Prevalence of rhabdomyolysis in sympathomimetic toxicity: a comparison of stimulants. J Med Toxicol. 2015;11(2):195–200 [C].

[66] emcdda.europa.eu [Internet]. Portugal: The European Monitoring Centre for Drugs and Drug Addiction; 2017. [cited 2017 March 22]. Available from, http://www.emcdda.europa.eu [S].

[67] drugabuse.gov [Internet]. Rockville, MD: National Institute on Drug Abuse; 2017. [cited 2017 March 22.]. Available from, http://www.drugabuse.gov [S].

[68] Rambod M, Elhanafi S, Mukherjee D. Brugada phenocopy in concomitant ethanol and heroin overdose. Ann Noninvasive Electrocardiol. 2015;20(1):87–90 [A].

[69] Deroux A, Buisson TT, Bernard C, et al. Acute interstitial pneumonia following heroin inhalation. Presse Med. 2015;44(1):119–21 [A].

[70] Bui DH, Pace J, Manjila S, et al. Heroin inhalation complicated by refractory hydrocephalus: a novel presentation. Neurology. 2015;84(20):2093–5 [A].

[71] Dastur CK, Chang GY. Heroin inhalation complicated by refractory hydrocephalus: a novel presentation. Neurology. 2015;85(23):2083 [r].

[72] Pirompanich P, Chankrachang S. Intravenous heroin-associated delayed spongiform leukoencephalopathy: case report and reviews of the literature. J Med Assoc Thai. 2015;98(7):703–8 [A].

[73] Woodcock EA, Lundahl LH, Burmeister M, et al. Functional mu opioid receptor polymorphism (OPRM1 A(118) G) associated with heroin use outcomes in Caucasian males: a pilot study. Am J Addict. 2015;24(4):329–35 [c].

[74] Center for Behavioral Health Statistics and Quality. Key substance use and mental health indicators in the United States: results from the 2015 National Survey on drug use and health (HHS publication no. SMA 16-4984, NSDUH series H-51), Retrieved from, http://www.samhsa.gov/data/; 2016 [MC].

[75] Rudd RA, Aleshire N, Zibbell JE, et al. Increases in drug and opioid overdose deaths—United States, 2000–2014. MMWR Morb Mortal Wkly Rep. 2016;64(50–51):1378–82 [MC].

[76] Ries R, Krupski A, West IIC, et al. Correlates of opioid use in adults with self-reported drug use recruited from public safety-net primary care clinics. J Addict Med. 2015;9(5):417–26 [C].

[77] Lev R, Petro S, Lee A, et al. Methadone related deaths compared to all prescription related deaths. Forensic Sci Int. 2015;257:347–52 [C].

[78] Davis CS, Johnston JE, Pierce MW. Overdose epidemic, prescription monitoring programs, and public health: a review of state laws. Am J Public Health. 2015;105(11):e9–e11 [c].

[79] Sgarlato A, deRoux SJ. Prescription opioid related deaths in New York city: a 2 year retrospective analysis prior to the introduction of the New York State I-STOP law. Forensic Sci Med Pathol. 2015;11(3):388–94 [MC].

[80] Vignali C, Stramesi C, Morini C, et al. Methadone-related deaths. A ten year overview. Forensic Sci Int. 2015;257:172–6 [c].

[81] Marteau D, McDonald R, Patel K. The relative risk of fatal poisoning by methadone or buprenorphine within the wider population of England and Wales. BMJ Open. 2015;5(5) e007629 [MC].

[82] Martins SS, Sampson L, Cerda M, et al. Worldwide prevalence and trends in unintentional drug overdose: a systematic review of the literature. Am J Public Health. 2015;105(11):e29–49 [R].

[83] Budnitz DS, Lovegrove MC, Sapiano MR, et al. Notes from the field: pediatric emergency department visits for buprenorphine/naloxone ingestion—United States, 2008–2015. MMWR Morb Mortal Wkly Rep. 2016;65(41):1148–9 [MC].

[84] Reisner A, Hayes LL, Holland CM, et al. Opioid overdose in a child: case report and discussion with emphasis on neurosurgical implications. J Neurosurg Pediatr. 2015;16(6):752–7 [A].

[85] Zawilska JB, Andrzejczak D. Next generation of novel psychoactive substances on the horizon—a complex problem to face. Drug Alcohol Depend. 2015;157:1–17 [r].

[86] Peterson AB, Gladden RM, Delcher C, et al. Increases in fentanyl-related overdose deaths—Florida and Ohio, 2013–2015. MMWR Morb Mortal Wkly Rep. 2016;65(33):844–9 [MC].

[87] Vo KT, van Wijk XM, Lynch KL, et al. Counterfeit Norco poisoning outbreak—San Francisco Bay Area, California, March 25–April 5, 2016. MMWR Morb Mortal Wkly Rep. 2016;65(16):420–3 [A].

[88] Lynch KL, Shapiro BJ, Coffa D, et al. Promethazine use among chronic pain patients. Drug Alcohol Depend. 2015;150:92–7 [C].

[89] Siddiqi S, Verney C, Dargan P, et al. Understanding the availability, prevalence of use, desired effects, acute toxicity and dependence potential of the novel opioid MT-45. Clin Toxicol (Phila). 2015;53(1):54–9 [r].

[90] Rhode Island Department of Health. Fatal drug overdoses, http://www.health.ri.gov/data/death/drugoverdoses/2013 [S].

[91] Rhode Island Department of Health. Fatal drug overdoses, http://www.health.ri.gov/data/death/drugoverdoses/2016 [S].

[92] Ayres WA, Starsiak MJ, Sokolay P. The bogus drug: three methyl & alpha methyl fentanyl sold as "China White". J Psychoactive Drugs. 1981;13(1):91–3 [A].

[93] Higashikawa Y, Suzuki S. Studies on 1-(2-phenethyl)-4-(N-propionylanilino) piperidine (fentanyl) and its related compounds. VI. Structure-analgesic activity relationship for fentanyl, methyl substituted fentanyls and other analogues. Forensic Toxicol. 2008;26(1):1–5 [E].

[94] Lozier MJ, Boyd M, Stanley C, et al. Acetyl fentanyl, a novel fentanyl analog, causes 14 overdose deaths in Rhode Island, March–May 2013. J Med Toxicol. 2015;11(2):208–17 [c].

[95] McIntyre IM, Trochta A, Gary RD, et al. An acute acetyl fentanyl fatality: a case report with postmortem concentrations. J Anal Toxicol. 2015;39(6):490–4 [A].

[96] McIntyre IM, Trochta A, Gary RD, et al. An acute butyr-fentanyl fatality: a case report with postmortem concentrations. J Anal Toxicol. 2016;40(2):162–6 [A].

[97] Cole JB, Dunbar JF, McIntire SA, et al. Butyrfentanyl overdose resulting in diffuse alveolar hemorrhage. Pediatrics. 2015;135(3):e740–3 [A].

[98] Bäckberg M, Beck O, Jonsson KD, et al. Opioid intoxications involving butyrfentanyl, 4-fluorobutyrfentanyl, and fentanyl from the Swedish STRIDA project. Clin Toxicol (Phila). 2015;53(7):609–17 [A].

[99] Helander A, Bäckberg M, Beck O. Intoxications involving the fentanyl analogs acetylfentanyl, 4-methoxybutyrfentanyl and furanylfentanyl: results from the Swedish STRIDA project. Clin Toxicol (Phila). 2016;54(4):324–32 [A].

[100] Hillman AD, Witenko CJ, Sultan SM, et al. Serotonin syndrome caused by fentanyl and methadone in a burn injury. Pharmacotherapy. 2015;35(1):112–7 [A].

[101] Robles LA. Serotonin syndrome induced by fentanyl in a child: case report. Clin Neuropharmacol. 2015;38(5):206–8 [A].

[102] MacDonald LE, Onsrud JE, Mullins-Hodgin R. Acute sensorineural hearing loss after abuse of an inhaled, crushed oxymorphone extended-release tablet. Pharmacotherapy. 2015;35(7):e118–21 [A].

[103] Flory JH, Wiesenthal AC, Thaler HT, et al. Methadone use and the risk of hypoglycemia for inpatients with cancer pain. J Pain Symptom Manage. 2016;51(1):79–87. e71 [C].

[104] Fournier JP, Azoulay L, Yin H, et al. Tramadol use and the risk of hospitalization for hypoglycemia in patients with noncancer pain. JAMA Intern Med. 2015;175(2):186–93 [MC].

[105] Gjedsted J, Dall R. Severe hypoglycemia during methadone escalation in an 8-year-old child. Acta Anaesthesiol Scand. 2015;59(10):1394–6 [A].

[106] Doris MK, Sandilands EA. Life-threatening opioid toxicity from a fentanyl patch applied to eczematous skin. BMJ Case Rep [Published online 4 April 2015], http://dx.doi.org/10.1136/bcr-2014-208945 [A].

[107] Eggleston W, Marraffa JM, Stork CM, et al. Notes from the field: cardiac dysrhythmias after loperamide abuse—New York, 2008–2016. MMWR Morb Mortal Wkly Rep. 2016;65(45):1276–7 [C].

[108] Spinner HL, Lonardo NW, Mulamalla R, et al. Ventricular tachycardia associated with high-dose chronic loperamide use. Pharmacotherapy. 2015;35(2):234–8 [A].

[109] Lasoff DR, Schneir A. Ventricular dysrhythmias from loperamide misuse. J Emerg Med. 2016;50(3):508–9 [A].

[110] Dierksen J, Gonsoulin M, Walterscheid JP. Poor man's methadone: a case report of loperamide toxicity. Am J Forensic Med Pathol. 2015;36(4):268–70 [A].

[111] Betts KS, McIlwraith F, Dietze P, et al. Can differences in the type, nature or amount of polysubstance use explain the increased risk of non-fatal overdose among psychologically distressed people who inject drugs? Drug Alcohol Depend. 2015;154:76–84 [MC].

[112] Jones CM, Baldwin GT, Manocchio T, et al. Trends in methadone distribution for pain treatment, methadone diversion, and overdose deaths—United States, 2002–2014. MMWR Morb Mortal Wkly Rep. 2016;65(26):667–71 [C].

[113] Swenson O. Accidental methadone intoxication masquerading as asthma exacerbation with respiratory arrest in a six-year-old boy. Del Med J. 2015;87(5):147–9 [A].

[114] Kruckow L, Linnet K, Banner J. Psychiatric disorders are overlooked in patients with drug abuse. Dan Med J. 2016;63(3): pii: A5207, [C].

[115] Simonsen KW, Christoffersen DJ, Banner J, et al. Fatal poisoning among patients with drug addiction. Dan Med J. 2015;62(10):A5147 [A].

[116] Bardy G, Cathala P, Eiden C, et al. An unusual case of death probably triggered by the association of buprenorphine at therapeutic dose with ethanol and benzodiazepines and with very low norbuprenorphine level. J Forensic Sci. 2015;60(Suppl 1):S269–71 [A].

[117] Swartzentruber GS, Richardson WH, Mack EH. Buprenorphine ingestion in a 23-month-old boy. Hosp Pediatr. 2015;5(3):164–6 [A].

[118] Federal Drug Administration. FDA announces enhanced warnings for immediate-release opioid pain medications related to risks of misuse, abuse, addiction, overdose and death. New safety warnings also added to all prescription opioid medications to inform prescribers and patients of additional risks related to opioid use. Released: 3/22/2016, https://www.fda.gov/NewsEvents/Newsroom/PressAnnouncements/ucm491739.htm; 2016 [S].

[119] Federal Drug Administration. FDA requires strong warnings for opioid analgesics, prescription opioid cough products, and benzodiazepine labeling related to serious risks and death from combined use. Action to better inform prescribers and protect patients as part of Agency's Opioids Action Plan, https://www.fda.gov/NewsEvents/Newsroom/PressAnnouncements/ucm518697.htm. Released: 9/1/2016 [S].

[120] Crist RC, Doyle GA, Nelson EC, et al. A polymorphism in the OPRM1 3'-untranslated region is associated with methadone efficacy in treating opioid dependence. Pharmacogenomics J. 2016; http://dx.doi.org/10.1038/tpj.2016.89. [Epub ahead of print] [C].

[121] Kharasch ED, Regina KJ, Blood J, et al. Methadone pharmacogenetics: CYP2B6 polymorphisms determine plasma concentrations, clearance and metabolism. Anesthesiology. 2015;123(5):1142–53 [c].

[122] Yang HC, Chu SK, Huang CL, et al. Genome-wide pharmacogenomic study on methadone maintenance treatment identifies SNP rs17180299 and multiple haplotypes on CYP2B6, SPON1, and GSG1L associated with plasma concentrations of methadone R- and S-enantiomers in heroin-dependent patients. PLoS Genet. 2016;12(3)e1005910 [C].

[123] Chidambaran V, Venkatasubramanian R, Zhang X, et al. ABCC3 genetic variants are associated with postoperative morphine-induced respiratory depression and morphine pharmacokinetics in children. Pharmacogenomics J. 2017;17(2):162–9 [c].

[124] Linares OA, Fudin J, Daly AL, et al. Individualized hydrocodone therapy based on phenotype, pharmacogenetics, and pharmacokinetic dosing. Clin J Pain. 2015;31(12):1026–35 [R].

[125] Fonseca S, Amorim A, Costa HA, et al. Sequencing CYP2D6 for the detection of poor-metabolizers in post-mortem blood samples with tramadol. Forensic Sci Int. 2016;265:153–9 [E].

[126] Parvaz Madadi P, Kelly LE, Ross CJ, et al. Forensic investigation of methadone concentrations in deceased breastfed infants. J Forensic Sci. 2016;61(2):576–80 [A].

[127] Zarobkiewicz MK, Wawryk-Gawda E, Woźniakowski MW, et al. Tobacco smokers and electronic cigarettes users among polish universities students. Rocz Panstw Zakl Hig. 2016;67(1): 75–80 [MC].

[128] Singh T, Arrazola RA, Corey CG, et al. Tobacco use among middle and high school students—United States, 2011–2015. MMWR Morb Mortal Wkly Rep. 2016;65:361–7 [MC].

[129] Bunnell RE, Agaku IT, Arrazola RA, et al. Intentions to smoke cigarettes among never-smoking US middle and high school electronic cigarette users: National Youth Tobacco Survey, 2011–2013. Nicotine Tob Res. 2015;17(2):228–35 [MC].

[130] Cho JH, Paik SY. Association between electronic cigarette use and asthma among high school students in South Korea. PLoS One. 2016;11(3)e0151022 [MC].

[131] Thrasher JF, Abad-Vivero EN, Barrientos-Gutíerrez I, et al. Prevalence and correlates of e-cigarette perceptions and trial among Mexican adolescents. J Adolesc Health. 2016;58(3):358–65 [MC].

[132] White J, Li J, Newcombe R, et al. Tripling use of electronic cigarettes among New Zealand adolescents between 2012 and 2014. J Adolesc Health. 2015;56(5):522–8 [MC].

[133] Kinnunen JM, Ollila H, Sel-T E-A, et al. Awareness and determinants of electronic cigarette use among Finnish adolescents in 2013: a population-based study. Tob Control. 2015;24(e4):e264–70 [MC].

[134] Hughes K, Bellis MA, Hardcastle KA, et al. Associations between e-cigarette access and smoking and drinking behaviours in teenagers. BMC Public Health. 2015;15:244 [MC].

[135] Goniewicz ML, Zielinska-Danch W. Electronic cigarette use among teenagers and young adults in Poland. Pediatrics. 2012;130(4):e879–85 [MC].

[136] Babineau K, Taylor K, Clancy L. Electronic cigarette use among Irish youth: a cross sectional study of prevalence and associated factors. PLoS One. 2015;10(5)e0126419 [C].

[137] Lotrean LM. Use of electronic cigarettes among Romanian university students: a cross-sectional study. BMC Public Health. 2015;15:358 [C].

[138] Leventhal AM, Strong DR, Sussman S, et al. Psychiatric comorbidity in adolescent electronic and conventional cigarette use. J Psychiatr Res. 2016;73:71–8 [C].

[139] Syamlal G, Jamal A, King BA, et al. Electronic cigarette use among working adults—United States, 2014. MMWR Morb Mortal Wkly Rep. 2016;65:557–61 [MC].

[140] Harrold TC, Maag AK, Thackway S, et al. Prevalence of e-cigarette users in New South Wales. Med J Aust. 2015;203(8):326 [MC].

[141] Rogers JS, Rehrer SJ, Hoot NR. Acetylfentanyl: an emerging drug of abuse. J Emerg Med. 2016;50(3):433–6 [A].

[142] Chen BC, Bright SB, Trivedi AR, et al. Death following intentional ingestion of e-liquid. Clin Toxicol (Phila). 2015;53(9):914–6 [A].

[143] Durmowicz EL, Rudy SF, Chen IL. Electronic cigarettes: analysis of FDA adverse experience reports in non-users. Tob Control. 2016;25(2):242 [c].

[144] Ordonez JE, Kleinschmidt KC, Forrester MB. Electronic cigarette exposures reported to Texas poison centers. Nicotine Tob Res. 2015;17(2):209–11 [C].

[145] Forrester MB. Pediatric exposures to electronic cigarettes reported to Texas poison centers. J Emerg Med. 2015;49(2):136–42 [C].

[146] Tan AS, Bigman CA, Mello S, et al. Is exposure to e-cigarette communication associated with perceived harms of e-cigarette secondhand vapour? Results from a national survey of US adults. BMJ Open. 2015;5(3)e007134 [MC].

[147] Hiratsuka VY, Avey JP, Trinidad SB, et al. Views on electronic cigarette use in tobacco screening and cessation in an Alaska native healthcare setting. Int J Circumpolar Health. 2015;74:27794 [c].

[148] Geiss O, Bianchi I, Barahona F, et al. Characterisation of mainstream and passive vapours emitted by selected electronic cigarettes. Int J Hyg Environ Health. 2015;218(1):169–80 [E].

[149] O'Connell G, Colard S, Cahours X, et al. An assessment of indoor air quality before, during and after unrestricted use of e-cigarettes in a small room. Int J Environ Res Public Health. 2015;12(5):4889 [c].

[150] Hartmann-Boyce J, McRobbie H, Bullen C, et al. Electronic cigarettes for smoking cessation. Cochrane Database Syst Rev. 2016;14:9 [M].

[151] Kalkhoran S, Glantz SA. E-cigarettes and smoking cessation in real-world and clinical settings: a systematic review and meta-analysis. Lancet Respir Med. 2016;4(2):116–28 [R].

[152] Cravo AS, Bush J, Sharma G, et al. A randomised, parallel group study to evaluate the safety profile of an electronic vapour product over 12 weeks. Regul Toxicol Pharmacol. 2016;81 (Suppl 1):S1–14 [MC].

[153] Walele T, Sharma G, Savioz R, et al. A randomized, crossover study on an electronic vapour product, a nicotine inhalator and a conventional cigarette. Part B: safety and subjective effects. Regul Toxicol Pharmacol. 2016;74:193–9 [c].

[154] Yan XS, D'Ruiz C. Effects of using electronic cigarettes on nicotine delivery and cardiovascular function in comparison with regular cigarettes. Regul Toxicol Pharmacol. 2015;71(1):24–34 [c].

[155] Russo C, Cibella F, Caponnetto P, et al. Evaluation of post cessation weight gain in a 1-year randomized smoking cessation trial of electronic cigarettes. Sci Rep. 2016;6:18763 [C].

[156] Hecht SS, Carmella SG, Kotandeniya D, et al. Evaluation of toxicant and carcinogen metabolites in the urine of e-cigarette users versus cigarette smokers. 2015;17(6):704–9 [c].

[157] Kosmider L, Sobczak A, Fik M, et al. Carbonyl compounds in electronic cigarette vapors: effects of nicotine solvent and battery output voltage. Nicotine Tob Res. 2014;16:1319–26 [E].

[158] Schweitzer KS, Chen SX, Law S, et al. Endothelial disruptive proinflammatory effects of nicotine and e-cigarette vapor exposures. Am J Physiol Lung Cell Mol Physiol. 2015;309:L175–87 [E].

[159] Shepperd CJ, Newland N, Eldridge A, et al. Changes in levels of biomarkers of exposure and biological effect in a controlled study of smokers switched from conventional cigarettes to reduced-

toxicant-prototype cigarettes. Regul Toxicol Pharmacol. 2015;72(2):273–91 [C].

[160] Haziza C, de La Bourdonnaye G, Skiada D, et al. Evaluation of the tobacco heating system 2.2. Part 8: 5-day randomized reduced exposure clinical study in Poland. Regul Toxicol Pharmacol. 2016;81(Suppl 2):S139–50 [C].

[161] Morris DS, Fiala SC. Online electronic cigarette retailers can do more to prevent accidental poisonings. Tob Control. 2015;24(4):415–6 [c].

[162] Buettner-Schmidt K, Miller DR, Balasubramanian N. Electronic cigarette refill liquids: child-resistant packaging, nicotine content, and sales to minors. J Pediatr Nurs. 2016;31(4):373–9 [E].

[163] Salt Lake County Health Department. Analysis of nicotine content in E-liquid samples, Salt Lake County Health Department, 2014. Accessed 20 March 2017. http://health.utah.gov/opha/publications/hsu/1501_HPV.pdf; 2015 [E].

[164] Goniewicz ML, Gupta R, Lee YH, et al. Nicotine levels in electronic cigarette refill solutions: a comparative analysis of products from the U.S., Korea, and Poland. Int J Drug Policy. 2015;26(6):583–8 [E].

[165] European Commission-Press release Brussels May 20 2016. "10 Key changes for tobacco products sold in the EU" [S].

5

Hypnotics and Sedatives

Tina C. Beck[1], Jason A. Garcia-Trevino, Brittney A. Ramirez

University of the Incarnate Word Feik School of Pharmacy, San Antonio, TX, United States

[1]Corresponding author: tclee@uiwtx.edu

HYPNOTICS

General Information

Review

A review article specifically looked at the elderly population to assess the safety and efficacy of various sleep medications [1R]. Benzodiazepines are still a popular class of medication. Various studies cited in this review article mention known adverse effects of benzodiazepines to be daytime drowsiness, dizziness, and decrease in cognitive function. The nonbenzodiazepine receptor agonists such as zolpidem, zopiclone, eszopiclone, and zaleplon have observational studies that showed adverse effects such as dementia, delirium, sleepwalking, serious fractures, and increase risk of cancer (zolpidem). These agents are also Schedule IV controlled substances, making them a concern for potential abuse, especially in people with a history of substance abuse. Like benzodiazepines, FDA recommends these agents for short-term use to treat insomnia. Ramelteon is a melatonin agonist that showed longer half-life in the elderly, and this is believed to be caused by reduced phase I metabolism that in the elderly. However, having ramelteon linger in the body was not associated with more adverse reactions or requiring dosing changes. There are drug interactions with CYP1A2 drugs and the combination of ramelteon and inhibitors of CYP1A2 medications such as ciprofloxacin should be avoided. Suvorexant is an orexin receptor antagonist that was approved in 2014 for the treatment of insomnia, and clinical studies show mild adverse effects such as somnolence, fatigue, headache, and dry mouth. Serious adverse effects were seen to be dose related that affected women more than men, such as excessive daytime sleepiness, driving impairment, sleep paralysis, and falls. However, there is lack of clinical experience with suvorexant. The conclusion of the review article showed that the elderly population is more vulnerable to the adverse effects of benzodiazepines and should be avoided in this population. The nonbenzodiazepine receptor agonists should also be limited in the elderly population. Ramelteon has a lower side effect profile than the other classes and may be an option to treat insomnia in the elderly.

A systematic review and meta-analysis were also released in 2016 that showed that mortality was associated with anxiolytic and hypnotic drugs [2M]. Prior to this review, there were inconsistent results when evaluating mortality associated with hypnotics and anxiolytics. The primary outcome of the meta-analysis was all-cause mortality associated with hypnotics and anxiolytics, and secondary outcomes were sex-stratified mortality risk and mortality associated with benzodiazepines or Z-drugs use only. Twenty-five studies (cohorts and case-control study) were included in the final analysis. For the primary outcome, the pooled adjusted hazard ratio for mortality among hypnotic and anxiolytic users was statistically significantly higher compared to non-users. Patients that used hypnotics or anxiolytics had a 43% higher risk of mortality compared to non-users. After removing six studies for higher heterogeneity, users had a 21% higher risk of mortality compared to non-users. The secondary outcome looking sex-stratified mortality risk, similar increase risk of mortality was seen in both men and women (HR: 1.6, 95% CI: 1.29–1.99 vs HR: 1.68, 95% CI: 1.38–2.04, respectively). For benzodiazepine users, there was a 60% increased risk of mortality compared to non-users (95% CI: 1.03–2.49). Although Z-drug users showed a 73% increased risk of mortality, the effect was not statistically significant (95% CI: 0.95–3.16). Not all studies looked at the specific cause of death for hypnotic and anxiolytic users, but 12 studies reported mortality associated with suicides, cardiovascular and cancer-related deaths as common causes. The authors suggest that future studies evaluate the

ISSN: 0378-6080

http://dx.doi.org/10.1016/bs.seda.2017.07.008

underlying mechanism for increased risk of mortality among patients using hypnotics and anxiolytics.

NEUROMUSCULAR FUNCTION

Fall-Related Injury

In the United States, the elderly population is associated with higher incidence of insomnia, which is associated with increased risk of morbidity, mortality, and lower quality of life. A crossover study was conducted to determine the risk of hospitalization for hip fracture or traumatic brain injury in patients using nonbenzodiazepine sedative hypnotic (eszopiclone, zaleplon, and zolpidem) users among Medicare beneficiaries [3C]. The authors evaluated the differences between Medicare beneficiaries that used the nonbenzodiazepine sedative hypnotics in the 30 days prior to hospitalization and non-users in the control periods of 3, 6, 9, and 12 months prior to injury in 2007–2009. Each patient served as their own control to minimize bias. For traumatic brain injury, 15 031 patients met the inclusion criteria, and out of these patients, 3.3% ($n = 491$) used one of the sedatives in the previous 30 days prior to injury, and these patients were more likely to have used the sedative at least once before compared non-users. Looking at specific sedatives for traumatic brain injury, zolpidem use during the 30 days prior to the injury was associated with a statistically significant risk of hospitalization for traumatic brain injury (OR: 1.87, 95% CI: 0.56–2.25). However, eszopiclone and zaleplon were not associated with an increased risk of traumatic brain injury (OR: 0.67, 95% CI: 0.4–1.13 vs OR: 0.85, 95% CI: 0.21–3.34, respectively). In regards to hip fractures, 37 833 patients met inclusion criteria and 3.2% ($n = 1192$) used a sedative 30 days prior to hospitalization. Again, when analyzing individual sedatives, zolpidem use 30 days prior to injury was associated with increased risk for hospitalization for a hip fracture (OR: 1.59, 95% CI: 1.41–1.79) while eszopiclone and zaleplon were not. It is interesting to note that for both traumatic brain injury and hip fracture, zaleplon use did not have enough sample size to meet power to make an accurate assessment on the primary outcome. The authors conclude that eszopiclone may be a safer alternative to zolpidem for elderly patients needing pharmacotherapy treatment for insomnia.

ESZOPICLONE

Psychiatric

A 48-year-old male developed parasomnia and tried to commit suicide while taking eszopiclone [4A]. The patient had a remote depressive episode in the past but resolved without treatment. Besides this remote history, the patient denied any prior mental health history. He specifically denied any history of suicidal ideations. The patient did develop a profound depression after being laid off 4 weeks prior to presentation but denied any suicidal or morbid ideations. His primary care physician prescribed sertraline 50 mg and eszopiclone 2 mg, both at bedtime, 2 days prior to the episode. After 2 days of taking the medications, he went to bed at 10:00 pm and woke up abruptly 2.5 hours later agitated, paranoid, and fidgeting. He believed someone was after him. The patient sliced his own neck with a box cutter after his agitation continued to escalate. Patient survived after emergent tracheotomy and blood transfusion. After a psychiatry consultation, it was determined that the events that led to the patient's presenting condition were likely due to the medications and did not represent a suicide attempt related to his ongoing depression. Many drugs like sertraline (serotonin reuptake inhibitors-SSRIs) are known to inhibit CYP450 drug metabolism. Eszopiclone is metabolized by CYP3A4 and CYP2E1, and the combination with sertraline may have increased levels of eszopiclone, increasing the risk of adverse effects. There is one other case report specifically related to eszopiclone and potential psychiatric episode of severe formication. With several reports with zolpidem and suicide attempts, the authors conclude that there is increased risk of adverse effects from benzodiazepine-like hypnotics and concomitant administration with drugs like SSRIs.

ZOLPIDEM

Psychiatric

A case report was published of acute delirium after a small one time dose of zolpidem 5 mg [5A]. Most case reports involving zolpidem use more than the recommended dose (>10 mg). This reaction was seen in an 81-year-old male patient with no prior history of psychiatric or substance abuse. The patient presented to the emergency department after passing out while standing and walking around. He had been complaining of non-postural dizziness for 3 or 4 days. There was no head trauma, seizure bowel or bladder incontinence during syncopal episode. A pacemaker was placed for symptomatic bradycardia. The patient complained of difficulty sleeping during his inpatient stay. The patient reported prior use of zolpidem without side effects. He was ordered 5 mg of zolpidem, and 1 hour later the patient started experiencing confusion, restlessness and visual hallucinations. His vitals were stable, but he was combative and not oriented to person. After administration of haloperidol IV and soft restraints, the patient returned to normal mental function in 8 hours. Case reports of zolpidem causing delirium have been reported, but are usually seen in patients with a history of psychiatric illness and taking more than 10 mg of zolpidem. This case report shows that even a small dose in a patient with no psychiatric history may be at risk of developing delirium on zolpidem.

Urinary Tract

In Taiwan, a case-control study was completed to determine the risk of zolpidem use and the development of acute pyelonephritis in women [6MC]. A previously conducted experimental study demonstrated zolpidem to be an inflammatory mediator, and it may increase the risk of infection. There is no current evidence linking zolpidem to acute pyelonephritis, which is why the authors decided to conduct this study. Female participants aged 20–84 years who received a diagnosis of acute pyelonephritis from January 1, 2000 to December 31, 2011 were identified for the case group. For every patient found in the case group, two women with no history of acute pyelonephritis would be randomly selected into the control group. Participants with chronic pyelonephritis, pregnancy, renal transplant and HIV/AIDS were excluded. Definitions of current zolpidem use was within 7-day period from diagnosis, while early zolpidem use was one tablet use 8–14 days before diagnosis, and late zolpidem use was using one tablet >15 days before diagnosis. Over 3000 female participants were included in the case group, and over 6000 females were in the control group. Patients with current zolpidem use had statistically significant different adjusted OR compared to non-users of acute pyelonephritis (OR = 2.2, 95% CI = 1.7–2.8). However, when looking at the early and late zolpidem use, there was no statistical difference (early: AOR = 1.4, 95% CI = 0.8–2.5; late: AOR = 1.1, 95% CI = 0.9–1.2). The results of the study show that an increased risk of acute pyelonephritis may occur within the first 7 days after the end of treatment, but more research needs to be conducted to prove causal link of zolpidem and acute pyelonephritis. The authors conclude that physicians and pharmacists need to be more cautious with prescribing and dispensing zolpidem in women.

Cancer Risk

There is some evidence of zolpidem increasing the risk of cancer. A cohort study in Taiwan, looked at zolpidem usage on the risk of cancer over a 3 year follow-up [7MC]. Using health insurance database that enrolls up to 99% of Taiwan's population, patients were identified using sleep disorder diagnostic codes in 2002. The dosage, supply days, and total numbers of pills of zolpidem were obtained through the outpatient pharmacy database. Almost 7000 patients were enrolled in the cohort (zolpidem $n = 1728$, without zolpidem $n = 5196$), and 56 patients reported cancer (zolpidem $n = 26$, without zolpidem $n = 30$). After adjusting for gender, age, comorbidities, other medications, it was found that zolpidem users had a 1.75 times (95% CI = 1.02–3.02) higher risk of cancer events than those that did not use zolpidem in a 3 year follow-up period. It was also noted that total daily doses >10 mg and >2 months of zolpidem use were associated with 3.74 times 995% CI = 1.42–9.83, $P = 0.008$) higher risk of cancer. The mechanism of how zolpidem increases the risk of cancer is still unknown and more research is necessary to determine the mechanism. Authors conclude that risks and benefits of zolpidem should be explained to patients, and cognitive behavioral therapy may be more beneficial than use of hypnotics.

BENZODIAZEPINES

Central Nervous System

The elderly population, especially in residential facilities, is associated with decreased sleep quality and length due to altered circadian rhythms. Benzodiazepines are a common class prescribed to the residents of these facilities. A cross-sectional study [8C] showed that the use of as needed benzodiazepines had an association with longer daytime napping, while regular long-acting benzodiazepine use were associated with higher nighttime sleep quality. The study included 383 residents of six Australian residential aged care facilities. The study included patients over the age of 65 and used a validated questionnaire to determine sleep quality. The results showed that benzodiazepine users had a higher prevalence of diagnosed insomnia (21.3% vs 4.9%, $P < 0.01$) and depression (68% vs 53.2%, $P < 0.01$) compared to the non-users. There was also a statistically significant difference in the prevalence of agitation and aggression compared to non-users (34.3% vs 19.5%, $P < 0.01$). In regards to the sleep quality questionnaire, there was no statistical difference between benzodiazepine users and non-users until analysis adjusted for the use of long-acting vs short-acting benzodiazepines. A correlation between short-acting PRN (as needed) benzodiazepines and lower nighttime sleep quality was shown to be not statistically significant (AOR = 0.59, 95% CI = 0.34–1.02). However, when looking at long-acting benzodiazepines, there was a statistical significance associated with higher nighttime sleep quality (AOR = 4.00, 95% CI = 1.06–15.15). There was no statistical difference in daytime drowsiness between users and non-users, which is a different finding compared to previous reports of excessive daytime drowsiness. The findings also showed a relationship between the use of PRN only benzodiazepines and long daytime napping (AOR = 1.77, 95% CI = 1.01–3.08), although there was no significant difference in mean daytime napping time between benzodiazepine users and non-users overall (3.03 hours vs 3.01 hours per week, $P = 0.97$). The study did not specify dose and duration of benzodiazepine, making it hard to extrapolate findings to all residential facility residents. The authors of the study discuss the possibility of future studies researching the effect of dose and duration on sleep quality.

Interactions

Drug–Drug Interaction

A French cross-sectional study aimed to estimate the overall prevalent use of benzodiazepine users and to quantify in these users the prevalence of comorbidities and concurrent medications that increase the risk of adverse drug reactions [9MC]. Using a French reimbursement claims database, benzodiazepine users were considered anyone in 2013 that had at least one reimbursement for all benzodiazepines (except those used for anticonvulsants: clonazepam and midazolam, and as muscle relaxants: tetrazepam) or zolpidem and zopiclone. In 2013, France saw a prevalence of 13.8% benzodiazepine use, specifically more women were to use benzodiazepines and an increased prevalence in the elderly population. The type of benzodiazepine used was broken down to 10.6% for anxiolytic use and 6.1% for hypnotic use. Almost half of the benzodiazepine users had an increased risk for adverse drug reaction, with drug–drug interactions with opioids being the leading cause (39.3% of users). It was also found that 11.3% of users had a comorbidity that increased the risk of adverse respiratory effect (13.9% in the 65- to 79-year-old patients), and 7% had comorbidities that increased the risk of falls/fractures. This study shows still high use of benzodiazepine users (in France), particularly the elderly population that are more vulnerable for polypharmacy and adverse reactions related to the medications.

CLONAZEPAM

Endocrine

There was no association of clonazepam causing thyroid dysfunction reported in the literature until a case report of a 50-year-old woman who developed subclinical hypothyroidism while on clonazepam [10A]. The patient had no history of comorbidities until she suffered from a clavicle fracture in March 2015 that led to an attempted suicide attempt due to severe shoulder pain in June 2015. Her previous history and laboratory values indicated her to be euthyroid. After her attempted suicide, she was initiated on oral duloxetine 20 mg and clonazepam 0.5 mg once daily. She underwent surgical treatment for her should pain. Due to her psychiatric history, a detailed examination was completed in August 2015. Her thyroid lab values indicated subclinical hypothyroidism, but she did not display any signs of symptoms of hypothyroidism. As her depression and insomnia worsened, her clonazepam dose was increased to 1 mg daily and duloxetine increased to 40 mg daily. After the dosage increase, her labs were repeated and showed increasing TSH levels. There is no literature evidence to indicate duloxetine as a plausible cause. Her home medications of cefepime, paracetamol, pantoprazole, zolpidem, amitriptyline, and vitamin D3 are not likely to be attributed to her altered thyroid hormone levels. There are several animal studies that looked at the mechanism of how benzodiazepines can affect thyroid hormones, but no human studies show an exact mechanism.

DIAZEPAM

Pediatrics

A prospective cohort study of 18 090 patients was used to differentiate the safety profiles of midazolam, diazepam, or a combination when used during third molar extractions in adolescents [11MC]. More than 18 000 patients met the inclusion criteria. The most common perioperative complications were vomiting without aspiration, peripheral vascular injury, and syncope. After adjusting for patient demographics, perioperative factors, and additional anesthetics used, the multiple regression showed adverse complications for patients receiving diazepam were increased by 50% over the midazolam group (AOR = 1.5, 95% CI = 1.05–2.16, $P = 0.027$). However, the group that received the combination midazolam and diazepam did not have an increased risk of anesthetic complication. Although a 50% increase risk of adverse complications was seen in the diazepam group, only a small number of perioperative complications were seen in general (1.4% over sample).

FLUMAZENIL

Although flumazenil is an antidote for benzodiazepine overdose, the chemical structure is similar to benzodiazepine. The review was conducted to show the safety of flumazenil use in benzodiazepine overdose patients [12M]. Thirteen studies were included in this study, and all of them were randomized, double blinded, placebo-controlled prospective trials. Adverse events were significantly associated with flumazenil treated group compared to no-intervention group (RR = 2.85,

95% CI=2.11–3.84, $P<0.00001$). The common adverse effects were agitation, anxiety, and gastrointestinal symptoms. The flumazenil group was also associated with serious adverse events compared to placebo group such as supraventricular arrhythmia, unspecified tachycardia, convulsions, multiple ventricular beats, and sudden hypotension (RR=3.81, 95% CI=1.28–11.39, $P=0.02$). There were no deaths in either groups.

The study also noted other adverse events such as aggressive behavior, nausea/vomiting, anxiety/distress. The results are similar to a previous meta-analysis published in 2007. Authors conclude that using flumazenil in the emergency department setting for suspected or known benzodiazepine overdose is significantly associated with increased risk of serious adverse events compared to placebo, and should not be routinely used.

MIDAZOLAM

Interaction

Drug–Drug Interaction

Clarithromycin is drug metabolized by cytochrome (CYP)3A4 that can cause auto-inhibition of metabolism and competitive inhibitor of P-glycoprotein. Midazolam, metabolized by CYP3A4, and digoxin, metabolized by P-glycoprotein, were paired with clarithromycin to predict physiological based pharmacokinetic (PBPK) model to drug–drug interactions [13E]. The models showed that during a co-treatment of oral clarithromycin 250–500 mg twice daily, oral midazolam dose should be reduced by 74%–88% to ensure constant midazolam exposure. Steady state of oral clarithromycin 500 mg twice daily showed IV midazolam dose needed to be reduced by 62% to achieve similar exposure as without co-treatment. Although these are model predictions and the main objective was not to determine dosing adjustments of midazolam, practitioners may need to consider that using midazolam with a CYP3A4 inhibitor may require lower doses of midazolam to get the same affect.

TETRAZEPAM

Immunologic

Common adverse reactions to tetrazepam are more neurological or gastrointestinal. It is rare to have cutaneous reactions to tetrazepam. A case series looked at tetrazepam cutaneous allergic reactions at an allergy clinic [14A]. The 10 year retrospective series showed a total of 8 patients were found to have an allergy to tetrazepam in this particular allergy clinic. The reactions were classified as Type IV sensitivity reactions and all but one of the

reactions were described as mild cutaneous, with the last being described as an erythema multiforme-like exanthema. All the reactions subsided without sequelae after stopping tetrazepam. These eight cases add to the 16 cutaneous cases that were published since 2002. Diazepam is structurally similar to tetrazepam but only one case report exists that show a cross-reactivity to diazepam after tetrazepam reaction. Other benzodiazepines may still be an option for patients that react to tetrazepam.

TRIAZOLAM

Infection Risk and Trauma

A retrospective cohort study in Japan was conducted to find the clinically relevant adverse effect of triazolam in an elderly population, specifically pneumonia, trauma, and pressure ulcers [15MC]. Due to increased risk of sedation and psychomotor performance impairment in the elderly, it is believed that the elderly population is at an increased risk of pneumonia due to aspiration, trauma possibly due to motor impairment and falls, and pressure ulcers may be from impairment of psychomotor performance leading to long-term confinement to a bed and malnutrition. Patients included in the study had used triazolam for ≥180 days in 2011 compared those that did not receive any hypnotics in that time period. Using variables for propensity score matching such as age, gender, primary disease, medications, and other clinical factors, the two groups were matched. After the propensity score matching, cohort 1 had over 13 000 patients, and cohort 2 had almost 13 000 patients. The results showed that triazolam users had an increased risk (after adjusting for all variables) for pneumonia by 40% (AOR=1.41, CI=1.31–1.52, $P<0.001$), trauma by 30% (AOR=1.30, CI 1.23–1.36, $P<0.001$), and pressure ulcer formation by almost 30% (AOR=1.29, CI=1.14–1.45, $P<0.001$). The authors concluded that physicians try cognitive behavioral therapy to manage insomnia in older patients instead of prescribing triazolam.

SEDATIVES

Cardiovascular

The use of opioids and sedatives can cause respiratory depression. A retrospective analysis was conducted to investigate the association of opioid therapy (with or without sedatives) and in-hospital cardiopulmonary resuscitation [16MC]. The cohorts were divided into received opioid and sedatives, opioid only, sedative only, and neither opioid or sedative. The highest incidence of cardiopulmonary resuscitation was in the opioids and sedatives together group compared to the other groups. It was associated with a 3.47-fold increase risk (95% CI = 3.40–3.54, $P < 0.0001$) compared to the opioid only group which was associated with 1.81-fold increase risk (95% CI = 1.77–1.85, $P < 0.0001$). The sedatives only group was found to have similar results as opioid only group. No specific sedative was implicated in the study.

DEXMEDETOMIDINE

Psychiatric

Postoperative delirium after a cardiac surgery can be as high as 50%, and the elderly population is at the greatest risk of developing postoperative delirium. There has been conflicting evidence about using dexmedetomidine in critically ill patients and the decreased risk of delirium. A large prospective, randomized control trial was conducted comparing dexmedetomidine and propofol-based postoperative sedation in elderly patients that underwent cardiac surgery [17C]. Patients received dexmedetomidine bolus of 0.4 µg/kg followed by a continuous infusion of 0.2–0.7 µg/kg/hour or propofol infusion 25–50 µg/kg/min. If the patient required more than 24 hours of intubation after surgery, the facility protocol was to switch dexmedetomidine to propofol. Both medications were titrated to achieve light sedation that was assessed using the Sedation Agitation Scale (SAS). Patients were evaluated perioperatively (baseline) and postoperatively at 12 hour intervals or as needed for the patient's condition for delirium. A total of 183 patients were analyzed, and postoperative delirium was present in 16 out of 91 patients in the dexmedetomidine group vs 29 out of 92 in the propofol group (OR = 0.46, 95% CI: 0.23–0.92, $P = 0.028$, NNT = 7.1) Dexmedetomidine use was also associated with delayed onset and shorter duration of delirium compared to propofol in patients that did get delirious postoperatively after a cardiac surgery.

KETAMINE

Neuromuscular Function

A case describes ketamine-induced muscle rigidity in the lower extremities in a 70-year-old female [18A]. The patient had a past medical history of end stage renal disease, renal transplant, diabetes, hypothyroidism, and osteoporosis. She required an orthopedic procedure for her right ankle fracture and received a 1.5 mg/kg (125 mg) IV ketamine dose. Two minutes after the IV ketamine, the patient began experiencing bilateral lower extremity muscle rigidity. The patient did not experience any muscle rigidity to the upper extremities, torso, neck,

or seizure-like activity. There were no changes in the patient's respiratory status. An injection of 2 mg midazolam mitigated the side effect. There are other case reports of ketamine-associated muscle rigidity but of the upper extremities. This is the first case of lower extremity rigidity after ketamine usage. The mechanism and true cause and effect relationship cannot be determined.

PEDIATRICS

Cardiovascular

There is an established correlation of ketamine-induced hypertension and tachycardia, yet there were no current studies reporting this effect in pediatric patients. A prospective study was conducted on pediatric patients presenting to the emergency department for orthopedic surgery [19c]. Sixty children were included in the study, but only 50 were included in the analysis. The average systolic blood pressure (SBP) was 130 mm Hg, average diastolic blood pressure (DBP) was 75 mm Hg, and average heart rate (HR) was 92 beats/min prior to procedures. During sedation, there was a statistically significant but modest increase in SBP (8 mm Hg higher), DBP (4 mm Hg higher) and HR (13 beats/min higher). There was a statistical difference of SBP (3 mm Hg) and DBP (4 mm Hg) during sedation compared to recovery. However, manipulation during the procedure increased SBP by 5 mm Hg and DBP by 7 mm Hg ($P < 0.001$). There is a possibility some of the changes are due to failure of ketamine dissociation, and the pain from manipulations may affect blood pressure change. This study demonstrates that compared to the adult population, pediatric population may have a milder increase in blood pressure and heart rate with ketamine use.

PROPOFOL

Susceptibility Factors: Sex

In a retrospective observation study in Japan, women needed higher infusion rates of propofol compared to men to achieve appropriate sedation for oral implant-related surgery [20C]. The authors looked at potential predictor variables such as age, sex, body weight, treatment time, and amount of midazolam when looking at the average infusion rate of propofol. The study had 125 patients (36 males, 89 females) and statistically found a difference that females required higher infusion rates (mean ± SD) of propofol (54.7 ± 19.8 µg/kg/min vs 44.1 ± 16 µg/kg/min). Conflicting study results show that women have lower plasma concentration levels of propofol compared to men, but the exact mechanism of why is not clear. The study cites weaknesses such as there are more females enrolled than men due to the hours of operation of the facility, and men were more likely to be working during the study time. It was also noted that females are more likely to want oral implant surgery than men. Continued research on gender differences with propofol and appropriate sedation will need to be continued, but important to note that this study showed that gender might affect the amount of drug infused to appropriately sedate patients.

References

[1] Schroek JL, Ford J, Conway EL, et al. Review of safety and efficacy of sleep medicine in older adults. Clin Ther. 2016;38(11):2340–72 [R].

[2] Parsaik AK, Mascarenhas SS, Khosh-Chashm D, et al. Mortality associated with anxiolytic and hypnotic drugs—a systematic review and meta-analysis. Aust N Z J Psychiatry. 2016;50(6):520–33 [M].

[3] Tom SE, Wickwire EM, Park Y, et al. Nonbenzodiazepine sedative hypnotics and risk of fall-related injury. Sleep. 2016;39(5):1009–14 [C].

[4] Pennington JG, Guina J. Eszopiclone-induced parasomnia with suicide attempt: a case report. Innov Clin Neurosci. 2016;13(9–10):44–8 [A].

[5] Tahir H, Saleemi MA, Wolfe C, et al. Acute delirium caused by single small dose of zolpidem. Am J Case Rep. 2016;4(4):137–9 [A].

[6] Hsu FG, Sheu MJ, Lin CL, et al. Use of zolpidem and risk of acute pyelonephritis in women: a population-based case-control study in Taiwan. J Clin Pharmacol. 2016;57(3):376–81 [MC].

[7] Lin SC, Su YC, Huang YS, et al. Zolpidem increased cancer risk in patients with sleep disorder: a 3-year follow-up study. J Med Sci. 2016;36(2):68–74 [MC].

[8] Chen L, Bell JS, Visvanathan R, et al. The association between benzodiazepine use and sleep quality in residential aged care facilities: a cross-sectional study. BMC Geriatr. 2016;16(1):196 [C].

[9] Bénard-Laribière A, Noize P, Pambrun E, et al. Comorbidities and concurrent medications increasing the risk of adverse drug reactions: prevalence in French benzodiazepine users. Eur J Clin Pharmacol. 2016;72(7):869–76 [MC].

[10] Gill R, Bhattacharjee D, Patil NA, et al. Clonazepam associated hypothyroidism: aforethought on a concealed dilemma. J App Pharm Sci. 2016;6(10):222–5 [A].

[11] Inverso G, Resnick CM, Gonzalez ML, et al. Anesthesia complications of diazepam use for adolescents receiving extraction of third molars. J Oral Maxillofac Surg. 2016;74(6):1140–4 [MC].

[12] Penninga EI, Graudal N, Ladekarl MB, et al. Adverse events associated with flumazenil treatment for the management of suspected benzodiazepine intoxication—a systematic review with meta-analyses of randomised trials. Basic Clin Pharmacol Toxicol. 2016;118(1):37–44 [M].

[13] Moj D, Hanke N, Britz H, et al. Clarithromycin, midazolam, and digoxin: application of PBPK modeling to gain new insights into drug–drug interactions and co-medication regimens. AAPS J. 2017;19(1):298–312. Epub 2016 Nov 7 [E].

[14] Huseynov I, Wirtz M, Hunzelmann N. Tetrazepam allergy: a case series of cutaneous adverse events. Acta Derm Venereol. 2016;96(1):110–1 [A].

[15] Maeda T, Babazono A, Nishi T, et al. Quantification of adverse effects of regular use of triazolam on clinical outcomes for older people with insomnia: a retrospective cohort study. Int J Geriatr Psychiatry. 2016;31(2):186–94 [MC].

[16] Overdyk FJ, Dowling O, Marino J, et al. Association of opioids and sedatives with increased risk of in-hospital cardiopulmonary arrest from an administrative database. PLoS One. 2016;11(2). e0150214 [MC].

[17] Djaiani G, Silverton N, Fedorko L, et al. Dexmedetomidine versus propofol sedation reduces delirium after cardiac surgery: a randomized controlled trial. Anesthesiology. 2016;124(2):362–8 [C].

[18] Vien A, Chhabra N. Ketamine-induced muscle rigidity during procedural sedation mitigated by intravenous midazolam. Am J Emerg Med. 2017;35(1). 200.e3–e4 [A].

[19] Patterson AC, Wadia SA, Lorenz DJ, et al. Changes in blood pressure and heart rate during sedation with ketamine in the pediatric ED. Am J Emerg Med. 2016;35(2):322–5 [c].

[20] Maeda S, Tomoyasu Y, Higuchi H, et al. Female patients require a higher propofol infusion rate for sedation. Anesth Prog. 2016;63:67–70 [C].

6

Antipsychotic Drugs

Pierre S. Chue*,1, Arno G. Siraki†

*Canadian Consortium for Early Intervention in Psychosis, University of Alberta, Edmonton, AB, Canada
†University of Alberta, Edmonton, AB, Canada
1Corresponding author: pierre.chue@epicanada.org

GENERAL [SEDA-15, 2438; SEDA-32, 83; SEDA-33, 39; SEDA-34, 51; SEDA-35, 85; SEDA-36, 59; SEDA-37, 63; SEDA-38; 35]

Comparative Studies

A 24-week, randomised controlled trial (RCT) in schizophrenia ($n=149$) with second-generation antipsychotics (SGAs) compared to first-generation antipsychotics (FGAs) found that there were more *adverse events* (*AEs*) with SGAs [1C]. *Weight gain* was significantly greater with SGAs, while the most common *AEs* for FGAs were *nervous system disorders*.

A RCT comparing brexpiprazole to aripiprazole in acute schizophrenia ($n=97$) found the incidence of *akathisia* to be 9.4% and 21.2%, respectively [2c].

A 6-month RCT comparing clozapine ($n=53$) to risperidone ($n=54$) in schizophrenia found that *salivation*, *sweating* and *tachycardia* were significantly greater with clozapine [3C].

A RCT in agitated schizophrenia ($n=80$) found greater *sedation* with olanzapine intramuscular (im) compared with aripiprazole im [4c].

A 24-week, RCT of aripiprazole compared to blonanserin ($n=46$) found the most common *AEs* (equal incidence) to be *anxiety*, *akathisia*, *insomnia* and *tremor* [5c].

A 5-day RCT in antipsychotic (AP)-naïve patients with acute psychosis ($n=60$) compared haloperidol im with levosulpiride im and found higher rates of *akathisia* and *extrapyramidal symptoms* (*EPS*) with haloperidol [6c].

A RCT comparing risperidone and olanzapine in schizophrenia ($n=71$) found no differences in *EPS* or *metabolic parameters*, but greater *prolactin elevation* with risperidone [7c].

An 8-week RCT in children and adolescents with tic disorder ($n=36$) found that *sedation* for twice weekly aripiprazole was half that of daily aripiprazole [8c].

Observational Studies

A study comparing aripiprazole to risperidone ($n=44$) for ADHD in children with autistic spectrum disorder (ASD) found increased *prolactin* levels with risperidone [9c].

A study of AP-naïve youth ($n=327$) found that discontinuation due to *sedation* was greatest with quetiapine followed by olanzapine, risperidone, and aripiprazole [10C]. Overall, higher rates of *activation* were noted with aripiprazole and lower rates with olanzapine; all APs reduced *insomnia* and increased *hypersomnia*.

A 36-month study in schizophrenia ($n=220$) reported *EPS* significantly more frequently with haloperidol compared with olanzapine, while *weight gain* was greater with the latter [11C].

A study of *AEs* in children ($n=184$) switched from risperidone to aripiprazole or a FGA found that 130 patients experienced an *AE*, which more prevalent with aripiprazole [12C].

A study of patients initiating quetiapine ($n=4658$), olanzapine ($n=5856$) or risperidone ($n=7229$) found quetiapine was associated with lower *EPS*, but higher *suicide attempt rates* compared to risperidone; and lower *EPS* and *DM* rates compared to olanzapine [13C]. A study ($n=18\,869$) of adults initiated on APs for any reason found that quetiapine was associated with more *emergency department mental and physical health event visits*, for all age groups [14C].

A study ($n=6671$) of bipolar disorder found that compared to lithium, there was more *weight gain* (>15%) with olanzapine and quetiapine, and more *hypertension* with olanzapine [15MC].

Systematic Reviews

A systematic review and meta-analysis (56 reports; $n=10\,177$) in schizophrenia found fluphenazine decanoate, haloperidol, haloperidol decanoate and tri-fluoperazine produced more *EPS* than olanzapine or quetiapine, while olanzapine was associated with more *weight gain* than other APs [16M].

A systematic review and meta-analysis (7 studies; $n = 1016$) of long-acting injectable (LAIs) APs in bipolar disorder found risperidone LAI was associated with a higher incidence of *prolactin-related AEs* than oral medication or placebo, and *weight gain* vs placebo [17M].

A systematic review and meta-analysis (5 studies; $n = 1022$) of LAIs in first episode psychosis (FEP) found that LAIs were associated with a higher incidence of at least 1 *AE*, and *tremor*, compared with oral APs [18M].

CARDIOVASCULAR

A study ($n = 3505$) found signals of disproportionate reporting for *Torsade de Pointes (TdP)-related events* for amisulpride, aripiprazole, haloperidol, olanzapine, risperidone, and a new signal for flupentixol [19MC].

Two studies ($n = 2411$; $n = 725$) evaluating *QTc prolongation* found that AP polypharmacy and cumulative dose increased risk, as well as haloperidol combined with antidepressants (ADs); aripiprazole was associated with a lower risk [20MC,21C].

A study in schizophrenia ($n = 147$) found significantly increased risks of developing *acute coronary syndrome* within the first 30 days for haloperidol and chlorpromazine (both duration-dependent), and aripiprazole (duration- and dose-dependent) [22C].

A study in schizophrenia and bipolar disorder ($n = 96$) treated with quetiapine, risperidone, olanzapine, or aripiprazole found an increase in *pulse wave velocity* (PWV), which is a marker of *arterial stiffness* and *arteriosclerosis* [23c].

A study ($n = 225$) found that olanzapine followed by clozapine, quetiapine and risperidone were associated with *QT prolongation* [24C]. However, a study ($n = 173$; 43% AP-naïve) of risperidone, olanzapine, quetiapine, and ziprasidone in acute psychosis found no statistically significant *QTc prolongation* with any AP [25C].

A study ($n = 18319$) did not find any difference in *cardiovascular disease* risk between olanzapine and either risperidone or quetiapine [26MC].

A study ($n = 216$) of AP-naïve or quasi-naïve children and adolescents found no differences in *QTc* between risperidone, olanzapine or quetiapine; only baseline overweight correlated with *QTc prolongation* [27C]. *Heart rate* decreased during follow-up, with the exception of quetiapine, compared with risperidone.

ELECTROLYTES

A study of patients (≥65 years) found that use of SGAs ($n = 58008$) compared to non-use ($n = 58008$) was associated with an increased risk of hospitalisation with *hyponatremia* within 30 days [28MC].

RESPIRATORY

A study in hospitalised schizophrenic patients with pneumonia ($n = 494$) found that only clozapine was associated with a risk for *recurrent pneumonia* vs controls; the risk was greater with higher dose, re-exposure to clozapine and for females [29C].

A study found that APs were associated with a higher risk of *pneumonia* in patients with ($n = 60584$) and without Alzheimer's disease ($n = 60584$); there was no difference between quetiapine, risperidone and haloperidol [30MC].

NERVOUS SYSTEM

A study of the Japanese Adverse Drug Event Report (JADER) database (370000 reports) found no significant differences in frequency or median time to onset of *EPS* between FGAs and SGAs [31MC]. Time to onset (cumulative incidence rate) was shortest for paliperidone and longest for olanzapine for the SGAs; and shortest for haloperidol and longest for chlorpromazine of the FGAs.

A study of *AP-related seizures* ($n = 288397$; 550 events) found FGAs had higher risk than SGAs in the first 12 months of treatment [32MC]. Clozapine, thioridazine, chlorprothixene, and haloperidol had higher risks than risperidone; aripiprazole had a slightly lower risk.

A study of patients with delirium ($n = 56$) found the most common *AE* was *QTc prolongation*, and the most severe AEs were with haloperidol [33c].

Two cases of *pica*, in a 44-year-old female on olanzapine and a 50-year-old female on risperidone, are reported [34A].

SENSORY SYSTEMS

A study ($n = 1274$) of *intraoperative floppy-iris syndrome* (IFIS) identified quetiapine, benzodiazepines and hypertension as risk factors for IFIS [35MC].

Three cases of *IFIS* with APs in a 39-year-old male, a 63-year-old male and a 65-year-old female are reported [36A].

PSYCHIATRIC

A study ($n = 495$) of patients with schizophrenia or bipolar disorder found serum concentrations risperidone and quetiapine was correlated with worse *verbal memory* and *verbal fluency* for [37C].

ℛ *Insomnia is prevalent in schizophrenia, and typically involves an increase of sleep latency (SL), and decrease in total sleep time (TST) and sleep efficiency (SE). Non-rapid-eye-movement (NREM) sleep, slow wave sleep (SWS) and rapid-eye-movement (REM) sleep latency are decreased, but REM sleep tends to remain unchanged.*

A review of the effects of SGAs on sleep variables found that quetiapine *increased SL, wake time after sleep onset* (WASO) and *REM sleep latency,* and *reduced SWS* and *REM sleep* patients with schizophrenia [38r].

A review of AP-induced *somnolence* classified clozapine as *high somnolence,* olanzapine, perphenazine, quetiapine, risperidone, ziprasidone as *moderate somnolence;* and aripiprazole, asenapine, haloperidol, lurasidone, paliperidone, cariprazine as *low somnolence* [39r].

A study of the WHO pharmacovigilance database (11 million reports) found an association between *sleep apneas* and quetiapine and clozapine for individual drugs, and for APs as a class [40MC].

ENDOCRINE

A study of aripiprazole, blonanserin, olanzapine, paliperidone, quetiapine, and risperidone ($n = 245$) found the greatest elevations of *macroprolactin* and *prolactin* with risperidone and paliperidone; *sexual dysfunction* was reported in 36%, but not correlated with total prolactin level [41C].

A study of psychiatric inpatients ($n = 1364$) found *hyperprolactinemia* was more likely to be associated with risperidone than clozapine or aripiprazole [42MC]. The frequency of *hyperprolactinemia* was 61.3%; 15.1% of patients reported moderately severe *breast symptoms* and *lactation,* and 53.9% reported moderate or severe *discomfort;* 30.4% of females reported moderate *menstrual changes* and 24.2% of males reported moderate *erectile dysfunction.*

A study of *bone mineral density* (BMD) in males with schizophrenia (18–55 years) on APs for 12 months found that *BMD* and *T-scores* were lower for prolactin-raising (*hyperprolactinemia* = 65.2%) APs vs prolactin-sparing (*hyperprolactinemia* = 15.8%) APs, and healthy controls, and were consistent with *osteopenia* [43c].

A systematic review (11 studies) of *prolactin-related AEs* in children with schizophrenia found that risperidone, olanzapine, and paliperidone were associated with increased *prolactin* levels [44M].

A systematic review and meta-analysis (13 studies, $n = 185\,105$) of youth exposed to APs found an increased cumulative *type 2 diabetes mellitus* (DM) risk compared with healthy controls and psychiatric controls; risk was associated with longer follow-up, olanzapine and male sex [45M].

A study of AP-associated *DKA* found the following cases: olanzapine ($n = 9$), aripiprazole ($n = 6$), risperidone ($n = 6$), clozapine ($n = 3$) and quetiapine ($n = 1$); 9 patients were diagnosed with *type 1 DM* [46M].

A 1-year study of patients with schizophrenia ($n = 300$) found no significant differences in the rate of metabolic syndrome (*MetS*) between aripiprazole, olanzapine, or haloperidol [47C].

A study of children and adolescents (2–17 years) exposed ($n = 4922$) to APs compared with non-exposed ($n = 299\,593$) found an increased prevalence of *antidiabetic* and *antilipidemic* medication use with AP use [48MC]. Risperidone and quetiapine users had lower odds than olanzapine users of receiving *antidiabetic* medication, but there were no differences between the odds of receiving *antilipidemic* medication among the different APs.

A chart review ($n = 273$) of patients initiated on a SGA in the ICU ($n = 50$) found 45% of patients experienced at least 1 *hyperglycemic* episode; 60% experienced multiple *hyperglycemic* episodes [49C]. Patients with a higher Acute Physiology and Chronic Health Evaluation II (APACHE II) score and females were significantly more likely to have multiple *hyperglycemic* episodes.

METABOLISM

A study in ASD found risperidone, aripiprazole, and olanzapine, but not ziprasidone and quetiapine, had a significant increase in *BMI* z-score; olanzapine had a significantly greater increase in *BMI* z-score compared to other APs [50c].

A study of psychiatric ($n = 121$) and general practice patients ($n = 80$) found olanzapine was associated with the lowest *BMI* and aripiprazole the highest *BMI*; thought to be due to channeling bias [51C].

A study ($n = 6517$) of adolescents in care found that quetiapine and clozapine increased the risk of morbid *obesity* more than 2.5 times, and polypharmacy increased the risk five times [52MC].

GASTROINTESTINAL

A study of psychiatric inpatients found that 80% of clozapine patients had a *colonic hypomotility* and *median colonic transit time* that was four times longer than any other AP (olanzapine, risperidone, paliperidone, aripiprazole, zuclopenthixol, haloperidol) [53C].

A study ($n = 20$) of colitis due to APs (cyamemazine, loxapine, haloperidol, alimemazine) requiring surgery found high *morbidity* with *transparietal necrosis* and *colonic perforation* and a *mortality rate* of 15% [54c].

LIVER

A 3-year study ($n = 191$) of *cardiometabolic risk* and *non-alcoholic fatty liver disease* in AP-naïve schizophrenia spectrum disorder treated with aripiprazole, risperidone, quetiapine, or ziprasidone found that 25.1% of subjects showed a *fatty liver index* (FLI) score ≥60, which is a predictor of *steatosis* [55C]. A FLI score ≥60 at endpoint was also associated with a ≥7% in *BMI*, increased *triglyceride* levels and *waist circumference*, decreased *HDL* levels, and *hypertension*.

PANCREAS

A review of 41 case reports of AP-related (olanzapine, risperidone, quetiapine, aripiprazole, ziprasidone) *acute pancreatitis* found an association with polypharmacy [56r].

MUSCULOSKELETAL

A study ($n = 1\,540\,915$) of AP-naïve elderly (≥65 years) found an association for all APs with *fractures* (highest in the first 30 days), which was greatest with haloperidol and least with chlorprothixene [57MC].

SEXUAL FUNCTION

A case of a 16-year-old male with intermittent *priapism* on risperidone, olanzapine and quetiapine, but not with amisulpride is reported [58A]. A case of *priapism* in a 13-year-old male with chlorpromazine, risperidone and methylphenidate, and also quetiapine and methylphenidate, is reported [59A].

TERATOGENICITY

A study of *congenital malformations* from the WHO Global Individual Case Safety Report (ICSR) database (1977–2014) detected signals of disproportionate reporting for *palate, oesophageal, and anorectal disorders* for phenothiazines with a piperazine side-chain, risperidone, and aripiprazole [60C].

SUSCEPTIBILITY FACTORS

A study ($n = 113$) of 202 single-nucleotide polymorphisms (SNPs) in 31 candidate genes in FEP treated with amisulpride, paliperidone, risperidone or ziprasidone found 4 SNPs in different genes (*DRD2, SLC18A2, HTR2A* and *GRIK3*) contributed significantly to the risk of *EPS* [61C].

A study ($n = 569$) of functional polymorphism of the prolactin (*PRL*) gene -1149 G/T (rs1341239) in schizophrenia found a significantly higher frequency of the G allele in patients with *hyperprolactinemia* [62C]. A systematic review and meta-analysis (15 studies; $n = 1485$) in schizophrenia found that *prolactin* levels were significantly higher in *DRD2* gene Taq1A A1 carriers [63M].

A study ($n = 722$) of patients with schizophrenia on SGA monotherapy found that the rs11654081 T-allele of the *SREBF1* gene was significantly associated with an increased risk for *MetS* [64C]. A study in schizophrenia of females ($n = 48$) on SGAs (risperidone, clozapine, quetiapine, olanzapine) investigated the association between the $-759C > T$ functional polymorphism of the *HTR2C* gene and *weight gain* [65c]. Patients ($n = 11$) with the T allele at position -759 (TT or CT) gained less *weight* vs patients without ($n = 37$).

Another 14-week study ($n = 218$) of patients with schizophrenia treated with clozapine or olanzapine and a 190 day replication analysis found 2 *HTR2C* SNPs (rs3134701 AA-genotype, rs12662510 AA-genotype) were nominally associated with *weight gain* in those of European ancestry [66C].

PREGNANCY

A study of major *congenital malformations* of APs ($n = 9991$) in early pregnancy ($n = 1\,341\,715$) did not find a significant risk overall; risperidone was associated with a small increased risk [67MC].

LACTATION

A systematic review (37 reports; $n = 206$) of APs in breastfeeding found *somnolence, irritability, tremor* and *insomnia* with olanzapine [68M]. Mild *neurodevelopmental delays* were reported with low-dose quetiapine (and concomitant ADs). *Agranulocytosis, drowsiness* and *delayed speech* were reported with clozapine (also with exposure in utero).

DEATH

A study ($n = 81\,313$) of patients prescribed APs reported the highest *mortality rates* were found with FGAs, followed by FGAs and SGAs (in combination), clozapine, and SGAs [69MC].

A study ($n=137\,713$) of new AP-users (≥ 65 years) reported a higher risk of *death* for haloperidol, levomepromazine, zuclopenthixol and melperone, compared with risperidone [70MC]. Levomepromazine and chlorprothixene were only associated with a higher risk of *death* in patients aged ≥ 80 years, and with dementia.

A study ($n=1544$) found that clozapine, olanzapine, and quetiapine were most frequently associated with *unintentional fatal poisoning* [71MC].

A study found that levomepromazine and chlorpromazine–promethazine–phenobarbital had a high risk of *fatal overdose* [72C].

A study of new initiations found that the *mortality rates* for chlorpromazine, haloperidol, quetiapine, and risperidone were 17.4%, 45.5%, 26.8%, and 25.9%, respectively; with the *mortality risk* for haloperidol being highest in the first 30 days [73C].

A study ($n=7877$) in Parkinson's disease found AP use was associated with more than twice the hazard ratio (HR) of *death* vs no use [74MC]. The HR was lower for SGAs vs FGAs; and lowest for quetiapine followed by risperidone and olanzapine.

A systematic review and meta-analysis (53 studies; $n=17\,416$) regarding *all-cause death* found no significant difference between LAIs (aripiprazole, fluphenazine, haloperidol, olanzapine, paliperidone, risperidone, zuclopenthixol) and placebo or oral APs [75M].

MONITORING THERAPY

A study of patients measuring drug concentrations and C-reactive protein (CRP) levels found *elevated levels of CRP* were significantly associated with clozapine and risperidone [76c].

INDIVIDUAL DRUGS

Amisulpride [SEDA-32, 92; SEDA-33, 99; SEDA-34, 60; SEDA-35, 85; SEDA-36, 59; SEDA-37, 67; SEDA-38, 38]

Controlled Studies

Two RCTs ($n=689$) of amisulpride intravenous (iv) compared to placebo for postoperative nausea and vomiting (PONV) found no differences in safety, and less *nausea* with amisulpride [77C].

Observational Studies

A 6-week, switch study ($n=37$) found that most common *AEs* included *insomnia* and *cognitive decline*, followed

by *dry mouth, headache,* and *constipation; weight* decreased significantly [78c].

An 8-week study ($n=316$) found that the most common *AEs* were *neurological (EPS, akathisia, dystonia),* followed by *hyperprolactinemia* [79C].

CARDIOVASCULAR

A RCT ($n=40$) of amisulpride iv found a plasma concentration-dependent effect on *QTc prolongation* [80c].

A case of *bradycardia* and *hypotension* in a 41-year-old female 10 days after commencing amisulpride is reported [81A].

NERVOUS SYSTEM

Two cases of *EPS* in a 30-year-old and a 48-year-old male are reported within 24 days of switching to amisulpride from olanzapine[82A].

HEMATOLOGIC

A case of *agranulocytosis* in a 47-year-old female on amisulpride for 2 years is reported [83A].

SUSCEPTIBILITY

A study of AP-naïve patients ($n=69$) found that *weight gain* was predicted by low baseline reward-related activity in the right-sided putamen; and predisposition for amisulpride-induced *weight gain* was due to reward activity in the dorsal striatum [84c].

A 12-week study ($n=185$) of 14 SNPs of the *COMT* gene found that *prolactin* increase was associated with the A-allele carriers of rs4680 [85C].

Aripiprazole [SEDA-32, 93; SEDA-33, 99; SEDA-34, 60; SEDA-35, 96; SEDA-36, 59; SEDA-37, 68; SEDA-38, 38]

Controlled Studies

A 12-week RCT ($n=622$) in schizophrenia found *metabolic-related AEs* occurred in 2.4%, 1.4%, and 2.4% of patients in the aripiprazole lauroxil 441 mg, aripiprazole lauroxil 882 mg, and placebo groups, respectively [86C].

Observational Studies

A study in FEP ($n=73$) found 44% experienced a >7% *weight gain* [87c]. A study in children and adolescents found that in patients ($n=14$) with non-psychotic disorders *AEs* included *sleep disturbance, parkinsonism, behavioral changes, hallucinations, dizziness* and *weight gain* [88c]. In patients ($n=5$) with psychotic disorders, *AEs* included *anxiety, convulsions*, and *neuroleptic malignant syndrome (NMS)*.

Systematic Reviews

A Cochrane review (3 studies) in ASD found increased *weight gain, sedation* and *tremor* vs placebo [89M]. A meta-analysis (10 studies, $n=302$) of children with Tourette's disorder (mean age = 11.6 years) found *drowsiness, nausea,* and *headache* were the most common *AEs* [90M]. Another systematic review and meta-analysis (6 studies, $n=528$) of children with Tourette's disorder found less *EPS* than haloperidol (1.5% vs 43.5%), and no difference in *nausea, vomiting, dizziness,* and *dry mouth* compared with tiapride [91M]. A meta-analysis (41 studies; $n=1446$) in children and adolescents found a mean *EPS* incidence of 17.1% with aripiprazole, which was significantly greater than placebo [92M].

CARDIOVASCULAR

A single-dose study ($n=157$) of *cardiovascular* effects in healthy volunteers found that aripiprazole decreased *BP* and increased *HR* and *QTc* [93C]. Subjects with higher AUC and higher plasma concentrations, and females experienced more *AEs*; the latter including more *gastrointestinal AEs*.

A case of 14-year-old male with *Raynaud's phenomenon* after 1 week on aripiprazole is reported [94A].

EAR, NOSE, THROAT

A case of 12-year-old male with factor VII deficiency who developed *nasal* and *gingival bleeding* with aripiprazole, but not haloperidol, is reported [95A].

NERVOUS SYSTEM

A study found an increased odds ratio for *EPS* (5242 cases; 50 532 controls) for aripiprazole as well as an increased risk of *dyskinesia* [96MC].

Two cases of *acute dystonia* in a 17-year-old male and a 13-year-old female switched to low-dose aripiprazole from atomoxetine are reported [97A]. A case of *dyskinesia* in a 53-year-old male after discontinuation of aripirazole is reported [98A].

A case of 17-year-old female who developed recurrent *hiccups* within a few hours of taking aripiprazole is reported [99A].

PSYCHIATRIC

A case of a 60-year-old male with bipolar disorder who developed *hypersexuality* with no features of mania, after 1 month on aripiprazole is reported [100A].

A case of *gambling* and *hypersexuality* in a 27-year-old male is reported [101A].

A case of a 32-year-old male who experienced increased *hallucinations* but improved *catatonia* is reported [102A].

ENDOCRINE

A study of psychiatric patients ($n=25$) found that 44% had decreased *prolactin* [103c].

METABOLISM

Three cases of *hyperlipidemia* in a 27-year-old male, 33-year-old male and 36-year-old male are reported [104A].

ELECTROLYTE BALANCE

A case of a 35-year-old female who developed *hyponatremia* after 1 month on aripiprazole is reported [105A].

HEMATOLOGIC

A case of a *transient morning pseudoneutropenia* in an 11-year-old male is reported [106A].

SKIN

A case of *cutaneous leukocytoclastic vasculitis* in a 28-year-old female 5 days after commencing aripiprazole is reported [107A].

Asenapine [SEDA-37, 69; SEDA-38, 39]

Controlled Studies

A RCT ($n=311$) in acute schizophrenia found higher incidences of *oral hypoesthesia* and *dysgeusia* with asenapine, and greater *weight gain* with olanzapine [108C].

A 6-week RCT ($n=532$) in acute schizophrenia reported more *EPS, akathisia* and *weight gain* for asenapine vs placebo [109C].

Observational Studies

A 50-week study ($n=321$) in pediatric patients with bipolar disorder found the most common *AE* was *somnolence/sedation/hypersomnia* (42.4%) followed by *oral hypoesthesia/dysgeusia* (7.5%); 34.8% experienced $\geq7\%$ weight gain [110C].

A 3-week study ($n=25$) in geriatric mania (>60 years) reported 7 discontinued due to *AEs* [111c].

Systematic Review

A systematic review and meta-analysis (8 studies; $n=3765$) found that asenapine caused less clinically significant *weight gain* or increases in *triglycerides* than olanzapine, but was more likely to cause *EPS* [112M].

NERVOUS SYSTEM

A case of a 17-year-old male who developed *acute dystonia* after 4 weeks on asenapine is reported [113A].

Brexpiprazole [SEDA-38, 40]

Observational Studies

A 6-week study ($n=61$) in major depressive disorder (MDD) found the most common *AE* was *fatigue* (14.8%); *akathisia* was reported by 8.2% of patients [114c].

A 12-week study of young adults with MDD found the most common *AEs* were *headache* (21.3%), *weight increase* (17.0%), and *somnolence* (17.0%), followed by *akathisia* (6.4%); *weight gain* ($\geq7\%$) occurred in 10.5% of patients [115c].

A 6-week study ($n=37$) of adjunctive treatment in MDD with anxiety symptoms found the most frequent *AEs* were *increased appetite* (13.5%) and *diarrhea, dry mouth*, and *dizziness* (all 10.8%) [116c].

A 16-week study ($n=49$) in FEP found the most common *AEs* were *insomnia* (14.3%), *somnolence* (8.2%), *sedation, weight increase*, and *nausea* (6.1%) [117c].

Review

A review of pooled safety data from 4 studies in schizophrenia did not find any reports of *AEs* with an incidence $\geq5\%$ and two times placebo in patients treated with brexpiprazole [118r]. In the long-term studies *AEs* ($\geq5\%$) included *schizophrenia* (10.7%), *insomnia* (8.0%), *weight increase* (7.7%), *headache* (6.0%), and *agitation* (5.2%). *Akathisia* rates were 5.8% and 4.6% in the short- and long-term studies, respectively; *sedation* rates were 2.3% and 0.9% in the short- and long-term studies, respectively, while mean *weight increase* was 1.1 kg in both short- and long-term studies.

Cariprazine (SEDA-38, 40)

Controlled Studies

A 6-week study of low-dose (1.5–4.5 mg/day) and high-dose (6–12 mg/day) cariprazine in acute schizophrenia found that the most common *AEs* ($\geq5\%$ and twice the rate of placebo) were *akathisia, restlessness, tremor, back pain*, and *EPS* [119C].

A long-term study (up to 97 weeks; $n=765$) in schizophrenia found that *akathisia* (19.2%), *insomnia* (14.4%), and *headache* (12.0%) were reported in $\geq10\%$ of patients, during open-label treatment (20 weeks; $n=264$) [120C].

An 8-week study ($n=571$) in bipolar depression found the most common *AEs* ($\geq10\%$) were *akathisia* and *insomnia; weight gain* was slightly higher with cariprazine than with placebo [121C].

An 8-week RCT ($n=819$) of adjunctive cariprazine treatment in MDD found *AEs* reported in $\geq10\%$ of patients on cariprazine included *akathisia* (22.3%), *insomnia* (13.6%), and *nausea* (12.8%) [122C].

Systematic Review

A meta-analysis (9 studies; $n=4324$) found that compared to placebo, cariprazine was associated with higher risk of *EPS* (*akathisia, tremor, restlessness*) and *weight gain*, but not *CVS-related* events [123M].

Chlorpromazine [SEDA-35, 85; SEDA-36, 59; SEDA-37, 69; SEDA-38, 40]

Systematic Review

A Cochrane review (71 studies) found significantly more *EPS* with chlorpromazine compared to quetiapine, but not compared to risperidone [124M].

SENSORY SYSTEMS

A case of a 66-year-old female with *pigmentary depositions* on both corneas after 13 years on chlorpromazine, but only detected when switched to olanzapine, is reported [125A].

DRUG–DRUG INTERACTIONS

A case of a 67-year-old male who developed severe *agranulocytosis* after concomitant chlorpromazine and trimethoprim–sulfamethoxazole is reported [126A].

Clozapine [SEDA-32, 94; SEDA-33, 102; SEDA-34, 6; SEDA-35, 99; SEDA-36, 59; SEDA-37, 69; SEDA-38, 40]

Observational Studies

A chart review (n = 37) in autistic and non-autistic children and adolescents found the most frequently observed AE was *hypersalivation* (54.1%); there was one case of *neutropenia* [127c].

A 2-year study (n = 316) found that 45% discontinued clozapine and AEs accounted for >50% of discontinuations; *sedation* was the most common AE [128C].

CARDIOVASCULAR

A study (n = 18) in schizophrenia found significant increases in *heart rate* and number of patients with *hypertension*, and a non-significant increase in *systolic BP* [129c]. Two cases of *pericarditis* in a 22-year-old and a 28-year-old female, detected by elevations of *pro-brain natriuretic peptide*, are reported [130A]. A case of 33-year-old male developing *myocarditis* after 18 days of clozapine, detected by an increase in *CRP* with *fever* and *tachycardia*, is reported [131A]. Another case of a male in his early 20s who experienced a *tachycardia*, 3 days and a *fever* 10 days, after clozapine initiation, but normal ECG and blood tests, is reported [132A]. On day 12, he collapsed and *myocarditis* was confirmed with an echocardiogram and with elevated *cardiac enzymes*. A case of a 57-year-old female who developed *fever* and elevated *CRP* (both dose-dependent) after 12 days on clozapine is reported [133A]. A case of *cardiac arrest* and *ventricular tachycardia* in a patient with long QT syndrome with clozapine and olanzapine is reported [134A]. Two cases of *myocarditis* are reported in a 22-year-old and a 41-year-old male with concurrent gastroenteritis [135A]. Another case in a 37-year-old male who developed *myocarditis* and positive influenza titre after 3 weeks of clozapine is reported [136A]. A case of a 20-year-old male who developed *myocarditis* after 11 days on clozapine, but was successfully rechallenged, is reported [137A]. A case of a 71-year-old male with *myocarditis*, after 11 days of clozapine, is reported [138A]. A case of a 50-year-old male who *died* from *myocarditis* after 15 days of clozapine, having received a total dose of 1625 mg, is reported [139A]. A case of *perimyocarditis* and *parenchymal lung disease* in a 23-year-old male after 7 days on clozapine is reported [140A]. A case of a 31-year-old female who developed *pulmonary embolism* after 18 days on clozapine is reported; she was successfully maintained on treatment [141A]. A case of a 40-year-old male who developed *pulmonary embolism* and *died* within 24 hours of reinstatement of clozapine is reported [142A]. A case of *cerebral venous thrombosis* in a Parkinson's disease patient with low-dose clozapine is reported [143A]. A case of a 40-year-old female with a dose-dependent *supraventricular tachycardia* with 2 separate trials of clozapine (concomitantly with olanzapine) is reported [144A].

RESPIRATORY

A case of a 26-year-old female who developed *necrotizing pneumonia* with elevated clozapine levels is reported [145A]. A case of a 56-year-old male who developed *aspiration pneumonia* after 13 days on clozapine is reported [146A]. A case of a 26-year-old male who developed *aspiration pneumonia* secondary to *sialorrhoea* after 5 days on clozapine is reported [147A].

NERVOUS SYSTEM

Two cases of *restless legs syndrome* (RLS) in a 32-year-old and a 45-year-old female on clozapine are reported [148A]. A case of a 67-year-old male who developed atypical *NMS*, diagnosed as a urinary tract infection, on clozapine is reported [149A].

A case of a 32-year-old male who developed *delirium* after 22 days of clozapine is reported, despite slow titration and previous long-term tolerability; a central *anticholinergic toxicity* was hypothesized [150A].

SENSORY SYSTEMS

A study of patients with schizophrenia and on clozapine (n = 30) found significantly decreased *tear production* and *corneal thickness* compared to healthy controls (n = 30) [151c].

PSYCHIATRIC

A study (n = 70) in schizophrenia found increased *OCD* and *OCS* with clozapine vs other SGAs [152c].

A case of a 42-year-old male with a worsening of *OCD*, misdiagnosed as psychosis, is reported [153A].

A 2-year observational study (n = 133) found that 64.7% of patients *slept ≥9 hours* daily; for monotherapy patients (n = 30) this correlated with norclozapine levels [154C].

ENDOCRINE

A study (mean follow-up = 12.3 years) of clozapine (≥5 years; n = 91) in schizophrenia vs matched controls

($n=91$) found a cumulative incidence of *new onset DM* of 22.3% [155c].

A case of *DKA* and *hypertriglyceridemia* is reported [156A].

A case of *pseudopheochromocytoma* is reported [157A].

METABOLIC

A 6-month study ($n=13$) of children and adolescents found a prevalence of *MetS* at baseline of 23%, which increased to 38.5% by 6 months [158c]. Other AEs included *hypersalivation* (100%) and (69%).

A case of 51-year-old female who lost 26% of her *body weight* (21 kg) after starting clozapine is reported [159A].

HEMATOLOGIC

A study in schizophrenia found 34 cases of *neutropenia* with clozapine ($n=201$; mean follow-up$=9.2$ years) [160C], of which 24 were mild (1500–1900 neutrophils/mm^3); of the more severe (500–1400/mm^3) 1 developed *agranulocytosis*. Patients on other APs ($n=410$) had an equal risk of neutropenia. An 18-week study ($n=55$) of patients initiated on clozapine found an incidence rate of *neutropenia* of 1.82%; there were no cases of *leukopenia* or *agranulocytosis* [161c]. A chart review ($n=26$) of patients with benign *neutropenia*, prior to receiving clozapine, found that there were fewer occurrences of mild and moderate *neutropenia* and no cases of severe *neutropenia* after clozapine initiation compared with prior [162c]. A study ($n=19$) of clozapine rechallenge after *neutropenia* or *leucopenia* found that one-third of patients developed a *blood dyscrasia*; occurring more rapidly but less severely [163c]. A chart review ($n=193$) of clozapine-treated patients who experienced a *leukopenic/neutropenic* event found that Caucasians, males and those aged 40–49 years had the most events [164C].

Case Reports
A case of a 28-year-old male who developed *eosinophilia* and successfully rechallenged is reported [165A]. A case of a 37-year-old male who developed late-onset *agranulocytosis* after 11 years on clozapine and successfully treated with granulocyte stimulating factor (GSF) is reported [166A]. A case of a 61-year-old male with *neutropenia* after 20 weeks of clozapine who developed *cellulitis* 4 days after recommencing clozapine against medical advice, is reported [167A]. Three cases of a 25-year-old, 44-year-old and a 51-year-old female developing *neutropenia* but successfully managed with concomitant lithium treatment are reported [168A]. A further case of a 42-year-old female who developed *neutropenia* that

responded to concomitant lithium treatment, but was unable to tolerate the lithium leading to discontinuation and recurrence of *neutropenia*, is reported [169A].

SALIVARY GLANDS

A study ($n=98$) in schizophrenia found that 92% had clozapine-induced *hypersalivation*; *nocturnal hypersalivation* was more prevalent compared to *daytime hypersalivation* and had a negative impact on *quality of life* in 15% [170c].

GASTROINTESTINAL

A meta-analysis (32 studies) found that the prevalence of *constipation* with clozapine was three times that of other APs and highest in inpatient settings [171M]. A case of an 18-year-old male with 20% body *weight loss* due to *dysphagia* is reported [172A]. A case of 58-year-old male who developed *esophagitis* is reported [173A]. A case of a 58-year-old female with *paralytic ileus*, which resolved with conservative management is reported [174A].

URINARY TRACT

A case of a 47-year-old female who developed refractory *urinary incontinence*, which responded to bethanechol and aripiprazole, is reported [175A].

HAIR

A case of a 38-year-old female with *alopecia areata monolocularis* associated with clozapine-induced *hypereosinophilia*, which resolved on discontinuation, is reported [176A].

IMMUNOLOGIC

A 5-year study of *selective immunoglobulin M immunodeficiency (SIgMD)* found an increased frequency of *SIgMD* among clozapine-treated patients [177C].

A case of a 39-year-old male who developed a life-threatening *lupus-like syndrome* 9 days after initiating clozapine is reported [178A]. A case of a 25-year-old male with previous history of clozapine-induced *myocarditis* who developed a *systemic inflammatory response* with *pyrexia*, *tachycardia* and elevated *C-reactive protein*, but no *eosinophilia* or *myocarditis* on rechallenge, is reported [179A]. A case of a 30-year-old male who developed a *systemic inflammatory response syndrome* 2 weeks after initiating clozapine, and successfully rechallenged, is reported [180A].

BODY TEMPERATURE

A 60-year-old male with *heat stroke*, initially diagnosed as *NMS*, is reported [181A].

SUSCEPTIBILITY FACTORS

A genome-wide association study found a significant association of the *HLA* B*59:01 (rs1800625) gene with clozapine-induced *agranulocytosis* ($n = 22$) and/or *granulocytopenia* ($n = 28$), vs healthy controls ($n = 2905$) [182MC]. Another genome-wide association study and a meta-analysis (cases $= 163$, controls $= 7970$) found associations with clozapine-induced *neutropenia* and rs149104283 (intronic to transcripts of *SLCO1B3* and *SLCO1B7*), variants in *UBAP2* and *STARD9*, and a variant in HLA-DQB1 [183MC]. A study ($n = 310$) of clozapine patients vs controls found that for *neutropenia* ($n = 38$), *ABCB1* 3435TT and homozygosity for *GSTT1*^{null} were more frequent; while for *agranulocytosis* ($n = 31$) *NQO2* 1541AA and *ABCB1* 3435TT were more frequent [184C]. Finally, a study of patients with previous clozapine-induced *agranulocytosis* ($n = 10$) found that the *ABCB1* all-variant haplotype (TT-TT-TT) was not present, in contrast to 12% of treated controls ($n = 91$) [185c].

A case of a 32-year-old male with *agranulocytosis* after 35 months of clozapine was hypothesized to be related to *HLA DR4* status [186A].

A cross-sectional study ($n = 60$) of patients on clozapine found *MetS* was significantly associated with clozapine level and *CYP2C19*2* and *LEPR* c.668 A/G and G/G alleles [187c]. A study found that obestatin may be involved in clozapine-induced changes in *glucose metabolism* [188c].

DRUG–DRUG INTERACTIONS

A case of a 59-year-old female with elevated *plasma clozapine/norclozapine ratio* after urinary tract infection treatment is reported. This was hypothesized to be due to cytokine upregulation of *α1-acid glycoprotein* and possibly cotrimoxazole inhibition of CYP2C9 [189A].

A case of 28-year-old female who experienced *fatal acute clozapine toxicity* 2 days after the addition of ciprofloxacin to clozapine (stable dose for 3 years) is reported [190A].

A case of a 43-year-old male stable for 8 months on clozapine who experienced *neutropenia* associated with concomitant topiramate therapy is reported [191A].

A systematic review ($n = 241$) of adjunctive fluvoxamine found decreased *metabolic AEs* hypothesized to be due to changes in clozapine: *N*-desmethylclozapine ratios [192M].

Droperidol [SEDA-36, 59; SEDA-37, 71; SEDA-38, 42]
Systematic Review

A Cochrane review (4 studies) found that droperidol did not cause more *cardiovascular arrhythmia* and *airway obstruction* than placebo, more *hypotension* than haloperidol, or more *respiratory hypoxia* than midazolam [193M].

Fluphenazine [SEDA-37, 71]
Systematic Review

A Cochrane review of fluphenazine (4 studies; $n = 202$) found that more people required concomitant *anticholinergic* medication compared to amisulpride, but there was no difference in incidence of *akathisia* compared to olanzapine [194M].

Haloperidol [SEDA-35, 107; SEDA-36, 59; SEDA-37, 72; SEDA-38, 42]
Observational Study

A study ($n = 101$) of acutely agitated psychiatric patients found 2 cases of *acute dystonia* following haloperidol short-acting injections [195C].

NERVOUS SYSTEM

Two cases of *acute dystonia*, in a 49-year-old female and a 29-year-old male, following single exposure to haloperidol, are reported [196A]. A case of a 37-year-old female who developed *NMS* 2 months after the addition of haloperidol to clozapine is reported [197A].

DEATH

Two cases of *sudden death* following high-dose haloperidol, in a 27-year-old male and a 42-year-old female (also given ziprasidone and paliperidone palmitate), are reported [198A].

DRUG–DRUG INTERACTIONS

A case of a 27-year-old male with head injury who developed *inappropriate antidiuretic hormone syndrome* (*SIADH*) with high-dose haloperidol (and quetiapine) is reported [199A].

Iloperidone [SEDA-33, 103; SEDA-35, 109; SEDA-36, 59; SEDA-37, 72; SEDA-38, 43]

Comparative Study

A RCT ($n = 303$) of relapse-prevention found the most common *AEs* included *dizziness* (11.6%), *somnolence* (8.3%), and *dry mouth* (6.8%); rates of *EPS* or *akathisia* were 2.5% and 3.7%, respectively [200C].

NERVOUS SYSTEM

Two cases of a 55-year-old and a 54-year-old male who developed *tardive dyskinesia* after 3 months and 7 months, respectively, are reported [201A].

SEXUAL FUNCTION

A case series of 5 males (19–34 years) experiencing *dry orgasms* with iloperidone, attributed to α1-adrenergic receptor antagonism, is reported [202A].

LEVOSULPIRIDE [SEDA-37, 72; SEDA-38, 43]

Nervous System

A case series of 6 patients (4 males; 2 females; mean age 68.7 years) treated with levosulpiride for dyspepsia (3 in combination with a proton pump inhibitor) who developed *parkinsonism*, is reported [203A]. A case of 78-year-old female who developed *parkinsonism and neck flexion (dropped head)* is reported [204A]. A case of 63-year-old female who developed *hemichorea* is reported [205A].

Lurasidone [SEDA-37, 72; SEDA-38, 43]

Controlled Studies

In a 6-week RCT of lurasidone ($n = 180$) or placebo ($n = 176$) added to a mood stabiliser for bipolar depression, the most frequent *AEs* ($\geq$5% of patients) were *akathisia, somnolence, EPS, nausea* and *diarrhea* [206C]. In a RCT for relapse prevention ($n = 676$) in schizophrenia the most

common *AEs* ($\geq$10% of patients) were *akathisia, headache* and *nausea* [207C]. In a 6-week RCT of lurasidone ($n = 109$) vs placebo ($n = 100$) in MDD with mixed features, the most frequent *AEs* ($\geq$5% of patients) were *somnolence* and *nausea* [208C]. A 6-week RCT of lurasidone ($n = 50$) vs placebo ($n = 49$) in young patients (6–17 years) with ASD found the most common *AEs* ($\geq$5% of patients) were *vomiting* and *somnolence* [209c].

Observational Studies

In a 22-month study ($n = 251$) in schizophrenia, *AEs* in $\geq$10% of patients included *schizophrenia, akathisia,* and *somnolence;* and 19.2% reported at least one *movement disorder-related AE* [210C]. In a post-hoc analysis of two 6-week RCTs ($n = 142$) in older adults ($\geq$55 years) with bipolar depression the most common *AEs* ($\geq$10% of patients) were *nausea* and *somnolence* in the monotherapy group, and *akathisia* and *insomnia* in the adjunctive group [211C]. In a 24-week study ($n = 813$) in patients with bipolar depression the most frequent *AE* ($\geq$10% of patients) reported was *parkinsonism* [212C]. A study ($n = 49$) in patients with treatment resistant bipolar disorder reported *overactivation* (*insomnia, irritability, agitation, anxiety*) as the most common *AE* [213c].

NERVOUS SYSTEM

A case of a 71-year-old female who developed *RLS* after switching from aripiprazole is reported [214A].

DRUG–DRUG INTERACTION

A case of an atazanavir-precipitated *drug–drug interaction* that led *to elevated serum concentrations* of lurasidone is reported [215A].

Olanzapine [SEDA-32, 99; SEDA-33, 104; SEDA-34, 66; SEDA-35, 108; SEDA-36, 59; SEDA-37, 73; SEDA-38, 43]

Controlled Studies

A 6-week, RCT ($n = 210$) in bipolar depression reported significant mean *weight increase, total* and *LDL-cholesterol* and proportion of patients with *weight gain* ($\geq$7%) for olanzapine (24.1%) vs placebo (1.4%) [216C].

Observational Studies

A 52-week study of youth (13–17 years) with schizophrenia or bipolar disorder on olanzapine receiving either standard ($n = 101$) or intense weight counseling ($n = 102$) [217C]. In the standard group: *weight* and *BMI* increased by +12.1 kg and +3.6 kg/m^2, respectively, and 40% had *weight gain* $\geq$15%; and in the intense group by +9.6 kg and +2.8 kg/m^2, respectively, and 33% had *weight gain ≥15%*.

A study comparing olanzapine iv ($n=289$) to im ($n=485$) found *respiratory depression* occurred in 3.7% and 2.0%, and *non-respiratory complications* in 2% and 0.4%, in the respective groups [218C]. Two patients in the former and 5 patients in the latter group required *intubation*; there were 2 episodes of *bradycardia* were noted.

A retrospective study ($n=713$) of olanzapine iv reported 3 *intubations* "likely or possibly" related to olanzapine [219C].

Systematic Review

In a systematic review (7 studies) of olanzapine in PONV the most common AEs were *fatigue, drowsiness,* and *disturbed sleep* [220M].

CARDIOVASCULAR

Two cases of a 36-year-old and a 39-year-old male and *sudden death* due to *eosinophilic myocarditis* after olanzapine (high-dose) are reported [221A]. A case of a 28-year-old male who developed *dilated cardiomyopathy* with *eosinophilia* after 10 years of olanzapine is reported [222A].

NERVOUS SYSTEM

A case of a 17-year-old male with anorexia who developed *NMS* within 48 hours of initiating olanzapine is reported [223A]. A case of a 47-year-old male with history of seizures who developed repetitive *focal motor seizures* and *lingual dystonia*, after olanzapine was added, is reported [224A]. A case of a female in her 60s with hepatitis C and cirrhosis who developed *catatonia*, after being switched from sertraline and paliperidone, to olanzapine is reported [225A]. A case of a 42-year-old male who developed *stuttering* after 4 days of olanzapine is reported [226A].

Three cases including a 33-year-old male, 53-year-old female and 48-year-old male, who developed *OCS* after 3, 2 and 10 years, respectively, on olanzapine, are reported [227A].

A case of a 57-year-old female who developed *postinjection delirium syndrome (PDSS)* after 2 years on olanzapine LAI is reported [228A]. A case of a 32-year-old female who developed *PDSS* within 20 minutes of her 8th injection of olanzapine LAI is reported [229A]. A case of a 56-year-old male treated for 3 years who developed severe *PDSS* with olanzapine LAI is reported [230A].

A case of a 34-year-old male switched from risperidone who developed *camptocormia* is reported [231A].

HEMATOLOGIC

A case of a 32-year-old female who developed *thrombocytopenia* after 6 weeks of olanzapine is reported [232A]. A case of a 40-year-old female who developed *eosinophilia* after 2 weeks on olanzapine is reported [233A].

METABOLIC

A case of 66-year-old male who developed *hypertriglyceridemia* resulting in *necrotizing pancreatitis* after 6 weeks of olanzapine is reported [234A].

GASTROINTESTINAL

A case of a 38-year-old male with severe *ischemic colitis* requiring surgery after 5 years treatment with olanzapine (concomitant medications included melperone and biperiden) is reported [235A]. Another case of 38-year-old female who developed *ischemic colitis* after 4 months on olanzapine (added to quetiapine) is reported [236A].

MOUTH AND TEETH

A case of 70-year-old male with *black hairy tongue* after 2 months with olanzapine (and fluoxetine) is reported [237A].

ENDOCRINE

A study ($n=35$) of a 2-hour oral glucose tolerance test (OGTT) in olanzapine-treated nondiabetic patients with schizophrenia or schizoaffective disorder found 7 cases of*DM* [238c].

Case Reports

A case of a 38-year-old female who developed a *splenial lesion syndrome, hyperosmolar hyperglycemic state* and *NMS* after 4 months on olanzapine is reported [239A]. A case of a 45-year-old male who developed *DKA* after 3 months on olanzapine is reported [240A]. A case of elevation of *amylase* and *lipase* is reported [241A]. A case of a 27-year-old pregnant female with life-threatening *DKA* at 28 weeks gestation after 8 weeks of olanzapine is reported [242A].

MUSCULOSKELETAL

A case a 62-year-old male of *delayed-onset rhabdomyolysis* after 2 years on olanzapine is reported [243A].

SUSCEPTIBILITY FACTORS

In a 3-day study of healthy subjects with a genotype of *TCF7L2* rs7903146 CC ($n = 10$) or CT ($n = 7$), olanzapine caused *body weight gain, increased triglycerides* and *uric acid, reduced HDL-cholesterol, decreased total protein, albumin* and *hemoglobin* in both groups (CC group had lower *triglycerides* than CT at baseline) [244c]. The CT group had a greater *insulin* $AUC_{0-2\,hour}$ during OGTT compared to the CC group, before and after olanzapine treatment. *Uric acid* levels were increased and *HDL-C* was decreased with olanzapine, but neither was significantly associated with TCF7L2 genotype.

Another study in healthy subjects treated with olanzapine found low *TSH* levels were associated with *weight* gain, and greater *weight* reduction with adjunctive topiramate [245c].

A study in schizophrenia ($n = 31$) of olanzapine monotherapy (≤ 12 months) reported a mean increase in *BMI* of 2.1 ± 2.7 kg/m^2; there was a negative correlation with baseline *leptin* levels in female patients [246c].

BODY TEMPERATURE

A case of *fever* is reported [247A].

Paliperidone [SEDA-33, 108; SEDA-35, 85; SEDA-36, 59; SEDA-37, 74; SEDA-38, 44]

Controlled Studies

In a 15-month RCT ($n = 444$) in schizophrenia comparing paliperidone LAI to oral FGAs and SGAs, the incidence of *EPS* was lowest for oral paliperidone/risperidone, followed by oral SGAs, paliperidone LAI and oral FGAs [248C]. The incidence of *prolactin-related AEs* was lowest for oral SGAs and for oral paliperidone/risperidone, followed by oral FGAs, and highest with paliperidone LAI. The incidence of $\geq 7\%$ *weight increase* was lowest for the oral FGAs, followed by oral SGAs, oral paliperidone/ risperidone, and highest with paliperidone LAI.

In a 48-week RCT comparing paliperidone LAI 1-monthly and 3-monthly the most common AE was *weight gain* (equal incidence = 21%) [249C].

Observational Studies

In an 8-week study ($n = 75$) of paliperidone ER in FEP the most frequent *AEs* were *akathisia, somnolence, anxiety,* and *sedation*. There were modest increases in *weight* and *lipids* and significant increases in *prolactin* levels [250c].

In a 6-month study ($n = 667$) of paliperidone LAI in schizoaffective disorder the most common *AEs* were *akathisia, injection-site pain,* and *insomnia* [251C].

In a study ($n = 396$) of patients switched from olanzapine to paliperidone ER there was a significant decrease

in *EPS* and average *weight* decreased by 0.8 ± 5.2 kg; $\geq 7\%$ *weight gain* occurred in 8.0% of patients [252C].

In a 24-week study ($n = 106$) in schizophrenia the most common *AEs* reported with paliperidone ER were *akathisia, somnolence, nasopharyngitis,* and *constipation* [253C]; 1 patient had worsening of *psychosis* and 1 completed *suicide*.

CARDIOVASCULAR

A case of a 23-year-old female who developed severe *tachycardia* but no *QTc* changes, after an overdose of paliperidone ER, is reported [254A].

NERVOUS SYSTEM

A case of 37-year-old male who developed *pisa syndrome* after 3 months with paliperidone ER is reported [255A]. A case of a 22-year-old male who developed *tardive dyskinesia* and *dystonia* after 1.5 years on paliperidone LAI is reported [256A]. Another case of a 28-year-old female who developed *tardive dystonia*, after 10 months of paliperidone LAI, is reported [257A].

A case of a 28-year-old female who developed *catatonia*, after 6 weeks with paliperidone ER, is reported [258A].

A case of 61-year-old male who developed *NMS* with paliperidone LAI, after being switched from risperidone, is reported [259A]. A case of a 35-year-old male who developed *NMS, SIADH* with *seizures*, and *rhabdomyolysis* 2 days after paliperidone LAI is reported [260A].

A case of a 90-year-old male with dementia who developed *delirium* after 3 days of aliperidone ER is reported [261A]. A case of a 17-year-old female who developed *serotonin syndrome* with paliperidone ER and recurrence with re-exposure) is reported [262A].

ENDOCRINE

In a RCT in schizophrenia of females with *prolactin* elevation after 4 weeks with oral risperidone or paliperidone ($n = 60/66$), those subsequently randomised to 4 weeks with add-on aripiprazole experienced a *prolactin* decrease [263c].

A 12-month study ($n = 22$) in patients switched from risperidone LAI or 1 paliperidone ER to paliperidone LAI found no change in *prolactin* levels, except in males switched from risperidone LAI who showed a decrease [264c]. A case of a 15-year-old male who developed *hyperprolactinaemia, tremors, weight gain,* and *impaired fasting glycaemia* with paliperidone ER (reversed with bromocriptine), is reported [265A].

METABOLIC

A 12-month study ($n = 60$) of paliperidone LAI found that the proportion of patients with *MetS* at baseline did not significantly change at endpoint (33% vs 29.5%) [266c]. There was a slight but significant increase in *BMI* and of *waist circumference; weight gain* occurred in 15% of patients.

A case of a 41-year-old female who developed *hypoglycemia* on paliperidone ER and DM after discontinuation is reported [267A].

HEMATOLOGIC

A case of a 50-year-old female who developed *leukopenia* and *neutropenia* with paliperidone ER, treated with lithium, is reported [268A].

GASTROINTESTINAL

A case of a 38-year-old male who developed *ileus* with paliperidone LAI and biperiden, and previous history of ileus, is reported [269A].

URINARY TRACT

A case of a 26-year-old female with *urinary incontinence* after initiating paliperidone LAI is reported [270A].

SKIN

A case of a 24-year-old male who developed *toxic epidermal necrolysis* with paliperidone LAI, after successful tolerability of paliperidone ER, is reported [271A].

SEXUAL FUNCTION

A case of *retrograde ejaculation* with paliperidone LAI is reported [272A].

DEATH

A review of patients treated with paliperidone LAI in Japan ($n = 10962$) identified 32 cases of *death* [273MC]. This elevated *mortality rate* was attributed to factors including the reporting program, age (>50 years), greater physical and cardiovascular comorbidity and polypharmacy.

DRUG–DRUG INTERACTIONS

In a 6-month PK study, the *bioavailability* of paliperidone ER was increased by an estimated 51% (*Cmax*) and 51%–52% (*AUCs*) when coadministered with sodium divalproex ER [274c].

Prochlorperazine [SEDA-35, 85; SEDA-36, 59; SEDA-37, 74; SEDA-38, 45]

Systematic Review

In a systematic review and meta-analysis (49 studies, $n = 758$) of prochlorperazine in children the most common *AEs* reported were *EPS* and *sedation* [275M]. Serious *AEs* were rarely associated with prochlorperazine use in children; 5 *fatalities* were reported (no causal relationship established).

Quetiapine [SEDA-32, 104; SEDA-33, 110; SEDA-34, 69; SEDA-35, 85; SEDA-36, 59; SEDA-37, 74; SEDA-38, 45]

Controlled Studies

A 12-week, RCT ($n = 119$) of quetiapine IR in PTSD found the most common *AEs* were *dry mouth, somnolence* and *sedation* [276C].

An 8-week RCT ($n = 279$) of quetiapine XR in bipolar depression reported *somnolence, dizziness, dry mouth, constipation* and *fatigue* were the most common *AEs* vs placebo [277C]. An 8-week, RCT ($n = 23$) of quetiapine XR in MDD with GAD reported *somnolence, dizziness, dry mouth, constipation* and *fatigue* as the most common *AEs* [278c].

Observational Study

A study in older (>65) patients ($n = 1784$) found the most frequent *AEs* were *nervous system disorders*, followed by *psychiatric disorders, abnormal investigations* and *general disorders*, and *gastrointestinal* and *skin disorders* [279MC]. *Hyponatremia, decreased mobility, orthostatic hypotension* and *swollen tongue* were significantly greater in older than younger patients. *Skin* and *subcutaneous tissue disorders* and *hepatobiliary disorders* were more common in younger patients.

Systematic Review

A systematic review (69 studies) in older adults found the most common *AEs* to be *somnolence* (25%–39%), *dizziness* (15%–27%), *headache* (10%–23%), *postural hypotension* (6%–18%) and *weight gain* (11%–30%) [280M]. Quetiapine was associated with significantly greater *cognitive impairment, falls* and *injury* and *mortality* in patients with parkinsonism, but not in patients with dementia, compared with placebo. Quetiapine had a significantly lower risk of *mortality*, *metabolic disorders* and *cerebrovascular events* and increased *falls* and *injury* compared with olanzapine; but higher risk of *metabolic disorders* compared with risperidone.

CARDIOVASCULAR

A study ($n = 94$) evaluating *heart rate variability (HRV)* in psychiatric patients found that quetiapine caused a decrease in *HRV*, in combination with an AD [281c]. Another study ($n = 40$) in healthy volunteers found that quetiapine IR and escitalopram caused dose-dependent *QT prolongation* [282c].

Case Reports

A case of 53-year-old male with dose-dependent *QTc prolongation* with quetiapine (also on citalopram) is reported [283A]. A case of 32-year-old pregnant female who developed *QTc prolongation* (515 ms) after ingesting 6000 mg of quetiapine is reported; mother and fetus survived [284A]. A case of a 37-year-old female who developed *cardiomyopathy* is reported [285A]. A case of 62-year-old male with an inferior-lead *brugada-like ECG* with quetiapine (also on citalopram) is reported [286A]. A case of 72-year-old male who developed *symptomatic bradycardia* and *hypotension* after 1 month on quetiapine [287A].

NERVOUS SYSTEM

A case of 67-year-old female with Parkinson's disease who developed *NMS* within 24 hours of starting quetiapine is reported [288A]. The patient received 1 injection of haloperidol and subsequently *died* from *multiorgan failure*. Another case of *NMS* with quetiapine after withdrawal of olanzapine and donepezil is reported [289A].

A case of a 73-year-old female with dementia who developed *seizures* after initiation of quetiapine (and sertraline is reported) [290A].

A case of a 46-year-old male with dementia who developed *RLS* within 24 hours of a dose increase of quetiapine (also on escitalopram and lithium started 3 weeks prior) is reported [291A]. Another case of a patient developing *RLS* after 1 dose of quetiapine is reported [292A].

PSYCHIATRIC

A case of a 55-year-old female who developed *REM sleep behavior disorder*, within 1 week of initiating quetiapine, is reported [293A].

ELECTROLYTE BALANCE

A case of a 65-year-old female who developed *SIADH* presenting as *seizures* after 3 months of quetiapine is reported [294A].

HEMATOLOGIC

A case of a 24-year-old male who developed *thrombotic thrombocytopenic purpura* after initiating quetiapine (also on lithium and oxcarbazepine) is reported [295A]. A case of a 69-year-old male who developed *neutropenia* and *thrombocytopenia* due to quetiapine-induced *bone marrow* suppression is reported; 21 case reports of quetiapine-induced *blood dyscrasias* (1998–2015) are also reviewed [296A].

MOUTH

A case of a 65-year-old female who developed *edema* of her upper lip 24 hours after initiating quetiapine is reported [297A].

PANCREAS

A case of a 42-year-old male with *DM* who experienced 5 episodes of *hypertriglyceridemia-induced pancreatitis* and worsening of his *DM* is reported [298A].

SKIN

A case of a 68-year-old female who developed *cutaneous vasculitis* following initiation of quetiapine is reported [299A]. A case of a 61-year-old male who developed an *interstitial granulomatous cutaneous reaction*, after 1 month of quetiapine, is reported [300A].

IMMUNOLOGIC

A 6-week study ($n = 27$) in schizophrenia found quetiapine response correlated with increased *CD3+* and *CD16+* *lymphocytes*, and a decrease in *IgA* levels [301c].

A case of a 36-year-old male who developed *angioedema* after 3 days on quetiapine is reported [302A]. A case of a 34-year-old female who developed *pedal edema* is reported [303A].

DRUG–DRUG INTERACTIONS

A study ($n=101$) in acquired brain injury found the incidence of *neutropenia* was significantly higher in those receiving quetiapine and valproate in combination, than those receiving monotherapy [304C].

Risperidone [SEDA-32, 107; SEDA-33, 111; SEDA-34, 70; SEDA-35, 85; SEDA-36, 59; SEDA-37, 75; SEDA-38, 46]

Controlled Studies

An 8-week RCT ($n=101$) of children with ASD (5–17 years) found no difference in mean *QTc* change between risperidone and placebo [305C].

In an 8-week RCT of once-monthly risperidone subcutaneous injection (RBP-7000) in schizophrenia the most frequently reported *AEs* compared with placebo were *somnolence*, *weight gain*, and *akathisia* [306C].

Observational Studies

A study of adult females treated with APs (2006–2012) found no evidence of increased *breast cancer* risk for risperidone ($n=22\,908$) compared with SGAs ($n=24\,524$) or FGAs ($n=844$) [307MC].

In a study of risperidone LAI in schizophrenia the most frequently reported *AEs* were *injection site pain, somnolence/sedation*, and *anxiety*; 33% of patients experienced *prolactin* increase [308c].

Systematic Review

A Cochrane review (15 studies; $n=2428$) found greater *EPS* than placebo [309M].

CARDIOVASCULAR

A case of a 40-year-old female who developed *benign intracranial hypertension* causing *visual loss* after 12 months on risperidone is reported [310A].

RESPIRATORY

A case of acute *respiratory distress* in an adolescent with ASD is reported [311A].

NERVOUS SYSTEM

A case of a 44-year-old male who developed *Meige's syndrome* after 1 year on risperidone, which improved after switching to paliperidone, is reported [312A].

EYES

A case of a 27-year-old male who developed *bilateral cataracts* is reported [313A]. A case of a 28-year-old female who developed *xanthopsia* after 2 days on risperidone is reported [314A].

PSYCHIATRIC

A case of a 16-year-old female who developed a *sleep-related eating disorder* after 3 days on risperidone is reported [315A].

ENDOCRINE

A 1-year RCT ($n=374$) of female patients with schizophrenia found 15.8% of *prolactin-related symptoms* at baseline; these decreased over the study correlated with dose reduction [316C]. A study ($n=103$) of children and adolescents with ASD found *prolactin* levels were significantly correlated with 9-hydroxyrisperidone levels, especially in those with *hyperprolactinaemia* [317C].

A case of severe *hypoglycemia* is reported [318A].

MOUTH AND TEETH

A case of an 11-year-old male who developed *gingival bleeding* after 1 week on risperidone, following dose increase, is reported [319A].

BLADDER

A case of a 28-year-old male who developed dose-dependent *nocturnal enuresis* after several weeks on risperidone, and responding to reboxetine, is reported [320A].

SEXUAL FUNCTION

A case of 12-year-old male who developed *priapism* after initiating risperidone is reported [321A].

BODY TEMPERATURE

A case of 75-year-old female who developed *hypothermia* leading to *cardiac arrest* is reported [322A]. A case of mild *hypothermia* in a child with low-dose risperidone is reported [323A].

SUSCEPTIBILITY FACTORS

A study ($n = 201$) of *ABCB1* gene polymorphisms in schizophrenia treated with risperidone or paliperidone found C allele carriers of rs1128503 and GT/GA carriers of rs2032582 had a higher total *EPS* incidence rate than TT carriers and other genotype carriers (AA/GG/AT/TT) [324C]. The *tremor* incidence rate was higher in C-G-C haplotype carriers (rs1045642–rs2032582–rs1128503) than in non-carriers. C allele (CT+CC) carriers of rs2235048 had a smaller degree of *prolactin* increase, and T-A-T haplotype (rs1045642–rs2032582–rs1128503) carriers had lower *prolactin* levels.

In a study ($n = 147$) in children and youth (3–19 years) with ASD treated with risperidone the median *prolactin* level in patients with *DRD2* Taq1A A2A2 was significantly higher than A1A2 and A1A1 [325C].

A study of patients with ($n = 97$) and without ($n = 398$) *AEs* found a relationship between 9-hydroxyrisperidone and *AEs*, but not with risperidone or active moiety (risperidone + 9-hydroxyrisperidone) [326C]. However, another study found an association of *EPS* with the active moiety, but not with risperidone or 9-hydroxyrisperidone [327C].

DRUG–DRUG INTERACTIONS

A case of a 53-year-old male who developed *neurotoxicity*, *nephrotoxicity* and *NMS-like symptoms* with risperidone added to lithium, and re-occurring on rechallenge, is reported [328A].

Ziprasidone [SEDA-32, 111; SEDA-33, 114; SEDA-34, 74; SEDA-35, 85; SEDA-36, 59; SEDA-37, 75; SEDA-38, 47]

Controlled Studies

An 8-week RCT ($n = 139$) of adjunctive ziprasidone to escitalopram in adults with MDD found a significantly increase in global *akathisia* scores and *weight*, and a non-significant increase in *QTc* vs placebo [329C].

PSYCHIATRIC

A case of a 28-year-old male who developed *sleep walking* and *sleep eating* after 6 months on ziprasidone, and after a dose increase, is reported [330A].

HYPERSENSITIVITY

A case of a 38-year-old male who developed *Kounis syndrome* (*type 1*) with ziprasidone im is reported [331A].

A case of an 89-year-old female who developed subacute cutaneous *lupus erythematosus* after 4 weeks on ziprasidone is reported [332A].

Acknowledgements

The authors thank Jonathan D. Chue BSc for his editorial assistance.

References

[1] Gründer G, Heinze M, Cordes J, et al. Effects of first-generation antipsychotics versus second-generation antipsychotics on quality of life in schizophrenia: a double-blind, randomised study. Lancet Psychiatry. 2016;3(8):717–29 [C].

[2] Citrome L, Ota A, Nagamizu K, et al. The effect of brexpiprazole (OPC-34712) and aripiprazole in adult patients with acute schizophrenia: results from a randomized, exploratory study. Int Clin Psychopharmacol. 2016;31(4):192–201 [c].

[3] Schooler NR, Marder SR, Chengappa KN, et al. Clozapine and risperidone in moderately refractory schizophrenia: a 6-month randomized double-blind comparison. J Clin Psychiatry. 2016;77(5):628–34 [C].

[4] Kittipeerachon M, Chaichan W. Intramuscular olanzapine versus intramuscular aripiprazole for the treatment of agitation in patients with schizophrenia: a pragmatic double-blind randomized trial. Schizophr Res. 2016;176(2–3):231–8 [c].

[5] Kishi T, Matsuda Y, Matsunaga S, et al. A randomized trial of aripiprazole vs blonanserin for the treatment of acute schizophrenia and related disorders. Neuropsychiatr Dis Treat. 2016;12:3041–9 [c].

[6] Lavania S, Praharaj SK, Bains HS, et al. Efficacy and safety of levosulpiride versus haloperidol injection in patients with acute psychosis: a randomized double-blind study. Clin Neuropharmacol. 2016;39(4):197–200 [c].

[7] Suresh Kumar PN, Anish PK, Rajmohan V. Olanzapine has better efficacy compared to risperidone for treatment of negative symptoms in schizophrenia. Indian J Psychiatry. 2016;58(3):311–6 [c].

[8] Ghanizadeh A. Twice-weekly aripiprazole for treating children and adolescents with tic disorder, a randomized controlled clinical trial. Ann Gen Psychiatry. 2016;15(1):21 [c].

[9] Lamberti M, Siracusano R, Italiano D, et al. Head-to-head comparison of aripiprazole and risperidone in the treatment of ADHD symptoms in children with autistic spectrum disorder and ADHD: a pilot, open-label, randomized controlled study. Paediatr Drugs. 2016;18(4):319–29 [c].

[10] Al-Dhaher Z, Kapoor S, Saito E, et al. Activating and tranquilizing effects of first-time treatment with aripiprazole, olanzapine, quetiapine, and risperidone in youth. J Child Adolesc Psychopharmacol. 2016;26(5):458–70 [C].

[11] Buoli M, Kahn RS, Serati M, et al. Haloperidol versus second-generation antipsychotics in the long-term treatment of schizophrenia. Hum Psychopharmacol. 2016;31(4):325–31 [C].

[12] Rafaniello C, Pozzi M, Pisano S, et al. Second generation antipsychotics in 'real-life' paediatric patients. Adverse drug reactions and clinical outcomes of drug switch. Expert Opin Drug Saf. 2016;15(2):1–8 [C].

[13] Heintjes EM, Overbeek JA, Penning-van Beest FJ, et al. Post authorization safety study comparing quetiapine to risperidone and olanzapine. Hum Psychopharmacol. 2016;31(4):304–12 [C].

[14] Vanasse A, Blais L, Courteau J, et al. Comparative effectiveness and safety of antipsychotic drugs in schizophrenia treatment:

a real-world observational study. Acta Psychiatr Scand. 2016;134(5):374–84 [C].

[15] Hayes JF, Marston L, Walters K, et al. Adverse renal, endocrine, hepatic, and metabolic events during maintenance mood stabilizer treatment for bipolar disorder: a population-based cohort study. PLoS Med. 2016;13(8):e1002058 [MC].

[16] Zhao YJ, Lin L, Teng M, et al. Long-term antipsychotic treatment in schizophrenia: systematic review and network meta-analysis of randomised controlled trials. BJPsych Open. 2016;2(1):59–66 [M].

[17] Kishi T, Oya K, Iwata N. Long-acting injectable antipsychotics for prevention of relapse in bipolar disorder: a systematic review and meta-analyses of randomized controlled trials. Int J Neuropsychopharmacol. 2016;19(9). http://dx.doi.org/10.1093/ijnp/pyw038 pii:pyw038, [M].

[18] Kishi T, Oya K, Iwata N. Long-acting injectable antipsychotics for the prevention of relapse in patients with recent-onset psychotic disorders: a systematic review and meta-analysis of randomized controlled trials. Psychiatry Res. 2016;246:750–5 [M].

[19] Raschi E, Poluzzi E, Salvo F, et al. The contribution of national spontaneous reporting systems to detect signals of torsadogenicity: issues emerging from the ARITMO Project. Drug Saf. 2016;39(1):59–68 [MC].

[20] Nosè M, Bighelli I, Castellazzi M, et al. Prevalence and correlates of QTc prolongation in Italian psychiatric care: cross-sectional multicentre study. Epidemiol Psychiatr Sci. 2016;25(6):532–40 [MC].

[21] Barbui C, Bighelli I, Carrà G, et al. Antipsychotic dose mediates the association between polypharmacy and corrected QT interval. PLoS One. 2016;11(2)e0148212 [C].

[22] Liu HC, Yang SY, Liao YT, et al. Antipsychotic medications and risk of acute coronary syndrome in schizophrenia: a nested case-control study. PLoS One. 2016;11(9):e0163533 [C].

[23] Fındıklı E, Gökçe M, Nacitarhan V, et al. Arterial stiffness in patients taking second-generation antipsychotics. Clin Psychopharmacol Neurosci. 2016;14(4):365–70 [c].

[24] Rodríguez-Leal CM, López-Lunar E, Carrascosa-Bernáldez JM, et al. Electrocardiographic surveillance in a psychiatric institution: avoiding iatrogenic cardiovascular death. Int J Psychiatry Clin Pract. 2017;21:64–6 [C].

[25] Olsen RE, Kroken RA, Bjørhovde S, et al. Influence of different second generation antipsychotics on the QTc interval: a pragmatic study. World J Psychiatry. 2016;6(4):442–8 [C].

[26] Osborn D, Marston L, Nazareth I, et al. Relative risks of cardiovascular disease in people prescribed olanzapine, risperidone and quetiapine. Schizophr Res. 2017;183:116–23. [MC].

[27] Alda JA, Muñoz-Samons D, Tor J, et al. Absence of change in corrected QT interval in children and adolescents receiving antipsychotic treatment: a 12 month study. J Child Adolesc Psychopharmacol. 2016;26(5):449–57 [C].

[28] Gandhi S, McArthur E, Reiss JP, et al. Atypical antipsychotic medications and hyponatremia in older adults: a population-based cohort study. Can J Kidney Health Dis. 2016;3:21 [MC].

[29] Hung GC, Liu HC, Yang SY, et al. Antipsychotic reexposure and recurrent pneumonia in schizophrenia: a nested case-control study. J Clin Psychiatry. 2016;77(1):60–6 [C].

[30] Tolppanen AM, Koponen M, Tanskanen A, et al. Antipsychotic use and risk of hospitalization or death due to pneumonia in persons with and those without Alzheimer disease. Chest. 2016;150(6):1233–41 [MC].

[31] Kose E, Uno K, Hayashi H. Evaluation of the expression profile of extrapyramidal symptoms due to antipsychotics by data mining of Japanese Adverse Drug Event Report (JADER) Database. Yakugaku Zasshi. 2017;137(1):111–20 [MC].

[32] Wu CS, Wang SC, Yeh IJ, et al. Comparative risk of seizure with use of first- and second-generation antipsychotics in patients with schizophrenia and mood disorders. J Clin Psychiatry. 2016;77(5): e573–9 [MC].

[33] Hale GM, Kane-Gill SL, Groetzinger L, et al. An evaluation of adverse drug reactions associated with antipsychotic use for the treatment of delirium in the intensive care unit. J Pharm Pract. 2016;29(4):355–60 [c].

[34] Chawla N, Charan D, Kumar S, et al. Pica associated with initiation of atypical antipsychotic drugs: report of two cases. Psychiatry Clin Neurosci. 2016;70(8):363–4 [A].

[35] Chatziralli IP, Peponis V, Parikakis E, et al. Risk factors for intraoperative floppy iris syndrome: a prospective study. Eye (Lond). 2016;30(8):1039–44 [MC].

[36] Matsuo M, Sano I, Ikeda Y, et al. Intraoperative floppy-iris syndrome associated with use of antipsychotic drugs. Can J Ophthalmol. 2016;51(4):294–6 [A].

[37] Steen NE, Aas M, Simonsen C, et al. Serum levels of second-generation antipsychotics are associated with cognitive function in psychotic disorders. World J Biol Psychiatry. 2017;18(6): 471–82 [C].

[38] Monti JM, Torterolo P, Pandi Perumal SR. The effects of second generation antipsychotic drugs on sleep variables in healthy subjects and patients with schizophrenia. Sleep Med Rev. 2017;33:51–7 [r].

[39] Fang F, Sun H, Wang Z, et al. Antipsychotic drug-induced somnolence: incidence, mechanisms, and management. CNS Drugs. 2016;30(9):845–67 [r].

[40] Linselle M, Sommet A, Bondon-Guitton E, et al. Can drugs induce or aggravate sleep apneas? A case non case study in Vigibase(®), the WHO Pharmacovigilance Database. Fundam Clin Pharmacol. 2017;31:359–66 [MC].

[41] Park YM, Lee SH, Lee BH, et al. Prolactin and macroprolactin levels in psychiatric patients receiving atypical antipsychotics: a preliminary study. Psychiatry Res. 2016;239:184–9 [C].

[42] An FR, Yang R, Wang ZM, et al. Hyperprolactinemia, prolactin-related side effects and quality of life in Chinese psychiatric patients. Compr Psychiatry. 2016;71:71–6 [MC].

[43] Bulut SD, Bulut S, Atalan DG, et al. The effect of antipsychotics on bone mineral density and sex hormones in male patients with schizophrenia. Psychiatr Danub. 2016;28(3):255–62 [c].

[44] Druyts E, Zoratti MJ, Toor K, et al. Prolactin-related adverse events and change in prolactin levels in pediatric patients given antipsychotics for schizophrenia and schizophrenia spectrum disorders: a systematic review. BMC Pediatr. 2016;16(1):181 [M].

[45] Galling B, Roldán A, Nielsen RE, et al. Type 2 diabetes mellitus in youth exposed to antipsychotics: a systematic review and meta-analysis. JAMA Psychiat. 2016;73(3):247–59 [M].

[46] Polcwiartek C, Vang T, Bruhn CH, et al. Diabetic ketoacidosis in patients exposed to antipsychotics: a systematic literature review and analysis of Danish adverse drug event reports. Psychopharmacology (Berl). 2016;233(21–22):3663–72 [M].

[47] Parabiaghi A, Tettamanti M, D'Avanzo B, et al. Metabolic syndrome and drug discontinuation in schizophrenia: a randomized trial comparing aripiprazole olanzapine and haloperidol. Acta Psychiatr Scand. 2016;133(1):63–75 [C].

[48] Varghese D, Kirkwood CK, Carroll NV. Prevalence of antidiabetic and antilipidemic medications in children and adolescents treated with atypical antipsychotics in a Virginia Medicaid Population. Ann Pharmacother. 2016;50(6):463–70 [MC].

[49] Bishara A, Phan SV, Young HN, et al. Glucose disturbances and atypical antipsychotic use in the intensive care unit. J Pharm Pract. 2016;29(6):534–8 [C].

[50] Yoon Y, Wink LK, Pedapati EV, et al. Weight gain effects of second-generation antipsychotic treatment in autism spectrum disorder. J Child Adolesc Psychopharmacol. 2016;26(9):822–7 [c].

[51] McAvoy S, Cordiner M, Kelly J. Body mass index and blood glucose in psychiatric and general practice populations. BJPsych Bull. 2016;40(3):127–31 [C].

[52] Allaire BT, Raghavan R, Brown DS. Morbid obesity and use of second generation antipsychotics among adolescents in foster care: evidence from Medicaid. Child Youth Serv Rev. 2016;67:27–31 [MC].

[53] Every-Palmer S, Nowitz M, Stanley J, et al. Clozapine-treated patients have marked gastrointestinal hypomotility, the probable basis of life-threatening gastrointestinal complications: a cross sectional study. EBioMedicine. 2016;5:125–34 [C].

[54] Abdalla S, Brouquet A, Lazure T, et al. Outcome of emergency surgery for severe neuroleptic-induced colitis: results of aprospective cohort. Colorectal Dis. 2016;18(12):1179–85 [c].

[55] Morlán-Coarasa MJ, Arias-Loste MT, Ortiz-García de la Foz V, et al. Incidence of non-alcoholic fatty liver disease and metabolic dysfunction in first episode schizophrenia and related psychotic disorders: a 3-year prospective randomized interventional study. Psychopharmacology (Berl). 2016;233(23–24):3947–52 [C].

[56] Silva MA, Key S, Han E, et al. Acute pancreatitis associated with antipsychotic medication: evaluation of clinical features, treatment, and polypharmacy in a series of cases. J Clin Psychopharmacol. 2016;36(2):169–72 [r].

[57] Torstensson M, Leth-Møller K, Andersson C, et al. Danish register-based study on the association between specific antipsychotic drugs and fractures in elderly individuals. Age Ageing. 2017;46:258–64 [MC].

[58] Sinha P, Garg A. Use of amisulpride in treating adolescent onset schizophrenia associated with stuttering priapism induced by multiple antipsychotics. Asian J Psychiatr. 2016;19:85–6 [A].

[59] Baytunca MB, Kose S, Ozbaran B, et al. Risperidone, quetiapine and chlorpromazine may have induced priapism in an adolescent. Pediatr Int. 2016;58(1):61–3 [A].

[60] Montastruc F, Salvo F, Arnaud M, et al. Signal of gastrointestinal congenital malformations with antipsychotics after minimizing competition bias: a disproportionality analysis using data from Vigibase(®). Drug Saf. 2016;39(7):689–96 [C].

[61] Mas S, Gassó P, Lafuente A, et al. Pharmacogenetic study of antipsychotic induced acute extrapyramidal symptoms in a first episode psychosis cohort: role of dopamine, serotonin and glutamatecandidate genes. Pharmacogenomics J. 2016;16(5):439–45 [C].

[62] Ivanova SA, Osmanova DZ, Boiko AS, et al. Prolactin gene polymorphism (-1149 G/T) is associated with hyperprolactinemia in patients with schizophrenia treated with antipsychotics. Schizophr Res. 2017;182:110–4 [C].

[63] Miura I, Zhang JP, Hagi K, et al. Variants in the DRD2 locus and antipsychotic-related prolactin levels: a meta-analysis. Psychoneuroendocrinology. 2016;72:1–10 [M].

[64] Yang L, Chen J, Li Y, et al. Association between SCAP and SREBF1 gene polymorphisms and metabolic syndrome in schizophrenia patients treated with atypical antipsychotics. World J Biol Psychiatry. 2016;17(6):467–74 [C].

[65] Daray FM, Rodante D, Carosella LG, et al. -759C > T Polymorphism of the HTR2C Gene is associated with second generation antipsychotic-induced weight gain in female patients with schizophrenia. Pharmacopsychiatry. 2017;50:14–8 [c].

[66] Tiwari AK, Brandl EJ, Zai CC, et al. Association of orexin receptor polymorphisms with antipsychotic-induced weight gain. World J Biol Psychiatry. 2016;17(3):221–9 [C].

[67] Huybrechts KF, Hernández-Díaz S, Patorno E, et al. Antipsychotic use in pregnancy and the risk for congenital malformations. JAMA Psychiat. 2016;73(9):938–46 [MC].

[68] Uguz F. Second-generation antipsychotics during the lactation period: a comparative systematic review on infant safety. J Clin Psychopharmacol. 2016;36(3):244–52 [M].

[69] Zagozdzon P, Goyke B, Wrotkowska M. Mortality rates in users of typical and atypical antipsychotics: a database study in Poland. Drugs Real World Outcomes. 2016;3(3):345–51 [MC].

[70] Schmedt N, Kollhorst B, Enders D, et al. Comparative risk of death in older adults treated with antipsychotics: a population-based cohort study. Eur Neuropsychopharmacol. 2016;26(9):1390–400 [MC].

[71] Handley S, Patel MX, Flanagan RJ. Antipsychotic-related fatal poisoning, England and Wales, 1993-2013: impact of the withdrawal of thioridazine. Clin Toxicol (Phila). 2016;54(6):471–80 [MC].

[72] Hikiji W, Okumura Y, Matsumoto T, et al. Identification of psychotropic drugs attributed to fatal overdose—a case–control study by data from the Tokyo Medical Examiner's Office and prescriptions. Seishin Shinkeigaku Zasshi. 2016;118(1):3–13 [C].

[73] Wang LJ, Lee SY, Yuan SS, et al. Risk of mortality among patients treated with antipsychotic medications: a nationwide population-based study in Taiwan. J Clin Psychopharmacol. 2016;36(1):9–17 [C].

[74] Weintraub D, Chiang C, Kim HM, et al. Association of antipsychotic use with mortality risk in patients with Parkinson disease. JAMA Neurol. 2016;73(5):535–41 [MC].

[75] Kishi T, Matsunaga S, Iwata N. Mortality risk associated with long-acting injectable antipsychotics: a systematic review and meta-analyses of randomized controlled trials. Schizophr Bull. 2016;42(6):1438–45 [M].

[76] Hefner G, Shams ME, Unterecker S, et al. Inflammation and psychotropic drugs: the relationship between C-reactive protein and antipsychotic drug levels. Psychopharmacology (Berl). 2016;233(9):1695–705 [c].

[77] Gan TJ, Kranke P, Minkowitz HS, et al. Intravenous amisulpride for the prevention of postoperative nausea and vomiting: two concurrent, randomized, double-blind, placebo-controlled trials. Anesthesiology. 2017;126:268–75 [C].

[78] Kim Y, Wang SM, Kwak KP, et al. Amisulpride switching in schizophrenic patients who showed suboptimal effect and/or tolerability to current antipsychotics in a naturalistic setting: an explorative study. Clin Psychopharmacol Neurosci. 2016;14(4):371–7 [c].

[79] Liang Y, Cao C, Zhu C, et al. The effectiveness and safety of amisulpride in Chinese patients with schizophrenia: an 8-week, prospective, open-label, multicenter, single-arm study. Asia Pac Psychiatry. 2016;8(3):241–4 [C].

[80] Täubel J, Ferber G, Fox G, et al. Thorough QT study of the effect of intravenous amisulpride on QTc interval in Caucasian and Japanese healthy subjects. Br J Clin Pharmacol. 2017;83(2):339–48 [c].

[81] Su CH, Chen CS, Huang MF. Asymptomatic bradycardia and hypotension associated with amisulpride: a case report. Asia Pac Psychiatry. 2016;8(2):175 [A].

[82] Kumar PN, Gopalakrishnan A. Extrapyramidal side effects with low dose amisulpride: a report of two cases. Indian J Psychol Med. 2016;38(5):480–2 [A].

[83] Pickard L, Fordham N, Koh M. Amisulpride induced agranulocytosis: a case report. Ann Hematol. 2016;95(7):1193–5 [A].

[84] Nielsen MØ, Rostrup E, Wulff S, et al. Striatal reward activity and antipsychotic-associated weight change in patients with schizophrenia undergoing initial treatment. JAMA Psychiat. 2016;73(2):121–8 [c].

[85] Chen CY, Yeh YW, Kuo SC, et al. Catechol-O-methyltransferase gene variants may associate with negative symptom response and plasma concentrations of prolactin in schizophrenia after amisulpride treatment. Psychoneuroendocrinology. 2016;65:67–75 [C].

[86] Nasrallah HA, Newcomer JW, Risinger R, et al. Effect of aripiprazole lauroxil on metabolic and endocrine profiles and related safety considerations among patients with acute schizophrenia. J Clin Psychiatry. 2016;77(11):1519–25 [C].

[87] Malla A, Mustafa S, Rho A, et al. Therapeutic effectiveness and tolerability of aripiprazole as initial choice of treatment in first episode psychosis in an early intervention service: a one-year outcome study. Schizophr Res. 2016;174(1–3): 120–5 [c].

[88] Jakobsen KD, Bruhn CH, Pagsberg AK, et al. Neurological, metabolic, and psychiatric adverse events in children and adolescents treated with aripiprazole. J Clin Psychopharmacol. 2016;36(5):496–9 [c].

[89] Hirsch LE, Pringsheim T. Aripiprazole for autism spectrum disorders (ASD). Cochrane Database Syst Rev. 2016;6: CD009043 [M].

[90] Liu Y, Ni H, Wang C, et al. Effectiveness and tolerability of aripiprazole in children and adolescents with tourette's disorder: a meta-analysis. J Child Adolesc Psychopharmacol. 2016;26(5):436–41 [M].

[91] Zheng W, Li XB, Xiang YQ, et al. Aripiprazole for Tourette's syndrome: a systematic review and meta-analysis. Hum Psychopharmacol. 2016;31(1):11–8 [M].

[92] Bernagie C, Danckaerts M, Wampers M, et al. Aripiprazole and acute extrapyramidal symptoms in children and adolescents: a meta-analysis. CNS Drugs. 2016;30(9):807–18 [M].

[93] Belmonte C, Ochoa D, Román M, et al. Evaluation of the relationship between pharmacokinetics and the safety of aripiprazole and its cardiovascular effects in healthy volunteers. J Clin Psychopharmacol. 2016;36(6):608–14 [C].

[94] Camkurt MA, Gunes S, Tecimer E. Aripiprazole-induced Raynaud's phenomenon: an adolescent case. J Child Adolesc Psychopharmacol. 2016;26(10):953–4 [A].

[95] Hoşoğlu E, Bayram Ö, Hergüner S. Nasal and gingival bleeding during aripiprazole but not haloperidol treatment. J Child Adolesc Psychopharmacol. 2016;26(10):950–1 [A].

[96] Etminan M, Procyshyn RM, Samii A, et al. Risk of extrapyramidal adverse events with aripiprazole. J Clin Psychopharmacol. 2016;36(5):472–4 [MC].

[97] Başay Ö, Basay BK, Öztürk Ö, et al. Acute dystonia following a switch in treatment from atomoxetine to low-dose aripiprazole. Clin Psychopharmacol Neurosci. 2016;14(2): 221–5 [A].

[98] Mahgoub Y, Hameed A, Francis A. Covert dyskinesia with aripiprazole: a case report. Prim Care Companion CNS Disord. 2016;18(3). http://dx.doi.org/10.4088/PCC.15l01889 [A].

[99] Bilgiç A, Yılmaz S, Yılmaz E. Hiccups associated with aripiprazole in an adolescent with bipolar disorder. J Child Adolesc Psychopharmacol. 2016;26(7):656–7 [A].

[100] Bulbena-Cabré A, Bulbena A. Aripiprazole-induced hypersexuality. Prim Care Companion CNS Disord. 2016;18(6). http://dx.doi.org/10.4088/PCC.16l01983 [A].

[101] Mété D, Dafreville C, Paitel V, et al. Aripiprazole, gambling disorder and compulsive sexuality. Encéphale. 2016;42(3):281–3 [A].

[102] Lin CH, Tsai YF, Huang WL. Aripiprazole relieves catatonia but worsens hallucination in a patient with catatonic schizophrenia. Asia Pac Psychiatry. 2016;8(2):176 [A].

[103] Sogawa R, Shimomura Y, Minami C, et al. Aripiprazole-associated hypoprolactinemia in the clinical setting. J Clin Psychopharmacol. 2016;36(4):385–7 [c].

[104] Tarraf C, Naja WJ. Aripiprazole-induced hyperlipidemia: an update. Prim Care Companion CNS Disord. 2016;18(4). http://dx.doi.org/10.4088/PCC.16r01958 [A].

[105] Lin MW, Chang C, Yeh CB, et al. Aripiprazole-related hyponatremia and consequent valproic acid-related hyperammonemia in one patient. Aust N Z J Psychiatry. 2017;51:296–7 [A].

[106] Pinnaka S, Roberto AJ, Giordano A, et al. Aripiprazole-induced transient morning pseudoneutropenia in an 11-year-old male. J Child Adolesc Psychopharmacol. 2016;26(9):858–9 [A].

[107] Keshavarz-Akhlaghi AA, Abdollahpour E, Seddigh R. A case of cutaneous leukocytoclastic vasculitis associated with aripiprazole. Prim Care Companion CNS Disord. 2016;18(4). http://dx.doi.org/10.4088/PCC.15l01898 [A].

[108] Landbloom R, Mackle M, Wu X, et al. Asenapine for the treatment of adults with an acute exacerbation of schizophrenia: results from a randomized, double-blind, fixed-dose, placebo-controlled trial with olanzapine as an active control. CNS Spectr. 2017;22(4):333–41 [C].

[109] Kinoshita T, Bai YM, Kim JH, et al. Efficacy and safety of asenapine in Asian patients with an acute exacerbation of schizophrenia: a multicentre, randomized, double-blind, 6-week, placebo-controlled study. Psychopharmacology (Berl). 2016;233(14):2663–74 [C].

[110] Findling RL, Landbloom RL, Mackle M, et al. Long-term safety of asenapine in pediatric patients diagnosed with bipolar I disorder: a 50-week open-label, flexible-dose trial. Paediatr Drugs. 2016;18(5):367–78 [C].

[111] Barak Y, Finkelstein I, Pridan S. The geriatric mania asenapine study (GeMS). Arch Gerontol Geriatr. 2016;64:111–4 [c].

[112] Orr C, Deshpande S, Sawh S, et al. Asenapine for the treatment of psychotic disorders: a systematic review and meta-analysis. Can J Psychiatry. 2017;62:123–37 [M].

[113] Bhuyan D, Ghosh S, Bhattacharya A, et al. Asenapine-induced acute dystonia in an adolescent male. J Child Adolesc Psychopharmacol. 2016;26(10):955–6 [A].

[114] Fava M, Okame T, Matsushima Y, et al. Switching from inadequate adjunctive or combination treatment options to brexpiprazole adjunctive to antidepressant: an open-label study on the effects on depressive symptoms and cognitive and physical functioning. Int J Neuropsychopharmacol. 2017;20:22–30 [c].

[115] Weisler RH, Ota A, Tsuneyoshi K, et al. Brexpiprazole as an adjunctive treatment in young adults with major depressive disorder who are in a school or work environment. J Affect Disord. 2016;204:40–7 [c].

[116] Davis LL, Ota A, Perry P, et al. Adjunctive brexpiprazole in patients with major depressive disorder and anxiety symptoms: an exploratory study. Brain Behav. 2016;6(10)e00520 [c].

[117] Malla A, Ota A, Nagamizu K, et al. The effect of brexpiprazole in adult outpatients with early-episode schizophrenia: an exploratory study. Int Clin Psychopharmacol. 2016;31(6):307–14 [c].

[118] Kane JM, Skuban A, Hobart M, et al. Overview of short- and long-term tolerability and safety of brexpiprazole in patients with schizophrenia. Schizophr Res. 2016;174(1–3):93–8 [r].

[119] Durgam S, Litman RE, Papadakis K, et al. Cariprazine in the treatment of schizophrenia: a proof-of-concept trial. Int Clin Psychopharmacol. 2016;31(2):61–8 [C].

[120] Durgam S, Earley W, Li R, et al. Long-term cariprazine treatment for the prevention of relapse in patients with schizophrenia: a randomized, double-blind, placebo-controlled trial. Schizophr Res. 2016;176(2–3):264–71 [C].

[121] Durgam S, Earley W, Lipschitz A, et al. An 8-week randomized, double-blind, placebo-controlled evaluation of the safety and efficacy of cariprazine in patients with bipolar I depression. Am J Psychiatry. 2016;173(3):271–81 [C].

[122] Durgam S, Earley W, Guo H, et al. Efficacy and safety of adjunctive cariprazine in inadequate responders to antidepressants: a randomized, double-blind, placebo-controlled study in adult patients with major depressive disorder. J Clin Psychiatry. 2016;77(3):371–8 [C].

[123] Lao KS, He Y, Wong IC, et al. Tolerability and safety profile of cariprazine in treating psychotic disorders, bipolar disorder and major depressive disorder: a systematic review with meta-analysis of randomized controlled trials. CNS Drugs. 2016;30(11):1043–54 [M].

[124] Saha KB, Bo L, Zhao S, et al. Chlorpromazine versus atypical antipsychotic drugs for schizophrenia. Cochrane Database Syst Rev. 2016;4:CD010631 [M].

[125] Choy BN, Ng AL, Shum JW, et al. A case report: anti-psychotic agents related ocular toxicity. Medicine (Baltimore). 2016;95(15) e3360 [A].

[126] Jha A, Ghoz H, James N. Severe agranulocytosis following simultaneous administration of chlorpromazine and trimethoprim-sulfamethoxazole in a patient with sepsis: a possible toxic combination. Case Rep Med. 2016;2016:5653497 [A].

[127] Yalcin O, Kaymak G, Erdogan A, et al. A retrospective investigation of clozapine treatment in autistic and nonautistic children and adolescents in an inpatient clinic in turkey. J Child Adolesc Psychopharmacol. 2016;26(9):815–21 [c].

[128] Legge SE, Hamshere M, Hayes RD, et al. Reasons for discontinuing clozapine: a cohort study of patients commencing treatment. Schizophr Res. 2016;174(1–3):113–9 [C].

[129] Norman SM, Sullivan KM, Liu F, et al. Blood pressure and heart rate changes during clozapine treatment. Psychiatr Q. 2017;88(3):545–52 [c].

[130] Prisco V, Monica P, Fiore G, et al. Brain natriuretic peptide as a biomarker of asymptomatic clozapine-related heart dysfunction: a criterion for a more cautious administration. Clin Schizophr Relat Psychoses. 2016. http://dx.doi.org/10.3371/CSRP. PRMO.112316 [Epub ahead of print] [A].

[131] Fehily SR, Forlano R, Fitzgerald PB. C-reactive protein: an early critical sign of clozapine-related myocarditis. Australas Psychiatry. 2016;24(2):181–4 [A].

[132] Earnshaw CH, Powell L, Haeney O. Lessons learned and questions raised by an atypical case of clozapine-induced myocarditis. Case Rep Psychiatry. 2016;2016:4159081 [A].

[133] Buist NC, Schauer CK. Fever and elevated CRP-related to clozapine dose. Aust N Z J Psychiatry. 2016;50(2):182–3 [A].

[134] Woloszyn E, Whig N, Trigoboff E, et al. Cardiac arrest with clozapine and olanzapine: revealing long QT syndrome. Clin Schizophr Relat Psychoses. 2016. http://dx.doi.org/10.3371/ CSRP.WOWH.112316 [A].

[135] Szema AM, Marboe C, Fritz P, et al. Clozapine-associated cardiac dysfunction during a gastroenteritis outbreak. J Community Hosp Intern Med Perspect. 2016;6(6):32683 [A].

[136] Munjal S, Ferrando S. Myocarditis in a patient on clozapine: what did it? Clin Schizophr Relat Psychoses. 2016. http://dx.doi.org/ 10.3371/CSRP.MUFE.070816 [A].

[137] Ittasakul P, Archer A, Kezman J, et al. Rapid rechallenge with clozapine following pronounced myocarditis in a treatment-resistant schizophrenia patient. Clin Schizophr Relat Psychoses. 2016;10(2):120–2 [A].

[138] Swart LE, Koster K, Torn M, et al. Clozapine-induced myocarditis. Schizophr Res. 2016;174(1–3):161–4 [A].

[139] Chopra N, de Leon J. Clozapine-induced myocarditis may be associated with rapid titration: a case report verified with autopsy. Int J Psychiatry Med. 2016;51(1):104–15 [A].

[140] Bugge E, Nissen T, Wynn R. Probable clozapine-induced parenchymal lung disease and perimyocarditis: a case report. BMC Psychiatry. 2016;16(1):438 [A].

[141] Goh JG, John AP. A case report of clozapine continuation after pulmonary embolism in the context of other risk factors for thromboembolism. Aust N Z J Psychiatry. 2016;50(12): 1205–6 [A].

[142] Gami RK, Mishra P, Sedlak T. Pulmonary embolism and clozapine use: a case report and literature review. Psychosomatics. 2017;58(2):203–8 [A].

[143] Colin O, Quillet A, Benatru I, et al. Cerebral venous thrombosis in a Parkinson's disease patient: an unusual case report with low-dose clozapine. Therapie. 2016;71(5):521–4 [A].

[144] Basu S. Dose-dependent clozapine-induced supraventricular tachycardia. Prim Care Companion CNS Disord. 2016; 18(3). http://dx.doi.org/10.4088/PCC.15l01867 [A].

[145] Leung JG, Nelson S, Barreto JN, et al. Necrotizing pneumonia in the setting of elevated clozapine levels. J Clin Psychopharmacol. 2016;36(2):176–8 [A].

[146] Gurrera RJ, Parlee AC, Perry NL. Aspiration pneumonia: an underappreciated risk of clozapine treatment. J Clin Psychopharmacol. 2016;36(2):174–6 [A].

[147] Saenger RC, Finch TH, Francois D. Aspiration pneumonia due to clozapine-induced sialorrhea. Clin Schizophr Relat Psychoses. 2016;9(4):170–2 [A].

[148] Kumar V, Venkatasubramanian G. Gabapentin treatment in clozapine-induced restless legs syndrome: two cases and a review of the literature. Ther Adv Psychopharmacol. 2017;7(1):42–7 [A].

[149] Cherry S, Siskind D, Spivak V, et al. Fever, confusion, acute kidney injury: is this atypical neuroleptic malignant syndrome following polypharmacy with clozapine and risperidone? Australas Psychiatry. 2016;24(6):602–3 [A].

[150] Khanra S, Sethy RR, Munda SK, et al. An unusual case of delirium after restarting clozapine. Clin Psychopharmacol Neurosci. 2016;14(1):107–8 [A].

[151] Ceylan E, Ozer MD, Yilmaz YC, et al. The ocular surface side effects of an anti-psychotic drug, clozapine. Cutan Ocul Toxicol. 2016;35(1):62–6 [c].

[152] Schreiter S, Hasan A, Majic T, et al. Obsessive-compulsive symptoms in a sample of patients with chronic schizophrenia under clozapine treatment. Fortschr Neurol Psychiatr. 2016;84(11):675–81 [c].

[153] Leung JG, Palmer BA. Psychosis or obsessions? Clozapine associated with worsening obsessive-compulsive symptoms. Case Rep Psychiatry. 2016;2016:2180748 [A].

[154] Perdigués SR, Quecuti RS, Mané A, et al. An observational study of clozapine induced sedation and its pharmacological management. Eur Neuropsychopharmacol. 2016;26(1):156–61 [C].

[155] Schulte PF, Bocxe JT, Doodeman HJ, et al. Risk of new-onset diabetes after long-term treatment with clozapine in comparison to other antipsychotics in patients with schizophrenia. J Clin Psychopharmacol. 2016;36(2):115–9 [c].

[156] Hepburn K, Brzozowska MM. Diabetic ketoacidosis and severe hypertriglyceridaemia as a consequence of an atypical antipsychotic agent. BMJ Case Rep. 2016;2016. http://dx. doi.org/10.1136/bcr-2016-215413 pii: bcr2016215413, [A].

[157] López-Sánchez G, Reyna-Villasmil E. Pseudopheochromocytoma caused by clozapine. Med Clin (Barc). 2016;146(12):562–3 [A].

[158] Grover S, Hazari N, Chakrabarti S, et al. Metabolic disturbances, side effect profile and effectiveness of clozapine in adolescents. Indian J Psychol Med. 2016;38(3):224–33 [c].

[159] Tungaraza TE. Significant weight loss following clozapine use, how is it possible? A case report and review of published cases and literature relevant to the subject. Ther Adv Psychopharmacol. 2016;6(5):335–42 [A].

[160] Ingimarsson O, MacCabe JH, Haraldsson M, et al. Neutropenia and agranulocytosis during treatment of schizophrenia with clozapine versus other antipsychotics: an observational study in Iceland. BMC Psychiatry. 2016;16(1):441 [C].

[161] Capllonch A, de Pablo S, de la Torre A, et al. Rev Psiquiatr Salud Ment. 2016 May 3. pii: S1888-9891(16)30002-7 [c].

[162] Richardson CM, Davis EA, Vyas GR, et al. Evaluation of the safety of clozapine use in patients with benign neutropenia. J Clin Psychiatry. 2016;77(11):e1454–9 [c].

[163] Prokopez CR, Armesto AR, Gil Aguer MF, et al. Clozapine rechallenge after neutropenia or leucopenia. J Clin Psychopharmacol. 2016;36(4):377–80 [c].

[164] Demler TL, Morabito NE, Meyer CE, et al. Maximizing clozapine utilization while minimizing blood dyscrasias: evaluation of patient demographics and severity of events. Int Clin Psychopharmacol. 2016;31(2):76–83 [C].

[165] McArdle PA, Siskind DJ, Kolur U, et al. Successful rechallenge with clozapine after treatment associated eosinophilia. Australas Psychiatry. 2016;24(4):365–7 [A].

[166] Comacchio C, Dusi N, Lasalvia A. Successful use of single doses of granulocyte-colony stimulating factor (G-CSF) in the treatment of late-onset agranulocytosis associated with clozapine in a patient with treatment-resistant schizophrenia: a case report. J Clin Psychopharmacol. 2016;36(2):173–4 [A].

[167] Yaylaci S, Yilmaz EU, Guclu E, et al. Clozapine-induced febrile neutropenia and cellulitis. Turk J Emerg Med. 2016;14(1):41–3 [A].

[168] Aydin M, Ilhan BC, Calisir S, et al. Continuing clozapine treatment with lithium in schizophrenic patients with neutropenia or leukopenia: brief review of literature with case reports. Ther Adv Psychopharmacol. 2016;6(1):33–8 [A].

[169] Dumas R, Bardin P, Vedie C. Long-term treatment of clozapine-induced leukopenia with lithium: fast-onset agranulocytosis following lithium discontinuation. Prim Care Companion CNS Disord. 2016;18(1). http://dx.doi.org/10.4088/PCC.15l01841 [A].

[170] Maher S, Cunningham A, O'Callaghan N, et al. Clozapine-induced hypersalivation: an estimate of prevalence, severity and impact on quality of life. Ther Adv Psychopharmacol. 2016;6(3):178–84 [c].

[171] Shirazi A, Stubbs B, Gomez L, et al. Prevalence and predictors of clozapine-associated constipation: a systematic review and meta-analysis. Int J Mol Sci. 2016;17(6). pii E863, http://dx.doi.org/10.3390/ijms17060863.

[172] Osman M, Devadas V. Clozapine-induced dysphagia with secondary substantial weight loss. BMJ Case Rep. 2016; 2016. pii: bcr2016216445, http://dx.doi.org/10.1136/bcr-2016-216445.

[173] Javelot H, Michel B, Kumar D, et al. Clozapine-induced esophagitis at therapeutic dose: a case report. Rev Bras Psiquiatr. 2016;38(2):177 [A].

[174] Castillo-García IM, Maestro G, Puerta S, et al. Clozapine-induced paralytic ileus. Actas Esp Psiquiatr. 2016;44(1):44–5 [A].

[175] Dadlani N, Austin M. Bethanechol and aripiprazole for the management of refractory urinary incontinence in a patient on clozapine. Aust N Z J Psychiatry. 2016;50(2):182 [A].

[176] Jha S, Khanna A. Alopecia areata monolocularis in clozapine-induced hypereosinophilia. Indian J Psychol Med. 2016;38(1):84–5 [A].

[177] Lozano R, Marin R, Santacruz MJ, et al. Effect of clozapine on immunoglobulin M plasma levels. Ther Adv Psychopharmacol. 2016;6(1):58–60 [C].

[178] Buzina N, Eterović M. Life-threatening lupus-like syndrome associated with clozapine. J Clin Psychopharmacol. 2016;36(5):532–4 [A].

[179] Davey P, Gee S, Shergill SS. Inflammatory response to clozapine in the absence of myocarditis: case report. BJPsych Open. 2016;2(3):244–6 [A].

[180] Ramasamy RS, Bronson B, Lerman M. Systemic inflammatory response syndrome associated with clozapine and successful rechallenge: a case report. J Clin Psychopharmacol. 2016;36(1):93–5 [A].

[181] Hoffmann MS, Oliveira LM, Lobato MI, et al. Heat stroke during long-term clozapine treatment: should we be concerned about hot weather? Trends Psychiatry Psychother. 2016;38(1):56–9 [A].

[182] Saito T, Ikeda M, Mushiroda T, et al. Pharmacogenomic study of clozapine-induced agranulocytosis/granulocytopenia in a Japanese population. Biol Psychiatry. 2016;80(8):636–42 [MC].

[183] Legge SE, Hamshere ML, Ripke S, et al. Genome-wide common and rare variant analysis provides novel insights into clozapine-associated neutropenia. Mol Psychiatry. 2016, July 12. http://dx.doi.org/10.1038/mp.2016.97 [MC].

[184] van der Weide K, Loovers H, Pondman K, et al. Genetic risk factors for clozapine-induced neutropenia and agranulocytosis in a Dutch psychiatric population. Pharmacogenomics J. 2016, May 10. http://dx.doi.org/10.1038/tpj.2016.32 [C].

[185] Anıl Yağcıoğlu AE, Yoca G, Ayhan Y, et al. Relation of the allelic variants of multidrug resistance gene to agranulocytosis associated with clozapine. J Clin Psychopharmacol. 2016;36(3):257–61 [c].

[186] Singh A, Grover S, Malhotra P, et al. Late onset agranulocytosis with clozapine associated with HLA dr4 responding to treatment with granulocyte colony-stimulating factor: a case report and review of literature. Clin Psychopharmacol Neurosci. 2016;14(2):212–7 [A].

[187] Vasudev K, Choi YH, Norman R, et al. Genetic determinants of clozapine-induced metabolic side effects. Can J Psychiatry. 2017;62:138–49 [c].

[188] Wysokiński A. Obestatin may be involved in clozapine-induced changes in glucose metabolism. Schizophr Res. 2016;176(2–3):201–2 [c].

[189] Lee LH, White RF, Barr AM, et al. Elevated clozapine plasma concentration secondary to a urinary tract infection: proposed mechanisms. J Psychiatry Neurosci. 2016;41(4):E67–8 [A].

[190] Meyer JM, Proctor G, Cummings MA, et al. Ciprofloxacin and clozapine: a potentially fatal but underappreciated interaction. Case Rep Psychiatry. 2016;2016:5606098 [A].

[191] Sharma P, Davis J, Rachamallu V, et al. Concomitant use of topiramate inducing neutropenia in a schizophrenic male stabilized on clozapine. Case Rep Psychiatry. 2016;2016:6086839 [A].

[192] Polcwiartek C, Nielsen J. The clinical potentials of adjunctive fluvoxamine to clozapine treatment: a systematic review. Psychopharmacology (Berl). 2016;233(5):741–50 [M].

[193] Khokhar MA, Rathbone J. Droperidol for psychosis-induced aggression or agitation. Cochrane Database Syst Rev. 2016;12: CD002830 [M].

[194] Sampford JR, Sampson S, Li BG, et al. Fluphenazine (oral) versus atypical antipsychotics for schizophrenia. Cochrane Database Syst Rev. 2016;7:CD010832 [M].

[195] Bauer JØ, Stenborg D, Lodahl T, et al. Treatment of agitation in the acute psychiatric setting. An observational study of the effectiveness of intramuscular psychotropic medication. Nord J Psychiatry. 2016;70(8):599–605 [C].

[196] Angelis MV, Giacomo RD, Muzio AD, et al. A subtle mimicker in emergency department: illustrated case reports of acute drug-induced dystonia. Medicine (Baltimore). 2016;95(41) e5137 [A].

[197] Cheng M, Gu H, Zheng L, et al. Neuroleptic malignant syndrome and subsequent clozapine-withdrawal effects in a patient with refractory schizophrenia. Neuropsychiatr Dis Treat. 2016;12:695–7 [A].

[198] Wahidi N, Johnson KM, Brenzel A, et al. Two sudden and unexpected deaths of patients with schizophrenia associated with intramuscular injections of antipsychotics and practice guidelines to limit the use of high doses of intramuscular antipsychotics. Case Rep Psychiatry. 2016;2016:9406813 [A].

[199] Kenes MT, Hamblin SE, Tumuluri SS, et al. Syndrome of inappropriate antidiuretic hormone in a patient receiving high-dose haloperidol and quetiapine therapy. J Neuropsychiatry Clin Neurosci. 2016;28(2):e29–30 [A].

[200] Weiden PJ, Manning R, Wolfgang CD, et al. A randomized trial of iloperidone for prevention of relapse in schizophrenia: the REPRIEVE study. CNS Drugs. 2016;30(8):735–47 [C].

[201] Naglich AC, Nelson LA, Hornstra Jr R. Two cases of iloperidone-related tardive dyskinesia. J Clin Psychopharmacol. 2016;36(6):742–3 [A].

[202] Ravani NN, Katke PH. Iloperidone-induced ejaculatory dysfunction: a case series. Indian J Psychiatry. 2016;58(1):87–9 [A].

[203] Mathew T, Nadimpally US, Prabhu AD, et al. Drug-induced Parkinsonism on the rise: beware of levosulpiride and its combinations with proton pump inhibitors. Neurol India. 2017;65(1):173–4 [A].

[204] Cho SH, Lee D, Ahn TB. Dropped head syndrome after minor trauma in a patient with levosulpiride-aggravated vascular parkinsonism. J Mov Disord. 2016;9(2):126–8 [A].

[205] Lee HC, Hwang SH, Kang SY. Levosulpiride-associated hemichorea. Yonsei Med J. 2016;57(3):803–5 [A].

[206] Suppes T, Kroger H, Pikalov A, et al. Lurasidone adjunctive with lithium or valproate for bipolar depression: a placebo-controlled trial utilizing prospective and retrospective enrolment cohorts. J Psychiatr Res. 2016;78:86–93 [C].

[207] Correll CU, Cucchiaro J, Silva R, et al. Long-term safety and effectiveness of lurasidone in schizophrenia: a 22-month, open-label extension study. CNS Spectr. 2016;21(5):393–402 [C].

[208] Sajatovic M, Forester BP, Tsai J, et al. Efficacy of lurasidone in adults aged 55 years and older with bipolar depression: post hoc analysis of 2 double-blind, placebo-controlled studies. J Clin Psychiatry. 2016;77(10):e1324–31 [C].

[209] Ketter TA, Sarma K, Silva R, et al. Lurasidone in the long-term treatment of patients with bipolar disorder: a 24-week open-label extension study. Depress Anxiety. 2016;33(5):424–34 [c].

[210] Tandon R, Cucchiaro J, Phillips D, et al. A double-blind, placebo-controlled, randomized withdrawal study of lurasidone for the maintenance of efficacy in patients with schizophrenia. J Psychopharmacol. 2016;30(1):69–77 [C].

[211] Suppes T, Silva R, Cucchiaro J, et al. Lurasidone for the treatment of major depressive disorder with mixed features: a randomized, double-blind, placebo-controlled study. Am J Psychiatry. 2016;173(4):400–7 [C].

[212] Loebel A, Brams M, Goldman RS, et al. Lurasidone for the treatment of irritability associated with autistic disorder. J Autism Dev Disord. 2016;46(4):1153–63 [C].

[213] Schaffer CB, Schaffer LC, Nordahl TE, et al. An open trial of lurasidone as an acute and maintenance adjunctive treatment for outpatients with treatment-resistant bipolar disorder. J Clin Psychopharmacol. 2016;36(1):88–9 [c].

[214] Ghori AK, Sajatovic M, Tampi RR. A case of emergent restless legs syndrome with lurasidone therapy. J Clin Psychopharmacol. 2016;36(3):293–4 [A].

[215] Naccarato M, Hall E, Wai A, et al. A case of a probable drug interaction between lurasidone and atazanavir-based antiretroviral therapy. Antivir Ther. 2016;21(8):735–8 [A].

[216] Wang G, Cheng Y, Wang JN, et al. Efficacy and safety of olanzapine for treatment of patients with bipolar depression: Chinese subpopulation analysis of a double-blind, randomized, placebo-controlled study. Neuropsychiatr Dis Treat. 2016;12:2077–87 [C].

[217] Detke HC, DelBello MP, Landry J, et al. A 52-week study of olanzapine with a randomized behavioral weight counseling intervention in adolescents with schizophrenia or bipolar I disorder. J Child Adolesc Psychopharmacol. 2016;26(10):922–34 [C].

[218] Cole JB, Moore JC, Dolan BJ, et al. A prospective observational study of patients receiving intravenous and intramuscular olanzapine in the emergency department. Ann Emerg Med. 2017;69:327–36. e2. pii: S0196-0644(16)30466-8 [C].

[219] Martel ML, Klein LR, Rivard RL, et al. A large retrospective cohort of patients receiving intravenous olanzapine in the emergency department. Acad Emerg Med. 2016;23(1):29–35 [C].

[220] Chow R, Chiu L, Navari R, et al. Efficacy and safety of olanzapine for the prophylaxis of chemotherapy-induced nausea and vomiting (CINV) as reported in phase I and II studies: a systematic review. Support Care Cancer. 2016;24(2):1001–8 [M].

[221] Vang T, Rosenzweig M, Bruhn CH, et al. Eosinophilic myocarditis during treatment with olanzapine - report of two possible cases. BMC Psychiatry. 2016;16:70 [A].

[222] Puttegowda B, Theodore J, Basappa R, et al. Olanzapine induced dilated cardiomyopathy. Malays J Med Sci. 2016;23(2): 82–84 [A].

[223] Ayyıldız H, Turan ⬛, Gülcü D, et al. Olanzapine-induced atypical neuroleptic malignant syndrome in an adolescent man with anorexia nervosa. Eat Weight Disord. 2016;21(2):309–11 [A].

[224] Anzellotti F, Capasso M, Frazzini V, et al. Olanzapine-related repetitive focal seizures with lingual dystonia. Epileptic Disord. 2016;18(1):83–6 [A].

[225] Kalivas BC, Goodwin AJ. A woman in her 60s with fever and altered mental status in a psychiatric hospital. Chest. 2016;150(6): e171–4 [A].

[226] Lasić D, Cvitanović MŽ, Krnić S, et al. Olanzapine induced stuttering: a case report. Psychiatr Danub. 2016;28(3):299–300 [A].

[227] Figueiredo T, Segenreich D, Mattos P. Fluoxetine adjunctive therapy for obsessive-compulsive symptoms associated with olanzapine in schizophrenic patients. J Clin Psychopharmacol. 2016;36(4):389–91 [A].

[228] Bengtsson C, Nilsson BM, Bodén R. Postinjection delirium syndrome associated with olanzapine long-acting injectable. J Clin Psychopharmacol. 2016;36(4):388–9 [A].

[229] Sarangula SM, Mythri SV, Sanjay Y, et al. Postinjection delirium/sedation syndrome with olanzapine depot injection. Indian J Psychol Med. 2016;38(4):366–9 [A].

[230] Descusse A, Chebili S, Artiges E. Post-injection syndrome and olanzapine pamoate: a severe case report. Encéphale. 2017;43(4):405 [A].

[231] González-Pablos E, Valles-de la Calle JM, Iglesias-Santa Polonia F, et al. A case report of camptocormia coinciding with olanzapine use. J Clin Psychopharmacol. 2016;36(2):183–4 [A].

[232] Sahoo S, Singla H, Spoorty M, et al. Thrombocytopenia associated with olanzapine: a case report and review of literature. Indian J Psychiatry. 2016;58(3):339–41 [A].

[233] Tournikioti K, Douzenis A, Antoniadou A, et al. Eosinophilia associated with olanzapine. J Clin Psychopharmacol. 2016;36(2):180–1 [A].

[234] Buszek SM, Roy-Chaudhury P, Yadlapalli G. Olanzapine-induced hypertriglyceridemia resulting in necrotizing pancreatitis. ACG Case Rep J. 2016;3(4)e104 [A].

[235] Oliveira E, Velosa J, Araújo-Correia L, et al. Severe ischemic colitis following olanzapine use—a case report. Rev Esp Enferm Dig. 2016;108(9):595–8 [A].

[236] Sáez González E, Díaz Jaime FC, Blázquez Martínez MT, et al. Olanzapine-induced ischemic colitis. Rev Esp Enferm Dig. 2016;108(8):507–9 [A].

[237] Jhaj R, Gour PR, Asati DP. Black hairy tongue with a fixed dose combination of olanzapine and fluoxetine. Indian J Pharmacol. 2016;48(3):318–20 [A].

[238] Guina J, Gupta A, Langleben DD, et al. Clinical correlates of oral glucose tolerance test performance in olanzapine-treated patients with schizophrenia or schizoaffective disorder. J Clin Psychiatry. 2016;77(12):e1650–1.F [c].

[239] Kaino K, Kumagai R, Furukawa S, et al. Reversible splenial lesion syndrome with a hyperosmolarhyperglycemic state and neuroleptic malignant syndrome caused by olanzapine. J Diabetes Investig. 2017;8(3):392–4 [A].

[240] Agrawal Y, Lingala K, Tokala H, et al. Antipsychotic therapy-induced new onset diabetic ketoacidosis. Am J Ther. 2016;23(6): e1944–5 [A].

[241] Ustohal L, Mayerova M, Valkova B, et al. Asymptomatic elevation of amylase and lipase after olanzapine treatment. J Clin Psychopharmacol. 2016;36(2):181–3 [A].

[242] Frise C, Attwood B, Watkinson P, et al. Life-threatening ketoacidosis in a pregnant woman with psychotic disorder. Obstet Med. 2016;9(1):46–9 [A].

[243] Lee YF, Mao WC, Tai YM, et al. Delayed-onset rhabdomyolysis related to olanzapine: a case report. Singapore Med J. 2016;57(5):279 [A].

[244] Li Q, Guo D, Yang H, et al. Metabolic response to olanzapine in healthy Chinese subjects with rs7093146 polymorphism in transcription factor 7-like 2 gene (tcf7l2): a prospective study. Basic Clin Pharmacol Toxicol. 2017;120(6):601–9 [c].

[245] Evers SS, van Vliet A, van Vugt B, et al. A low TSH profile predicts olanzapine-induced weight gain and relief by adjunctive topiramate in healthy male volunteers. Psychoneuroendocrinology. 2016;66:101–10 [c].

[246] Tsuneyama N, Suzuki Y, Sawamura K, et al. Effect of serum leptin on weight gain induced by olanzapine in female patients with schizophrenia. PLoS One. 2016;11(3)e0149518 [c].

[247] Georges A, Fitz-Gerald MJ. Reconsidering olanzapine as a possible culprit for drug fever, defying "incomplete neuromalignant syndrome" J La State Med Soc. 2016;168(4):123–4 [A].

[248] Kim E, Correll CU, Mao L, et al. Once-monthly paliperidone palmitate compared with conventional and atypical daily oral antipsychotic treatment in patients with schizophrenia. CNS Spectr. 2016;21(6):466–77 [C].

[249] Savitz AJ, Xu H, Gopal S, et al. Efficacy and safety of paliperidone palmitate 3-month formulation for patients with schizophrenia: a randomized, multicenter, double-blind, noninferiority study. Int J Neuropsychopharmacol. 2016, July 5;19(7). http://dx.doi.org/10.1093/ijnp/pyw018 pii: pyw018 [C].

[250] Kang NI, Koo BH, Kim SW, et al. Efficacy and tolerability of paliperidone extended-release in the treatment of first-episode psychosis: an eight-week, open-label, multicenter trial. Clin Psychopharmacol Neurosci. 2016;14(3):261–9 [c].

[251] Fu DJ, Turkoz I, Simonson RB, et al. Paliperidone palmitate once-monthly injectable treatment for acute exacerbations of schizoaffective disorder. J Clin Psychopharmacol. 2016;36(4):372–6 [C].

[252] Kotler M, Dilbaz N, Rosa F, et al. A flexible-dose study of paliperidone ER in patients with nonacute schizophrenia previously treated unsuccessfully with oral olanzapine. J Psychiatr Pract. 2016;22(1):9–21 [C].

[253] Zhang H, Li H, Liu Y, et al. Safety and efficacy of paliperidone extended-release in Chinese patients with schizophrenia: a 24-week, open-label extension of a randomized, double-blind, placebo-controlled study. Neuropsychiatr Dis Treat. 2016;12:69–77 [C].

[254] Wong LY, Greene SL, Odell M, et al. Severe prolonged posture-evoked tachycardia after massive overdose of paliperidone. Clin Toxicol (Phila). 2016;54(6):535 [A].

[255] Tsou CC, Huang SY. Olanzapine as a possible replacement choice for paliperidone-induced Pisa syndrome: a case report. Australas Psychiatry. 2016;24(6):545–7 [A].

[256] Singh S, Gupta A, Kuppili PP, et al. Paliperidone palmitate-associated severe refractory tardive dyskinesia with tardive dystonia: management and six-months follow-up. J Clin Psychopharmacol. 2016;36(4):391–3 [A].

[257] Ma CH, Chien YL, Liu CC, et al. A case of tardive dystonia associated with long-acting injectable paliperidone palmitate. Eur Neuropsychopharmacol. 2016;26(7):1251–2 [A].

[258] Tu CY, Chien YL, Huang WL. Case of catatonia associated with paliperidone. Psychiatry Clin Neurosci. 2016;70(8):366 [A].

[259] Langley-DeGroot M, Joshi Y, Lehman D, et al. Atypical neuroleptic malignant syndrome associated with paliperidone long-acting injection: a case report. J Clin Psychopharmacol. 2016;36(3):277–9 [A].

[260] Kaur J, Kumar D, Alfishawy M, et al. Paliperidone inducing concomitantly syndrome of inappropriate antidiuretic hormone, neuroleptic malignant syndrome, and rhabdomyolysis. Case Rep Crit Care. 2016;2016:2587963 [A].

[261] Tsai MC, Chang PT, Yang CH, et al. The delirium related to oral paliperidone in dementia: a case report. J Clin Psychopharmacol. 2016;36(2):184–5 [A].

[262] Yang CH, Juang KD, Chou PH, et al. A case report of probable paliperidone ER-induced serotonin syndrome in a 17-year-old Taiwanese female with new onset psychosis. Medicine (Baltimore). 2016;95(9)e2930 [A].

[263] Qiao Y, Yang F, Li C, et al. Add-on effects of a low-dose aripiprazole in resolving hyperprolactinemia induced by risperidone or paliperidone. Psychiatry Res. 2016;237:83–9 [c].

[264] Nakamura M, Nagamine T, Sato G, et al. Prolactin levels after switching to paliperidone palmitate in patients with schizophrenia. Innov Clin Neurosci. 2016;13(5–6):28–30 [c].

[265] Naguy A, Al-Tajali A. Bromocriptine mitigated paliperidone metabolic and neuro-hormonal side effects and improved negative domain in a case of early onset schizophrenia. Nord J Psychiatry. 2016;70(4):318–9 [A].

[266] Rosso G, Pessina E, Martini A, et al. Paliperidone palmitate and metabolic syndrome in patients with schizophrenia: a 12-month observational prospective cohort study. J Clin Psychopharmacol. 2016;36(3):206–12 [c].

[267] Omi T, Riku K, Fukumoto M, et al. Paliperidone induced hypoglycemia by increasing insulin secretion. Case Rep Psychiatry. 2016;2016:1805414 [A].

[268] Matsuura H, Kimoto S, Harada I, et al. Lithium carbonate as a treatment for paliperidone extended-release-induced leukopenia and neutropenia in a patient with schizoaffective disorder; a case report. BMC Psychiatry. 2016;16:161 [A].

[269] Can SS, Kabadayı E. A case of ileus in a patient with schizophrenia under paliperidone palmitate treatment. Psychiatry Investig. 2016;13(6):665–7 [A].

[270] Karslıoğlu EH, Özalp E, Çayköylü A. Paliperidone palmitate-induced urinary incontinence: a case report. Clin Psychopharmacol Neurosci. 2016;14(1):96–100 [A].

[271] Struye A, Depuydt C, Abdel Sater E, et al. Toxic epidermal necrolysis related to paliperidone palmitate: first case report. J Clin Psychopharmacol. 2016;36(3):279–82 [A].

[272] Madan R, Langenfeld RJ, Ramaswamy S. Paliperidone palmitate induced retrograde ejaculation. Clin Schizophr Relat Psychoses. 2016. http://dx.doi.org/10.3371/csrp.MALA.123015 [A].

[273] Pierce P, Ghopal S, Savitz A, et al. Paliperidone palmitate: Japanese postmarketing mortality results in patients with schizophrenia. Curr Med Res Opin. 2016;32(10):1–9 [MC].

[274] Remmerie B, Ariyawansa J, De Meulder M, et al. Drug-drug interaction studies of paliperidone and divalproex sodium

extended-release tablets in healthy participants and patients with psychiatric disorders. J Clin Pharmacol. 2016;56(6):683–92 [c].

[275] Lau Moon Lin M, Robinson PD, Flank J, et al. The safety of prochlorperazine in children: a systematic review and meta-analysis. Drug Saf. 2016;39:509–16 [M].

[276] Villarreal G, Hamner MB, Cañive JM, et al. Efficacy of quetiapine monotherapy in posttraumatic stress disorder: a randomized, placebo-controlled trial. Am J Psychiatry. 2016;173(12):1205–12 [C].

[277] Li H, Gu N, Zhang H, et al. Efficacy and safety of quetiapine extended release monotherapy in bipolar depression: a multi-center, randomized, double-blind, placebo-controlled trial. Psychopharmacology (Berl). 2016;233(7):1289–97 [C].

[278] Li R, Wu R, Chen J, et al. A randomized, placebo-controlled pilot study of quetiapine-xr monotherapy or adjunctive therapy to antidepressant in acute major depressive disorder with current generalized anxiety disorder. Psychopharmacol Bull. 2016;46(1):8–23 [c].

[279] El-Saifi N, Jones C, Moyle W. Quetiapine adverse events in older adults in Australia. Australas J Ageing. 2016;35(4):281–4 [MC].

[280] El-Saifi N, Moyle W, Jones C, et al. Quetiapine safety in older adults: a systematic literature review. J Clin Pharm Ther. 2016;41(1):7–18 [M].

[281] Huang WL, Liao SC, Kuo TB, et al. The effects of antidepressants and quetiapine on heart rate variability. Pharmacopsychiatry. 2016;49(5):191–8 [c].

[282] Kim A, Lim KS, Lee H, et al. A thorough QT study to evaluate the QTc prolongation potential of two neuropsychiatric drugs, quetiapine and escitalopram, in healthy volunteers. Int Clin Psychopharmacol. 2016;31(4):210–7 [c].

[283] Melada A, Krčmar T, Vidović A. A dose-dependent relationship between quetiapine and QTc interval. Int J Cardiol. 2016;222:893–4 [A].

[284] B AK, Usha G, Sravan G, et al. A case of quetiapine poisoning in antenatal woman. J Assoc Physicians India. 2016;64(1):143 [A].

[285] Smolders DM, Smolders WA. Case report and review of the literature: cardiomyopathy in a young woman on high-dose quetiapine. Cardiovasc Toxicol. 2016, November 1;1–4 [A].

[286] Brunetti ND, Ieva R, Correale M, et al. Inferior ST-elevation acute myocardial infarction or an inferior-lead Brugada-like electrocardiogram pattern associated with the use of pregabalin and quetiapine? Am J Ther. 2016;23(4):e1057–9 [A].

[287] Nakamura M, Seki M, Sato Y, et al. Quetiapine-induced bradycardia and hypotension in the elderly-a case report. Innov Clin Neurosci. 2016;13(1–2):34–6 [A].

[288] Schattner A, Kitroser E, Cohen JD. Fatal neuroleptic malignant syndrome associated with quetiapine. Am J Ther. 2016;23(5): e1209–10 [A].

[289] López Pardo P, Jiménez Rojas C, Ortiz Pascual A, et al. Neuroleptic malignant syndrome associated with quetiapine after withdrawal of olanzapine and donepezil, with EEG differential diagnosis of Creutzfeldt-Jakob disease. Rev Esp Geriatr Gerontol. 2016;51(5):301–2 [A].

[290] Shao SC, Wu WH, Yang YK, et al. Quetiapine-induced absence seizures in a dementia patient. Geriatr Gerontol Int. 2016;16(10):1168–71 [A].

[291] Chen PH. Restless leg syndrome induced by escitalopram and lithium combined with quetiapine treatment in Bipolar II Disorder: a case report. Clin Neuropharmacol. 2016;39(2):118–9 [A].

[292] Soyata AZ, Celebi F, Yargc LI. Restless legs syndrome after single low dose quetiapine administration. Curr Drug Saf. 2016;11(2):172–3 [A].

[293] Tan L, Zhou J, Liang B, et al. A case of quetiapine-induced rapid eye movement sleep behavior disorder. Biol Psychiatry. 2016;79(5):e11–2 [A].

[294] Koufakis T. Quetiapine-induced syndrome of inappropriate secretion of antidiuretic hormone. Case Rep Psychiatry. 2016;2016:4803132 [A].

[295] Husnain M, Gondal F, Raina AI, et al. Quetiapine associated thrombotic thrombocytopenic purpura: a case report and literature review. Am J Ther. 2016;0(1). http://dx.doi.org/10.1097/MJT.0000000000000456 [A].

[296] Arslan FC, Aykut DS, Ince C, et al. Neutropenia and thrombocytopenia induced by quetiapine monotherapy: a case report and review of literature. Klinik Psikofarmakoloji Bülteni-Bull Clin Psychopharmacol. 2016;26(3):319–23 [A].

[297] Aguglia A, Maina G. Can quetiapine extended release (ER) induce labial edema in a female patient with treatment-resistant major depressive episode? Aging Clin Exp Res. 2016;28(4):791–3 [A].

[298] Alastal Y, Hasan S, Chowdhury MA, et al. Hypertriglyceridemia-induced pancreatitis in psychiatric patients: a case report and review of literature. Am J Ther. 2016;23(3):e947–9 [A].

[299] Chew J, Cheong S, Tay L. Quetiapine-induced cutaneous vasculitis: diagnostic challenges and therapeutic implications. J Am Geriatr Soc. 2016;64(5):1137–8 [A].

[300] Tan ES, Robson A, Lai-Cheong JE, et al. Interstitial granulomatous drug reaction induced by quetiapine. Clin Exp Dermatol. 2016;41(2):210–1 [A].

[301] Vetlugina TP, Lobacheva OA, Semke AV, et al. An effect of quetiapine on the immune system of patients with schizophrenia. Zh Nevrol Psikhiatr Im S S Korsakova. 2016;116(7):55–8 [c].

[302] Tuman TC, Tuman BA, Çereflican B, et al. Quetiapine associated with angioedema. J Clin Psychopharmacol. 2016;36(3):289–90 [A].

[303] Munshi S, Mukherjee S, Saha I, et al. Pedal edema associated with atypical antipsychotics. Indian J Pharmacol. 2016;48(1):88–90 [A].

[304] Park HJ, Kim JY. Incidence of neutropenia with valproate and quetiapine combination treatment in subjects with acquired brain injuries. Arch Phys Med Rehabil. 2016;97(2):183–8 [C].

[305] Vo LC, Snyder C, McCracken C, et al. No apparent cardiac conduction effects of acute treatment with risperidone in children with autism spectrum disorder. J Child Adolesc Psychopharmacol. 2016;26(10):900–8 [C].

[306] Nasser AF, Henderson DC, Fava M, et al. Efficacy, safety, and tolerability of rbp-7000 once-monthly risperidone for the treatment of acute schizophrenia: an 8-week, randomized, double-blind, placebo-controlled, multicenter phase 3 study. J Clin Psychopharmacol. 2016;36(2):130–40 [C].

[307] Reutfors J, Wingård L, Brandt L, et al. Risk of breast cancer in risperidone users: a nationwide cohort study. Schizophr Res. 2017;182:98–103 [MC].

[308] Llaudó J, Anta L, Ayani I, et al. Phase I, open-label, randomized, parallel study to evaluate the pharmacokinetics, safety, and tolerability of one intramuscular injection of risperidone ISM at different dose strengths in patients with schizophrenia or schizoaffective disorder (PRISMA-1). Int Clin Psychopharmacol. 2016;31(6):323–31 [c].

[309] Rattehalli RD, Zhao S, Li BG, et al. Risperidone versus placebo for schizophrenia. Cochrane Database Syst Rev. 2016;12: CD006918 [M].

[310] Alexander ST, Kattula D, Mannam P, et al. Risperidone induced benign intracranial hypertension leading to visual loss. Indian J Psychol Med. 2016;38(3):249–51 [A].

[311] Chen F. Risperidone-induced acute respiratory distress in an adolescent with autism. J Child Adolesc Psychopharmacol. 2016;26(9):851–2 [A].

[312] Yoshimura R, Hori H, Katsuki A, et al. Marked improvement of Meige syndrome in a japanese male patient with schizophrenia after switching from risperidone to paliperidone: a case report. J UOEH. 2016;38(3):233–6 [A].

[313] Patel E, Gallego JA. Bilateral cataracts in a young patient with bipolar disorder on treatment with risperidone. Aust N Z J Psychiatry. 2016;50(12):1210 [A].

[314] Camkurt MA, Gülpamuk B. Acute onset of xanthopsia associated with risperidone. J Clin Psychopharmacol. 2016;36(3):288–9 [A].

[315] Güneş S, Camkurt MA. Sleep-related eating disorder associated with risperidone: an adolescent case. J Clin Psychopharmacol. 2016;36(3):286–8 [A].

[316] Bo Q, Dong F, Li X, et al. Prolactin related symptoms during risperidone maintenance treatment: results from a prospective, multicenter study of schizophrenia. BMC Psychiatry. 2016;16(1):386 [C].

[317] Ngamsamut N, Hongkaew Y, Vanwong N, et al. 9-Hydroxyrisperidone-induced hyperprolactinaemia in Thai children and adolescents with autism spectrum disorder. Basic Clin Pharmacol Toxicol. 2016;119(3):267–72 [C].

[318] Nagamine T. Severe hypoglycemia associated with risperidone. Psychiatry Clin Neurosci. 2016;70(9):421 [A].

[319] Hergüner S, Özayhan HY, Erdur EA. Risperidone-induced gingival bleeding in a pediatric case: a dose-dependent side effect. Clin Psychopharmacol Neurosci. 2016;14(2):210–1 [A].

[320] Mergui J, Jaworowski S. Risperidone-induced nocturnal enuresis successfully treated with reboxetine. Clin Neuropharmacol. 2016;39(3):152–3 [A].

[321] Aabbassi B, Benali A, Asri F. Risperidone-induced priapism in an autistic child: a case report. J Med Case Rep. 2016;10: 164 [A].

[322] Nagamine T. Complete recovery from cardiac arrest caused by risperidone-induced hypothermia. Innov Clin Neurosci. 2016;13(11–12):28–31 [A].

[323] Grau K, Plener PL, Gahr M, et al. Mild hypothermia in a child with low-dose risperidone. Z Kinder Jugendpsychiatr Psychother. 2017;45(4):335–7 [A].

[324] Mi W, Liu F, Liu Y, et al. Association of ABCB1 gene polymorphisms with efficacy and adverse reaction to risperidone or paliperidone in Han Chinese schizophrenic patients. Neurosci Bull. 2016;32(6):547–9 [C].

[325] Sukasem C, Hongkaew Y, Ngamsamut N, et al. Impact of pharmacogenetic markers of CYP2D6 and DRD2 on prolactin response in risperidone-treated Thai children and adolescents with autism spectrum disorders. J Clin Psychopharmacol. 2016;36(2):141–6 [C].

[326] Schoretsanitis G, Stegmann B, Hiemke C, et al. Pharmacokinetic patterns of risperidone-associated adverse drug reactions. Eur J Clin Pharmacol. 2016;72(9):1091–8 [C].

[327] Schoretsanitis G, Haen E, Hiemke C, et al. Risperidone-induced extrapyramidal side effects: is the need for anticholinergics the consequence of high plasma concentrations? Int Clin Psychopharmacol. 2016;31(5):259–64 [C].

[328] Hsu CW, Lee Y, Lee CY, et al. Neurotoxicity and nephrotoxicity caused by combined use of lithium and risperidone: a case report and literature review. BMC Pharmacol Toxicol. 2016;17(1):59 [A].

[329] Mischoulon D, Shelton RC, Baer L, et al. Ziprasidone augmentation of escitalopram for major depressive disorder: cardiac, endocrine, metabolic, and motoric effects in a randomized, double-blind, placebo-controlled study. J Clin Psychiatry. 2017;78(4):449–55 [C].

[330] Das P. A case of sleepwalking with sleep-related eating associated with ziprasidone therapy in a patient with schizoaffective disorder. J Clin Psychopharmacol. 2016;36(4):393–4 [A].

[331] Hamera L, Khishfe BF. Kounis syndrome and ziprasidone. Am J Emerg Med. 2017;35(3):493–4. pii: S0735-6757(16)30896-8 [A].

[332] Codina MQ, Vila LC, Ninot GM, et al. Ziprasidone-induced sub acute cutaneous lupus erythematosus. Lupus. 2017;26(7):785–6. [A].

7

Antiepileptics

Robert D. Beckett*,[1], Nora Klemke[†], Matthew Bessesen*, Sidhartha D. Ray*

*Manchester University College of Pharmacy, Natural and Health Sciences, Fort Wayne, IN, United States
[†]Lutheran Health Network, Fort Wayne, IN, United States
[1]Corresponding author: rdbeckett@manchester.edu

ANTIEPILEPTIC DRUGS (AEDs) WITH POTENTIAL GABA MECHANISM OF ACTION

Gabapentin

A meta-analysis of 9 randomized-controlled trials, comprising 588 participants treated with gabapentin for tonsillectomy procedures (i.e., cold or thermal, no other nasal or otologic surgery), was conducted to assess the efficacy of gabapentin for improving the patient (adult and pediatric) experience via the evaluation of pain scores, postoperative analgesic requirements, time to first analgesia, and adverse effects [1M]. Adverse events (AEs) were analyzed via standard mean difference (SMD) or log odds ratio (OR) for the studies that reported the events. Postoperative nausea and vomiting was significantly lower in the gabapentin group than in the control group (Log OR = −0.49; CI [−0.87 to −0.10]). The degree of sedation (SMD = 0.10; CI [−0.17 to 0.38]), dizziness (Log OR = −0.41; CI [−1.04 to 0.22]), and headache (Log OR = 0.14; CI [−0.39 to 0.68]) during the postoperative period was not significantly different in the gabapentin group compared to the control group.

A retrospective case series, of 11 neurologically impaired term and preterm infants treated with gabapentin for visceral hyperalgesia was conducted to assess clinical response and adverse events (AEs) [2c]. All infants were receiving multiple sedative and analgesic medications when gabapentin was initiated. Adverse events were reported in 5 of the 8 preterm infants and in 0 of the 3 term infants. Three of the 5 reported AEs were related to abrupt discontinuation of gabapentin due to nil per os (NPO) status. These 3 infants experienced episodic tachycardia, emesis, and increased irritability, which resolved after re-initiation of gabapentin, suggesting the existence of gabapentin withdrawal syndrome. The remaining 2 AEs occurred in twin infants, who experienced episodes of bradycardia within 24 hours of initiation of gabapentin (1 twin restarted lower dose gabapentin [5 mg/kg/12 h] titrated to 2.5 mg/kg/12 h] with no further bradycardia).

A phase IV, multicenter, randomized, open-label, parallel group, noninferiority study, consisting of 270 patients, was conducted to assess the efficacy and safety of concomitant gabapentin, vitamin B1, and B12 compared to pregabalin in patients with moderate to severe diabetic neuropathy [3C]. During this 12 week, 6 visit study, 147 patients received gabapentin/B1 (100 mg)/B12 (0.20 mg), starting at 300 mg gabapentin at visit 1 (day 1) and ending with 3600 mg gabapentin at visits 4 and 5. Adverse events occurred in 43% of patients treated with gabapentin/B1/B12. The most common AEs were somnolence (27%), lightheadedness (24.1%), dizziness (17%), headache (7.5%), and vertigo (3.2%). Although influence of vitamin B1 and B12 cannot be ruled out, considering the study design, both agents are generally well tolerated at the administered doses. Pregabalin was initiated in 123 patients, starting at 75 mg at visit 1 (day 1) and ending with 600 mg at visits 4 and 5. Adverse events (AEs) occurred in 44% of patients treated with pregabalin. The most common AEs were dizziness (24%), somnolence (23%), vertigo (4%) and headache (3%). The findings from this study suggest the combination of gabapentin/B1/B12 have synergistic effects that allow for pain control at lower doses of gabapentin which are associated with less AEs.

Pregabalin

A multicenter, double-blind, randomized, placebo-controlled study treated 233 patients receiving palliative

---

radiotherapy for cancer-induced bone pain (CIBP) with pregabalin 75 mg every 12 hours ($n=116$) or placebo ($n=117$) [4C]. The safety population included all patients who received any dose of the trial medication, and AE reporting was monitored through contacting the patients every 2–3 days and continued until 30 days after trial completion. Common AEs that were reported in the pregabalin arm included: cognitive disturbance (9%), nausea (6%), fatigue (4%), vomiting (3%), pain (3%) and common adverse events reported in the placebo group included: cognitive disturbance (3%), nausea (8%), fatigue (3%), vomiting (3%), and pain (4%).

A meta-analysis of six randomized-controlled trials, including 769 patients, assessed visual analogue scale (VAS), cumulative morphine consumption, and safety endpoints after a total knee arthroplasty (TKA) to compare pregabalin vs control (placebo or nothing) [5M]. Adverse events were reported as relative risk (RR), probability (P), and number needed to harm (NNH). Pregabalin was shown to reduce the occurrence of nausea (RR=0.73; 95% CI=0.61–0.88; $P=0.001$) and vomiting (RR=0.55; 95% CI=0.38–0.78; $P=0.001$). Pregabalin increased the risk of dizziness (RR=1.49; 95% CI= 1.08–2.05; $P=0.014$; NNH=14) and sedation (RR=1.84; 95% CI=1.42–2.39; $P<0.001$; NNH=4.38).

A randomized, double-blinded, placebo-controlled study, including 100 patients aged 18–70 years, evaluated the efficacy of pregabalin (150 mg), celecoxib (400 mg), and their combination in the management of acute postoperative pain in patients undergoing laparoscopic cholecystectomy [6c]. Sedation and postoperative nausea and vomiting (PONV) scores were rated according to hospital practice and other AEs were reported throughout the study period. No significant difference was identified in the incidence of sedation, PONV, or other AEs of headache, diplopia, lightheadedness, drowsiness, pruritus, difficulty walking or concentrating, dry mouth, and confusion between all four groups. Statistically significant increases in drowsiness (OR=3.07; 95% CI= 1.105–8.98; $P=0.04$) and lightheadedness (OR=3.93; 95% CI=1.25–12.35; $P=0.019$) were seen in the pregabalin alone group as compared to placebo. It is unclear whether these AEs were higher in the pregabalin only, but not the combination group as there were no differences across the three treatment groups in terms of postoperative opioid requirements.

A randomized, multicenter, double-blinded, 14-week, crossover study (with 2-week washout period) of 301 patients with painful diabetic peripheral neuropathy (DPN) using nonsteroidal anti-inflammatory drug (NSAID) for non-DPN-related pain, evaluated the safety and efficacy of pregabalin (150–300 mg/day) vs placebo in reduction of pain [7C]. The per protocol population of 272 patients treated with pregabalin and 276 patients treated with placebo were included in the analysis

of AEs. Fifty-four percent of patients treated with pregabalin reported an AE (34.2% were deemed treatment related by investigators) as compared to 43.1% in the placebo group (21.7% deemed treatment related). The most common (≥5% pregabalin group) AEs were dizziness (10.3% vs 1.4%), somnolence (5.1% vs 2.5%), and fatigue (5.1% vs 1.4%) pregabalin vs placebo respectfully. No serious AEs were deemed treatment related, however, 6.6% discontinued treatment and 5.5% reduced therapy in the pregabalin group due to AEs and 6.9% discontinued treatment and 4.3% reduced therapy in the placebo group.

VALPROIC ACID/DIVALPROEX SODIUM

A prospective cohort, multicenter, observational study of women enrolled in the North American Antiepileptic Drug (AED) Pregnancy Registry investigated the neurodevelopmental effects of 252 children (ages 3–6 years old) exposed prenatally to lamotrigine ($n=104$), sodium valproate ($n=51$), or carbamazepine ($n=97$) to determine if prenatal exposure to these monotherapies would be associated with adaptive behavior impairments and if these outcomes were dose dependent [8C]. Adaptive behavior was measured using the Vineland-II Adaptive Behavior Scales, administered by phone. Mean Adaptive Behavior Composite (ABC); domain standard scores for communication, daily living, socialization, and motor skills; and adaptive levels were analyzed across drug groups and correlated with first trimester drug dose. Lower Vineland-II scores indicate greater impairment. After adjusting for maternal age, education, epilepsy type, prenatal seizures, folate use, cigarette and alcohol exposure, gestational age, and birth weight, the mean ABC score for valproate-exposed children was 95.6 (95% CI 91–101), vs 100.8 (95% CI 98–103) and 103.5 (95% CI 101–106) for carbamazepine and lamotrigine, respectively ($P=0.017$). Higher valproate dose was associated with significantly lower ABC ($P=0.020$), socialization ($P=0.009$), and motor ($P=0.041$) scores before adjusting for cofounders. No dose effect was observed for carbamazepine or lamotrigine.

A multicenter, open-label, prospective, observational study was conducted to evaluate the safety ($n=489$) and effectiveness ($n=468$) of divalproex sodium XR containing regimen in patients with bipolar disorder (BPD) who were in continuation phase [9C]. The mean duration of BPD was 69.2 ± 82.2 months and the mean dose of divalproex sodium XR was 907.9 ± 316.1 and 883.5 ± 300.8 mg/day during visits 2 and 3, respectively. A total of 66 AEs were observed in 56 patients (11.5%, $n=489$). Of the total 66 AEs, 89.0% were mild, 10.9% were moderate, and no serious AEs occurred. The AEs included: tremors (1.4%), somnolence (1.4%), weight gain (1.4%), headache (1.2%), constipation (1.0%), gastritis (0.8%), nausea, peripheral edema, pyrexia, appetite disorder, increased appetite (0.4%), and vomiting, insomnia, amenorrhea, rhinitis, upper respiratory tract infection (0.2%).

A case series of sodium valproate-induced Fanconi's syndrome was described for three patients age ranging from 5 to 12 years [10c]. The first case was a 6-year-old Caucasian-British boy, diagnosed with Mowat–Wilson syndrome, developed atypical absent seizures and was treated with valproate and topiramate at age 2. At age 6 he was admitted for hypophosphatemia and pathological fractures, he weighed 13.8 kg and was on 35 mg/kg/day valproate. The second case was a 12-year-old Asian-British boy, at age 1 he was diagnosed with tonic seizure and failed therapy with phenobarbital and phenytoin and switched to valproate and topiramate. At age 12 he was admitted for lethargy and generally not well, his dose of valproate was 17 mg/kg/day. The final case is of a 5-year-old Asian-British boy, he was admitted for puffiness and swelling of face and lower limbs, his dose of valproate was 35 mg/kg/day. The most important diagnostic features for valproate sodium-induced Fanconi's syndrome hypophosphatemia, glycosuria and proteinuria were noted in the three cases. After tapering valproate sodium to discontinuation, the patient's serum urine biochemistry returned to normal, which was also the ultimate resolution of the first two cases.

A retrospective cohort study of 329 patients receiving a continuous infusion of valproic acid, aged 1 month to 85 years, was conducted to assess therapeutic response, common AEs, and pharmacokinetic parameters of valproic acid continuous infusion [11C]. Patients received a 20–40 mg/kg loadings dose of valproic acid infused over 30–60 minutes followed by a 1 mg/kg/h continuous infusion. A valproic acid serum concentration was obtained approximately 4 hours after the loading dose and then again 24 hours after initiating the continuous infusion. The infusion rate was adjusted proportionally based on the 24-hours concentration to achieve target serum concentrations (typically within 50–100 μg/mL). Continuous infusion valproic acid was well tolerated overall, and documented adverse events were similar to published data. Gastrointestinal complaints were documented in 7.3% of patients (typically dyspepsia or diarrhea). Hyperammonemia (ammonia concentration greater than 50 mg/dL) occurred in 3.6% of patients, and elevated liver enzymes (three times upper limit of normal) were detected in 1.2% of all patients. Concurrent neurological changes were not reported in hyperammonemic patients, and none had other symptoms of hepatic dysfunction. Prevalence of other factors, including critical illness, malnutrition, and prolonged treatment, were attributed to cases of hyperammonemia by the investigators. Thrombocytopenia was rare, with only 1.8% of patients having a minimum platelet count of <100000/mL. No other obvious adverse effects related to valproic acid therapy were documented.

A case report described an 18-month-old girl with Lennox–Gastaut syndrome of unknown cause, who developed hepatic dysfunction in association with the combined use of valproic acid and the ketogenic diet (KD) [12A]. At 18 months, after failure of multiple anticonvulsant medication regimens, the child was started on a ketogenic diet. At the time of initiation, she was stable (in terms of medications and dosing) on and continued to take topiramate (2.5 mg/kg/day divided twice daily), valproic acid (20 mg/kg/day divided twice daily), and clobazam (0.75 mg/kg/day divided twice daily). After 3 days of therapy, the patient began experiencing respiratory symptoms. She was diagnosed with pneumonia, remained febrile, and was admitted to the intensive care unit with an elevated alanine aminotransferase (ALT) of 924 IU/L among other abnormal laboratory findings. Valproic acid and ketogenic were stopped at this time. After stopping valproic acid and AST and ALT had reduced to 38 and 132 U/L, respectively, ketogenic diet was restarted, her liver enzymes returned to normal and she achieved markedly improved seizure control and quality of life. The investigators noted that hepatic dysfunction has previously been reported with the combination of valproic acid and ketogenic diet, but that this case illustrates ketogenic may be safely restarted prior to complete reversal of hepatic effects.

A retrospective review was conducted to assess the safety of combined KD and valproic acid therapy in 75 patients with drug-resistant epilepsy aged 6 months to 9 years. Of the 75 patients, only 2 experienced AEs [13c]. One was a 4-year-old girl with severe psychomotor retardation and refractory epilepsy resulting from perinatal asphyxia. She was treated with a 4:1 KD (4 parts fat to 1 part carbohydrates and protein combined) along with valproic acid and zonisamide treatment. After 6 months seizure free she was titrated off of zonisamide and after 2 years seizure free was gradually titrated off of valproic acid (50 mg every 2 weeks). By the final removal of valproate a sharp increase in ketosis (maximum serum b-OH butyrate 3.7 mg/dL) was observed accompanied by clinical signs (somnolence, apathy). By changing the KD ratio of 4:1 down to 2.5:1, the patient returned to her former condition. The second patient who experiences an AE was a 4-year-old girl with drug resistant epilepsy that was on a 4:1 KD with topiramate, zonisamide, and valproic acid as drug therapy. Topiramate and zonisamide were titrated off without AE, but after valproate cessation an increase in the level of ketosis (maximum serum b-OH butyrate 3.9 mg/dL) was observed with accompanying clinical signs, including dry mouth with ketotic breath, lack of hunger, fatigue and somnolence.

After adjustment of KD ratio to 2:1, the adverse clinical signs resolved. The majority of co-administered valproic acid and KD seem to be safe and it should be noted that if a patient is over-ketotic when valproic acid is titrated down, lowering KD ratio seems to decrease ketosis to desired levels.

AEDs WITH OTHER MECHANISMS OF ACTION

Brivaracetam

An indirect meta-analysis compared randomized-controlled trials of adjunctive brivaracterm, eslicarbazepine, lacosamide, and perampanel for treatment of focal epilepsy (i.e., complex focal, simple focal, or secondary generalized tonic–clonic seizures) in adults or pediatrics [14M]. Safety endpoints assessed included proportions of patients who experienced a treatment-emergent adverse event (TEAE) and a TEAE that led to study discontinuation. Brivaracetam 50 mg was associated with reduced risk for TEAE compared to perampanel 8 mg (RR 0.54, 95% CI 0.33–0.90); brivaracetam 200 mg was associated with reduced risk for TEAE compared to perampanel 12 mg (RR 0.33, 95% CI 0.20–0.56) and eslicarbazepine 1200 mg (RR 0.63, 95% CI 0.40–0.97). No additional comparisons were statistically significant in either direction, and impact on TEAEs leading to study discontinuation was no different across treatment groups. It should be noted that specific AEs were not reported. Heterogeneity results were not reported and no direct comparisons between agents were identified in the authors' literature search.

A Phase I, open-label, pharmacokinetic study assessed the addition of brivaractetam 50 mg twice daily titrated over 22 days to 100 mg twice daily and continued for 1 week in patients receiving carbamazepine ($n=9$) or carbamazepine plus valproate in combination ($n=9$) [15c]. Compared to prior to addition of brivaracetam, serum trough concentrations of carbamazepine epoxide were elevated throughout the duration of treatment in patients on monotherapy (highest geometric least-squares means ratio 2.20, 90% CI 1.65–2.92) and combination (highest geometric least-squares means ratio 2.24, 90% CI 1.98–2.53). Serum trough concentrations of carbamazepine and carbamazepine diol were unaffected by addition of brivaracetam. There was at least one TEAE reported by 83% of participants, with the most frequent being constipation, convulsion, dizziness, fatigue, headache, nasopharyngitis, and somnolence. Three patients experienced serious TEAEs leading to hospitalization: abnormal feeling, aggression, and increased seizures. These results are consistent with known inhibition of epoxide hydrolase by brivaracetam; however, the implications of altered carbamazepine epoxide remain unclear.

Ethosuximide

In an open-label pilot study, 7 adult patients with essential tremor received ethosuximide 250 mg daily increased to 250 mg twice daily [16c]. There was no benefit on clinician-assessed motor task performance or daily living activities, and no impact on patient-assessed symptoms or global appraisal; however, 2 patients discontinued the study due to AEs, including anxiety, dizziness, headache, and nervousness.

In a cross-sectional study, 61 patients (mean age 9.4 ± 2.7 years) receiving ethosuximide as monotherapy (mean total daily dose 686 ± 245 mg) were administered a set of neuropsychological tests in order to describe the cognitive profile of ethosuximide in this population [17c]. Scores across attentional (i.e., activation, alertness), intelligence, and visuomotor function demonstrated impairment compared to population averages; however, clinical relevance of these findings is not clear due to ethosuximide's role as a first-line agent for pediatric absence seizures, and lack of a control group.

Levetiracetam

A prospective, multicenter, observational study, including 101 patients aged 1–11 months, was conducted to evaluate the safety of levetiracetam and its impact on epilepsy severity in infants with different seizure types [18C]. Of 101 patients who started, 75 completed the study and 26 discontinued prematurely. Seven patients discontinued due to AEs, and three were lost to follow-up. Overall 55 of patients experienced a TEAE at any time during the study, 5 of whom experienced a TEAE judged by the investigators to be related to levetiracetam. Twelve patients had a least one severe TEAE and 6 patient deaths were reported, of which none were related to the study drug according to investigators. The most common TEAEs reported ($\geq 5\%$) were bronchitis (10), convulsion (10), pyrexia (8), and diarrhea (6).

A retrospective cohort of 46 patients aged 20–65 years, treated with levetiracetam for epilepsy for at least 1 year, were assessed for bone mineral density (BMD) measurements [19c]. Seven patients (15.2%) were found to have osteopenia and no patient was identified with osteoporosis. Separate gender analyses disclosed that men in the long treatment group (>5.5 years of levetiracetam therapy) have better bone health than men in the short treatment group, although not statistically significant. However, women in the long treatment group have worse bone health than women in the short treatment group (specific statistical analysis not reported).

A single-center, pragmatic, open-label, comparative trial 84 patients who had failed initial monotherapy with an older AED (carbamazepine, valproate sodium, or phenytoin) were randomized to receive to substitution monotherapy of levetiracetam (LEV) (1000 mg/day) or an older AED (carbamazepine 400 mg/day or valproate sodium 1000 mg/day, whichever had not been failed) to assess the effects on bone health [20c]. Patients were adults, with 21%–29% premenopausal and 10%–18% postmenopausal females depending on the treatment group. Areal BMD and content at lumbar spine (LS), total hip (TH), forearm (FA), and femoral neck (FN), radial and tibial peripheral quantitative compute tomography and serum one turnover markers, were assessed at 3 and 15 months. Of the 84 patients randomized, 70 completed assessments (40 in the levetiracetam group and 30 in the older AED group). Analysis showed statistically significant decreases in BMD at the LS (−9.0% vs −9.8%), FA (−1.46% vs −0.96%) and radial trabecular (−1.46% vs −2.31%) fracture sites in levetiracetam group and old AED group respectfully. In conclusion, use of both levetiracetam and older AEDs was associated with bone loss over 1 year at clinically relevant fracture sites and a reduction in bone turnover.

A retrospective cohort of 186 patients, aged 13–44 years, diagnosed with juvenile myoclonic epilepsy (JME) reviewed the long-term use of AEDs [21C]. Over the course of follow-up, 76 AED monotherapy schedules produced intolerable side-effects that required a change in therapy. Aggression was the most common cause for withdrawal in the levetiracetam group (4/12 patients treated with levetiracetam monotherapy). Overall, 92% of patients were able to obtain remission with AED treatment, despite adverse drug reactions or need to change therapy.

A retrospective chart of the 19-item Liverpool Adverse Event Profile (LAEP) of 841 patient aged ≥16 years, with epilepsy for ≥12 months, was analyzed to identify independent predictors for specific AEs of AEDs [22C]. One-hundred fifty-one patients identified on levetiracetam monotherapy (with standardized daily dosage using a defined daily dose of 1500 mg) were analyzed along with several other AEDs against LAEP outcomes using logistic regression to assess the independent contribution of individual AEDs to frequent occurrence of specific AEs. Levetiracetam was found to be independently associated with anger/aggression (OR 7.3), nervousness/agitation (OR 5.4), upset stomach (OR 5.4), depression (3.02), and sleep disturbance (2.4).

Two reported pediatric cases with epilepsy that developed diurnal frequent urination after levetiracetam administration [23A]. One case reported a 6-year-old male patient who experienced increased daytime urinary frequency and urgency after his third day of adjunctive levetiracetam therapy (titrated up to 25 mg/kg/day).

Symptoms worsened as the dose was increased (more than 20 times daily, though total volume remained the same) and laboratory tests and auxiliary examination did not reveal evidence of an organic disease. Levetiracetam dose was cut in half and urinary frequency reduced to 10 times daily. Levetiracetam was discontinued due to parenteral concerns and urinary frequency returned to normal. Another case reported a 13-year-old female with similar symptoms of urinary frequency after the initiation of levetiracetam. Symptoms were increased during times of stress, to the point where urgent wetting reach, at most, seven to eight times daily. Other causes for micturition were ruled out; therefore, the dose of levetiracetam was reduced to one-third the initial dose (3000–1000 mg/day). This yielded a 60% reduction in frequency of urination.

A multicenter, open-label, follow-up study of extended-release levetiracetam was conducted in patients with partial-onset seizures (POS) in order to assess the long-term safety of extended-release levetiracetam monotherapy in patient with POS [24C]. Patients ($n = 189$), who successfully completed the titration up to extended-release levetiracetam 2000 mg/day from the previous trial, were enrolled and 166 patients completed the study. TEAEs occurred in 66.7% of patients; most were mild to moderate severity. The most common TEAEs were headache (13.8%), nasopharyngitis (7.9%), somnolence (7.9%), influenza (7.4%), and dizziness (5.3%). Five patients (2.6%) experience a TEAE that lead to treatment discontinuation (convulsion, psychotic disorder, drowning, and pregnancy). Thirty percent of patients experienced drug-related TEAEs; of these, somnolence (6.9%) was the only event that occurred in ≥5% of patients.

A case report of a 9-year-old girl, with a 2-month history of intracranial space occupying mass-related seizures was initiated with levetiracetam monotherapy. The patient developed pharyngitis accompanied by exudative membrane, bilateral cervical lymphadenopathy, tender hepatomegaly, skin rash, and fever after 19 days of therapy [25A]. Laboratory findings revealed leukocytosis, lymphocytosis with an atypical lymphocytosis, eosinophilia, thrombocytopenia, and elevated serum transaminases. The patient was diagnosed with drug reaction with eosinophilia and systemic symptoms syndrome and antiepileptic therapy was immediately discontinued. The patient's systemic signs and symptoms improved after administration of systemic steroids and antihistamine therapy. Levetiracetam is a commonly used and usually well-tolerated antiepileptic in pediatric patients. This present pediatric case report shows the potential severe hypersensitivity reactions of levetiracetam therapy.

A case was reported of a 43-year-old female who presented 8 hours post ingestion of 60–80 g of levetiracetam, 10 g of paracetamol, 600 mg of codeine, and unknown quantity of alcohol presented with mild central nervous system depression, bradycardia, hypotension, and oliguria [26A]. Her levetiracetam concentration was 463 mcg/mL 8 hours post ingestion (therapeutic range 10–40 mcg/mL, proposed by investigators). Her cardiovascular toxicity did respond to atropine and intravenous fluids and she made a complete recovery after 48 hours with normal left and right ventricular contractility.

Rufinamide

A meta-analysis of 5 double blind, randomized, placebo-controlled trials, including 1512 patients, was conducted to evaluate the clinical efficacy and safety of rufinamide (200–3200 mg/day) in drug-resistant epilepsy [27M]. Regardless of dose, rufinamide increased withdrawal rate due to AEs and severe AEs (RR=2.3; 95% CI 1.5–3.5; $P < 0.001$). The rate of at least one AE (RR=1.1; 95% CI=1.0–1.2; $P < 0.001$) also increased in the rufinamide group, but it did not increase the rate of severe AEs (RR=1.5; 95% CI=0.9–2.2; $P = 0.090$). Individual AEs were significantly higher in the rufinamide group: headache (RR=1.3; 95% CI=1.0–1.6; $P = 0.028$), dizziness (RR=2.1; 95% CI=1.2–3.3; $P < 0.001$), fatigue (RR=1.5; 95% CI=1.1–2.2; $P = 0.021$), somnolence (RR=1.9; 95% CI=1.4–2.6; $P < 0.001$), nausea (RR=1.8; 95% CI=1.0–3.2; $P = 0.001$), diplopia (RR=5.4; 95% CI=3.0–10.0; $P < 0.001$) and vomiting (RR=3.3; 95% CI=1.8–6.3; $P < 0.001$).

An interim analysis from a phase III, multicenter, randomized, active-controlled, open-label study, of 37 subjects, was conducted to evaluate the safety and age group-specific pharmacokinetics of rufinamide in patients less than 4 years of age with Lennox–Gastaut syndrome [28c]. The safety results showed that TEAEs were similar between the rufinamide (n=22) and control group (n=9). The control AED was selected at the clinician's discretion, and included lamotrigine (n=5), clobazam (n=2), and phenobarbital, topiramate, valproic acid, and zonisamide (n=1 for each). The most frequently reported TEAEs (occurring in at least 10% of subjects) in the rufinamide group were vomiting (24.0%), upper respiratory tract infection (20.0%), diarrhea and somnolence (16.0% each), and constipation, cough, bronchitis, rash, and decreased appetite (12.0% each). In the any-other-AED group, they were diarrhea and upper respiratory tract infection (27.3% each), and convulsion (18.2%). Eight (32.0%) subjects in the rufinamide group and 3 (27.3%) subjects in the any-other-AED group had TEAEs requiring study drug dose adjustment or interruption.

A multicenter, retrospective chart review of 58 patients, prescribed adjunctive rufinamide therapy, at seven Spanish epilepsy centers was conducted to evaluate long-term effectiveness in the management of Lennox–Gastaut syndrome and other epileptic diseases [29c]. The mean daily rufinamide dose was 32.0 mg/kg (range 12.5–66.7 mg/kg) in children and 24.7 mg/kg (range 5.0–47.0 mg/kg) in adults. Side effects were reported in 36.2% patients: nausea, vomiting and weight loss were most frequent. Treatment was withdrawn in 8.6% of these patients due to AEs. Adverse events resolved with no changes to rufinamide dose in 15.5% patients and with dose reduction or slower rufinamide titration in 12.1%. Most of the AEs were considered to be mild and were similar in type and frequency to previously reported studies.

A case study described a 12-year-old-boy with intractable epilepsy had tonic and atonic seizures despite treatment with valproic acid (3000 mg/day), levetiracetam (3000 mg/day), and clobazam (40 mg/day) [30A]. Rufinamide was added as adjunctive therapy for 2 weeks, starting at 100 mg/day and was titrated up 50 mg every 3 days up to 250 mg/day. The patient began to experience atonic seizure worsening and the frequency of epileptic discharges increased. The increase in seizure frequency and epileptiform discharges resolved when rufinamide was discontinued.

SODIUM CHANNEL BLOCKERS

Carbamazepine

A retrospective cohort, single-center, 12-week analysis of 196 patients treated for vestibular paroxysmia (VP) with carbamazepine (n=73), carbamazepine plus betahistine mesilate tablets (n=65), or oxcarbazepine plus betahistine mesilate tablets (n=58) was conducted to evaluate the frequency of vertigo, vertigo duration, vertigo score, response rate and side effects between the three treatment groups to assess efficacy and acceptability [31C]. The average dose of carbamazepine, oxcarbazepine, and betahistine mesilate was 351, 726 and 34 mg/day, respectively. The age of patients ranged from 45 to 73 years, mean duration of vertigo was 1.48 ± 0.45 years, and the mean age of onset of vertigo attacks was 56.9 ± 8.63 years. Various AEs included drowsiness, erythema, dry mouth, dizziness, ataxia, and nausea. The incidence of side effects was highest in carbamazepine (30.1%), second in the carbamazepine+betahistine mesilate (18.5%) and lowest in oxcarbazepine+betahistine mesilate group (8.6%). Two patients receiving carbamazepine withdrew due to severe side effects of erythema and ataxia. The mild side effects disappeared with dose reduction.

A case report described a 64-year-old male who presented with a fever and systemic erythrodermic eruptions 7 weeks after being initiated on carbamazepine for diabetic neuropathy [32A]. Laboratory data showed liver dysfunction (AST 36 U/L, ALT 90 U/L, ALP 505 U/L), a high serum C-reactive protein level (CRP 3.34 mg/dL), and eosinophilia (2192/mcL), without leukocytosis or atypical lymphocytes. Chest radiography showed no abnormal findings. The eruptions and lab data improved after carbamazepine discontinuation and initiating oral prednisolone (30 mg/day). The patient later developed oral ulcerations and viral pneumonia consistent with CMV reaction likely due to corticosteroid therapy. This case met the diagnostic criteria for atypical drug-induced hypersensitivity caused by carbamazepine.

A case was reported of an 88-year-old female who was on low dose (200 mg/day) of carbamazepine for trigeminal neuralgia, presented to the emergency department experiencing syncope while in sitting position, with no complaints of chest pain or dyspnea [33A]. Her electrocardiogram showed advanced degree heart block (Mobitz type I AV block and 2:1 AV block). Her carbamazepine serum concentration was 2.7 mcg/mL (reference 4–12 mcg/mL). Her carbamazepine was discontinued despite normal levels and she returned to normal sinus rhythm. Carbamazepine has been previously reported to cause AV node dysfunction, and investigators advocate considering it as a potential reversible cause prior to invasive procedures.

Eslicarbazepine Acetate

An open-label, multicenter, prospective, non-interventional study assessed retention, tolerability, safety, efficacy and effects on quality of life with eslicarbazepine acetate as an add-on treatment over 6 months in an adult population with partial-onset seizures ($n = 247$) on baseline antiepileptic drugs [34C]. The most frequent eslicarbazepine target dose was 800 mg/day. Levetiracetam ($n = 83$), lamotrigine ($n = 54$), valproate ($n = 30$), and carbamazepine ($n = 14$) were the most commonly reported base-line antiepileptic drugs. Overall 109 AEs were reported in 57 patients (26%). One death occurred, in a 78-year-old male with history of cardiac myxoma surgery and was not related to eslicarbazepine treatment. The majority of the AEs were considered to be related to eslicarbazepine treatment (84 AE in 49 patients). The most frequently reported events were dizziness (4.6%), headache (3.2%), convulsion (3.2%), and fatigue (2.7%); all other events were reported for less than six patients.

Lacosamide

In order to evaluate risk for cardiovascular and psychiatric TEAEs associated with adjunctive AEDs, an observational cohort study of 1004 patients 16 years of age or older who received lacosamide ($n = 511$) or another AED ($n = 493$, specific AEDs not specified) [35C]. Patients on lacosamide were more likely to receive concomitant AEDs compared to the control group (60.9% vs 52.5%) and less likely to receive a single concomitant AED (14.7% vs 31.4%). The most common concomitant AEDs were levetiracetam (48.9% vs 39.8%), lamotrigine (42.5% vs 33.9%), carbamazepine (26.4% vs 22.7%), oxcarbazepine (24.1% vs 17.0%), and valproate sodium (19.6% vs 20.1%). Median duration of exposure was similar between groups (324.5 vs 321 days), and the most common lacosamide total daily dose was 400 mg by 12 months of treatment. At baseline, about 3.7% and 20% of patients had a concomitant cardiac or psychiatric disorder, respectively, in each group. The rate of cardiovascular TEAEs was similar between groups (0.8% vs 0.8%); cardiovascular TEAEs in the lacosamide group included 2 cases of sinus bradycardia, and single cases of AV block and bradycardia. The rate of psychiatric TEAEs was also similar (4.1% vs 5.5%), with fewer events judged to be treatment related (2.2% vs 3.7%). The most common psychiatric events were depression (2.9% vs 4.3%) and depressed mood (0.8% vs 1.0%). Overall, investigators concluded that risk for cardiac and psychiatric AEs with lacosamide is low.

In a double-blind, randomized, controlled clinical trial, 548 adult Chinese and Japanese patients with uncontrolled focal, partial-onset seizures were randomized to receive 24-weeks of adjunctive treatment with lacosamide 200 mg per day, lacosamide 400 mg per day, or placebo [36C]. Lacosamide doses were titrated from an initial dose of 100 mg per day in weekly intervals of 100 mg per day. The most common concomitant AEDs were carbamazepine (47.6%), valproate (45.4%), levetiracetam (23.9%), and lamotrigine (21.7%). Rates of any TEAE, serious TEAE, and discontinuation due to TEAE were higher with lacosamide 400 mg (79.4%, 5.0%, 15.6%, respectively) compared to lacosamide 200 mg (65.0%, 1.1%, 4.4%) and placebo (69.6%, 1.6%, 6.5%). Overall, the most common TEAEs with placebo, lacosamide 200 mg, and lacosamide 400 mg were dizziness (9.2% vs 16.4% vs 35.6%, respectively), nasopharyngitis (12.5% vs 13.7% vs 15.0%), somnolence (3.8% vs 9.8% vs 10.6%), and headache (6.0% vs 8.2% vs 10.6%). Of the serious TEAEs, 5 were judged by investigators to be related to lacosamide: one case each of dizziness, liver injury, pneumonia, suicide attempt, upper gastrointestinal bleed.

In an open-label extension study 322 patients who received lacosamide monotherapy or adjunctive therapy in a previous clinical trial continued treatment; 65.2% of patients completed the entire 2-year treatment period [37C]. The most common daily doses received at onset were 300–400 mg (33.2%), 400–500 mg (21.1%) and 500–600 mg (20.2%), and 87.6% received lacosamide as monotherapy. Overall, 91.0% of patients reported a TEAE, and 83.9% of patients on monotherapy reported a TEAE. TEAEs were generally dose related with 59.6% of patients on 300–400 mg, 61.4% of patients on 400–500 mg, and 66.7% of patients on 500–600 mg experiencing a TEAE. The most common TEAEs were dizziness (17.5%), headache (15.1%), upper respiratory tract infection (10.6%), nausea (10.3%), fall (9.6%), nasopharyngitis (8.9%), and fatigue (8.2%). Dizziness and headache appeared to be dose related. A total of 17.4% of patients and 12.0% of patients on monotherapy reported serious TEAEs, with convulsion (2.7%) and syncope (0.7%) being the most common. TEAEs reportedly led to discontinuation for 7.1% of patients.

In a single-center, retrospective, observational study, 106 adult patients with partial-onset seizures initiated on lacosamide (50 mg twice daily titrated in 100 mg weekly intervals as needed) were classified according to whether they experienced planned reduction of a concomitant AED ($n=59$) or not ($n=47$) based on provider documentation [38c]. TEAEs occurred in 49.2% of patients with compared to 68.1% of patients without planned AED reduction; ultimate discontinuation of lacosamide also occurred less often in the planned reduction group (22.0% vs 40.4%). In an adjusted logistic regression model, the odds for planned AED reduction was lower for patients who experienced a TEAE (OR 0.36, 95% CI 0.016–0.84, $P=0.019$) and lacosamide discontinuation (OR 0.40, 95% CI 0.17–0.96, $P=0.040$).

In a multicenter, retrospective observational study, 105 adult patients with brain tumor-related epilepsy treated with lacosamide were assessed considering data from baseline, month 3, and month 6 of treatment [39c]. The majority of patients (54.3%) had previously been treated with AEDs (87.6% of these with levetiracetam), and about 80% were receiving one or two concomitant AEDs (75.2% of these with levetiracetam). AEs were reported in 34.3% of patients at 3 months and 41.9% of patients by 6 months. Similar to previous reports, at 6 months, the most common AEs were somnolence/fatigue (21.0%), dizziness (12.4%), unsteadiness (8.6%), blurred vision/diplopia (6.7%), mental slowness (2.9%), anxiety (1.9%), and rash (1.9%).

In a single-group, open-label, multicenter clinical trial, 86 patients with non-lesional temporal lobe epilepsy non-responsive to the first agent received adjunctive (67.4%) or monotherapy (32.6%) with lacosamide [40c]. Lacosamide doses were titrated from 50 mg weekly up to 200–400 mg per day for a median treatment duration of 18 months (range 6–46 months). Although minimal safety results were provided, there were reported to be 3 patients who experienced mild AEs of confusion, itching, and swelling that did not require discontinuation.

In a single-center, retrospective chart review, 47 patients less than 12 years of age (median age 6.5 years) were treated with IV lacosamide as adjunctive therapy in combination with at least 2 AEDs [41c]. IV administration was most commonly used for acute exacerbation of seizure frequency and severity ($n=18$, median initial dose 4.5 mg/kg, range 1–11 mg/kg), inability to take oral medications ($n=15$, median dose 4 mg/kg, range 2–10 mg/kg), and status epilepticus ($n=11$, median dose 7.2 mg/kg, range 4–11 mg/kg). There were 5 documented cases of sedation as an AE that all resolved, and no other documented AEs, including none in the 18 patients less than 3 years of age.

In a 38-patient pilot study, lacosamide 200–400 mg IV loading dose, followed by 200–400 mg daily was administered to patients with seizure emergencies (i.e., seizure clusters [$n=15$], status epilepticus [$n=23$]) [42c]. Safety assessments included ECG, metabolic panel, hemogram, and blood levels of concomitant AEDs. No relevant changes related to these safety assessments were not described. Two cases of dizziness were reported, both of which occurred in patients with established status epilepticus, and most patients experienced some level of sedation, although none of the latter were described as AEs.

In a prospective, open-label, single-group study, 34 adult patients were treated with lacosamide (50 mg twice daily titrated as needed to 200 mg twice daily) for 24 weeks in order to assess effects on cognition, mood, and quality of life [43c]. There was no change in cognitive, mood, or quality of life scores at the end of study compared to baseline in a univariate analysis and when changes in seizure frequency was accounted for in a linear model. Reported AEs were similar to previous studies, and included, most commonly, headache ($n=10$), dizziness ($n=7$), tiredness ($n=7$), attention or memory concern ($n=4$), irritability ($n=3$), and depression ($n=3$).

In a Phase IIIb, multicenter, open-label trial, 11 otherwise healthy male patients (mean age 31.5 ± 5.9 years, 63.6% BMI at least 25 kg/m^2) with focal seizures were switched from adjunctive carbamazepine to lacosamide and assessed for changes in hormone and lipid levels following 12 weeks of treatment [44c]. Median sex hormone binding globulin (SHBG) decreased from a baseline of 61.7 nmol/L (range 43.3–80.6 nmol/L) to 47.5 nmol/L (range 32.5–85.5 nmol/L, $P=0.027$). Median free androgen index (i.e., $100\times$ testosterone/SHBG) increased from 25.4 (range 11.8–34.6) to 36.4 (range 18.3–55.9, $P=0.002$). Median total cholesterol increased from 5.5 mmol/L (range 3.6–6.3 mmol/L) to 4.9 mmol/L (range 3.6–6.2 mmol/L, $P=0.012$). There were no other statistically significant changes from baseline in other reproductive hormones (i.e., testosterone, progesterone), thyroid hormones, or other lipid values. There were 10 TEAEs, including aggression, attention disturbance, bronchitis, convulsion, fatigue, hot flash, influenza, paresthesia, partial seizures, and tremor.

A retrospective chart review assessed 9 pediatric patients (5 females, mean age 5.7 years, range 3 months to 16 years) who were treated with IV lacosamide for status epilepticus [45c]. Patients received a mean loading dose of 8.7 mg/kg (range 3.3–10 mg/kg), with 7 patients receiving 10 mg/kg; the mean dose received during the first 24 hours of treatment was 13.8 mg/kg (range 4.3–15 mg/kg). Treatment was effective for 7 of 9 patients, and the only reported AE was a single case of bradycardia.

In a double-blind, double-dummy, randomized, crossover study, 60 healthy subjects received lacosamide 150 mg twice daily and immediate release carbamazepine 200 mg three times daily in separate treatment periods [46c]. Doses were titrated in weekly increments of 100 and 200 mg, respectively, for 3 weeks followed by 4-week maintenance periods, and treatment periods were separated by a 24-day washout period. TEAEs (60.0% vs 75.4%), drug-related TEAEs (22% vs 49%) and withdrawals due to TEAEs (4% vs 14%) were less common with lacosamide. Similar to previous studies, the most common TEAEs were headache (10.0% vs 24.6%), fatigue (8.0% vs 12.3%), upper respiratory tract infection (8.0% vs 7.0%), nasopharyngitis (8.0% vs 3.5%), excoriation (6.0% vs 5.3%), memory impairment (6.0% vs 5.3%), disturbance in attention (6.0% vs 1.8%), cough (6.0% vs 1.8%), nausea (4.0% vs 8.8%), and somnolence (4.0% vs 7.0%).

Lamotrigine

A case report of a 14-year-old girl started on lamotrigine after antiepileptic treatment failure for partial seizure disorder discovered that 9 weeks post treatment, she was admitted to the hospital with a history of rash, fever, and cough [47A]. At this time she discontinued treatment with lamotrigine. Her condition deteriorated with clinical features suggestive of anticonvulsant hypersensitivity syndrome (ACHS) (including fever, rash, hypereosinophilia, and multiple organ involvement) complicated with bronchiolitis obliterans organizing pneumonia (BOOP) secondary to lamotrigine treatment. The patient was treated with pulse methylprednisolone and experienced gradual improvement, reduction of fever, and was discharged on an oral prednisone taper. At 4 weeks the patient was seen in clinic with normal spirometry.

A case report described a female, in her mid-thirties, on a stable dose of lamotrigine 200 mg for 3 months who developed a severe rash on her right rib cage a week after switching to another prescribed brand. She was not taking any other medication at the time of the occurrence [48A]. A week later she developed swollen neck glands, headaches and sensitivity to artificial light. The rash spread to her trunk with some blistering symptoms indicative of Stevens–Johnson syndrome. She discontinued

lamotrigine and the rash completely disappeared over the next week.

Oxcarbazepine

A case of eyelid nystagmus induced by oxcarbamazepine was reported in a 59-year-old man presenting to the emergency department with daily episodes of dizziness and unsteady gait lasting 3–5 hours every afternoon [49A]. He was on amitriptyline (50 mg/day), phenytoin (350 mg/day, serum levels not reported), levetiracetam (2500 mg/day), and oxcarbazepine (1800 mg/day). The attacks occurred 30 minutes after taking the second dose of oxcarbazepine. A reduction of oxcarbazepine to 1500 mg caused complete remission of the episodes.

A prospective cohort study recruited children and adolescents ($n = 59$; age range 3–16 years) with primary seizure disorder and evaluated the effect of oxcarbamazepine ($n = 26$) monotherapy on growth patterns compared with the effect of valproate monotherapy ($n = 33$) [50c]. Eight months post-oxcarbazepine therapy, body weight and BMI increased significantly and the percentage of overweight/obese children climbed from 23% to 38.5% an increase of 15.4%.

Phenytoin

Phenytoin has been associated with the severe dermatological reactions Stevens–Johnson Syndrome (SJS) and toxic epidermal necrolysis (TEN). Symptoms most commonly present within 28 days of initiation of treatment, but may also present later. Increased susceptibility has been linked to Asian ancestry, particularly in patients with the HLA-B*1502 genotype (also linked to SJS and TEN for patients taking carbamazepine). The approved phenytoin labeling does not currently recommend screening for HLA-B*1502 due to lack of consistent evidence. The objective of the following study was to assess HLA genotypes associated with SJS or TEN.

Sixty patients with phenytoin-related severe cutaneous adverse reactions, 39 with SJS or TEN and 21 with drug reactions with eosinophilia and systemic symptoms (DRESS), were compared to the control group of phenytoin-tolerant patients ($n = 92$) [51c]. The genotypes of HLA class I and CYP2C9 were determined. Six HLA alleles including HLA-A*33:03, HLA-B*38:02, HLA-B*51:01, HLA-B*56:02, HLA-B*58:01, and HLA-C*14:02 were significantly associated with phenytoin-related SJS/TEN, whereas only the HLA-B*51:01 were significantly associated with phenytoin-related DRESS. The odds ratios of phenytoin-related SJS/TEN in the patients who carried one of these alleles ranged from 4- to 10-fold. The frequencies of patients who carried the HLA-B*15:02 in the SJS/TEN (12.82%) or the DRESS (9.52%) groups were not significantly different from that of the controls (14.13%). The higher risk of phenytoin-related SJS/TEN was observed in the patients with

CYP2C9*3 (odds ratio=4.30, 95% confidence interval= 1.41–13.09, P<0.05). Neither SJS/TEN nor DRESS caused by phenytoin was significantly associated with the HLA-B*15:02. The CYP2C9*3 variant was significantly associated with phenytoin-related SJS/TEN, but not DRESS. Certain alleles of HLA, particularly HLA-B*56:02, were significantly associated with phenytoin-related SCAR in the study population.

A case reported the clinical history of a boy diagnosed with early onset epileptic encephalopathy, with mutations in the *STXBP1* gene and variants of the *CYP2C9 gene*, experienced an episode of phenytoin neurotoxicity [52A]. At 10-days-old, the child showed clonic movements of four limbs in clusters. Electroencephalography (EEG) recordings showed a suppression-burst pattern due to clonic seizures. At age 7, because of seizure persistence, phenytoin was added to background therapy consisting of topiramate (3 mg/kg/24 h) and clobazam (1 mg/kg/24 h), initially at 0.5 mg/kg followed by increments of 0.5 mg/kg each 5 days, up to 2.6 mg/kg/day after 2 weeks. The child showed marked lethargy, coma and plasma phenytoin levels with unexpected values of 23.1 mcg/mL (it was not specified whether this was a total or free phenytoin, no additional phenytoin or albumin levels were provided). His serum acid–base balance, ammonium, lactate, creatinine and liver function, were normal. Phenytoin was thus discontinued and the patient quickly recovered.

In a case report, a 2-month-old Thai infant developed phenytoin toxicity resulting from *CYP2C9* gene polymorphism [53A]. The patient had VACTERL association (vertebral anomalies, anal atresia, cardiac defects, tracheo-esophageal fistula, renal and radial anomalies, and limb defects. He was admitted to the hospital for diarrhea and septicemia. A week after admission he experienced a focal tonic–clonic seizure and received a loading dose of IV phenytoin 20 mg/kg with an IV maintenance dose of 7 mg/kg/day. Blood phenytoin levels were evaluated (not provided) in response to two successive left-sided focal seizures and intravenous phenytoin 10 mg/kg was given. Maintenance dose was increased to 10 mg/kg/day. The patient became lethargic and was found to have trough phenytoin levels of 50.22 and 53.63 mcg/mL (it was not noted whether these were free or total phenytoin, and albumin levels were not provided). Phenytoin was discontinued and lethargy symptoms improved within 4 days.

In a case report, a 39-year-old African American male was referred for evaluation of dyspnea [54A]. Six years earlier he was diagnosed with seizure disorder and placed on phenytoin 400 mg/day. He reported progressive shortness of breath, but denied cough, fever, chills, hemoptysis, leg swelling, palpitations, syncope, and chest pain. He denied taking any other medications. On examination, there was jugular vein distention, but no edema or skin lesions. The chest computed tomography revealed mosaic attenuation involving both lungs and no evidence of pulmonary embolism. A video assisted thoracoscopic lung biopsy revealed granulomatous vasculitis of muscular pulmonary arteries. The diagnosis was consistent with changes reported in phenytoin-associated vasculitis. Phenytoin was switched to zonisamide and he was initiated on prednisone 40 mg orally daily. Two months after phenytoin was discontinued he reported improvement with shortness of breath on exertion.

Zonisamide

In a multicenter, single-arm, prospective study, 655 adult patients with generalized, partial, or combined seizures were treated with zonisamide as adjunctive ($n=518$) or first line monotherapy ($n=137$) with a median total daily dose of 200 mg for a total of 24 weeks [55C]. The most common concomitant AEDs were carbamazepine (25.7%), valproate (24.7%), and phenytoin (24.1%). The most common seizure types were generalized tonic–clonic (30.5%), complex (27.3%), and secondary generalized tonic–clonic (18.9%). Of 112 subjects (17.1%) who experienced at least one AE, the most common were loss of appetite (7.3%), weight loss (3.5%), sedation (2.1%), dizziness (2.0%), and irritability (1.1%). Six patients discontinued treatment due to AEs, but there were no serious AEs. At week 24, 93.8% of patients rated zonisamide tolerability as "good" or "excellent."

GLUTAMATE BLOCKERS

Felbamate

A single-center, retrospective cohort, evaluated the safety and efficacy of felbamate in children, adolescents, and adults with epilepsy ($n=103$) [56C]. The range of felbamate dose was 300–4500 mg (mean 1800 ± 900 mg). The duration of therapy ranged from 1 month to 20 years (mean duration 35 ± 45 months). Eighteen (17.5%) subjects experienced adverse events including insomnia, nausea ($n=6$), vomiting ($n=6$), decreased appetite, weight loss, gastric discomfort ($n=6$), diarrhea ($n=6$), mood and behavioral problems ($n=1$), high blood pressure ($n=1$), headache ($n=1$), abnormal CBC ($n=4$), and elevated liver enzymes ($n=1$). Out of these, 6 (5.9%) patients discontinued felbamate (A 3-year-old male for vomiting, 9-year-old male for loss of appetite and diarrhea, a 25-year-old female for nausea, vomiting and loss of appetite, a 61-year-old female for migraine type headache, high blood pressure, and hyponatremia, a 55-year-old male for increased liver enzymes, and an

11-year-old male for unknown adverse event). No hepatic failure or agranulocytosis was observed.

Perampanel

A pooled post-hoc analysis of three Phase III studies (*n* = 1478) demonstrating efficacy and tolerability of perampanel in partial seizures in patients aged at least 12 years was conducted to determine the efficacy and tolerability based on the number of concomitant antiepileptic drugs (AEDs) at baseline and examine which baseline characteristics were predictors of efficacy [57MC]. At baseline, 13.9%, 50.7%, and 35.4% patients were on 1, 2, or 3 AEDs, respectively, and were included in this analysis. Carbamazepine, lamotrigine, levetiracetam, oxcarbazepine, topiramate, and valproic acid were the most common co-administered AEDs at baseline (at least 10% of patients in the total population) in all Phase III studies. The most common TEAEs included dizziness, somnolence, headache, fatigue, and irritability, which were found in all AED groups. The TEAEs of fall and upper respiratory tract infection were observed at a rate of at least 5% only in total perampanel-treated patients on 3 AEDs at baseline (6.1% and 5.0%, respectively), and at a lower rate in placebo-treated groups (3.7% for each). Patients treated with perampanel 8 and 12 mg had a higher incidence of treatment-related TEAEs compared to placebo, regardless of the number of AEDs at baseline. No deaths occurred in any treatment group.

A pooled post-hoc analysis of three Phase III studies demonstrating safety and efficacy of perampanel in partial seizures in patients aged at least 12 years was conducted to determine the impact of perampanel on concomitant AED pharmacokinetics [58MC]. A total of 2272 patients were included in the analysis. Depending on the concomitant AED, mean weight ranged from 67.9 ± 17.3 to 75.0 ± 19.9 kg, and the most commonly represented racial or ethnic groups were white (63.3%–84.0%) and Asian (4.9%–27.2%). Clonazepam, levetiracetam, phenobarbital, phenytoin, topiramate, and zonisamide were not altered by perampanel. Carbamazepine, clobazam, lamotrigine, and valproate had minor alterations in clearance that were not considered clinically relevant. The only AED that underwent significant alteration in clearance was oxcarbazepine (26% decreased clearance, adjusted reduction 0.26, 95% CI 0.13–0.39), but perampanel impact on oxcarbazepine active metabolites was not measured and the implications of this finding remain unclear.

A prospective cohort study evaluated the effectiveness and safety of perampanel as add-on treatment in patients (*n* = 22) with severe refractory focal epilepsy [59c]. Perampanel was initiated at 2 mg/day at bedtime and was titrated up by 2 mg/day every 2–4 weeks at the discretion of the treating physician according to medical needs, occurrence of side effects, and concomitant medications. Thirteen (59.1%) reported side effects; tiredness in 8, behavioral changes (aggression) in 4, difficulty in finding words in 3, lack of concentration in 2, depression in 2, and tremor in 1. Side effects were less common in patients with the slowest titration rate (2 mg every 4 weeks). PER was withdrawn in 7 patients due to intolerable side effects such as tiredness, aggression (*n* = 3), and dizziness. The mean dosage in this subgroup with side effects was 5.5 mg (range 4–8 mg). Duration of side effects and duration of PER treatment were related.

A prospective cohort study evaluated the preliminary outcomes of perampanel as add-on therapy for patients age at least 12 years old (*n* = 54; age range 21–65 years old) with primary generalized tonic–clonic seizures [60c]. At baseline, patients were taking a median of 2 other antiepileptic drugs (AEDs) [range 1–4 drugs], with refractory epilepsy. Patients were initiated on 2 mg perampanel in the evening with most increasing by 2 mg every 2 weeks, aiming for a daily maintenance dose of 6–12 mg. Overall, 21 patients discontinued perampanel due to side effects. Mean perampanel dosage in these patients was 4 mg/day with a range of 2 mg to 12 mg/day. The common problems were nausea/vomiting (*n* = 4), ataxia (*n* = 4), dizziness (*n* = 3), and somnolence (*n* = 3). Three withdrew due to depression and 3 due to irritability and/or aggression; therefore, only 6 patients reported neuropsychiatric symptoms resulting in discontinuation.

Topiramate

A prospective, non-interventional study assessed (1) the magnitude and reversibility of transience of decreased urinary citrate excretion in patients (*n* = 12) just starting topiramate 100–200 mg and (2) the effects of alkali replacement on topiramate-induced hypocitraturia (*n* = 22) [61c]. After starting topiramate for headache remediation, urinary citrate excretion dropped significantly by 30 days and 62% of patients had hypocitraturia (citrate less than 320 mg/day). At 60 days, urine citrate was even lower than baseline and 86% of patients developed hypocitraturia. 85% of patients were hypocitraturic on topiramate alone vs 40% after adding potassium citrate.

A study re-analyzed data from a 12 week, double-blind, randomized, placebo-controlled trial of topiramate (25 mg/day gradually increased to 200 mg/day) in 138 heavy drinkers who were randomized 1:1 to receive topiramate (*n* = 67) or placebo (*n* = 71) [62C]. Most patients were male (placebo: *n* = 41, topiramate: *n* = 45). The genotype distribution among EAs was as follows: 21 topiramate-treated patients were rs2832407*C homozygotes and 30 were A-allele carriers (i.e., either heterozygotes or A-allele homozygotes) and the comparable numbers in the placebo group were 35 and 36, respectively. Patients reported at least one adverse event, including 96% of the topiramate group and 86% of the placebo group ($P = 0.053$). Although most adverse events were rated as mild, the mean severity rating was, greater in the topiramate group (1.3 ± 0.4) than in the placebo group (1.1 ± 0.5), $P = 0.003$. Among topiramate patients, 78% reported at least one adverse event of moderate or greater severity compared to 48% for placebo. A severe or greater adverse event was reported in 16% for topiramate and 3% for placebo. Adverse events reported as topiramate vs placebo and include numbness/tingling (53.7% vs 14.1%), change in taste (37.3% vs 8.45%), tiredness (26.9% vs 22.5%), difficulty with memory (23.9% vs 22.5%), loss of appetite (23.9% vs 2.8%), headache (22.4% vs 19.7%), diarrhea (20.9% vs 14.1%), weight loss (19.4% vs 2.8%), difficulty concentrating (17.9% vs 5.63%), dry mouth (16.4% vs 5.63%).

A single-center observational study of 200 children (mean age 4.1 ± 2.5 years) with epilepsy, treated for 3 months, were randomized into an observation group given topiramate ($n = 100$) initiated at 0.5–1 mg/kg/day twice daily, then added 0.5–1 mg/kg/day weekly until titrated to a maintenance dose of 4–8 mg/kg/day after 4–8 weeks or a control group given phenobarbital ($n = 100$) initiated orally at 2–3 mg/kg/day once or twice daily and titrated up to 3–5 mg/kg/day by the second week [63C]. Adverse events reported in the topiramate group included: somnolence (15%), anorexia (2%), fatigue (2%), weight loss (2%), cool response (1%); all adverse events were alleviated through slow titration and taking with meals during additional medicine dose periods. Specific adverse events in the control group were not reported; it was just reported that the differences between the two groups were statistically significant ($P < 0.05$) and adverse events in the topiramate groups were less than in the phenobarbital group.

A case report of spermatorrhea accompanied by loss of libido was described in a 39-year-old Chinese man with complex partial seizures and secondarily generalized tonic–clonic seizures diagnosed 1 year before presenting to a clinic [64A]. He was diagnosed with partial epilepsy and treated with topiramate 100 mg/day. After 11 days of therapy with topiramate, he was awakened by the sensation of emission of semen without orgasm or erection at night. He complained of spermatorrhea every 2–3 days lasting for a period of 2 months, accompanied by loss of libido, lack of energy, lassitude, weakness, poor appetite, frequent urination, and nocturia. The patient was not on any other medications and this adverse event affected his quality of life. When topiramate was discontinued, spermatorrhea occurred once in the first week but then stopped. All other symptoms disappeared and he was switched to valproate.

A prospective pilot study examined changes in the eyes of 15 patients (mean age of the patients was 42.4 ± 12.54 years (range, 28–56 years) recently diagnosed with migraine and scheduled to begin topiramate [65c]. The objective was to investigate the acute effects of topiramate on the anterior chamber angle (ACA) and choroidal thickness of the eye. None of the patients experienced any pain or discomfort in the eye during the first week of topiramate therapy. The mean baseline ACA was 40.34 ± 7.06 degrees, which decreased to 36.89 ± 6.87 degree at the first week ($P = 0.001$). Also, the mean baseline choroidal thickness increased significantly at all measurement points at the first week of topiramate therapy ($P = 0.01$ for all). None of the patients demonstrated an acute increase in intraocular pressure. The mean intraocular pressures were 13.15 ± 2.82 mm Hg (median 14.50 mm Hg; range 10–18 mm Hg) and 13.24 ± 2.75 mm Hg (median 14.00 mm Hg; range 10–19 mm Hg) before and at the first week of starting topiramate therapy, respectively. There were no reports of blurred vision. It was concluded that the carbonic anhydrase potential of topiramate did not impact intraocular pressure.

An observational study was conducted with the objective of comparing the frequency of topiramate-induced paresthesia in migraine headache ($n = 160$; mean age 34.5 ± 9.9 years and range of 12–61) to epileptic patients ($n = 160$; mean age 28.9 ± 13 years and range of 7–61) [66C]. Patients with migraine without aura and epilepsy were enrolled. The migraine group was 92.5% female and epilepsy group 40% female. Duration of treatment for migraine was 8 months vs 10.2 months for epilepsy. Topiramate dose in migraine group was 33.2 ± 12.7 mg vs 62.3 ± 30 mg in the epilepsy group. Paresthesia occurred in 53% of migraine patients vs 15% in epilepsy patients ($P < 0.05$). The odds ratio of developing topiramate-induced paresthesia in migraine compared to epilepsy is 6.4 (95% CI 3.76–10.95, $P < 0.0001$). After adjusting for confounding factors, the odds ratio was reduced to 3.4 (95% CI 1.58–7.5, $P = 0.002$). Female sex was associated with topiramate-induced paresthesia (odds ratio 2.1, 95% CI 1.0–4.38, $P = 0.04$); topiramate 50 mg dose was associated with decreased odds for paresthesia (odds ratio 0.3, 95% CI .11–0.94; $P = 0.03$).

A case report of topiramate-induced severe heatstroke was described in a 57-year-old Caucasian man who was admitted to the emergency room in a febrile comatose state after working in an unusually hot environment for 3 days [67A]. He had a past medical history of hypertension, type II diabetes mellitus, dyslipidemia, and essential tremor for which he was prescribed 6 weeks earlier an initial dose of 25 mg/day progressively titrated to 50 mg twice a day. Other medications included citalopram, clonazepam, allopurinol, ibuprofen, mefenamic acid, metformin, esomeprazole, propranolol, losartan, torsemide, and hydrochlorothiazide. His temperature on admission was 40.4°C, he was in a comatose state, Glasgow Coma Score (GCS) of 3, tachypneic (55 breaths/min), blood pressure was 110/62 mm Hg, heart rate 89 beats/min, and tympanic temperature was 41°C (105.8°F), reaching the maximal scale of the thermometer. He received 4 L of 0.9% sodium chloride and norepinephrine. A complete workup ruled out usual etiologies of such condition (e.g. meningoencephalitis) leaving the assumption of topiramate-induced heatstroke.

A randomized, double-blind, placebo-controlled study of amitriptyline 1 mg/kg/day ($n = 132$), topiramate 2 mg/kg/day ($n = 130$), and placebo ($n = 66$) in children and adolescents (age 8–17 years old) with migraines was conducted to determine which medication was superior in the prevention of headache of pediatric migraine [68c]. The patients ($n = 361$) were randomized in 2:2:1 ratio to receive one of the medications or placebo. A total of 852 adverse events were reported (301 with amitriptyline, 419 with topiramate, and 132 with placebo), in 272 patients, with no reports of death. Adverse events that occurred significantly more often in the topiramate group than in the placebo group were paresthesia (31% vs 8%, $P < 0.001$) and decreased weight (8% vs 0%, $P = 0.02$). Other commonly occurring adverse events with topiramate were fatigue (25%), dry mouth (18%), memory impairment (17%), aphasia (16%), cognitive disorder (16%), and upper respiratory tract infection (12%). One serious adverse event in the topiramate group included a suicide attempt (0.8%).

GABA RECEPTOR AGONISTS

Clobazam

Patients ($n = 200$) aged 2–60 years with Lennox–Gastaut syndrome enrolled in an open-label extension study assessing 2 years of treatment with adjunctive clobazam (0.5 mg/kg/day up to 40 mg per day titrated up to 2 mg/kg/day, maximum daily dose 80 mg) were assessed for development of tolerance in a post-hoc analysis [69c]. Tolerance, defined as a 40% or greater dose increase due to loss of response, was assessed in patients who had responded to treatment, and according to degree of response. Overall, tolerance occurred in 11.8% of patients, including 5.6% of 100% responders, 17.1% in 75%–100% responders, and 7.7% in 50%–75% responders. No data regarding tolerability or AEs were reported.

Clonazepam

No relevant publications from the review period were identified.

Diazepam

No relevant publications from the review period were identified.

Lorazepam

No relevant publications from the review period were identified.

Phenobarbital

A single-arm cohort study contained 7231 patients within an epilepsy management program receiving phenobarbital and was designed to investigate the rate of adverse effects in a rural, indigent population [70C]. Phenobarbital was started at 60 mg daily at bedtime and increased by 30 mg per day based on seizure control to a maximum dose of 240 mg per day, per protocol. Pediatric patients (i.e., age less than 15 years or weight less than 30 kg) received 2 mg/kg/day increased by 1 mg/kg/day to a maximum dose of 5 mg/kg/day. The most common adverse effects were classified as mild: drowsiness (49%), dizziness (41%), headache (26%), anxiety (22%), gastrointestinal complaints (19%), ataxia (18%), hyperactivity (14%), and skin rash (10%). Additionally, the following common adverse effects were rated as moderate severity: drowsiness (4%), dizziness (4%), anxiety (2%), ataxia (2%), and hyperactivity (2%). No serious adverse events in the listed domains occurred in 1% or more of patients. Patients receive doses between 180 and 240 mg were more likely to experience mild (RR 1.22, 95% CI 1.13–1.30) and moderate (RR 1.27, 95% CI 1.06–1.53) adverse effects compared to lower dose patients. Patients on multiple antiepileptic medications were more likely to experience serious (RR 2.52, 95% CI 1.63–3.89), moderate (RR 1.55, 95% CI 1.23–1.94), and mild (RR 1.12, 1.01–1.24) adverse effects compared to patients on phenobarbital monotherapy.

A retrospective cohort study of patients aged less than 15 years ($n = 15$) with focal seizures examined the effects of high-dose phenobarbital (i.e., 0.5–2 mg/kg/day titrated by 0.5–2 mg/kg/day every 2–4 weeks to a total daily dose greater than 5 mg/kg and a concentration of 40 mcg/mL or greater) for at least 6 months [71c]. Nine patients (60%) experienced drowsiness (transient and always rated as mild). There were no other reported adverse effects, or discontinuations due to adverse effects.

Pediatric patients with epilepsy were randomized to receive topiramate ($n = 100$, total daily dose 0.5–1 mg/kg titrated by 0.5–1 mg/kg per day in weekly increments to a maximum daily dose of 4–8 mg/kg) or phenobarbital ($n = 100$, total daily dose 2–3 mg/kg increased to 3–5 mg/kg) [72c]. The most common adverse effects were somnolence (15% vs 34%) and rise in aminotransferase (0% vs 4%) ($P < 0.05$). No other adverse effects occurred in more than 2 patients.

Primidone

No relevant publications from the review period were identified.

GABA REUPTAKE INHIBITORS

Tiagabine

The National Poison Data System was reviewed for tiagabine-related events ($n = 2147$) in a retrospective cross-sectional analysis reported from 2000 to 2012 [73C]. The majority of reports were submitted from 2002 through 2005. Most patients were adults (72%, mean age 30.7 years), and the majority were female (59%). The most common adverse effects reported (other than seizures) were drowsiness/lethargy (27%), agitation (19%), confusion (12%), tachycardia (10%), dizziness (5%), coma (5%), hypertension (4%), vomiting (3%), and mydriasis (2%). Approximately 35% of patients experienced events with a major or moderate medical outcome, but there were no deaths in patients who had only been taking tiagabine. Over 70% of events with a major outcome and about 50% of events with a moderate outcome (precise numbers not reported) were due to a suicide attempt.

GABA TRANSAMINASE INHIBITORS

Vigabatrin

A retrospective cross-sectional analysis described outcomes of patients enrolled in a Risk Evaluation Mitigation Strategy (REMS)-mandated registry for vigabatrin as of August 2014 ($n = 6823$) [74C]. Median patient age was 32.3 years (range 17.0–82.7 years), with 50% males, 86% naïve to vigabatrin, and 88% treated for refractory complex partial seizures. Overall, 789 patients (12%) discontinued the registry. Concern for side effects and non-visual adverse events were occasional reasons for discontinuation (4.8% and 4.1%, respectively). Visual field defects were the reason for discontinuation in an additional 1.0% of patients.

NEURONAL POTASSIUM CHANNEL OPENERS

Ezogabine (Retigabine)

In a multi-center, retrospective, single-arm cohort study, the outcomes for patients ($n = 195$) with refractory

focal epilepsy receiving ezogabine were described [75C]. Patients had a mean age of 37.6 ± 13.3 years, duration of epilepsy of 23 ± 12.8 years, and were receiving ezogabine at a total daily dose of 701.8 ± 283.5 mg. A total of 149 patients (76%) experienced an adverse event; the most common event types were neuropsychiatric ($n = 115$), urinary ($n = 28$), hepatic ($n = 25$), vegetative (e.g., diarrhea, headache, pain; $n = 16$), and weight gain or loss ($n = 10$). The most common types of neuropsychiatric events, other than seizures, were effects on alertness (27% of total population), impaired balance, coordination, etc. (19%), impaired speech (15%), cognitive effects (11%), mood or behavioral effects (8%), and visual impairment (8%). No additional adverse event types occurred in more than 2% of patients.

References

[1] Hwang SH, Park IJ, Cho YJ, et al. The efficacy of gabapentin/pregabalin in improving pain after tonsillectomy: a meta-analysis. Laryngoscope. 2016;126(2):357–66 [M].
[2] Edwards L, Demeo S, Hornik CD, et al. Gabapentin use in the neonatal intensive care unit. J Pediatr. 2016;169:310–2 [c].
[3] Mimenza A, Aguilar S. Clinical trial assessing the efficacy of gabapentin plus B complex (B1/B12) versus pregabalin for treating painful diabetic neuropathy. J Diabetes Res. 2016;2016:4078695 [C].
[4] Fallon M, Hoskin PJ, Colvin LA, et al. Randomized double-blind trial of pregabalin versus placebo in conjunction with palliative radiotherapy for cancer-induced bone pain. J Clin Oncol. 2016;34(6):550–6 [C].
[5] Dong J, Li W, Wang Y. The effect of pregabalin on acute postoperative pain in patients undergoing total knee arthroplasty: a meta-analysis. Int J Surg. 2016;34:148–60 [M].
[6] Gurunathan U, Rapchuk IL, King G, et al. The effect of pregabalin and celecoxib on the analgesic requirements after laparoscopic cholecystectomy: a randomized controlled trial. J Anesth. 2016;30(1):64–71 [c].
[7] Raskin P, Huffman C, Yurkewicz L, et al. Pregabalin in patients with painful diabetic peripheral neuropathy using an NSAID for other pain conditions: a double-blind crossover study. Clin J Pain. 2016;32(3):203–10 [C].
[8] Deshmukh U, Adams J, Macklin EA, et al. Behavioral outcomes in children exposed prenatally to lamotrigine, valproate, or carbamazepine. Neurotoxicol Teratol. 2016;54:5–14 [C].
[9] Shah N, Reddy MS, Vohra S, et al. Safety and effectiveness of divalproex sodium extended release containing regimen in Indian patients with bipolar I disorder in continuation phase: results of EASED registry. Asian J Psychiatr. 2016;20:32–8 [C].
[10] Knights M, Thekkekkara T, Morris A, et al. Sodium valproate-induced Fanconi type proximal renal tubular acidosis. BMJ Case Rep. 2016. http://dx.doi.org/10.1136/bcr-2015-213418 [c].
[11] Cook AM, Zafar MS, Mathias S, et al. Pharmacokinetics and clinical utility of valproic acid administered via continuous infusion. CNS Drugs. 2016;30(1):71–7 [C].
[12] Stevens CE, Turner Z, Kossoff EH. Hepatic dysfunction as a complication of combined valproate and ketogenic diet. Pediatr Neurol. 2016;54:82–4 [A].
[13] Spilioti M, Pavlou E, Gogou M, et al. Valproate effect on ketosis in children under ketogenic diet. Eur J Paediatr Neurol. 2016;20(4):555–9 [c].
[14] Brigo F, Bragazzi NL, Nardone R, et al. Efficacy and tolerability of brivaracetam compared to lacosamide, eslicarbazepine acetate, and perampanel as adjunctive treatments in uncontrolled focal

epilepsy: results of an indirect comparison meta-analysis of RCTs. Seizure. 2016;42:29–37 [M].

[15] Stockis A, Sargentinin-Maier ML, Brodie MJ. Pharmacokinetic interaction of brivaracetam on carbamazepine in adult patients with epilepsy, with and without valproate co-administration. Epilepsy Res. 2016;128:163–8 [c].

[16] Gironell A, Marin-Lahoz J. Ethosuximide for essential tremor: an open-label trial. Tremor Other Hyperkinet Mov (N Y). 2016;6:378. http://dx.doi.org/10.7916/D8FQ9WN0 [c].

[17] IJff DM, van Veenendaal TM, Debeij-van Hall MH, et al. The cognitive profile of ethosuximide in children. Paediatr Drugs. 2016;18(5):379–85 [c].

[18] Arzimanoglou A, Lösch C, Garate P, et al. Safety of levetiracetam among infants younger than 12 months—results from a European multicenter observational study. Eur J Paediatr Neurol. 2016;20(3):368–75 [C].

[19] Artemiadis AK, Lambrinoudaki I, Voskou P, et al. Preliminary evidence for gender effects of levetiracetam monotherapy duration on bone health of patients with epilepsy. Epilepsy Behav. 2016;55:84–6 [c].

[20] Hakami T, O'brien TJ, Petty SJ, et al. Monotherapy with levetiracetam versus older AEDs: a randomized comparative trial of effects on bone health. Calcif Tissue Int. 2016;98(6):556–65 [c].

[21] Chowdhury A, Brodie MJ. Pharmacological outcomes in juvenile myoclonic epilepsy: support for sodium valproate. Epilepsy Res. 2016;119:62–6 [C].

[22] Kowski AB, Weissinger F, Gaus V, et al. Specific adverse effects of antiepileptic drugs—a true-to-life monotherapy study. Epilepsy Behav. 2016;54:150–7 [C].

[23] Ju J, Zou LP, Shi XY, et al. Levetiracetam: probably associated diurnal frequent urination. Am J Ther. 2016;23(2):e624–7 [A].

[24] Chung S, Ceja H, Gawłowicz J, et al. Levetiracetam extended release for the treatment of patients with partial-onset seizures: a long-term, open-label follow-up study. Epilepsy Res. 2016;120:7–12 [C].

[25] Bayram AK, Canpolat M, Çınar SL, et al. Drug reaction with eosinophilia and systemic symptoms syndrome induced by levetiracetam in a pediatric patient. J Emerg Med. 2016;50(2):e61–6 [A].

[26] Page CB, Mostafa A, Saiao A, et al. Cardiovascular toxicity with levetiracetam overdose. Clin Toxicol (Phila). 2016;54(2):152–4 [A].

[27] Xu Z, Zhao H, Chen Z. The efficacy and safety of rufinamide in drug-resistant epilepsy: a meta-analysis of double-blind, randomized, placebo controlled trials. Epilepsy Res. 2016;120:104–10 [M].

[28] Arzimanoglou A, Ferreira JA, Satlin A, et al. Safety and pharmacokinetic profile of rufinamide in pediatric patients aged less than 4 years with Lennox–Gastaut syndrome: an interim analysis from a multicenter, randomized, active-controlled, open-label study. Eur J Paediatr Neurol. 2016;20(3):393–402 [c].

[29] Jaraba S, Santamarina E, Miró J, et al. Rufinamide in children and adults in routine clinical practice. Acta Neurol Scand. 2017;135(1):122–8 [c].

[30] Bektaş G, Çalışkan M, Aydın A, et al. Aggravation of atonic seizures by rufinamide: a case report. Brain Dev. 2016;38(7):654–7 [A].

[31] Yi C, Wenping X, Hui X, et al. Efficacy and acceptability of oxcarbazepine vs carbamazepine with betahistine mesilate tablets in treating vestibular paroxysmia: a retrospective review. Postgrad Med. 2016;128(5):492–5 [C].

[32] Hase I, Arakawa H, Sakuma H, et al. Bronchoscopic investigation of atypical drug-induced hypersensitivity syndrome showing viral lung involvement. Intern Med. 2016;55:2691–6 [A].

[33] Can I, Tholakanahalli V. Carbamazepine-induced atrioventricular block in an elderly woman. Turk Kardiyol Dern Ars. 2016;44(1):68–70 [A].

[34] Holtkamp M, McMurray R, Bagul M, et al. Real-world data on eslicarbazepine acetate as add-on to antiepileptic monotherapy. Acta Neurol Scand. 2016;134:76–82 [C].

[35] Steinhoff BJ, Eckhardt K, Doty P, et al. A long-term noninterventional safety safety study of adjunctive lacosamide therapy in patients with epilepsy and uncontrolled partial-onset seizures. Epilepsy Behav. 2016;58:35–43 [C].

[36] Hong Z, Inoue Y, Liao W, et al. Efficacy and safety of adjunctive lacosamide for the treatment of partial-onset seizures in Chinese and Japanese adults: a randomized, double-blind, placebo-controlled study. Epilepsy Res. 2016;127:267–75 [C].

[37] Vossler DG, Weschsler RT, Williams P, et al. Long-term exposure and safety of lacosamide monotherapy for the treatment of partial-onset (focal) seizures: results from a multicenter, openlabel trial. Epilepsia. 2016;57(10):1625–33 [C].

[38] Foldvary-Schaefer N, Fong JS, Morrison S, et al. Lacosamide tolerability in adult patients with partial-onset seizures: impact of planned reduction and mechanism of action of concomitant antiepileptic drugs. Epilepsy Behav. 2016;57:155–60 [c].

[39] Villanueva V, Saiz-Diaz R, Toledo M, et al. NEOPLASM study: real-life use of lacosamide in patients with brain tumor-related epilepsy. Epilepsy Behav. 2016;65:25–32 [c].

[40] Borzi G, Di Gennaro G, Schmitt FC, et al. Lacosamide with temporal lobe epilepsy: an observational muticentric open-label study. Epilepsy Behav. 2016;58:111–4 [c].

[41] Arkilo D, Gustafson M, Ritter FJ. Clinical experience of intravenous lacosamide in infants and young children. Eur J Paediatr Neurol. 2016;20(2):212–7 [c].

[42] d'Orsi G, Pascarella MG, Martino T, et al. Intravenous lacosamide in seizure emergencies: observations from a hospitalized in-patient adult population. Seizure. 2016;42:20–8 [c].

[43] Lancman ME, Fertig EJ, Tobliger RW, et al. The effects of lacosamide of cognition, quality-of-life measures, and quality of life in patients with refractory partial epilepsy. Epilepsy Behav. 2016;61:27–33 [c].

[44] Elger CE, Rademacher M, Brandt C, et al. Changes in hormone and lipid levels in male patients with focal seizures when switched from carbamazepine to lacosamide as adjunctive treatment to levetiracetam: a small phase IIIb, prospective, multicenter, open-label trial. Epilepsy Behav. 2016;62:1–5 [c].

[45] Poddar K, Sharma R, Ng Y-T. Intravenous lacosamide in pediatric status epilepticus: an open-label efficacy and safety study. Pediatr Neurol. 2016;61:83–6 [c].

[46] Meador KJ, Loring DW, Boyd A, et al. Randomized double-blind comparison of cognitive and EEG effects of lacosamide and carbamazepine. Epilepsy Behav. 2016;62:267–75 [c].

[47] Ghandourah H, Bhandal S, Brundler M, et al. Bronchiolitis obliterans organising pneumonia associated with anticonvulsant hypersensitivity syndrome induced by lamotrigine. BMJ Case Rep. 2016. http://dx.doi.org/10.1136/bcr-2014-207182 [A].

[48] Parker G. Development of an incipient Stevens–Johnson reaction while on a stable dose of lamotrigine. Australas Psychiatry. 2016;24(2):193–4 [A].

[49] Matarazzo M, Sánchez-Seco VG, Méndez-Guerrero AJ, et al. Drug-related eyelid nystagmus: two cases of a rare clinical phenomenon related to carbamazepine and derivatives. Clin Neuropharmacol. 2016;39(1):49–50 [A].

[50] Garoufi A, Vartzelis G, Tsentidis C, et al. Weight gain in children on oxcarbazepine monotherapy. Epilepsy Res. 2016;122:110–3 [c].

[51] Tassaneeyakul W, Prabmeechai N, Sukasem C, et al. Associations between HLA class I and cytochrome P450 2CP genetic polymorphisms and phenytoin-related severe cutaneous adverse reactions in a Thai population. Pharmacogenet Genomics. 2016;26:225–34 [c].

[52] Guacci A, Chetta M, Rizzo R, et al. Phenytoin neurotoxicity in a child carrying new STXBP1 and CYP2C9 gene mutations. Seizure. 2016;34:26–8 [A].

[53] Veeravigrom M, Jaroonvanichkul V, Netbaramee W, et al. Phenytoin toxicity in two-month-old Thai infant with CYP2C9 gene polymorphism—a case report. Brain Dev. 2016;38:136–8 [A].

[54] Kheir F, Daroca P, Lasky J. Phenytoin-associated granulomatous pulmonary vasculitis. Am J Ther. 2016;23:e311–4 [A].

[55] Dash A, Ravat S, Srinivasan AV, et al. Evaluation of safety and efficacy of zonisamide in adult patients with partial, generalized, and combined seizures: an open labeled, noncomparative, observational Indian study. Ther Clin Risk Manag. 2016;12:327–34 [C].

[56] Shah Y, Singh K, Friedman D, et al. Evaluating the safety and efficacy of felbamate in the context of a black box warning: a single center experience. Epilepsy Behav. 2016;56:50–3 [C].

[57] Glauser T, Laurenza A, Yang H, et al. Efficacy and tolerability of adjunct perampanel based on number of antiepileptic drugs at baseline and baseline predictors of efficacy: a phase III post-hoc analysis. Epilepsy Res. 2016;119:34–40 [MC].

[58] Majid O, Laurenza A, Ferry J, et al. Impact of perampanel on pharmacokinetics of concomitant antiepileptics in patients with partial-onset seizures: pooled analysis of clinical trials. Br J Clin Pharmacol. 2016;82:422–30 [MC].

[59] Juhl S, Rubboli G. Perampanel as add-on treatment in refractory focal epilepsy. The Dianalund experience. Acta Neurol Scand. 2016;134:374–7 [c].

[60] Brodie M, Stephen L. Prospective audit with adjunctive perampanel: preliminary observations in focal epilepsy. Epilepsy Behav. 2016;54:100–3 [c].

[61] Jhagroo RA, Wertheim M, Penniston KL. Alkali replacement raises urinary citrate excretion in patients with topiramate-induced hypocitraturia. Br J Clin Pharmacol. 2015;81(1):131–6 [c].

[62] Feinn R, Curtis B, Kranzler HR. Balancing risk and benefit in heavy drinkers treated with topiramate: implications for personalized care. J Clin Psychiatry. 2016;77(3):e278–82 [C].

[63] Wang YY, Wang MG, Yao D, et al. Comparison of impact on seizure frequency and epileptiform discharges of children with epilepsy from topiramate and phenobarbital. Eur Rev Med Pharmacol Sci. 2016;20:993–7 [C].

[64] Wu M, Hao N, Zhou D. Spermatorrhea and loss of libido induced by topiramate: first case report and review of literature. Clin Neuropharmacol. 2016;39(6):1 [A].

[65] Karalezli A, Koktekir BE, Celik G. Topiramate-induced changes in anterior chamber angle and choroidal thickness. Eye Contact Lens. 2016;42(2):120–3 [c].

[66] Sedighi B, Shafiei K, Azizpour I. Topiramate-induced paresthesia is more frequently reported by migraine than epileptic patients. Neurol Sci. 2016;37:585–9 [C].

[67] Canel L, Zisimopoulou S, Besson M, et al. Topiramate-induced severe heatstroke in an adult patient: a case report. J Med Case Reports. 2016;10:95 [A].

[68] Powers SW, Coffey CS, Chamberlin LA, et al. Trial of amitriptyline, topiramate, and placebo for pediatric migraine. N Engl J Med. 2017;376(2):115–24 [c].

[69] Gidal BE, Wechsler RT, Sankar R, et al. Deconstructing tolerance with clobazam: post hoc analyses from an open-label extension study. Neurology. 2016;87:1806–12 [c].

[70] Wang Y-Y, Wang M-G, Yao D, et al. Comparison of impact on seizure frequency and epileptiform discharges of children with epilepsy from topiramate and phenobarbital. Eur Rev Med Pharmacol Sci. 2016;20(5):993–7 [C].

[71] Si Y, Liu L, Tian L, et al. A preliminary observation of the adverse effects of phenobarbital among patients with convulsive epilepsy in rural West China. Epilepsy Behav. 2016;54:65–70 [c].

[72] Okumura A, Nakahara E, Ikeno M, et al. Efficacy and tolerability of high-dose phenobarbital in children with focal seizures. Brain Dev. 2016;38(4):414–8 [c].

[73] Spiller HA, Wiles D, Russell JL, et al. Review of toxicity and trends in the use of tiagabine as reported to US poison centers from 2000 to 2012. Hum Exp Toxicol. 2016;35(2):109–13 [C].

[74] Krauss G, Faught E, Foroozan R, et al. Sabril® registry 5-year results: characteristics of adult patients treated with vigabatrin. Epilepsy Behav. 2016;56:15–9 [C].

[75] Nass RD, Kurth C, Kull A, et al. Adjunctive retigabine in refractory focal epilepsy: postmarketing experience at four tertiary epilepsy care centers in Germany. Epilepsy Behav. 2016;56:54–8 [C].

8

Opioid Analgesics and Narcotic Antagonists

Michael G. O'Neil*,1, Justin G. Kullgren†

*South College School of Pharmacy, Knoxville, TN, United States
†The Ohio State University Wexner Medical Center, Columbus, OH, United States
1Corresponding author: moneil@Southcollegetn.edu*

INTRODUCTION OF DESIGNER OPIOID ANALGESICS INTO THE PUBLIC WITH LETHAL CONSEQUENCES

Opioid analgesics are commonly used pharmacotherapeutic agents for moderate-to-severe acute and chronic pain. Although the efficacy in the management of acute pain is well supported throughout the literature, published data supporting efficacy and safety in the treatment of chronic, malignant and nonmalignant pain are limited [1M,2R]. Despite limited long-term treatment outcomes for chronic, nonmalignant pain, opioid analgesics are commonly prescribed prescription analgesics for chronic pain. Experts have suggested that overprescribing of opioids is partially to blame for the largest opioid epidemic the world has ever faced [3S,4S]. The introduction of excessive opioids into communities has fueled the abuse and addiction of traditional prescription opioids such as oxycodone and hydrocodone and has propagated resurgence in heroin addiction resulting in the largest number of opioid overdose-related deaths ever known [5S,6S]. Demand of opioid products such as oxycodone and heroin has led to increased trafficking of traditional opioids and introduction of newer designer opioids [5S]. The high incidence of opioid misuse, abuse, and addiction coupled with the profits gained from illegal synthesis and distribution of these products has led to a surge of illegal opioid production subsequently contributing to opioid overdoses and deaths [5S,6S].

Designer opioids may be defined as synthetic analogs of legally controlled substances that are not regulated by traditional medical or law enforcement policies [7S,8S]. The transfer of these designer opioid products, commonly from countries such as China, avoids traditional shipping and import regulations of controlled substances [5S]. The synthesis of opioid analog products frequently produces substances that are significantly more potent than the base products utilized in the process. Potency in these formulations has been reported to be up to 100 times more potent than traditional products [5S,6S]. These synthetic opioids are commonly added to heroin or counterfeit pills to add or intensify the euphoric effects [5S,6S]. Adverse effects of opioids include sedation, euphoria, dysphoria, constipation, respiratory depression and death. Due to the illegality of this activity and since there are no quality assurance measures in the production or distribution of these extremely potent products, lethal consequences are inevitable.

In August of 2016, in less than 4 hours, 26 opioid-related overdoses were reported in a single community in Huntington, WV [9r]. While heroin was the primary product users were intending to purchase, many of the products sold contained the synthetic opioid carfentanil [9r]. Carfentanil, also known as 4-methoxycarbonylfentanyl, is a potent synthetic opioid developed in 1974 by Janssen Pharmaceuticals with a reported potency that is 10000 times greater than morphine and 100 times greater than fentanyl [5S,6S,10S]. Carfentanil is a registered drug solely approved as a tranquilizer in animals. Other potent fentanyl analogs being reported illegally in the United States, Canada, and Europe include uranyl fentanyl, 3-methyl fentanyl, acetyl fentanyl and W-18 [11S,12S,13S,14A]. These fentanyl derivatives are produced in clandestine laboratories primarily in China and shipped through various routes for distribution [5S,13S].

The introduction of illegal opioid analogues into the mainstream of opioid addicted communities has led to one of the most serious reports of opioid-related overdoses in the United States [4S]. The demand for potent opioids remains high due to the increased incidence of opioid addiction and profits to be gained through

Side Effects of Drugs Annual, Volume 39
ISSN: 0378-6080
http://dx.doi.org/10.1016/bs.seda.2017.06.023

diversion of these substances. The potency of these illegally produced substances predictably produces unwarranted consequences including respiratory depression and death.

Opioid Receptor Agonists

Fentanyl (SEDA-38, 71–76)
ANALGESIA

Twenty-one healthy male volunteers participated in a double-blinded randomized controlled trial of low-dose (1 µg/kg) or high-dose (10 µg/kg) fentanyl. Volunteers were assessed using intercutaneous electrical stimulation and cold temperature pain tolerance. High-dose infusions of fentanyl led to significantly decreased pain scores as measured by the numeric rating scale. High-dose fentanyl also had increased cold pressor pain threshold and tolerance. Researchers concluded higher dosages of fentanyl led to a decrease in pain scores. However, areas of increased hyperalgesia were noted [15c].

Hydromorphone
VASCULAR

This is a case report of a 37-year-old male that presented with respiratory symptoms for several days. The patient reported routine crushing and injecting a new formulation of sustained release hydromorphone. Laboratory indices were consistent for Mycoplasma IgM antibodies, anemia, and renal insufficiency. Due to persistent elevations in serum creatinine with an unknown etiology, a renal biopsy was performed. Biopsy results were consistent with thrombotic microangiopathy. Other known potential causes of thrombotic microangiopathy were excluded. Thrombotic thrombocytopenic purpura-like syndrome or thrombotic microangiopathy due to intravenous sustained release hydromorphone was initially suspected so plasmapheresis was initiated. The authors postulated that this toxicity may be associated with components of the sustained release hydromorphone matrix [16A].

DERMATOLOGICAL

This is a case report of a 34-year-old female presenting to the emergency room for treatment of reoccurring deep vein thrombosis. The patient was administered hydromorphone 2 mg IV for pain. Within 1 hour, the patient developed throat discomfort, oropharynx erythema, swelling of the tongue and uvula, and inflammation of the oral mucosa consistent with angioedema. Following treatment of diphenhydramine and famotidine, the patient developed dysarthria and respiratory distress requiring emergent intubation. She was treated with epinephrine, methylprednisolone, and dexamethasone.

Other medications and causes associated with angioedema were excluded. It was theorized that possible stimulation of bradykinin receptors or upregulation of the kallikrein system may have predisposed the patient to this adverse event [17A].

Methadone (SEDA-37, 107–114; SEDA-38, 71–76)
NEUROLOGICAL

This is a case report of a 14-year-old male presenting to the emergency room after being found unresponsive. The patient failed to respond to treatment with naloxone. Physical exam revealed decerebrate posturing, miosis, elevated blood pressure, tachycardia, respiratory depression and fever. Head CT and EEGs revealed significant anomalies in the cerebellum. A comprehensive drug screen was negative for everything except methadone and caffeine. Methadone levels were later reported as 210 mg/mL, which may be associated with methadone overdose. Other laboratory exams and studies were consistent for renal, liver and cardiac damage. The patient regained consciousness 2 days later. He maintained significant neurologic deficits consistent with cerebellar injury prior to discharge to a rehabilitation center. The authors concluded that although cerebellar toxicity and end organ damage secondary to hypoxia could not be excluded, methadone overdose should be considered in patients presenting with the findings discussed earlier [18A].

ENDOCRINE/METABOLIC

This is a retrospective observational study in inpatient cancer patients admitted for greater than 48 hours between November 1, 2011 and October 20, 2013. Patients were divided into 2 groups: patients receiving methadone vs other nonmethadone opioid medications. Medication doses were evaluated as were any reports of hypoglycemia defined as blood glucose less than 70 mg/dL. Researchers reported an increased risk of hypoglycemia when doses of methadone were greater than 40 mg per day. Nonmethadone opioid medications were not associated with hypoglycemia [19C].

Morphine (SEDA-37, 107–114; SEDA-38, 71–76)
DRUG INTERACTION

Twelve normal volunteers were randomized and administered 60 mg of prasugrel with either placebo or 5 mg intravenous morphine in a crossover study. Pharmacokinetic parameters and pharmacodynamic effects of prasugrel on platelet activity were evaluated. Researchers concluded that morphine did not significantly decrease AUC or delay absorption of prasugrel. Morphine did reduce the Cmax, and there was a slight delay in onset of maximal inhibition of platelet plug formation [20c].

Tapentadol (SEDA-38, 71–76)

OVERDOSE/INTOXICATION

This is a case report of a 41-year-old female found deceased in her home. Autopsy results were consistent with aspiration pneumonia and pulmonary edema. Postmortem laboratory analysis indicated tapentadol and oxycodone. The cause of death was reported as a mixed drug overdose. While the literature does not report any documented postmortem tapentadol drug concentrations, the authors describe post-mortem tapentadol concentrations in blood, liver, vitreous humor, and stomach with the intent to provide reference points that may be helpful in future overdose cases [21A].

NEUROLOGICAL

This is a case report of a 48-year-old male that was found unresponsive after an intentional witnessed overdose of tapentadol. He was successfully resuscitated with 1 mg intramuscular naloxone by emergency service personnel and became combative requiring restraints. Concurrent ingested medications included duloxetine, amitriptyline, atenolol and enalapril. Other physical symptoms included hyperreflexia, tremor and fever leading clinicians to suspect serotonin syndrome. After contacting a poison control center, the patient was treated with intravenous lorazepam, intravenous diphenhydramine and intramuscular haloperidol. The patient's clinical signs and symptoms improved, and the patient was admitted to the medical intensive care unit (MICU) without further consequences [22A].

Partial Opioid Receptor Agonists

Buprenorphine (SEDA-37, 107–114)

PSYCHIATRIC

This is a case report of a 20-year-old male admitted to a treatment center for opioid addiction. The patient had a history of polysubstance abuse including heroin, LSD, MDMA, benzodiazepines, and marijuana. Physical exam on admission was within normal limits except for symptoms consistent with mild opioid withdrawal. Urine toxicology screens were significant only for benzodiazepine and opioids. He was started on a standard buprenorphine treatment protocol of 2–4 mg sublingually. On day 2 of treatment the patient reported an "LSD-like trip" characterized by symptoms of heightened excitement, euphoria, visualizing radiant colors, trance music and visual hallucinations lasting 4–6 hours. Buprenorphine was withheld with resolution of symptoms. Reinitiating of buprenorphine produced similar but less intense symptoms [23A].

PHARMACOKINETICS

This is a case report of an 80-year-old male receiving chronic hemodialysis three times weekly for end-stage renal disease. The patient was receiving 5760 μg oral and transdermal buprenorphine daily for analgesia. Pharmacokinetic parameters evaluated before and after hemodialysis indicated a significant decrease in free buprenorphine concentrations post hemodialysis. Researchers concluded that supplemental dosages of buprenorphine during hemodialysis may be warranted [24A].

CARDIAC

Ninety-five youths, 15–21 years of age, were randomized to receive either buprenorphine–naloxone sublingually or an abstinence detoxication program without medication support. Patients were dosed to achieve clinical response and not to exceed 32 mg/day. Electrocardiograms were evaluated at baseline, week 4 and week 12 of treatment. Researchers reported that although there were some elevated QTc intervals in both groups, the findings were not thought to be clinically significant. This is the first report of QTc evaluation of youths receiving buprenorphine–naloxone treatment [25c].

Opioid Receptor Antagonist

Eluxadoline

PANCREATIC/BILIARY

In a randomized, double-blind, parallel-group, placebo-controlled study conducted at 263 primary and tertiary care centers in the United States, 2814 patients with irritable bowel disease with diarrhea were evaluated and 2776 patients were enrolled. Patients were randomized to eluxadoline 75 mg BID, 100 mg BID, or placebo for 12, 26, or 52 weeks. All adverse effects were evaluated. Ten Sphincter of Oddi Spasms (SOS) events were reported in the eluxadoline-treated group characterized by abdominal pain, elevated aminotransferases, elevated lipases or pancreatitis. Eight of ten patients were receiving higher doses of eluxadoline, and all events occurred within 1 week of initiating treatment. Two other events were associated with pancreatitis not thought to be SOS. The researchers concluded that eluxadoline may increase the risk of SOS especially at higher doses in patients without gallbladders. These patients may require closer monitoring [26C].

Naloxegol

PHARMACOKINETIC/PHARMACODYNAMIC

This is a double-blind, randomized, crossover study in healthy volunteers evaluating the pharmacokinetic and CNS distribution effect of quinidine on oral naloxegol and morphine-induced miosis. Data from 36 participants treated with naloxegol 25 mg plus placebo and 38 patients treated with 25 mg naloxegol plus 600 mg quinidine were evaluated. Coadministration of quinidine with naloxegol produced an increase in naloxegol's AUC and Cmax without antagonizing morphine-induced miosis. Coadministration of naloxegol with morphine or quinidine was reported to be safe and well tolerated [27c].

Naltrexone (SEDA-37, 107–114)

OCULAR

Twenty healthy volunteers were enrolled and divided into study groups to receive topical administration of escalating doses of naltrexone combined with moxifloxacin administered over a 24-hour period. The naltrexone dosages tested were $1 \times 10(-6)$ M (1 drop), $1 \times 10(-6)$ M (4 drops), $5 \times 10(-6)$ M (4 drops), $1 \times 10(-5)$ M (4 drops), and $5 \times 10(-5)$ M (4 drops). Drops were administered over a 24-hour period. Prior to, 24 hours after completing the study, and 1 week after completing the study, participants had comprehensive eye exams. No significant adverse effects were reported [28c].

References

[1] Noble M, Treadwell JR, Tregear SJ, et al. Long-term opioid management for chronic noncancer pain. Cochrane Database Syst Rev. 2010;1:CD006605 [M].

[2] Kissin Igor. Long-term opioid treatment of chronic nonmalignant pain: unproven efficacy and neglected safety? J Pain Res. 2013;6:513–29 [R].

[3] National Institute on Drug Abuse. America's addiction to opioids: heroin and prescription drug abuse, https://www.drugabuse.gov/about-nida/legislative-activities/testimony-to-congress/2016/americas-addiction-to-opioids-heroin-prescription-drug-abuse. Accessed Jan 10, 2017 [S].

[4] Centers for Disease control on Prevention. Understanding the epidemic, https://www.cdc.gov/drugoverdose/epidemic/. Accessed Jan 10, 2017 [S].

[5] Drug Enforcement Administration. DEA report: counterfeit pills fueling U.S. fentanyl and opioid crisis: problems resulting from abuse of opioid drugs continue to grow, https://www.dea.gov/divisions/hq/2016/hq072216.shtml. Accessed Jan 10, 2017 [S].

[6] Center for Disease Control and Prevention. Influx of fentanyl-laced counterfeit pills and toxic fentanyl-related compounds further increases risk of fentanyl-related overdose and fatalities, https://emergency.cdc.gov/han/han00395.asp. Accessed Jan 10, 2017 [S].

[7] Santos A, Drug enforcement Agency. Synthetic drug trafficking and abuse trends, https://www.deadiversion.usdoj.gov/mtgs/pharm_awareness/conf_2013/july_2013/asantos2.pdf. Accessed Jan 10, 2017 [S].

[8] National Institute of Drug Abuse. The science behind designer drugs, https://www.drugabuse.gov/news-events/latest-science/science-behind-designer-drugs. Accessed Jan 10, 2017 [S].

[9] Stuck T, herald-dispatch.com. 26 overdoses reported Monday evening. http://www.herald-dispatch.com/news/overdoses-reported-monday-evening/article_81990238-4a74-5431-9420-76e0f35c5cbf.html. Accessed Jan 10, 2017.

[10] PubChem Open Chemistry Database. Carfentanil, https://pubchem.ncbi.nlm.nih.gov/compound/carfentanil. Accessed Jan 10, 2017 [S].

[11] Center for Disease Control and Prevention. Notes from the field, https://www.cdc.gov/mmwr/volumes/65/wr/mm6537a6.htm; 2017. Accessed Jan 10, 2017 [S].

[12] Drug Enforcement Agency. Acetyl fentanyl, https://www.deadiversion.usdoj.gov/drug_chem_info/acetylfentanyl.pdf. Accessed Jan 10, 2017 [S].

[13] Drug Enforcement Agency. Counterfeit prescription pills containing fentanyls: a global threat, https://www.dea.gov/docs/Counterfeit%20Prescription%20Pills.pdf. Accessed Jan 10, 2017 [S].

[14] Hibbs J, Perper J, Winek CL. An outbreak of designer drug-related deaths in Pennsylvania. JAMA. 1991;265(8):1011–3 [A].

[15] Mauermann E, Filitz J, Dolder P. Does fentanyl lead to opioid-induced hyperalgesia in healthy volunteers? A double-blind, randomized, crossover trial. Anesthesiology. 2016;124(2):453–63 [c].

[16] Jabr FI, Yu L. Thrombotic microangiopathy associated with Opana ER intravenous abuse: a case report. J Med Liban. 2016;64(1):40–2 [A].

[17] Masson S, Villerot M, Dalal B. A rare case of hydromorphone-induced angioedema effectively managed by a difficult airway response team. A A Case Rep. 2016;7(9):188–9 [A].

[18] Rando J, Szari S, Kumar G. Methadone overdose causing acute cerebellitis and multi-organ damage. Am J Emerg Med. 2016;34(2):343 [A].

[19] Flory J, Wiesenthal A, Thaler H. Methadone use and the risk of hypoglycemia for inpatients with cancer pain. J Pain Symptom Manage. 2016;51(1):79–87 [C].

[20] Hobl E, Reiter B, Schoergenhofer C. Morphine interaction with prasugrel: a double-blind, cross-over trial in healthy volunteers. Clin Res Cardiol. 2016;105(4):349–55 [c].

[21] Cantrell FL, Mallett P, Aldridge L. A tapentadol related fatality: case report with postmortem concentrations. Forensic Sci Int. 2016;266:e1–3 [A].

[22] Walczyk H, Liu CH, Alafris A. Probable tapentadol-associated serotonin syndrome after overdose. Hosp Pharm. 2016;51(4):320–7 [A].

[23] Saddichha S, Subodh B, Chand P. Sublingual buprenorphine-induced psychomimetic effects. Am J Ther. 2016;23(1):e242–3 [A].

[24] Salili A, Müller D, Skendaj R. Breakthrough pain associated with a reduction in serum buprenorphine concentration during dialysis. Clin Ther. 2016;38(1):212–5 [A].

[25] Poole S, Pecoraro A, Subramaniam G. Presence or absence of QTc prolongation in buprenorphine-naloxone among youth with opioid dependence. J Addict Med. 2016;10(1):26–33 [c].

[26] Cash B, Lacy B, Schoenfeld P. Safety of eluxadoline in patients with irritable bowel syndrome with diarrhea. Am J Gastroenterol. 2017;112(2):365–74. http://dx.doi.org/10.1038/ajg.2016.542. Published online 2016 Dec 6 [C].

[27] Bui K, She F, Zhou D. The effect of quinidine, a strong P-glycoprotein inhibitor, on the pharmacokinetics and central nervous system distribution of naloxegol. J Clin Pharmacol. 2016;56(4):497–505 [c].

[28] Liang D, Sassani J, McLaughlin P. Topical application of naltrexone to the ocular surface of healthy volunteers: a tolerability study. J Ocul Pharmacol Ther. 2016;32(2):127–32 [c].

9

General Anesthetics and Therapeutic Gases

Joanna Fawkner-Corbett, Alison Hall[1]

Royal Liverpool Hospital, Liverpool, Merseyside, United Kingdom

[1]Corresponding author: alison.hall@rlbuht.nhs.uk

ANAESTHETIC VAPOURS

Desflurane

Psychiatric

Emergence delirium has again been described in children undergoing desflurane anesthesia [1c]. They described a 40.6% incidence of emergence delirium in children undergoing desflurane anesthesia. This study investigated the benefit of a single dose of dexmedetomidine or propofol in these cases. They prospectively investigated 100 ASA 1 or 2 children (2–8 years) undergoing elective infra-umbilical surgery under general anesthesia (GA) and caudal anesthesia anticipated to last 1 hour or less. Patients were randomized into 3 groups: dexmedetomidine (0.3 μg/kg administered 15 minutes prior to the end), propofol (1 mg/kg administered 5 minutes before the end) or control (0.9% saline administered). All injections were blinded. The validated pediatric anesthesia emergence delirium (PAED) scale was used in recovery to assess emergence delirium at 5, 10, 15, 20, 25, and 30 minutes after removal of the laryngeal mask. A score of >10 was considered as a diagnosis of emergence delirium and >15 severe. PAED scores were significantly higher in the control group (8.5 vs 3.0 $P = 0.038$) but dexmedetomidine significantly increased the transfer and awakening time compared to control. Most events were self-limiting and did not require treatment; however, three children in the propofol and five in the control group had PAED score >15 requiring pharmacological treatment.

Respiratory

A further randomized double-blind study compared recovery times and respiratory complications during emergence from varying depths of desflurane anesthesia [2c]. Patients were randomized to receive either deep anesthesia using either desflurane Minimum alveolar concentration (MAC) 1.5 ($n = 25$) or a lower concentration of desflurane (1 MAC) with remifentanil Target-Controlled Infusion (TCI) (1 ng/mL) ($n = 29$). Jaw thrust time, obey-command time, and time to Aldrete score 10 points (a score used to determine a patient's ability to be discharged from the recovery room (0–10 points)) were improved indicating quicker recovery times in the desflurane/remifentanil group ($P < 0.001$). During deep extubation in the desflurane group, 48% (12/25) subjects showed breath holding and coughing, whereas in the desflurane/remifentanil group only 3.4% (1/29) subjects coughed ($P < 0.001$), with no patients demonstrating breath holding. When extubation is performed during deep anesthesia, 1 MAC of desflurane with 1 ng/mL TCI of remifentanil significantly reduces recovery time and respiratory complications, compared with 1.5 MAC of desflurane alone.

Genotoxicity

Nogueira et al. conducted a small study ($n = 15$) to evaluate the genotoxicity of desflurane in healthy patients undergoing elective minor minimally invasive surgery scheduled to last at least 90 minutes [3E]. Following a standard IV induction, anesthesia was maintained using desflurane (Minimum alveolar concentration of 1.0) in 40% oxygen. Blood samples were drawn at 3 specified time points (on induction, 90 minutes and 24 hours post induction). Lymphocytes were isolated and were subjected the comet assay, a simple, rapid and sensitive method for measuring DNA damage in individual cells. There were no surgical or anesthetic complications. A significant increase in DNA damage was observed on the day following surgery compared with the baseline ($P < 0.05$). This study showed for the first time, that surgical patients anaesthetized with desflurane (6%) had increased DNA damage in lymphocytes.

Liver

A prospective randomized parallel clinical trial ($n=62$) compared the incidence of post reperfusion syndrome (PRS) during liver transplant between sevoflurane and desflurane [4c]. There was significantly more PRS in the desflurane group compared to the group receiving sevoflurane (77.4% vs 38.7% $P=0.004$), and more adrenaline required (45.2% vs 19.4% $P=0.030$). Multivariate analysis identified desflurane as the only risk factor (OR 7.314, $P=0.001$) for PRS. Only patients scheduled for living donor liver transplantation were enrolled in this study, and although the results were statistically significant the numbers were insufficient to identify differences in clinical outcomes and will likely have limited the results of the multivariate regression analysis for identifying risk factors for PRS.

Isoflurane

Neurological

A retrospective case note review studied a group of 200 surgical patients on the Intensive care unit (ICU) sedated either with isoflurane (ET_{ISO} 0.3%–0.8%) ($n=72$) or propofol (2–4mg/kg/h) and midazolam (0.05–0.2mg/kg/h) ($n=128$) [5c]. There were no differences in the characteristics of the two groups. Primary and secondary outcomes of hospital and 365 day mortality were analyzed. Patients receiving isoflurane had a lower risk of death in hospital (OR 0.39, 95% CI 0.22–0.71, $P=0.002$) and death within the first 365 days (OR 0.45, 95% CI 0.25–0.82, $P=0.009$) than those receiving propofol/midazolam in combination. They had more ventilator-free days at 60 days (32.5±29.2 vs 23.2±28.2 days, $P=0.03$) and more hospital-free days at 180 days (62.1±59.5 vs 44.1±64.8 days, $P=0.04$). The improvements in mortality were maintained after adjusting for potential confounders (Coronary heart disease, COPD, acute renal failure, creatinine, age and SAPS score on admission). Limitations of this non-randomized single-centre, retrospective study included the decision to initiate isoflurane being at the discretion of the on-call physician and only two sets of isoflurane delivery equipment being available thus limiting recruitment of patients. In addition, the study only included patients ventilated continuously for more than 96 hours thus excluding a large cohort of patients. This may have biased the results.

Immunological

Volatile anesthetics, isoflurane and sevoflurane, at clinically relevant concentrations have been shown to reduce the ability of leukocytes to adhere to inflamed vascular endothelial cells. It has been previously shown that isoflurane and sevoflurane bind to and inhibit leukocyte function-associated antigen-1 (LFA-1). Research by Jung and Yuki tested the hypothesis that these two volatiles would inhibit macrophage-1 antigen (MAC-1), a leukocyte adhesion molecule that plays a significant role in leukocyte crawling and phagocytosis [6E]. They demonstrated that isoflurane inhibited binding of MAC-1 to its ligand intercellular adhesion molecule-1 (ICAM-1), whereas sevoflurane did not. It is implied therefore that their effects on the immune system may differ.

Methoxyflurane

Urinary Tract

Clinical and anecdotal evidence indicate that methoxyflurane is a useful and effective analgesic agent. Past use in significantly higher anesthetic doses, has continued to raise concerns about its safety. Anesthetic use of methoxyflurane is associated with high-output renal dysfunction and dose-related renal failure. Methoxyflurane-induced nephrotoxicity is related to total dose (time and concentration) and rate of metabolism. Dayan conducted a thorough data review of all laboratory and clinical data relevant to nephrotoxicity and methoxyflurane to evaluate the risk of nephrotoxicity due to its analgesic use [7R]. The dose employed to produce analgesia (6mL/day of 0.1%–0.7%, 15mL/week, exposure 0.59 MAC-hours) is well below the reported level of risk (2 MAC-hours) and has not been associated with renal tubular toxicity.

Nervous System

A small single-centre randomized crossover pilot study ($n=8$) compared self-administered methoxyflurane inhalation via a Penthrox inhaler to ketamine–midazolam patient-controlled analgesia in patients undergoing changes of burns dressings [8c]. Patients were randomly allocated to one method for their initial procedure and then the other modality for the second. Methoxyflurane was preferred in 5/8 patients (easier administration, feeling of control, absence of hallucinations, greater ability to cooperate, better recovery). A subsequent series of 173 minor surgical and radiological procedures (123 patients) using methoxyflurane analgesia was prospectively audited to assess satisfaction (patient and surgical) and to monitor for adverse events. Methoxyflurane analgesia was unsuccessful in only 5/173 cases (citing insufficient analgesia, anxiety, agitation during a prolonged procedure as causes). The following adverse events were noted: hypotension (1.7%); oxygen desaturation (0.6%); cough (1.7%); nausea (0.6%); vomiting (1.2%); agitation (0.6%); headache (0.6%); over-sedation (0.6%).

SEVOFLURANE

Cardiovascular

The dorsalis pedis artery (DPA) is a good alternative to the radial artery (RA) for invasive blood pressure monitoring when the upper limb is not available. Understanding the pattern of pressure difference (overestimation or underestimation) between these two arteries during inhalational anesthesia is helpful for haemodynamic management and therapeutic decisions.

A prospective, single-centre, self-controlled, study was conducted at a teaching hospital to investigate the time-dependent variation of DPA/RA pressure gradient during sevoflurane anesthesia [9c]. All patients ($n = 30$) underwent scheduled neurosurgery under GA. The mean $\pm$ SD DPA/RA pressure gradient gradually decreased with time from 9.7 ± 8.8 to -1.8 ± 7.6 mmHg for systolic pressure, and -2.3 ± 2.7 to -3.7 ± 2.8 mmHg for diastolic pressure. The DPA/RA skin temperature gradient gradually reduced from $-3.6 \pm 2.4°C$ to $-1.1 \pm 1.3°C$. A greater increase in the inner cross-sectional area and blood flow from the baseline was observed at DPA compared with RA. The authors conclude that the blood pressure, temperature and inner cross-sectional area differences between DPA and RA reduced gradually during surgery. However, this small study did not investigate the impacts at times of anesthetic instability (induction of anesthesia, bleeding, shock, or vasopressors), nor age, hypertension, atherosclerosis, type of surgery or surgical position on the DPA–RA pressure gradient, nor the inner-cross sections and blow flow of RA and DPA in the process of neurosurgery.

A single-centre, prospective, small randomized controlled clinical trial aimed to demonstrate that sevoflurane during cardiopulmonary bypass (CPB) for pediatric patients undergoing congenital heart defect repair may have benefits in terms of clinical outcome and myocardial protection [10c]. Patients ($n = 103$) were randomized to either an anesthetic regimen with 2% sevoflurane or a total intravenous anesthesia (TIVA) midazolam regimen. A small but significant increase of arterial diastolic pressure immediately after CPB was seen with the sevoflurane group compared with the TIVA group (46.9 ± 9.3 mmHg vs 43.6 ± 8.9 mmHg; $P = 0.033$). The postoperative ventilation time was shorter in the sevoflurane group, but this was not reflected in the postoperative ICU time and hospital days. Regarding myocardial protection, the serial plasma troponin I concentrations (used as a marker) were not significantly different between the two groups.

Two case reports have been published of pediatric patients with congenital heart disease having arrhythmias with sevoflurane anesthesia.

Case Report 1 [11A]

A 14-year-old ASA II Caucasian female with long QT syndrome (LQTS) and intermittent 2nd degree heart block presented for pacemaker replacement and heart catheterisation. She had taken her prescribed atenolol pre-operatively. The patient declined intravenous induction, instead undergoing inhalational induction with sevoflurane. After successful induction, and while the planned propofol TIVA was started, VT in the form of Torsades de Pointes (TdP) occurred. Sevoflurane was stopped and shortly after there was spontaneous resolution of VT. Vital signs were stable, and the case continued uneventfully under propofol TIVA. Recovery was uneventful and the patient discharged. Although the list of medications known to be a risk factor for TdP is extensive, sevoflurane is the only anesthetic gas listed.

Case Report 2 [12A]

A 2-year old with trisomy 21 (weight 10.2 kg) presented for adenotonsillectomy. Past medical history includes small ventricular septal defect successfully closed at 6 months of age, gastrostomy, tympanostomy tubes, broncopulmonary dysplasia, hypotonia, conductive hearing loss and obstructive sleep apnea. An inhalational induction was carried out with 70% nitrous oxide (N_2O) followed by sevoflurane at an increasing concentration (maximum concentration 8%). N_2O concentration was then decreased to 50%. At this point the heart rate dropped abruptly from a baseline of 170–28bpm over 20 seconds with a BP of 60/30 mmHg (baseline 101/41). Inspired oxygen was increased to 100% and sevoflurane decreased to 2%. Atropine 0.2 mg was given without effect at which point adrenaline 10 mcg was administered. Heart rate and blood pressure returned rapidly to baseline. Oxygen saturations remained 100% throughout. Observations quickly normalized and the surgery completed uneventfully. Literature review found a higher incidence of bradycardia during anesthetic induction with sevoflurane to be well documented in pediatric trisomy 21 patients.

Respiratory

Post-operative airway reflex status is partly influenced by the choice of maintenance anesthetic in non-intubated patients (recovery is slower after sevoflurane than desflurane). Mckay et al. investigated whether this significant difference also applied to those receiving rocuronium for intubation or whether the neuromuscular blockade would obtund the difference between the two volatile agents [13c]. The study recruited 81 ASA I and

II patients undergoing scheduled surgery of 2–3 hours duration. All patients passed a pre-operative swallow test. Patients were randomly assigned to receive sevoflurane ($n = 41$) or desflurane ($n = 40$) following a standard intravenous (IV) induction (fentanyl and propofol). Thereafter, rocuronium was administered; neuromuscular block monitored using a quantitative train-of-four (TOF), and reversed according to a protocol. Time to first command and time to first ability to swallow was significantly longer in the sevoflurane group (540 vs 290 seconds, $P = 0.0001$ and 960 vs 540 seconds, $P = 0.007$, respectively). A significantly higher number of patients in the sevoflurane group were too somnolent to pass the swallow test at 2 minutes following response to first command. A number of patients in both groups were not tested due to somnolence and therefore this may have biased the results. In multivariate analysis, neuromuscular protocol adherence was independently associated with the ability to pass the swallow test. In 18/81 patients, the neuromuscular reversal protocol was not followed and therefore this may have cofounded the results.

Other Environmental Interactions

Anesthetic gases are a source of hospital environmental pollution as the anesthetic vapors are greenhouse gases. The amount of sevoflurane in exhaled gas of hospital visitors ($n = 45$) and hospital staff ($n = 24$), compared with external controls ($n = 31$) has been evaluated [14c]. Breath samples were studied and confirmed significantly higher levels of exhaled sevoflurane in staff members compared with visitors to the hospital (0.522 vs 0.196 parts per billion by volume (ppbv), respectively, $P = 0.00024$). Small amounts of sevoflurane could be detected in the exhaled breath of any person that has stayed for at least 30 minutes inside the hospital environment. Exposure levels were, however, well below the recommended exposure limit of 2.3 ppbv for staff and 0.9 ppbv for visitors.

Nervous System

A randomized controlled trial investigated the effect of Bispectral Index (BIS) guided sevoflurane anesthesia on severe emergence agitation in children undergoing ophthalmological surgery [15c]. Patients ($n = 40$) aged 2–8 years were randomized to either low-normal (BIS 40–45, deep) or high-normal (BIS 55–60, light) anesthesia groups. The primary outcome, post-anesthesia care unit (PACU) peak PAED scores (validated (0 − 20) score of children's behavior), showed little difference between the groups (light: 7.7 ± 4.6; deep: 8.6 ± 5.3; $P = 0.18$). At emergence, however, patients in the deep group had greater PAED scores (9.3 vs 4.8; $P = 0.03$) and Face, Legs, Activity, Cry and Consolability (FLACC) score (a validated children's pain score (0 − 10)) (3.5 vs 1.5,

$P = 0.04$) compared with subjects in the light group. The primary outcome was to identify severe emergence delirium in the recovery room, which was rare in this study. This study was not large enough to find a relationship between depth of anesthesia and emergence delirium.

A retrospective case note analysis has been carried out looking at 180 patients who underwent liver surgery [16c]. They compared the post-operative pain scores of patients who underwent maintenance anesthesia with either propofol (given using TIVA, $n = 95$) or sevoflurane ($n = 95$). Pain scores were measured using a verbal numeric rating scale (0–10). The sevoflurane group reported higher post-operative pain scores when coughing on day 1 (5.08 vs 4.3, $P = 0.0127$) and day 2 (4.56 vs 4.00, $P = 0.0472$). There was no difference on day 3. The sevoflurane group also consumed significantly more daily, accumulative and total morphine on all post-operative days. There were no differences in total duration of intravenous patient-controlled analgesia (PCA) morphine use and patient satisfaction. The sevoflurane group had a significantly increased incidence of pruritis (6.3% vs 0, $P = 0.029$). There were no differences in other side effects recorded (nausea, vomiting and dizziness).

OTHER VAPOURS

Nitrous Oxide

Gastrointestinal

Nitrous oxide (N_2O) is well known to be emetogenic and this has again been shown in a large multi-centre, internationally recruited randomized trial. They investigated 7112 patients over 45 years of age undergoing elective non-cardiac major surgery as a pre-planned secondary analysis from ENIGMA-II trial [17C]. Patients were randomized to receive 70:30 $N_2O:O_2$ or Air:O_2 with a primary hypothesis that there would be a correlation between severe Post-Operative Nausea and Vomiting (PONV) and patient outcomes including quality of recovery (QoR), fever, wound infection and hospital stay. Duration of surgery and anesthesia was similar between the two groups. 884 patients had severe PONV (12.4%) within 3 days of surgery. Female patients, non-smokers, patients undergoing gastrointestinal surgery and those having surgery with a duration of more than 2 hours and receiving N_2O were more likely to suffer severe PONV whether or not they received prophylactic anti-emetics. Avoiding N_2O reduced the risk of severe PONV (11% vs 15%; RR, 0.74 [95% CI, 0.63–0.84]; $P < 0.0001$) despite the fact that patients assigned to N_2O group were more likely to receive anti-emetic prophylaxis ($P < 0.001$). The emetogenic effect of N_2O was strongest in Asian patients (interaction $P = 0.004$; RR, 1.89 [95% CI 1.08–2.33]; $P < 0.001$) and in those receiving intraoperative morphine (RR, 1.72 [95% CI, 1.41–2.13], $P < 0.001$). Patients with severe PONV had lower QoR scores compared to those who did not (10.4 [95% CI, 10.2–10.7] vs 13.1 [95% CI, 13.0–13.2], $P < 0.0005$). Severe PONV was an independent predictor of post-operative fever (5% vs 20%; adjusted OR: 1.44 [95% CI 1.17–1.77]; $P = 0.001$). It was not, however, associated with wound infections (adjusted OR: 1.20 [95% CI 0.97–1.48]; $P = 0.093$). Patients with severe PONV had a longer hospital stay (median [interquartile range], 7.0 [4.9–12.1] days) compared with those who did not (6.0 [3.2–10.1] days; adjusted hazard ratio, 1.14 [95% CI 1.05–1.23]; $P = 0.002$).

Nervous System

N_2O is a safe, quick-acting and well-tolerated sedative agent with analgesic and anxiolytic properties that make it ideal for emergency department (ED) use. In a prospective, non-blinded observational study, patients presenting to ED ($n = 85$) with moderate to severe pain received a mixture of 50% N_2O and were assessed for reduction in baseline pain scores at 20, 30 and 60 minutes [18c]. There was a clinically and statistically significant reduction in mean pain scores from baseline to 20 minutes of N_2O administration. This was sustained through the 60-minute period. Sixty-five minor adverse events were experienced in 38 patients. Only 3 patients required intervention (1 verbal stimulation for drowsiness, 1 supplemental oxygen for agitation, 1 supplemental oxygen for desaturation). More than half the patients received additional analgesic agents but the study design meant that they were unable to evaluate differences in pain scores between patients who received N_2O alone and those who received N_2O+additional analgesics.

Switching from maintenance anesthesia with an ether anesthetic to maintenance with high-dose (concentration >50% and total gas flow rate >4 L per minute) N_2O can be used to facilitate emergence from GA. This transition is associated with a switch in site of anesthetic action. A small retrospective study ($n = 19$) investigated whether there is an electroencephalogram (EEG) marker of the transition between ether anesthetic to N_2O [19c]. They concluded that the administration of high-dose N_2O is associated with transient, large amplitude slow-delta oscillations. This is in contrast to the beta oscillations commonly observed with lower concentrations of N_2O (20%–40%). Pavone et al. postulate that these slow-delta oscillations may result from N_2O-induced blockade of major excitatory inputs from the brainstem to the thalamus and cortex, and that this may offer new insights into brain states during general anesthesia.

Cardiovascular

A report has identified two cases of sustained venous thromboembolic events associated with massive hyperhomocysteinaemia after prolonged but intermittent therapeutic use of inhaled nitrous oxide [20A].

Two women (aged 36 and 30 years old), both with sickle cell disease (SCD) taking hydroxyurea for recurrent vaso-occlusive disease, were admitted to ICU for treatment of severe acute pain. Pain was refractory to common treatments, and therefore inhaled 50% N_2O/O_2 premix was given frequently, intermittently and for 7–9 days. Both suffered deep vein thrombosis, and subsequent thrombophilia screening identified massive hyperhomocysteinaemia (153 and 99 $\mu mol\,L^{-1}$, respectively, normal value 5–15 $\mu mol\,L^{-1}$). Serum folic acid and vitamin B12 were normal. Homocysteine levels returned to normal after N_2O withdrawal and folic acid supplementation. The cases highlight the potential for transient massive hyperhomocysteinaemia, an independent risk factor for venous thrombosis. The authors suggest that prolonged 50% N_2O/O_2 premix in patients with SCD be used with caution and that homocysteinaemia should be monitored.

Xenon

Genetic Factors [21A]

Case Report

A 31-year-old male with a positive test for malignant hyperthermia underwent a laparotomy successfully using xenon for maintenance of anesthesia in a referral centre for xenon anesthesia. The noble gas xenon offers haemodynamic stability, and rapid induction and emergence from anesthesia regardless of its duration. Following induction with target-controlled infusion (TCI) propofol and remifentanil, xenon was administered to a concentration of 60%–70%. Propofol was then stopped. There was no intraoperative haemodynamic instability and post-operatively the patient did not show any signs of intolerance or adverse events.

Comparative Studies

A meta-analysis of randomized controlled trials on xenon anesthesia looked at 43 studies [22M]. A systematic review found a total of 31 studies comparing xenon ($n = 841$) with other inhaled agents ($n = 836$) and 12 studies comparing xenon ($n = 373$) with propofol ($n = 360$). Clinical outcomes such as intraoperative haemodynamics, emergence and PONV were evaluated. Xenon anesthesia provides a relatively more stable intraoperative blood pressure, lower heart rate, and faster emergence from anesthesia than volatile and propofol anesthesia. Xenon is, however, associated with a higher incidence of PONV (34.3% vs 19.9%; RR=1.72 [99% CI 1.10–2.69], risk difference 0.19 [99% CI 0.04–0.33]).

INTRAVENOUS AGENTS

Comparative Studies

A systematic review has been carried out looking at the adverse events of procedural sedations carried out in the emergency department [23M]. Fifty-five eligible articles were identified between January 2005 and January 2015 of which 25 were RCTs and the remainder observational studies. All procedures and all sedation regimes were included. There was some heterogeneity between the studies due to sample size and definitions of adverse events. Studies looking at apnea, bradycardia, intubation and laryngospasm had low heterogeneity, those looking at agitation, hypotension and vomiting, had moderate heterogeneity and hypoxia a high degree of heterogeneity. In total, 9652 sedations were investigated. The most common adverse events were hypoxia (40.2%), vomiting (16.4%), hypotension (15.2%) and apnea (12.4%). Severe adverse events requiring medical intervention were rare with laryngospasm, intubation and aspiration occurring in 14.2, 1.6 and 1.2/1000 sedations. When looking at isolated adverse events, agitation and vomiting were most common with ketamine sedations (164 and 170/1000 sedations), apnea with midazolam (51.4/1000 sedations), bradycardia with etomidate (4.02/1000 sedations) and hypotension and hypoxia with propofol sedation (19.1 and 19.1/1000 sedations). When the observational studies were excluded from the analysis, the incidence of adverse events increased and no single agent outperformed the rest. There was no comment on doses used or procedure success. Unfortunately, there were differences in the definition of hypoxia which will account for the heterogeneity.

Etomidate

Nervous System [24c]

A prospective trial investigated the effect of ketamine on etomidate induced myoclonus. They randomized 104 ASA 1 or 2 adult patients undergoing elective surgery under GA using etomidate to receive either low dose ketamine (0.5 mg/kg) or placebo prior to induction of anesthesia. The groups were observed for myoclonus defined as involuntary short muscle contractions which led to a short observable movement of body parts. Adverse events were also recorded before induction of anesthesia and 2 hours after recovery by a blinded observer. The incidence of myoclonus was significantly lower in the ketamine group (23.1% vs 75%, $P < 0.001$) and with severe myoclonic jerks observed in only 1% of

the ketamine group compared to 28% of the placebo group. The incidence of nausea and vomiting was low in both groups (approx. 0.5%), and there were no incidences of sedation, respiratory depression or hallucinations. Cardiovascular and respiratory parameters were similar between the two groups.

Ketamine

Nervous System

A prospective, randomized, double-blinded placebo-controlled trial has investigated dexmedetomidine and ketamine and their impact on post operative analgesia in spinal surgery [25c]. They randomized 66 ASA 1 and 2 adults to one of 3 groups: Group K: 0.25 μg/kg bolus ketamine followed by infusion at 25 μg/kg/h (co administered with midazolam 10 μg/kg), Group D: 0.5 μg/kg dexmedetomidine followed by infusion of 0.5 μg/kg/h, Group C: Control administered equal volumes of normal saline, all to be given in the post anesthesia care unit for a minimum of 24 hours. The pain-free period was significantly longer in groups D and K than group C (265 vs 580 (group D) vs 860 (group K) minutes, $P = 0.002$). The pain-free period was also longer individually between groups K and C and groups D and C, and it was comparable between groups K and D. Rescue morphine requirements were significantly higher in group C at all time points (21.08 mg vs 7.98 mg (group D) and 2.59 mg 9 group K, $P = 0.00$), but groups K and D were comparable. Heart rate was significantly decreased and blood pressure significantly higher in both treatment groups compared to control. Sedation scores differed significantly between the three groups, but unfortunately the data are missing; however, no patient required an airway maneuver for over-sedation. All other side effects measured (dizziness, hallucinations, nightmares and nausea and vomiting) were comparable between the 3 groups.

A prospective randomized, double-blind study investigated 120 ASA 1 and 2 patients (30–60 years) undergoing a total abdominal hysterectomy for fibroid uterus or uterine myomectomy [26C]. They studied the effect of ketamine (Group K), magnesium (Group M) and placebo (Group C) on the primary outcome of morphine use in the first post-operative 48 hours. They also observed pain scores at 2, 4, 6, 12, 24 and 48 hours and adverse events. The study used a validated numeric pain rating scale (0–10) to investigate pain scores. Induction of anesthesia was standardized and morphine 0.05 mg/kg was administered to all patients 20 minutes prior to the end of surgery. Once surgery was completed, a PCA device was given to each patient. Concurrently with commencing the PCA, Group K received 0.2 mg/kg bolus with an infusion of 0.05 mg/kg/h, Group M received 50 mg/kg magnesium followed by infusion of 10 mg/kg/h and

Group C received a bolus and infusion of normal saline. All study drugs were continued for 48 hours post operatively. There was a significant reduction in morphine consumption in Group K compared to Group M and C in the first 48 hours post-operatively (32.6 mg vs 58.9 mg and 65.7 mg, respectively, $P = 0.015$). Despite this, there were no differences in the pain scores between the three groups. Rescue analgesia was given to 40% of patients in Group C, 30% in Group M and 12.5% in Group K ($P < 0.05$). There were no differences in the incidence of adverse events with the exception that pruritis and nausea were increased in Group C.

A retrospective case note review of children with cerebral palsy undergoing ketamine-based sedation for botulinum toxin injection was carried out [27c]. 152 injections were performed in 87 children. 81.9% received ketamine and midazolam sedation with the remainder having ketamine used as a sole agent. 54% received a single injection with the remainder receiving multiple injections but no procedure had to be aborted for pain or side effects. 10 procedures (6.6%) were associated with an acute side effect. Four had a rash, 3 had nausea and vomiting, 1 had limb tremors and 1 had a mild headache. On follow-up review, one child reported nightmares on the evening of the procedure. There were no serious adverse events (laryngospasm, respiratory depression, emergence delirium, speech or swallowing difficulties or incontinence). The authors did not comment as to whether the patients with side effects had received combined sedation or ketamine alone. The study does admit to a stringent pre-procedure questionnaire to select appropriate cases for this procedure and therefore this may have biased the results.

A review article of 11 case reports ($n = 74$) has examined the use of ketamine infusions in critically ill infants and children [28c]. Although each individual case has small numbers, the authors conclude that ketamine infusions are safe to be used in the critically ill child for bronchospasm/status asthmaticus or respiratory distress although there was significant heterogeneity in the dosing regimens used. 10.8% of children experienced adverse effects. One child experiencing each of hypersalivation, hypertension and flushing, and two, nystagmus. None required treatment and all resolved on discontinuation of the drug. The reported incidence of emergence phenomenon is 12% but in this review only 4% of children experienced this known side effect, all of whom had received benzodiazepines in an attempt to alleviate this. Again, resolution was complete following withdrawal of ketamine.

A retrospective database review was carried out looking at procedural sedations in the emergency department over a 7-year period to investigate adverse events [29c]. 243 children (median age 4 years) were sedated, primarily for wound management, of whom 215 received ketamine. 87% received IV sedation and where ketamine was used the median initial dose was 1.25 mg/kg IV or 3.94 mg/kg IM. 9.8% had an adverse reaction. The most common were recovery agitation and apnea (each 4/21 cases). There was only one case who was risk stratified as moderate (paradoxical agitation requiring a general anesthetic), and all others were minor risk with no intervention required (paradoxical response, failed IV access, desaturation rash, vomiting, hypersalivation, airway repositioning required).

Psychiatric

Ketamine has long being known for its positive effect on treatment resistant depression (TRD) and is postulated to be secondary to a mismatch in the activity of the prefrontal cortex and the amygdala.

A prospective randomized single-centre trial investigated 48 TRD patients into receiving 0.5 mg/kg (Group A), 0.2 mg/kg (Group B) Ketamine or placebo and monitored the effect using Standardised uptake values (SUV) of glucose metabolism as measured by F-FDG positron emission tomography scans [30c]. Depressive symptoms were also recorded using the validated Hamilton Depression rating scale (HDRS). Observations were taken at 0, 40, 80, 120 and 240 minutes. This scan was used as a proxy measure for glutamate neurotransmission. In groups A and B there were significantly more responders at time points 40 and 80 minutes with significant reduction in HDRS scores at 40 minutes compared to Group C (-32.8% and -37.1% in groups A and B compared to -12% in Group C ($P < 0.005$)). The SUV in the prefrontal cortex was significantly increased in both ketamine groups ($P < 0.001$) and reduced in all groups in the amygdala. The ketamine group did have a significant increase in side effects with 8/16 patients in the high-dose group complaining of floating sensation compared to 1/16 and 0/16 in the low dose and placebo groups, respectively. There were no differences in the incidence of dizziness, nausea and chest tightness. This study concluded that the rapid alleviation of depressive symptoms with ketamine treatment involve the facilitation of glutaminergic transmission in the prefrontal cortex.

Ketamine has again been studied in the treatment of severe major depressive disorder (MDD) [31c]. A randomized, double-blind parallel group trial investigated 37 patients with MDD (as documented by a score of >24 on the Hamilton Rating scale for depression (HAMD)). After a 2-week drug washout period, patients were randomized to receive either Escitalopram and single-dose ketamine (0.5 mg/kg over 40 minutes) or placebo. Depressive symptoms were assessed using the Montgomery-Asberg Depression rating scale (MADRS) and Quick inventory of depressive symptomatology (QIDS-SR) scales. Adverse psychological effects were assessed using the Brief Psychiatric rating scale (BPRS), Young Mania rating scale (YRMS) and the clinician administered dissociative states scale. Scores were measured at a number of predefined time points, and a reduction of >50% of the MADRS score was considered clinically significant. At 4 weeks post treatment, the ketamine group had a superior response to treatment (cumulative figures 92% vs 57%, $P=0.04$) with cumulative remission in 76.9% vs 14.3% of placebo group ($P=0.01$). The time to respond was also quicker in the ketamine group (8.9 vs 28 days, $P=0.01$). At all individual time points between 2 hours and 2 weeks, the ketamine group has significantly lower MADRS and QIDS-SR scores. In the ketamine group, there was a significant increase in the YRMS score at 1 and 2 hours, indicating an increase in dissociative symptoms, but these became and remained non-significant thereafter. There were no other changes in the adverse event scores observed.

In contrast a case report has identified the onset of depressive symptoms on withdrawal of ketamine [32A].

Case Report

A 28-year-old male ketamine-dependent user of 12 years experienced euphoria and dissociation on use of the drug. He also developed urinary symptoms (well known to be associated with ketamine). He had no psychotic symptoms whilst on the drug and psychometric testing prior to a standard withdrawal programme revealed minimal mood-related symptoms. 6 hours after withdrawal, the patient started to experience fatigue and dysphoria which deteriorated to a peak at 1 week. There were no suicidal ideations. The symptoms started to improve after approximately 2 weeks and spontaneously remitted at 1 month post withdrawal.

Cardiovascular

Two studies have examined the effects of ketamine on cardiovascular dynamics in the pediatric congenital heart disease population.

This small observational study studied the effects of ketamine and etomidate in 22 children under 12 years with tetralogy of Fallot (TOF): Group A: moderate to severe cyanosis Sp02 <85% and Group B: Mild cyanosis Sp02 >85% [33c]. All children were undergoing intracardiac repair of their TOF, and anesthesia was induced using sevoflurane, rocuronium and fentanyl. After tracheal intubation a trans-oesophageal echo probe was inserted and children were mechanically ventilated. Post-induction, both groups were given separate doses of ketamine (2mg/kg) and etomidate (0.3mg/kg). Injections were given in a computer generated randomized fashion, 15 minutes apart and thus patients acted as their own controls. Clinicians were blinded to the drug choice. Cardiovascular, respiratory and arterial gas observations were taken at 1, 2, 4, 6, 8 and 15 minutes post injection.

Etomidate produced no significant changes in respiratory, arterial gas or echocardiographic parameters. Ketamine injection, however, in Group A had a significant reduction in Sp02 whilst those in group B had a significant rise in Sp02 vs baseline. Further divergent effects were observed with pulmonary blood flow increasing in children with mild cyanosis (group B) and reducing in those with moderate to severe cyanosis (group A).

The second study was a small observational study investigating 24 children (0.5–18 years) scheduled to undergo cardiac catheterisation for assessment of pulmonary hypertension [34c]. Following anesthetic induction with sevoflurane and rocuronium, a bolus of 2 mg/kg ketamine was injected over 2 minutes. Baseline clinical and cardiovascular parameters were measured prior and 2 minutes after ketamine bolus. Whilst there were small statistically significant increases in mean arterial pressure, pulmonary artery pressure and right atrial pressure, these were deemed not to be clinically significant and therefore the authors deemed ketamine a safe drug to use in this patient population as part of a balanced anesthetic technique.

Ketofol

Nervous System

A meta-analysis of studies that compared ketofol to propofol for procedural sedation in the emergency department has been undertaken [35M]. 18 trials met the inclusion criteria of 'RCT comparing the two drugs'. Ketofol showed a much improved side effect profile compared to propofol with fewer respiratory complications (RR 0.31, 95% CI 0.47–0.7, $P=0.001$, 14 trials) and cardiovascular complications (reduced hypotension (RR 0.11 95% CI 0.17–0.97, $P=0.04$, 9 trials) and bradycardia (RR0.47, 95% CI 0.28–0.72, $P=0.008$, 8 trials)). The incidence of psychotomimetic side effects, muscle rigidity and nausea and vomiting was not significantly different although only 2 of the included trials investigated muscle rigidity.

Propofol

Respiratory

Two studies have compared the effects of propofol and dexmedetomidine in drug-induced sleep endoscopy (DISE), a validated technique used to investigate patients with obstructive sleep apnea (OSA).

The first, a prospective, single-center observational trial ($n=50$) examined patients on consecutive treatments [36c]. They were given TCI propofol (starting effect site concentration 2μg/mL) or dexmedetomidine (1μg/kg followed by an infusion of 1μg/kg/h). All patients had standard monitoring with BIS depth of sedation monitoring. During the treatment where patients received propofol, there was a significant increase in airway narrowing at all depths of sedation. This was despite the number of sites of obstruction being the same in both groups. Also, there was an increase in the number of desaturations, with the minimum SpO_2 of 83.7% compared to 91.4%. The propofol group also had a significantly higher number of patients with SpO_2 <90% and 80% although unfortunately approximate numbers are only available from the graph. There were significantly more patients in the propofol group who developed cardiovascular instability with 52% vs 38% and 58% vs 38% having >20% change in baseline of blood pressure and heart rate, respectively. Unfortunately, this study excluded patients with a BMI of >30 kg/m^2 and therefore this may limit its relevance to the general OSA population.

The second was a retrospective single-centre case note review [37c]. They examined 52 patients undergoing DISE with propofol sedation and 164 with dexmedetomidine, all of whom had refused or failed CPAP treatment. The two groups were demographically and clinically similar. They looked specifically for the degree of anteroposterior base of tongue obstruction. They identified a significant increase in the incidence of complete obstruction (75% vs 42.7%) and partial or no obstruction (25% vs 57.3%, OR: 4, 95% CI 2–8.1, $P = 0.001$) in the propofol group compared to the dexmedetomidine group. Although this study was unblinded, it increases the information of these two drugs in this context with the optimal strategy, as yet, unknown.

Drug Administration

A recognized side effect of propofol administration is pain on injection.

Two studies have investigated different drugs to ameliorate this known side effect.

A prospective double-blind study investigated the effect of magnesium sulphate and lidocaine on this in 300 women undergoing elective hysteroscopy [38C]. Patients were randomized to receive either lidocaine (40 mg), magnesium sulphate 300 mg or both. All test drugs were the same volume and thus blinded the administration. Test drugs were administered 10 seconds prior to 50 mg propofol. Primary outcome was the 4 point pain score immediately on administration of propofol and secondary outcome was post-operative recall of the propofol administration. Significantly more patients exhibited no pain (27%) in the combined group compare with either lidocaine or magnesium alone (7% and 5%, respectively, $P < 0.01$). Fewer patients in the combined group exhibited moderate pain (5 vs 18 and 24 in the lidocaine and magnesium groups, respectively) and pain scores were significantly reduced (1/4 vs 2.88 and 2.77, respectively, $P < 0.01$). There were significantly fewer withdrawal movements in the group receiving both drugs. There

were no haemodynamic or other side effects reported in any group.

A meta-analysis of 8 RCTS investigating the effect of 5HT3 antagonists on propofol injection was carried out [39M]. The risk of bias was assessed by two independent practitioners and all studies deemed to be low risk of bias. Overall pain on injection was shown to be reduced by the pre-treatment with 5HT3 receptor antagonists (RR 0.43, 95% CI 0.33–0.56, $P < 0.05$). In addition, 5HT3 receptor antagonists were deemed to reduce the severity of pain on injection. Compared to the control group, 5HT3 receptor antagonists increased the number of patients with mild pain (RR 1.63, 95% CI 1.21–2.2, $P < 0.05$) and reduced those with moderate (RR 0.21, 95% CI 0.15–0.30, $P < 0.05$) and severe pain (RR 0.16, 95% CI 0.10–0.25, $P < 0.05$). No patient in the trial exhibited pain or discomfort from the 5HT3 inhibitor. There were no other significant side effects reported.

Nervous System

A small observational trial investigated 80 ASA 1–4 adults scheduled for elective upper gastrointestinal endoscopy under propofol TCI for swallowing impairment [40c]. Glottis videoendoscopy was used to assess swallowing and two validated but subjective scores (dysphagia severity score (DSS) 0–4 and penetration and aspiration score (PAS) 1–8. The scorer was not blinded to the TCI target. Severe impairment was identified as a DSS of 3 or PAS 7–8. Propofol TCI was commenced at 2 μg/mL and increased to 3 and 4 μg/mL (all effect site concentrations). Swallowing assessment was performed in all patients at all concentrations. The observer's assessment of alertness/sedation scale (OAAS) was used to assess sedation depth in all patients (5-awake: 1-does not respond to shaking or prodding). In the 2 μg/mL target group, the OAAS score was 2 in 26% and 1 in 73%. In the other target groups the OAAS was 1 in all patients. The 21 patients who had an OAAS of 2 all had normal swallowing. 24% of patients at the 3 μg/mL propofol target had severe swallowing impairment. PAS scores identified 23% and 58% with severe swallowing impairment in the 3 μg/mL and 4 μg/mL, respectively, compared to 6.25% in the 2 μg/mg propofol target group. Respiratory side effects were also evaluated and 15% in the 3 μg/mL target group ($n = 78$) and 77% patients in the 4 μg/mL ($n = 66$) had oxygen desaturation (>10% drop from baseline) following the swallowing assessment. In multivariate analysis, increasing age, BMI and TCI target were all independent risk factors for impaired swallowing using both swallowing assessment scores ($P < 0.05$ for all values).

A retrospective case note review of patients undergoing endoscopic resection of early gastric cancer under deep sedation has been carried out [41C]. 349 patients had their pre- and postprocedure chest radiographs reviewed to identify presence or absence of atelectasis. Deep sedation was defined as the loss of consciousness but the retention of spontaneous respiration and protective reflexes. To achieve this, midazolam 2–4 mg and propofol 0.5–1 mg/kg was administered. 19.5% (68 patients) had newly diagnosed atelectasis following the procedure. Following univariate analysis, atelectasis significantly correlated with BMI, smoking, diabetes mellitus, procedure duration, size of lesion and total amount of propofol given. Age, gender and other co-morbid conditions were not associated with atelectasis. In the multi-variate analysis, BMI, procedure duration and total propofol administered were all significant risk factors for atelectasis. Of these patients, 9/68 developed a fever and 6/68 patients displayed pneumonic infiltration.

A further retrospective study has investigated whether propofol sedation increased adverse events in colonoscopy [42c]. This study looked at 3 168 228 adults undergoing out-patient colonoscopy over 4 years, identifying patients using insurance records. The patient was assumed to have had the procedure under GA if anesthesia services were billed for on the same day. Further information on the type and depth of sedation is not available. Any increase in adverse events colonic (perforation/hemorrhage/pain), sedation related (pneumonia/infection/sedation complications) or cardiorespiratory event (hypotension/myocardial infarction/stroke) was recorded. 34.4% colonoscopies were performed with anesthesia services and the use of anesthesia increased the risk of perforation (OR 1.07), hemorrhage (OR 1.28), pain (OR 1.07) and complications secondary to anesthesia (OR 1.15). There were no quoted values for statistical significance. In addition, those having a polypectomy had a 26% increased risk of perforation. The clinical significance of this study is unclear due to the large amount of assumed and missing data.

A further study utilized a questionnaire to ascertain the use and side effects of propofol in Pediatric Intensive Care Units (PICU) in Israel [43c]. With an 86.6% response rate, they found that 100%, 70% and 12% of respondents used propofol for induction, procedural sedation and sedation, respectively. 88% used propofol for a limit of 24 hours but 40% used the drug with no specified upper limit. 25% of respondents encountered adverse events comprising self-limiting apnea, bradycardia and hypotension. There were two cases of suspected propofol infusion syndrome (PIS), both of whom were treated for more than 24 hours and above the recognized maximum dose of 4 mg/kg/h. Symptoms of PIS included metabolic acidosis, rhabdomyolysis and cardiac failure.

Drug Administration Route

A small study investigated whether TCI propofol could provide a better sedation quality for colonoscopy than manually controlled infusion (MCI) in training inexperienced anesthesiology residents [44c]. Eighteen residents were allocated into 2 groups receiving either TCI or MCI training in their first month of experience. Data

from the final 2 patients of each resident were analyzed. In the second month, TCI trained residents used MCI and vice versa and data from the final two patients again were analyzed. Endoscopists satisfaction was significantly higher in the TCI group (VAS 81.3 vs 74.2 $P = 0.003$) but patient satisfaction scores were similar. All patients successfully completed the procedure with no severe adverse events. The TCI group also exhibited a more stable cardiovascular (min MAP 72.9 mmHg vs 67.7 mmHg, max MAP 95.4 vs 100.3 $P < 0.05$) and respiratory profile (min SpO2 97.4% vs 95.6%, $P = 0.008$). Recovery time was also longer in the MCI group (11.3 vs 9.1 minutes $P < 0.001$) thus concluding that TCI is a safer technique than MCI in for colonoscopy patients.

A single-centre retrospective analysis of patients undergoing off-pump coronary artery bypass (OPCAB) surgery was carried out to ascertain any differences in outcome dependent on the type of anesthetic given [45c]. 192 patients underwent OPCAB surgery receiving propofol–remifentanil total intravenous anesthesia (TIVA), and they were propensity score matched to 662 patients who underwent Isoflurane anesthesia. There were no significant differences in the incidence of in-hospital major adverse events, defined as death, MI, coronary revascularization, stroke, renal failure or prolonged mechanical ventilation (OR 1.29 95%, CI 088–1.88, $P = 0.2$). There was no difference in the incidence of major adverse cardiovascular and cerebral events (OR 0.81, 95% CI 0.46–1.42, $P = 0.46$). This was consistent amongst all patients and sub-group analyses (old age (>70 year), high risk and diabetic patients). The risk of post-operative new arrhythmia including atrial fibrillation was, however, significantly increased in the TIVA group. One limitation of this study was that remifentanil infusion was only used in the propofol group, and therefore it does not directly compare propofol vs isoflurane.

References

[1] Makkar JK, Bhatia N, Bala I, et al. A comparison of single dose dexmedetomidine with propofol for the prevention of emergence delirium after desflurane anaesthesia in children. Anaesthesia. 2016;71:50–7 [c].

[2] Kim MK, Baek CW, Kang H, et al. Comparison of emergence after deep extubation using desflurane or desflurane with remifentanil in patients undergoing general anesthesia: a randomized trial. J Clin Anesth. 2016;28:19–25 [c].

[3] Nogueira FR, Braz LG, de Andrade LR, et al. Evaluation of genotoxicity of general anesthesia maintained with desflurane in patients under minor surgery. Environ Mol Mutagen. 2016;57:312–6 [E].

[4] Lee J, Yoo YJ, Lee JM, et al. Sevoflurane versus desflurane on the incidence of postreperfusion syndrome during living donor liver transplantation: a randomized controlled trial. Transplantation. 2016;100:600–6 [c].

[5] Bellgardt M, Bomberg H, Herzog-Niescery J, et al. Survival after long-term isoflurane sedation as opposed to intravenous sedation in critically ill surgical patients: retrospective analysis. Eur J Anaesthesiol. 2016;33:6–13 [c].

[6] Jung S, Yuki K. Differential effects of volatile anesthetics on leukocyte integrin macrophage-1 antigen. J Immunotoxicol. 2016;13:148–56 [E].

[7] Dayan AD. Analgesic use of inhaled methoxyflurane: evaluation of its potential nephrotoxicity. Hum Exp Toxicol. 2016;35:91–100 [R].

[8] Gaskell AL, Jephcott CG, Smithells JR, et al. Self-administered methoxyflurane for procedural analgesia: experience in a tertiary Australasian centre. Anaesthesia. 2016;71:417–23 [c].

[9] Chen Y, Cui J, Sun JJ, et al. Gradient between dorsalis pedis and radial arterial blood pressures during sevoflurane anaesthesia: a self-control study in patients undergoing neurosurgery. Eur J Anaesthesiol. 2016;33:110–7 [c].

[10] Xiong HY, Liu Y, Shu DC, et al. Effects of sevoflurane inhalation during cardiopulmonary bypass on pediatric patients: a randomized controlled clinical trial. ASAIO J. 2016;62:63–8 [c].

[11] Choromanski DW, Amin S, Zestos MM. Sevoflurane as a cause of torsade de pointes in patient with the long QT syndrome: case report. Middle East J Anaesthesiol. 2016;23:471–4 [A].

[12] Walia H, Ruda J, Tobias JD. Sevoflurane and bradycardia in infants with trisomy 21: a case report and review of the literature. Int J Pediatr Otorhinolaryngol. 2016;80:5–7 [A].

[13] McKay RE, Hall KT, Hills N. The effect of anesthetic choice (sevoflurane versus desflurane) and neuromuscular management on speed of airway reflex recovery. Anesth Analg. 2016;122:393–401 [c].

[14] Castellanos M, Xifra G, Fernandez-Real JM, et al. Breath gas concentrations mirror exposure to sevoflurane and isopropyl alcohol in hospital environments in non-occupational conditions. J Breath Res. 2016;10:016001 [c].

[15] Frederick HJ, Wofford K, de Lisle DG, et al. Randomized controlled trial to determine the effect of depth of anesthesia on emergence agitation in children. Anesth Analg. 2016;122:1141–6 [c].

[16] Chan AC, Qiu Q, Choi SW, et al. Effects of intra-operative total intravenous anaesthesia with propofol versus inhalational anaesthesia with sevoflurane on post-operative pain in liver surgery: a retrospective case-control study. PLoS One. 2016;11: e0149753 [c].

[17] Myles PS, Chan MT, Kasza J, et al. Severe nausea and vomiting in the evaluation of nitrous oxide in the gas mixture for anesthesia II trial. Anesthesiology. 2016;124:1032–40 [C].

[18] Herres J, Chudnofsky CR, Manur R, et al. The use of inhaled nitrous oxide for analgesia in adult ED patients: a pilot study. Am J Emerg Med. 2016;34:269–73 [c].

[19] Pavone KJ, Akeju O, Sampson AL, et al. Nitrous oxide-induced slow and delta oscillations. Clin Neurophysiol. 2016;127:556–64 [c].

[20] Faguer S, Ruiz J, Mari A. Massive hyperhomocysteinaemia as a complication of nitrous oxide inhalation. Br J Clin Pharmacol. 2016;81:391–2 [A].

[21] Carlomagno M, Esposito C, Marra A, et al. Xenon anaesthesia in a patient with susceptibility to malignant hyperthermia: a case report. Eur J Anaesthesiol. 2016;33:147–50 [A].

[22] Law LS, Lo EA, Gan TJ. Xenon anesthesia: a systematic review and meta-analysis of randomized controlled trials. Anesth Analg. 2016;122:678–97 [M].

[23] Bellolio MF, Gilani WI, Barrionuevo P, et al. Incidence of adverse events in adults undergoing procedural sedation in the emergency department: a systematic review and meta-analysis. Acad Emerg Med. 2016;23:119–34 [M].

[24] Wu GN, Xu HJ, Liu FF, et al. Low-dose ketamine pretreatment reduces the incidence and severity of myoclonus induced by etomidate: A randomized, double-blinded, controlled clinical trial. Medicine. 2016;95(6):e2701. http://dx.doi.org/10.1097/MD.0000000000002701 [c].

[25] Garg N, Panda NB, Gandhi KA, et al. Comparison of small dose ketamine and dexmedetomidine infusion for postoperative analgesia in spine surgery—a prospective randomized

[26] Arikan M, Aslan B, Arikan O, et al. But b comparison of the effects of magnesium and ketamine on postoperative pain and morphine consumption. A double-blind randomized controlled clinical study. Acta Cir Bras. 2016;31:67–73 [C].

[27] Chow C, Choong CT. Ketamine-based procedural sedation and analgesia for botulinum toxin A injections in children with cerebral palsy. Eur J Paediatr Neurol. 2016;20:319–22 [c].

[28] Golding CL, Miller JL, Gessouroun MR, et al. Ketamine continuous infusions in critically ill infants and children. Ann Pharmacother. 2016;50:234–41 [c].

[29] Kidd LR, Lyons SC, Lloyd G. Paediatric procedural sedation using ketamine in a UK emergency department: a 7 year review of practice. Br J Anaesth. 2016;116:518–23 [c].

[30] Li CT, Chen MH, Lin WC, et al. The effects of low-dose ketamine on the prefrontal cortex and amygdala in treatment-resistant depression: a randomized controlled study. Hum Brain Mapp. 2016;37:1080–90 [c].

[31] Hu YD, Xiang YT, Fang JX, et al. Single i.v. ketamine augmentation of newly initiated escitalopram for major depression: results from a randomized, placebo-controlled 4-week study. Psychol Med. 2016;46:623–35 [c].

[32] Lin PC, Lane HY, Lin CH. Spontaneous remission of ketamine withdrawal-related depression. Clin Neuropharmacol. 2016;39:51–2 [A].

[33] Jha AK, Gharde P, Chauhan S, et al. Echocardiographic assessment of the alterations in pulmonary blood flow associated with ketamine and etomidate administration in children with tetralogy of fallot. Echocardiography. 2016;33:307–13 [c].

[34] Friesen RH, Twite MD, Nichols CS, et al. Hemodynamic response to ketamine in children with pulmonary hypertension. Paediatr Anaesth. 2016;26:102–8 [c].

[35] Jalili M, Bahreini M, Doosti-Irani A, et al. Ketamine-propofol combination (ketofol) vs propofol for procedural sedation and analgesia: systematic review and meta-analysis. Am J Emerg Med. 2016;34:558–69 [M].

[36] Yoon BW, Hong JM, Hong SL, et al. A comparison of dexmedetomidine versus propofol during drug-induced sleep endoscopy in sleep apnea patients. Laryngoscope. 2016;126:763–7 [c].

[37] Capasso R, Rosa T, Tsou DY, et al. Variable findings for drug-induced sleep endoscopy in obstructive sleep apnea with propofol versus dexmedetomidine. Otolaryngol Head Neck Surg. 2016;154:765–70 [c].

[38] Sun J, Zhou R, Lin W, et al. Magnesium sulfate plus lidocaine reduces propofol injection pain: a double-blind, randomized study. Clin Ther. 2016;38:31–8 [C].

[39] Wang W, Zhou L, Wu LX, et al. 5-HT3 receptor antagonists for propofol injection pain: a meta-analysis of randomized controlled trials. Clin Drug Investig. 2016;36:243–53 [M].

[40] Gemma M, Pasin L, Oriani A, et al. Swallowing impairment during propofol target-controlled infusion. Anesth Analg. 2016;122:48–54 [c].

[41] Choe JW, Jung SW, Song JK, et al. Predictive factors of atelectasis following endoscopic resection. Dig Dis Sci. 2016;61:181–8 [C].

[42] Wernli KJ, Brenner AT, Rutter CM, et al. Risks associated with anesthesia services during colonoscopy. Gastroenterology. 2016;150:888–94. quiz e18 [c].

[43] Rosenfeld-Yehoshua N, Klin B, Berkovitch M, et al. Propofol use in Israeli PICUs. Pediatr Crit Care Med. 2016;17:e117–20 [c].

[44] Wang JF, Li B, Yang YG, et al. Target-controlled infusion of propofol in training anesthesiology residents in colonoscopy sedation: a prospective randomized crossover trial. Med Sci Monit. 2016;22:206–10 [c].

[45] Min JJ, Kim G, Lee JH, et al. Does the type of anesthetic technique affect in-hospital and one-year outcomes after off-pump coronary arterial bypass surgery? PLoS One. 2016;11:e0152060 [c].

10

Local Anesthetics

Sujana Dontukurthy, Allison Kalstein, Joel Yarmush[1]

New York Presbyterian—Brooklyn Methodist Hospital, Brooklyn, NY, United States

[1]Corresponding author: joelyarmush@gmail.com

GENERAL INFORMATION

Adverse events of local anesthetics are usually seen when (a) patients are hypersensitive to the drug administered in accepted safe therapeutic doses or when (b) the drug is administered and absorbed in doses that exceed safe levels. Local anesthetic systemic toxicity (LAST) usually manifests initially as neurotoxicity, including perioral tingling, change in sensorium and if severe, seizure activity. Cardiac toxicity symptoms are seen if the toxicity progresses. Cardiovascular symptoms manifest first as hypotension and tachycardia, followed by cardiovascular collapse. Many of the papers surveyed look at LAST.

Lipid emulsion is used to treat LAST and its use and mechanism of action are surveyed in several of the papers. The availability of lipid emulsion is a concern of several other papers surveyed. A clarion call to have lipid emulsion available whenever local anesthetics are used is made. One paper surveyed looked at the order of rescue drugs administered and found that lipid emulsion should probably precede epinephrine in LAST. This would imply that lipid emulsion should not only be readily available but rather immediately available when using local anesthetics.

But there are those papers surveyed that say that lipid emulsion therapy may be helpful but is certainly not proven. And lipid emulsion therapy is not without its own adverse effects. One paper surveyed stated that adverse events for acute administration used for other than local anesthetic toxicity were extensive and problematic.

Local anesthetics seem to cause cell toxicity when evaluated with in vitro studies. This is seen in many of the surveyed articles this year and years past. Most of these studies show that endogenous and exogenous substances reduce the cellular toxic effects caused by the local anesthetics. However, the clinical significance of local anesthetic cell toxicity is uncertain, at best.

A couple of studies that were surveyed show that despite in vitro toxicity there is no clinical in vivo consequence. One editorial suggests that single intraarticular of local anesthetics should be safe but that prolonged exposure to local anesthetics as seen in continuous intraarticular blocks may be problematic.

COMBINED OR NONSPECIFIC LOCAL ANESTHETICS

Cardiovascular and Central Nervous System Toxicity

Intralipid and Its Effect on LAST

This double blind crossover study [1C] was performed on 16 (i.e., 8 men and 8 women) healthy volunteers. Each volunteer was able to detect early nervous system toxicity with an intravenous lidocaine infusion as part of the inclusion criteria.

The volunteers then received 4 test intravenous infusions in a crossover fashion. The infusions contained 8 mg/min (maximum 120 mg) of either ropivacaine or levobupivacaine followed 2 minutes later by either 120 mL of 20% intralipid or normal saline over 1 minute. When signs of early toxicity were present the local anesthetic infusion was stopped (unless it was stopped previously because maximum dose had been achieved). Blood levels of local anesthetics and EKGs were obtained.

Blood pressure, heart rate, QRS duration and QTc interval increased significantly in all of the 4 groups without statistical differences between groups. The maximum concentration (Cmax) of local anesthetic was significantly reduced when intralipid was used compared to normal saline. The Cmax was also significantly lower in the levobupivacaine—saline group as compared to the ropivacaine—saline group. Time to local anesthetic toxicity was unaffected by intralipid for ropivacaine or levobupivacaine.

The authors concluded that while blood pressure, pulse, QRS and QTc were not affected by intralipid, the Cmax was decreased. They also pointed out that this study only looked at low to moderate toxic doses of ropivacaine or levobupivacaine.

A pharmacokinetic model was also developed which led the authors of the study to conclude that lipid emulsion works best if administered early.

An editorial [2r] on this study points out that the 'lipid sink' theory for lipid emulsion is, at least in part, correct.

Doses of Intralipid Needed to Treat LAST

This letter to the editor [3r] is concerned that the current 2012 [4R] standards of intralipid treatment are problematic because of the volume of drug needed. As an example: a bolus of 100 mL of intralipid is to be followed by 1000 mL/hour in a 70 kg person. If needed the infusion should be doubled to 2000 mL/hour. Given that intralipid is available in the author's institution in 250 mL bags, the author rightfully suggests that there may be hesitancy to give the proper dose. The author of the letter asks that any ambiguities of intralipid dose be addressed and that maximum doses of local anesthetics be added to the universal time-out to make sure the dose of intralipid that may be needed should be calculated and an adequate amount of the intralipid be available before any procedure is performed with local anesthetic use.

LAST Reviewed

This review [5M] looked at the current literature as it pertains to LAST and delineated, in a fairly comprehensive manner, the mechanisms and clinical presentations, risk factors, prevention, and treatment of LAST.

Clarification on LAST and Its Impact

An editorial [6r] and a letter to the editor [7r] on a retrospective review which was included in last year's chapter [8R] state that vigilance is necessary for LAST. The retrospective study was a 5-year single institutional review that addressed cardiac arrest and seizures after peripheral nerve blocks. The authors of the review suggested that the current state of the practice allows for these very infrequent events and implies that LAST is no longer to be feared. The editorial and the letter draw the opposite conclusion. The editorial states that the incidence of LAST is decreasing especially when ultrasound is used in institutions with significant experience in regional anesthesia but that greater care must be taken as the number of events is still high.

Lipid Emulsion Therapy in China

This study [9A] was a survey on the use of lipid emulsion in LAST after regional anesthesia in China. 36 of 41 orthopedic anesthesia academic institutions responded to the survey with only 8 institutions claiming to have readily available lipid emulsion. Findings included limited availability, limited use and limited knowledge of lipid emulsion therapy. There were 27 incidents of LAST in the year surveyed, only 12 of which were treated with lipid emulsion. Of the 12 patients, 11 survived and 1 did not.

Lipid Emulsion Therapy in Germany

This study [10A] was a survey on the availability of lipid emulsion in LAST in Germany. 509 of 1305 hospitals responded to the survey with 338 institutions claiming to have readily available lipid emulsion therapy. 132 hospitals had an incidence of LAST treated with lipid emulsion. 128 of these hospitals had success.

The authors conclusions that German hospitals are prepared for treatment of LAST is problematic as fewer than 40% of the hospitals surveyed responded.

Lipid Emulsion Treatment in LAST

This review [11M] found 75 human studies and 37 animal studies and 1 both human and animal study highlighted lipid emulsion therapy in LAST. The authors admitted that lipid emulsion seemed to be useful in LAST but found that the evidence was less than convincing. An editorial [12r] from the same group of authors used the above and other non surveyed papers to declare that evidence is lacking for lipid emulsion therapy in LAST and should not be necessarily thought of as first line therapy.

Lipid Emulsion Treatment and Adverse Effects

This review [13M] found 87 human studies and 27 animal studies which highlighted some of the adverse effects of rapid administration of acute lipid emulsion therapy when used for either treatment of acute poisoning or parenteral nutrition. These included acute kidney injury, cardiac arrest, ventilation perfusion mismatch, acute lung injury, venous thromboembolism, hypersensitivity, fat embolism, fat overload syndrome, pancreatitis, extracorporeal circulation machine circuit obstruction, allergic reaction, and increased susceptibility to infection. Adverse effects seem to be proportional to the rate of infusion as well as total dose received but more studies are needed.

Lipid Emulsion Attenuates Bupivacaine but Not Mepivacaine-Induced Toxicity

This in vitro study [14E] looked at a LAST model set up to evaluate local anesthetic-induced toxicity of rat aorta epithelium. They found that lipid emulsion lessened the effect seen with bupivacaine but not mepivacaine. They further suggest that this may be because of the relative lipid solubility of bupivacaine compared to mepivacaine. Similar findings by the same group were found using rat cardiomyoblast cells [15E].

Paravetebral Block Toxicity

This case study [16A] looked at a patient who had a continuous paravertebral block after a minithoracotomy under general anesthesia. Initially 0.25% bupivacaine was injected followed by a 0.2% ropivacaine infusion. The patient had convulsions successfully treated with lipid emulsion. The authors of the study state that the measured ropivacaine concentration was just shy of toxic levels.

The infusion concentration could and probably should have been decreased to a more reasonable level (i.e., 0.1%) of ropivacaine.

Cell Toxicity

Review of Local Anesthetic-Induced Neurotoxicity

This review [17M] looks at the incidence, risk factors, and mechanisms of local anesthetic-induced neurotoxicity especially related to regional anesthesia.

Cell Toxicity and Motor Function After Intraneural Injection

This in vivo animal study [18E] looked at intraneural injection of various amide local anesthetics into rat sciatic nerve. The study showed greater histopathologic changes than motor deficiency for bupivacaine, levobupivacaine and lidocaine with no significant differences between local anesthetics.

Genotoxicity of Bupivacaine and Levobupivacaine

This in vivo study [19E] demonstrated that bupivacaine and levobupivacaine did not exhibit genotoxicity in a Drosophila wing spot test. It also revealed that degradation products of levobupivacaine showed recombinogenic affects but bupivacaine did not.

Toxicity of Lidocaine and Ropivacaine

This in vitro study [20E] demonstrated that lidocaine, ropivacaine and a combination of lidocaine and ropivacaine caused toxicity when human melanoma cells were exposed to the local anesthetics.

Continuous Intraarticular Blocks May Be Problematic

This editorial [21r] suggests that single intraarticular injections of local anesthetic have been shown to be useful and should be safe to administer. Cell toxicity which usually increases with increased time of exposure to local anesthetics may become problematic and the authors of the study suggest that continuous intraarticular blocks should be avoided until further evidence of their safety has been studied.

Lidocaine and Ropivacaine May Help in Treating Cancer

This in vitro study [22E] looked at viability of human non-small cell lung cancer cells. The study determined that there was an increase in apoptosis when exposed to lidocaine and ropivacaine.

Amides Affect Human Fibroblasts

This in vitro study [23E] looked at four amide local anesthetics and their effect on human dermal fibroblasts (HFB). The authors found that lidocaine affected proliferation of aged HFB more than mepivacaine. Ropivacaine and bupivacaine did not significantly affect aged HFB. None of the amide local anesthetics affected young HFB.

Dermatologic

Not Every Allergy Has Local Anesthetic as an Allergen

This review article [24M] addresses the concept that adverse reactions to local anesthetics may be caused by substances other than the local anesthetic itself. Vascular absorption of epinephrine or allergies to preservatives may be the real cause of the adverse effect and the authors suggest that skin tests and provocative challenges be used.

A Potential In Vitro Test for Amide Local Anesthetic Hypersensitivity

This case study [25A] looked at a patient who developed a delayed cutaneous hypersensitivity reaction after receiving mepivacaine, lidocaine and bupivacaine. The authors of the study found that the whole-blood-derived eosinophilic cationic protein (ECP) was elevated when exposed in vitro to the amide anesthetics mentioned. They further suggest that measuring ECP might be useful to test for hypersensitivity.

Sensitivity to Most Local Anesthetics but Not Articaine

This case study [26A] involved a patient who seemed to be allergic to both ester and amide local anesthetics. Articaine, however, was found not to cause the delayed hypersensitivity reaction seen with other amides. As articaine has a thiopene rather than metaxylene aromatic moiety, the authors of the study suggest that metaxylene may be the antigenic factor.

Testing for Amide Allergies

This clinical study [27c] gave patch tests to amide local anesthetics (especially lidocaine) to 756 patients. The authors of the study found a 1.72% prevalence (i.e., positive patch test) in the population tested. Further testing with intradermal skin and subcutaneous injections were mostly negative and led to the conclusion that positive patch test does not necessarily prevent the safe use of those local anesthetics in the future.

Testing can be confusing as seen by 2 case studies [28A,29A]. In the first case a 12-year-old dental patient was found to be negative with prick and intradermal tests to articaine and mepivacaine but was positive to subcutaneous injections of both. This patient was subsequently found to be negative in all testing to prilocaine which was used for his dental surgery. In the second case, a 54-year-old woman was found to be negative with prick and intradermal tests to bupivacaine but was positive to subcutaneous injection only after an 18 hour delay. Testing with lidocaine and mepivacaine was negative with all tests.

Hypersensitivity to Local Anesthetics

This review article [30M] talks about hypersensitivity to local anesthetics in general. It maps out a plan to diagnose and treat hypersensitivity. Another review article [31M] talks about hypersensitivity to local anesthetics in dermatologic surgery.

BENZOCAINE

Hematologic

Methemoglobinemia

This case report [32A] reviews the topic of what the authors imply is a rare adverse event: namely, methemoglobinemia. It reveals that benzocaine was used as a topical local anesthetic to facilitate transesophageal echocardiography. It does not state the dose used.

Benzocaine topical spray allows for the safe application of the drug with a usual maximum of two 1-second puffs. This dose is often exceeded and an overdose was undoubtedly the cause of the methemoglobinemia.

BUPIVACAINE

Cardiovascular

LAST Seen With Bupivacaine for Penile Block

This study [33A] lists 7 cases of LAST in a 7-year period while performing pediatric penile blocks. The dose of bupivacaine used was at the upper extreme (i.e., 2.5 mg/kg) in all the cases. The occurrence of so many cases of LAST led to a change in policy for penile block redirecting the needle away from the vascular area and giving the dose as 1.25 mg/kg and if needed another 1.25 mg/kg after 30 minutes. No further cases of LAST have been seen in the 2 years since the change in policy.

Cardiac Arrest After Caudal Block

This case study [34A] described a complicated cardiac arrest after a caudal block with bupivacaine. The patient was treated aggressively with cardiopulmonary resuscitation utilizing cardiovascular drugs including amiodirone and epinephrine. A lipid emulsion was also used and the patient was eventually discharged home without obvious sequela.

The dose of bupivacaine used was nearly 3 mg/kg which was touted as being just below the toxic dose and the concentration of drug was 0.5%. The authors should have considered a more reasonable toxic dose (i.e., 2.5 mg/kg) which could have easily been achieved with the same volume of drug and the more often used concentration of 0.25%.

Occulocardiac Reflex and Bupivacaine

This case study [35A] looked at asystole immediately after a subcuticular injection of 1 mL of 0.25% bupivacaine with 1:200 000 epinephrine for chalazion incision. The asystole was attributed to the occulocardiac reflex. A second operation was uneventful after premedication with atropine.

Lipid Emulsion Should Be Given First

This in vivo animal study [36E] looked at the order of drugs given in bupivacaine-induced LAST in rats. The study found that lipid emulsion should be given before epinephrine.

High Dose Lipid Emulsion in Cardiotoxic Pigs

This in vivo animal study [37E] looked at high dose intralipid vs Ringer's acetate administered to pigs given toxic doses of bupivacaine. Of note is that intralipid administration resulted in a significant increase in systemic vascular resistance but no significant change in cardiac index and left ventricular ejection fraction. In addition mitochondrial respiration was elevated in biopsied myocardial cells from the intralipid group but not from the Ringer's acetate group.

Lipid Emulsion Normalizes the QRS Interval in Bupivacaine Toxicity

This in vitro animal study [38E] looked at the QRS lengthening seen in bupivacaine-induced toxicity in pigs. Lipid emulsion was found to significantly reduce the lengthening seen in this LAST model compared to normal saline.

Long- vs Long/Medium-Chain Emulsions to Treat Toxicity

This in vivo animal study [39E] looked at the difference between long-chain triglyceride and long/medium-chain triglyceride emulsion on bupivacaine-induced LAST in rats. The study concluded that long-chain emulsions were superior to long/medium-chain emulsions.

Insulin Metabolism and Intralipid

This in vivo animal study [40E] looked at the effect of bupivacaine on insulin metabolism especially as it concerned cardiac toxicity. The study showed that a lipid emulsion altered the insulin metabolic effect of bupivacaine and may partially explain the direct improvement of cardiac function.

Bupivacaine Toxicity in a Pediatric Burn Patient

This case study [41A] revealed a pediatric burn patient who suffered cardiac arrest under general anesthesia after subcutaneous infusion of 2.5 L of a 3.5 L Pitkin's solution. The Pitkin's solution contained 2 mg/L of epinephrine and 0.5% bupivacaine (3 mg/kg). The injection was over the entire back (to harvest skin) while the burn was over the lower extremities and buttocks. Intralipid was administered with apparent eventual recovery.

The authors of this study admit that LAST may have been possible but do not seem concerned that the dose albeit subcutaneous might have been toxic (i.e., >2.5 mg/kg). A more dilute solution in regards to bupivacaine might be warranted.

TAP Block in Neonates

This prospective observational study [42C] looked at blood levels of bupivacaine from TAP blocks in 10 neonates undergoing abdominal surgery. At the doses (i.e., 1 mL/kg of 0.125% solution) used, no toxic levels were reported.

Cell Toxicity

Bupivacaine Neurotoxicity Attenuated by Dexmedetomidine

This in vivo animal study [43E] looked at neuronal injury after sciatic nerve block in rats. Bupivacaine alone caused more neuronal injury than bupivacaine with dexmedetomidine. Both of the solutions were neurotoxic compared to saline control.

Bupivacaine Neurotoxicity and microRNA

This in vitro study [44E] demonstrated that bupivacaine-induced neurotoxicity in mouse dorsal root ganglia is affected by manipulation of microRNA (miR). Specifically the downregulation of miR-210 was shown to reduce the damage caused by bupivacaine.

In Vivo Study With No Bupivacaine Toxicity

This in vivo study [45E] looked at chondrocyte toxicity in healthy and arthritis-induced rat knees. Bupivacaine was injected once a week for 5 weeks and the chondrocytes were evaluated subsequently (i.e., 8, 16 and 24 weeks) after animal sacrifice. The study found that there was no toxicity or progression of osteoarthritis. The significance of the study was highlighted in an editorial [46r].

Bupivacaine Neurotoxicity and Caffeine

This in vitro study [47E] demonstrated that bupivacaine-induced myotoxicity in mouse muscle cell cultures is affected by calcium metabolism. Specifically dantrolene decreased cellular calcium levels and reduced myotoxicity and caffeine increased cellular calcium levels and increased myotoxicity. These effects were most pronounced at low bupivacaine levels.

Bupivacine Neurotoxicity via PI3K

This in vitro study [48E] looked at bupivacaine application to human neuroblastoma cells. The study isolated the expression protein, phosphatidy-3-kinase, as a central figure in bupivacaine-induced neurotoxicity.

Bupivacaine and Lipid Emulsion on Cardiomyocytocity

This in vitro study [49E] looked at the effect that bupivacaine and lipid emulsion had on apoptosis of rat cardiac myocytes. The study showed that lipid emulsion decreased bupivacaine-induced apoptosis. The mechanism was attributed to modulation of signaling pathways including involvement of PI3K.

Long Noncoding RNA Involved With Bupivacaine Toxicity

This in vitro study [50E] looked at the long noncoding RNA, BDNF-AS, influence on bupivacaine toxicity on mice dorsal ganglion neurons. BDNF-AS was upregulated with the bupivacaine neurotoxicity. Further, when BDNF-AS was artificially downregulated, the neurons were partially protected and even had neurite growth.

GM 1 Inhibits Bupivacaine Neurotoxicity

This in vitro study [51E] looked at bupivacaine-induced neurotoxicity on mouse neuroblastoma cells. The concentration and time-dependent neurotoxicity was found to be inhibited by GM1 a naturally occurring mammalian ganglioside.

Bupivacaine Toxicity Modified by Curcumin

This in vitro study [52E] looked at bupivacaine-induced toxicity on SH-SY5Y, a human neuroblastoma cell line. The study found that curcumin, a low molecular weight polyphenol, attenuated the bupivicaine-induced neurotoxicity.

Nervous System

Bupivacaine Toxicity After Thoracic Epidural Infusion

This case study [53A] discussed the postoperative course of a 12-month-old girl who underwent a resection of a giant omphalocele under general anesthesia and thoracic epidural. The position of the epidural was checked and the dose used was within reasonable range. On postoperative day 3 she developed seizures. The epidural was discontinued and the seizures treated with lorazepam with eventual resolution. The cause was attributed to liver dysfunction which led to bupivacaine toxicity despite seemingly sub toxic doses. No blood samples of bupivacaine were obtained.

LEVOBUPIVACAINE

Cardiovascular

Last With Ropivacaine

This case study [54A] looked at a woman who suffered cardiac arrest after intra-articular and subcutaneous injections of levobupivacaine. She was successfully treated with epinephrine. Further complications included pulmonary edema and renal failure. The authors admit that the dose may have been toxic but the late sequela (i.e., pulmonary edema and renal failure) are attributed to the epinephrine. No lipid emulsion was given.

Epinephrine Allows for Greater Levobupivacaine Doses

This pharmacokinetic study [55H] looked at levobupivacaine with and without epinephrine administered for TAP blocks. The authors of the study found that in order to prevent LAST, the dose of levobupivacaine without epinephrine should be no greater than 1.5 mg/kg.

Dextran as an Adjuvant May Decrease the Risk of Levobupivacaine Toxicity

This double blind prospective study [56C] looked at administering levobupivacaine in saline vs dextran for TAP block. The dextran group had lower blood levels (i.e., presumed less absorption) and seemingly better analgesia compared to the saline group. The use of dextran with local anesthetics needs to be further studied to see if can reduce the incidence of LAST.

Preacidification May Assist Lipid Emulsions in LAST

This in vivo study [57E] looked at a model of LAST in isolated rat aorta endothelium treated with levobupivacaine. They found that mild (i.e., pH 7.2) acidification of the lipid emulsion used in the model enhanced its effect on bupivacaine. The authors of the study postulated that the mechanism was associated with the lipid emulsion-mediated inhibition of nitric oxide.

Lipid Emulsion After Levobupivacaine Toxicity

This in vivo animal study [58E] looked at lipid emulsion vs Ringers acetate rescue after mepivacaine-induced toxicity in a pig model of LAST. The authors found that the lipid emulsion was not superior to the Ringer's acetate for the treatment of LAST.

Nervous

Retigabine Inhibits Levobupivacaine-Induced Seizures

This in vivo animal study [59E] looked at the effect of the anticonvulsant retigabine on levobupivaciane-induced seizures. The study found that retigabine successfully treated the seizures.

LIDOCAINE

Cardiovascular

Safety of Tumescent Lidocaine

This crossover study [60C] looked at lidocaine use with and without liposuction in 14 volunteers. The study used a very dilute solution of subcutaneous lidocaine and epinephrine in doses (range: 19.2–52 mg/kg) much higher than considered toxic (i.e., 7 mg/kg) when administered intravenously. The study found that the maximum concentration (Cmax) of serum lidocaine never exceeded the threshold concentration for toxic effects (i.e., 6 µg/mL). Further, the Cmax was greatly reduced for liposuction compared to no liposuction.

An editorial [61r] on this study made clear that not all applications of local anesthetic are the same. Injecting a potentially toxic dose into a highly vascular area may give very different results than injection into a non-vascular area. Nevertheless, potential toxicity must always be considered when using local anesthetics.

In Vivo and In Vitro Look at Lidocaine

This in vivo and in vitro animal study [62E] looked at intraarticular injection of 12 dogs under general anesthesia for elbow surgery. Half of the dogs received lidocaine with epinephrine (lidocaine 2% with 1:100000 epinephrine) (group LA) and half received saline (group S).

Volumes varied from 12–20 mL for group LA to 9–20 mL for group S. Blood samples were taken from the dogs at various times. The study also looked at exposure of chondrocytes from the harvested cartilage with differing concentrations of lidocaine alone and lidocaine with epinephrine.

There were no signs of LAST in either group. Signs of toxicity were evident in the in vitro part of the study in a time- and concentration-dependent manner. Adding epinephrine lessened this toxicity.

LAST With Dental Lidocaine

This study [63A] highlighted three cases of LAST after subcutaneous injection of toxic doses of lidocaine for dental extractions. The three healthy patients experienced seizures and were managed conservatively with valium. The authors suggest that maximum doses of local anesthetic be pre calculated and intralipid be available.

Cell Toxicity

Lidocaine May Help Suppress Cancer Gene Expression

This in vitro study [64E] looked at the effect lidocaine had on cell viability of breast, prostatic and ovarian cancer cells. At high lidocaine concentrations, lidocaine decreased cell viability. At low lidocaine concentrations cell invasion and migration seemed to be decreased.

Lidocaine Neurotoxicity May Be Inhibited via IGF2AS

This in vitro study [65E] looked at lidocaine exposed to mice dorsal root ganglion (DRG). They found that inhibiting IGF2AS, a cancer regulator may promote neuronal growth and protect local anesthetic-induced neurotoxicity.

Hyaluronan Inhibits Lidocaine-Induced Cell Toxicity

This in vitro study [66E] looked at lidocaine-induced toxicity in human and murine chondrocytes. They found that the addition of hyaluronan suppressed the toxicity.

Dermatolgic

Topical Lidocaine Causes Keratopathy

In this study [67A] two diabetic patients suffered retinal keratopathy after each had a single topical instillation of 4% lidocaine to the eyes. In both cases the corneal insult was reversed after 3 days with topical antibiotics. Both the lidocaine and antibiotics had methylparaben as a preservative eliminating it as the causative agent.

Lidocaine May Help Treat Atopic Dermatitis

This in vivo study [68E] looked at administering intravenous lidocaine in four patients and mice to see the effect on atopic dermatitis. The authors looked at T regulatory cells as well as RNA and protein expression. The net results were that the atopic dermatitis seems to have been ameliorated by the administration of the intravenous lidocaine.

Nervous System

Ocular Complication After Inferior Alveolar Nerve Block

This case study [69A] reports on a contralateral ocular complication after an inferior nerve block with an appropriate small dose of lidocaine. The paper reviews side effects in general and suggests the possible etiologies in this case in particular. As inferior nerve blocks were performed without any adverse events two times subsequently, the hypothesis that a partial, inadvertent intravascular (most likely arterial) injection was administered is probably correct.

Controversy Over a Low Dose Transforaminal Cervical Epidural Block

A letter to the editor [70r] questioned the practice of transforaminal cervical epidural block with low dose local anesthetic used in a recent double blind prospective study [71C]. Transforaminal cervical epidural block has a known complication involving intra-arterial injection. The study showed that a steroid containing compound could be delivered with a theoretically intra-arterial sub seizure inducing dose of lidocaine with good short-term results. The letter to the editor was critical of the study as it is unclear if an intra-arterial injection would be safe at any dose. The authors of the study responded [72r] by admitting that the procedure is risky but can be useful in certain circumstances and should be studied further.

Lidocaine and Hoigne Syndrome

This case study [73A] attempts to attribute Hoigne syndrome as an adverse event to local anesthetic injection. Hoigne syndrome is a psychiatric syndrome seen after local anesthetic injection characterized by ill feelings not related to local anesthetic dose. This patient had a total of 5 mg/kg lidocaine injected near the right iliac crest. This dose of lidocaine is possibly toxic and the patient may have experienced LAST as she developed tingling in her right leg and right ear as well as light headedness and other ill feelings. This cause of the adverse events is unclear, at best.

Intravenous Lidocaine at Safe Doses Causing Convulsions

This case report [74A] revealed that injection of an apparently safe dose of intravenous lidocaine can cause convulsions. The patient was under general anesthesia, and paralysis was reversed in anticipation of extubation. An intravenous dose of lidocaine (~1.3 mg/kg) was administered to minimize tracheal irritation. This dose is much less than the accepted toxic dose (i.e., ~5 mg/kg). Convulsions ensued which were treated and eventually resolved. The case authors stated that respiratory acidosis was a contributing factor to the seizures. Other causes were not discussed and should be examined.

Dexmedetomidine Delays Lidocaine-Induced Convulsions

This in vivo animal study [75E] looked at giving intravenous dexmedetomine vs saline before inducing convulsions in rabbits. The study showed that dexmedetomidine, in a dose-dependent manner, delayed the onset of convulsions and may have some positive effect on treating the convulsions.

MEPIVACAINE

Cardiovascular

Inadvertent Intravascular Injection Treated With Intralipid

This case study [76A] looked at a case where 2% mepivacaine was inadvertently injected intravascularly with resultant LAST. Intralipid was given and the symptoms resolved. The authors then delineated a protocol for treatment of LAST.

ROPIVACAINE

Cardiovascular

Ropivacaine Toxicity After Paravertebral Block

This pilot observational study [77C] was planned to look at bilateral paravertebral blocks after cardiac surgery using ropivacaine. The study was stopped after only 4 days and 8 patients as LAST symptoms were present. The initial ropivacaine bolus of 3 mg/kg followed by bilateral infusions of 0.25 mg/kg/hour was found to be too high and did not eliminate the need for supplemental narcotics.

Thermography as a Tool to Predict LAST

This in vivo rat study [78E] looked at thermographic changes with infrared imaging after inducing ropivacaine systemic toxicity. The study had mixed results. Future study to see if thermography can predict and or monitor LAST may be indicated.

Nervous System

Dexmedetomidine Attenuates Ropivacaine Toxicity

This in vivo animal study [79E] showed that dexmedetomidine, in a dose-dependent manner, prolonged the latency and lessened the duration of ropivacaine-induced seizures in mice.

Sub-Mammary Injections With Ropivacaine

This study [80A] discussed two separate cases of women who had delayed seizures after sub-mammary injection of ropivacaine for breast augmentation. Seizures started in both cases after ~1 hour and resolved spontaneously. No lipid emulsion therapy was given despite getting ropivacaine doses that were probably toxic (>3 mg/kg).

References

[1] Dureau P, Charbit B, Nicolas N, et al. Effect of intralipid® on the dose of ropivacaine or levobupivacaine tolerated by volunteers: a clinical and pharmacokinetic study. Anesthesiology. 2016;125(3):474–83 [C].
[2] Harvey M, Cave G. Lipid emulsion in local anesthetic toxicity: long-winded, rude, and right. Anesthesiology. 2016;125(3):451–3 [r].
[3] Thompson BM. Revising the 2012 American society of regional anesthesia and pain medicine checklist for local anesthetic systemic toxicity: a call to resolve ambiguity in clinical implementation. Reg Anesth Pain Med. 2016;41(1):117–8 [r].
[4] Neal JM, Mulroy MF, Weinberg GL. American society of regional anesthesia and pain medicine checklist for managing local anesthetic systemic toxicity: 2012 version. Reg Anesth Pain Med. 2012;37(1):16–8 [R].
[5] El-Boghdadly K, Chin KJ. Local anesthetic systemic toxicity: continuing professional development. Can J Anesth. 2016;63(3):330–49 [M].
[6] Weinberg G, Barron G. Local anesthetic systemic toxicity (LAST): not gone, hopefully not forgotten. Reg Anesth Pain Med. 2016;41(1):1–2 [r].
[7] Barrington MJ, Uda Y. We should fear the reaper: collaborating to understand local anesthetic systemic toxicity. Reg Anesth Pain Med. 2016;41(4):545–6 [r].
[8] Liu SS, Ortolan S, Sandoval MV, et al. Cardiac arrest and seizures caused by local anesthetic systemic toxicity after peripheral nerve blocks: should we still fear the reaper? Reg Anesth Pain Med. 2016;41(1):5–21 [R].
[9] Xu M, Jin S, Li Z, et al. Regional anesthesia and lipid resuscitation for local anesthetic systemic toxicity in China: results of a survey by the orthopedic anesthesia group of the Chinese society of anesthesiology. BMC Anesthesiol. 2016;16(1):1–7 [A].
[10] Rosenthal G, Wetsch WA, Neumann T. Padosch et al. Local anesthetic toxicity: who is ready for lipid resuscitation? A survey of German hospitals. Anaesthesist. 2016;65(4):267–73 [A].
[11] Hoegberg LC, Bania TC, Lavergne V, et al. Systematic review of the effect of intravenous lipid emulsion therapy for local anesthetic toxicity. Clin Toxicol (Phila). 2016;54(3):167–93 [M].

[12] Rosenberg PH. Current evidence is not in support of lipid rescue therapy in local anaesthetic systemic toxicity. Acta Anaesthesiol Scand. 2016;60(8):1029–32 [r].

[13] Hayes BD, Gosselin S, Calello DP, et al. Systematic review of clinical adverse events reported after acute intravenous lipid emulsion administration. Clin Toxicol (Phila). 2016;54(5):365–404 [M].

[14] Cho H, Ok SH, Kwon SC, et al. Lipid emulsion inhibits vasodilation induced by a toxic dose of bupivacaine by suppressing bupivacaine-induced PKC and CPI-17 dephosphorylation but has no effect on vasodilation induced by a toxic dose of mepivacaine. Korean J Pain. 2016;29(4):229–38 [E].

[15] Ok SH, Yu J, Lee Y, et al. Lipid emulsion attenuates apoptosis induced by a toxic dose of bupivacaine in H9c2 rat cardiomyoblast cells. Hum Exp Toxicol. 2016;35(9):929–37 [E].

[16] Tsang TM, Okullo AT, Field J, et al. Lipid rescue for treatment of delayed systemic ropivacaine toxicity from a continuous thoracic paravertebral block. BMJ Case Rep. 2016;2016: bcr2016215071 [A].

[17] Verlinde M, Hollmann MW, Stevens MF, et al. Local anesthetic-induced neurotoxicity. Int J Mol Sci. 2016;17:339.1–339.14 [M].

[18] Sen O, Sayilgan NC, Tutuncu AC, et al. Evaluation of sciatic nerve damage following intraneural injection of bupivacaine, levobupivacaine and lidocaine in rats. Braz J Anesthesiol. 2016;66(3):272–5 [E].

[19] Gürbüzel M, Karaca U, Karayilan N. Genotoxic evaluation of bupivacaine and levobupivacaine in the Drosophila wing spot test. Cytotechnology. 2016;68(4):979–86 [E].

[20] Kang DK, Zhao LY, Wang HL. Cytotoxic effects of local anesthesia through lidocaine/ropivacaine on human melanoma cell lines. Braz J Anesthesiol. 2016;66(6):594–602 [E].

[21] Yap G, Singh A. Should we reconsider the use of intra-articular local anaesthetics? Br J Hosp Med (Lond). 2016;77(1):58 [r].

[22] Wang HW, Wang LY, Jiang L, et al. Amide-linked local anesthetics induce apoptosis in human non-small cell lung cancer. J Thorac Dis. 2016;8(10):2748–57 [E].

[23] Ben Tov I, Damodarasamy M, Spiekerman C, et al. Lidocaine impairs proliferative and biosynthetic functions of aged human dermal fibroblasts. Anesth Analg. 2016;123(3):616–23 [E].

[24] Malinovsky JM, Chiriac AM, Tacquard C, et al. Allergy to local anesthetics: reality or myth? Presse Med. 2016;45(9):753–7 [M].

[25] Domínguez-Ortega J, Phillips-Angles E, González-Muñoz M, et al. Allergy to several local anesthetics from the amide group. J Allergy Clin Immunol Pract. 2016;4(4):771–2 [A].

[26] Ing Lorenzini K, Gay-Crosier Chabry F, Piguet C, et al. Meta-xylene: identification of a new antigenic entity in hypersensitivity reactions to local anesthetics. J Allergy Clin Immunol Pract. 2016;4(1):162–4 [A].

[27] Corbo MD, Weber E, DeKoven J. Lidocaine allergy: do positive patch results restrict future use? Dermatitis. 2016;27(2):68–71 [c].

[28] Ertoy Karagol I, Yilmaz O, Bakirtas A. Challenge-proven immediate type multiple local anesthetic hypersensitivity in a child. Eur Ann Allergy Clin Immunol. 2016;48(1):27–30 [A].

[29] Vega F, Argíz L, Bazire R, et al. Delayed urticaria due to bupivacaine: a new presentation of local anesthetic allergy. Allergol Int. 2016;65(4):498–500 [A].

[30] Grzanka A, Wasilewska I, Śliwczyńska M, et al. Hypersensitivity lo local anesthetics. Anaesthesiol Intensive Ther. 2016;48(2):128–34 [M].

[31] Fathi R, Serota M, Brown M. Identifying and managing local anesthetic allergy in dermatologic surgery. Dermatol Surg. 2016;42(2):147–56 [M].

[32] Panikkath R, Panikkath D, Wischmeyer J. An uncommon complication with use of topical local anesthetic agents: methemoglobinemia. Am J Ther. 2016;23(6):e1968–9 [A].

[33] Yu RN, Houck CS, Casta A, et al. Institutional policy changes to prevent cardiac toxicity associated with bupivacaine penile blockade in infants. A A Case Rep. 2016;7(3):71–5 [A].

[34] de Araújo Azi LM Torres, Figueroa DG, Simas AA. Cardiac arrest after local anaesthetic toxicity in a paediatric patient. Case Rep Anesthesiol. 2016;2016:7826280 [A].

[35] Katowitz WR, O'Brien M, Kiskis E, et al. An asystolic event after eyelid skin bupivicaine injection during chalazion surgery. J AAPOS. 2016;20(1):75–7 [A].

[36] Luo M, Yun X, Chen C, et al. Giving priority to lipid administration can reduce lung injury caused by epinephrine in bupivacaine-induced cardiac depression. Reg Anesth Pain Med. 2016;41(4):469–76 [E].

[37] Heinonen JA, Schramko AA, Skrifvars MB, et al. The effects of intravenous lipid emulsion on hemodynamic recovery and myocardial cell mitochondrial function after bupivacaine toxicity in anesthetized pigs. Hum Exp Toxicol. 2017;36:365–75. pii: 0960327116650010. [E].

[38] Zaballos M, Sevilla R, González J, et al. Analysis of the temporal regression of the QRS widening induced by bupivacaine after Intralipid administration. Study in an experimental porcine model. Rev Esp Anestesiol Reanim. 2016;63(1):13–21 [E].

[39] Tang W, Wang Q, Shi K, et al. The effect of lipid emulsion on pharmacokinetics of bupivacaine in rats: long-chain triglyceride versus long- and medium-chain triglyceride. Anesth Analg. 2016;123(5):1116–22 [E].

[40] Fettiplace MR, Kowal K, Ripper R, et al. Insulin signaling in bupivacaine-induced cardiac toxicity: sensitization during recovery and potentiation by lipid emulsion. Anesthesiology. 2016;124(2):428–42 [E].

[41] Musielak M, McCall J. Lipid rescue in a pediatric burn patient. J Burn Care Res. 2016;37(4):e380–2 [A].

[42] Suresh S, De Oliveira Jr. GS. Blood bupivacaine concentrations after transversus abdominis plane block in neonates: a prospective observational study. Anesth Analg. 2016;122(3):814–7 [C].

[43] Memari E, Hosseinian MA, Mirkheshti A, et al. Comparison of histolopathological effects of perineural administration of bupivacaine and bupivacaine-dexemetetomidine in rat sciatic nerve. Exp Toxicol Pathol. 2016;68(10):559–64 [E].

[44] Wang Y, Ni H, Zhang W, et al. Downregulation of miR-210 protected bupivacaine-induced neurotoxicity in dorsal root ganglion. Exp Brain Res. 2016;234(4):1057–65 [E].

[45] Iwasaki K, Sudo H, Kasahara Y, et al. Effects of multiple intra-articular injections of 0.5% bupivacaine on normal and osteoarthritic joints in rats. Arthroscopy. 2016;32(10):2026–36 [E].

[46] Milano G. Editorial commentary: New perspectives on the intraday-articulate use of local anesthetics: five weekly injections of 0.5 percent bupivicaine does not alter articulate cartilage. Arthroscopy. 2016;32(10):2037–8 [r].

[47] Plank C, Hofmann P, Gruber M, et al. Modification of bupivacaine-induced myotoxicity with dantrolene and caffeine In vitro. Anesth Analg. 2016;122(2):418–23 [E].

[48] Zhao W, Liu Z, Yu X, et al. iTRAQ proteomics analysis reveals that PI3K is highly associated with bupivacaine-induced neurotoxicity pathways. Proteomics. 2016;16(4):564–75 [E].

[49] Lv D, Bai Z, Yang L, et al. Lipid emulsion reverses bupivacaine-induced apoptosis of h9c2 cardiomyocytes: PI3K/Akt/GSK-3β signaling pathway. Environ Toxicol Pharmacol. 2016;42:85–91 [E].

[50] Zhang Y, Yan L, Cao Y, et al. Long noncoding RNA BDNF-AS protects local anesthetic induced neurotoxicity in dorsal root ganglion neurons. Biomed Pharmacother. 2016;80:207–12 [E].

[51] Liang Y, Ji J, Lin Y, et al. The ganglioside gm-1 inhibits bupivacaine-induced neurotoxicity in mouse neuroblastoma neuro2a cells. Cell Biochem Funct. 2016;34(6):455–62 [E].

[52] Fan YL, Li HC, Zhao W, et al. Curcumin attenuated bupivicaine induced neurotoxicity in sh-sy5y cell via activation of the Akt signaling pathway. Neurochem Res. 2016;41(9):2425–32 [E].

[53] Shapiro P, Schroeck H. Seizure after abdominal surgery in an infant receiving a standard-dose postoperative epidural bupivacaine infusion. A A Case Rep. 2016;6(8):238–40 [A].

[54] Tomita A, Satani M, Suzuki K, et al. A case of cardiac arrest following intra-articular administration of levobupivacaine during total knee arthroplasty. Masui. 2016;65(2):179–83 [A].

[55] Miranda P, Corvetto MA, Altermatt FR, et al. Levobupivacaine absorption pharmacokinetics with and without epinephrine during TAP block: analysis of doses based on the associated risk of local anesthetic toxicity. Eur J Clin Pharmacol. 2016;72(10):1221–7 [H].

[56] Hamada T, Tsuchiya M, Mizutani K, et al. Levobupivacaine-dextran mixture for transversus abdominis plane block and rectus sheath block in patients undergoing laparoscopic colectomy: a randomised controlled trial. Anaesthesia. 2016;71(4):411–6 [C].

[57] Ok SH, Kim WH, Yu J, et al. Effects of acidification and alkalinization on the lipid emulsion-mediated reversal of toxic dose levobupivacaine-induced vasodilation in the isolated rat aorta. Int J Med Sci. 2016;13(1):68–76 [E].

[58] Heinonen JA, Skrifvars MB, Haasio J, et al. Intravenous lipid emulsion for levobupivacaine intoxication in acidotic and hypoxaemic pigs. Anaesth Intensive Care. 2016;44(2):270–7 [E].

[59] Cheng Y, Li H, Li J, et al. Effectiveness of retigabine against levobupivacaine-induced central nervous system toxicity: a prospective, randomized animal study. J Anesth. 2016;30(1):109–15 [E].

[60] Klein JA, Jeske DR. Estimated maximal safe dosages of tumescent lidocaine. Anesth Analg. 2016;122(5):1350–9 [C].

[61] Weinberg G. Local anesthetic systemic toxicity and liposuction: looking back, looking forward. Anesth Analg. 2016;122(5):1250–2 [r].

[62] Di Salvo A, Chiaradia E, della Rocca G, et al. Intra-articular administration of lidocaine plus adrenaline in dogs: pharmacokinetic profile and evaluation of toxicity in vivo and in vitro. Vet J. 2016;208:70–5 [E].

[63] Jayanthi R, Nasser K, Monica K. Local anesthetic systemic toxicity. J Assoc Physicians India. 2016;64(3):92–3 [A].

[64] Jiang Y, Gou H, Zhu J, et al. Lidocaine inhibits the invasion and migration of TRPV6-expressing cancer cells by TRPV6 downregulation. Oncol Lett. 2016;12(2):1164–70 [E].

[65] Zhang X, Chen K, Song C, et al. Inhibition of long non-coding RNA IGF 2AS has profound effect on inducing neuronal growth and protecting local-anesthetic induced neurotoxicity in dorsal root ganglion neurons. Biomed Pharmacother. 2016;82:298–303 [E].

[66] Lee YJ, Kim SA, Lee SH. Hyaluronan suppresses lidocaine-induced apoptosis of human chondrocytes in vitro by inhibiting the p53-dependent mitochondrial apoptotic pathway. Acta Pharmacol Sin. 2016;37(5):664–73 [E].

[67] Kumar A. Diffuse epithelial keratopathy following a single instillation of topical lignocaine: the damaging drop. Cutan Ocul Toxicol. 2016;35(2):173–5 [A].

[68] Li H, Li C, Zhang H, et al. Effects of lidocaine on regulatory T cells in atopic dermatitis. J Allergy Clin Immunol. 2016;137(2):613–7 [E].

[69] Kempster C, Ghabriel M, Kaidonis G, et al. An unusual ocular complication following dental anaesthesia: case report. Aust Dent J. 2016;61:374–80 [A].

[70] Manchikanti L, Boswell MV, Kaye AD. Hirsch JA Cervical transforaminal with low-dose local anesthetic is not a safeguard for neurological complications. Pain Med. 2016;17(1):191–2 [r].

[71] Woo JH, Park HS. Cervical transforaminal epidural block using low-dose local anesthetic: a prospective, randomized, double-blind study. Pain Med. 2015;16:61–7 [C].

[72] Woo JH, Park HS. In response to letter to the editor: cervical transforaminal with low-dose local anesthetic is not a safeguard for neurological complications. Pain Med. 2016;17(1):192–3 [r].

[73] Thompson TM, Theobald JL. Hoigne syndrome: a little-known adverse effect of lidocaine. Am J Emerg Med. 2016;34(3):679 [A].

[74] Haldar R, Dubey M, Rastogi A, et al. Intravenous lignocaine to blunt extubation responses: a double-edged sword. Am J Ther. 2016;23(2):e646–8 [A].

[75] Wang XF, Luo XL, Liu WC, et al. Effect of dexmedetomidine priming on convulsion reaction induced by lidocaine. Medicine (Baltimore). 2016;95(43)e4781 [E].

[76] Valdivielso Cortázar E, Oteiza Olaso J, Etxeberría Lekuona D, et al. Acute toxicity due to local anesthetics. Rev Esp Anestesiol Reanim. 2016;63(1):58–60 [A].

[77] Ho AM, Karmakar MK, Ng SK, et al. Local anaesthetic toxicity after bilateral thoracic paravertebral block in patients undergoing coronary artery bypass surgery. Anaesth Intensive Care. 2016;44(5):615–9 [C].

[78] Carstens AM, Tambara EM, Colman D, et al. Infrared image monitoring of local anesthetic poisoning in rats. Braz J Anesthesiol. 2016;66(6):603–12 [E].

[79] Zhai MZ, Wu HH, Yin JB, et al. Dexmedetomidine dose-dependently attenuates ropivacaine-induced seizures and negative emotions via inhibiting phosphorylation of amygdala extracellular signal-regulated kinase in mice. Mol Neurobiol. 2016;53(4):2636–46 [E].

[80] Chiew A, Raos MP, Isbister GK. Sub-mammary injection of ropivacaine resulting in severe toxicity with seizures. Emerg Med Australas. 2016;28(2):246–7 [A].

11

Drugs That Affect Autonomic Functions or the Extrapyramidal System

Toshio Nakaki[1]

Teikyo University School of Medicine, Tokyo, Japan
[1]Corresponding author: nakaki@med.teikyo-u.ac.jp

DRUGS THAT STIMULATE BOTH α- AND β2-ADRENOCEPTORS [SEDA-33, 313; SEDA-34, 233; SEDA-35, 255; SEDA-36, 179; SEDA-37, 163; SEDA-38, 115]

Adrenaline and Noradrenaline [SEDA-32, 281; SEDA-33, 259; SEDA-34, 233; SEDA-35, 255; SEDA-36, 179; SEDA-37, 163; SEDA-38, 115]

Drug Administration Route

A study was designed to compare the effect of lignocaine alone or in combination with adrenaline injection, and with topical adrenalin on perioperative hemodynamic effect, hemorrhage and postoperative pain. It is suggested that the use of adrenaline infiltration during septal surgery is unnecessary and may subject the patient to the risk of cardiogenic side effects of systemic absorption [1c].

Cardiovascular: Serious adverse effects are commonly reported following adrenaline use for anaphylaxis, especially when given intravenously. These include hypertension, ventricular arrhythmias, myocardial infarction, and pulmonary edema. Due to the lack of adequate evidence supporting the use of adrenaline in patients with anaphylaxis, except in severe cases, the strength of recommendations should be carefully reconsidered, limiting administration to selected categories of patients [2R].

An association between adrenaline and Takotsubo syndrome has been suggested. It was pointed out several other interpretations of Takotsubo syndrome-related death: possible roles of preservatives used for adrenaline in causing anaphyraxis, and other medication used for the treatment of Takotsubo syndrome in patient's death [3r].

Noradrenaline vs terlipressin: The choice of vasopressor for treating cirrhosis with septic shock is unclear. This study compared the safety of noradrenaline and terlipressin in cirrhotics with septic shock. Therapy-related adverse effects were comparable in both the arms (40.5% vs 21.4%, $P = 0.06$), mostly minor (GradeII-88%) and reversible. Terlipressin appeared to provide early survival benefit and reduced the risk of variceal bleed [4c].

Pseudoephedrine [SEDA-33, 318; SEDA-34, 236; SEDA-35, 255; SEDA-36, 185]

Urological: Pseudoephedrine is a sympathomimetic drug widely used as a nasal decongestant and can cause adverse effects, such as voiding dysfunction. The International Prostate Symptom Score (IPSS) questionnaire was used to evaluate voiding function before and 1 week after the pseudoephedrine treatment. Most patients less than 52.8 years old exhibited no change or slight improvement in voiding function after the medication. By contrast, most patients older than 52.8 years exhibited deterioration in voiding function after the medication, and the difference increased with age. Throughout the study period, three of the 131 patients, aged 29, 51, and 62 years, respectively, experienced symptomatic dysuria and visited urological clinics. No patients experienced acute urinary retention during the survey. All dysuria symptoms improved after pseudoephedrine discontinuation [5C].

Droxidopa [SEDA-38, 117]

Review: Postural orthostatic tachycardia syndrome is a constellation of signs and symptoms that occur when a patient is upright and relieved by recumbence. Droxidopa is a drug for the treatment for postural orthostatic tachycardia syndrome. The most commonly reported side effect was nausea/vomiting in 6 patients which warranted stopping therapy in all of them. Other side effects included urinary symptoms (2 patients) and chest pain/palpitations (2 patients), weight gain (1 patient) and insomnia in 1 patient [6c].

Reivew: A study was performed to evaluate the long-term safety and durability of efficacy of the noradrenaline precursor droxidopa in patients with symptomatic neurogenic orthostatic hypotension. The most frequently reported adverse effects were falls, urinary tract infection, and headache. There was a low incidence ($\leq$2%) of cardiac adverse effects such as first-degree atrioventricular block and supraventricular extrasystoles [7C].

Systematic review: A systematic review and meta-analysis aimed to determine the efficacy and safety of droxidopa in the treatment of orthostatic hypotension. Of 224 identified records, four studies met eligibility, with a pooled sample size of 494. Study duration was between 1 and 8 weeks. Rates of adverse events were similar between droxidopa and control groups, including supine hypertension [odds ratio 1.93 (0.87, 4.25)] [8M].

Reivew: Droxidopa is converted to norepinephrine and thought to improve both blood pressure and symptoms in patients with orthostatic intolerance. Of total, 40.5% of patients stopped the treatment either due to side effects or ineffectiveness [6c].

DRUGS THAT PREDOMINATLY STIMULATE α₁-ADRENOCEPTORS
[SEDA-33, 318; SEDA-34, 236; SEDA-35, 257; SEDA-36, 186; SEDA-37, 163; SEDA-38, 117]

Phenylephrine [SEDA-15, 2808; SEDA-32, 283; SEDA-33, 318; SEDA-34, 236; SEDA-38,117]

Placebo-controlled studies: To evaluate the efficacy and safety of phenylephrine 30-mg modified-release tablets in patients with nasal congestion caused by allergic rhinitis in a multicenter, randomized, double-blinded, placebo-controlled, 2-arm, parallel-group study. Of 575 patients, 288 received the tablets and 287 received placebo. Overall, the organ system class with the most treatment-related emergency adverse events were nervous system disorders (23 of 575 [4.0%]), and the most common treatment-emergency adverse event in the group was headache, occurring in 17 of 575 patients

(3.0%): 9 of 288 (3.1%) in the phenylephrine group and 8 of 287 (2.8%) in the placebo group. No serious adverse events, deaths, or discontinuations because of adverse events were reported [9C].

Reproductive system: Ninety parturients showing acute fetal compromise during intrapartum period and taken up for cesarean delivery under spinal anesthesia were randomized to receive prophylactic infusion of ephedrine 2.5 mg/min or phenylephrine 30 µg/min. Incidence of maternal nausea and vomiting was higher with ephedrine than with phenylephrine (22.2% vs 4.4%; $P=0.02$). Maternal bradycardia was observed with phenylephrine ($P=0.02$) [10c].

Cardiovascular: A study investigated the incidence of serious bradycardia and identified risk factors associated with phenylephrine-induced serious bradycardia and other side effects of phenylephrine. Predelivery hypotension was treated by intravenous 100 µg phenylephrine. Incidence of serious bradycardia was 11% (95% CI: 8.0–14.0). A 1-bpm increment increase in pretherapeutic heart rate reduced this incidence by 4% (adjusted OR: 0.96; 95% CI: 0.94–0.98; $P<0.001$). As compared to age-predicted heart rate greater than 80 bpm, age-predicted heart rate of 61–80 bpm and a pretherapeutic heart rate of 60 bpm or lower increased the risk of serious bradycardia by 3.55 times and 12.81 times, respectively. Other risk factors were height (adjusted OR: 0.94; 95% CI: 0.89–0.98; $P=0.015$), baseline diastolic blood pressure (adjusted OR: 0.97; 95% CI: 0.94–0.99; $P=0.03$), and anesthetic level at first minute (adjusted OR: 1.13; 95% CI: 1.02–1.23; $P=0.02$). Benign and temporary abnormal ECG readings were noted [11C].

DRUGS THAT STIMULATE α₁-ADRENOCEPTORS [SEDA-33, 265; SEDA-34, 285; SEDA-35, 257; SEDA-36, 187; SEDA-37; SEDA-38, 117]

Methoxamine

Cardiovascular: Hypotension is a common complication of spinal anesthesia for cesarean delivery. A study was aimed to assess the effect of methoxamine–atropine therapy in treating spinal anesthesia hypotension for cesarean section. Women under spinal anesthesia for elective caesarean delivery received boluses of methoxamine 2 mg alone (Group M, $n=40$), or with addition of atropine 0.1 mg (Group MA1, $n=40$), atropine 0.2 mg (Group MA2, $n=40$) or atropine 0.3 mg (Group MA3, $n=40$) upon a maternal systolic pressure $\leq$80% of baseline. The incidences of bradycardia in Groups M and MA1 were significantly higher than those in Group MA2 and MA3 [12c].

DRUGS THAT STIMULATE β₂-ADRENOCEPTORS

Indacaterol [SEDA-33, 361-2; SEDA-34, 318; SEDA-36, 188; SEDA-37, 165; SEDA-38, 118]

Respiratory: A study assessed the effect of indacaterol/glycopyrronium fixed dose combination 110/50 µg once daily vs placebo in patients with moderate-to-severe COPD. The only suspected adverse event that occurred in more than one patient in either group was cough in 5 patients (2.6%) that were receiving indacaterol/glycopyrronium, and 1 patient (0.5%) receiving placebo. Overall, there was a low incidence of newly occurring or worsening of notable abnormal vital signs values with no clinically meaningful differences between the treatments [13C].

Respiratory: Most guidelines recommend either a long-acting β2-agonist plus an inhaled glucocorticoid, or a long-acting muscarinic antagonist as the first-choice treatment for patients with COPD who have a high risk of exacerbations. The incidence of adverse events and deaths was similar in the two groups. The incidence of pneumonia was 3.2% in the indacaterol–glycopyrronium group and 4.8% in the salmeterol–fluticasone group ($P = 0.02$) [14C].

Indacaterol vs tiotropium: To assess relative effects of the treatments described below on markers of exacerbations, symptoms, quality of life and lung function in patients with COPD. The treatment combinations were (1) tiotropium plus long-acting β2-agonists and inhaled corticosteroids vs tiotropium alone, (2) tiotropium plus long-acting β2-agonists and inhaled corticosteroids vs long-acting β2-agonists and inhaled corticosteroids. Randomised controlled trials lasting 3 months or longer were included to compare two combinations. A pooled estimate of these studies did not show a statistically significant difference in adverse events. Evidence is insufficient to support the benefit of tiotropium + long-acting β2-agonists and inhaled corticosteroids for mortality and exacerbations. Compared with the use of tiotropium plus placebo, tiotropium plus long-acting β2-agonists and inhaled corticosteroids-based therapy does not increase undesirable effects such as adverse events or serious non-fatal adverse events [15C].

Salbutamol [SEDA-21, 182; SEDA-22, 190; SEDA-35, 318; SEDA-36, 189; SEDA-37, 116]

Review: The aim of this study was to assess the perceived effect of salbutamol in adult patients with spinal muscular atrophy and to evaluate the usefulness of the World Health Organization Disability Assessment Schedule II and Fatigue Severity Scale for its measurement. Ten patients were interviewed and completed the above questionnaires to assess disability and fatigue. Patients were satisfied with the treatment as shown by decreased fatigue, improved functioning, and infrequent side effects [16c].

DRUGS THAT STIMULATE DOPAMINE RECEPTORS [SEDA-33, 266; SEDA-34, 283; SEDA-35, 262; SEDA-36, 190; SEDA-37, 167; SEDA-38, 118]

Cabergoline [SEDA-17, 169; SEDA-35, 262; SEDA-36, 190; SEDA-37, 167; SEDA-38, 118]

Cabergoline has been associated with adverse reactions consistent with other dopaminergic agonists including cardiovascular, gastrointestinal and neuropsychiatric effects. In this case, The first manic episode was reported, occurring after cabergoline use for hyperprolactinemia [17c].

A 26-year-old woman gave birth 15 months ago. A month ago, she was diagnosed with polycystic ovarian syndrome and subsequently treated with a levonorgestrel-containing intrauterine device. Cabergoline was started at 0.5 mg once per day to stop lactating. Two days after the first dose of cabergoline, the patient complained of irritation, insomnia, and a short temper. She locked her child and herself into a room and then removed everything that might hurt somebody at home. She started to talk to herself and then began arguing with her husband. She also began listening to music at high volume, laughing loudly, and spending much more money than usual. In the final week, she even began to neglect her child and her home. She began to think she had some special power. She was laughing loudly, having difficulty sleeping, talking too much, and harming her child in the last few days. The patient was admitted to an emergency room and hospitalized in a psychiatry clinic with the prediagnosis of manic episode with psychotic features. Her mental status examination revealed that the content of her thoughts revealed grandiose and paranoid delusions. She demonstrated psychomotor hyperactivity and her Young Mania Rating Scale score was calculated as 39. There were no abnormalities in her physical examination and laboratory results. Her cranial MRI was normal. Her dostinex treatment was stopped, and a new treatment was initiated of 20 mg/day of olanzapine, and 600 mg/day of carbamazepine was added as a mood stabilizer. At the end of the second week, the carbamazepine treatment was stopped because of carbamazepine-induced hyponatremia, and a 900 mg/day lithium treatment was started. The psychomotor hyperactivity, irritability, and grandiosity of the patient persisted, and her Young Mania Rating Scale score was 19. Her daily olanzapine dose was increased from 20 to 30 mg. At the end of third week, her Young Mania Rating Scale score was down to 6. An examination of her mental status showed that her mood was euthymic, her grandiose thoughts had disappeared, and her psychomotor activity was normal. Her elevated mood was significantly improved, as her adaptation to clinical conditions and medications was successful. She was discharged with a treatment regimen of 900 mg/day of lithium and 30 mg/day of olanzapine.

A case of bipolar patient treated with cabergoline has been described

A 34-year-old woman was admitted to a hospital, as she showed increased energy level, impulsivity, inflated self-esteem, increased goal-directed activity, including excessive involvement in gambling. Her ideation was characterized by delusional thoughts of being drugged with cocaine and controlled by her husband through the mobile phone. She also presented neuro-vegetative symptoms, such as increased appetite and decreased need of sleep. She had a positive family history for mood disorders and pathological gambling. Her father had been suffering from Tourette's syndrome since he was 7 years old. Her first contact with psychiatric services occurred at the age of 19. She received the diagnosis of post traumatic stress disorder, and she was treated exclusively with benzodiazepines. She developed the first manic episode at the age of 24, with mild behavioural disinhibition, mood elevation, and hyperactivity but she did not seek clinical attention although these symptoms significantly impact on her everyday functioning. She received her first pharmacological treatment few years later (fluoxetine 60 mg/day), after the occurrence of a depressive episode characterized by low mood, fatigue, hypersomnia, and hyperphagia. In the following years, she experienced hypomanic symptoms, including flight of ideas, logorrhea, irritability, and high level of energy. It is worth noting that, in that period, she was still on treatment with fluoxetine (60 mg/day), that she kept on taking without consulting any psychiatrist, and then stopped. She underwent several diagnostic tests due to a menstruation delay, after pregnancy had been excluded by a negative urine test. High prolactin level was detected and a MRI exam revealed a microprolactinoma. Three months later, she was started on cabergoline 0.5 mg orally once a week.

However, approximately 1 month later, it was stopped as she gradually developed mixed symptoms, including low mood, apathy, irritability, and verbal aggressiveness against her husband. Four months later, cabergoline was restarted at a lower dosage (0.25 mg/week), but rapidly discontinued in consultation with her outpatient endocrinologist, due to the gradual development of manic symptoms. After 2 weeks, she was admitted to an emergency room reporting manic symptoms, together with transient paranoid ideation. Drug screening confirmed she didn't assume alcohol or illicit substances. Upon admission, she underwent a psychiatric assessment and the psychometric scales, receiving the diagnosis of bipolar disorder. A pharmacological treatment with asenapine 5 mg/day, valproic acid 500 mg/day, and haloperidol 2 mg/day was started. Due to excessive sedation and akathisia, asenapine was soon substituted with aripiprazole up to 30 mg/day, and haloperidol was stopped. Valproic acid was then increased to 750 mg/day for mood stabilization. She showed a gradual improvement of symptoms, as confirmed by psychometric scales' scores. Two weeks after discharge, she reached substantial mood stability and good global functioning [18c].

Ropinirole [SEDA-36, 199; SEDA-38, 119]

Open-label study: Long-term safety of once-daily ropinirole extended/prolonged release was evaluated in patients with early and advanced Parkinson's disease. Subjects ($n = 419$) who completed one of three prior studies evaluating ropinirole for the treatment of Parkinson's disease were enrolled in this open-label, multicenter, extension study and were to be followed for up to 73 months. Levodopa and other nondopamine agonist medications were permitted. Most subjects (87%) reported at least one averse effect, with the most common ($\geq 10\%$) being, back pain (14%), hallucinations (13%), somnolence (11%) and peripheral edema (11%). Twenty-five percent of subjects discontinued the study prematurely due to an adverse event during the treatment period. Long-term treatment with ropinirole was not associated with any new or unexpected safety concerns in patients with early and advanced patients with Parkinson's disease [19c].

Rotigotine [SEDA-35, 264; SEDA-37, 167; SEDA-38, 119]

Clinical Study: The short- and long-term efficacy and tolerability of a cross-titration algorithm from oral dopamine agonists to the rotigotine transdermal patch in patients dissatisfied with their restless legs syndrome treatment. Seventy percent of patients reported at least one adverse effect during the first year. Somnolence was the most frequently reported, with nine patients experiencing it at some point during the study. Six patients reported a worsening of their restless legs syndrome symptoms during the cross-titration, five patients reported a skin reaction at the patch application site, three patients reported experiencing insomnia, two patients reported nausea, two patients reported experiencing a headache, and two patients reported fatigue. All adverse effects were judged to be of mild-to-moderate intensity [20c].

Placebo-controlled trials: Restless legs syndrome/Willis–Ekbom disease is a sensorimotor disorder characterized by unpleasant sensations in the legs accompanied by an urge to move them, typically occurs and tends to worsen in the evening/night or during period of inactivity. Standard medications include dopamine agonists. The most common adverse effects were application-site reactions, dose-dependent, more frequently reported in the first period of treatment [21c].

A randomized controlled trial investigated effects of rotigotine in patients with restless legs syndrome and end-stage renal disease. Thirty patients were randomly assigned (rotigotine, 20; placebo, 10); 25 (15; 10) completed the study with evaluable data. The most common adverse events (≥2 patients) were nausea (rotigotine, 4 [20%]; placebo, 0); vomiting (3 [15%]; 0); diarrhea (1 [5%]; 2 [20%]); headache (2 [10%]; 0); dyspnea (2 [10%]; 0); and hypertension (2 [10%]; 0) [22c].

A placebo-controlled trial was performed to evaluate the effects of rotigotine transdermal patch on daytime symptoms in patients with idiopathic restless legs syndrome. Application site reactions (rotigotine: 20 patients [19.8%]; placebo: 4 [8.2%]) and nausea (16 [15.8%]; 3 [6.1%]) were the most common adverse effects [23c].

Apomorphine [SEDA-37, 168]

There are not many data about the beneficial effect of nocturnal continuous subcutaneous apomorphine infusion over sleep disturbances in advanced Parkinson's disease. Evaluate the effect of the nocturnal continuous subcutaneous apomorphine infusion in sleeping problems and insomnia due to nocturnal hypokinesia in advanced Parkinson's disease. Nocturnal continuous subcutaneous apomorphine infusion was well tolerated with no major adverse effects were noticed [24c].

Management of adverse events: Key local and systemic adverse effects during apomorphine titration, initiation and long-term treatment were reviewed, and practical management strategies are discussed. Management of adverse events includes nausea and vomiting, orthostatic hypotension, arrhythmias, dyskinesia, sedation, local injection site adverse events, neuropsychiatric events, impulse control disorders, hemolytic anemia, and erectile dysfunction [25r].

Dopamine Receptor Agonists [SEDA-34, 242; SEDA-35, 261; SEDA-36, 191; SEDA-37, 169; SEDA-38, 119]

Piribedil [SEDA-35, 263; SEDA-37, 169; SEDA-38, 119]

Review: Piribedil acts as a non-ergot partial dopamine D2/D3-selective agonist, blocks α2-adrenoreceptors. The tolerability and safety profile of piribedil fits with that of the class of dopaminergic agonists. As for other non-ergot agonists, pneumo-pulmonary, retroperitoneal, and valvular fibrotic side effects are not a concern with piribedil [26c].

Pramipexole [SEDA-36, 193; SEDA-37, 168; SEDA-38, 124]

Psychiatric: The long-term clinical follow-up (83 ± 24 months) of seven patients with BH4 deficiency treated with pramipexole. After a period of good clinical compensation, different impulse control disorders (gambling, compulsive buying, and hypersexuality) were observed in three patients treated with high-dose pramipexole (0.030–0.033 mg/kg/day) beyond adolescence. These psychiatric adverse effects promptly disappeared after curtailing pramipexole dose by 50%–60%. Low-dose pramipexole therapy has been safe and effective in the long-term period in all treated patients (59 ± 9 months). High-dose pramipexole therapy in BH4 deficiency can be complicated, like in Parkinson disease, by psychiatric adverse effects [27c].

Cotard's syndrome is a relatively rare condition that involves a delusion of negation in which an individual believes he or she has lost his or her soul, is dead, or is without functional body systems. A case of Cotard's syndrome was reported in treatment-resistant major depression associated with abnormal behaviours that might be caused by pramipexole [28c].

> The patient's abnormal behaviours, such as eating other patients' food and taking her medicine before the scheduled time, might differ from typical compulsive behaviours induced by pramipexole, but they could be regarded as disinhibition. These abnormal behaviours gradually disappeared in about 2 months after the discontinuation of pramipexole. The existence of Lewy body pathology could facilitate the emergence of abnormal behaviours after treatment with pramipexole [28c].

Levodopa [SEDA-32, 285; SEDA-33, 320; SEDA-34, 286-8; SEDA-35, 259; SEDA-36, 192; SEDA-37, 169; SEDA-38, 122]

Levodopa-induced dyskinesia is a major adverse event. Many studies have been performed to find effective methods to manage the adverse events including dyskinesia. These include molecular research on genetic factors, non-invasive transcranial current or magnetic stimulation, blood concentration control of levodopa, analysis of factors influencing motor levodopa-induced complications, pharmacological intervention and intestinal infusion of levodopa/carbidopa gel.

Management of the adverse drug reactions: In late-stage Parkinson patients there is an unmet need for new treatments to adequately control motor complications, especially dyskinesias. One or multiple sessions of bilateral low frequency repetitive transcranial magnetic stimulation applied to the primary motor cortex were unable to reduce levodopa-induced dyskinesias in late-stage Parkinson patients [29c].

Transcranial direct current stimulation is a non-invasive technique for inducing prolonged functional changes in the human cerebral cortex. This simple and safe neurostimulation technique for modulating motor functions in Parkinson's disease could extend treatment option for patients with movement disorders. This study assessed whether transcranial direct current stimulation applied daily over the cerebellum and motor cortex improves motor and cognitive symptoms and levodopa-induced dyskinesias in patients with Parkinson's disease. Nine patients with idiopathic Parkinson's disease were recruited. After patients received anodal cerebellar transcranial direct current stimulation for 5 days, dyskinesias improved ($P < 0.001$). Conversely, sham transcranial direct current stimulation unchanged ($p > 0.05$). Despite the small sample size, this preliminary results show that anodal transcranial direct current stimulation applied for 5 consecutive days over the motor cortical areas and cerebellum improves parkinsonian patients' levodopa-induced dyskinesias [30c].

Levodopa-induced dyskinesia and impulse control disorders are suggested to share pathophysiological processes and may be related to alterations of the glutamatergic neurotransmission. Anti-glutamatergic interventions are therefore worth considering: several lines of evidence already indicate their beneficial effect. The kynurenine pathway offers the endogenous glutamate receptor antagonist kynurenic acid, which may act as a promising candidate for future drug development with the aim of assessment of the motor symptoms and therapy-related complications of Parkinson's disease [31r].

At baseline (before the start of levodopa–carbidopa intestinal gel therapy), 3/33 (9%) patients showed symptomatic polyneuropathy and 7/33 (21%) subclinical polyneuropathy. During a follow-up of 24.36 ± 12.18 months, 2/23 patients with normal baseline clinical-electrophysiological assessment developed a subacute polyneuropathy, 2/23 developed a chronic polyneuropathy and 7/23 developed a subclinical polyneuropathy. Levodopa–carbidopa intestinal infusion was immediately halted in the subacute cases, while the infusion therapy was not interrupted in chronic and subclinical forms. All patients with polyneuropathy were supplemented with vitamin B1 and B12, showing a clinical improvement and/or substantial stability at the following evaluations. Higher levodopa-equivalent daily dose (P: 0.024) and homocysteine levels (P: 0.041) were found in chronic polyneuropathy, while no correlations were observed with vitamin B12, folate and UPDRS values. One patient developed a symptomatic polyneuropathy associated with a relevant weight loss [32c].

Genetic factors: A molecular study using animals aimed at investigating whether leucine-rich repeat kinase 2 phosphorylation/function is involved in the molecular pathways downstream D1 dopamine receptor leading to levodopa-induced dyskinesias. Leucine-rich repeat kinase 2 phosphorylation level at serine 935 was shown to inversely correlate with levodopa-induced dyskinesia induction. The inhibition of leucine-rich repeat kinase 2 induces a significant increase in the dyskinetic score in levodopa-induced dyskinesia [33c].

A study was performed to investigate the relationship of dopamine receptor D2 and D3 gene polymorphisms with gastrointestinal symptoms induced by levodopa in patients with 217 Parkinson's disease. D2 rs1799732 and D3 rs6280 polymorphisms were genotyped by PCR-based methods. Multiple Poisson regression method with robust variance estimators was performed to assess the association between polymorphisms and gastrointestinal symptoms. The analyses showed that D2 Ins/Ins (prevalence ratio = 2.374, 95% CI: 1.105–5.100; P = 0.027) and D3 Ser/Ser genotypes (prevalence ratio = 1.677, 95% CI 1.077–2.611; P = 0.022) were independent and predictors of gastrointestinal symptoms associated with levodopa therapy [34c].

Susceptibility Factor: Factors influencing prevalence of motor levodopa-induced complications were investigated in 76 patients with Parkinson's disease. The mean disease duration was 10.33 years, and mean levodopa therapy duration was 8.65 years. The most common drug regimen was levodopa with ropinirole. The prevalence of motor levodopa-induced complications was 54% with their mean duration of 3.34 years. Motor levodopa-induced complications were influenced by higher levodopa equivalent dose, younger age at onset, younger age, longer disease duration, and longer levodopa therapy regardless of clinical subtype of Parkinson's disease. Although women had more advanced disease according to Hoehn and Yahr score, sex did not influence motor levodopa-induced complications [35c].

Food-drug interaction: Clinical records of 1037 Parkinson's disease patients were analyzed to determine the proportion of patients with motor fluctuations related to protein interaction with levodopa. Motor fluctuations due to protein interaction with levodopa were defined as dietary protein being associated with (i) longer time to levodopa effectiveness, (ii) reduced benefit or duration of benefit, (iii) dose failures or (iv) wearing off relatively sooner from a previously effective dose. Dose failures, sudden, painful or behavioral wearing-off periods, gait freezing, nausea, hallucinations, orthostasis, and dyskinesias were taken as markers of motor fluctuations, disease severity, and levodopa side effects potentially influenced by protein. Parkinson's disease patients (5.9%) on levodopa, and 12.4% with motor fluctuations on levodopa correlated their fluctuations with the relative timing of levodopa and protein intake. These patients were younger at disease onset, had worse motor fluctuations and had a higher incidence of family members with Parkinson's disease. Early wearing off or decreased dose efficacy were most commonly associated with protein interaction [36C].

Drug dosage regimens: A unique population pharmacokinetic/pharmacodynamic model in Parkinson's disease was identified to investigate the relationship and dissociability of motor response and dyskinesia. The model was developed using NONMEM software. Thirty parkinsonian patients (Hoehn and Yahr stages 3–4), treated with levodopa and suffering from peak-dose dyskinesia, were included in a prospective open-label study. They received a single dose of levodopa equal to 150% of their usual daily dose. In patients treated with levodopa and suffering from dyskinesia, the motor response and dyskinesia have close onsets and duration effects. Maximal motor response to levodopa tends to be inevitably associated with dyskinesia [37c].

Levodopa-induced dyskinesia may be encountered even within a few weeks or months after initiation of levodopa therapy. Based on the temporal pattern in relationship to levodopa dosing, the dyskinesia is divided into "peak-dose dyskinesia," "diphasic dyskinesia," and "wearing off" or "off-period" dyskinesia, of which peak-dose dyskinesia is the most common, followed by off-period, and then diphasic dyskinesia. Treatment strategy includes identifying the kind of dyskinesia and tailoring treatment accordingly. Peak-dose dyskinesia is treated mainly by reducing individual doses of levodopa and adding amantadine and dopamine agonists, whereas off-period dystonia often responds to baclofen and botulinum toxin injections. Diphasic dyskinesias, occurring particularly in patients with young-onset Parkinson's disease, are the most difficult to treat. While fractionation of levodopa dosage is the most frequently utilized strategy, many patients require deep brain stimulation to control their troublesome motor fluctuations and levodopa-induced dyskinesia [38c].

Drug formulations: To evaluate the safety and tolerability of the T-Port(®) for intestinal infusion of levodopa/carbidopa gel in patients with advanced Parkinson's disease.

The number of adverse device effects proved to be significantly lower as compared to the endoscopic gastrojejunostomy literature data [39c].

Motor symptoms, motor fluctuations, non-motor symptoms, quality of sleep, symptoms of depression and anxiety of 10 patients with advanced Parkinson's disease were evaluated just before initiation of intrajejunal levodopa/carbidopa therapy, and after 1 and 3 months of regular treatment. All aspects of mental and psychic symptoms are not alleviated within a short period of reduction of motor fluctuations [40c].

Levodopa–carbidopa is an oral extended-release therapy composed of microbeads designed to dissolve at various rates that allows for quick absorption and sustained levodopa release over an extended period. Levodopa–carbidopa therapy improved symptoms in patients with both early and advanced Parkinson's disease without worsening troublesome dyskinesias when compared to other levodopa formulations. Tolerability and safety were comparable to other formulations [41r].

A study was performed to assess the effect of levodopa–carbidopa intestinal gel in advanced Parkinson's disease with troublesome dyskinesia. The changes in "off" time, "on" time with and without troublesome dyskinesia, and the overall safety and tolerability of levodopa–carbidopa intestinal gel were analyzed. An increase in levodopa–carbidopa intestinal gel dose was not significantly correlated with increased "on" time with troublesome dyskinesia in either study (double-blind: $r=-0.073$, $P=0.842$; open-label: $r=-0.001$, $P=0.992$). Adverse events were usually mild to moderate in severity and related to the gastrointestinal procedure [42C].

A retrospective analysis of levodopa–carbidopa intestinal gel therapy was conducted in nine neurology centers in Romania. In the 113 patients included, there were few adverse effects and few cases of the therapy discontinuation [43c].

An open-label, 12-month prospective study of treatment with levodopa–carbidopa intestinal gel in 15 patients with advanced Parkinson's disease was conducted. The most common adverse event was reversible peripheral neuropathy secondary to vitamin $B12 \pm B6$ deficiency (40%), local tube problems (40%), and impulse control disorder (27%). No patient had stoma bleeding or peritonitis. All patients with impulse control disorder had a past psychiatric diagnosis of depression with or without anxiety and a higher daily levodopa intake at 6 and 12 months of levodopa–carbidopa intestinal gel infusion [44c].

Drug administraton route: Human experience with levodopa given intravenously was reviewed. Over 200 articles referring to i.v. levodopa were examined for details of adverse effects expected from clinical experience with oral levodopa and dopamine agonists. The authors identified 142 original reports, beginning with psychiatric research in 1959–1960 before the development of peripheral decarboxylase inhibitors. At least 2760 subjects received intravenous levodopa. Reported outcomes included parkinsonian signs, sleep variables, hormone levels, hemodynamics. Mean pharmacokinetic variables were summarized for 49 healthy subjects and 190 with Parkinson's disease. Side effects were those expected from clinical experience with oral levodopa and dopamine agonists. No articles reported deaths or induction of psychosis [45C].

Eighty-six patients used inhaled levodopa and placebo at an average frequency of 2.1 times per day. The most frequently reported adverse events in the inhaled levodopa group were dizziness, cough, and nausea, each in 7% (3 of 43 patients) [46c] (Fig. 1).

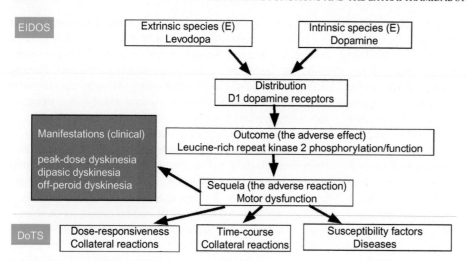

FIG. 1 The EIDOS and DoTS descriptions of levodopa-induced dyskinesia.

MISCELLANEOUS OTHER DRUGS THAT INCREASE DOPAMINE ACTIVITY

Amantadine [SEDA-37, 344]

Skin: Although livedo reticularis is a known adverse effect of amantadine, only limited studies have addressed this association. Livedo racemosa in contrast to livedo reticularis is characterized by a striking violaceous net-like pattern of the skin similar to livedo reticularis with a different histopathology and morphology (irregular, broken circular segments). Two cases of livedo racemosa and edema of lower extremities following amantadine treatment were reported.

A 57-year-old woman with Parkinson's disease received amantadine 200 mg daily. She was referred to the Dermatology Department due to asymptomatic rash on her knees within the first year after receiving amantadine. She had erythematous to violaceus net-like mottled patches on knees with irregular and broken segments, demonstrating a pattern of livedo racemosa. She also had bilateral swelling of lower extremities and associated burning sensation.
A cutaneous biopsy from the pallor area of the livedo racemosa demonstrated normal epidermis and partial thrombotic occlusion of blood vessels (arterioles) by blood red cells and fibrin in deep dermis and subcutis. The histopathological diagnosis of thrombotic vasculopathy was established. The neurology consult and a peripheral nerve biopsy showed enlargement of epineurum and perineurum by collagen fibers and the blood vessels (vasa nervorum) associated with hyaline deposition in the vessel walls. The number of myelinated fibers and axonal degeneration are reduced with lack of inflammatory infiltrate or vascular thrombosis. An extensive workup was performed to rule out differential diagnoses of livedo racemosa-related conditions, and a diagnosis of

amantadine-induced livedo racemosa was made. The only positive exam was rheumatoid factor 53.5 IU/mL (normal range < 20 IU/mL by nephelometric method). She denied using any other drugs, and she did not have any other joint symptoms. On follow-up 2 months after discontinuation of amantadine, the livedo racemosa faded.

A 54-year-old man with a past history of Parkinson's disease, on amantadine 300 mg daily, was referred to a dermatologist due to mottled discoloration of his legs typical of livedo racemosa. He also had bilateral swelling of the lower extremities. The patient noticed that his symptoms were present within the first 6 months of commencing amantadine. All blood tests were normal or negative. The level of lipoprotein(a) was elevated (89 mg/dL; normal range < 9 mg/dL, immunoturbidimetric method). Histopathology of pallor area of the livedo racemosa demonstrated hyaline microthrombi in blood vessel of superficial dermis. A diagnosis of amantadine-induced livedo racemosa was established [47A].

Psychiatric: Psychosis and delirium induced by amantadine have been previously reported among elderly patients with Parkinson's disease. The following case study presents a young male patient who showed a psychotic episode due to amantadine-containing OTC drug for a cold.

A 28-year-old man was admitted because of hallucinations and persecutory delusions, which lasted for 48 hours. When he was alone at home, he had auditory and visual hallucination. He did not report experiencing headache, fever, or convulsions. Prior to admission, he had been in excellent health and did not have a history of medical problems, psychiatric disorders, or substance abuse. He was a nonsmoker and did not drink alcohol habitually. His family history was negative for psychotic disorders. Five days prior to admission, he reported symptoms of a cold, including a runny nose, and had therefore started taking an over-the-counter cold medicine, which contained 250 mg of acetaminophen and 100 mg of amantadine hydrochloride. The patient took one capsule twice daily. Three days later, he began to experience hallucinations and delusions. During the mental status examination administered upon admission, the patient had obvious auditory and visual hallucinations. Although the patient acknowledged his own abnormal mental state, his insight was still partially impaired. Physical and neurologic examinations and laboratory studies did not identify any abnormalities. The patient was immediately treated with haloperidol (5 mg daily) and paliperidone extended release (3 mg daily), while the over-the-counter cold medicine administration was ceased. After 48 hours of treatment, auditory and visual hallucinations, as well as paranoid ideation, resolved completely. Haloperidol was used for 3 days, and the use of paliperidone extended release was maintained for 2 weeks to prevent relapse. After the 2-week treatment course, he had fully recovered and was discharged. Six months later, the patient reported of no subsequent psychotic experiences [48c].

Entacapone [SEDA-15, 1219; SEDA-32, 289; SEDA-33, 324; SEDA-34, 246; SEDA-38, 124]

Tolcapone [SEDA-32,289]

Liver: Tolcapone and entacapone are catechol-*O*-methyltransferase inhibitors developed as adjunct therapies for treating Parkinson's disease. While both drugs have been shown to cause mitochondrial dysfunction and inhibition of the bile salt export protein, liver injury has only been associated with the use of tolcapone [49r].

DRUGS THAT AFFECT THE CHOLIERGIC SYSTEM [SEDA-31, 272; SEDA-32, 290; SEDA-33, 324; SEDA-34, 290-1, 318; SEDA-35, 266; SEDA-36, 199; SEDA-37, 172; SEDA-38, 124]

Anticholinergic Drugs [SEDA-31, 273; SEDA-32, 290; SEDA-33, 324; SEDA-34, 290, 318; SEDA-35, 266; SEDA-36, 199; SEDA-37, 172; SEDA-38, 124]

Ipratropium [SEDA-35, 266; SEDA-36, 247; SEDA-37, 198; SEDA-38, 124]

Randomized controlled trial: Double-blind, crossover study was performed to evaluate whether ipratropium bromide/albuterol metered-dose inhaler provides more effective acute relief of bronchospasm in moderate-to-severe asthma than albuterol alone after 4 weeks in 226 patients with asthma. Adverse events were comparable across groups, including cough and asthma exacerbations [50C].

Tiotropium [SEDA-35, 319; SEDA-36, 247; SEDA-37, 199; SEDA-38, 124]

Systematic review: Tiotropium/olodaterol is a fixed-dose combination of the long-acting antimuscarinic agent tiotropium and the long-acting β2-adrenoreceptor agonist olodaterol delivered via an inhaler. It is indicated for the maintenance treatment of airflow obstruction in adults with COPD. The tolerability profile of tiotropium/olodaterol in the phase III studies was generally similar to that of the component monotherapies. The most common adverse events and serious adverse events during 52 weeks' therapy were respiratory in nature, with COPD exacerbation [51c].

A systematic literature review was performed to estimate the relative efficacy and safety of fixed-dose combination aclidinium/formoterol 400/12 μg twice daily compared to tiotropium 18 μg once daily in adult patients with moderate-to-severe chronic obstructive pulmonary disease. The results suggest similar safety profiles regarding adverse effects, serious adverse events and hospitalization [52M].

Randomized Controlled Trial: The efficacy and safety of once-daily tiotropium plus olodaterol maintenance treatment was demonstrated in the large, multinational, replicate, randomized studies in patients with moderate to very severe COPD. Adverse-event incidence was generally balanced across treatment groups [53C].

This 12-week, randomized, parallel-group, multicentre, open-label study was conducted in East Asia. After a 14-day run-in period during which patients received tiotropium 18 μg once daily, patients were randomized to tiotropium (18 μg once daily) plus budesonide/formoterol (160/4.5 μg 2 inhalations twice daily) or tiotropium alone (18 μg once daily). Incidence of adverse events was 26% for both groups. It should be noted the authors have conflicts of interest in relation to pharmaceutical companies selling those drugs [54C].

Fluticasone furoate/vilanterol is a novel, once-daily, inhaled corticosteroid/long-acting β2-agonist combination approved for the treatment of COPD and asthma. A randomized, blinded, double-dummy, parallel-group study compared the safety and efficacy of fluticasone furoate/vilanterol and tiotropium in subjects with moderate-to-severe COPD with greater risk for comorbid cardiovascular disease. Pneumonia occurred more frequently in the fluticasone furoate/vilanterol group, and two tiotropium-treated subjects died following cardiovascular events. Other safety measures were similar between groups, and cardiovascular monitoring did not reveal increased cardiovascular risk [55c].

Placebo-controlled trial: A double-blind, placebo-controlled trial was conducted employing adults with symptomatic asthma receiving low- to medium-dose inhaled corticosteroids. In total, 464 patients were randomized, and adverse events were comparable across the treatment groups [56c].

Drug administration route: There is a shortage of data to support the efficacy of long-acting inhaled anticholinergic agents in improving these adverse effects; however, they are known to have negative impact on clinical outcomes. A randomized, open-label, parallel-group trial was aimed to compare the tiotropium Respimat Soft Mist Inhaler and the HandiHaler in terms of their effects on sleeping oxygen saturation and sleep quality in patients with COPD. A total of 188 patients completed the trial. The patients using the Respimat had significantly better sleep-time with SaO_2 below 90 compared to those using the HandiHaler. Sleep disturbance was highly variable in these patients, but the sleep stage durations were significantly better in the Respimat group [57C].

Oxybutynin [SEDA-32, 266; SEDA-38, 125]

Drug administration route: Antimuscarinic medications are used to treat nonneurogenic overactive bladder refractory to nonpharmacologic therapy. Side effects such as dry mouth, constipation, blurred vision, dizziness, and impaired cognition limit the tolerability of therapy and are largely responsible for high discontinuation rates. Oxybutynin is a potent muscarinic receptor antagonist whose primary metabolite after first-pass hepatic metabolism is considered largely responsible for its associated anticholinergic side effects. Transdermal administration of medications bypasses hepatic processing. Specifically with oxybutynin, whose low-molecular weight permits transdermal administration, bioavailability of the parent drug with oral administration is less than 10%, whereas with transdermal delivery is a minimum of 80%. The result has been an improved side effect profile in multiple clinical trials with maintained efficacy relative to placebo; however, the drug may still be discontinued by patients due to anticholinergic side effects and application site reactions [58R].

Solifenacin [SEDA-35, 266; SEDA-38, 125]

Randomized Controlled Trial: Three hundred thirty-eight men 50+ years old (average age 58.4 years) diagnosed with benign prostatic hyperplasia and severe symptoms of overactive bladder were enrolled in the study. Patients of the main group, during 2 months, received treatment with daily combination of solifenacin 5 mg plus trospium 5 mg, simultaneously with

tamsulosin 0.4 mg. Patients of the control group were treated only with tamsulosin. Severity of side effects did not exceed the level which is common for antimuscarinic monotherapy [59C].

References

[1] Gunel C, Sari S, Eryilmaz A, et al. Hemodynamic effects of topical adrenaline during septoplasty. Indian J Otolaryngol Head Neck Surg. 2016;68(4):391–5 [c].

[2] Cervellin G, Sanchis-Gomar F, Lippi G. Adrenaline in anaphylaxis treatment. Balancing benefits and harms. Expert Opin Drug Saf. 2016;15(6):741–6 [R].

[3] Kounis NG, Soufras GD. Shoulder arthroscopy and atak (adrenaline, takotsubo, anaphylaxis, and kounis hypersensitivity-associated syndrome). Orthop Traumatol Surg Res. 2016;102(2):273–4 [r].

[4] Choudhury A, Kedarisetty CK, Vashishtha C, et al. A randomized trial comparing terlipressin and noradrenaline in patients with cirrhosis and septic shock. Liver Int. 2017;37(4):552–61 [c].

[5] Shao IH, Wu CC, Tseng HJ, et al. Voiding dysfunction in patients with nasal congestion treated with pseudoephedrine: a prospective study. Drug Des Devel Ther. 2016;10:2333–9 [C].

[6] Ruzieh M, Dasa O, Pacenta A, et al. Droxidopa in the treatment of postural orthostatic tachycardia syndrome. Am J Ther. 2017;24(2): e157–61 [c].

[7] Isaacson S, Shill HA, Vernino S, et al. Safety and durability of effect with long-term, open-label droxidopa treatment in patients with symptomatic neurogenic orthostatic hypotension (NOH303). J Parkinsons Dis. 2016;6(4):751–9 [C].

[8] Strassheim V, Newton JL, Tan MP, et al. Droxidopa for orthostatic hypotension: a systematic review and meta-analysis. J Hypertens. 2016;34(10):1933–41 [M].

[9] Meltzer EO, Ratner PH, McGraw T. Phenylephrine hydrochloride modified-release tablets for nasal congestion: a randomized, placebo-controlled trial in allergic rhinitis patients. Ann Allergy Asthma Immunol. 2016;116(1):66–71 [C].

[10] Jain K, Makkar JK, Subramani Vp S, et al. A randomized trial comparing prophylactic phenylephrine and ephedrine infusion during spinal anesthesia for emergency cesarean delivery in cases of acute fetal compromise. J Clin Anesth. 2016;34:208–15 [c].

[11] Anusorntanawat R, Uerpairojkit K, Thongthaweeporn N, et al. Safety of phenylephrine in antihypotensive treatment during spinal anesthesia for cesarean section. J Med Assoc Thai. 2016;99(2):188–96 [C].

[12] Luo XJ, Zheng M, Tian G, et al. Comparison of the treatment effects of methoxamine and combining methoxamine with atropine infusion to maintain blood pressure during spinal anesthesia for cesarean delivery: a double blind randomized trial. Eur Rev Med Pharmacol Sci. 2016;20(3):561–7 [c].

[13] Watz H, Mailander C, Baier M, et al. Effects of indacaterol/glycopyrronium (QVA149) on lung hyperinflation and physical activity in patients with moderate to severe COPD: a randomised, placebo-controlled, crossover study (the move study). BMC Pulm Med. 2016;16(1):95 [C].

[14] Wedzicha JA, Banerji D, Chapman KR, et al. Indacaterol-glycopyrronium versus salmeterol-fluticasone for COPD. N Engl J Med. 2016;374(23):2222–34 [C].

[15] Rojas-Reyes MX, Garcia Morales OM, Dennis RJ, et al. Combination inhaled steroid and long-acting β(2)-agonist in addition to tiotropium versus tiotropium or combination alone for chronic obstructive pulmonary disease. Cochrane Database Syst Rev. 2016;(6):Cd008532 [C].

[16] Giovannetti AM, Pasanisi MB, Cerniauskaite M, et al. Perceived efficacy of salbutamol by persons with spinal muscular atrophy: a mixed methods study. Muscle Nerve. 2016;54(5):843–9 [c].

[17] Yuksel RN, Elyas Kaya Z, Dilbaz N, et al. Cabergoline-induced manic episode: case report. Ther Adv Psychopharmacol. 2016;6(3):229–31 [c].

[18] Rovera C, Cremaschi L, Thanju A, et al. Cabergoline can induce mania with psychotic features in bipolar I disorder: a case report. Asian J Psychiatr. 2016;22:94–5 [c].

[19] Makumi CW, Asgharian A, Ellis J, et al. Long-term, open-label, safety study of once-daily ropinirole extended/prolonged release in early and advanced Parkinson's disease. Int J Neurosci. 2016;126(1):30–8 [c].

[20] Winkelman JW, Mackie SE, Mei LA, et al. A method to switch from oral dopamine agonists to rotigotine in patients with restless legs syndrome and mild augmentation. Sleep Med. 2016;24:18–23 [c].

[21] Ferini-Strambi L, Marelli S, Galbiati A. Clinical pharmacology and efficacy of rotigotine (Neupro® patch) in the treatment of restless leg syndrome. Expert Opin Drug Metab Toxicol. 2016;12(8):967–75 [c].

[22] Dauvilliers Y, Benes H, Partinen M, et al. Rotigotine in hemodialysis-associated restless legs syndrome: a randomized controlled trial. Am J Kidney Dis. 2016;68(3):434–43 [c].

[23] Garcia-Borreguero D, Allen R, Hudson J, et al. Effects of rotigotine on daytime symptoms in patients with primary restless legs syndrome: a randomized, placebo-controlled study. Curr Med Res Opin. 2016;32(1):77–85 [c].

[24] Fernandez-Pajarin G, Sesar A, Ares B, et al. Evaluating the efficacy of nocturnal continuous subcutaneous apomorphine infusion in sleep disorders in advanced Parkinson's disease: the apo-night study. J Parkinsons Dis. 2016;6(4):787–92 [c].

[25] Bhidayasiri R, Garcia Ruiz PJ, Henriksen T. Practical management of adverse events related to apomorphine therapy. Parkinsonism Relat Disord. 2016;33(Suppl 1):S42–8 [r].

[26] Perez-Lloret S, Rascol O. Piribedil for the treatment of motor and non-motor symptoms of Parkinson disease. CNS Drugs. 2016;30(8):703–17 [c].

[27] Porta F, Ponzone A, Spada M. Long-term safety and effectiveness of pramipexole in tetrahydrobiopterin deficiency. Eur J Paediatr Neurol. 2016;20(6):839–42 [c].

[28] Maruo H, Haraguchi Y, Tateishi H, et al. Abnormal behaviours during pramipexole treatment for cotard's syndrome: a case report. Psychogeriatrics. 2016;16(4):283–6 [c].

[29] Flamez A, Cordenier A, De Raedt S, et al. Bilateral low frequency rTMS of the primary motor cortex may not be a suitable treatment for levodopa-induced dyskinesias in late stage Parkinson's disease. Parkinsonism Relat Disord. 2016;22:54–61 [c].

[30] Ferrucci R, Cortese F, Bianchi M, et al. Cerebellar and motor cortical transcranial stimulation decrease levodopa-induced dyskinesias in Parkinson's disease. Cerebellum. 2016;15(1):43–7 [c].

[31] Majlath Z, Toldi J, Fulop F, et al. Excitotoxic mechanisms in non-motor dysfunctions and levodopa-induced dyskinesia in Parkinson's disease: the role of the interaction between the dopaminergic and the kynurenine system. Curr Med Chem. 2016;23(9):874–83 [r].

[32] Merola A, Romagnolo A, Zibetti M, et al. Peripheral neuropathy associated with levodopa-carbidopa intestinal infusion: a long-term prospective assessment. Eur J Neurol. 2016;23(3):501–9 [c].

[33] Stanic J, Mellone M, Cirnaru MD, et al. LRRK2 phosphorylation level correlates with abnormal motor behaviour in an experimental model of levodopa-induced dyskinesias. Mol Brain. 2016;9(1):53 [c].

[34] Rieck M, Schumacher-Schuh AF, Altmann V, et al. Association between DRD2 and DRD3 gene polymorphisms and gastrointestinal symptoms induced by levodopa therapy in Parkinson's disease. Pharmacogenomics J. 2016; [c].

[35] Michalowska M, Fiszer U, Szatanowski T. Motor levodopa-induced complications in Parkinson's disease. Pol Merkur Lekarski. 2016;40(240):357–61 [c].

[36] Virmani T, Tazan S, Mazzoni P, et al. Motor fluctuations due to interaction between dietary protein and levodopa in Parkinson's disease. J Clin Mov Disord. 2016;3:8 [C].

[37] Simon N, Viallet F, Boulamery A, et al. A combined pharmacokinetic/pharmacodynamic model of levodopa motor response and dyskinesia in Parkinson's disease patients. Eur J Clin Pharmacol. 2016;72(4):423–30 [c].

[38] Vijayakumar D, Jankovic J. Drug-induced dyskinesia, part 1: treatment of levodopa-induced dyskinesia. Drugs. 2016;76(7):759–77 [c].

[39] van Laar T, Nyholm D, Nyman R. Transcutaneous port for levodopa/carbidopa intestinal gel administration in Parkinson's disease. Acta Neurol Scand. 2016;133(3):208–15 [c].

[40] Bellante F, Dethy S, Zegers de Beyl D. Depression, anxiety and non-motor symptoms on initiation of intrajejunal levodopa/carbidopa therapy. Acta Neurol Belg. 2016;116(1):39–41 [c].

[41] Dhall R, Kreitzman DL. Advances in levodopa therapy for Parkinson disease: review of RYTARY (carbidopa and levodopa) clinical efficacy and safety. Neurology. 2016;86(14 Suppl 1):S13–24 [r].

[42] Antonini A, Fung VS, Boyd JT, et al. Effect of levodopa-carbidopa intestinal gel on dyskinesia in advanced Parkinson's disease patients. Mov Disord. 2016;31(4):530–7 [C].

[43] Bajenaru O, Ene A, Popescu BO, et al. The effect of levodopa-carbidopa intestinal gel infusion long-term therapy on motor complications in advanced Parkinson's disease: a multicenter Romanian experience. J Neural Transm (Vienna). 2016;123(4):407–14 [c].

[44] Chang FC, Kwan V, van der Poorten D, et al. Intraduodenal levodopa-carbidopa intestinal gel infusion improves both motor performance and quality of life in advanced Parkinson's disease. J Clin Neurosci. 2016;25:41–5 [c].

[45] Siddiqi SH, Abraham NK, Geiger CL, et al. The human experience with intravenous levodopa. Front Pharmacol. 2015;6:307 [C].

[46] LeWitt PA, Hauser RA, Grosset DG, et al. A randomized trial of inhaled levodopa (CVT-301) for motor fluctuations in Parkinson's disease. Mov Disord. 2016;31(9):1356–65 [c].

[47] Criado PR, Alavi A, Valente NY, et al. Amantadine-induced livedo racemosa. Int J Low Extrem Wounds. 2016;15(1):78–81 [A].

[48] Xu WJ, Wei N, Xu Y, et al. Does amantadine induce acute psychosis? A case report and literature review. Neuropsychiatr Dis Treat. 2016;12:781–3 [c].

[49] Longo DM, Yang Y, Watkins PB, et al. Elucidating differences in the hepatotoxic potential of tolcapone and entacapone with DILIsym®, a mechanistic model of drug-induced liver injury. CPT Pharmacometrics Syst Pharmacol. 2016;5(1):31–9 [r].

[50] Donohue JF, Wise R, Busse WW, et al. Efficacy and safety of ipratropium bromide/albuterol compared with albuterol in patients with moderate-to-severe asthma: a randomized controlled trial. BMC Pulm Med. 2016;16(1):65 [C].

[51] Dhillon S. Tiotropium/olodaterol: a review in COPD. Drugs. 2016;76(1):135–46 [c].

[52] Medic G, Lindner L, van der Weijden M, et al. Efficacy and safety of aclidinium/formoterol versus tiotropium in COPD: results of an indirect treatment comparison. Adv Ther. 2016;33(2):379–99 [M].

[53] Ichinose M, Taniguchi H, Takizawa A, et al. The efficacy and safety of combined tiotropium and olodaterol via the Respimat® inhaler in patients with COPD: results from the Japanese sub-population of the Tonado® studies. Int J Chron Obstruct Pulmon Dis. 2016;11:2017–27 [C].

[54] Lee SD, Xie CM, Yunus F, et al. Efficacy and tolerability of budesonide/formoterol added to tiotropium compared with

tiotropium alone in patients with severe or very severe COPD: a randomized, multicentre study in East Asia. Respirology. 2016;21(1):119–27 [C].

[55] Covelli H, Pek B, Schenkenberger I, et al. Efficacy and safety of fluticasone furoate/vilanterol or tiotropium in subjects with COPD at cardiovascular risk. Int J Chron Obstruct Pulmon Dis. 2016;11:1–12 [c].

[56] Paggiaro P, Halpin DM, Buhl R, et al. The effect of tiotropium in symptomatic asthma despite low- to medium-dose inhaled corticosteroids: a randomized controlled trial. J Allergy Clin Immunol Pract. 2016;4(1). 104–13.e2. [c].

[57] Bouloukaki I, Tzanakis N, Mermigkis C, et al. Tiotropium respimat soft mist inhaler versus handihaler to improve sleeping oxygen saturation and sleep quality in COPD. Sleep Breath. 2016;20(2):605–12 [C].

[58] Cohn JA, Brown ET, Reynolds WS, et al. An update on the use of transdermal oxybutynin in the management of overactive bladder disorder. Ther Adv Urol. 2016;8(2):83–90 [R].

[59] Kosilov KV, Loparev SA, Ivanovskaya MA, et al. Effectiveness of solifenacin and trospium for managing of severe symptoms of overactive bladder in patients with benign prostatic hyperplasia. Am J Mens Health. 2016;10(2):157–63 [C].

12

Dermatological Drugs, Topical Agents, and Cosmetics

Adrienne T. Black[1]

3E Company, Warrenton, VA, United States
[1]Corresponding author: adrienne159@gmail.com

INTRODUCTION

This chapter provides a concise overview of drug-induced skin reactions or side effects reported in the literature from January 2016 to December 2016. The effects include those resulting from medications used to treat dermal disorders such as melanoma and psoriasis as well as drug-associated cutaneous reactions by antibiotics, antivirals, neurological treatments and chemotherapy. The information presented includes case reports, clinical trial results, pooled clinical trial analyses and literature reviews.

Cutaneous T-Cell Lymphoma

Quisinostat

A multicenter phase 2 trial evaluated the safety and efficacy of oral quisinostat, a histone deacetylase inhibitor, for previously treated cutaneous T-cell lymphoma. Patients ($n=26$) received quisinostat (8 or 12 mg) orally on days 1, 3 and 5 of each week in 21-day treatment cycles. Common adverse events included nausea, diarrhea, asthenia, hypertension, thrombocytopenia and vomiting. More serious adverse events (grade 3) were hypertension, lethargy, pruritus, chills, hyperkalemia and pyrexia [1C].

Melanoma

BRAF and MEK Inhibitors: Vemurafenib, Dabrafenib, Trametinib

Inactivation of the mitogen-activated protein (MAP) kinase pathway has been shown to be an effective treatment option for metastatic melanoma patients with a BRAF mutation. Vemurafenib and dabrafenib are selective BRAF inhibitors and have been proven effective in clinical trials for treatment of BRAF-mutated metastatic melanoma. The addition of trametinib, a mitogen-activated protein kinase kinase (MEK) inhibitor, to the combination therapy was used to increase the length of survival in cases of drug resistance in these types of patients. A 4-year retrospective observational study in Spain evaluated the skin adverse effects associated with BRAF and MEK inhibitors (vemurafenib, dabrafenib or a combination of dabrafenib and trametinib). A total of 23 patients with BRAF-mutated metastatic melanoma received vemurafenib ($n=11$), dabrafenib ($n=6$) or a combination of dabrafenib and trametinib ($n=6$) for an average duration of 11 months. Adverse effects with vemurafenib and dabrafenib monotherapy were generally mild (grade 1 or 2) and included arthralgia, alopecia, asthenia, photosensitivity, hyperkeratosis, dry skin and vitiligo. Treatment discontinuation occurred in 10% of these patients due to a grade 3 or higher adverse effects. Serious adverse events with vemurafenib alone included 1 case each of photosensitivity (grade 3), immediate and delayed QT interval prolongation, basal cell carcinoma, hand–foot syndrome (grade 3), fluid retention (grade 3), facial nerve paralysis and delayed autoimmune thyroiditis (grade 3). Dabrafenib monotherapy resulted in 1 severe adverse effect: delayed hand–foot syndrome (grade 3). The combination of dabrafenib with trametinib treatment group reported fewer adverse events and all were of lesser toxicity (all grade 1 or 2) than those with the other treatments; these effects included diarrhea, dry skin, liver enzyme and electrolyte disturbances and diminished renal function [2c].

Ipilimumab

Ipilimumab is an anti-cytotoxic T-lymphocyte antigen-4 monoclonal antibody commonly used for treatment of melanoma. Recent case reports, however, have described the development of adverse cutaneous events following ipilimumab administration. In the first report, a 50-year-old man with metastatic melanoma treated with ipilimumab developed edematous erythema with sterile pustules 2 weeks after starting treatment. This reaction was diagnosed as acute generalized exanthematous pustulosis based on histology. Ipilimumab was discontinued and the symptoms resolved within 25 days [3A]. In the second report, a 73-year-old man received ipilimumab for metastatic melanoma and developed a widespread polymorphic papulovesicular dermatosis 5 weeks after starting treatment. A skin biopsy showed acantholytic dermatosis, confirming the diagnosis of a Grover's disease-like drug eruption [4A].

Nivolumab

Nivolumab, a humanized monoclonal anti-programmed cell death 1 (PD-1) antibody for treatment of metastatic melanoma, has been associated with the development of a grade 3 or 4 skin rash. A case report described a 64-year-old female with ipilimumab-refractory metastatic melanoma who developed a widespread maculopapular skin rash with bullae and skin detachment following 2 doses of nivolumab. A skin biopsy showed dermatitis with a lymphocytic infiltrate and areas of complete epidermal necrosis, confirming a toxic epidermal necrolysis reaction. The symptoms were initially treated with steroids and immunoglobulin but improved with cyclosporine and high-dose prednisone administration [5A].

Pembrolizumab

Anti-PD1 antibodies such as pembrolizumab have shown improved progression-free and overall survival in patients with advanced melanoma. A 3-year review was conducted of 124 hospitalized patients treated with pembrolizumab for advanced melanoma with 3 cases of bullous pemphigoid reported. The authors suggest that, as no cases of bullous pemphigoid have been reported with BRAF inhibitor therapy, this adverse event may be associated with the use of the PD-1 antibody treatment as opposed to the presence of metastatic melanoma itself [6c].

Vemurafenib

Vemurafenib, a BRAF inhibitor for treatment of melanoma, is known to cause severe dermal side effects. A retrospective study in 131 patients with melanoma was conducted over 4 years to determine the rate of vemurafenib treatment discontinuation due to skin side effects. Treatment with vemurafenib resulted in grade 3–4 skin effects in 26% of the patients. Within this group, 44% of the patients discontinued vemurafenib due to development of Stevens–Johnson syndrome and drug reaction with eosinophilia and systemic symptoms (DRESS) syndrome while the remaining patients (56%) continued vemurafenib in spite of the grade 3–4 effects (rash, photosensitivity). Interestingly, the development of severe skin toxicity was significantly associated with prolonged survival if these adverse skin effects occurred within the first 4–8 weeks of treatment [7c].

A safety study was conducted in 13 patients treated with vemurafenib (960 mg) twice daily for BRAF V600-mutated metastatic melanoma in the outpatient clinic. Adverse dermal effects occurred in all patients with the most common being hyperkeratotic perifollicular rash (69%) and photosensitivity (15%) with the rashes occurring primarily in the first month of treatment. Serious adverse events included the development of squamous cell carcinoma in 38% of the patients and occurred more frequently in women than in men (60% and 25%, respectively) [8c].

Psoriasis

Brodalumab

A literature review of three phase 3 trials (AMAGINE-1, NCT01708590; AMAGINE-2, NCT01708603; and AMAGINE-3, NCT01708629) evaluated the efficacy and safety profile of brodalumab, a monoclonal antibody interleukin-17 (IL-17) inhibitor for psoriasis treatment. Patients (AMAGINE-1, $n=661$; AMAGINE-2, $n=1831$; AMAGINE-3, $n=1881$) received brodalumab (140 or 210 mg) or placebo subcutaneously on day 1 and then once per week for weeks 1, 2, 4, 6, 8, and 10 for a duration of 12 weeks to 1 year. The analysis evaluated the pooled results from the trials at 12 weeks of treatment. Adverse events occurred with 210 mg brodalumab (57.6% of patients), 140 mg brodalumab (55.6% of patients) and placebo (51.0% of patients); the most common adverse effects were nasopharyngitis, upper respiratory tract infection, headache, and arthralgia. Serious adverse events included neutropenia and occurred more frequently with either dose of brodalumab than with placebo. In addition, two successful suicides were reported in the brodalumab group after 1 year of treatment, although it is unclear if these occurrences were treatment related [9R].

Methotrexate

Several case reports have described cutaneous adverse effects following overdoses of methotrexate, a commonly used medication for the treatment of psoriasis. The first report described cutaneous and mucosal adverse effects due to noncompliance with methotrexate use. A 58-year-old woman with psoriasis was prescribed methotrexate (10 mg) orally once per week supplemented with folic acid (5 mg) three times per week. She developed oral mucosal ulcerations and psoriatic plaques after daily oral use of 10 mg methotrexate for 10 days as opposed to the prescribed weekly dose and did not take the folic acid supplementation as directed [10A]. In the second case, a 43-year-old man was diagnosed with psoriasis and received oral methotrexate, 25 mg for 3 days and then 10 mg daily. After 10 days of treatment, ulcerated erythematous lesions developed across his body in addition to oral and genital erosions. Although folic acid supplementation was taken as directed, it was thought that the concurrent ingestion of 100 mg aspirin daily may have decreased the clearance rate of methotrexate, resulting in the accumulation of a toxic concentration of the drug [11A].

Etanercept

Etanercept, a tumor necrosis factor-alpha (TNF-α) inhibitor, is a widely used treatment for immunological diseases including rheumatoid and psoriatic arthritis, polyarticular juvenile idiopathic active, ankylosing spondylitis, and plaque psoriasis. A report described the development of figurate urticaria in a 65-year-old man following etanercept treatment for psoriasis. The patient initially received etanercept (50 mg) subcutaneously for 90 days with a substantial improvement in the symptoms causing the patient to discontinue the medication. The remaining lesions then worsened, resulting in hospitalization and re-administration of etanercept. An urticarial rash occurred 10 days after treatment was restarted; etanercept was discontinued and the rash was resolved [12A].

Infliximab

A retrospective cross-sectional study evaluated the adverse effects resulting from IV infusions of infliximab, a TNF-α inhibitor, for treatment of psoriasis. A total of 168 patients were separated into 2 groups: those with psoriasis ($n=24$) and those with arthritis or another chronic inflammatory disease such as rheumatoid arthritis, ankylosing spondylitis, Crohn's disease or ulcerative colitis ($n=144$). Severe adverse events requiring infliximab discontinuation occurred in 2 (8.3%) of the psoriasis patients and included a lupus-like reaction and an anaphylactic reaction. In the chronic inflammation group, sever adverse events causing treatment continuation occurred in 6 (4.2%) of the patients and included a lupus-like reaction, hyperemia, papular rash and an anaphylactic reaction [13C].

A meta-analysis of 13 controlled trials of 1816 patients assessed the efficacy and safety of IV infliximab (3 or 5 mg/kg) for the treatment of psoriasis vulgaris. The most common adverse events were pain, abnormal liver function tests, and infusion reactions; secondary infections including hepatitis and fungal disease frequently followed the initial effects [14M].

Ixekizumab

The safety and efficacy of ixekizumab, a recently approved monoclonal IL-17A antibody treatment for psoriasis, were evaluated in three phase 3 trials: UNCOVER-1 (1296 patients; NCT01474512), UNCOVER-2 (1224 patients; NCT01597245), and UNCOVER-3 (1346 patients; NCT01646177). In each trial, patients were divided into three groups: a 2-week dosing ixekizumab group (160 mg initially and then 80 mg every 2 weeks); a 4-week dosing ixekizumab group (160 mg initially and then 80 mg every 4 weeks); or placebo. Additional patients in the UNCOVER-2 and UNCOVER-3 trials received etanercept (50 mg) twice per week. All doses were given via subcutaneous injections and the treatment durations lasted for 60 weeks. The most common adverse events with ixekizumab treatment were nasopharyngitis, injection site reaction, neutropenia, *Candida* infection, and inflammatory bowel disease and occurred with greater frequency in the ixekizumab groups than in the placebo groups (54.8%–58.8% vs 46.8%, respectively). It was noted that the safety of ixekizumab beyond 60 weeks of administration is not known [15MC,16MC].

Secukinumab

A literature review of four phase 3 trials (NCT01365455, NCT01358578, NCT01555125, and NCT01636687) evaluated the efficacy and safety of secukinumab, a monoclonal IL-17A inhibitor recently approved for the treatment of psoriasis. The individual trial data were pooled for further analysis. A total 2075 patients with moderate-to-severe psoriasis received secukinumab (150 mg, $n=692$; or 300 mg, $n=691$) or placebo ($n=692$) subcutaneously once per week for weeks 1–3 and then once every 4 weeks for weeks 4–48. Adverse events were reported with 150 and 300 mg secukinumab (81.2% and 83.3%, respectively) and included nasopharyngitis, headache, diarrhea and upper respiratory tract infection. Serious adverse effects occurred in 6.9% and 7.0% of patients receiving 150 and 300 mg secukinumab, respectively; drug discontinuation occurred in 3.6% and 3.0% of the 150 and 300 mg groups, respectively [17R].

A second analysis evaluated the pooled data from 10 phase 2 and 3 trials to determine the safety of secukinumab treatment for moderate to severe plaque psoriasis. Patients ($n=3993$) received secukinumab (150 or 300 mg) or etanercept for 1 year. The adjusted incidence rates for total adverse events were similar between treatments (236.1, 239.9, and 243.4, respectively). Serious adverse events also occurred at similar incidence rates (7.4, 6.8, and 7.0, respectively) and included serious infections, malignant or unspecified tumors and major cardiovascular events [18R].

A case report described a 62-year-old man who received secukinumab for treatment of psoriasis that was unresponsive to other medications. Erosions and ulcers developed on the lower lip less than 1 week after starting secukinumab. The patient continued with secukinumab treatment due to improved psoriasis symptoms but the oral lesions continued for 3 months, at which time, secukinumab was discontinued. A biopsy of the oral lesions indicated a severe, ulcerative, lichenoid mucositis [19A].

Vitiligo

Azathioprine

A case report described a 52-year-old man treated with azathioprine (50 mg/day) for acral vitiligo who developed a high-grade fever, headache and painful vesicular skin rash 8 days after starting treatment. Leukocytosis with neutrophilia was found with clinical testing and a skin biopsy showed dense neutrophilic infiltration of dermis without signs of vasculitis. These results indicated a probable diagnosis of Sweet's syndrome. Azathioprine was discontinued, and the symptoms and skin lesions were resolved within 72 hours with high-dose oral prednisolone [20A].

Cutaneous Side Effects From Antibiotic Medications

Ceftaroline

A retrospective review of health records was completed of 96 hospitalized patients (median age=57 years) who received ceftaroline for methicillin-resistant cutaneous *Staphylococcus aureus* infections. Adverse events ($n=31$) occurred in 20 of these patients and included 15 hematologic and 9 cutaneous events. Hypersensitivity reactions were also reported (1 mucosal rash with lesions; 1 skin rash with desquamation; 2 possible organ-specific reactions). It was reported that the adverse reactions occurred in patients receiving a greater number of ceftaroline doses (median number=46) than those patients without reactions (median number=21) [21c].

Dalbavancin

Dalbavancin is a recently available antibiotic for treatment of acute bacterial skin and skin structure infections (ABSSSI) due to Gram-positive bacteria. This drug has a half-life of 14.4 days so it is possible that a single dose may be as effective as multiple dosing. A randomized, double-blind trial compared the safety and efficacy of dalbavancin given as a single IV dose or as the standard two doses (NCT02127970). A total of 698 patients with an

ABSSSI received IV dalbavancin infusion as a single dose (1500 mg; $n=349$) or in a weekly 2 dose regimen (1000 mg on day 1 and 500 mg 1 week later; $n=349$). Similar adverse effects at similar frequencies were reported with single dalbavancin dose (20.1%) and 2-dose dalbavancin (19.9%) and included nausea, headache and vomiting. Drug discontinuation due to adverse effects occurred with 6 patients receiving the single dose and with 5 patients in the 2-dose group [22C].

The safety of dalbavancin and comparative antibiotics was assessed in a pooled analysis of 14 phase 2 and 3 clinical trials. Patients ($n=3002$) received either dalbavancin ($n=1778$) or other antibiotics including vancomycin, linezolid, cefazolin, nafcillin, or oxacillin ($n=1224$). Adverse effects (nausea, headache, diarrhea, constipation, vomiting, rash, urinary tract infection, pruritus, and insomnia) were similar in both groups: dalbavancin (799 events; 44.9%) and comparative antibiotics (573 events; 46.8%). Serious adverse events ($n=3$) following dalbavancin treatment were cellulitis progression, leukopenia and an anaphylactoid reaction. For the comparative antibiotics, the serious adverse events ($n=9$) included acute renal failure, cellulitis, edema, pancytopenia, thrombocytopenia and pancreatitis [23R].

Levofloxacin

A 74-year-old woman, hospitalized for pneumonia, was treated with levofloxacin, a fluoroquinolone antibiotic. Erythematous macules developed within 6 hours of the first dose and purpuric lesions on 85% of her body were present by the next day. Levofloxacin was discontinued, and the symptoms were resolved with administration of omalizumab and prednisolone. A biopsy and clinical laboratory results indicated toxic epidermal necrolysis [24A].

Moxifloxacin

A 25-year-old woman with tuberculosis (TB) was hospitalized and treated with moxifloxacin, isoniazid, ethambutol, and pyrazinamide upon admission. Symptoms of a drug reaction with eosinophilia and systemic syndrome (DRESS) developed 10 days later; the symptoms improved with immunoglobulin and prednisolone treatment and the anti-TB therapy was changed to isoniazid, ethambutol, pyrazinamide, cycloserine, and streptomycin. This combination also caused a skin rash with itching, elevated liver enzymes and eosinophil counts. Although the anti-TB treatment was changed again to cycloserine, streptomycin, ethionamide, and *para*-aminosalicylic acid, the symptoms continued. At this time, all medications were discontinued except for streptomycin which was then changed to moxifloxacin. The patient then developed erythematous pustules with desquamation, fissures, and swelling which was diagnosed as moxifloxacin-induced acute generalized exanthematous pustulosis (AGEP) [25A].

Nitrofurantoin

A case of drug reaction with eosinophilia and systemic symptom (DRESS) was reported in a 34-year-old woman after receiving nitrofurantoin (100 mg) three times per day for 6 days for treatment of an urinary tract infection. Nitrofurantoin was discontinued and the patient fully recovered in a few weeks with intensive supportive treatment [26A].

Piperacillin and Tazobactam

A case report described a 74-year-old woman received a combination piperacillin and tazobactam antibiotic treatment for pneumonia upon hospitalization. Acute generalized exanthematous pustulosis (AGEP) in conjunction with drug-related rash with eosinophilia and systemic symptoms (DRESS) developed 9 days after start of the therapy. The symptoms responded to steroid administration but the patient expired due to worsening of the pneumonia [27A].

Vancomycin

A literature review analyzed the extent of vancomycin-induced hypersensitivity reactions. The analysis comprised of 57 articles that described 71 hypersensitivity cases due to vancomycin treatment, and the reactions were divided into those of immediate onset and those that were nonimmediate or delayed. Immediate reactions included 7 cases of anaphylaxis. Nonimmediate reactions (64 cases) were also reported and included linear IgA bullous dermatosis ($n = 34$), drug rash eosinophilia and systemic symptoms (DRESS) syndrome ($n = 16$), acute interstitial nephritis ($n = 8$), and Stevens–Johnson syndrome/toxic epidermal necrolysis ($n = 6$). The median duration of vancomycin therapy prior to the nonimmediate reactions was 7–26 days. A total of 4 deaths (6%) were attributed to occurrence of hypersensitivity reactions [28R].

Cutaneous Side Effects From Antiviral Medications

Interferon-Alpha and Ribavirin

A 50-year-old man received pegylated interferon-alpha and ribavirin treatment for a recently diagnosed acute hepatitis C infection. Red scaly papular skin lesions developed 3 weeks later and progressed to severe erythrodermia in spite of steroid treatment. Psoriasis vulgaris was diagnosed via skin biopsy. The interferon-alpha and ribavirin treatment was stopped, and the steroid levels were increased [29A].

Nevirapine

Nevirapine is an antiretroviral medication for the treatment of HIV and is known to be associated with severe skin reactions. A case–control study was conducted in a South African hospital to quantify this association between nevirapine treatment and severe skin reactions. Patients (n = 91 with previous reactions; n = 361 matched controls) received nevirapine for 120 days; 169 severe skin reactions (Stevens–Johnson syndrome/toxic epidermal necrolysis, 49%; drug hypersensitivity syndrome, 36%) were reported. Development of a severe skin reaction was independently associated with nevirapine treatment with an adjusted odds ratio of 7.6 [30c].

A case report described a 72-year-old HIV-positive man was hospitalized with a diffuse, erythematous and maculopapular skin rash over 100% of his body after 3 weeks of a combination therapy: zidovudine (300 mg), lamivudine (150 mg) and nevirapine (200 mg). Toxic epidermal necrolysis was diagnosed using clinical symptoms, a positive Nikolsky's sign and skin histology. In spite of aggressive treatment and discontinuation of the combination therapy, the patient died 7 days after admission. Nevirapine was identified as the causative agent using the Naranjo algorithm (Naranjo score = 8) and the WHO-UMC standardized case causality assessment criteria [31A].

Telaprevir

The incidence of adverse dermal effects associated with use of the antiviral telaprevir in the treatment of chronic hepatitis C has reportedly increased. A prospective study determined the frequency of skin reactions associated with telaprevir in 60 hospitalized hepatitis C patients. Telaprevir-related skin reactions were found in 48.3% of the patients (29/60) while 31 patients did not have any reactions. The skin reactions started an average of 9 weeks from the start of treatment and were characterized by eczematous reactions and spongiotic dermatitis. Severe reactions (grade 3) were reported in 8 patients, and telaprevir was discontinued in 6 patients [32c].

Cutaneous Side Effects From Cancer Medications

Afatinib

Afatinib, an epidermal growth factor receptor (EGFR) inhibitor for the treatment of non-small-cell lung cancers positive for EGFR mutations, is known to frequently cause cutaneous adverse effects. A case report described a 39-year-old woman who received afatinib treatment for a newly diagnosed EGFR-mutation-positive inoperative lung adenocarcinoma. A rapidly worsening severe papulopustular eruption developed over the next several days in conjunction with significant tumor reduction. Afatinib treatment was discontinued, and the skin effects were resolved with oral and topical corticosteroids, oral antibiotics, and oral antihistamines [33A].

Aflibercept

Aflibercept, an engineered humanized anti-vascular endothelial growth factor (VEGF) treatment for colorectal cancer, has been associated with severe infections. A meta-analysis of 10 phase 2 and 3 prospective clinical trials was conducted to determine the risk of aflibercept-associated infections in 4310 cancer patients with solid tumors. Aflibercept-associated severe infections were reported in 7.3% of the patients with a relative risk of 1.87. Fatal infections occurred in up to 6.7% of the patients with a 2.2% mortality rate; the occurrence of fatal infections had an odds ratio of 2.16. The analysis also found that the risk of infection was significantly greater with aflibercept treatment than with bevacizumab, another anti-VEGF agent used to treat colorectal cancer [34M].

Cabozantinib

A meta-analysis determined the incidence and risk of hand–foot skin reactions associated with cabozantinib, an oral multikinase inhibitor used to treat metastatic medullary thyroid cancer. The analysis included 8 phase 2 and 3 clinical trials with a total of 831 patients treated with cabozantinib (100–175 mg) for solid tumor cancers. The overall incidence of cabozantinib-associated hand–foot skin reactions was 35.3% (relative risk = 27.3) and 9.5% for high-grade reactions (relative risk = 28.1) [35M].

Capecitabine

Capecitabine is an oral fluoropyrimidine used for treatment of metastatic breast and colon cancer and is known to cause adverse skin reactions. A report described the development of diffuse scleroderma in an 86-year-old woman treated with capecitabine for metastatic colorectal cancer. It was noted that the development of scleroderma was not accompanied by a hand-and-foot reaction as in previous cases of capecitabine-induced disease [36A].

Enzalutamide

Enzalutamide is an inhibitor of the androgen receptor signaling pathway used for the treatment of metastatic castration-resistant prostate cancer. A report described the development of acute generalized exanthematous pustulosis (AEGP) in a 62-year-old man with metastatic prostatic adenocarcinoma who received enzalutamide treatment. A skin reaction with plaques and pustules developed 10 days after starting treatment; enzalutamide was discontinued and the lesions were completely resolve in 4 weeks with supportive care. An evaluation of the criteria listed by the European Study of Severe Cutaneous Adverse Reactions resulted in an AEGP score of 7, indicating that the patient had experienced enzalutamide-induced AGEP [37A].

Erlotinib

Erlotinib, an epidermal growth factor receptor (EGFR) inhibitor for treatment of non-small-cell lung cancer, is frequently associated with papulopustular eruptions. It was reported that a 73-year-old woman who was treated with erlotinib for 3 months for lung adenocarcinoma developed a rash with nonpruritic papules and pustules over her body after 2 months. The pustules contained methicillin-sensitive S. aureus and histological analysis of the papules showed cellular damage and inflammatory cell infiltration. Erlotinib was discontinued and the rash was resolved with azithromycin [38A].

Regorafenib

A clinical study in 5 French cancer hospitals evaluated the safety and efficacy of regorafenib, a multikinase inhibitor treatment for chemotherapy-refractory metastatic colorectal cancer. Patients ($n = 29$) with colorectal tumors and refractory to standard chemotherapies received oral regorafenib (80, 120 or 160 mg per day) for a median duration of 2.5 months. Cutaneous adverse events (generally hand–foot skin reactions) occurred in 20% of the patients. Stevens–Johnson syndrome/toxic epidermal necrolysis occurred in 1 patient receiving 120 mg regorafenib per day [39c].

Sorafenib

Sorafenib, an oral multitargeted kinase inhibitor, is frequently used for the treatment of hepatocellular and metastatic renal cell carcinomas. However, multiple clinical trials and postmarketing surveillance studies have shown that sorafenib treatment was directly linked to drug-induced cutaneous reactions. A large, international, prospective, observational study (GIDEON; Global Investigation of Therapeutic Decisions in Hepatocellular Carcinoma and of its Treatment with Sorafenib; NCT0082175) reported that the most common adverse skin effect of once daily sorafenib treatment (800 mg) was hand–foot skin reaction, occurring in approximately 50% of patients. Study results were reported for the Chinese cohort ($n = 338$) [40C], the Korean cohort ($n = 482$) [41C] and the Japanese cohort ($n = 508$) [42C]. In addition, a prospective postmarketing all-patient surveillance study (NCT01411436) in Japan of 1109 patients treated with sorafenib (400 mg) twice daily for unresectable hepatocellular carcinoma found that 44.5% of the patients had discontinued treatment due to the development of adverse events including hand–foot skin reaction [43C].

Cutaneous Side Effects From Neurological Medications

Lamotrigine

Several case reports describe the development of drug rash with eosinophilia and systemic symptoms (DRESS) syndrome following administration of lamotrigine, an antiepileptic drug. The first report described a 37-year-old woman who developed DRESS after taking lamotrigine for treatment of limbic encephalitis. She also had a concurrent reactivation of the Epstein–Barr virus (EBV), resulting in an autoimmune reaction. Lamotrigine was discontinued and the symptoms improved with methylprednisolone and IV immunoglobulin [44A]. The second report described a 30-year-old woman with a diagnosis of DRESS after receiving lamotrigine (50 mg per day) for 40 days. A skin biopsy also showed characteristics of a cutaneous CD30+ lymphoma. The symptoms were resolved with oral prednisolone [45A].

Oxcarbazepine

Oxcarbazepine, an antiepileptic drug for the treatment of seizures, has been known to cause severe adverse skin reactions including Stevens–Johnson syndrome, toxic epidermal necrolysis, DRESS and maculopapular eruption reactions. A case report described a 35-year-old man who developed DRESS syndrome 3 weeks after using oxcarbazepine for a seizure disorder. Oxcarbazepine was discontinued and the symptoms gradually improved with oral and topical corticosteroids [46A].

Several studies have investigated the relationship between the human leukocyte antigen (HLA) genotype and risk of oxcarbazepine-induced severe adverse skin reactions. A prospective trial of 50 patients with previously reported oxcarbazepine-induced reactions found a significant association between the HLA-B*15:02 allele and the occurrence of the drug-induced reactions (odds ratio of 27.90) while no association was found for HLA-A*31:01 [47c].

Phenytoin

Phenytoin, an anti-convulsant, is known to induce severe skin reactions including Stevens–Johnson syndrome (SJS), toxic epidermal necrolysis (TEN), and drug reactions with eosinophilia and systemic symptoms (DRESS). The association between HLA or cytochrome (CYP) P450 genotype and phenytoin-induced drug reactions has been investigated in several studies. A case–control study of 152 Thai patients (60 with phenytoin-related reactions and 92 controls) found significant associations (odds ratio range of 4–10) between phenytoin-related SJS and TEN and 6 HLA alleles (HLA-A*33:03, HLA-B*38:02, HLA-B*51:01, HLA-B*56:02, HLA-B*58:01, and HLA-C*14:02). The HLA-B*51:01 allele, however, was significantly associated only with

phenytoin-related DRESS. No significant association was found with the HLA-B*15:02 allele and any phenytoin-induced reactions. The CYP2C9*3 polymorphism also showed a greater risk of phenytoin-related SJS or TEN (odds ratio of 4.30) but no significant association with DRESS development [48C]. A similar case–control study in Malay individuals (phenytoin-induced reactions, $n=16$; phenytoin-tolerant controls, $n=32$; healthy controls, $n=300$) found significant associations between HLA-B*15:13 and phenytoin-related SJS/TEN (odds ratio of 11.28) and phenytoin-related DRESS (odds ratio of 59). HLA-B*15:02 was also associated with phenytoin-induced reactions (odds ratio of 5.71) [49C].

Sulthiame

A report described a 10-year-old girl with anti-epileptic drug resistance who received sulthiame treatment for greater seizure control. A fever with a diffuse erythematous maculopapular rash, elevated transaminases and atypical lymphocytes developed 5 weeks after administration of sulthiame; thrombocytopenia, hepatosplenomegaly, and pneumonitis developed 3 days later. Sulthiame was discontinued and complete resolution of the symptoms occurred within 30 days with methylprednisolone treatment. Sulthiame-induced drug reaction with eosinophilia and systemic symptoms (DRESS) syndrome was diagnosed based on laboratory and skin histology results [50A].

Individual Medications

Acetaminophen

A case of toxic epidermal necrolysis (TEN) was reported in a 43-year-old Japanese woman with poorly controlled ulcerative colitis treated with high doses of prednisolone, infliximab, acetaminophen and lansoprazole. Targetoid erythematous and bullous lesions appeared 9 days after starting acetaminophen treatment; these lesions spread rapidly, resulting in skin detachment over almost 100% of her body within 3 weeks and was diagnosed as TEN. Acetaminophen was identified as the causative drug via a high stimulation index in lymphocyte transformation tests; no positive results were reported with the other drugs [51A].

Allopurinol

Allopurinol, a xanthine oxidase inhibitor, is commonly used for the treatment of hyperuricemia and gout. Several recent case reports have described the development of severe skin adverse events associated with allopurinol treatment. The first report described development of Sweet's syndrome in an 87-year-old woman following treatment with allopurinol for hyperuricemia. The symptoms developed 8 days after the treatment started and included fever, painful edema in the extremities with non-pruritic erythematous plaques and pus-filled skin blisters, conjunctivitis, splenomegaly and joint pain. Treatment with IV methylprednisolone during hospitalization resulted in rapid resolution of all symptoms. A likely association between the development of Sweet's syndrome and allopurinol treatment was indicated via the Naranjo adverse drug reaction probability scale [52A]. A second report described skin rash, eosinophilia, and renal impairment in a 62-year-old man with chronic kidney disease, hypertension and gout after receiving allopurinol for 2 weeks. The patient was mistakenly taking a 1200 mg daily dose as opposed to the prescribed 300 mg daily dose. The symptoms resolved when allopurinol was discontinued and high-dose steroids administered; allopurinol-induced drug-induced rash with eosinophilia and systemic symptoms (DRESS) syndrome was diagnosed based on patient history and laboratory values [53A].

Several studies investigated previous reports that the human leukocyte antigen (HLA) HLA-B*58:01 genotype is associated with allopurinol-induced severe cutaneous adverse reactions. A correlation study of 146 patients with severe allopurinol-induced dermal adverse reactions and 285 patients tolerant to allopurinol found that the HLA-B*58:01 allele was significantly associated with severe skin reactions (odds ratio of 44.0) and disease severity (odds ratio of 44.0). The risk of allopurinol-induced severe skin effects was also dependent upon the heterozygosity of the HLA-B*58:01 allele with an odds ratios of 15.25 for heterozygotes and 72.45 for homozygotes. In addition, the risk of drug-induced reactions was increased with severe renal impairment in HLA-B*58:01 patients [54C]. A retrospective and prospective case–control study compared patients with severe allopurinol-induced skin reactions ($n = 30$), patients tolerant to allopurinol ($n = 100$), and a general population ($n = 1095$). Genotype analysis showed that 96.7% of the patients who experienced allopurinol-induced reactions were at least heterozygous for the HLA-B*58:01 allele as compared to 4.0% of the allopurinol-tolerant patients. This analysis showed that allopurinol-induced severe skin reactions were significantly associated with the HLA-B*58:01 allele with an odds ratio of 696.0 [55C].

Daclizumab

A multicenter, randomized, double-blind, active-controlled phase 3 trial (DECIDE; NCT01064401) assessed the frequency and type of adverse skin effects caused by administration of daclizumab high-yield process (HYP), a humanized anti-CD25 antibody for treatment of multiple sclerosis. A total of 1841 patients with relapsing multiple sclerosis received either daclizumab HYP (150 mg; $n = 919$) subcutaneously every 4 weeks or interferon beta-1a (30 mcg; $n = 922$) intramuscularly once

per week. The treatment duration for both drugs was 96–144 weeks. The majority of adverse effects were mild or moderate for daclizumab and interferon (37% and 19%, respectively); the most common effects with both drugs were dermatitis, rash and eczema. Serious cutaneous adverse events occurred in 14 (2%) of the daclizumab HYP patients and in 1 (<1%) interferon beta-1a patient, resulting discontinuation of daclizumab (2% of patients) and interferon (0.8% of patients) [56MC].

A phase 1, open-label study also assessed the occurrence of cutaneous adverse events associated with administration of daclizumab HYP (NCT01143441). A total of 31 patients were divided into two groups: previous treatment with IV daclizumab HYP ($n = 16$) and no anti-CD25 treatment ($n = 15$). Adverse events were observed in 77% of patients; the majority was eczema that required no treatment. A serious adverse event was the development of a moderate to severe rash in 6 daclizumab HYP patients (19%), resulting in drug discontinuation in 4 patients [57C].

Etoricoxib

A report described a 74-year-old woman who developed widespread erythematous lesions on her body and recurrent blistering on the fingers within several hours of taking etoricoxib, a non-steroid, anti-inflammatory drug (NSAID). The symptoms were resolved with topical betamethasone and fusidic acid although residual pigmentation was present 6 weeks later. Etoricoxib was confirmed as the causative agent with a skin patch [58A].

Fexofenadine

It was reported that a 40-year-old woman developed fever with multiple erythematous nonfollicular pustules 2 days after starting the oral antihistamine fexofenadine (180 mg) for treatment of rhinitis. Fexofenadine-induced acute generalized exanthematous pustulosis (AGEP) was identified based on the clinical symptoms, histopathology and a Naranjo adverse drug reaction probability score of 9. Fexofenadine was discontinued and the symptoms resolved within 8–10 days [59A].

Ibuprofen

A report described a 22-year-old man who developed Stevens–Johnson syndrome and toxic epidermal necrolysis after 3 doses of ibuprofen (400 mg) orally every 8 hours. Ibuprofen was discontinued and the symptoms were resolved with antibiotics and IV corticosteroids [60A].

Methotrexate

A retrospective cohort study determined the risk of a second nonmelanoma skin cancer in rheumatoid arthritis (RA) and inflammatory bowel disease (IBD) patients receiving treatment with methotrexate, anti-tumor necrosis factor (anti-TNF) or thiopurines after an initial skin cancer diagnosis. A total of 9460 Medicare patients (RA, $n = 6841$; IBD, $n = 2788$) were enrolled in the study. The average incidence rate of a second skin cancer per 1000 person-years was 58.2 and 58.9 for RA and IBD patients, respectively. Methotrexate, when used concurrently with other medications, was associated with an increased risk of a second skin cancer (hazard ratio of 1.60) for RA patients. The addition of anti-TNF drugs also showed an increased risk (hazard ratio of 1.49). No increased risk of secondary skin cancer was found with the other medications, abatacept and rituximab [61MC].

Pirfenidone

A severe phototoxic reaction was reported in a 64-year-old man treated for 30 days with pirfenidone, an oral antifibrotic agent, for treatment of idiopathic pulmonary fibrosis. The symptoms included a strong generalized exfoliative erythema and intense itching with fatigue and mild fever after 5 days strong sun exposure. Laboratory analysis showed increased levels of inflammatory markers and a lymphocytic inflammatory infiltrate was evident upon skin biopsy. Pirfenidone was discontinued and resolution of the lesions occurred within 20 days with oral and topical steroid and oral antihistamine administration [62A].

Strontium Ranelate

Strontium ranelate, a treatment for postmenopausal osteoporosis, has been associated with the development of drug rash with eosinophilia and systemic symptoms (DRESS) syndrome as described in two case reports. First, a woman with postmenopausal osteoporosis developed DRESS syndrome with a generalized maculopapular rash, eosinophilia, dyspnea, bilateral cervical lymphadenopathy, and reactivation of the Epstein–Barr virus (EBV) with liver damage 3 weeks after starting strontium ranelate treatment. Autoimmune hepatitis developed 6 months after resolution of the dermal symptoms [63A]. In the second case, the DRESS symptoms occurred 3 weeks after starting strontium ranelate and involved reactivation of a systemic human herpes virus (HHV)-7 infection. The symptoms included a maculopapular skin rash with fever and leukocyte and liver abnormalities. Strontium ranelate was discontinued but the symptoms worsened and the patient did not survive [64A].

TUMOR NECROSIS FACTOR (TNF) INHIBITORS

A population-based cohort study characterized the risk of squamous cell and basal cell skin cancer development associated with TNF inhibitor treatment for rheumatoid arthritis. The analysis included several cohorts of patients from Swedish health registry data: the first cohort ($n = 46\,409$) included patients with rheumatoid arthritis without prior TNF inhibitor treatment, the second cohort ($n = 12\,558$) patients with rheumatoid arthritis who received TNF inhibitor treatment and the third cohort consisted of matched general population individuals. A greater hazard ratio (HR) for development of basal cell cancer was associated with rheumatoid arthritis without TNF inhibitor treatment; $HR = 1.22$ for TNF inhibitor-naive rheumatoid arthritis patients vs the general population while the HR was 1.14 for TNF inhibitor-treated patients as compared to those without treatment. The results for squamous cell cancer were similar; $HR = 1.88$ for no inhibitor treatment vs the general population and $HR = 1.30$ for TNF inhibitor treatment vs no inhibitor treatment. It was also found that the use of TNF inhibitors in individuals with a history of squamous cell or basal cell cancer did not create any further risks for recurrence of these diseases [65R].

References

[1] Child F, Ortiz-Romero PL, Alvarez R, et al. Phase II multicentre trial of oral quisinostat, a histone deacetylase inhibitor, in patients with previously treated stage IB-IVA mycosis fungoides/Sézary syndrome. Br J Dermatol. 2016;175(1):80–8 [C].

[2] Cebollero A, Puértolas T, Pajares I, et al. Comparative safety of BRAF and MEK inhibitors (vemurafenib, dabrafenib and trametinib) in first-line therapy for BRAF-mutated metastatic melanoma. Mol Clin Oncol. 2016;5(4):458–62 [c].

[3] Hwang SJ, Carlos G, Wakade D, et al. Ipilimumab-induced acute generalized exanthematous pustulosis in a patient with metastatic melanoma. Melanoma Res. 2016;26(4):417–20 [A].

[4] Koelzer VH, Buser T, Willi N, et al. Grover's-like drug eruption in a patient with metastatic melanoma under ipilimumab therapy. J Immunother Cancer. 2016;4:47 [A].

[5] Nayar N, Briscoe K, Fernandez Penas P. Toxic epidermal necrolysis-like reaction with severe satellite cell necrosis associated with nivolumab in a patient with ipilimumab refractory metastatic melanoma. J Immunother. 2016;39(3):149–52 [A].

[6] Hwang SJ, Carlos G, Chou S, et al. Bullous pemphigoid, an autoantibody-mediated disease, is a novel immune-related adverse event in patients treated with anti-programmed cell death 1 antibodies. Melanoma Res. 2016;26(4):413–6 [c].

[7] Peuvrel L, Quéreux G, Saint-Jean M, et al. Profile of vemurafenib-induced severe skin toxicities. J Eur Acad Dermatol Venereol. 2016;30(2):250–7 [c].

[8] Nowara E, Huszno J, Slomian G, et al. Skin toxicity in BRAF(V600) mutated metastatic cutaneous melanoma patients treated with vemurafenib. Postepy Dermatol Alergol. 2016;33(1):52–6 [c].

[9] Farahnik B, Beroukhim K, Abrouk M, et al. Brodalumab for the treatment of psoriasis: a review of phase III trials. Dermatol Ther (Heidelb). 2016;6(2):111–24 [R].

[10] Souza CF, Suarez OM, Silva TF, et al. Ulcerations due to methotrexate toxicity in a psoriasis patient. An Bras Dermatol. 2016;91(3):375–7 [A].

[11] Knoll K, Anzengruber F, Cozzio A, et al. Mucocutaneous ulcerations and pancytopenia due to methotrexate overdose. Case Rep Dermatol. 2016;8(3):287–93 [A].

[12] Sessa M, Sullo MG, Mascolo A, et al. A case of figurate urticaria by etanercept. J Pharmacol Pharmacother. 2016;7(2):106–8 [A].

[13] Antonio JR, Sanmiguel J, Cagnon GV, et al. Infliximab in patients with psoriasis and other inflammatory diseases: evaluation of adverse events in the treatment of 168 patients. An Bras Dermatol. 2016;91(3):306–10 [C].

[14] Wang J, Zhan Q, Zhang L. A systematic review on the efficacy and safety of infliximab in patients with psoriasis. Hum Vaccin Immunother. 2016;12(2):431–7 [M].

[15] Gordon KB, Blauvelt A, Papp KA, et al. Phase 3 trials of ixekizumab in moderate-to-severe plaque psoriasis. N Engl J Med. 2016;375(4):345–56 [MC].

[16] Farahnik B, Beroukhim K, Zhu TH, et al. Ixekizumab for the treatment of psoriasis: a review of phase III trials. Dermatol Ther (Heidelb). 2016;6(1):25–37 [MC].

[17] Kircik L, Fowler J, Weiss J, et al. Efficacy of secukinumab for moderate-to-severe head and neck psoriasis over 52 weeks: pooled analysis of four phase 3 studies. Dermatol Ther (Heidelb). 2016;6(4):627–38 [R].

[18] van de Kerkhof PC, Griffiths CE, Reich K, et al. Secukinumab long-term safety experience: a pooled analysis of 10 phase II and III clinical studies in patients with moderate to severe plaque psoriasis. J Am Acad Dermatol. 2016;75(1):83–98.e4 [R].

[19] Thompson JM, Cohen LM, Yang CS, et al. Severe, ulcerative, lichenoid mucositis associated with secukinumab. JAAD Case Rep. 2016;2(5):384–6 [A].

[20] Biswas SN, Chakraborty PP, Gantait K, et al. Azathioprine-induced bullous Sweet's syndrome: a rare association. BMJ Case Rep. 2016;2016. http://dx.doi.org/10.1136/bcr-2016-215192 [A].

[21] Blumenthal KG, Kuhlen Jr. JL, Weil AA, et al. Adverse drug reactions associated with ceftaroline use: a 2-center retrospective cohort. J Allergy Clin Immunol Pract. 2016;4(4):740–6 [c].

[22] Dunne MW, Puttagunta S, Giordano P, et al. A randomized clinical trial of single-dose versus weekly dalbavancin for treatment of acute bacterial skin and skin structure infection. Clin Infect Dis. 2016;62(5):545–51 [C].

[23] Dunne MW, Talbot GH, Boucher HW, et al. Safety of dalbavancin in the treatment of skin and skin structure infections: a pooled analysis of randomized, comparative studies. Drug Saf. 2016;39(2):147–57 [R].

[24] Uzun R, Yalcin AD, Celik B, et al. Levofloxacin induced toxic epidermal necrolysis: successful therapy with omalizumab (anti-IgE) and pulse prednisolone. Am J Case Rep. 2016;17:666–71 [A].

[25] Kim H, Bang ES, Lim SK, et al. DRESS syndrome and acute generalized exanthematous pustulosis induced by antituberculosis medications and moxifloxacin: case report. Int J Clin Pharmacol Ther. 2016;54(10):808–15 [A].

[26] Singh J, Dinkar A, Atam V, et al. Drug reaction with eosinophilia and systemic symptoms syndrome associated with nitrofurantoin. J Res Pharm Pract. 2016;5(1):70–3 [A].

[27] Kim TI, Jeong KH, Shin MK, et al. Piperacillin/tazobactam-associated hypersensitivity syndrome with overlapping features of acute generalized exanthematous pustulosis and drug-related rash with eosinophilia and systemic symptoms syndrome. Ann Dermatol. 2016;28(1):98–101 [A].

[28] Minhas JS, Wickner PG, Long AA, et al. Immune-mediated reactions to vancomycin: a systematic case review and analysis. Ann Allergy Asthma Immunol. 2016;116(6):544–53 [R].

[29] Lemmenmeier E, Gaus B, Schmid P, et al. A case of erythrodermia from exacerbated psoriasis vulgaris due to treatment of acute hepatitis C. BMC Dermatol. 2016;16(1):5 [A].

[30] Stewart A, Lehloenya R, Boulle A, et al. Severe antiretroviral-associated skin reactions in South African patients: a case series and case-control analysis. Pharmacoepidemiol Drug Saf. 2016;25(11):1313–9 [c].

[31] Paik S, Sen S, Era N, et al. Fatal nevirapine-induced toxic epidermal necrolysis in a HIV infected patient. J Clin Diagn Res. 2016;10(3):FD03–6 [A].

[32] Carrascosa R, Capusan TM, Llamas-Velasco M, et al. High frequency of severe telaprevir-associated skin eruptions in clinical practice. Acta Derm Venereol. 2016;96(1):97–9 [c].

[33] Osborn LP, Cohen PR. Afatinib-associated cutaneous toxicity: a correlation of severe skin reaction with dramatic tumor response in a woman with exon 19 deletion positive non-small-cell lung cancer. Cureus. 2016;8(9)e763 [A].

[34] Zhang X, Ran Y, Shao Y, et al. Incidence and risk of severe infections associated with aflibercept in cancer patients: a systematic review and meta-analysis. Br J Clin Pharmacol. 2016;81(1):33–40 [M].

[35] Belum VR, Serna-Tamayo C, Wu S, et al. Incidence and risk of hand-foot skin reaction with cabozantinib, a novel multikinase inhibitor: a meta-analysis. Clin Exp Dermatol. 2016;41(1):8–15 [M].

[36] Saif MW, Agarwal A, Hellinger J, et al. Scleroderma in a patient on capecitabine: is this a variant of hand-foot syndrome? Cureus. 2016;8(6)e663 [A].

[37] Alberto C, Konstantinou MP, Martinage C, et al. Enzalutamide induced acute generalized exanthematous pustulosis. J Dermatol Case Rep. 2016;10(2):35–8 [A].

[38] Akoglu G, Yavuz SO, Metin A. Erlotinib-induced purpuric papulopustular eruption treated with pulsed azithromycin. Indian J Pharmacol. 2016;48(3):324–6 [A].

[39] Calcagno F, Lenoble S, Lakkis Z, et al. Efficacy, safety and cost of regorafenib in patients with metastatic colorectal cancer in French clinical practice. Clin Med Insights Oncol. 2016;10:59–66 [c].

[40] Ye SL, Chen X, Yang J, et al. Safety and efficacy of sorafenib therapy in patients with hepatocellular carcinoma: final outcome from the Chinese patient subset of the GIDEON study. Oncotarget. 2016;7(6):6639–48 [C].

[41] Kim DY, Kim HJ, Han KH, et al. Real-life experience of sorafenib treatment for hepatocellular carcinoma in Korea: from GIDEON data. Cancer Res Treat. 2016;48(4):1243–52 [C].

[42] Kudo M, Ikeda M, Takayama T, et al. Safety and efficacy of sorafenib in Japanese patients with hepatocellular carcinoma in clinical practice: a subgroup analysis of GIDEON. J Gastroenterol. 2016;51(12):1150–60 [C].

[43] Kaneko S, Ikeda K, Matsuzaki Y, et al. Safety and effectiveness of sorafenib in Japanese patients with hepatocellular carcinoma in daily medical practice: interim analysis of a prospective postmarketing all-patient surveillance study. J Gastroenterol. 2016;51(10):1011–21 [C].

[44] Ozisik L, Tanriover MD, Saka E. Autoimmune limbic encephalitis and syndrome of inappropriate antidiuretic hormone secretion associated with lamotrigine-induced drug rash with eosinophilia and systemic symptoms (DRESS) syndrome. Intern Med. 2016;55(10):1393–6 [A].

[45] Stephan F, Haber R, Kechichian E, et al. Lamotrigine-induced hypersensitivity syndrome with histologic features of CD30+ lymphoma. Indian J Dermatol. 2016;61(2):235 [A].

[46] Saha M, Gorai S, Madhab V. Oxcarbazepine-induced drug rash with eosinophilia and systemic symptoms syndrome presenting as exfoliative dermatitis. J Pharmacol Pharmacother. 2016;7(3):142–5 [A].

[47] Moon J, Kim TJ, Lim JA, et al. HLA-B*40:02 and DRB1*04:03 are risk factors for oxcarbazepine-induced maculopapular eruption. Epilepsia. 2016;57(11):1879–86 [c].

[48] Tassaneeyakul W, Prabmeechai N, Sukasem C, et al. Associations between HLA class I and cytochrome P450 2C9 genetic polymorphisms and phenytoin-related severe cutaneous adverse reactions in a Thai population. Pharmacogenet Genomics. 2016;26(5):225–34 [C].

[49] Chang CC, Ng CC, Too CL, et al. Association of HLA-B*15:13 and HLA-B*15:02 with phenytoin-induced severe cutaneous adverse reactions in a Malay population. Pharmacogenomics J. 2016;17(2): 170–3.

[50] Fong CY, Hashim N, Gan CS, et al. Sulthiame-induced drug reaction with eosinophilia and systemic symptoms (DRESS) syndrome. Eur J Paediatr Neurol. 2016;20(6):957–61 [A].

[51] Watanabe H, Kamiyama T, Sasaki S, et al. Toxic epidermal necrolysis caused by acetaminophen featuring almost 100% skin detachment: acetaminophen is associated with a risk of severe cutaneous adverse reactions. J Dermatol. 2016;43(3):321–4 [A].

[52] Polimeni G, Cardillo R, Garaffo E, et al. Allopurinol-induced Sweet's syndrome. Int J Immunopathol Pharmacol. 2016;29(2):329–32 [A].

[53] Jmeian A, Hawatmeh A, Shamoon R, et al. Skin rash, eosinophilia, and renal impairment in a patient recently started on allopurinol. J Family Med Prim Care. 2016;5(2):479–81 [A].

[54] Ng CY, Yeh YT, Wang CW, et al. Impact of the HLA-B(*)58:01 allele and renal impairment on allopurinol-induced cutaneous adverse reactions. J Invest Dermatol. 2016;136(7):1373–81 [C].

[55] Sukasem C, Jantararoungtong T, Kuntawong P, et al. HLA-B (*) 58:01 for allopurinol-induced cutaneous adverse drug reactions: implication for clinical interpretation in Thailand. Front Pharmacol. 2016;7:186 [C].

[56] Krueger JG, Kircik L, Hougeir F, et al. Cutaneous adverse events in the randomized, double-blind, active-comparator DECIDE study of daclizumab high-yield process versus intramuscular interferon beta-1a in relapsing-remitting multiple sclerosis. Adv Ther. 2016;33(7):1231–45 [MC].

[57] Cortese I, Ohayon J, Fenton K, et al. Cutaneous adverse events in multiple sclerosis patients treated with daclizumab. Neurology. 2016;86(9):847–55 [C].

[58] Sousa AS, Cardoso JC, Gouveia MP, et al. Fixed drug eruption by etoricoxib confirmed by patch test. An Bras Dermatol. 2016;91(5):652–4 [A].

[59] Gupta T, Garg VK, Sarkar R, et al. Acute generalized exanthematous pustulosis induced by fexofenadine. Indian J Dermatol. 2016;61(2):235 [A].

[60] Angadi SS, Karn A. Ibuprofen induced Stevens-Johnson syndrome—toxic epidermal necrolysis in Nepal. Asia Pac Allergy. 2016;6(1):70–3 [A].

[61] Scott FI, Mamtani R, Brensinger CM, et al. Risk of nonmelanoma skin cancer associated with the use of immunosuppressant and biologic agents in patients with a history of autoimmune disease and nonmelanoma skin cancer. JAMA Dermatol. 2016;152(2):164–72 [MC].

[62] Papakonstantinou E, Prasse A, Schacht V, et al. Pirfenidone-induced severe phototoxic reaction in a patient with idiopathic lung fibrosis. J Eur Acad Dermatol Venereol. 2016;30(8):1354–6 [A].

[63] di Meo N, Gubertini N, Crocè L, et al. DRESS syndrome with autoimmune hepatitis from strontium ranelate. Cutis. 2016;97(5): E22–6 [A].

[64] Drago F, Cogorno L, Broccolo F, et al. A fatal case of DRESS induced by strontium ranelate associated with HHV-7 reactivation. Osteoporos Int. 2016;27(3):1261–4 [A].

[65] Raaschou P, Simard JF, Asker Hagelberg C, et al. Rheumatoid arthritis, anti-tumour necrosis factor treatment, and risk of squamous cell and basal cell skin cancer: cohort study based on nationwide prospectively recorded data from Sweden. BMJ. 2016;352:i262 [R].

13

Antihistamines (H1 Receptor Antagonists)

Tyler S. Dougherty[1]

South College School of Pharmacy, Knoxville, TN, United States

[1]Corresponding author: tdougherty@southcollegetn.edu

BILASTINE (SEDA-36, 233; SEDA-37, 185; SEDA-38, 143)

Nervous System, Gastrointestinal

Researchers prospectively evaluated the pharmacokinetics, pharmacodynamics, and safety of bilastine in a randomized, placebo-controlled, single-blinded study. Sixty healthy male volunteers between 20 and 39 years old participated in a two part trial. Thirty-six participants received either 10, 20, or 50 mg of bilastine or placebo for 1 day in part one (9 active:3 placebo for each dosing group). In part two, 24 participants received either 20 or 50 mg of bilastine, or placebo daily for 14 days (9 active:3 placebo for each dosing group). In part one, 2/9 (22.2%) participants in the 20 mg bilastine group developed dizziness, while 1/9 (11.1%) participants in the 50 mg group developed diarrhea. Zero participants reported adverse events in the placebo or 10 mg dose groups. In part two of the trial, 5/9 (55.6%) participants in the 20 mg bilastine dose, 4/9 (44.4%) participants in the 50 mg bilastine dose group, and 4/6 (66.6%) participants in the placebo group reported adverse events. The most notable adverse event was moderate gastroenteritis in the 20 mg bilastine group, resulting in the participant being withdrawn from the trial on day 4. Diarrhea (1/9, 11.1%) and stomatitis (1/9, 11.1%) were noted in the bilastine 20 mg group, while eczema (1/9, 11.1%), glossitis (1/9, 11.1%), and epistaxis (1/9, 11.1%) were reported in the 50 mg bilastine group through day 14 of the trial [1c].

CHLORPHENIRAMINE (SEDA-36, 233; SEDA-37, 185; SEDA-38, 143)

Cardiovascular, Drug–Drug Interaction

A 35-year-old male had been taking propranolol 20 mg daily for anxiety and essential tremor for many years. In this case report, the patient began taking 4 mg chlorpheniramine for an upper respiratory tract infection when he began to develop chest pain and palpitation approximately 1 hour after the second dose of chlorpheniramine. The patient had no history of heart disease or arrhythmias, and did not present with any electrolyte abnormalities. An electrocardiogram displayed ST-segment depression and no QTc prolongation. In addition, an echocardiogram demonstrated normal systolic heart function with normal coronary arteries. After 2 days of hospitalization, the patient exhibited polymorphic ventricular tachycardia, eventually resulting in ventricular fibrillation. The patient was defibrillated leading to full restoration of sinus rhythm [2A]. Chlorpheniramine has been reported in the literature to cause QTc prolongation and torsades de pointes [3]. This is a unique case report resulting in the development of torsades de pointes while on propranolol without prolongation of the QTc interval [2A].

CYPROHEPTADINE

Drug Misuse

People in sub-Saharan Africa recognize obesity as a display of social status. Particularly, in Kinshasa, Democratic Republic of Congo, a "C4 phenomenon" has developed where cyproheptadine is used to increase weight and obtain a look of bodily "roundness". In this cross-sectional study, 499 participants in Kinshasa were surveyed on their use of cyproheptadine and combination of drugs with cyproheptadine. Seventy-three percent (364/499) of patients surveyed reported using cyproheptadine within the past 6 months for appetite stimulation, with more than 50% of subjects using for greater than 12 months. Females were statistically more likely to use cyproheptadine than males (88.9% vs 34.7%, chi-square = 154.5, df = 1). In addition, participants between the ages of 13 and 19 were more likely to use the appetite stimulant than participants aged 36–55 (77.8% vs 43.5%, chi-square = 33.2, df = 3). Twenty-two percent (80/364) of participants reported using cyproheptadine for anorexia, whereas 78.0% (284/364) of participants reported using cyproheptadine to increase weight. Participants reported that friends, media, and relatives were the most common source of recommendation for using cyproheptadine. Concurrent dexamethasone use was reported in 87.6% (197/364) of cyproheptadine users. Finally, 96.7% (352/364) of participants reported being aware of side effects of cyproheptadine abuse, along with 77.2% (281/364) expressing fear of addiction. The authors concluded the Kinshasa people misuse cyproheptadine for the purpose of weight gain and mate attraction, thus increasing their risk of obesity and, subsequently, non-communicable diseases [4C].

Gastrointestinal, Psychological

A retrospective chart review evaluated 39 patients under the age of 3 years old being treated with cyproheptadine for feeding intolerance. Feeding intolerance included discomfort during feeds, abdominal distention, or vomiting. The median age of patients starting the medication was 17.6 months, with an average starting dose of 0.227 mg/kg/day. Side effects reported were considered mild. Ten percent (4/39) of patients exhibited increased sleepiness, 7.6% (3/39) of patients had increased constipation, and 5.1% (2/39) of patients showed behavioral changes. These behavioral changes were listed as "behavioral problems" and "increased tantrums", in each respective patient. The families of the two patients exhibiting behavioral changes elected to discontinue the drug. The patients who demonstrated increased sleepiness and constipation experienced a decrease in these side effects with decreasing doses [5c].

DIMENHYDRINATE

Nervous System

A randomized, double-blind, clinical trial studied dimenhydrinate for the treatment of vomiting in acute gastroenteritis. The trial consisted of 200 pediatric patients between the ages of 1 and 12 years. Patients received either placebo or dimenhydrinate (1 mg/kg, max 200 mg) every 6 hours. In the dimenhydrinate group, 36 patients (36%) experienced sedation, 16 patients (16%) had increased sleepiness, and 1 patient (1%) showed increased excitement. Zero patients in the placebo group experienced adverse effects [6C].

FEXOFENADINE

A 40-year-old female patient was taking fexofenadine and developed acute generalized exanthematous pustulosis (AGEP). In this case report, the patient had ingested two doses of fexofenadine 180 mg orally over the course of 2 days for rhinitis. Upon presentation, the patient had a fever great than 38°C with "1–2 mm nonfollicular pustules on an erythematous base" located on her torso and arms. Pertinent patient labs included: elevated white blood cell count with neutrophilia, negative Gram's stain, and negative culture growth. The histopathology demonstrated "subcorneal pustules with epidermal spongiosis along with scattered neutrophils and eosinophils in the dermis." The patient mistakenly took another dose of fexofenadine 180 mg orally, which resulted in a similar event. The adverse drug reaction was also evaluated using the Naranjo scale, resulting in a score of 9. The authors noted this being the first reported case of AGEP by fexofenadine in the literature [7A].

KETOTIFEN (SEDA-38, 143)

Nervous System

Many therapies have been used to treat uremic pruritus in hemodialysis patients, including ketotifen and gabapentin. However, limited research has been done comparing ketotifen and gabapentin in the treatment of uremic pruritus [8]. In this randomized, double-blind trial, 52 patients were randomized to receive either ketotifen or gabapentin for the treatment of uremic pruritus in hemodialysis patients. Patients either received ketotifen 1 mg twice daily for 2 weeks or gabapentin 100 mg daily for 2 weeks. The frequency of drowsiness reported in the gabapentin and ketotifen groups was the same at 15.4% (4/26 participants in each group). Dizziness was also reported at the same rate in both the gabapentin and ketotifen groups at 3.8% (1/26 participants in each group) [9c].

LEVOCETIRIZINE (SEDA-36, 233; SEDA-37, 185; SEDA-38, 143)

Immunologic

A 49-year-old male patient was being treated for scabies and developed a fixed drug eruption. In this case report, the patient took a one-time dose of ivermectin 12 mg, 150 mg ranitidine twice daily, and 5 mg of levocetirizine once daily for 3 days. The patient had a previous history of fixed drug eruption while being treated with topical permethrin and cetirizine, the racemic mixture of levocetirizine and dextrocetirizine. The patient started ivermectin and ranitidine on day 1 with no reaction. On day 2, the patient started the levocetirizine and, within 1 hour of ingestion, developed "several bullae formations with generalized itching and multiple erythematous macules" on the lower left extremity, bottom of the right foot, genitalia, and right middle finger. This presentation was similar to the patient's experience with cetirizine. The patient was prescribed clobetasol cream for the skin areas and desloratadine, while levocetirizine was halted. The erupted skin areas resolved within 7 days with "faint lingering hyper-pigmentation". Case reports for fixed drug eruptions with cetirizine or levocetirizine are rare. The authors noted the uniqueness of this case report because the patient was accidentally prescribed levocetirizine, even though the patient had a previous fixed drug eruption with cetirizine [10A].

Liver

A 48-year-old male was being treated with levocetirizine and developed acute hepatitis. In this case report, the patient was being treated with levocetirizine 5 mg for prurigo nodularis for 2 months. The patient had no previous history of liver disease, reported taking no other medications, and consumed approximately 57 g of ethanol per week. Upon presentation, the patient had a physical exam positive for "jaundice with icteric sclera", but no other physical signs of liver disease. Abnormal labs included an international normalized ratio 0.88, alkaline phosphatase 184 μ/L, aspartate aminotransferase 1208 IU/L, alanine aminotransferase 2043 IU/L, and total bilirubin 8.68 mg/dL. After an X-ray and abdominal sonography demonstrated no evidence of liver injury, a liver biopsy was performed via percutaneous ultrasonography. This biopsy revealed "portal inflammation and hepatitis with apoptotic hepatocytes." Upon discontinuation of levocetirizine, all of the patient's liver enzymes normalized after 3 weeks. The patient was then diagnosed with idiosyncratic drug-induced liver injury secondary to levocetirizine. The authors noted the uniqueness of this case report because it is the first case of levocetirizine-induced liver injury with confirmed histopathology [11A].

RUPATADINE (SEDA-36, 233; SEDA-37, 185; SEDA-38, 143)

Neurologic

In a placebo-controlled, randomized, double-blind study, 27 healthy participants received either placebo or rupatadine 10, 20, or 40 mg. The purpose of the study was to develop a pharmacokinetic and safety profile of rupatadine in Japanese patients. Patients were also assessed for cognition change by various methods. One participant (1/21, 5%) reported mild somnolence approximately 2 hours after taking 10 mg rupatadine that lasted for approximately 47 hours. No other subjects in the rupatadine group reported any adverse events leading to the discontinuation of the drug. Adverse events were only collected for 11 days, which was the end of the study [12c].

References

[1] Togawa M, Hidetoshi Y, Monica R, et al. Pharmacokinetics, pharmacodynamics and population pharmacokinetic/pharmacodynamics modelling of bilastine, a second-generation antihistamine, in healthy Japanese subjects. Clin Drug Investig. 2016;36:1011–21 [c].

[2] Osken A, Yelgec NS, Zehir R, et al. Torsades de pointes induced by concomitant use of chlorpheniramine and propranolol: an unusual presentation with no qt prolongation. Indian J Pharmacol. 2016;48(4):462–5 [A].

[3] Nia AM, Fuhr U, Gassanov N, et al. Torsades de pointes tachycardia induced by common cold compound medication containing chlorpheniramine. Eur J Clin Pharmacol. 2010;66(11):1173–5.

[4] Lulebo AM, Bavuidibo CD, Mafuta EM, et al. The misuse of cyproheptadine: a non-communicable disease risk behavior in Kinshasa population, Democratic Republic of Congo. Subst Abuse Treat Prev Policy. 2016;11(7):1–7 [C].

[5] Merhar SL, Pentiuk SP, Mukkada VA, et al. A retrospective review of cyproheptadine for feeding intolerance in children less than three years of age: effects and side effects. Acta Paediatr. 2016;105:967–70 [c].

[6] Gheini S, Ameli S, Hoseini J. Effect of oral dimenhydrinate in children with acute gastroenteritis: a clinical trial. Oman Med J. 2016;31(1):18–21 [C].

[7] Gupta T, Garg V, Sarkar R, et al. Acute generalized exanthematous pustulosis induced by fexofenadine. Indian J Dermatol. 2016;61(2):235 [A].

[8] Manenti L, Tansinda P, Vaglio A. Uraemic pruritus: clinical characteristics, pathophysiology and treatment. Drugs. 2009;69:251–63.

[9] Amirkhanlou S, Rashedi A, Taherian J, et al. Comparison of gabapentin and ketotifen in treatment of uremic pruritus in hemodialysis patients. Pak J Med Sci. 2016;32(1):22–6 [c].

[10] Jhaj R, Asati DP, Chaudhary D. Fixed drug eruption due to levocetirizine. J Pharmacol Pharmacother. 2016;7(2):109–11 [A].

[11] Jung MC, Kim KM, Cho JY, et al. A case of levocetirizine-induced liver injury. Clin Mol Hepatol. 2016;22(4):495–8 [A].

[12] Taubel J, Ferber G, Fernandes S, et al. Pharmacokinetics, safety and cognitive function profile of rupatadine 10, 20, and 40 mg in healthy Japanese subjects: a randomized placebo-controlled trial. PLoS One. 2016;15(9):1–15 [c].

14

Drugs that Act on the Respiratory Tract

Joy Creaser-Thomas*, Vignaresh Rajasundaram†, Gwyneth A Davies‡,1

*Institute of Life Science 1, Swansea University, Swansea, United Kingdom
†Abertawe Bro Morgannwg University Health board, Singleton Hospital, Swansea, United Kingdom
‡School of Medicine, Swansea University, Swansea, United Kingdom
1Corresponding author: gwyneth.davies@swansea.ac.uk

INHALED GLUCOCORTICOIDS [SEDA-36, 241; SEDA-37, 195; SEDA-38, 153]

Inhaled corticosteroids (ICS) are widely used in the management of asthma and chronic obstructive pulmonary disease (COPD). Adverse events (AEs) associated with ICS use can be local, including dysphonia and oral candidiasis at low doses or systemic including pneumonia and hyperglycemia at higher doses. These are well documented in the literature and more recently reviewed in detail in SEDA-38 (p. 153). The most common inhaled corticosteroids used in the management of obstructive airway diseases are beclomethasone, budesonide, ciclesonide, fluticasone, and mometasone.

ICS are often combined with other drug classes such as long-acting bronchodilators (LABA) for the management of more complex obstructive airway disease. Due to the recognised AE profile of ICS, interest remains in moving towards combination therapy such as LABA with long-acting muscarinic antagonists (LAMA) in COPD.

A recent retrospective pooled analysis combined data from ILLUMINATE [1C] and LANTERN [2C] studies to explore the efficacy and safety of indacaterol/glycopyrronium (IND/GLY) [3M]. In both studies, symptomatic COPD patients were randomized to once-daily IND/GLY 110/50 µg or twice-daily salmeterol/fluticasone (SFC) 50/500 µg. Similar percentage of AEs were reported in both groups (44.1% vs 53.2%) but the incidence of pneumonia was lower with IND/GLY (IND/GLY, 3 patients; SFC, 14 patients ($P = 0.0074$)). COPD (worsening) was the most commonly reported serious adverse event (SAE) occurring more frequently in the SFC group (IND/GLY, 17.9%; SFC, 27.6%). Maximum number of discontinuations due to AE was observed in the SFC cohort. Deaths occurred in both studies but were deemed not treatment related.

A recent Cochrane review evaluated whether ICS and LABA/LAMA combination in patients with stable COPD had any benefit/increased side effects over LABA/LAMA alone [4M]. The review concluded there were insufficient studies addressing this. Another Cochrane review evaluated the effects of vilanterol (VI) and fluticasone furoate (FF) in combination vs placebo or vs other ICSs and/or LABAs on acute exacerbations of asthma in adults and children [5M]. Five studies included reported no increased incidence of SAEs in VI/FF 100/25 µg when compared to placebo. Data on AEs could not be combined.

A 12-week, randomized, double-blind, parallel group study was performed to compare the efficacy and safety of beclomethasone/formoterol fumarate (BDP/FF) 200/6 µg with BDP 100 µg monotherapy, in a population of 376 randomized adult asthmatics [6C]. There was similar reporting of AEs between the groups (15.3% BDP/FF vs 16.7% BDP) and included asthma, dysphonia and throat irritation.

Ongoing interest also remains in the AE profile of individual glucocorticoids at differing doses. Specifically, a recent meta-analysis reviewed safety data from 10 parallel-group, randomised, double blind phase II and III studies, as part of the fluticasone furoate global clinical development programme in asthma [7M]. A total of 3345 patients received at least one dose of fluticasone furoate at doses 50, 100 and 200 µg. The most frequently reported AEs were headache, dysphonia and oral/oropharyngeal candidiasis. Upper respiratory tract infections were reported at a higher incidence at the higher steroid doses (FF 100 and 200 µg).

The incidence of drug-related AEs increased with the dose administered (2% with FF 50 μg, 6% with FF 100 and 200 μg for once-daily administration, 8% with twice-daily FP 250 μg and FP 500 μg). Reporting of local steroid AEs (oral and oropharyngeal candidiasis) also increased with the dose, 80.8 PYs (Patient Years) (placebo), 103.4 PYs (FF 100 μg) and 283.8 PYs (FF 200 μg). However, two longer-term studies included in the meta-analysis reported no increased incidence of AEs after 6 months of therapy. Using adjusted means analysis, the authors also concluded that the overall incidence of pneumonia was higher in the FF 200 μg group (23.6 PYs) but the severity of the pneumonia was comparable between groups (FF 100 μg 4.2 PYs, FF 200 μg 5.9 PYs and placebo 5.4 PYs). No statistical difference was observed in 24 hour urinary cortisol excretion from baseline to treatment end between each FF group.

Adding to this, a recent Cochrane review evaluated 8 RCTs ($n = 1669$) to determine the clinical effectiveness and safety of increased vs stable doses of ICS during an acute exacerbation of asthma [8M]. The authors concluded that increased dose of ICS during acute exacerbations was not associated with increased risk of SAEs (OR 1.69, 95% CI 0.77–3.71; participants = 394; two studies) or general AE (OR 2.15, 95% CI 0.68–6.73; participants = 142; two studies) compared with keeping the dose stable. The odds of occurrence of specific AEs including oral irritation, headaches, psychiatric disturbance, gastrointestinal discomfort, dysphonia and change in appetite were not significantly higher in the increased ICS vs stable dose groups.

In addition to fluticasone, beclomethasone and budesonide, mometasone furoate (MF), is a treatment option for pediatric patients with asthma [9C]. Amar et al. conducted a 12-week double-blind, placebo-controlled trial randomising 578 patients aged 5–11 years to receive mometasone furoate (MF) 50 μg, MF 100 μg and MF 200 μg or placebo to evaluate change in Forced Expiratory volume in 1 second (FEV1). No significance in reporting of AEs was seen between groups despite variable doses of MF.

Although well studied in COPD and asthma, a recent observational study of 120 patients with non-Cystic Fibrosis Bronchiectasis reviewed the efficacy and safety of salmeterol–fluticasone (SF) combined inhaled therapy [10C]. Patients received either routine non-pharmacological therapy or SF (100/500 μg daily) combined inhaled therapy. AEs were few (15.52% vs 8.77%, $P = 0.269$) with no significant differences between the 2 groups. Oropharyngeal discomfort, dental ulcers and dysphonia were of marginally greater prevalence in the SF group. Furthermore, a recent Cochrane review identified 13 studies evaluating the use of ICS (beclomethasone and fluticasone) in 506 people with cystic fibrosis aged between 6 and 55 years [11M]. SAEs were reported in 5 of the trials included.

Respiratory

Pneumonia: ICS have a recognised association with increased risk of pneumonia. A recent meta-analysis of 29 RCTs and 9 observational studies evaluated the effects of pneumonia incidence and mortality in COPD patients [12M]. There was an increased risk of pneumonia in the RCTs (RR 1.61; 95% CI 1.35–1.93, $P < 0.001$), as well as in observational studies (OR 1.89; 95% CI 1.39–2.58, $P < 0.001$) when receiving ICS therapy. Of the studies included, 6 RCTS and 9 observational studies did not identify a statistically significant pneumonia-associated mortality (RR 0.91; 95% CI 0.52–1.59, $P = 0.74$; and OR 0.72; 95% CI 0.59–0.88, $P = 0.001$, respectively). No overall increase in mortality was identified.

In addition, the nested case–control IMPACT study, evaluated the association between ICS exposure patterns and the risk of pneumonia in COPD patients [13MC]. A total of 51 739 patients including 19 838 cases of pneumonia were matched to 74 849 controls from a cohort of COPD patients. They concluded that the use of ICS was associated with an increased pneumonia risk (OR = 1.25 95% confidence interval [CI] = 1.20–1.30), with a dose dependent increase in the OR as the average ICS dose increased. In particular fluticasone/salmeterol, fluticasone, and either fluticasone/salmeterol or fluticasone were associated with a higher risk of pneumonia (OR = 1.35, 95% CI = 1.28–1.41; OR = 1.22, 95% CI = 1.10–1.35; and OR = 1.33, 95% CI = 1.27–1.39, respectively) in contrast to budesonide/formoterol or budesonide monotherapy where no statistical association was found. This prompts the need for comparative studies between glucocorticoids for pneumonia risk.

SUMMIT, a double-blind randomised controlled trial conducted across 1368 centres, aimed to assess whether combined fluticasone furoate and vilanterol (FF/VI) could improve survival when compared with placebo in patients with moderate COPD and heightened cardiovascular CV risk [14MC].

Participants were randomised to receive placebo ($n = 4111$), FF ($n = 4135$), VI ($n = 4118$) or FF/VI combination ($n = 4121$). Combination therapy was not associated with increased risk of pneumonia or adverse cardiac events. In contrast, a 52-week randomised, double-blind, double-dummy trial assessed annual rate of COPD exacerbations when taking indacaterol/glycopyrronium combination vs fluticasone/salmeterol [15MC]. Though the incidence of AEs was similar between the two groups, an increased incidence of pneumonia was observed in the salmeterol/fluticasone group (4.8% vs 3.2% $P = 0.02$).

A retrospective cohort study of 163 514 applied the quasi-cohort analysis to estimate the risk ratio of sepsis in patients with COPD on ICS and oral corticosteroids [16MC]. ICS use was not associated with an increased risk ratio of sepsis 0.98 (95% CI=0.84–1.14).

Ear, Nose and Throat: A recent review article evaluating the effects of ICS on voice concluded that the prevalence of dysphonia was less common with ciclesonide and beclomethasone [17R]. The authors concluded that comparative investigation between available ICS is needed to have a better understanding on epidemiology, predisposing factors, mechanisms, prevention, and treatment of voice problems attributed to ICS.

Eyes: A recent randomised, double-masked, placebo-controlled trial of 22 adults with well-controlled open-angle glaucoma or ocular hypertension randomised participants to receive a 6-week course of twice weekly fluticasone propionate 250-µg metered-dose inhaler or saline placebo metered-dose inhaler [18c]. There were no statistically significant differences in intra-ocular pressure between groups at baseline (14.3 ± 3.0 and 15.6 ± 3.6 mm Hg in steroid and placebo groups, respectively, $P=0.39$) or at week 6 (14.7 ± 2.4 and 14.8 ± 3.8 mm Hg in steroid and placebo groups, respectively, $P=0.92$). The small sample size limits generalisability.

Endocrine: There is convincing evidence that high dose ICS therapies significantly suppress cortisol levels and there is a dose-dependent effect, particularly in children, as noted in previous editions (SEDA-38, p. 154). A recent systematic review evaluated 64 studies and applied a multivariate regression model to determine dose-dependent effects of different ICS on cortisol suppression [19M]. The greatest suppression of urinary cortisol was observed with beclomethasone (8.4% per 100 µg; $P=0.029$), followed by fluticasone (3.2% per 100 µg; $P<0.001$), and budesonide (3.1% per 100 µg; $P=0.001$). No significant urinary cortisol suppression was associated with ciclesonide treatment (1.8% per 100 µg; $P=0.267$). The authors concluded that novel Freon-free delivery devices for ICS do not eliminate the adverse adrenal suppression of cortisol secretion.

Metabolism: A recent matched retrospective cohort study evaluated the effect of ICS therapy in patients with COPD and comorbid type 2 diabetes mellitus (T2DM) on diabetic control [20C]. Increases in HbA1c were significantly greater in those prescribed ICS when compared with those on non-ICS therapies; (0.16% (95% confidence interval [CI]: 0.05%–0.27%) in all COPD patients, however, risk associated with individual ICS was not evaluated.

Musculoskeletal: ICS therapies are recognized to decrease bone mineral density and thus predispose to osteoporosis and increased fracture risk. This risk increases further with age and in post-menopausal women, as detailed in previous annuals [SEDA-37, 195; SEDA-38, 157].

A recent retrospective cohort and population-based study in post-menopausal women assessed the incidence of osteoporosis in COPD [21MC]. A total of 10 723 patients with COPD including ICS users ($n=812$) were included. Increased ICS dose was associated with lower incidence of osteoporosis (doses ≤ 20 mg, HR: 0.84, 95% CI: 0.69–1.04; >20 to ≤ 60 mg, HR: 0.78, 95% CI: 0.59–1.04; and >60 mg, HR: 0.72, 95% CI: 0.55–0.96; P for trend$=0.0023$). However, the proportion of participants on ICS therapy was very low and likely to have contributed to the unexpected result.

Second-Generation Effects

Pregnancy: There are some concerns regarding the AEs of ICS therapies in pregnancy. Limited literature exists in this field and has been limited by small sample sizes [22c]. Two nested case–control studies reviewed the incidence of pregnancy-induced hypertension (PIH) and gestational diabetes (GDM) in those taking ICS therapies [23C]. When other concomitant drugs use during pregnancy was adjusted, ICS use was associated with an increased rate of PIH (adjusted odds ratio, 1.40 [95% CI, 1.05–1.870]). However, the statistical significance was not found in other models. In both unadjusted and adjusted multivariable models, ICS use was not associated with increase in the risk of GDM. The author concluded that further observational studies were needed.

BETA₂-ADRENOCEPTOR AGONISTS [SEDA-36, 245; SEDA-37, 197; SEDA-38, 153]

Previous editions have evaluated the safety of beta₂-adrenoceptor agonists and noted well-recognized AEs including tachycardia, hypertension and myocardial ischemia in the cardiovascular system. Other well-recognized AEs include headaches, hypokalemia and fine tremors [SEDA-36, 245; SEDA-37, 197; SEDA-38, 153].

Combination Therapies: The significant AE profile associated with long-term ICS use has encouraged a move towards dual bronchodilator therapies (LABA/LAMA) in COPD. The long-term AE profile of these newer agents is of ongoing interest, particularly as the patients receiving them often have other comorbidities.

Cardiovascular: A retrospective cohort study of 3458 patients in Taiwan compared the cardiovascular and cerebrovascular safety of long-acting bronchodilators in patients with COPD [24MC]. The primary analysis focused on patients treated with a LAMA or LABA alone who experienced their first admission due to cardiovascular or cerebrovascular disease. Similar risks were observed when comparing LABA to long-acting muscarinic antagonist (LAMA) with a hazard ratio

(HR) of 1.09; 95% CI; 0.87–1.37. The HR of a LABA/LAMA combination therapy with LAMA alone was 1.13 (95% CI; 0.60–2.13). A secondary analysis for patients who had changed treatment showed slightly higher HRs for LABA/LAMA combinations against LAMA alone (HR 1.26; 95% CI; 0.74–2.15). This indicates that the use of a LABA/LAMA combination exhibits a similar cardiovascular and cerebrovascular safety profile compared to the monotherapies.

Formoterol

A recent multi-center, double-blind, 26-week study evaluated whether adding formoterol to budesonide maintenance therapy increased the risk of serious asthma-related events [25MC]. Patients were randomized to receive budesonide–formoterol ($n = 5846$) or budesonide monotherapy ($n = 5847$). The risk of a serious asthma-related event was similar between groups (HR, 1.07; 95% CI, 0.70–1.65). The author concluded that treatment with combined therapy with formoterol was associated with a lower risk of asthma exacerbation than BDP monotherapy (HR 0.84; 95% CI, 0.74–0.94; $P = 0.002$) with no statistical difference in the risk of serious asthma-related events.

Comparative Studies

Formoterol vs Salmeterol: A post-hoc analysis of a subgroup of the RELIEF study in East Asia compared the efficacy and safety of formoterol against salbutamol [26C]. 2834 patients were randomized; 1418 in the formoterol group and 1416 in the salbutamol group. The OR for non-asthma-related AEs between formoterol and salbutamol was 1.10 (95% CI; 0.90, 1.34. $P = 0.347$). Cardiovascular-related AEs OR was 0.58 (95% CI; 0.23, 1.47. $P = 0.250$) and non-cardiovascular AEs OR was 1.05 (95% CI; 0.87, 1.26. $P = 0.633$). There was no significant difference between the two beta-agonist therapies in the reporting of SAEs or AEs suggesting a similar safety profile.

Olodaterol

A recent meta-analysis evaluated the impact of olodaterol on the risk of mortality and SAEs in patients with COPD and asthma [27M]. A total of 26 studies were included; 8 parallel trials and 18 crossover trials of 16591 patients. Olodaterol was compared with placebo in 17 trials and tiotropium in the remaining 9 at doses between 2 and 20 μg. The total risk of AE was equivocal between olodaterol and placebo arms (Peto fixed OR 1.00; 95% CI 0.93–1.08) in addition to the risk of non-fatal SAE (Peto fixed OR 1.03; 95% CI 0.91–1.15). Twelve trials recorded the incidence of treatment-related AEs

concluding no difference between the interventions (Peto fixed OR 0.93; 95% CI 0.78–1.11).

Regarding mortality, olodaterol vs placebo was associated with an increased OR for death; however, no statistical difference in death rates were reported (Peto fixed OR 1.31; 95% CI 0.90–1.89). No association between risk of SAEs and treatment duration or olodaterol dosage was established. Several limitations were identified by the authors including lack of standardised definition of SAEs and treatment-related AEs, possibility of confounding between severity of disease and use of ICS in COPD patients and the wide range of study duration included. They favoured the need for longer-term large clinical trials to address safety concerns regarding olodaterol.

Susceptibility Factors: Two trials examined the effect of hepatic and renal impairment on olodaterol's pharmacokinetic effect [28c]. The first trial matched 16 healthy subjects with 8 subjects with mild and moderate hepatic impairment each. No significant AEs were reported during the trial. Two of the patients with moderate hepatic impairment experienced a decrease in serum potassium which resolved with treatment. The second trial matched 14 subjects with normal renal function to 8 subjects with severe renal impairment (creatinine clearance <30 millilitres per minute). None of the patients with renal impairment in this trial experienced AEs. Three individuals in the healthy group experienced four AEs which are associated with LABAs: myalgia, cough and headache. Impaired hepatic or renal function did not translate into a clinically relevant change of systemic exposure to olodaterol compared to normal subjects.

Salbutamol (Albuterol)

The safety of salbutamol (180 μg dose) in a multi-dose dry powder inhaler (MDPI) was evaluated [29C]. Data was pooled from two 12-week double-blind, parallel-group RCT, the 12-week double-blind phase of a 52-week trial along and the safety data from a 40-week open-label phase of the 52-week trial. Patients were randomized to placebo (MDPI) ($n = 333$) or albuterol MDPI ($n = 321$). The incidence of β2-agonist-related events (excluding headache) during the pooled 12-week dosing periods was low (≤1%) in both groups. Upper respiratory tract infection (URTI) (11% vs 10%), nasopharyngitis (6% vs 5%) and headache (6% vs 4%) were the most frequently reported AE with no statistical differences between groups across the 40-week phase. The study concluded a favorable safety profile for salbutamol 180 μg MDI.

Salmeterol

A recent RCT evaluated the effect of adding salmeterol to fluticasone propionate in asthmatic children on the risk of a serious asthma exacerbation requiring oral glucocorticoids [30MC]. 6028 children aged 4–11 were randomised to receive either salmeterol/fluticasone or fluticasone alone over 26 weeks. The HR with salmeterol/fluticasone vs fluticasone alone was 1.28 (95% confidence interval [CI], 0.73–2.27) concluding no statistically significant increase in the risk of serious asthma-related events ($P = 0.006$).

Vilanterol

A phase IIb, randomized, double-blind, parallel-group, placebo-controlled study looked at the effect of adding vilanterol (VI) to fluticasone furoate (FFU) once daily on improving asthma control in children [31C]. Patients were assigned to a placebo group or a group on varying doses of vilanterol (6.25, 12.5 and 25 μg). Drug-related AEs were only reported in the VI 6.25 μg (3%) and the VI 12.5 μg groups (2%) and included headache, nasopharyngitis.

A study compared the effectiveness of the combination LAMA/LABA therapies against the monotherapies in patients with COPD [32C]. Two randomized, double-blind, three-way complete-block, cross over studies randomized patients to 1 of 6 sequences. Patients received once-daily umeclidinium (UM) 62.5 μg, vilanterol (VI) 25 μg, and umeclidinium/vilanterol (UM/VI) 62.5/25 μg (one treatment/14-day period; 10–14-day washout). The overall incidence of AEs in each study was similar across all treatment groups. The most common AEs reported were nasopharyngitis and headache reported at increased frequency in VI and UM/VI groups. Overall, all treatments were tolerated well in both arms with the combination therapy having the greatest efficacy.

Cardiovascular: As described earlier, the SUMMIT trial, a double-blind RCT across 1368 centers aimed to assess whether combined fluticasone furoate and vilanterol (FF/VI) could improve survival when compared with placebo in patients with moderate COPD and heightened CV risk [14MC]. Participants were randomised to receive placebo ($n = 4111$), FF ($n = 4135$), VI ($n = 4118$) or FF/VI combination ($n = 4121$). The incidence of overall cardiovascular AEs was similar across groups (17%–18%), as was the reporting of cardiac arrhythmias (placebo group 229 (6%), FF 224 (5%), VI 209 (5%)). There was no significant difference in the reporting of β-adrenoceptor agonist-related AE including tremor and hypokalaemia across groups.

ANTICHOLINERGIC DRUGS [SEDA-36, 245; SEDA-37, 197; SEDA-38, 153]

Anticholinergic drugs act on the muscarinic acetylcholine receptors inhibiting the parasympathetic nervous system and the long-acting muscarinic antagonists (LAMAs) are widely used in COPD and have recently been included in guidelines on the management of asthma.

Glycopyrronium Bromide

A multicenter, double-blind, randomized, placebo-controlled, crossover study aimed to determine the dose–response of the LAMA, glycopyrronium bromide (GB) at doses 12.5, 25 or 50 μg when combined with BDP/FF in COPD patients [33C]. A total of 178 patients were randomized to GB 12.5 μg + BDP/FF, GB 25 μg + BDP/FF, GB 50 μg + BDP/FF or placebo + BDP/FF. There was no significant difference in the reporting of AEs between groups.

TRILOGY, a randomized, parallel group, double-blind, active-controlled study evaluated the effects of triple therapy of BDP/FF/GB (12.5 μg) compared to BDP/FF in improving FEV1 in COPD patients [34MC]. 1368 patients received either BDP/FF/GB ($n = 687$) or BDP/FF ($n = 681$). A similar proportion of treatment emergent AEs (54% vs 56%) and SAEs (15% vs 18%) were reported between groups. However, there was an increased incidence of the treatment-related AEs, oral candidiasis, muscle spasms and dry mouth in the BDP/FF/GB group.

Cardiovascular: There was similar incidence of treatment-emergent cardiovascular AEs between groups ($\leq 1\%$ vs 2%). However, one treatment-related SAE of atrial fibrillation was reported in the BDP/FF/GB group. It lasted 15 days and was self-limited. No differences in mean change in blood pressure, heart rate or corrected QT interval were observed between the groups.

Drug–Drug Interactions: A case of QTc prolongation was reported in a 78-year-old female with moderate COPD presenting with syncope [35A]. The patient was also taking tamoxifen for breast cancer. Cardiac monitoring confirmed QTc prolongation >600 ms which resolved on stopping both medications. The authors concluded the need for future studies to identify high-risk populations at potential risk of life-threatening arrhythmias and any potential interaction with tamoxifen.

Tiotropium Bromide

A recent Cochrane review evaluated the effect of adding tiotropium (of either 5 or 18 mcg dose) to LABA/ICS combination therapy in adults with asthma. A total of 1197 patients in three RCTs of 12-weeks duration were included [36M]. The authors could not conclude that adding tiotropium to LABA/ICS therapy reduced the incidence of SAEs but did deduce an overall reduction in the incidence of any type of AE in the population included (OR 0.70, 95% CI 0.52–0.94).

A phase III, double-blind trial evaluated the efficacy and safety of once daily tiotropium at doses of 2.5 and 5 µg s in comparison to the placebo in 464 adults with symptomatic asthma [37C]. In each group, 2 patients (1.3%) had a drug-related AE including headache and dysphonia (5 µg tiotropium dose), asthma and hematuria (2.5 µg tiotropium dose) and hematuria and dry mouth (placebo group). No SAEs reported were deemed treatment related and no deaths were reported.

Comparative Studies

Tiotropium vs Aclidinium: A systematic review used Baysesian indirect comparison to evaluate the safety and efficacy of aclidinium/formoterol (400/12 µg twice daily) in comparison to tiotropium (18 µg once daily) [38M]. It demonstrated a marked improvement in efficacy when using aclidinium/formoterol treatment over tiotropium (OR 1.51; 95% CI 1.11–2.06) but an indirect treatment comparison suggested similar safety profiles.

Umeclidinium Bromide

The effectiveness and safety of umeclidinium (UM) when added to fluticasone propionate (FP) and salmeterol combination therapy in COPD patients was evaluated [39MC]. Two 12-week double-blind parallel studies compared umeclidinium at doses of 62.5 and 125 µg to fluticasone/salmeterol treatment (250/50 µg) for a total of 1084 patients. Headache and nasopharyngitis were the most commonly reported AEs. The incidence of drug-related AE was highest at the 125 µg UM dose (6%, 12%) compared to the 62.5 µg dose (6%, 8%) and placebo (8%, 3%). Overall, the efficacy of the umeclidinium when added to the combination therapy was significant.

The long-term safety of umeclidinium 125 µg once daily was evaluated in 52 week, multi-centre, open-label study of 152 Japanese patients with COPD [40C]. The incidence of AEs did not increase with prolonged exposure. SAEs were reported in 17 patients (13%). One case of angina pectoris was deemed related to the pharmacological effects of LAMAs. Authors concluded that a higher dose of umeclidinium bromide (up to 125 µg) had a reassuring long-term safety profile.

Comparative Studies

Umeclidinium Bromide vs Tiotropium Bromide: A randomized, blinded study evaluated the efficacy and safety of umeclidinium compared with tiotropium in patients with COPD [41MC]. 1017 patients were randomized to receive umeclidinium bromide 62.5 µg once daily ($n = 489$) or tiotropium bromide 18 µg once daily ($n = 487$). The overall incidence of AEs was similar in both groups (umeclidinium 165 (32%), tiotropium 153 (30%)). Headache (6% both groups) and nasopharyngitis (5% both groups) were the most commonly reported, in keeping with previous studies on anticholinergics. Drug-related AEs were reported in 17 patients (3%) on umeclidinium and 8 patients (2%) on tiotropium. The authors concluded that umeclidinium was a more effective treatment and had comparable rates of AEs with tiotropium.

LEUKOTRIENE MODIFIERS [SEDA-36, 245; SEDA-37, 197; SEDA-38, 153]

Montelukast

Psychiatric: A retrospective analysis of Individual Case Safety Reports (ICSRs) was conducted in the WHO database (vogibase) to investigate whether montelukast was associated with psychiatric disorders [42MC]. A total of 2630 psychiatric ICSRs for montelukast were reported in those less than 18 years. Using a Bayesian Confidence Propagation Neural Network (BCPNN) approach, symptoms reported were sleep disorders (children aged less than 2 years), depression/anxiety (aged 2–11) and suicidal behaviour with depression/anxiety (12–17 years). The onset of AR following commencing montelukast varied depended on the specific effect (days to years: a few days in relation to sleep disorders, agitation and nervousness, and months to years in relation to depression and suicide-related behaviour). The authors admitted several limitations including the lack of information on any pre-existing psychiatric disease, thus could not conclusively associate the reporting of such AEs with montelukast directly.

Pranlukast

An RCT evaluated reducing doses of ICS against a switch to pranlukast hydrate as step down therapy for patients with well-controlled asthma [43c]. 20 adult patients were randomized to each arm and reported no AE in the pranlukast hydrate group. The small sample size limits generalizability. Authors concluded the need for further larger scale studies evaluating LTRA as a step down therapy for controlled asthma.

Immunologic: A case of pranlukast anaphylaxis was reported in a 56-year-old woman presenting with generalized urticaria, angioedema, collapse and loss of consciousness [44A]. The authors confirmed with positive skin prick testing suggesting an IgE-dependent pathway mediating the reaction. Only 2 previous anaphylaxis cases specific to pranlukast have been reported.

PHOSPHODIESTERASE INHIBITORS
[SEDA-35, 321; SEDA-36, 252; SEDA-37, 201; SEDA-38, 153]

Rofumilast

Two recent meta-analyses have reviewed the efficiency and safety of roflumilast in patients with COPD. One reviewed its combination with LABAs in 5746 patients, including 6 RCTs and 2 smaller trials concluding a significant reduction in exacerbations of COPD (RR, 0.77; 95% CI, 0.69–0.86; $P < 0.00001$; $I^2 = 0\%$) [45M]. Compared to placebo and LABA, roflumilast and LABA combination was associated with severe back pain (RR 1.53; 95% CI 1.12–2.10), diarrhoea (RR 3.03; 95% CI 2.44–3.76), headache (RR 2.23; 95% CI 1.62–3.08), insomnia (RR 2.36; 95% CI 1.61–3.44), nausea (RR 3.09; 95% CI 2.26–4.23) and significantly decreased appetite (RR 6.60; 95% CI 3.87–11.24) and weight (RR 3.35; 95% CI 3.03–4.90). Roflumilast did not significantly increase the incidence of influenza (RR 1.04; 95% CI 0.70–1.53), nasopharyngitis (RR 0.96; 95% CI 0.80–1.15), or respiratory tract infection (RR 0.63; 95% CI 0.63–1.05).

A second meta-analysis comparing roflumilast with placebo concluded AEs were observed in seven articles and nine RCT studies [46M]. Cumulative incidence was 54.2% in the roflumilast group and 48.2% in the placebo group (OR = 1.36, 95% CI = 1.13–1.65) with no statistical significance between the two groups. Similar profiles of AEs were observed and included diarrhoea (7.2% and 1.8% of patients in the roflumilast and placebo groups, respectively; OR = 4.49, 95% CI = 3.16–6.38), nausea (3.6% and 1.1% of patients in the roflumilast and placebo groups, respectively; OR = 3.82, 95% CI = 2.16–4.53), and nasopharyngitis (7.6% and 5.6% of patients in the roflumilast and placebo groups, respectively; OR = 0.96, 95% CI = 0.83–1.12).

The JADE study, a double blinded placebo controlled, phase III trial in Korea recruited 260 patients with COPD [47C]. Patients were randomised to receive roflumilast 500 μg ($n = 102$) or placebo ($n = 105$) over 12 weeks with an interest in the mean change in post bronchodilator FEV1 from baseline. Contrary to the previous meta-analysis a higher cumulative incidence of AEs was observed in the Roflumilast arm compared with placebo (69.95% vs 45.7%). In addition, there was increased incidence of SAEs when compared with placebo (8.8% vs 1%). Similar results were seen in the RE²SPOND (Roflumilast Effect on Exacerbations in Patients on Dual [LABA/ICS] Therapy) trial, a double-blind placebo-controlled phase IV trial of patients with moderate/severe COPD [48C]. Adverse event-related discontinuations occurred in 11.7% roflumilast-treated and 5.4% placebo-treated participants. Deaths occurred in 2.5%

roflumilast and 2.1% placebo participants but not attributed to treatment.

Though the use of roflumilast in COPD is well studied there is limited evidence for its use in asthma. In a phase II, randomized, double-blind, placebo-controlled, multiple-dose, 2-sequence, crossover study, 64 patients were randomized to receive 500 μg of roflumilast plus montelukast followed by placebo plus 10 mg of montelukast (sequence AB) or placebo plus 10 mg of montelukast followed by 500 μg of roflumilast plus 10 mg of montelukast (sequence BA) [49c]. Mean durations for sequence AB and BA were 83.1 days and 78.4 days, respectively. A total of 41 patients (64.1%) reported at least 1 treatment-emergent AE. The majority were mild or moderate with headache (8.2% of those receiving roflumilast plus montelukast) the most commonly reported. There were three cases of discontinuation due to neuralgia (roflumilast plus montelukast), abdominal pain and pneumonia (placebo plus montelukast). No SAEs or deaths occurred. This study was the first exploring the interaction between PDE4 inhibitors and leukotriene modulators in asthma but the AE were consistent with those recognised with roflumilast therapy.

Metabolism: Weight loss in patients taking roflumilast remains of particular interest. As outlined earlier, one recent meta-analysis of 5746 patients, 6RCTs and 2 smaller trials reported increased nausea (RR 3.09; 95% CI 2.26–4.23) and significantly decreased appetite (RR 6.60; 95% CI 3.87–11.24) and weight (RR 3.35; 95% CI 3.03–4.90). The JADE study concluded a mean change in body weight from baseline to last study visit was −2.0 (2.4) kg in the roflumilast group and +0.1 (2.0) kg in the placebo group (LSMean difference, −2.07, $P < 0.001$) [48C]. The precise mechanism of weight loss has not yet been identified and potential mechanisms have been reviewed [50R]. The gastro-intestinal side effects of anorexia and diarrhoea are also thought to contribute.

IMMUNOLOGICAL THERAPIES
[SEDA-38, 153]

Omalizumab

Omalizumab (Xolair©) is a recombinant monoclonal anti-IgE antibody that binds to the Fc portion of IgE, thus reducing circulating levels of free IgE and is licensed for the management of patients with severe persistent allergic asthma refractory to high dose ICS and LABA treatments [51R]. Recent studies have examined long-term safety profile, including examination of cardiovascular events.

A recent multi centre, double blind, placebo-controlled, randomised withdrawal study of 176 patients compared the risks and benefits of continuing omalizumab vs switching to placebo over a period of 52 weeks [52C]. In total 33 subjects transitioned from placebo to omalizumab; therefore, AE were calculated per exposure time. They reported no statistical difference in the reporting of AEs (placebo 425.9/100 patient years (PYs) vs omalizumab 413.2/100 PYs) or SAEs (placebo 9.1/100 PYs vs omalizumab 8.3/100 PYs) between placebo and omalizumab groups. Similar results were seen in another phase III randomised placebo-controlled study in Chinese patients [53C]. One death was reported in the omalizumab arm thought attributable to instability of disease not omalizumab treatment. An observational study [54c] evaluating the long-term safety and efficacy of omalizumab in 19 consecutive patients aged 65 and over with severe asthma concluded that no significant adverse events were reported. One case of myalgia and one local site reaction were reported.

An observational study of 179 asthmatics patients listed on the Australian Xolair Register reviewed the risk/benefits of Xolair at within range dosing (300–600 mg) and above dose range (650 mg, 750 mg) [55C]. The incidence of AEs was poorly reported but three above-range participants reported 3 AEs leading to discontinuation including one case of anaphylaxis. This is comparable to two patients from the within dosing range who discontinued omalizumab due to AEs, one of which was anaphylaxis.

A multicentre observational study evaluated omalizumab treatment outcomes and predictors of response in patients with multiple co-morbidities such as rhinitis (485), obesity (45%) and cardiovascular disease (23%). A total of 42 serious AEs for 36 participants receiving a median initial dose of 450 mg per month over 6 months was reported [56C]. Asthma exacerbations accounted for 27 AEs reported. Seven AEs were suspected due to omalizumab and included anaphylactoid reactions ($n = 4$), headaches ($n = 2$), chest pains ($n = 1$) and local reactions ($n = 1$). The APEX II study [57C] evaluated mean reduction of oral corticosteroid (OCS) dose pre- and postomalizumab. Mean duration of treatment was 304 days (SD 104). 43 omalizumab-related AEs were reported in 24 patients, including 19 SAEs. In total 9 SAEs lead to discontinuation of treatment including anaphylaxis ($n = 1$), hypersensitivity reaction ($n = 1$) and anaphylactoid reactions (wheezing $n = 1$, urticaria $= 1$, oral paraesthesia $n = 1$). Two deaths occurred in the study (pneumonia, respiratory arrest), but not attributed to treatment.

Cardiovascular: A multicentre post marketing observational study assessed the long-term safety of omalizumab with respect to cardiovascular (CV) events [58MC]. EXCELS focused on a subset of arterial thromboembolic disease (ATE) comprising CV death, myocardial infarction, ischemic stroke, transient ischemic attack, and unstable angina. EXCELS reported a higher incidence of cardiovascular SAEs in the omalizumab group (13.4 per 1000 person years [PYs]) than the non-omalizumab-treated patients (8.1 per 1000 PYs). The ATE rates per 1000 PYs were 6.66 (101 patients/15 160 PYs) in the omalizumab cohort and 4.64 (46 patients/9904 PYs) in the non-omalizumab cohort. After control for available confounding factors, the hazard ratio was 1.32 (95% CI, 0.91–1.91). When critically evaluating, although the demographics of the groups were similar, there was a higher incidence of hypertension, type 2 diabetes mellitus, hypercholesterolemia and coronary artery disease in the omalizumab group. Furthermore, the authors concluded that differences in asthma severity between cohorts likely contributed but could not exclude an increased risk.

INTERLEUKIN-5 MONOCLONAL ANTIBODIES

IL-5 humanized monoclonal antibodies selectively inhibit interleukin-5 (IL-5) by blocking it from binding to the α-chain of the IL-5 receptor complex on the eosinophil cell surface [59R]. IL-5 is the main cytokine involved in eosinophil activation that mediates airway eosinophil recruitment and hyper responsiveness and thus selective inhibition leads to reduced exacerbation rates in asthma. Over the last few years, multiple trials have evaluated the role of biologics targeting IL-5 in asthma with particular focus on reducing exacerbation rates, with more recent interest on longer-term safety.

Mepolizumab

Mepolizumab (Nucala) is indicated as an add-on treatment for severe eosinophilic asthma, on the basis of its clinical benefit in reducing exacerbation rates in the placebo-controlled trials MENSA, DREAM and SIRIUS [60C,61C,62C]. In the randomised, placebo-controlled trials the incidence of adverse events was similar between mepolizumab 100 mg SC and 75 mg IV compared to placebo, 79% and 83% vs 82%, respectively. The most commonly reported adverse events were headache (20%, 23% and 18%), nasopharyngitis (16%, 23% and 19%) and asthma (5.7%, 9.3% and 15%). After adjustment for differences between the studies and duration of exposure, mepolizumab was associated with a relative risk greater than two compared to placebo for three adverse events: eczema, nasal congestion and dyspnoea. MENSA, a multicentre randomised, placebo-controlled, double-dummy phase III trial reported the incidence of injection-site reactions was more frequent in the subcutaneous mepolizumab group (9%) than in the intravenous-mepolizumab group or the placebo group (3% in both groups) [60C].

A Cochrane meta-analysis published in 2015 of mepolizumab vs placebo in severe asthma included 8 clinical trials of 1707 patients ages 12 and over [63M]. The conclusion was that mepolizumab leads to a reduction in asthma exacerbation rates for people with severe eosinophilic asthma randomised to receive mepolizumab compared to placebo. The analysis of serious adverse events indicated a significant difference favouring mepolizumab (risk ratio 0.49, 95% CI 0.30–0.80; participants =1441; studies=5; $I^2 = 0$%). Deaths occurring during the studies occurred in the placebo arms. More recently a single-blind randomised control trial also found similar reporting of AEs when receiving mepolizumab 750 mg IV vs placebo (71% and 67%, respectively) [64c].

COSMOS, a 52-week open-label extension study recruited patients from previous mepolizumab vs placebo trials and 691 received subcutaneous mepolizumab [65C]. Median cumulative exposure was 17.6 months and AEs were reported in 558 (86%). Most common AEs were nasopharyngitis (30%), upper respiratory tract infection (16%), and worsening or exacerbation of asthma (14%). SAEs were reported in 94 patients with two patients experiencing SAEs considered related to the study treatment (type IV hypersensitivity reaction, which was resolved, and spontaneous abortion). No fatal SAEs were reported during the study. Systemic and local reactions were reported in 2% and 4% patients but there were no cases of anaphylaxis.

There is a pregnancy exposure registry that monitors pregnancy outcomes in women exposed to NUCALA during pregnancy. Clinical trial data on safety in pregnancy are insufficient.

Reslizumab (Cinqair)

Reslizumab (Cinquair) was approved by the FDA in 2016. This decision was supported by the results from two duplicate, multicentres, double blind, parallel group, randomised placebo-controlled, phase III trials evaluating effect on asthma exacerbations [66C]. 953 Asthma patients (aged 12–75 years) were randomly assigned to receive placebo or reslizumab (2.0 mg/kg) IV every 4 weeks for 1 year. Lower incidence of AE events were reported in the reslizumab arm when compared with placebo. However, two cases of anaphylaxis were reported in the reslizumab study (N=2) leading to patient withdrawal. A recent double blind, placebo-controlled Phase III study evaluating the effects of reslizumab stratified by baseline eosinophil counts also reported 2 cases of anaphylaxis leading to discontinuation of therapy [67C].

More recently a randomised phase III trial evaluated the efficacy and safety of different doses of reslizumab (0.3mk/kg and 3.0 mg/kg) vs placebo [68C]. A lower proportion of patients receiving reslizumab 0.3 mg/kg (n=59 [57%]) and 3.0 mg/kg (n=61 [59%]) experienced ≥1 AE compared with placebo (n=66 [63%]). Though a higher incidence of SAEs was reported in reslizumab 3 mg/kg group none were attributable to treatment.

Finally, one meta-analysis compared 21 RCTs of anti-IL-5 s including reslizumab, mepolizumab and benralizumab [69M]. Subgroup analysis highlighted that compared with placebo, treatment with reslizumab was associated with a trend of lower AE incidence (RR=0.88, 95% CI: 0.81–0.96, P=0.003), while no significant differences were found for mepolizumab groups (RR=0.95, 95% CI: 0.89–1.01, P=0.12).

References

[1] Vogelmeier CF, Bateman ED, Pallante J, et al. Efficacy and safety of once-daily QVA149 compared with twice-daily salmeterol-fluticasone in patients with chronic obstructive pulmonary disease (ILLUMINATE): a randomised, double-blind, parallel group study. Lancet Respir Med. 2013;1(1):51–60 [C].

[2] Zhong N, Wang C, Zhou X, et al. LANTERN: a randomized study of QVA149 versus salmeterol/fluticasone combination in patients with COPD. Int J Chron Obstruct Pulmon Dis. 2015;10:1015–26 [C].

[3] Vogelmeier C, Zhong N, Humphries M, et al. Indacaterol/glycopyrronium in symptomatic patients with COPD (GOLD B and GOLD D) versus salmeterol/fluticasone: ILLUMINATE/LANTERN pooled analysis. Int J Chron Obstruct Pulmon Dis. 2016;11:3189–319 [M].

[4] Tan DJ, White CJ, Walters JAE, et al. Inhaled corticosteroids with combination inhaled long-acting beta-agonists and long-acting muscarinic antagonists for chronic obstructive pulmonary disease. Cochrane Database Syst Rev. 2016;(11)CD011600. http://dx.doi.org/10.1002/14651858.CD011600.pub2 [M].

[5] Dwan K, Milan SJ, Bax L, et al. Vilanterol and fluticasone furoate for asthma. Cochrane Database Syst Rev. 2016;9:CD010758 [M].

[6] Paggiaro P, Corradi M, Latorre M, et al. High strength extrafine pMDI beclometasone/formoterol (200/6 µg) is effective in asthma patients not adequately controlled on medium-high dose of inhaled corticosteroids. BMC Pulm Med. 2016;16:180 [C].

[7] O'Byrne P, Jacques L, Goldfrad C. Integrated safety and efficacy analysis of once-daily fluticasone furoate for the treatment of asthma. Respir Res. 2016;17:157 [C].

[8] Kew K, Quinn M, Quon BS, et al. Increased versus stable doses of inhaled corticosteroids for exacerbations of chronic asthma in adults and children. Cochrane Database Syst Rev. 2016;(6)CD007524. http://dx.doi.org/10.1002/14651858.CD007524.pub4 [M].

[9] Amar NJ, Shekar T, Varnell TA, et al. Mometasone furoate (MF) improves lung function in pediatric asthma: a double-blind, randomized controlled dose-ranging trial of MF metered-dose inhaler. Pediatr Pulmonol. 2017;52:310–8. http://dx.doi.org/10.1002/ppul.23563 [C].

[10] Wei P, Yang JW, Lu HW, et al. Combined inhaled corticosteroid and long-acting β2-adrenergic agonist therapy for non-cystic fibrosis bronchiectasis with airflow limitation: an observational study. Medicine (Baltimore). 2016;95(42)e5116 [C].

[11] Balfour-Lynn IM, Welch K. Inhaled corticosteroids for cystic fibrosis. Cochrane Database Syst Rev. 2016;(8). CD001915. http://dx.doi.org/10.1002/14651858.CD001915.pub5 [M].

[12] Festic E, Bansal V, Gupta E, et al. Association of inhaled corticosteroids with incident pneumonia and mortality in COPD patients; systematic review and meta-analysis. COPD. 2016;13(3):312–26 [M].

[13] Wang C-Y, Lai C-C, Yang W-C, et al. The association between inhaled corticosteroid and pneumonia in COPD patients: the improvement of patients' life quality with COPD in Taiwan (IMPACT) study. Int J Chron Obstruct Pulmon Dis. 2016;11:2775–83 [MC].

[14] Vestbo J, Anderson JA, Brook RD, et al. Fluticasone furoate and vilanterol and survival in chronic obstructive pulmonary disease with heightened cardiovascular risk (SUMMIT): a double-blind randomised controlled trial. Lancet. 2016;387(10030): 1817–26 [MC].

[15] Wedzicha JA, Banerji D, Chapman KR, et al. Indacaterol-glycopyrronium versus salmeterol-fluticasone for COPD. N Engl J Med. 2016;374(23):2222–34 [MC].

[16] Ernst P, Coulombe J, Brassard P, et al. The risk of sepsis with inhaled and oral corticosteroids in patients with COPD. COPD. 2016;23:1–6 [MC].

[17] Spantideas N, Drosou E, Bougea A, et al. Inhaled corticosteroids and voice problems. What is new? J Voice. 2017;31:384.e1–7. S0892-1997(16)30266-1. [R].

[18] Moss EB, Buys YM, Low SA, et al. A randomized controlled trial to determine the effect of inhaled corticosteroid on intraocular pressure in open-angle glaucoma and ocular hypertension: the ICOUGH study. J Glaucoma. 2017;26:182–6 [c].

[19] Kowalski ML, Wojciechowski P, Dziewonska M, et al. Adrenal suppression by inhaled corticosteroids in patients with asthma: a systematic review and quantitative analysis. Allergy Asthma Proc. 2016;37(1):9–17 [M].

[20] Price D, Russell R, Mares R, et al. Metabolic effects associated with ICS in patients with COPD and comorbid type 2 diabetes: a historical matched cohort study. PLoS One. 2016; 11(9). e0162903 [C].

[21] Liu SF, Kuo HC, Liu GH, et al. Inhaled corticosteroids can reduce osteoporosis in female patients with COPD. Int J Chron Obstruct Pulmon Dis. 2016;11:1607–14 [MC].

[22] Martel MJ, Rey E, Beauchesne MF, et al. Use of inhaled corticosteroids during pregnancy and risk of pregnancy induced hypertension: nested case–control study. BMJ. 2005;330:230 [PMC free article]. [c].

[23] Lee CH, Kim J, Jane E, et al. Inhaled corticosteroids use is Not associated with an increased risk of pregnancy-induced hypertension and gestational diabetes mellitus. Two nested case–control studies. Medicine (Baltimore). 2016;95(22)e3627 [C].

[24] DongYH Chang CH, Gagane JJ, et al. Comparative cardiovascular and cerebrovascular safety of inhaled long-acting bronchodilators in patients with chronic obstructive pulmonary disease: a population-based cohort study. Pharmacotherapy. 2016;36(1):26–37 [MC].

[25] Peters SP, Bleecker ER, Canonica GW, et al. Serious asthma events with budesonide plus formoterol vs. budesonide alone. N Engl J Med. 2016;375(9):850–60 [MC].

[26] Cheng QJ, Huang S, Chen YZ, et al. Formoterol as reliever medication in asthma: a post-hoc analysis of the subgroup of the RELIEF study in East Asia. BMC Pulm Med. 2016;16:8–15 [C].

[27] Lee HW, Kim HJ, Lee CH, et al. The impact of olodaterol on the risk of mortality and serious adverse events: a systematic review and meta-analysis. Br J Clin Pharmacol. 2017;83:1166–75. http://dx.doi.org/10.1111/bcp.13210 [M].

[28] Kunz C, Luedtke D, Unseld A, et al. Pharmacokinetics and safety of olodaterol administered with the respimat soft mist inhaler in subjects with impaired hepatic or renal function. Int J Chron Obstruct Pulmon Dis. 2016;11:585–95 [c].

[29] Raphael G, Taveras H, Iverson H, et al. Twelve- and 52-week safety of albuterol multidose dry powder inhaler in patients with persistent asthma. J Asthma. 2016;53(2):187–93 [C].

[30] Stempel DA, Szefler SJ, Pedersen S, et al. Safety of adding salmeterol to fluticasone propionate in children with asthma. N Engl J Med. 2016;375(9):840–9 [MC].

[31] Oliver AJ, Covar RA, Caroline H, et al. Randomised trial of once-daily vilanterol in children with asthma on inhaled corticosteroid therapy. Respir Res. 2016;5(17):37–43 [C].

[32] Donohue JF, Singh D, Munzu C, et al. Magnitude of umeclidinium/vilanterol lung function effect depends on monotherapy responses: results from two randomized controlled trials. Respir Med. 2016;112:65–74 [C].

[33] Singh D, Schröder-Babo W, Cohuet G, et al. The bronchodilator effects of extrafine glycopyrronium added to combination treatment with beclomethasone dipropionate plus formoterol in COPD: a randomized crossover study (the TRIDENT study). Respir Med. 2016;114:84–90 [C].

[34] Singh D, Papi A, Corradi M, et al. Single inhaler triple therapy versus inhaled corticosteroid plus long-acting β2-agonist therapy for chronic obstructive pulmonary disease (TRILOGY): a double-blind, parallel group, randomized controlled trial. Lancet. 2016;388(10048):963–73 [M].

[35] Chiu M, Al-Majed N, Stubbins R, et al. A case report of QT prolongation with glycopyrronium bromide in a patient with chronic tamoxifen use. BMC Res Notes. 2016;9:310 [A].

[36] Kew KM, Dahri K. Long-acting muscarinic antagonists (LAMA) added to combination long-acting beta₂-agonists and inhaled corticosteroids (LABA/ICS) versus LABA/ICS for adults with asthma. Cochrane Database Syst Rev. 2016;(1) CD01172 [M].

[37] Paggiaro P, Halpin DM, Buhl R, et al. The effect of tiotropium in symptomatic asthma despite Low- to medium-dose inhaled corticosteroids: a randomized controlled trial. J Allergy Clin Immunol Pract. 2016;4(1):104–13 [C].

[38] Medic G, Lindner L, van der Weijden M, et al. Efficacy and safety of aclidinium/formoterol versus tiotropium in COPD: results of an indirect treatment comparison. Adv Ther. 2016;33(3):379–99 [M].

[39] Siler TM, Kerwin E, Singletary K, et al. Efficacy and safety of umeclidinium added to fluticasone propionate/salmeterol in patients with COPD: results of two randomized, double-blind studies. COPD. 2016;13(1):1–10 [MC].

[40] Yamagata E, Soutome T, Hashimoto K, et al. Long-term (52 weeks) safety and tolerability of umeclidinium in Japanese patients with chronic obstructive pulmonary disease. Curr Med Res Opin. 2016;32(5):967–73 [C].

[41] Feldman G, Maltias F, Khindri S, et al. A randomized, blinded study to evaluate the efficacy and safety of umeclidinium 62.5 µg compared with tiotropium 18 µg in patients with COPD. Int J Chron Obstruct Pulmon Dis. 2016;11:719–30 [MC].

[42] Perona A, Garcia-Saiz M, Alvarez E. Psychiatric disorders and montelukast in children: a disproportionality analysis of the VigiBase®. Drug Saf. 2016;39(1):69–78 [MC].

[43] Harada S, Harada N, Itoigawa Y, et al. Evaluation of switching low-dose inhaled corticosteroids to pranlukast for step-down therapy in well-controlled patients with mild persistent asthma. J Asthma. 2016;53(2):207–12 [c].

[44] Kim S, Lee JN. A case of pranlukast-induced anaphylactic shock. Allergy Asthma Immunol Res. 2016;8(3):276–8 [A].

[45] Luo P, Li S, Chen Y, et al. Efficiency and safety of roflumilast combined with long-acting bronchodilators on moderate-to-severe stable chronic obstructive pulmonary disease patients: a meta-analysis. J Thorac Dis. 2016;8(9):2638–45 [M].

[46] Yuan L, Dai X, Yang M, et al. Potential treatment benefits and safety of roflumilast in COPD: a systematic review and meta-analysis. Int J Chron Obstruct Pulmon Dis. 2016;11:1477–83 [M].

[47] Lee JS, Hong YK, Part TS, et al. Efficacy and safety of roflumilast in Korean patients with COPD. Yonsei Med J. 2016;57(4):928–35 [C].

[48] Martinez FJ, Rabe KF, Sethi S, et al. Effect of roflumilast and inhaled corticosteroid/long-acting β2-agonist on chronic obstructive pulmonary disease exacerbations (RE(2)SPOND). a randomized clinical trial. Am J Respir Crit Care Med. 2016;194(5):559–67 [C].

[49] Bateman ED, Goehring UM, Richard F, et al. Roflumilast combined with montelukast versus montelukast alone as add-on treatment in patients with moderate-to-severe asthma. J Allergy Clin Immunol. 2016;138(1):142–9 [c].

[50] Rabe K. Update on roflumilast, a phosphodiesterase 4 inhibitor for the treatment of chronic obstructive pulmonary disease. Br J Pharmacol. 2011;163(1):53–67 [R].

[51] Al Efraij K, FitzGerald J. Current and emerging treatments for severe asthma. J Thorac Dis. 2015;7(11):522–5 [R].

[52] Ledford D, Busse W, Trzaskoma B, et al. A randomized, multicenter study evaluating xolair® persistency of response after long-term therapy (XPORT). J Allergy Clin Immunol. 2016;150(1):162–9 [Available online 5 November 2016]. [C].

[53] Li J, Kang J, Wang C, et al. Omalizumab improves quality of life and asthma control in Chinese patients with moderate to severe asthma: a randomized phase III study. Allergy Asthma Immunol Res. 2016;8(4):319–28 [C].

[54] Tat TS, Cilli A. Evaluation of long-term safety and efficacy of omalizumab in elderly patients with uncontrolled allergic asthma. Ann Allergy Asthma Immunol. 2016;117(5):546–9 [C].

[55] Hew M, Gillman A, Sutherland M, et al. Real-life effectiveness of omalizumab in severe allergic asthma above the recommended dosing range criteria. Clin Exp Allergy. 2016;46(11):1407–15 [C].

[56] Gibson PG, Reddel H, Mcdonald VM, et al. Effectiveness and response predictors of omalizumab in a severe allergic asthma population with a high prevalence of comorbidities: the Australian xolair registry. Intern Med J. 2016;46(9):1054–62 [C].

[57] Niven RM, Saralaya D, Chaudhuri R, et al. Impact of omalizumab on treatment of severe allergic asthma in UK clinical practice: a UK multicentre observational study (the APEX II study). BMJ Open. 2016;6:e011857 [C].

[58] Iribarren C, Rahmaoui A, Long AA, et al. Cardiovascular and cerebrovascular events among patients receiving omalizumab: results from EXCELS, a prospective cohort study of moderate-to-severe asthma. J Allergy Clin Immunol. 2017;139:1489–96 S0091-6749(16)30961-7. [MC].

[59] Smith D, Minthorn E, Beerahee M. Pharmacokinetics and pharmacodynamics of mepolizumab, an anti-interleukin-5 monoclonal antibody. Clin Pharmacokinet. 2011;50(4):215–27 [R].

[60] Ortega HG, Liu MC, Parvord ID, et al. Mepolizumab treatment in patients with severe eosinophilic asthma. N Engl J Med. 2014;371(13):1198–207.

[61] Pavord ID, Korn S, Howarth P, et al. Mepolizumab for severe eosinophilic asthma (DREAM): a multicentre, double-blind, placebo-controlled trial. Lancet. 2012;380:651 [C].

[62] Bel E, Wenzel S, Thompson P, et al. Oral glucocorticoid-sparing effect of Mepolizumab in eosinophilic asthma. N Engl J Med. 2014;371:1189–97 [C].

[63] Powell C, Milan SJ, Dwan K, et al. Mepolizumab versus placebo for asthma. Cochrane Database Syst Rev. 2015;7:CD010834 [M].

[64] Tsukamotot N, Takahashi N, Itoh H, et al. Pharmacokinetics and pharmacodynamics of mepolizumab, an anti-interleukin 5 monoclonal antibody in healthy Japanese male subjecys. Clin Pharmacol Drug Dev. 2016;5(2):102–8 [c].

[65] Lugogo N, Domingo C, Chanez P, et al. Long-term efficacy and safety of mepolizumab in patients with severe eosinophilic asthma: a multi-center, open-label, phase IIIb study. Clin Ther. 2016;38(9):2058–70 [C].

[66] Castro M, Zangrilli J, Wechsler M, et al. Reslizumab for inadequately controlled asthma with elevated blood eosinophil counts: results from two multicentre, parallel, double-blind, randomised, placebo-controlled, phase 3 trials. Lancet. 2015;3(5):355–66 [C].

[67] Corren J, Weinstein S, Janka L. Phase 3 study of reslizumab in patients with poorly controlled asthma: effects across a broad range of eosinophil counts. Chest. 2016;150(4):799–810 [C].

[68] Bjermer L, Lemiere C, Maspero J, et al. Reslizumab for inadequately controlled asthma with elevated blood eosinophil levels: a randomized phase 3 study. Chest. 2016;150(4):789–98 [M].

[69] Wang FP, Liu T, Lan Z, et al. Efficacy and safety in anti-interleukin-5 therapy in patients with asthma: a systemic review and meta-analysis. PLoS One. 2016;11(11). e0166833 [C].

15

Positive Inotropic Drugs and Drugs Used in Dysrhythmias

Cassandra Maynard[1], Jingyang Fan

SIUE School of Pharmacy, Edwardsville, IL, United States

[1]Corresponding author: cmaynar@siue.edu

CARDIAC GLYCOSIDES [SED-16, 117; SEDA-35, 327; SEDA-36, 257; SEDA-37, 205]

Digoxin

Skin

- A 91-year-old woman, initially admitted after a fall, developed cardiac decompensation as a result of rapid atrial fibrillation (AF) and was started on digoxin (unknown dose or route). Eight days after initiation of digoxin, the patient developed multiple skin afflictions, including a non-itchy and non-painful rash on her back and trunk and later bullous lesions and ulcerations on her lower extremities. A skin biopsy revealed leukocytoclasic vasculitis with necrosis. The skin rash resolved once digoxin was discontinued [1A].

Susceptibility Factors: Age, Comorbidities

In an Australian study looking at the extent of polypharmacy in elderly patients (65 years or older) with AF, 30.2% of 367 patients were using digoxin. In addition, 20% of the patients who took 10 or more medications (major polypharmacy) were taking digoxin. The authors cautioned clinicians on the potential inappropriate use of digoxin, compounded by the risk of older age, multiple comorbidities, and drug interactions. All these can lead to an increased risk of adverse effects from digoxin thus increased attention should be paid to any patient, particularly the elderly, that is prescribed digoxin [2C].

Drug–Drug Interaction

An in vitro study showed that when digoxin was added, cancer cells were noted to be resistant to the effect of cisplatin. However, digoxin sensitized cancer cells to the effect of etoposide. Although not evaluated in clinical settings, digoxin may decrease the effectiveness of cisplatin when patients receive both. The authors also suggested that co-administration of digoxin may allow a lower dose of etoposide thus minimizing adverse effects of etoposide [3E]. Of course, the clinical relevance of these observations needs to be evaluated in in vivo studies.

ANTIDYSRYTHMIC DRUGS

Amiodarone [SED-16, 255; SEDA-35, 332; SEDA-36, 259; SEDA-37, 208]

Cardiovascular

- A 58-year-old female developed an acute brachial artery occlusion following the administration of 300 mg of intravenous amiodarone into the artery. Immediately following the injection, the patient's arm became painful and pale. Angiography confirmed the presence of an acute thrombus at the site of injection. The thrombus was aspirated and medications (vasodilators, heparin and glycoprotein 2b3a inhibitor) were given with success to restore blood flow; however, she still developed compartment syndrome necessitating surgery [4A].

This case demonstrates that amiodarone, when injected inappropriately, can have direct toxicity to the vessel wall. This can result in vascular inflammation which led to acute thrombus formation requiring immediate treatment. While this adverse effect resulted from an administration error, it is critical to be aware of the potential harm from intra-arterial administration of amiodarone as this will require emergent attention.

ISSN: 0378-6080
http://dx.doi.org/10.1016/bs.seda.2017.06.008

Liver

Hepatotoxicity is a well known yet poorly understood adverse effect of amiodarone. Although hepatotoxicity from amiodarone has been previously reported, the following case illustrates the potential for not only acute liver dysfunction but also the possibility for patients to experience issues with one formulation and not another of amiodarone.

- A 57-year-old Asian male was initiated on oral amiodarone for atrial fibrillation. He received 100 mg of oral amiodarone for 2 days before treatment was switched to intravenous (150 mg followed by a continuous infusion). After 24 hours, the patient's AST and ALT were found to be 4374 and >2500, respectively (increased from a baseline of 29 and 77). Amiodarone was discontinued and his LFTs declined to normal values within 2 weeks. There was no recurrence in hepatotoxicity noted. Other potential causes of hepatotoxicity were ruled out. The patient was subsequently re-initiated on oral amiodarone 100 mg daily without any increase in liver enzymes noted [5A].

In this case the patient appeared to tolerate the oral amiodarone without incident and only developed liver dysfunction when the intravenous form was initiated. It has been theorized in other cases, and likewise in this one, that the possible cause for the hepatotoxicity was the polysorbate 80 in the diluent [6A,7A].

Multiorgan

Toxicities that involve more than one organ may occur in patients receiving amiodarone.

- A 65-year-old white male developed acute liver and renal failure within 12 hours of initiation of intravenous amiodarone. The patient was initiated on IV amiodarone 150 mg followed by 1 mg/min for 6 hours, then 0.5 mg/min for 18 hours for control of supraventricular tachycardia which was leading to AICD shocks. His labs were reported as normal upon admission with normal blood pressure (140/88). Upon starting amiodarone, he became hypotensive (90/60) with the blood pressure only resolving 2 hours after amiodarone was discontinued. The patient's AST increased to 8981 and ALT to 4450 within 24 hours. Additionally, his serum creatinine and potassium increased while the urine output decreased necessitating dialysis. Work-up for other potential causes was negative. The patient was hospitalized for 5 days and follow-up labs at 6 months were within normal limits [8A].

There have been several case reports of acute hepatotoxicity with amiodarone while nephrotoxicity is rare.

In this case, it is likely that the hypotension led to a reduction in liver and renal perfusion resulting in acute injury. Even short infusions of amiodarone necessitate monitoring of blood pressure, liver function tests and renal function.

- A 13-year-old male with congenital heart disease was initiated on amiodarone for atrial flutter 6 years prior. He presented to an outpatient center with blue-gray facial skin and pulmonary nodules on a chest X-ray. The presence of foamy macrophages on bronchoscopy confirmed a diagnosis of amiodarone-induced pulmonary toxicity. Following discontinuation of amiodarone, the patient's skin tone returned to normal but the pulmonary nodules were still present 2 years later [9A].

While pulmonary fibrosis is the most common occurrence of amiodarone-induced pulmonary toxicity, other manifestations have been reported. It has been postulated that pulmonary masses arise from selective accumulation of the drug within a pre-existing lung lesion. It is difficult to discern if the above child had any pre-existing lung issues; however, it is recommended that patients obtain a baseline chest X-ray prior to initiating amiodarone therapy. Additionally close monitoring for potential long-term adverse effects, particularly serious ones, is necessary to avoid any delay in management.

Susceptibility Factors: Age, Concurrent Illness

Amiodarone is well known for causing thyroid dysfunction, both hypo- and hyperthyroidism. Understanding which patients are at greater risk of developing these adverse effects may help to improve monitoring, prevention and rapid treatment of this complication.

- A 2-year retrospective cohort study from 2012 to 2013 in Japanese patients who were treated with oral amiodarone sought to identify what, if any, risk factors for amiodarone-induced thyroid dysfunction were present in those developing this adverse reaction. This study identified 30 patients (9.5%) that developed amiodarone-induced hyperthyroidism while 60 patients (18.9%) were found to have amiodarone-induced hypothyroidism. Hypothyroidism was most likely to develop early in therapy (at less than 1 year of treatment) and in those with altered baseline thyroid function tests prior to initiation of amiodarone. Positive predictors for the development of hyperthyroidism were identified as younger age, presence of dilated cardiomyopathy, and presence of cardiac sarcoidosis [10C].

It is not only beneficial to understand which patients may be at increased risk, but also whether there are certain patients which may have more difficulty in recovering from these adverse effects.

- Patients in Taiwan experiencing amiodarone-induced hypothyroidism (AIH) were evaluated to determine if any factors could be identified which impacted their recovery from AIH. Of the 314 patients evaluated that were receiving amiodarone, 97 patients were found to have hypothyroidism. Amiodarone was discontinued in 33 patients, with 24 patients initiated on levothyroxine while the remaining 9 did not receive any treatment for AIH. All 9 non-treatment patients and 23 of the 24 levothyroxine patients had a return to baseline of their thyroid function within 3 years. Those with the quickest recovery, within 3 months, were patients that did not receive levothyroxine. Elderly patients (age >70 years) also tended to have a slower recovery time compared to those less than 70. There did not appear to be any discrepancy in recovery from AIH based on gender [11C].

In this analysis, patients with higher TSH levels tended to receive treatment with levothyroxine. Therefore, it is possible that it is the severity of the TSH elevation that is more likely to contribute to the recovery time period as opposed to the usage of levothyroxine in and of itself.

Both of these reports were specific to Asian patients and as such can only be used to discern risk in this population. However, the more information which is available to both identify those at risk and the likely recovery time involved upon drug discontinuation is valuable and may be relatable to other ethnicities.

DOFETILIDE [SED-16, 1060; SEDA-35, 338; SEDA-37, 209; SEDA-38, 170]

Drug Overdose

Although well known for causing QT prolongation and torsades de pointes (TdP), there has been limited literature on the clinical course and outcomes from dofetilide overdose. A retrospective cohort study evaluated overdose cases that were reported to a poison center from January 2002 to January 2016. Of the 27 overdose cases, 10 patients (37%) were treated at home, while 9 (33%) were managed in the emergency departments without being admitted and 8 (30%) were admitted for inpatient management. All, except one case, were unintentional ingestions which led to mild overdose. The most notable adverse effect was QTc prolongation which occurred without significant clinical effects. Most of these patients only required cardiac monitoring and electrolyte replacement. The one case of intentional overdose involved a patient that took 90 times his usual dose and exhibited an 8-beat run of non-sustained ventricular tachycardia, frequent multifocal premature ventricular beats and ventricular bigeminy. He recovered after treatment with magnesium sulfate and potassium replacement [12c].

This case series suggested that some cases of mild dofetilide overdose may be managed at home or with cardiac monitoring and electrolyte replacement with or without gastrointestinal decontamination. However, it is also important to keep in mind that even a single extra dose had been reported to lead to ventricular fibrillation [13S]. Therefore, it is important to triage patients based on the amount of overdose, patient's renal function, electrolytes, presence of additional QTc prolonging medications, and other high-risk comorbidities.

FLECAINIDE [SED-16, 327; SEDA-35, 339; SEDA-36, 262]

Cardiovascular

- A 65-year-old female patient, with a history of paroxysmal AF and intolerance to amiodarone, presented to the hospital with AF. She was started on flecainide 50 mg every 12 hours and bisoprolol 2.5 mg every 12 hours, after spontaneously converting to normal sinus rhythm. At some point during the hospitalization, the patient developed a pruriginous rash on the lower extremities, for which she received loratadine 10 mg daily and hydroxyzine 25 mg daily. Four days after the initiation of concomitant H_1 antagonists, the patient developed TdP which deteriorated into ventricular fibrillation. She received defibrillation six times and regained a pulse after 15 minutes. The patient made a full recovery and received only bisoprolol for rate control when her AF returned. Although H_1 antagonists have been associated with QTc prolongation and TdP, its synergistic effect with flecainide in QTc prolongation has rarely been reported. This case demonstrated that concurrent use of flecainide and H_1 antagonists should be avoided if possible [14A].

- A white female patient in her 50s presented to the emergency department with palpitations. She was receiving flecainide 100 mg twice daily for rhythm control of her paroxysmal AF. She denied any changes in her flecainide dose. The EKG initially showed wide complex tachycardia at a rate of 214 bpm; then after administration of IV bicarbonate, the rhythm became atrial flutter at a rate of 214 bpm with 2:1 ventricular response. The authors postulated that the wide complex tachycardia on the first EKG was actually atrial flutter with 1:1 AV conduction. They hypothesized that flecainide slowed AF into slower flutter, which then resulted in fast ventricular response in the absence of an AV nodal blocking agent. And the effect of flecainide on intraventricular conduction delays was potentiated by the fast heart rates, resulting in a wide complex QRS. The authors expressed caution in using flecainide without AV nodal blocking agents and encouraged flecainide dose adjustment with exercise testing to increase the heart rate. The patient was taken off of flecainide and successfully cardioverted to sinus rhythm. She received metoprolol for rate control and apixiban for stroke prevention with plans for catheter ablation [15A].

- An 89-year-old man, with AF and heart failure with preserved ejection fraction, presented with acute heart failure. He was receiving flecainide 100 mg twice daily, in addition to aspirin, perindopril, furosemide and simvastatin. His EKG showed QTc prolongation at 562 s with QRS widening, which is consistent with class Ic antiarrhythmic toxicity. The authors attributed patient's worsening heart failure to flecainide, which was precipitated by worsening renal function. The patient's heart failure and renal function improved after flecainide was discontinued. He was discharged home with bisoprolol for rate control [16A]. Extreme caution should be exercised when using flecainide in the elderly as this population is more at risk of having renal dysfunction which can adversely affect antiarrhythmic therapy.

Urinary Tract

- A 24-year-old pregnant woman was started on flecainide 200 mg per day (unsure if it was 100 mg twice daily) for fetal tachycardia in her 36th week of gestation. After 10 days of flecainide therapy, it was discontinued upon her admission for a planned C-section. A serum level 24 hours after the last flecainide dose showed therapeutic level at 391 ng/mL (therapeutic range 300–1000 ng/mL). On her delivery day (day 1 of hospitalization), the patient received ibuprofen 600 mg and diclofenac 100 mg one time. Five days after delivery (day 6), the patient's serum creatinine went from 0.34 to 3.13 mg/dL; it continued to rise to 4.65 mg/dL on day 7. A renal biopsy on day 10 confirmed acute interstitial nephritis (AIN). Within 4 days, her renal function improved without any steroid treatment and she was discharged on day 13 of hospitalization. The authors speculated that flecainide, in combination with NSAIDs, was the culprit of her biopsy-proven AIN. They also argued that the flecainide serum level 24 hours after the last dose was "well within" the therapeutic range of 300–1000 ng/mL, which was suggestive of potential overdose [17A].

Although a possibility, this case cannot definitively conclude that flecainide was responsible for the AIN. A previous case described a 76-year-old patient who received flecainide 200 mg per day for 3 years and developed acute kidney injury after receiving concurrent indomethacin [18A]. These two cases both involved NSAIDs

use, which is a known cause of AIN. Whether flecainide potentiated this adverse effect cannot be determined based on the information given. In addition, the authors suggested a potential overdose of flecainide based on the serum level. Considering the half-life of flecainide ranges from 12 to 27 hours [19S], it is not surprising to have a serum level of 391 ng/mL 24 hours of the last flecainide dose. Regardless, it is important for the clinicians to be vigilant of the potential drug interactions between flecainide and NSAIDs, avoid the combination whenever possible, and monitor renal function closely if the combination cannot be avoided.

POSITIVE INOTROPES

Omecamtiv mecarbil, formerly identified as CK-1827452, is a novel agent currently being investigated for the management of congestive heart failure. It is a positive inotrope with a unique mechanism of action. It is the first in its class of cardiac-specific myosin activators. Omecamtiv increases myocardial contraction via an increase in myosin cross-bridge formation resulting in an increase in the force of the contraction without increasing intracellular calcium levels. It has been shown to increase systolic ejection time and systolic function [20R,21R].

Published in 2016, the Chronic Oral Study of Myosin Activation to Increase Contractility in Heart Failure (COSMIC-HF) was a phase 2 pharmacokinetic study designed to evaluate the ability of a dose titration schedule of oral omecamtiv mecarbil to attain adequate plasma levels. Patients aged 18–85 years of age with systolic heart failure were divided into 3 groups: placebo (149 patients), a fixed-dose of oral omecamtiv at 25 mg twice daily (150 patients) and an omecamtiv titration-dose group (149 patients). The titration dose group was started at 25 mg twice daily and increased to 50 mg twice daily based upon plasma levels. A little over half of the patients (78/146) received the maximum dose of 50 mg with no patients exceeding the maximum recommended plasma levels of 1000 ng/mL. Patients receiving omecamtiv experienced the following adverse events at a rate of 5% or more (total of 296 patients): dyspnea (8.1%; 24 patients), fatigue (7.7%; 23 patients), and dizziness (6%; 18 patients). Angina occurred in 3 patients (2%) in the fixed dose group, 1 patient (1%) in the titration dose group and no patients in the placebo group [22C].

Omecamtiv mecarbil has been shown to reduce heart rate [23E,24c,25c]. In this trial, while patients in the fixed-dose group did have a decrease in heart rate compared to placebo, it was not found to be statistically significant. However, those in the titration-dose group did have a statistically significant change in heart rate compared to placebo, an approximate 2.5 beat/min reduction vs a 0.5 beat/min increase, respectively, although it would likely not be considered clinically significant [22C].

The Acute Treatment with Omecamtiv Mecarbil to Increase Contractility in Acute Heart Failure (ATOMIC-AHF) Study investigated various dosing arms of intravenous omecamtiv compared to placebo over a 48-hour period [26C]. Patients were separated into three groups with titrating doses to achieve plasma concentrations of 115 ng/mL (103 patients), 230 ng/mL (99 patients) and 310 ng/mL (101 patients). Each group was matched 1:1 with a placebo group. At 30 days, there were 10 deaths in the pooled placebo group compared to 8 in pooled omecamtiv arms. While at 6 months, the mortality rate appeared to narrow to almost equivalency between the groups, 12.9% (39 patients) in placebo and 12.5% (38 patients) receiving omecamtiv.

Similar to the COSMIC-HF trial, omecamtiv mecarbil led to a greater decrease in heart rate and systolic blood pressure with increasing omecamtiv plasma concentrations; however, these adverse effects were not found to be symptomatic. Patients receiving omecamtiv experienced the following side effects at a rate greater than 5% in the ATOMIC-AHF trial: hypokalemia (6.6%; 20 patients) and hypotension (7.9%, 24 patients). Cardiac failure was reported in 15.2% (46) of patients receiving omecamtiv although this compared to 17.5% (53) of placebo and as such is more likely a reflection of the drug's efficacy in the management of chronic heart failure and not a true side effect of the drug.

Omecamtiv mecarbil has been shown to have an increased incidence of myocardial ischemia and with that an increase cardiac troponin I (cTnI) levels [24c,25c]. Both trials measured cTnI at baseline and during treatment. Each study found a greater increase in cTnI levels in patients receiving omecamtiv compared to placebo. In COSMIC-HF, no patients were determined to have experienced any myocardial ischemia or infarction by the clinical events committee, whereas 7 patients receiving omecamtiv in ATOMIC-AHF were found to have had a myocardial infarction (compared to only 3 patients in the placebo group). Additionally, no correlation was found between omecamtiv dosing and the potential for myocardial damage. Current evidence suggests that omecamtiv does not increase myocardial oxygen demand; however, the increase in troponin level is concerning [23E]. It is suspected that the prolongation of the systolic ejection time is the cause of myocardial ischemia. More studies are warranted to elucidate the exact mechanism.

The COSMIC-HF and ATOMIC-AHF trials have been short (20 weeks and 48 hours, respectively) and were dose-finding in nature. These were small, initial trials and neither study was powered to evaluate clinical outcomes. Omecamtiv mecarbil requires further study to elicit the full safety profile of the drug including but not limited to those adverse effects which may occur in low incidence and thus would only be identified in a large clinical trial setting. Additionally, in total, more than 80% of those enrolled in these trials have been white males. It is prudent to evaluate the drug in women and those of other racial backgrounds to insure safety across all populations. Of particular concern will be the incidence of myocardial infarction and resultant cardiovascular mortality of patients exposed to the medication.

References

[1] Ludwig-Béal S, Vernier N, Popitean L, et al. Digoxin-related leukocytoclastic vasculitis in a very elderly woman: a case report. J Mal Vasc. 2016;41:220–3 [A].

[2] Wang Y, Singh S, Bajorek B. Old age, high risk medication, polypharmacy: a "trilogy" of risks in older patients with atrial fibrillation. Pharm Pract (Granada). 2016;14:1–12 [C].

[3] Kulikov AV, Slobodkina EA, Alekseev AV, et al. Contrasting effects of cardiac glycosides on cisplatin-and etoposide-induced cell death. Biol Chem. 2016;397:661–70 [E].

[4] Witkowski M, Mochmann H-C, Rauch U, et al. Acute thrombotic occlusion of the left brachial artery after intra-arterial administration of amiodarone. Crit Care Med. 2016;44: e227–30 [A].

[5] Chen C-C, Wu C-C. Acute hepatotoxicity of intravenous amiodarone: case report and review of the literature. Am J Ther. 2014;263:2014–7 [A].

[6] Stratton A, Fenderson J, Kenny P, et al. Severe acute hepatitis following intravenous amiodarone: a case report and review of the literature. Acta Gastroenterol Belg. 2015;78:233–9 [A].

[7] Rhodes A, Eastwood JB, Smith SA. Early acute hepatitis with parenteral amiodarone: a toxic effect of the vehicle? Gut. 1993;34:565–6 [A].

[8] Paudel R, Dogra P, Suman S, et al. Acute liver and renal failure: a rare adverse effect exclusive to intravenous form of amiodarone. Case Rep Crit Care. 2016;2016:1–4 [A].

[9] Paech C, Wagner F, Suchowerskyj P, et al. The blue child—amiodarone-induced blue-gray skin syndrome and pulmonary mass in a child. Clin Case Reports. 2016;4:276–8 [A].

[10] Kinoshita S, Hayashi T, Wada K, et al. Risk factors for amiodarone-induced thyroid dysfunction in Japan. J Arrhythmia. 2016;32:474–80 [C].

[11] Huang JH, Lin YK, Hsieh MH, et al. Age and thyroid hormone replacement delays the recovery from amiodarone-induced hypothyroidism. Int J Cardiol. 2016;202:561–3 [C].

[12] Hieger MA, Maskell KF, Moss MJ, et al. Dofetilide in overdose: a case series from poison center data. Cardiovasc Toxicol. 2016;1–4 [c].

[13] Tikosyn® [package insert]. New York, NY: Pfizer Inc.; 2016 [S].

[14] Acosta-Materán C, Díaz-Oliva E, Fernández-Rodríguez D, et al. QT interval prolongation and torsade de pointes: synergistic effect of flecainide and H1 receptor antagonists. J Pharmacol Pharmacother. 2016;7:102–5 [A].

[15] Hegde S, Kumar V. Wide complex tachycardia in a patient with a history of atrial fibrillation. JAMA Intern Med. 2016;176:386–8 [A].

[16] McKenzie GAG, Porter B, Kaprielian R. An 89-year-old man presents with worsening heart failure. Heart. 2016;102:633 [A].

[17] Schmidt JJ, Ramazan L, Bockemeyer C, et al. Acute interstitial nephritis due to flecainide therapy in the 38th week of pregnancy. BMC Nephrol. 2016;17:28 [A].

[18] Meurin P, Larrazet F, Weber H, et al. Iatrogenic acute renal failure caused by overdosage of flecainide acetate. Presse Med. 1998;27:1473–5 [A].

[19] Flecainide [package insert]. Jacksonville, FL: Ranbaxy Pharmaceuticals Inc.; 2003 [S].

[20] Nanasi PJ, Vaczi K, Papp Z. The myosin activator omecamtiv mecarbil: a promising new inotropic agent. Can J Physiol Pharmacol. 2016;94:1033–9 [R].

[21] Teerlink JR. A novel approach to improve cardiac performance: cardiac myosin activators. Heart Fail Rev. 2009;14:289–98 [R].

[22] Teerlink JR, Felker GM, McMurray JJV, et al. Chronic Oral Study of Myosin Activation to Increase Contractility in Heart Failure (COSMIC-HF): a phase 2, pharmacokinetic, randomized, placebo-controlled trial. Lancet. 2016;388:2895–903 [C].

[23] Shen Y-T, Malik FI, Zhao X, et al. Improvement of cardiac function by a cardiac Myosin activator in conscious dogs with systolic heart failure. Circ Heart Fail. 2010;3:522–7 [E].

[24] Teerlink JR, Clarke CP, Saikali KG, et al. Dose-dependent augmentation of cardiac systolic function with the selective cardiac myosin activator, omecamtiv mecarbil: a first-in-man study. Lancet. 2011;378:667–75 [c].

[25] Cleland JGF, Teerlink JR, Senior R, et al. The effects of the cardiac myosin activator, omecamtiv mecarbil, on cardiac function in systolic heart failure: a double-blind, placebo-controlled, crossover, dose-ranging phase 2 trial. Lancet. 2011;378:676–83 [c].

[26] Teerlink JR, Felker GM, McMurray V JJ, et al. Acute treatment with omecamtiv mecarbil to increase contractility in acute heart failure: the ATOMIC-AHF study. J Am Coll Cardiol. 2016;67:1444–55 [C].

16

Drugs Acting on the Cerebral and Peripheral Circulations

Arduino A. Mangoni[1]

School of Medicine, Flinders University and Flinders Medical Centre, Bedford Park, SA, Australia
[1]Corresponding author: arduino.mangoni@flinders.edu.au

DRUGS USED IN THE TREATMENT OF ARTERIAL DISORDERS OF THE BRAIN AND LIMBS AND IN THE TREATMENT OF MIGRAINE

Cilostazol [SEDA-36, 275–276]

Cardiovascular System

Clinical reports suggest that donepezil-mediated cardiotoxicity can occur after concomitant treatment with cilostazol. However, the mechanisms responsible for this interaction are unknown. An in vitro study investigated whether cilostazol affects the efflux transporters P-glycoprotein (ABCB1) and breast cancer resistance protein (BCRP, ABCG2) in Madin–Darby canine kidney cells and rat heart slices [1E]. At clinical concentrations, cilostazol inhibited BCRP-mediated, but not P-glycoprotein-mediated, transport of donepezil. When isolated rat heart slices were incubated with donepezil in the presence of cilostazol, the accumulation of donepezil was significantly higher. These results suggest that cilostazol may cause increased accumulation of donepezil in the heart by inhibiting BCRP. The latter might explain, at least in part, the increased risk of cardiotoxicity when donepezil is co-administered with cilostazol.

Ginkgo biloba [SEDA-37, 274]

Cardiovascular, Nervous, and Gastrointestinal

Self-reported adverse effects with the use of food supplements containing botanicals were collected during the European PlantLIBRA Plant Food Supplements Consumer Survey 2011–2012. This survey, involving 2359 participants, was followed by a critical assessment of the plausibility and causality of the symptoms reported, using data from the literature and the PlantLIBRA Poisons Centre's survey [2C]. There were five cases of G. biloba-related adverse events: dizziness ($n=1$), insomnia ($n=3$) and constipation ($n=1$). In each case, G. biloba was the only botanical in the food supplements reported by the participants. Causality was considered possible in all reported cases.

Vitamin E

Hematologic, Urinary Tract, and Tumorigenicity

A systematic review investigated the association between use of herbal and dietary supplements and risk of hemolysis in subjects with glucose-6-phosphate dehydrogenase deficiency in studies published in 14 electronic databases from their inception to November 2015 [3M]. A total of 32 publications, reporting on 10 herbal and dietary supplements, met the inclusion criteria. A qualitative analysis of these studies did not show any plausible association between the use of either G. biloba (1 study) or vitamin E (7 studies) and hemolysis.

A 6-week study in male and female mice investigated the safety of high-dose vitamin E supplementation (recommended daily intake $\times$ 25:550 mg/kg diet), considered close to the upper limit to toxicity [4E]. High-dose vitamin E induced significant changes in biomarkers of inflammation and toxicity (alkaline phosphatase, aspartate aminotransferase, biological antioxidant potential, monocyte chemoattractant protein-1, interkeukin-6, tumor necrosis factor alpha, and plasminogen activator inhibitor-1) in kidney tissue of male, but not female, mice.

The effects of 100–200 mg/kg vitamin E daily for 7–14 days on redox homeostasis and carcinogen metabolizing enzymes were studied in male Sprague-Dawley rats [5E].

ISSN: 0378-6080
http://dx.doi.org/10.1016/bs.seda.2017.06.004

In the liver, vitamin E treatment did not cause significant changes in phase-I and phase-II enzyme activities, whereas it increased antioxidant enzyme activities. By contrast, in the kidney vitamin E treatment induced a significant increase in phase-I, but not phase-II, carcinogen bio-activating enzymes, and a reduction in antioxidant enzyme activities. This was associated with a significant increase in concentrations of reactive oxidant species in kidney tissue. These results might provide a mechanistic explanation of the suggested increase in cancer risk with high-dose vitamin E supplementation.

Isoxsuprine

Cardiovascular System

A retrospective study investigated the possible causes of fetal ductus arteriosus constriction and closure in 45 consecutive cases between 1987 and 2013 [6c]. One case documented the use of intravenous isoxsuprine 10 mg for premature labor (gestational age: 34 weeks). An echocardiogram showed the presence of right ventricular dilatation and moderate tricuspid regurgitation. The delivery was uneventful; however, there was no further follow-up.

DRUGS USED IN THE TREATMENT OF VENOUS DISORDERS

Benzbromarone [SEDA-37, 274–275]

Drug–Drug Interactions

CYP2C9 and CYP3A4 activities were assessed in human liver microsomes, following pre-incubation with benzbromarone with or without the reduced form of nicotinamide adenine dinucleotide phosphate (NADPH) [7E]. Benzbromarone significantly inhibited both CYP2C9 and CYP3A4 activity. The magnitude of benzbromarone CYP3A4 inhibition, which was time-dependent, was greater after co-incubation with NADPH. The time-dependent inhibition of CYP3A4 suggests the generation of a chemically reactive metabolite during the oxidative metabolism of benzbromarone. By contrast, NADPH did not influence the effects of benzbromarone on CYP2C9 activity. These results suggest a possible involvement of CYP450 inhibition in the occurrence of idiosyncratic hepatotoxicity reported in the literature.

Diosmin [SEDA-37, 274]

Drug–Drug Interactions

An open-label, two-period, study was conducted in 12 healthy male volunteers to investigate whether diosmin affects the pharmacokinetics of fexofenadine through P-glycoprotein inhibition [8c]. Treatment with diosmin significantly increased fexofenadine Cmax (+49.2%) and AUC (+64.4%) vs control. This was associated with a significant reduction in apparent oral clearance (−41.3%). There were no significant changes in Tmax, $T_{1/2}$, and renal clearance. These results suggest that the intake of diosmin, or dietary supplements containing diosmin, might increase the absorption and/or bioavailability of fexofenadine.

An open-label, two-period, study was conducted in 12 healthy male volunteers to investigate whether diosmin affects the pharmacokinetics and metabolism of carbamazepine through a CYP3A4-mediated interaction [9c]. Treatment with diosmin caused a significant increase in carbamazepine Cmax (+57.6%), AUC (+43.8%) and $T_{1/2}$ (+44.4%) vs control. Furthermore, diosmin decreased the apparent oral clearance and elimination rate constant of carbamazepine, as well as the metabolite to parent ratios of Cmax and AUC, suggesting a reduced metabolism of carbamazepine to carbamazepine 10,11-epoxide through CYP3A4.

DRUGS USED IN THE TREATMENT OF MIGRAINE

Triptans

Liver

An in vitro sought to identify the mechanisms involved in triptan-induced hepatotoxicity using isolated rat hepatocytes [10E]. Rizatriptan (5 mM) caused a time-dependent cytotoxicity, characterized by increased synthesis of reactive oxidative species, lipid peroxidation, mitochondrial depolarization, and loss of integrity of lysosome membranes. This was associated with a significant reduction in cellular glutathione reservoirs with an increased concentration of oxidized glutathione. These cytotoxic effects were mediated by different CYP450 inducers and were prevented by the administration of reactive oxidative species scavengers, antioxidants, endocytosis inhibitors, and adenosine triphosphate regenerators. These results suggest that rizatriptan-induced hepatotoxicity is mediated by oxidative stress and mitochondrial and lysosomal damage.

OTHER PERIPHERAL VASODILATORS

Phosphodiesterase Type 5 Inhibitors [SEDA-37, 275–276]

Sensory Systems, Skin, and Nervous System

A 32-year-old woman with no history of eye problems noticed a decline in central vision in her left eye 1 month after commencing treatment with oral sildenafil 20 mg three times daily for a recently diagnosed primary pulmonary hypertension [11A]. Concomitant medications included topiramate, norethindrone, ambrisentan, tramadol, furosemide, spironolactone and digoxin. Although her symptoms progressed she did not seek medical attention for the following 5 years, when an optometrist documented a retinal abnormality. Visual acuity was 20/20 in the right and 20/100 in the left eye. On funduscopic examination, the left macula showed para-foveal retinal pigment epithelial mottling and atrophy in a ring-like configuration. Spectral domain optical coherence tomography documented mild hypoautofluorescence in the foveal center with an irregular autofluorescence pattern in the parafovea of the left eye. Her cardiologist considered treatment with sildenafil as the possible cause. Following treatment discontinuation her vision stabilized. Although this is the first report of outer macular atrophy with long-term use of sildenafil for pulmonary hypertension, the symptoms started a few weeks after treatment was initiated.

A 49-year-old male with HIV, on treatment with tenofovir, emtricitabine, atazanavir and ritonavir, was referred to the allergy clinic because of recent onset of pruritus and erythema in the palms and feet [12A]. There were no other abnormal symptoms and signs. He received treatment with ceftriaxone for syphilis 2 months earlier. Although cetirizine was prescribed the symptoms worsened and he returned after 24 hours with generalized pruritus and maculopapular rash. Physical examination revealed a single target lesion in his right palm and oral mucosal lesions, causing a tingling sensation. A diagnosis of erythema multiforme was set. On further questioning, the patient reported taking a table of sildenafil 100 mg 5 days before the onset of the initial rash. After further 7-day treatment with cetirizine and a cream containing polidocanol and urea the skin lesions and symptoms significantly improved. A patch test performed 6 months later, using sildenafil at 10% in petrolatum, resulted positive, confirming a cell-mediated drug allergy. This is the first reported case of erythema multiforme associated with sildenafil.

The potential mechanisms involved in the pro-convulsant effects of sildenafil were investigated in a pentylenetetrazole-induced seizure animal model [13E]. Sildenafil, at a dose of 10–40 mg/kg or higher, significantly reduced the seizure threshold. This was associated with a significant increase in oxytocin concentrations in the hippocampus. Administration of atosiban, an oxytocin receptor antagonist, significantly reversed the pro-convulsant effects of oxytocin and sildenafil, by inhibiting phosphorylation of cyclic AMP response element-binding protein (CREB). These results demonstrate for the first time that the pro-convulsant effects of sildenafil are mediated by oxytocin and CREB.

References

[1] Takeuchi R, Shinozaki K, Nakanishi T, et al. Local drug-drug interaction of donepezil with cilostazol at breast cancer resistance protein (ABCG2) increases drug accumulation in heart. Drug Metab Dispos. 2016;44(1):68–74 [E].

[2] Restani P, Di Lorenzo C, Garcia-Alvarez A, et al. Adverse effects of plant food supplements self-reported by consumers in the PlantLIBRA survey involving six European countries. PLoS One. 2016;11(2)e0150089 [C].

[3] Lee SW, Lai NM, Chaiyakunapruk N, et al. Adverse effects of herbal or dietary supplements in G6PD deficiency: a systematic review. Br J Clin Pharmacol. 2017;83(1):172–9 [M].

[4] Jansen E, Viezeliene D, Beekhof P, et al. Tissue-specific effects of vitamin E supplementation. Int J Mol Sci. 2016;17(7):E1166 [E].

[5] Vivarelli F, Canistro D, Franchi P, et al. Disruption of redox homeostasis and carcinogen metabolizing enzymes changes by administration of vitamin E to rats. Life Sci. 2016;145:166–73 [E].

[6] Lopes LM, Carrilho MC, Francisco RP, et al. Fetal ductus arteriosus constriction and closure: analysis of the causes and perinatal outcome related to 45 consecutive cases. J Matern Fetal Neonatal Med. 2016;29(4):638–45 [c].

[7] Masubuchi Y, Kondo S. Inactivation of CYP3A4 by benzbromarone in human liver microsomes. Drug Metab Lett. 2016;10(1):16–21 [E].

[8] Bedada SK, Boga PK, Kotakonda HK. The effect of diosmin on the pharmacokinetics of fexofenadine in healthy human volunteers. Xenobiotica. 2016;1–6 [c].

[9] Bedada SK, Boga PK. Influence of diosmin on the metabolism and disposition of carbamazepine in healthy subjects. Xenobiotica. 2016;1–6 [c].

[10] Fard JK, Hamzeiy H, Sattari M, et al. Triazole rizatriptan induces liver toxicity through lysosomal/mitochondrial dysfunction. Drug Res (Stuttg). 2016;66(9):470–8 [E].

[11] Sajjad A, Weng CY. Vision loss in a patient with primary pulmonary hypertension and long-term use of sildenafil. Retin Cases Brief Rep. 2016. in Press [A].

[12] Pitsios C. Erythema multiforme caused by sildenafil in an HIV(+) subject. Eur Ann Allergy Clin Immunol. 2016;48(2):58–60 [A].

[13] Khoshneviszadeh M, Rahimian R, Fakhfouri G, et al. Oxytocin is involved in the proconvulsant effects of sildenafil: possible role of CREB. Toxicol Lett. 2016;256:44–52 [E].

17

Antihypertensive Drugs

Katie Traylor*,1, Holly Gurgle*, Kyle Turner*, Anna Woods*, Kezia Brown*, Sidhartha D. Ray†

*University of Utah College of Pharmacy, Salt Lake City, UT, United States
†Manchester University College of Pharmacy, Natural and Health Sciences, Fort Wayne, IN, United States
1Corresponding author: katie.traylor@pharm.utah.edu

ANGIOTENSIN-CONVERTING ENZYME INHIBITORS

Benazepril

Hematology

Medications are common causes of drug-induced agranulocytosis. Among angiotensin-converting enzyme inhibitors (ACEIs), captopril has been described as a cause of agranulocytosis. Hashmini et al. described a case report of drug-induced agranulocytosis following treatment with benazepril, the first such report published in a patient treated with benazepril. White blood cell counts quickly recovered after benazepril was discontinued. Authors recommend prompt discontinuation of benazepril following recognition of agranulocytosis [1A].

Lisinopril

Endocrinology

Kataria et al. described a case report of a heart failure patient with lisinopril-induced alopecia. While others have previously reported alopecia induced by other ACEIs (enalapril and captopril), this was the first such report with lisinopril in particular. Alopecia improved 4 weeks after discontinuation of lisinopril in this case report. Clinicians should consider lisinopril as a causative factor for unexplained alopecia [2A].

Ramipril

Transplant

Mandelbrot et al. described the effects of ramipril on urinary protein excretion in maintenance renal transplant patients converted from a calcineurin inhibitor to sirolimus. After 1 year, ramipril was effective at preventing urinary protein excretion and did not increase adverse events associated with sirolimus. Statistically significant treatment-emergent adverse events included increased serum creatinine (16.1% vs 8.6%) and leukopenia (12.3% vs 4.3%) when comparing ramipril ($n = 155$) to placebo ($n = 140$), though these are known side effects associated with ACE inhibitor use [3C].

ANGIOTENSIN RECEPTOR BLOCKERS/ ANGIOTENSIN II RECEPTOR ANTAGONISTS

Azilsartan

General Information

The efficacy and safety of azilsartan, a new angiotension II receptor blocker (ARB), was compared to olmesartan and valsartan in patients with prediabetes or type 2 diabetes. All medications were similar in terms of efficacy and safety outcome. Authors conclude that this new, well-tolerated ARB is an option for patients with hypertension in the setting of type 2 diabetes [4M].

Fimasartan

General Information

Fimasartan is a new angiotensin II type 1 receptor blocker recently approved in Korea. A derivative of losartan, fimasartan has a longer duration and higher potency than losartan. Lee et al. conducted a candesartan-controlled parallel group trial of fimasartan in Korean patients with hypertension. Efficacy and safety outcomes of fimasartan 60 or 120 mg and candesartan 8 mg were similar [5C]. Youn et al. conducted a Phase III clinical trial comparing fimasartan 30 mg vs valsartan 80 mg and also found no statistically significant differences in efficacy or safety of the two ARBs [6C]. Authors of both articles concluded that fimasartan appears safe with comparable clinical outcomes to other available ARBs [5C, 6C].

Losartan

Urinary Tract

The PREVER-treatment randomized trial compared chlorthalidone/amiloride vs losartan for blood pressure control in patients with stage I hypertension ($n = 655$). While rates of reported adverse events in this trial did not differ significantly between study groups, authors noted a trend towards increased incidence of microalbuminuria in the losartan group (15.5 mg/L vs 16.2 mg/L, $P = 0.822$). Significant findings included lower serum cholesterol, LDL-cholesterol, triglycerides, and serum uric acid in the losartan group ($P \leq 0.001$). Authors note that increased lipid levels have previously been associated with amiloride, but that this adverse effect is unlikely to outweigh the beneficial lowering of blood pressure seen with the medication [7C].

Olmesartan

Gastrointestinal

Several cases of olmesartan-induced sprue-like enteropathy have been reported since 2012, although the potential mechanism of this rare adverse effect is not understood. Patients with suspected olmesartan-induced enteropathy usually have severe diarrhea, dehydration, or renal failure and have been taking olmesartan for several months or years [8A]. Testing for celiac disease is usually negative, and gluten-free diets are ineffective, but symptoms resolve with discontinuation of olmesartan [9A]. Basson et al. conducted an observational cohort study in the French National Health Insurance database to evaluate whether olmesartan compared to other ARBs or ACEIs increased the likelihood of enteropathy. Two hundred and eighteen events were observed in this observational study ($n = 4546680$; or 9010303 person-years), and olmesartan was associated with an increased risk of hospitalization for intestinal malabsorption ($P < 0.0001$) and hospitalization for enteropathy ($P < 0.0001$). No association with this adverse effect was found for other ARBs [10MC]. Healthcare providers should consider olmestartan as a cause of enteropathy, even after months or years of use.

Telmisartan

Drug–Drug Interaction

ARBs and statins are medications commonly co-administered to reduce the risk of cardiovascular events and death. Hu et al. described a drug–drug interaction between telmisartan and rosuvastatin. Co-administration of telmisartan and rosuvastatin to healthy subjects for 14 days significantly increased the maximum plasma concentration (Cmax) of rosuvastatin by 71% and the area under the plasma concentration time curve (AUC) of rosuvastatin by 26%. The mechanism of interaction was demonstrated to be inhibition of ATP-binding cassette transporter G2 (ABCG2)-mediated efflux of rosuvastatin. While further studies are needed to characterize the extent of this interaction, authors suggest considering a reduced dose of rosuvastatin in Chinese patients also taking telmisartan, which may help to avoid side effects of increased rosuvastatin plasma concentration [11c].

R ANGIOTENSIN II RECEPTOR BLOCKER; ANGIOTENSIN RECEPTOR NEPRILYSIN INHIBITOR

Valsartan/Sacubitril

General Information

Valsartan/sacubitril is a novel cardiovascular therapy, combining an ARB with an angiotensin receptor neprilysin inhibitor (ARNI). The PARIDIGM-HF trial found an exciting reduction in heart failure deaths and hospitalizations in patients with reduced ejection fraction treated with valsartan/sacubitil compared to enalapril [12MC]. The TITRATION trial published by Senna et al. evaluated the safety of two up-titration strategies, one condensed and the other more conservative, for starting valsartan/sacubitril in patients with heart failure ($n = 498$) and titrating to a target dose of 200 mg twice daily used in the PARIDIGM-HF trial. No significant differences in safety outcomes (serum creatinine, hypotension, hyperkalemia) were observed between the two titration regimens. Increased tolerability of optimized doses (200 mg twice daily) was reported among patients on lower doses of ACEI/ARB at baseline in the more conservation titration arm [13C].

BETA BLOCKERS

Atenolol

Skin

Several medication classes have been known to cause pityriasis rosea-like reactions; however, atenolol has not been generally thought of as a causative agent. One case study describes a 56-year-old female who presented to an outpatient clinical setting with itchy, scaly, bright red/violet skin patches on her neck, abdomen, axilla and upper limbs over the course of 1 week. Three weeks prior to the eruption, this patient had started atenolol for treatment of hypertension. In clinic, she had negative blood tests but a biopsy was consistent with the diagnosis of pityriasis rosea-like reaction. This appears to be the first case of this reaction related to atenolol use. Clinicians should consider atenolol as a potential cause of pityriasis rosea-like reactions [14A].

Propranolol

Mouth and Teeth

One case report identified a 32-year-old woman who presented to an oral specialty center with a 2-year duration of abnormal growth of her upper and lower gums. Her comorbid conditions included 6 years of hypertension and a congenital cardiac condition for which propranolol was prescribed as treatment. Given her clinical presentation of specific musculoskeletal, dermal, facial and developmental abnormalities, she was diagnosed with Nager syndrome. The medical team concluded that the abnormal gum development, not necessarily seen in Nager syndrome, was propranolol-induced gingival hyperplasia, a rare occurrence in beta blockers that is more closely associated with calcium channel blockers [15A].

Cardiovascular

In a case report, a 35-year-old male with a history of smoking who was otherwise healthy reportedly suffered from cardiac arrest due to Torsades de pointes without QT prolongation manifesting on his EKG following a medication combination of chlorpheniramine (prescribed for upper respiratory tract infection symptoms) and propranolol (prescribed for essential tremor and anxiety). He displayed no other abnormal findings on laboratory evaluations. The authors suggest that although both chlorpheniramine and propranolol have been known to cause arrhythmias, this is the first known case of a combination of these medications leading to cardiac arrest without electrical changes [16A].

Propranolol is considered first-line treatment for infantile hemangiomas and has demonstrated relative safety in populations including preterm neonates and those with congenital heart disease; however, adverse effects including bradycardia, hypotension, and hypoglycemia have been known to occur with this treatment. Tran et al. performed a novel case series to study the safety and efficacy of propranolol in nine patients with genital infantile hemangiomas. At doses increased to 2 mg/kg daily, no abnormal changes in blood pressure, heart rate, or blood glucose were noted. One patient was taken off propranolol treatment due to exacerbated peripheral cyanosis, though the effects were deemed neither harmful nor painful to the patient [17A].

CALCIUM CHANNEL BLOCKERS

Amlodipine

Respiratory

Hu et al. published a study comparing perindopril arginine 4 mg plus amlodipine 5 mg and monotherapy of each of these two medications. One treatment-emergent adverse event occurred in the perindopril/amlodipine group when a patient experienced diaphragmatic eventration requiring surgical intervention. After successful recovery, the patient finished the study [18C].

Drug Formulations

In a study comparing amlodipine besylate and amlodipine orotate, researchers investigated safety, efficacy and bioequivalence of the two different amlodipine salt forms paired with olmesartan. There was no significant difference in mild or moderate adverse effects with no severe effects reported. The study concluded that these two salt forms of amlodipine appear to be similar in both safety and bioequivalence and authors suggest that this new formulation could be utilized as an effective amlodipine salt [19c].

Nimodipine

Cardiovascular

Hanggi et al. compared enteral nimodipine and a sustained-release intraventricular form of the medication in patients suffering an aneurism-induced subarachnoid hemorrhage. This new dosage form is thought to reduce hypotensive effects of enteral dosing and increase cerebral spinal fluid concentrations, leading to increased efficacy. In this study, it lead to similar rates of overall adverse effects and fewer serious side effects in the intraventricular group. There were 3 cases of hypotension related to the study medication in the enteral nimodipine group ($n=18$) and none in the intraventricular group ($n=54$). The authors suggest that this new formulation may reduce the potential for adverse effects [20c].

Verapamil

Drug–Drug Interaction

In a case report, a 68-year-old man who was being treated with ibrutinib for relapsed mantle cell lymphoma was seen in the emergency department after losing consciousness with comorbid dizziness, nausea, severe diarrhea and malaise. After intensive review of his condition and his medication regimen from a clinical pharmacist, the team determined that his verapamil, in a combination product with trandolapril, resulted in CYP3A4 inhibition leading to ibrutinib toxicity. While other antihypertensive medications had been prescribed to this patient, including an ARB, the clinical effects were thought to be due to the verapamil drug interaction. Prescribers must take caution when utilizing ibrutinib in the presence of CYP3A4 inhibitors. In this case the patient was subsequently prescribed another calcium channel blocker that did not undergo metabolism through this pathway. Clinicians should consider avoiding verapamil in patients being treated with ibrutinib [21A].

DRUGS THAT ACT ON THE SYMPATHETIC NERVOUS SYSTEM

Clonidine

Respiratory

Clonidine was studied by El-Ebiary et al. as an adjuvant in the management of acute anticholinesterase pesticide poisoning. In 60 adult patients, moderate doses of clonidine did not significantly impact clinical outcomes following anticholinesterase pesticide poisoning, but did significantly impact patients' vital signs. In addition to lowering pulse rate ($P=0.0002$), clonidine was shown to decrease oxygen saturation ($P=0.0262$) and increase time to normalization of vital signs ($P=0.0067$) compared to placebo. Authors suggest that clonidine may not improve clinical outcomes significantly when used in the setting of anticholinesterase pesticide poisoning. Caution must be taken with this treatment due to high incidence of hypotension, though this may be beneficial for patients presenting with hypertension and tachycardia following these poisoning events [22c].

A case report described a clonidine overdose in a 22-month-old girl as a result of an unintentional oral exposure to a compounded topical cream containing clonidine, camphor, gabapentin, ketoprofen, and lidocaine. Serum analyses revealed undetectable levels of all ingredients except clonidine, which was slightly elevated at 2.6 ng/mL (reference range 0.2–2 ng/mL at steady state). Results of this overdose, as noted in the emergency department approximately 1 hour after ingestion, included intermittent excitation, altered consciousness, miosis, apnea requiring endotracheal intubation, hypothermia, bradycardia, first-degree heart block, and hypotension. After approximately 14 hours of supportive care,

the patient was successfully extubated. The authors of this case report urge healthcare providers and parents to be alert to the potential dangers associated with pediatric ingestion of compounded medications [23A].

Ketanserin

Drug–Drug Interactions

Valle et al. performed a placebo-controlled trial to explore the relationship between the psychotropic plant ayahuasca and the serotonergic 5-HT2A receptor. Ketanserin was utilized for the study based on its known mechanism as an antagonist of this receptor. Analysis of 12 healthy study participants confirmed that ketanserin attenuated the neurophysiological and psychotropic effects of ayahuasca; however, authors noted it was unexpected to see only partial blockade of these effects. Authors offered a possible explanation for this partial blockade regarding ayahuasca agonism at other serotonergic receptors, particularly the 5-HT1A receptor, implicating this receptor for the marked sedation displayed in participants who received the ketanserin/ayahuasca combination [24c].

Reserpine

Death

A case report from Gicquel et al. described the death of a 30-year-old woman related to consumption of a mislabeled powder supplement found to contain reserpine. In this case, a powder intended to treat opiate withdrawal was analyzed, along with autopsy findings. The powder, which was sold online as *Tabernatnthe iboga*, did not contain the labeled ibogaine, but rather contained several toxic alkaloids—ajmaline, yohimbine, and reserpine; of these three alkaloids found in *Rauvolfia* plant species, reserpine is described as the most potent. Blood and bile analyses revealed amounts of reserpine below therapeutic concentrations, in combination with therapeutic concentrations of ajmaline and yohimbine, as well as low concentrations of cannabinoids and oxazepam. The patient's death was deemed a consequence of exposure to a combination of substantial *Rauvolfia* concentrations (including reserpine) and concomitant drug withdrawal. While cases regarding *Rauvolfia* alkaloids have been described separately, the authors of this case note this is the first report of death related to the simultaneous consumption of all three. The authors also call attention to safety concerns surrounding counterfeit medications and supplements purchased over the Internet [25A].

References

[1] Hashmi HR, Jabbour R, Schreiber Z, et al. Benazepril-induced agranulocytosis: a case report and review of the literature. Am J Case Rep. 2016;17:425–8 [A].

[2] Kataria V, Wang H, Wald JW, et al. Lisinopril-induced alopecia: a case report. J Pharm Pract. 2016;1–5 [A].

[3] Mandelbrot DA, Alberú J, Barama A, et al. Effect of ramipril on urinary protein excretion in maintenance renal transplant patients converted to sirolimus. Am J Transplant. 2015;15(12):3174–84 [C].

[4] White WB, Cuadra RH, Lloyd E, et al. Effects of azilsartan medoxomil compared with olmesartan and valsartan on ambulatory and clinic blood pressure in patients with type 2 diabetes and prediabetes. J Hypertens. 2016;34(4):788–97 [M].

[5] Lee JH, Yang DH, Hwang JY, et al. A randomized, double-blind, candesartan-controlled, parallel group comparison clinical trial to evaluate the antihypertensive efficacy and safety of fimasartan in patients with mild to moderate essential hypertension. Clin Ther. 2016;38(6):1485–97 [C].

[6] Youn JC, Ihm SH, Bae JH, et al. Efficacy and safety of 30-mg fimasartan for the treatment of patients with mild to moderate hypertension: an 8-week, multicenter, randomized, double-blind, phase III clinical study. Clin Ther. 2014;36(10):1412–21 [C].

[7] Fuchs FD, Scala LC, Vilela-Martin JF, et al. Effectiveness of chlorthalidone/amiloride versus losartan in patients with stage I hypertension: results from the PREVER-treatment randomized trial. J Hypertens. 2016;34(4):798–806 [C].

[8] Galanopoulos M, Varytimiadis L, Tsigaridas A, et al. Small bowel enteropathy associated with olmesartan medoxomil treatment. Ann Gastroenterol. 2017;30(1):131–3 [A].

[9] Rishi A, Garland K. Unusual severe side effect of a commonly used drug. J Clin Hypertens (Greenwich). 2016;18(4):363 [A].

[10] Basson M, Mezzarobba M, Weill A, et al. Severe intestinal malabsorption associated with olmesartan: a French nationwide observational cohort study. Gut. 2016;65(10):1664–9 [MC].

[11] Hu M, Lee HK, To KK, et al. Telmisartan increases systemic exposure to rosuvastatin after single and multiple doses, and in vitro studies show telmisartan inhibits ABCG2-mediated transport of rosuvastatin. Eur J Clin Pharmacol. 2016;72(12):1471–8 [c].

[12] McMurray JJ, Packer M, Desai AS, et al. Angiotensin-neprilysin inhibition versus enalapril in heart failure. N Engl J Med. 2014;371(11):993–1004 [MC].

[13] Senni M, McMurray JJ, Wachter R, et al. Initiating sacubitril/valsartan (LCZ696) in heart failure: results of TITRATION, a double-blind, randomized comparison of two uptitration regimens. Eur J Heart Fail. 2016;18(9):1193–202 [C].

[14] Güleç AI, Albayrak H, Kayapinar O, et al. Pityriasis rosea-like adverse reaction to atenolol. Hum Exp Toxicol. 2016;35(3):229–31 [A].

[15] Raheel SA, Kujan OB, Tarakji B, et al. Propranolol-induced gingival hyperplasia with Nager syndrome: a rare adverse drug reaction. J Adv Pharm Technol Res. 2016;7(2):64–8 [A].

[16] Ösken A, Yelgeç NS, Zehir R, et al. Torsades de pointes induced by concomitant use of chlorpheniramine and propranolol: an unusual presentation with no QT prolongation. Indian J Pharmacol. 2016;48(4):462–5 [A].

[17] Tran C, Tamburro J, Rhee A, et al. Propranolol for treatment of genital infantile hemangioma. J Urol. 2016;195(3):731–7 [A].

[18] Hu D, Sun Y, Liao Y, et al. Efficacy and safety of fixed-dose perindopril arginine/amlodipine in hypertensive patients not adequately controlled with amlodipine 5 mg or perindopril tert-butylamine 4 mg monotherapy. Cardiology. 2016;134(1):1–10 [C].

[19] Lee SY, Kim JR, Jung JA, et al. Bioequivalence evaluation of two amlodipine salts, besylate and orotate, each in a fixed-dose combination with olmesartan in healthy subjects. Drug Des Devel Ther. 2015;9:2811–7 [c].

[20] Hänggi D, Etminan N, Aldrich F, et al. Randomized, open-label, phase 1/2a study to determine the maximum tolerated dose of intraventricular sustained release nimodipine for subarachnoid hemorrhage (NEWTON [Nimodipine microparticles to enhance recovery while reducing toxicity after subarachnoid hemorrhage]). Stroke. 2017;48(1):145–51 [c].

[21] Lambert Kuhn E, Levêque D, Lioure B, et al. Adverse event potentially due to an interaction between ibrutinib and verapamil: a case report. J Clin Pharm Ther. 2016;41(1):104–5 [A].

[22] El-Ebiary AA, Gad SA, Wahdan AA, et al. Clonidine as an adjuvant in the management of acute poisoning by anticholinesterase pesticides. Hum Exp Toxicol. 2016;35(4):371–6 [c].

[23] Cates AL, Wheatley SM, Katz KD. Clonidine overdose in a toddler due to accidental ingestion of a compounding cream. Pediatr Emerg Care. 2016;1–3 [A].

[24] Valle M, Maqueda AE, Rabella M, et al. Inhibition of alpha oscillations through serotonin-2A receptor activation underlies the visual effects of ayahuasca in humans. Eur Neuropsychopharmacol. 2016;26(7):1161–75 [c].

[25] Gicquel T, Hugbart C, Le Devehat F, et al. Death related to consumption of Rauvolfia sp. powder mislabeled as Tabernanthe iboga. Forensic Sci Int. 2016;266:e38–42 [A].

18

Diuretics

Sarah Quick*,†,1, Dustin Linn*

*Manchester University College of Pharmacy, Natural, and Heath Sciences, Fort Wayne, IN, United States
†Lutheran Hospital of Indiana, Fort Wayne, IN, United States
1Corresponding author: squick@lutheran-hosp.com

LOOP DIURETICS [SEDA-36, 290; SEDA-37, 237; SEDA-38, 185]

Renal Function and Clinical Outcomes in Heart Failure

The relationship between loop diuretic dose, changes in renal function, and clinical outcomes were assessed from the controlled Rosuvastatin Multinational Study in Heart Failure (CORONA) trial. The CORONA trial randomized patients who were ≥60 years of age with symptomatic heart failure and a reduced ejection fraction to either rosuvastatin or placebo. This analysis included patients with both a baseline serum creatinine and at least one follow-up measurement. The primary outcome was the first occurrence of a composite of cardiovascular death or re-hospitalization owing to heart failure. Patients were followed for a median of 32.8 months. Propensity score matching was utilized for the probability of receiving a loop diuretic at baseline. This resulted in 2114 matched patients for any use of a loop diuretic vs no loop diuretic use. The change in estimated glomerular filtration rate (eGFR) was found to be -8.6 ± 10 mL/min/1.73 m^2 in those not treated with a loop diuretic and -9.4 ± 10 mL/min/1.73 m^2 in those treated with a loop diuretic ($P < 0.05$). No difference in the slope of eGFR was noted in those that received low- and middle-doses of loop diuretics; however, the decrease in eGFR with high dose loop diuretic use was significantly greater than with the matched no loop diuretic group. In the matched patient population more patients who received loop diuretics compared to no diuretics experienced the composite outcome of cardiovascular death or re-hospitalization due to heart failure (33% vs 24%; HR 1.63, 95% CI 1.35–1.96, $P = 0.009$). Use of loop diuretics was associated with both an increased risk of all-cause mortality and hospitalization due to heart failure. The risk of poor clinical outcome was increased for higher loop diuretic doses. For each 40 mg increase in furosemide equivalent, the hazard ratio for poor clinical outcome was 1.11 (95% CI 1.08–1.14, $P < 0.001$). Because this was a retrospective analysis of a randomized, controlled trial, unmeasured confounders may account for the study findings. The authors concluded that the use of the lowest diuretic dose possible should be utilized to achieve euvolemia [1MC].

Furosemide

High-Dose vs Low-Dose

A post-hoc analysis of a prospective, randomized, open-label, double-blind study that compared continuous with intermittent infusion of furosemide in patients with a diagnosis of acute heart failure was conducted to evaluate the effect of diuretic dosing strategies on decongestion, worsening renal function, and outcomes. Mean furosemide daily doses ≥125 mg daily was defined as high loop diuretic dose. Worsening renal function, defined as a rise in serum creatinine ≥0.3 mg/dL or an estimated glomerular filtration rate (eGFR) decrease of more than 25%, occurred more frequent in those who received high dose loop diuretics (65% vs 29%; $P < 0.001$). The method of infusion (continuous vs intermittent) did not affect the occurrence of worsening renal function; however, in those who received high-dose furosemide, worsening renal function was more common when furosemide was administered as a continuous infusion as opposed to intermittently (42% vs 23%; $P < 0.05$) [2c].

Acute Kidney Injury

Fabiano et al. reported a case of acute kidney injury (AKI) occurring in a 7-month-old infant receiving the combination of furosemide and enalapril for the treatment of congestive cardiac failure (CCF). The infant started receiving oral furosemide at a dose of 2 mg/kg/day at the age of 5 months because of ultrasonographic findings of pulmonary hyperafflux and left ventricle dilatation with left atrium and septal hypokinesis. One month later, following incomplete response, oral enalapril 1.8 mg/kg/day was added and the oral furosemide dose was reduced to 1.7 mg/kg/day. Three months later the infant was admitted to the hospital with fever, feeding refusal, and mild dehydration. The infant developed AKI with a blood urea concentration of 168 mg/dL and a serum creatinine of 1.1 mg/dL. Furosemide and enalapril were discontinued on admission and an infusion of normal saline was initiated over the course of 72 hours with resolution of signs and symptoms and normalization of blood urea and creatinine values. Once resolution had been obtained furosemide and enalapril were restarted at doses of 0.85 and 1.3 mg/kg/day, respectively. This was followed 48 hours later by an increase in the blood urea and creatinine concentration. Furosemide and enalapril were discontinued and blood urea and creatinine concentrations subsequently returned to normal values. Because AKI could have occurred from either medication, it is difficult to distinguish if furosemide or enalapril was greater contributors to the development of AKI in this infant. Doses of enalapril generally employed in pediatric patients are in the neighborhood of 0.5–1 mg/kg/day and this study highlights the risks associated with high dose enalapril in combination with furosemide [3A].

Eruption of Hemorrhagic Bullae

Furosemide has been associated rarely with severe dermatologic reactions which may result from chlorine in the chemical structure leading to photosensitive skin reactions. Sladden et al. reported a case of furosemide-induced eruption of hemorrhagic bullae on the fingers. A 79-year-old male was admitted for coronary artery bypass surgery and aortic valve replacement. The patient presented to the hospital 1 week after discharge and furosemide was initiated due to lower limb pitting edema. The patient was subsequently discharged and presented again the following week with hemorrhagic bullous lesions on the second to fifth digits of the right hand and on the dorsum of the left little finger. The lesions were painless, non-pruritic, and had developed over the course of 3–4 days after which they began to ulcerate and bleed on contact. After not responding to initial treatment with ciprofloxacin and topical steroids an excision skin biopsy was performed. The biopsy revealed necrotic skin cells, eosinophil infiltration, and thrombosed dermal vessels with negative immunofluorescence which was suggestive of a drug reaction. Furosemide was discontinued and after 4 days the lesions had dried up [4A].

Topical Furosemide to Reduce the Recurrence of Polyps After Sinus Surgery

Hashemian et al. conducted a triple-blind randomized clinical trial of adults with chronic rhinosinusitis associated with polyposis undergoing endoscopic sinus surgery. Patients were randomized to receive intranasal furosemide 300 mcg per day for 2 months (n=46) or a placebo intranasal spray for 2 months (n=46). All patients received 30 mg of oral prednisone, 400 mg of oral cefixime, and fluticasone spray 2 puffs twice daily in each nostril for 10 days postoperatively. All patients also received fluticasone 2 puffs twice daily for 1 month and then 1 puff daily for 5 months. During 6 months of follow-up no clinically significant adverse effects were seen in either group. Among patients receiving furosemide, 1 reported nasal irritation, 2 reported constipation, and 1 reported headache. The authors concluded that topical furosemide is a safe drug with no important adverse effects and can be used to reduce the rate of relapse and severity of polyposis after surgery [5c].

QTc Interval Prolongation

Keller et al. conducted a prospective, observational, longitudinal cohort study to evaluate ECG changes induced by medications to determine the frequency of drug-induced QT interval prolongation in clinical practice. Patients were included in the analysis if they were at least 18 years of age, were treated exclusively at participating health centers in Argentina, and were receiving one or more drugs for a limited period of time that allows for the electrocardiographic monitoring of QTc interval. An electrocardiogram was performed on each patient at baseline, during treatment after at least five elimination half-lives, and after at least five half-lives after the end of treatment. Four criteria for QTc prolongation were defined: (1) Absolute value of QTc greater than 450 ms (males) or 470 ms (females); (2) Change in QTc greater than 30 ms; (3) Absolute value of QTc greater than 500 ms; (4) Change in QTc greater than 60 ms. Furosemide was prescribed to 69 patients in the cohort. A multiple logistic regression analysis was performed to control for several baselines and clinical variables that may impact the development of QTc prolongation. After multivariate regression, furosemide was significantly associated (OR: 6.50; 95% CI: 1.56–27.05 $P < 0.01$) with QTc prolongation (>450/470 ms) [6C].

CARBONIC ANHYDRASE INHIBITORS
[SEDA-36, 289; SEDA-37, 237; SEDA-38, 197]

Acetazolamide

Iris-Lens Diaphragm Displacement and Acute Angle Closure

Llovet-Rausell et al. reported a case of acetazolamide-induced acute angle closure induced by an anterior displacement of the irido-lentricular complex. The case involved a 44-year-old female who presented to an emergency department with decreased visual acuity (VA) in both eyes that had developed over the course of 4 hours. In the 24 hours prior to presentation the patient had begun treatment with naproxen 500 mg orally every 12 hours and acetazolamide 250 mg orally every 8 hours. Ocular findings revealed 4D myopia, corrected VA of 0.96, increased intraocular pressure (IOP) of 26 and 28 mm Hg, shiny and transparent corena without edema, and anterior chamber (AC) Shaffer grade II. Iris-lens displacement secondary to acetazolamide was suspected and acetazolamide was discontinued. Topical treatment with timolol, brimonidine, prednisolone, and cycloprentolate was initiated. Over the course of a 2-week follow-up, a gradual reduction in myopia and lens thickness was observed as well as AC expansion. The mechanism of this complication is unclear; however, the authors note that acetazolamide stimulates synthesis of prostaglandin E2, causing vasodilation and increase uveal vascular permeability potentially leading to adverse ocular consequences. The authors recommend that acetazolamide be prescribed with caution and that ophthalmological checks should be initiated to diagnose and treat complications at an early stage [7A].

Post-NIV Metabolic Alkalosis

The effects of acetazolamide on post-noninvasive ventilation (NIV) metabolic alkalosis in patients with acute exacerbation of chronic obstructive pulmonary disease (AECOPD) were evaluated in a prospective, observational study compared to a historical control group. Eleven patients received a dose of acetazolamide 500 mg orally for 2 consecutive days. In patients who received acetazolamide after 1 day of therapy $PaCO_2$ decreased from 63.9 ± 9.8 to 54.9 ± 8.3 mm Hg, ($P = 0.01$) serum pH from 7.46 ± 0.06 to 7.41 ± 0.06 ($P = 0.004$), and HCO_3 from 43.5 ± 5.9 to 36.1 ± 5.4 mmol/L ($P = 0.005$). No drug-related adverse effects were reported in patients who received acetazolamide [8c].

Safety During Treatment of Idiopathic Intracranial Hypertension

Acetazolamide is used in the management of idiopathic intracranial hypertension (IIH) where it is thought to lower intracranial pressure, intraocular pressure, and lead to diuresis through inhibition of carbonic anhydrase and formation of bicarbonate and hydrogen ions. Doses requires to lower IIH are much higher than those often used for other indications. The Idiopathic Intracranial Hypertension Treatment Trial (IIHTT) was a randomized, double-blind, placebo-controlled study of acetazolamide in patients with idiopathic intracranial hypertension who met modified Danby criteria and had reproducible mild visual loss. Patients in the acetazolamide group received 250 mg orally twice daily with subsequent dose increases of 250 mg twice daily to a maximum of 4 g daily (i.e. 2 g orally twice daily). A follow-up analysis evaluated reported adverse events that occurred during the study period. Adverse events were collected during routine clinical evaluations that were performed at screening, baseline, and at 1, 2, 3, 4.5, and 6 months after baseline and by questioning participants regarding the occurrence of any untoward events since their last visit. Of the 86 patients who received acetazolamide, 38 (44.2%) tolerated the maximum daily dosage of 4 g/day. Thirty-nine patients (45.3%) tolerated between 1 and 3.75 g as their maximum daily dosage while the remaining 9 patients (10.5%) tolerated between 0.125 and 0.75 g as their maximum daily dosage.

A total of 676 adverse events were reported during this trial, 480 in patients who received acetazolamide. Nine serious adverse events occurred including 6 in patients who received acetazolamide. The median number of adverse events was 5 in the acetazolamide group and 3 in the placebo group. Patients who received acetazolamide were more likely to report adverse effects within the nervous, gastrointestinal, renal, ear, skin, and psychiatric systems. Metabolic disturbances were more commonly reported in patients who received acetazolamide. Fifty-four patients (62.8%) who received acetazolamide reported 106 neurologic adverse effects including paresthesia ($n = 54$), dysgeusia ($n = 13$), headache ($n = 17$), dizziness ($n = 10$), and other ($n = 17$). Thirty-eight patients (44.2%) who received acetazolamide reported 89 gastrointestinal adverse effects including nausea ($n = 30$), diarrhea ($n = 14$), vomiting ($n = 12$), acid reflux ($n = 12$), dry mouth ($n = 3$), constipation ($n = 2$), and other ($n = 16$). Fifteen patients (17.4%) who received acetazolamide reported 19 skin adverse effects including rash ($n = 8$), hives ($n = 3$), acne ($n = 2$), pruritis ($n = 2$), and other ($n = 4$). Psychiatric adverse events occurred in 12 patients (14%), renal adverse events in 7 patients (8.1%), and ear adverse events in 13 patients (15.1%) who received acetazolamide. Seventeen patients (19.8%) who received acetazolamide experienced 23 metabolic adverse effects including metabolic acidosis ($n = 6$), loss of appetite ($n = 6$), hyperchloremia ($n = 4$), hypokalemia ($n = 4$), dehydration ($n = 2$), and other ($n = 1$). Serious adverse events that led to the discontinuation of acetazolamide and thought to be probably and possibly related to study medication included decreased kidney function, transaminitis, and allergic reaction [9C].

OSMOTIC DIURETICS [SEDA-36, 294; SEDA-37, 241, SEDA-38, 202]

Mannitol

Intraoperative Mannitol for Brain Relaxation

Seo et al. prospectively evaluated intraoperative use of mannitol for brain relaxation in patients undergoing craniotomy for resection of supratentorial brain tumor. Patients were randomized to one of four groups based on the mannitol dose administered. The doses administered in each of the four groups were 0.25 g/kg (Group A), 0.5 g/kg (Group B), 1 g/kg (Group C), and 1.5 g/kg (Group D) based on the total body weight. Mannitol was administered over 15–20 minutes at the time of skin incision. Four patients in the 0.25 g/kg group received additional mannitol for brain relaxation. Adverse effects occurring were generally transient with only two patients requiring potassium replacement secondary to hypokalemia. Serum osmolality was higher at 30 minutes in Group D than in the other groups 315 vs 303, 303, and 306 mOsm/kg in group A, B, and C ($P < 0.001$, respectively). The incidence of hyponatremia (serum Na $+ < 135$ mmol/L) occurred more frequently in Group D (80.6%) than in Groups A (25.8%) and B (45.2%). Moderate hyponatremia (Serum Na +125 to ≤130 mmol/L) also occurred more commonly in Group D (38.7%) than on the other groups (0%, 9.7%, 12.9% for groups A, B, and C, respectively). The serum potassium concentration 30 minutes after drug administration was higher in Group D than in Group A (4.1 vs 3.7 mmol/L) and at 60 minutes was higher in Group D than in Group A and B (4.2 vs 3.9 and 3.9, respectively). Adverse effects occurring were generally transient with only two patients (1 in Group C and 1 in Group D) requiring potassium replacement secondary to hypokalemia [10C].

THIAZIDE AND THIAZIDE-LIKE DIURETICS [SEDA-36, 292; SEDA-37, 239; SEDA-38, 199]

Hydrochlorothiazide

Review of Bilateral Secondary Angle-Closure Glaucoma (ACG) Case Reports

A PubMed literature review was done to identify relevant bilateral secondary angle-closure glaucoma (ACG) case reports. The Naranjo adverse drug reaction probability scale was used to assess each case for causality. Cases were given a score of −4 to +13 and the reaction was considered definite if the score was ≥9, probable if 5 to 8, possible if 1 to 4, and doubtful if ≤0. No drugs had a definite score, but hydrochlorothiazide and hydrochlorothiazide in combination with triamterene had a Naranjo score that was considered a probable association for ACG [11R].

Hydrochlorothiazide Used in Combination With Telmisartan

Higaki et al. evaluated the efficacy and safety with the addition of hydrochlorothiazide 12.5 mg to telmisartan 80 mg/amlodipine 5 mg when hypertension was uncontrolled on dual therapy. This 8-week, multicenter, randomized, double-blind, active-control, parallel-group comparative phase III clinical study enrolled Japanese patients 20 or older if they had essential hypertension and were already taking two or three antihypertensives. More overall adverse events were noted in the triple therapy group at 41.6% vs 28.1% in group not receiving hydrochlorothiazide. Of the adverse events, 23.5% of them were categorized as drug-related adverse events vs 3.8% in the group not receiving hydrochlorothiazide. The most common adverse events reported were increased blood uric levels, nasopharyngitis and hyperuricemia. Adverse events experienced were mild or moderate with no severe events or deaths reported in either group. Two patients withdrew from the triple therapy group due to atrial fibrillation and tachycardia (one patient) and hypotension (one patient). One patient withdrew from dual therapy due to ventricular extrasystoles. Overall the authors concluded, the addition of hydrochlorothiazide to telmisartan/amlodipine was well tolerated and improved blood pressure control [12MC].

Kondo et al. also studied the efficacy and safety of telmisartan/amlodipine vs telmisartan/hydrochlorothiazide in the treatment of uncontrolled hypertension in the Japanese population. Patients were randomly assigned to fixed dose telmisartan/amlodipine ($n = 36$) or telmisartan/hydrochlorothiazide ($n = 39$) with blood pressure monitored in the office at baseline and at 12 weeks. Serum potassium and beta-natriuretic peptide levels were decreased in the telmisartan/hydrochlorothiazide group, while uric acid and hemoglobin A1C levels were increased. Uric acid increased 0.5 ± 0.9 ($P < 0.01$) from baseline with hemoglobin A1C increasing 0.1 ± 0.3 ($P < 0.05$) from baseline. Also noted was a slight but significant decrease in the glomerular filtration rate in the telmisartan/hydrochlorothiazide group. One patient in the telmisartan/hydrochlorothiazide group withdrew due to photosensitivity. The authors concluded that both groups led to efficient blood pressure control and no serious adverse effects were noted [13c].

Meta-Analyses of Glycemic Changes With Use of Thiazide Diuretics

Glycemic changes during treatment with thiazide diuretics were noted in a meta-analysis reviewing 368 publications. Included for analysis were 13 parallel-designed randomized controlled trials involving 720 patients comparing the metabolic effects of hydrochlorothiazide vs non-hydrochlorothiazide treatment for hypertension in non-insulin-dependent diabetic patients. Several medications combinations were assessed with the addition of high-dose hydrochlorothiazide (>25 mg) and low-dose hydrochlorothiazide (<25 mg). In those treated with hydrochlorothiazide, there was a significant increase in fasting glucose (SMD = 0.27, 95% CI 0.11–0.43) and hemoglobin A1C (HbA1C) (SMD = 1.09, 95% CI 0.47–1.72). While a decrease in high-density lipoprotein (HDL) cholesterol (SMD = −0.44, 95% CI −0.81 to 0.08) was seen in those treated with low-dose hydrochlorothiazide. It had been suggested that the optimal dose of hydrochlorothiazide may be less than 25 mg, but glycemic changes were seen even in low-dose treatment groups. It should be noted that there was a high degree of heterogeneity of HbA1c and HDL results, with less heterogeneity in results pertaining to fasting glucose. However, the authors concluded low-dose hydrochlorothiazide be utilized preferentially to higher doses if utilized for patients with type 2 diabetes [14M].

Glycemic changes were also analyzed in hypertensive patients being treated with thiazide-type diuretics by another meta-analysis reviewing 1369 publications, finding 26 studies involving 16162 subjects. An increase in fasting glucose was seen in patients receiving thiazide-type diuretics that seemed to be dose dependent. The mean difference in fasting plasma glucose was 0.27 mmol/L [4.86 mg/dL]; 95% confidence interval [CI], 0.15–0.39, with patients receiving lower doses of thiazide (hydrochlorothiazide or chlorthalidone ≤25 mg daily) having less of a difference (mean change 0.15 mmol/L [2.7 mg/dL]; 95% CI, 0.03–0.27) than those receiving higher doses (MD, 0.60 mmol/L [10.8 mg/dL]; 95% CI, 0.39–0.82). No changes were noted in postprandial glucose results or hemoglobin A1C. The results suggest lower doses of hydrochlorothiazide may result in less glycemic abnormalities, but further research is needed to determine the clinical impact [15M].

Hyponatremic Encephalopathy With Life-threatening Seizures

A case report described seizures with life-threatening hyponatremic encephalopathy during use of duloxetine and hydrochlorothiazide. Duloxetine was added and titrated over several days to the medication regimen of a patient on a stable dose of triamterene/hydrochlorothiazide 37.5/25 mg daily for treatment of hypertension.

The patient had a normal physical exam and baseline sodium of 144 mEq/L prior the addition of duloxetine. The authors found this combination caused the patient to experience SIADH due to duloxetine in addition to sodium depletion due to the hydrochlorothiazide. The patient's sodium was 103 mEq/L, urine osmolarity of 134 mOsm/kg H_2O, and urine sodium 12 mEq/L. Prompt identification and treatment with hypertonic saline in accordance with current guidelines allowed the patient to improve over several days resulting in no permanent neurological damage. The authors concluded, caution should be used when prescribing multiple medications that put the patient at risk for dilutional hyponatremia [16A].

ALDOSTERONE RECEPTOR ANTAGONISTS [SEDA-36, 293; SEDA-37, 240; SEDA-38, 201]

Spironolactone

Use in Chronic Dialysis Patients

Lin et al. looked at the long-term efficacy, over 2 years, of spironolactone among 253 non-heart failure dialysis patients. Potassium levels increased in the spironolactone group during the 2-year follow-up, but not significantly compared with the control group. Three patients had increases in plasma potassium to 6–6.5 mmol/L and seven patients had increases from 5.5 to 6 mmol/L. No patients needed to stop the study due to hyperkalemia. Other adverse events observed were nonphysiologic gynecomastia, breast tenderness and nausea. These adverse effects led to therapy discontinuation by 8 patients, 5 patients due to the nonphysiologic gynecomastia, 1 patient due to breast tenderness and 2 patients because of nausea [17MC].

Intermenstrual Bleeding in Patients With Polycystic Ovarian Syndrome

A small study looked at the use of spironolactone 100 mg daily in 30 patients with polycystic ovary syndrome (PCOS) for association with intermenstrual abnormalities, specifically bleeding. It was found that half of the patients showed intermenstrual bleeding during treatment and patients were further analyzed as a bleeding group vs non-bleeding group. Hormonal values (estrogen, progesterone, follicle-stimulating hormone and luteinizing hormone) and endometrial thickness were measured at baseline, and days 14 and 16 of the cycle for all patients. Patients with bleeding had significantly lower estradiol values before and after treatment with spironolactone. Endometrial thickness was lower in the bleeding group but only on day 16 of the cycle. The authors concluded that spironolactone reduces estradiol levels in PCOS patients at both the 14th and the 16th day of the cycle, but bleeding appeared only in women with lower estrogen concentrations before treatment [18c].

Nonresolving Central Serous Chorioretinopathy With Chronic Epitheliopathy

Daruich et al. evaluated the efficacy and safety of oral mineralocorticoid-receptor antagonist (MRa) therapy in three clinical presentations of nonresolving central serous chorioretinopathy (CSCR) with chronic epitheliopathy. This study looked at 50 patients with 20 patients receiving spironolactone and 30 patients receiving eplerenone. Treatment-related side effects were noted in 6 of the patients. In patients receiving spironolactone there were 4 events, 1 case of gynecomastia that resolved by switching to eplerenone, 1 case a drop in systolic blood pressure to less than 100 mg Hg that resolved by switching to eplerenone, and 2 cases of hyperkalemia that resolved without treatment or by switching to eplerenone. In the eplerenone group, there were 2 cases of hyperkalemia that resolved without treatment or by interrupting therapy. In conclusion, no patient discontinued therapy for any reason before 3 months [19c].

Eplerenone

Safety in Kidney Transplant Recipients

A small study evaluated 31 kidney transplant recipients with impaired renal function (eGFR 30–50 mL/min/1.73 m^2) on eplerenone 25 mg daily who were also receiving cyclosporine A. During the study, 9 patients experienced at least one episode of mild hyperkalemia (>5 mmol), but there was only one episode of moderate hyperkalemia (>5.5 mmol/L). Three other patients experienced adverse effects: diarrhea, sweats and acute kidney injury not requiring specific management. Baseline characteristics of elevated potassium at baseline and lower serum bicarbonate at baseline were associated with a higher risk of developing hyperkalemia. The authors concluded that eplerenone could be safely given to kidney transplant recipients on cyclosporine A with impaired renal function, if potassium is monitored closely. Recommendations were also made for an adequately powered prospective randomized control trial to further study potential benefits of eplerenone and other mineralocorticoid receptor antagonists in this population [20c].

Chronic Central Serous Chorioretinopathy

A sample of 24 patients with treatment resistant central serous chorioretinopathy were monitoring over 4 months of treatment with eplerenone 25 mg daily, titrated to 50 mg daily after 1 week. Treatment was stopped in three patients because of mild bowel irritation, myotonia, and hyperkalemia. None of these events were listed as a serious adverse event [21c].

References

Loop Diuretics

[1] Damman K, Kjekshus J, Wikstrand J, et al. Loop diuretics, renal function, and clinical outcomes in patients with heart failure and reduced ejection fraction. Eur J Heart Fail. 2016;18:328–36 [MC].

[2] Palazzuoli A, Testani JM, Ruocco G, et al. Different diuretic dose and response in acute decompensated heart failure: clinical characteristics and prognostic significance. Int J Cardiol. 2016;224:213–9 [c].

[3] Fabiano V, Carnovale C, Gentili M, et al. Enalapril associated with furosemide induced acute kidney injury in an infant with heart failure. A case report, a revision of the literature and a pharmacovigilance database analysis. Pharmacology. 2016;97:38–42 [A].

[4] Sladden D, Mizzi S, Casha AR, et al. Furosemide-induced eruption of haemorrhagic bullae on the fingers. Br J Hosp Med. 2016;77:428–9 [A].

[5] Hashemian F, Ali Ghorbanian M, Hashemia F, et al. Effect of topical furosemide on rhinosinusal polyposis relapse after endoscopic surgery: a randomized clinical trail. JAMA Otolaryngol Head Neck Surg. 2016;142:1045–9 [c].

[6] Keller GA, Alvarez PA, Ponte ML, et al. Drug-induced QTc interval prolongation: a multicenter study to detect drugs and clinical factors involved in every day practice. Curr Drug Saf. 2016;11:86–98 [C].

Carbonic Anhydrase Inhibitors

[7] Llovet-Rausell A, Tolosa FR, Kudsieh B. Severe ocular side effect with acetazolamide: case report. Arch Soc Esp Oftalmol. 2016;91:543–6 [A].

[8] Fontana A, Santinelli S, Internullo M, et al. Effect of acetazolamide on post-NIV metabolic alkalosis in acute exacerbated COPD patients. Eur Rev Med Pharmcol Sci. 2016;20:37–43 [c].

[9] ten Hove MR, Friedman DI, Patel AD, et al. Safety and tolerability of acetazolamide in the idiopathic intracranial hypertension treatment trial. J Neuroophthalmol. 2016;36:13–9 [C].

Osmotic Diuretics

[10] Seo H, Kim E, Jung H, et al. A prospective randomized trial of the optimal dose of mannitol for intraoperative brain relaxation in patients undergoing craniotomy for supratentorial brain tumor resection. J Neurosurg. 2017;126:1839–46 [C].

Thiazide Diuretics

[11] Murphy R, Bakir B, O'Brien C, et al. Drug-induced bilateral secondary angle-closure glaucoma: a literature synthesis. J Glaucoma. 2016;25:e99–e105 [R].

[12] Higaki J, Komuro I, Shiki K, et al. Effect of hydrochlorothiazide in addition to telmisartan/amlodipine combination for treating hypertensive patients uncontrolled with telmisartan/amlodipine: a randomized, double-blind study. Hypertens Res. 2016;40:251–8 [MC].

[13] Kondo K, Toh R, Ishida T, et al. Comparison of telmisartan/amlodipine and telmisartan/hydrochlorothiazide in the treatment of Japanese patients with uncontrolled hypertension: the TAT-Kobe study. Blood Press Monit. 2016;21:171–7 [c].

[14] Lin J, Chang H, Ku C, et al. Hydrochlorothiazide hypertension treatment induced metabolic effects in type 2 diabetes: a

meta-analysis of parallel-design RCTs. Eur Rev Med Pharmacol Sci. 2016;20:2926–46 [M].

[15] Zhang X, Zhao Q. Association of thiazide-type diuretics with glycemic changes in hypertensive patients: a systematic review and meta-analysis of randomized controlled clinical trials. J Clin Hypertens. 2016;18:342–51 [M].

[16] Siegel AJ, Forte SS, Na Bhatti, et al. Drug-related hyponatremic encephalopathy: rapid clinical response averts life-threatening acute cerebral Edema. Am J Case Rep. 2016;17:150–3 [A].

Aldosterone Receptor Antagonists

[17] Lin C, Zhang Q, Zhang H, et al. Long-term effects of low-dose spironolactone on chronic dialysis patients: a randomized placebo-controlled study. J Clin Hypertens. 2016;18:121–8 [MC].

[18] Sabbadin C, Andrisani A, Zermiani M, et al. Spironolactone and intermenstrual bleeding in polycystic ovary syndrome with normal BMI. J Endocrinol Invest. 2016;39:1015–21 [c].

[19] Daruich A, Matet A, Dirani A, et al. Oral mineralocorticoid-receptor antagonists: real-life experience in clinical subtypes of nonresolving central serous chorioretinopathy with chronic epitheliopathy. Transl Vis Sci Technol. 2016;5:2 [c].

[20] Bertocchio JP, Barbe C, Lavaud S, et al. Safety of eplerenone for kidney-transplant recipients with impaired renal function and receiving cyclosporine A. PLoS One. 2016;11(4) e0153635 [c].

[21] Cakir B, Fischer F, Ehlken C, et al. Clinical experience with eplerenone to treat chronic central serous chorioretinopathy. Graefes Arch Clin Exp Ophthalmol. 2016;254:2151–7 [c].

19

Metals and Metal Antagonists

Joshua P. Gray*,1, *Natalia Suhali-Amacher*†, *Sidhartha D. Ray*‡

*United States Coast Guard Academy, New London, CT, United States
†Manchester University College of Pharmacy, Fort Wayne, IN, United States
‡Manchester University College of Pharmacy, Natural and Health Sciences, Fort Wayne, IN, United States
1Corresponding author: joshua.p.gray@uscga.edu

COMBINATION THERAPIES

Multiple chelation therapies are often used simultaneously to treat disorders of metal overload in the body. Studies investigating the side effects of these therapies are discussed in this section. A large review compares anticopper agents including D-penicillamine, trientine, sodium dimercaptosuccinate, dimercaptosuccinic acid, zinc, and tetrathiomolybdate [1R].

DEFERASIROX, DEFERIPRONE, AND DESFEROXAMINE

Deferasirox, deferiprone, and desferoxamine are iron chelators often given in combination; side effects resulting from their use as monotherapies are discussed in a subsequent section. Several publications compared and contrasted the use of these three drugs in 2016 [2R,3r]. A meta-analysis compared the safety of deferasirox, deferiprone, and desferoxamine in 2040 patients from 34 studies. Gastrointestinal disorders were observed with deferiprone (3.7%–18.4%) and deferasirox (5.8%–18.8%) [4M]. A major review discusses the toxicity associated with all three of the drugs [5R]. One review discusses how MRI has changed the understanding of the metabolic processes involved in iron deposition and shown that iron deposition is not uniform throughout the organs of the body [6R]. This review also explores the relative toxicity of non-transferrin bound iron vs injected iron, excess levels of iron in tissues causing toxicity, and the role of iron chelation on iron absorption. A review article discusses the use of iron chelators in the prevention of cancer growth [7R]. An experimental study compared the use of deferasirox and desferrioxamine for the removal of thallium

from rats. Deferoxamine was more effective than deferasirox in increasing urinary thallium excretion [8E].

Sensory Systems

Ototoxicity was observed only in patients receiving deferoxamine ($n=15$) in a comparative study of 55 patients treated with either deferoxamine, deferiprone, or deferasirox for thalassemia. The incidence of ototoxicity upon treatment with deferoxamine (<50 mg/kg/day) was 27.3% [9c].

Gastrointestinal

Gastrointestinal upset occurred more frequently with deferasirox than deferoxamine ($P=0.254$) in a prospective randomized study of 60 patients with β-thalassemia major over the course of 1 year [10c].

Skin

Skin rash occurred more frequently with deferasirox than deferoxamine ($P=0.254$) in a prospective randomized study of 60 patients with β-thalassemia major over the course of 1 year [10c].

Endocrine

The effect of long-term treatments with iron chelators on endocrinopathy (diabetes mellitus, hypothyroidism, or hypogonadism) was examined in 165 adults with β-thalassemia major. Endocrinopathy was decreased in patients treated with deferasirox, not changed with deferiprone and deferoxamine co-treatment, and increased with deferoxamine and deferiprone ($P=0.015$). Endocrinopathy was associated with serum ferritin above

1300 ng/mL ($P=0.025$) while reversal of endocrinopathy was associated with serum ferritin below 200 ng/mL ($P=0.147$) [11c].

AMMONIUM TETRATHIOMOLYBDATE

Ammonium tetrathiomolybdate, well known as a treatment for Wilson's disease, is increasingly used as an anti-cancer therapy; however, not all of its effects are attributed to copper chelation [12E].

Immunologic

Neutropenia (3.7%) was the most frequent side effect in a phase 2 clinical trial ($n=51$) of ammonium tetrathiomolybdate for the prevention of breast cancer recurrence [13c].

CADMIUM

Cadmium is a toxic heavy metal that may produce effects in the liver, kidneys, lungs, cardiovascular system, immune system, and reproductive systems (reviewed in Refs. [14r,15r,16r]). Soil, water, air, and food are sources of cadmium exposure. Cadmium has a long half-life (kidney $t_{1/2}=6–38$ years, liver $t_{1/2}=4–19$ years). There are three major routes of absorption: GI tract ingestion and absorption, pulmonary inhalation, and dermal absorption. Since cadmium has been identified as a human carcinogen, early detection of susceptibility to cancer using biomarkers is of importance to public health. According to German law, the permissible cadmium value exposed to workers is 15 µg/L; non-smokers show an average cadmium blood concentration of 0.5 µg/L whereas an average smoker has an intake of 30 µg/day in addition to daily intake of cadmium from food and drink.

Respiratory

The liver produces metallothionein (MT) which chelates cadmium for secretion by the kidney. Cadmium-induced MT acts as a negative regulator of apoptosis in the lung by both altering intracellular bioavailability and degree of oxidative stress. Cadmium-induced oxidative stress appears to play a leading role in mediating the negative effects of Cd in the lung in relation to both asthma and pulmonary fibrosis. This may be due in part to the activation of lung fibroblasts. Intestinal MT may play an important role in absorption, transport, and distribution of dietary cadmium to the kidney [17E]. If this mechanism is in operation, dietary Cd would be deposited directly in the kidneys since cadmium in MT-bound forms (Cd7MT and Cd5Zn2MT) has been shown to be taken up largely by the kidney.

Urinary Tract

Proteinuria is a biomarker of cadmium-induced tubule cell toxicity in kidneys. Urinary excretion of the protein markers, albumin, beta-2 microglobulin, retinol-binding protein and NAG/NAGB were elevated in persons with urinary Cd concentrations above 2 µg Cd/g creatinine and at lower urinary cadmium concentrations for NAGB relative to unexposed adults [18c]. The study observed that people who have been exposed to cadmium during childhood appeared to have more pronounced effects on renal tubular reabsorption than people who only have been exposed in adulthood. A study of Swedish women found that relatively low environmental exposures to Cadmium (median of 0.67 µg Cd/g creatinine) showed a positive association between urinary Cd concentrations and increased urinary excretion of NAG [19c]. Additionally, alterations occurred in glomerular function (GFR, creatinine clearance) at mean urinary cadmium concentrations of 0.8 µg Cd/g and cadmium potentiated diabetes effects on renal function. Increased risk of renal stone formation has also been found in people who have been exposed to cadmium.

Cancer

The underlying mechanism of cadmium as a human carcinogen appears to be related to cadmium-induced oxidative stress with DNA damage that is mediated in part by anti-oxidative cellular defense systems, such as glutathione. Battery workers in Japan had increased urinary excretion of 8-hydroxyguanine (8OH-G) [20c]. Cadmium and nickel were each associated with urinary (8OH-G) independently but the combined exposure produced effects that were greater than additive. The formation of 8OH-G and its presence in the urine sample of exposed workers suggests the use of this adduct as a potential biomarker for Cd-induced DNA damage in relation to cancer.

COPPER

Copper is an essential nutrient for human enzymes and involved in a number of vital biological processes. Normally bound to proteins, copper may be released and become free to catalyze the formation of highly reactive hydroxyl radicals through redox chemistry involving both oxidation states of Cu. Copper-rich foods include oyster, liver, nuts, legumes, whole grains, and dried fruit. Drinking water has a mean concentration of 4–10 µg Cu/L with most of the copper bound to organic matter. The U.S. Environmental Protection Agency's maximum contaminant level for copper in drinking water is 1.3 mg Cu/L.

Liver

Chronic copper toxicity primarily affects the liver because it is the first site of copper deposition after it enters the blood. The lethal dose of copper in an untreated adult is approximately about 10–20 g. Cu toxicity is typically marked by the development of liver cirrhosis with episodes of hemolysis and damage to renal tubules, brain, and other organs. Symptoms can progress to coma, hepatic necrosis, vascular collapse, and death. Certain medical conditions predispose the patient to increased copper concentration particularly those involving obstructive bile excretion such as primary biliary cirrhosis, obstructive hepatobiliary disease, extrahepatic biliary atresia, neonatal hepatitis, choledochal cysts and alpha-1-antitrypsin deficiency [21r].

The effects of increased cellular copper upon growth and viability of human hepatoma cells were investigated using the HepG2 line [22E]. Cellular copper content, acid vesicles, lysosomal function, proliferation, viability and cell cycle kinetics were measured up to 72 hours after the addition of copper (I) sulfate from 4 to 64 μM. HepG2 cells were also exposed to Cu^{2+} (up to 64 μM) for 8 weeks, and their replicative capacity was measured using a colony forming efficiency assay. Concentrations of 16 μM Cu^{2+} led to a 125-fold increase in cellular copper content. The study has demonstrated the link between sequestration of copper and progressive loss of replicative capacity and cell viability. Eventually, it leads to the release of pro-inflammatory molecules from dying cells and that may promote fibrosis and diminish the regenerative capacity of hepatocytes.

DEFERASIROX

Deferasirox is used to treat iron accumulation in patients with β-thalassemia. More recently, it has been used to treat cancers.

Cardiovascular

The use of deferasirox in non-thalassemic patients experiencing elevated ferritin levels after allogenic hematopoietic stem cell transplantation was investigated [23c]. Adverse effects included increased blood creatinine (26.5%), nausea (9.0%), abdominal discomfort (8.3%), with 54 patients (71.1%) experiencing drug-related adverse effects in a dose-dependent manner.

Neuromuscular Function

Proximal muscular atrophy and weakness were observed in two monozygotic twins under treatment with deferasirox for β-thalassemia [24A].

Sensory Systems

Bilateral central serous retinopathy occurred in a 76-year-old patient with paroxysmal nocturnal hemoglobinuria 4 days following the start of treatment with deferoxamine for iron overload secondary to blood transfusions [25A]. The symptoms resolved following withdrawal of deferoxamine treatment.

Gastrointestinal

A multicenter, retrospective, observational study of 44 elderly patients treated with deferasirox for myelodysplastic syndrome found that the most common side effects were diarrhea and serum creatinine resulting in discontinuation of treatment in approximately 10% of the patients [26c]. Anorexia occurred in 4 of 6 patients treated with deferasirox (30 mg/kg/day) for hepatocellular carcinoma [27c].

Urinary Tract

A clinical trial of 60 adult patients investigating the correlation between deferasirox concentration in the serum and pharmacological outcomes found that serum creatinine was positively correlated over 24 hours with serum creatinine and with the dose of administered drug and negatively correlated over 24 hours with serum ferritin and drug half-life [28c]. The authors suggest that adjustment of the dose of the drug may allow less to be administered, minimizing the chance of side effects. A longitudinal retrospective, observational study of at one hospital of 31 adults 18 and over under treatment with deferasirox for iron overload following treatment with regular blood transfusions for myelodysplastic syndrome found that the most common reasons for treatment discontinuation were renal toxicity (35%) and patient's death (25%) [29c].

Proteinuria spontaneously resolved in all 37 patients treated with deferasirox for either β-thalassemia major ($n=36$) or intermedia ($n=1$) [30c]. A higher risk of proteinuria occurred in patients above 29 mg/kg/day ($P=0.004$) and below the age of 23 years ($P=0.019$). Elevated serum creatinine occurred in 4 of 6 patients treated with deferasirox (30 mg/kg/day) for hepatocellular carcinoma, resolving upon withdrawal of the treatment [27c]. Decreased renal creatinine clearance was the most common adverse event in a study of 99 patients with myelodysplastic syndrome who were treated with deferasirox (15–20 mg/kg/day) [31c].

Hypercalciuria (~fourfold increase in the urine calcium to creatinine ratio) occurred in 91.9% of 152 patients under treatment with deferasirox for a variety of diseases including β-thalassemia major (81.5%), sickle cell disease (8%), thalassemia intermedia (2%), HbH disease (6.5%), and E/b thalassemia (2%) [32c].

Immunologic

A 17-year-old male with relapsed acute lymphocytic leukemia and iron overload due to repeat blood transfusions experienced a pruritic maculopapular rash after an increased dose of deferasirox from 500 mg/day for 1 month prior to 1000 mg/day and withdrawal of treatment with dexamethasone [33A]. His parents withheld deferasirox for 2 days, upon which the rash cleared without treatment. He resumed deferasirox at 1000 mg/day 8 days later, upon which a pruritic maculopapular rash developed 8–12 hours later and was marked with a fever of 102°F. He began a deferasirox desensitization protocol that resulted in increased tolerance of the drug for 9 months without problem, after which time he stopped medication.

A 4-year-old girl was similarly desensitized to deferasirox following an adverse skin reaction. The girl commenced oral deferasirox at age 2 (125 mg/100 mL water) and developed widespread erythema multiforme major, after which treatment was halted and the rash disappeared over a week [34A]. She was rechallenged and developed mouth ulcers and swelling 1 day following readministration of the drug. A desensitization regimen was performed beginning with 1.25 mg and escalation at small increments every 4 days, completing desensitization within 25 days.

SECOND-GENERATION EFFECTS

Pregnancy

Although contraindicated during pregnancy, deferasirox prior to unplanned pregnancy did not negatively impact the successful birth of nine children to six Greek thalassemic women [35c].

SUSCEPTIBILITY FACTORS

Genetic

Genetic differences in the *ugt1a1* were associated with different serum concentrations of deferasirox, potentially impacting the dose of drug required in individuals [36c].

Pediatric

A letter to the editor discusses the safety of deferasirox in children [37A]. The authors conclude that transient increases in transaminases are common, that monthly evaluation of serum creatinine and urine protein levels are necessary, and that reduction or stopping of deferasirox may be necessary to prevent kidney injury.

A 3-year-old girl with major thalassemia experienced three admissions for fever, vomiting, metabolic acidosis, azotemia, and dehydration following commencement of deferasirox (33 mg/kg day) [38A]. The patient was a carrier of *ugt1a1* and *abcc2* polymorphisms which the authors hypothesized resulted in decreased metabolism and greater burden of deferasirox (186 mg/mL, normal range is 0.16–40 mg/mL). Symptoms of renal tubular injury also occurred.

Acute liver failure and Fanconi syndrome occurred in a 3-year-old girl with β-thalassemia undergoing treatment with deferasirox [39A]. Fanconi syndrome developed in two pediatric patients with Diamond–Blackfan anemia treated with deferasirox for transfusion-related iron overload [40A]. A clinical study investigating the association of endocrinopathies in 89 adolescents receiving chelation therapy with oral deferiprone found short stature (55%), delayed puberty and/or hypogonadism (54.1%), impaired glucose tolerance or diabetes mellitus (13.0%), hypoparathyroidism (10.1%), and primary hypothyroidism (subclinical) 8.9%, with at least 44 patients (49.4%) presenting with at least one endocrinopathy [41c].

GENE THERAPY

A double knockout Atp7b (−/−) Wilson disease mouse model was transduced with an adeno-associated vector serotype 8 encoding the human ATP7B cDNA under transcriptional control of the liver-specific alpha1-antitrypsin promoter [42E]. Six months following administration of the adenoviral vector, no histological alterations were found and symptoms of Wilson's disease were reversed.

HYDROXYUREA

Hydroxyurea is used to increase the concentration of fetal hemoglobin in patients with sickle cell disease. The mechanism of action remains speculative [43r], but is usually attributed to inhibition of ribonucleotide reductase [44r].

Cardiovascular

Reversible cytopenias occurred in 22% of patients 133 patients under hydroxyurea treatment for sickle cell disease [45c]. Higher rate of thrombosis was found in treatments treated with hydroxyurea with three or more phlebotomies per year compared with 0–2 phlebotomies per year (20.5% vs 5.3% at 3 years; $P < 0.0001$) [46c]. Patients requiring more phlebotomies were those less responsive to hydroxyurea. The authors conclude that those patients with a higher phlebotomy requirement under hydroxyurea therapy have a higher risk of thrombosis and polycythemia vera [46c]. Vaso-occlusive pain (11 events in five (8%) of patients) was the most common side effect observed in a clinical trial of 159 patients comparing transfusion ($n = 61$) to hydroxyurea ($n = 60$) [47c].

Nervous System

Excessive daytime sleepiness was observed in a patient on long-term treatment with hydroxyurea; the symptoms resolved upon withdrawal of hydroxyurea [48A].

Skin

A squamous cell carcinoma and dermatomyosite-like eruption occurred in a sickle-cell patient on long-term hydroxyurea treatment [49A]. Chronic cutaneous lupus occurred in response to chronic hydroxyurea treatment [50A]. Hydroxyurea-induced squamous dysplasia was successfully treated with ingenol mubutate in a small clinical trial [51c]. Malleolar ulcers of the lower limb were concluded to be due to hydroxyurea therapy in chronic myeloproliferative disorders [52A].

Keratotic papules, psoriasiform plaques, and keratoderma occurred in a 69-year-old woman under treatment with hydroxyurea for 4 years which resolved following halting of treatment [53A]. Following initial diagnosis of hand and foot psoriasis, symptomatic treatment failed and the lesions subsequently ulcerated. The authors concluded that halting of hydroxyurea treatment sooner would have prevented the progression of the lesions.

Gastrointestinal

Persistent oral ulcerations occurred in a patient on long-term hydroxyurea treatment; the ulcerations resolved after treatment with topical and systemic corticosteroids followed by low-level laser therapy [54A].

Adipose

Panniculitis occurred in a patient on hydroxyurea therapy for the treatment of myeloproliferative disease [55A].

SECOND-GENERATION EFFECTS

Teratogenicity

Hydroxyurea-induced transcriptome changes during organogenesis within a murine embryo, activating pathways specific to DNA damage and oxidative stress [56E].

SUSCEPTIBILITY FACTORS

Genetic Factors

Variance in response to hydroxyurea was observed in patients treated for β-thalassemia or sickle cell disease; those with particular SIN3A genomic variants experienced greater efficacy from hydroxyurea [57c].

Age

An erratum found that there was no significant increase in constipation or neutrophil count in pediatric patients treated with hydroxyurea [58c].

LITHIUM

Cardiovascular

One case reported cardiotoxic effects of lithium overdose [59A]. A 62-year-old woman was admitted to the emergency room for weaknesses and acute chest pain. She had no history of any chronic diseases, except being put on lithium 400 mg/day and duloxetine 20 mg/day, a week earlier, due to bipolar disorder. Tremors and bilateral nystagmus were indicated in her physical examination. The patient's blood lithium level was measured as 2.3 mM (TR: 0.5–0.8 mM), and her troponin I level was 0.892 ng/mL (N: 0–0.01 ng/mL). A subsequent coronary angiography performed within an hour of admission provided a normal result. A resolution of ECG abnormalities accompanied by lithium elimination suggested her acute chest pain was due to lithium-associated cardiotoxic effects (threefold serum lithium concentration above normal range) which include QTc prolongation, AV block, sinus arrest, and ventricular dysrhythmias.

Nervous System

Lithium is approved by the American FDA for the treatment of patients that suffer from bipolar disorder and manic episode. A study compared the efficacy of lithium as an adjunct therapy to treat moderate to severe HIV-associated neurocognitive disorder (HAND) [60c]. The lithium dose used was 250 mg and titrated up to achieve blood lithium concentration of between 0.6 and 1.0 mM. The primary endpoint was the change in the Global Deficit Score (GDS) from baseline to 24 weeks in the placebo arm compared to the lithium arm. The improvement in GDS was not different between the lithium arm and the placebo arm, −0.57 and −0.56, respectively, with a mean difference of −0.054; $P = 0.716$. Adverse events considered relevant to lithium therapy include QTc prolongation, T-wave changes, hypothyroidism, weight gain, symptoms of nephrogenic diabetes, abdominal cramps, lower limb tremor, daytime somnolence, and insomnia. The previous study found that lithium improved the GDS from impaired to normal after 12 weeks in 8 participants. Moreover, there was another study found a decrease in glutamate with glutamine metabolites in the frontal gray matter, however, no neurocognitive improvement after 10 weeks in 13 participants.

A retrospective cohort study of lithium intoxication indicated that patients with serum lithium concentration level >2.50 mM had the highest risk of experiencing confusion, disorientation, and somnolence ($P < 0.05$) [61c]. Less likely to occur in an acute overdose setting were tremor ($P < 0.05$), vomiting, diarrhea, and ataxia or falls ($P < 0.001$). Lithium is exclusively eliminated by the kidneys. Therefore impaired renal function increases the risk of lithium retention and hence for lithium toxicity. The study confirmed a higher level of creatinine during intoxication ($P < 0.01$). The median change in GFR was 0 mL/min for all episodes. Thus kidney function did not differ before and after intoxication. Acute lithium exposure can lead to overt diabetes insidious and consequently to dehydration. This may explain a transient increase in serum creatinine during the acute intoxication period. In literature review between 1964 and 2004, syndrome of irreversible lithium-effectuated neurotoxicity (SILENT) revealed in 90 patients, presenting with persistent cerebellar dysfunction, extrapyramidal symptoms, brainstem dysfunction or dementia with varying degree of mental syndromes. However, SILENT of lithium intoxication seems rare.

MANGANESE

Manganese is an essential trace element found in dietary sources, including nuts, meat, fish, legumes, poultry, seeds, tea, whole grains, and leafy green vegetables. Manganese is involved in normal immune function, bone growth, regulation of blood glucose, cellular energy, and it is an essential component of manganese superoxide dismutase (MnSOD). Deficiency is very rare in human because the requirements are very low. However, deficiency of manganese may lead to osteoporosis, anemia, and symptoms of premenstrual syndrome (PMS). Manganese inhalation has been associated with neuropsychological and neurological symptoms in exposed workers. These symptoms include motor efficiency and speed, tremor, postural sway and rigidity (similar to Parkinson's disease), mood disturbances, and cognitive impairment. According to several studies, exposure to the air-manganese concentration ranging from 0.003 to 5.86 $\mu g/m^3$ increase ratios to reduced coordination and declines in motor function.

Nervous System

An increased risk of abnormal Unified Parkinson's Disease Rating Scale (UPDRS) motor findings for bradykinesia and the Computerized Adaptive Testing System (CATSYS) postural sway performance was found in residents exposed to manganese through inhalation in two small towns Mn processing facilities [62c]. The UPDRS and CATSYS findings might indicate subclinical effects of manganese exposure. Modeled air-Mn (M = 0.18 µg/m3; SD = 0.130, blood Mn (M = 9.65 µg/L; SD = 3.21), distance from smelter (M = 4.75 miles; SD = 1.64) and length of residence (M = 36.1 years; SD = 15.8) were found to significantly elevate generalized anxiety. Reduced performance on UPDRS motor function and bradykinesia were related to the high score of anxiety, and tremor and motor function were correlated with higher exposure to airborne Mn.

A 62-year-old man with acute pancreatitis and intestinal insufficiency was admitted to the intensive care unit (ICU) [63A]. He required parenteral nutrition (PN) solution throughout his stay because of fistulating celiac disease. Standard manganese supplementation was given in the multi-trace element (MTE) preparation Additrace® consisting of manganese, zinc, copper, chromium, and selenium, providing 270 µg of manganese per day. After 2 1/2 months of PN, he developed a short-lived, intermittent bilateral tremor start at rest lasting for 15–30s, initially distally and bilaterally then spreading to all four limbs. A non-contrast CT scan of his brain was reported normal. However, his blood Mn was significantly increased at 429 nmol/L (reference range 72.8–218.5 nmol/L) at the time the tremors developed. Hypermanganesemia and neurotoxicity can occur in patients on long-term PN therapy, especially if there is liver disease. Accumulation may be slow and the development of neurotoxicity subtle and insidious. Due to its long half-life of elimination, high manganese levels may take months to return to normal.

Endocrine

Plasma manganese levels and type 2 diabetes (T2D) were correlated in a population-based study in China [64c]. The study showing the association between plasma Mn and T2D followed a U-shaped curve; both low and high plasma levels of plasma manganese were associated with higher odds ratios (ORs) of newly diagnosed T2D. Compared with the middle tertile, the multivariate-adjusted ORs (95% confidence interval [CI]) of T2D associated with the lowest tertile and the highest tertile of plasma manganese were 1.89 (95% CI: 1.53–2.33) and 1.56 (95% CI: 1.23–1.97), respectively. U-shaped association was observed between plasma manganese and T2D ($P < 0.01$ for nonlinearity in the spline regression analysis). They found the levels of manganese could affect the metallation and activity of MnSOD (insufficient levels of Manganese), hence increased mitochondrial reactive oxygen species (ROS) formation, which may directly cause macromolecular damage or might indirectly result in oxidative stress by activating stress-sensitive pathways such as the NFKB, p38 MAPK, JNK/SPAK, and hexosamine pathways. Activation of these pathways has been shown to lead to significant deterioration of glucose-stimulated insulin secretion (GSIS), mitochondrial dysfunction, and B-cell dysfunction.

PENICILLAMINE

Autoimmune disease developed in six of 235 Wilson disease patients under long-term treatment with D-penicillamine for Wilson disease [65c]. Immunological side effects seen in Wilson disease patients include SLE, myasthenia gravis, polymyositis, elastosis perforans serpiginosa, pemphigus, and pemphigoid. In these six cases, ulcerative colitis, SLE, multiple sclerosis, morbus Werlhof, seronegative polyarthritis, and psoriasis arthritis developed. Interestingly, all patients who developed autoimmune disorders were administered D-penicillamine (6 of 91), and none of the patients receiving trientine ($n = 58$) or zinc ($n = 58$) developed an autoimmune disorder.

POLYSTYRENE SULFONATES

Polystyrene sulfonates are chelating agents used to treat hyperkalemia and are administered in the GI system. In 2016, two new gastrointestinal potassium chelators underwent clinical trials in the United States: patiromer sorbitex calcium (Veltassa) and sodium zirconium cyclosilicate (ZS-9). Patiromer sorbitex calcium, approved by the U.S. FDA in 2016, is a polymer resin and sorbitol complex that exchanges calcium for potassium. ZS-9 is a non-absorbed, selective inorganic cation exchanger that exchanges sodium and hydrogen for potassium [66R]. Both drugs are primarily associated with mild gastrointestinal side effects [67r,68r]. A review compares the efficacy and safety of older hyperkalemia medications with two new agents, patiromer and ZS-9 [69r].

PATIROMER

Patiromer is a non-absorbable synthetic polymer made of smooth spherical 100 µm beads [69r]. It does not swell when exposed to water and does not require a laxative to reach the distal colon. It exchanges calcium ions for potassium ions as it traverses the gastrointestinal system. The most common side effect is hypomagnesemia developed in the first month of therapy in 8.6% of patients, which responds to magnesium supplementation. The mechanism of action and pharmacology of patiromer was investigated in rat and dog animal models and in humans [70E]. 14C radiolabeled patiromer was used to show that the drug is not systemically absorbed, decreases serum potassium via increased fecal excretion, and is stable in the GI tract in all three organisms.

A review of many potassium chelators discusses the mechanism of action of patiromer [71R]. Patiromer is a polymer that exchanges calcium for potassium that acts primarily in the distal colon. Patiromer functions by increasing potassium excretion in the feces. Side effects included constipation, diarrhea, nausea, vomiting, and flatulence [72c,73c], with constipation occurring in 4.6% of patients and diarrhea occurring in 2.7% of patients [74c].

A meta-analysis concluded that constipation was the most common adverse effect seen with patiromer [75M]. A clinical trial of patiromer found that 47% of patients in the initial treatment phase had 1 adverse effect, with serious adverse effects in three patients in the initial treatment phase, although none were attributable to patiromer [76c]. Other clinical trials similarly found no treatment-related adverse effects [77c,78c] or only mild gastrointestinal effects [79c].

Although patiromer was originally approved in the United States in October of 2015 with a black box warning recommending patients take the drug 6 hours before or after other oral medications due to interactions in absorption, the U.S. Food and Drug Administration approved a supplemental New Drug Application [80A]. The new warning was moved from a black box warning to the Clinical Pharmacology section of the label and now recommends that no other drugs be taken within 3 hours before or after taking patiromer.

POLYSTYRENE SULFONATES (SODIUM AND POTASSIUM SALTS)

In a letter to the editor, an author argues that kayexalate-induced intestinal necrosis is quite rare (0.05%–0.14%) and that its decreased use will result in higher mortality [81r].

Gastrointestinal

A retrospective review of 156 pediatric patients with acute hyperkalemia found that an adverse gastrointestinal event in 24 (15%) of patients [82c]. Patients who received the medication via the rectal route were more likely to require additional intervention. The authors conclude that sodium polystyrene sulfonate may not be appropriate as a first-line agent in patients with severe acute hyperkalemia who require more than a 25% reduction in serum potassium levels or those at high risk for cardiac arrhythmias. A retrospective study of sodium polystyrene sulfate for treatment of hyperkalemia of 501 patients found two cases of bowel necrosis [83c].

Elevated concentration of resin in patients with renal failure may result in renin's activation of angiotensin II, subsequent splanchnic vasoconstriction, and non-occlusive mesenteric ischemia which predisposes the colonic mucosa to injury following dramatic electrolyte and fluid shifts (reviewed in Ref. [84r]).

Colon perforation occurred in a 55-year-old Caucasian female following kayexalate administration. 3 days following uncomplicated right total hip arthroplasty performed for avascular necrosis of the femoral head secondary to chronic steroid use, she presented to a hospital wherein she was diagnosed with Pseudomonas aeruginosa and Klebsiella oxytoca bacteremia. Kidney injury worsened on day 11 and resulted in hyperkalemia, for which she was treated with a single 30 g dose of oral kayexalate without sorbitol. On day 13, she experienced bloody diarrhea with increased abdominal distension, and on day 19 ischemic necrosis of the bowel was identified. Kayexalate-induced colon ischemia and necrosis were subsequently diagnosed [85A].

A 64-year-old male diabetic patient with ESRD on hemodialysis treated with 30 g of kayexalate twice per week experienced rectal bleeding followed by non-specific colitis diagnosed by colonoscopy. Histologic analysis found crystals of kayexalate in the colonic mucosa. 14 months later, kayexalate crystals were found in a new case of rectal bleeding, and the patient subsequently died of intestinal infarction [86A].

A 10-mm linear esophageal ulcer in the distal esophagus was diagnosed in a 59-year-old man with a 2-day history of coffee-ground emesis. Sodium polystyrene sulfonate crystals were identified in a histological specimen. Following discontinuation of sodium polystyrene sulfonate treatment, the symptoms resolved [87A].

Six cases of colitis induced by sodium polystyrene sulfonate in sorbitol were reviewed, discussing the pattern of injury to the colon and characteristic crystals [88A].

SODIUM ZIRCONIUM CYCLOSILICATE (ZS-9)

ZS-9 is a crystal that is highly selective for potassium and ammonium ions [89c]. It chelates potassium and ammonium after they shed their hydration shells, upon which they enter the crystal and form hydrogen bonds to the surrounding oxygen atoms in the crystal structure.

Other ions are too small and do not form stable bonds. Side effects in patients included edema in 6% of patients taking 10 g/day and 14% taking 15 g/day, compared to 2% of control subjects [89c]. Several reviews of ZS-9 discuss the mechanism of action of ZS-9, which eliminates excess potassium rather than acting via intracellular translocation [90r,91R,69R,71R]. The orally administered drug is not absorbed systemically and is eliminated in the feces. Rates of gastrointestinal events were similar between ZS-9 and placebo groups [89c,92c]. Hypokalemia was another side effect observed in the two studies [89c,92c].

TRIENTINE (TRIETHYLENETETRAMINE)

Trientine is a copper chelating drug excreted in the urine that is used to treat Wilson's disease. Pancytopenia is one adverse effect noted with trientine [1r].

ZINC

The use of zinc salts, typically given together with a copper chelation agent, to treat Wilson's disease by blocking intestinal copper absorption was reviewed [93R]. Evidence for efficacious treatment of osteoporosis in patients with β-thalassemia was reviewed [94r]. A meta-analysis investigating the treatment of osteoporosis in patients with β-thalassemia that reviewed four trials concluded that zinc sulfate supplementation increased bone mineral density at the lumbar spine and hip without incidence of side effects [95M].

Immunologic

Antinuclear antibodies sometimes develop in patients receiving treatment for Wilson disease; antinuclear antibody titers were not significantly increased in patients receiving zinc (7/58; 12.1%) [65c].

Readers are advised to refer to an extensive meta-analysis study on cadmium published in 2015 [96M]. Additional recent literature and case studies on metals and metal antagonists can be found in SEDA-38: 193–204, 2016 and SEDA-38: 205–210, 2016 [97M].

References

[1] Li WJ, Chen C, You ZF, et al. Current drug managements of Wilson's disease: from west to east. Curr Neuropharmacol. 2016;14(4):322–5. PubMed PMID: 26639459; PMCID: PMC4876588. [R].
[2] Mobarra N, Shanaki M, Ehteram H, et al. A review on iron chelators in treatment of iron overload syndromes. Int J Hematol Oncol Stem Cell Res. 2016;10(4):239–47. PubMed PMID: 27928480; PMCID: PMC5139945 [R].

[3] Taher AT, Porter JB, Kattamis A, et al. Efficacy and safety of iron-chelation therapy with deferoxamine, deferiprone, and deferasirox for the treatment of iron-loaded patients with nontransfusion-dependent thalassemia syndromes. Drug Des Devel Ther. 2016;10:4073–8. http://dx.doi.org/10.2147/DDDT.S117080. PubMed PMID: 28008230; PMCID: PMC5170616 [r].

[4] Botzenhardt S, Li N, Chan EW, et al. Safety profiles of iron chelators in young patients with haemoglobinopathies. Eur J Haematol. 2017;98(3):198–217. http://dx.doi.org/10.1111/ejh.12833. PubMed PMID: 27893170 [M].

[5] Kontoghiorghe CN, Kontoghiorghes GJ. Efficacy and safety of iron-chelation therapy with deferoxamine, deferiprone, and deferasirox for the treatment of iron-loaded patients with non-transfusion-dependent thalassemia syndromes. Drug Des Devel Ther. 2016;10:465–81. http://dx.doi.org/10.2147/DDDT.S79458. PubMed PMID: 26893541; PMCID: PMC4745840 [R].

[6] Kontoghiorghe CN, Kontoghiorghes GJ. New developments and controversies in iron metabolism and iron chelation therapy. World J Methodol. 2016;6(1):1–19. http://dx.doi.org/10.5662/wjm.v6.i1.1. PubMed PMID: 27019793; PMCID: PMC4804243 [R].

[7] Takami T, Yamasaki T, Saeki I, et al. Supportive therapies for prevention of hepatocellular carcinoma recurrence and preservation of liver function. World J Gastroenterol. 2016;22(32):7252–63. http://dx.doi.org/10.3748/wjg.v22.i32.7252. PubMed PMID: 27621572; PMCID: PMC4997645 [R].

[8] Saljooghi AS, Babaie M, Mendi FD, et al. Chelation of thallium by combining deferasirox and desferrioxamine in rats. Toxicol Ind Health. 2016;32(1):83–8. http://dx.doi.org/10.1177/0748233713498442. PubMed PMID: 24021432 [E].

[9] Derin S, Azik FM, Topal Y, et al. The incidence of ototoxicity in patients using iron chelators. J Int Adv Otol. 2016;13:136–9. http://dx.doi.org/10.5152/iao.2016.1852. PubMed PMID: 27879229 [c].

[10] Hassan MA, Tolba OA. Iron chelation monotherapy in transfusion-dependent beta-thalassemia major patients: a comparative study of deferasirox and deferoxamine. Electron Physician. 2016;8(5):2425–31. http://dx.doi.org/10.19082/2425. PubMed PMID: 27382454; PMCID: PMC4930264 [c].

[11] Poggi M, Sorrentino F, Pugliese P, et al. Longitudinal changes of endocrine and bone disease in adults with beta-thalassemia major receiving different iron chelators over 5 years. Ann Hematol. 2016;95(5):757–63. http://dx.doi.org/10.1007/s00277-016-2633-y. PubMed PMID: 26957357 [c].

[12] Hyvonen MT, Ucal S, Pasanen M, et al. Triethylenetetramine modulates polyamine and energy metabolism and inhibits cancer cell proliferation. Biochem J. 2016;473(10):1433–41. http://dx.doi.org/10.1042/BCJ20160134. PubMed PMID: 27001865 [E].

[13] Chan N, Willis A, Kornhauser N, et al. Influencing the tumor microenvironment: a phase II study of copper depletion using tetrathiomolybdate in patients with breast cancer at high risk for recurrence and in preclinical models of lung metastases. Clin Cancer Res. 2017;23(3):666–76. http://dx.doi.org/10.1158/1078-0432.CCR-16-1326. PubMed PMID: 27769988. [c].

[14] Satarug S, Haswell-Elkins MR, Moore MR. Safe levels of cadmium intake to prevent renal toxicity in human subjects. Br J Nutr. 2000;84(6):791–802. PubMed PMID: 11177195 [r].

[15] Godt J, Scheidig F, Grosse-Siestrup C, et al. The toxicity of cadmium and resulting hazards for human health. J Occup Med Toxicol. 2006;1:22. http://dx.doi.org/10.1186/1745-6673-1-22. PubMed PMID: 16961932; PMCID: PMC1578573 [r].

[16] Fowler BA. Monitoring of human populations for early markers of cadmium toxicity: a review. Toxicol Appl Pharmacol. 2009;238(3):294–300. http://dx.doi.org/10.1016/j.taap.2009.05.004. PubMed PMID: 19433102 [r].

[17] Elsenhans B, Strugala GJ, Schafer SG. Small-intestinal absorption of cadmium and the significance of mucosal metallothionein. Hum Exp Toxicol. 1997;16(8):429–34. http://dx.doi.org/10.1177/096032719701600803. PubMed PMID: 9292282 [E].

[18] Trzcinka-Ochocka M, Jakubowski M, Razniewska G, et al. The effects of environmental cadmium exposure on kidney function: the possible influence of age. Environ Res. 2004;95(2):143–50. http://dx.doi.org/10.1016/j.envres.2003.10.003. PubMed PMID: 15147919 [c].

[19] Akesson A, Lundh T, Vahter M, et al. Tubular and glomerular kidney effects in Swedish women with low environmental cadmium exposure. Environ Health Perspect. 2005;113(11):1627–31. PubMed PMID: 16263522; PMCID: PMC1310929 [c].

[20] Yoshioka N, Nakashima H, Hosoda K, et al. Urinary excretion of an oxidative stress marker, 8-hydroxyguanine (8-OH-Gua), among nickel-cadmium battery workers. J Occup Health. 2008;50(3):229–35. PubMed PMID: 18408348 [c].

[21] Beshgetoor D, Hambidge M. Clinical conditions altering copper metabolism in humans. Am J Clin Nutr. 1998;67(5 Suppl):1017S–21S. PubMed PMID: 9587145 [r].

[22] Aston NS, Watt N, Morton IE, et al. Copper toxicity affects proliferation and viability of human hepatoma cells (HepG2 line). Hum Exp Toxicol. 2000;19(6):367–76. http://dx.doi.org/10.1191/096032700678815963. PubMed PMID: 10962511 [E].

[23] Jaekel N, Lieder K, Albrecht S, et al. Efficacy and safety of deferasirox in non-thalassemic patients with elevated ferritin levels after allogeneic hematopoietic stem cell transplantation. Bone Marrow Transplant. 2016;51(1):89–95. http://dx.doi.org/10.1038/bmt.2015.204. PubMed PMID: 26367238 [c].

[24] Vill K, Muller-Felber W, Teusch V, et al. Proximal muscular atrophy and weakness: an unusual adverse effect of deferasirox iron chelation therapy. Neuromuscul Disord. 2016;26(4–5):322–5. http://dx.doi.org/10.1016/j.nmd.2016.02.011. PubMed PMID: 27068298 [A].

[25] Vahdani K, Makrygiannis G, Kaneshyogan H, et al. Bilateral central serous retinopathy in a patient with paroxysmal nocturnal hemoglobinuria treated with deferoxamine. Eur J Ophthalmol. 2016;26(6):e152–4. http://dx.doi.org/10.5301/ejo.5000840. PubMed PMID: 27445073 [A].

[26] Del Corso L, Biale L, Parodi EL, et al. Multidisciplinary evaluation at baseline and during treatment improves the rate of compliance and efficacy of deferasirox in elderly myelodysplastic patients. Int J Clin Oncol. 2017;22(2):380–6. http://dx.doi.org/10.1007/s10147-016-1042-5. PubMed PMID: 27771776 [c].

[27] Saeki I, Yamamoto N, Yamasaki T, et al. Effects of an oral iron chelator, deferasirox, on advanced hepatocellular carcinoma. World J Gastroenterol. 2016;22(40):8967–77. http://dx.doi.org/10.3748/wjg.v22.i40.8967. PubMed PMID: 27833388; PMCID: PMC5083802 [c].

[28] Allegra S, De Francia S, Cusato J, et al. Deferasirox pharmacokinetic and toxicity correlation in beta-thalassaemia major treatment. J Pharm Pharmacol. 2016;68(11):1417–21. http://dx.doi.org/10.1111/jphp.12638. PubMed PMID: 27672004 [c].

[29] Escudero-Vilaplana V, Garcia-Gonzalez X, Osorio-Prendes S, et al. Impact of medication adherence on the effectiveness of deferasirox for the treatment of transfusional iron overload in myelodysplastic syndrome. J Clin Pharm Ther. 2016;41(1):59–63. http://dx.doi.org/10.1111/jcpt.12348. PubMed PMID: 26778738 [c].

[30] Bayhan T, Unal S, Unlu O, et al. The questioning for routine monthly monitoring of proteinuria in patients with beta-thalassemia on deferasirox chelation. Hematology. 2017;22(4):248–51. http://dx.doi.org/10.1080/10245332.2016.1252004. PubMed PMID: 27809710 [c].

[31] Bruch HR, Dencausse Y, Hessling J, et al. CONIFER—Non-interventional study to evaluate therapy monitoring during deferasirox treatment of iron toxicity in myelodysplastic syndrome patients with transfusional iron overload. Oncol Res Treat. 2016;39(7–8):424–31. http://dx.doi.org/10.1159/000447035. PubMed PMID: 27486873 [c].

[32] Wong P, Polkinghorne K, Kerr PG, et al. Deferasirox at therapeutic doses is associated with dose-dependent hypercalciuria. Bone. 2016;85:55–8. http://dx.doi.org/10.1016/j.bone.2016.01.011. PubMed PMID: 26802257 [c].

[33] Bruner KE, White KM. Deferasirox desensitization. J Allergy Clin Immunol Pract. 2016;4(1):171–2. http://dx.doi.org/10.1016/j.jaip.2015.09.007. PubMed PMID: 26489716 [A].

[34] Davies GI, Davies D, Charles S, et al. Successful desensitization to deferasirox in a paediatric patient with beta-thalassaemia major. Pediatr Allergy Immunol. 2017;28(2):199–201. http://dx.doi.org/10.1111/pai.12677. PubMed PMID: 27797415 [A].

[35] Diamantidis MD, Neokleous N, Agapidou A, et al. Iron chelation therapy of transfusion-dependent beta-thalassemia during pregnancy in the era of novel drugs: is deferasirox toxic? Int J Hematol. 2016;103(5):537–44. http://dx.doi.org/10.1007/s12185-016-1945-y. PubMed PMID: 26861970 [c].

[36] Cusato J, Allegra S, De Francia S, et al. Role of pharmacogenetics on deferasirox AUC and efficacy. Pharmacogenomics. 2016;17(6):561–72. http://dx.doi.org/10.2217/pgs-2015-0001. PubMed PMID: 27043265 [c].

[37] Origa R, Zappu A, Foschini ML, et al. Deferasirox and children: from clinical trials to the real world. Am J Hematol. 2016;91(6):E304–5. http://dx.doi.org/10.1002/ajh.24353. PubMed PMID: 26950047 [A].

[38] Marano M, Bottaro G, Goffredo B, et al. Deferasirox-induced serious adverse reaction in a pediatric patient: pharmacokinetic and pharmacogenetic analysis. Eur J Clin Pharmacol. 2016;72(2):247–8. http://dx.doi.org/10.1007/s00228-015-1956-2. PubMed PMID: 26403473 [A].

[39] Ramaswami A, Rosen DJ, Chu J, et al. Fulminant liver failure in a child with beta-thalassemia on deferasirox: a case report. J Pediatr Hematol Oncol. 2017;39(3):235–7. http://dx.doi.org/10.1097/MPH.0000000000000654. PubMed PMID: 27479018 [A].

[40] Papneja K, Bhatt MD, Kirby-Allen M, et al. Fanconi syndrome secondary to deferasirox in Diamond–Blackfan anemia: case series and recommendations for early diagnosis. Pediatr Blood Cancer. 2016;63(8):1480–3. http://dx.doi.org/10.1002/pbc.25995. PubMed PMID: 27082377 [A].

[41] Sharma R, Seth A, Chandra J, et al. Endocrinopathies in adolescents with thalassaemia major receiving oral iron chelation therapy. Paediatr Int Child Health. 2016;36(1):22–7. http://dx.doi.org/10.1179/2046905514Y.0000000160. PubMed PMID: 25311879 [c].

[42] Murillo O, Luqui DM, Gazquez C, et al. Long-term metabolic correction of Wilson's disease in a murine model by gene therapy. J Hepatol. 2016;64(2):419–26. http://dx.doi.org/10.1016/j.jhep.2015.09.014. PubMed PMID: 26409215 [E].

[43] Ferrone FA. Sickle cell disease: its molecular mechanism and the one drug that treats it. Int J Biol Macromol. 2016;93(Pt A):1168–73. http://dx.doi.org/10.1016/j.ijbiomac.2016.09.073. PubMed PMID: 27667542 [r].

[44] Singh A, Xu YJ. The cell killing mechanisms of hydroxyurea. Genes (Basel). 2016;7(11):E99. http://dx.doi.org/10.3390/genes7110099. PubMed PMID: 27869662; PMCID: PMC5126785 [r].

[45] Luchtman-Jones L, Pressel S, Hilliard L, et al. Effects of hydroxyurea treatment for patients with hemoglobin SC disease. Am J Hematol. 2016;91(2):238–42. http://dx.doi.org/10.1002/ajh.24255. PubMed PMID: 26615793 [c].

[46] Alvarez-Larran A, Perez-Encinas M, Ferrer-Marin F, et al. Risk of thrombosis according to need of phlebotomies in patients with polycythemia vera treated with hydroxyurea. Haematologica. 2017;102(1):103–9. http://dx.doi.org/10.3324/haematol.2016.152769. PubMed PMID: 27686377; PMCID: PMC5210240 [c].

[47] Ware RE, Davis BR, Schultz WH, et al. Hydroxycarbamide versus chronic transfusion for maintenance of transcranial doppler flow velocities in children with sickle cell anaemia-TCD With Transfusions Changing to Hydroxyurea (TWiTCH): a multicentre, open-label, phase 3, non-inferiority trial. Lancet. 2016;387(10019):661–70. http://dx.doi.org/10.1016/S0140-6736(15)01041-7. PubMed PMID: 26670617 [c].

[48] Revol B, Joyeux-Faure M, Albahary MV, et al. Severe excessive daytime sleepiness induced by hydroxyurea. Fundam Clin Pharmacol. 2016;31:367–8. http://dx.doi.org/10.1111/fcp.12260. PubMed PMID: 27998000 [A].

[49] Mokni S, Fetoui Ghariani N, Aounallah A, et al. Dermatologic complications of long-term hydroxyurea therapy. Therapie. 2016;72:391–4. http://dx.doi.org/10.1016/j.therap.2016.05.009. PubMed PMID: 27912970 [A].

[50] Yanes DA, Mosser-Goldfarb JL. A cutaneous lupus erythematosus-like eruption induced by hydroxyurea. Pediatr Dermatol. 2017;34(1):e30–1. http://dx.doi.org/10.1111/pde.13018. PubMed PMID: 27813209 [A].

[51] Grandi V, Delfino C, Pimpinelli N. Ingenol mebutate in the treatment of 'Hydroxyurea-induced Squamous Dysplasia': a single centre experience. J Eur Acad Dermatol Venereol. 2016;30(7):1129–32. http://dx.doi.org/10.1111/jdv.13616. PubMed PMID: 27072602 [c].

[52] Aparicio Julian MA, Mayorga Baca MS, Morato Garcia C, et al. Malleolar ulcers associated to hydroxyurea treatment. Rev Enferm. 2016;39(4):42–4. PubMed PMID: 27349062 [A].

[53] Worley B, Glassman SJ. Acral keratoses and leucocytoclastic vasculitis occurring during treatment of essential thrombocythaemia with hydroxyurea. Clin Exp Dermatol. 2016;41(2):166–9. http://dx.doi.org/10.1111/ced.12708. PubMed PMID: 26269121 [A].

[54] Cabras M, Cafaro A, Gambino A, et al. Laser photobiomodulation for a complex patient with severe hydroxyurea-induced oral ulcerations. Case Rep Dent. 2016;2016:9810480. http://dx.doi.org/10.1155/2016/9810480. PubMed PMID: 27957350; PMCID: PMC5121453 [A].

[55] Ogawa Y, Akiyama M. Non-infectious panniculitis during hydroxyurea therapy in a patient with myeloproliferative disease. Acta Derm Venereol. 2016;96(4):566–7. http://dx.doi.org/10.2340/00015555-2292. PubMed PMID: 26576655 [A].

[56] El Husseini N, Schlisser AE, Hales BF. Editor's highlight: hydroxyurea exposure activates the P53 signaling pathway in murine organogenesis-stage embryos. Toxicol Sci. 2016;152(2):297–308. http://dx.doi.org/10.1093/toxsci/kfw089. PubMed PMID: 27208086; PMCID: PMC4960909 [E].

[57] Gravia A, Chondrou V, Kolliopoulou A, et al. Correlation of SIN3A genomic variants with beta-hemoglobinopathies disease severity and hydroxyurea treatment efficacy, Pharmacogenomics. 2016; http://dx.doi.org/10.2217/pgs-2016-0076. https://www.futuremedicine.com/doi/abs/10.2217/pgs-2016-0076?url_ver=Z39.88-2003&rfr_id=ori%3Arid%3Acrossref.org&rfr_dat=cr_pub%3Dpubmed. PubMed PMID: 27767389 [c].

[58] Thornburg CD, Files BA, Luo Z, et al. Impact of hydroxyurea on clinical events in the BABY HUG trial. Blood. 2012;120(22):4304–10. http://dx.doi.org/10.1182/blood-2016-10-748764. Blood. 2016; 128(24): 2869. PubMed PMID: 27979871; PMCID: PMC5159708 [c].

[59] Asim K, Selman Y, Suleyman Y, et al. Heart attack in the course of lithium overdose. Iran Red Crescent Med J. 2016;18(7):e21731. http://dx.doi.org/10.5812/ircmj.21731. PubMed PMID: 27703795; PMCID: PMC5027627 [A].

[60] Decloedt EH, Freeman C, Howells F, et al. Moderate to severe HIV-associated neurocognitive impairment: a randomized placebo-controlled trial of lithium. Medicine (Baltimore). 2016;95(46):e5401. http://dx.doi.org/10.1097/MD.0000000000005401. PubMed PMID: 27861379; PMCID: PMC5120936 [c].

[61] Ott M, Stegmayr B, Salander Renberg E, et al. Lithium intoxication: incidence, clinical course and renal function—a population-based retrospective cohort study. J Psychopharmacol. 2016;30(10):1008–19. http://dx.doi.org/10.1177/0269881116652577. PubMed PMID: 27307388; PMCID: PMC5036078 [c].

[62] Bowler RM, Beseler CL, Gocheva VV, et al. Environmental exposure to manganese in air: associations with tremor and motor function. Sci Total Environ. 2016;541:646–54. http://dx.doi.org/10.1016/j.scitotenv.2015.09.084. PubMed PMID: 26437342; PMCID: PMC4803294 [c].

[63] Walter E, Alsaffar S, Livingstone C, et al. Manganese toxicity in critical care: case report, literature review and recommendations for practice. J Intensive Care Soc. 2016;17(3):252–7. http://dx.doi.org/10.1177/1751143715622216. [A].

[64] Shan Z, Chen S, Sun T, et al. U-shaped association between plasma manganese levels and type 2 diabetes. Environ Health Perspect. 2016;124(12):1876–81. http://dx.doi.org/10.1289/EHP176. PubMed PMID: 27258818; PMCID: PMC5132633 interests [c].

[65] Seessle J, Gotthardt DN, Schafer M, et al. Concomitant immune-related events in Wilson disease: implications for monitoring chelator therapy. J Inherit Metab Dis. 2016;39(1):125–130. http://dx.doi.org/10.1007/s10545-015-9866-0. PubMed PMID: 26067812 [c].

[66] Packham DK, Kosiborod M. Potential new agents for the management of hyperkalemia. Am J Cardiovasc Drugs. 2016;16(1):19–31. http://dx.doi.org/10.1007/s40256-015-0130-7. PubMed PMID: 26156040 [R].

[67] Henneman A, Guirguis E, Grace Y, et al. Emerging therapies for the management of chronic hyperkalemia in the ambulatory care setting. Am J Health Syst Pharm. 2016;73(2):33–44. http://dx.doi.org/10.2146/ajhp150457. PubMed PMID: 26721532 [r].

[68] Vu BN, De Castro AM, Shottland D, et al. Patiromer: the first potassium binder approved in over 50 years. Cardiol Rev. 2016;24(6):316–23. http://dx.doi.org/10.1097/CRD.0000000000000123. PubMed PMID: 27548687 [r].

[69] Sterns RH, Grieff M, Bernstein PL. Treatment of hyperkalemia: something old, something new. Kidney Int. 2016;89(3):546–54. http://dx.doi.org/10.1016/j.kint.2015.11.018. PubMed PMID: 26880451 [r].

[70] Li L, Harrison SD, Cope MJ, et al. Mechanism of action and pharmacology of patiromer, a nonabsorbed cross-linked polymer that lowers serum potassium concentration in patients with hyperkalemia. J Cardiovasc Pharmacol Ther. 2016;21(5):456–65. http://dx.doi.org/10.1177/1074248416629549. PubMed PMID: 26856345; PMCID: PMC4976659 [E].

[71] Chaitman M, Dixit D, Bridgeman MB. Potassium-binding agents for the clinical management of hyperkalemia. P T. 2016;41(1):43–50. PubMed PMID: 26765867; PMCID: PMC4699486 [R].

[72] Weir MR, Bakris GL, Bushinsky DA, et al. Patiromer in patients with kidney disease and hyperkalemia receiving RAAS inhibitors. N Engl J Med. 2015;372(3):211–21. http://dx.doi.org/10.1056/NEJMoa1410853. PubMed PMID: 25415805 [c].

[73] Pitt B, Anker SD, Bushinsky DA, et al. Investigators P-H. Evaluation of the efficacy and safety of RLY5016, a polymeric potassium binder, in a double-blind, placebo-controlled study in patients with chronic heart failure (the PEARL-HF) trial. Eur Heart J. 2011;32(7):820–8. http://dx.doi.org/10.1093/eurheartj/ehq502. PubMed PMID: 21208974; PMCID: PMC3069389 [c].

[74] Pitt B, Bushinsky D, Garza D, et al. 1-Year safety and efficacy of patiromer for hyperkalemia in heart failure patients with chronic kidney disease on renin-angiotensin-aldosterone system inhibitors. J Am Coll Cardiol. 2015;65(10 Suppl):A855. http://dx.doi.org/10.1016/S0735-1097(15)60855-5. [c].

[75] Montaperto AG, Gandhi MA, Gashlin LZ, et al. Patiromer: a clinical review. Curr Med Res Opin. 2016;32(1):155–64. http://dx.doi.org/10.1185/03007995.2015.1106935. PubMed PMID: 26456884 [M].

[76] Weir MR, Bakris GL, Gross C, et al. Treatment with patiromer decreases aldosterone in patients with chronic kidney disease and hyperkalemia on renin-angiotensin system inhibitors. Kidney Int. 2016;90(3):696–704. http://dx.doi.org/10.1016/j.kint.2016.04.019. PubMed PMID: 27350174 [c].

[77] Kim ES, Deeks ED. Patiromer: a review in hyperkalaemia. Clin Drug Investig. 2016;36(8):687–94. http://dx.doi.org/10.1007/s40261-016-0432-9. PubMed PMID: 27380495 [c].

[78] Bushinsky DA, Spiegel DM, Gross C, et al. Effect of patiromer on urinary ion excretion in healthy adults. Clin J Am Soc Nephrol. 2016;11(10):1769–76. http://dx.doi.org/10.2215/CJN.01170216. PubMed PMID: 27679518; PMCID: PMC5053784 [c].

[79] Bushinsky DA, Rossignol P, Spiegel DM, et al. Patiromer decreases serum potassium and phosphate levels in patients on hemodialysis. Am J Nephrol 2016;44(5):404–10. http://dx.doi.org/10.1159/000451067. PubMed PMID: 27784004 [c].

[80] FDA approves supplemental new drug application for veltassa removing boxed warning regarding drug-drug interactions: relypsa; 2016 [cited 2017 4/11], 2016. Available from http://www.relypsa.com/newsroom/press-releases/112716/. [A].

[81] Abuelo JG. Moving away from Kayexalate, sodium polystyrene sulfate. Am J Emerg Med. 2016;34(8):1716. http://dx.doi.org/10.1016/j.ajem.2016.06.017. PubMed PMID: 27318747 [r].

[82] Lee J, Moffett BS. Treatment of pediatric hyperkalemia with sodium polystyrene sulfonate. Pediatr Nephrol. 2016;31(11):2113–7. http://dx.doi.org/10.1007/s00467-016-3414-5. PubMed PMID: 27215929 [c].

[83] Hagan AE, Farrington CA, Wall GC, et al. Sodium polystyrene sulfonate for the treatment of acute hyperkalemia: a retrospective study. Clin Nephrol. 2016;85(1):38–43. http://dx.doi.org/10.5414/CN108628. PubMed PMID: 26587776 [c].

[84] Rogers FB, Li SC. Acute colonic necrosis associated with sodium polystyrene sulfonate (Kayexalate) enemas in a critically ill patient: case report and review of the literature. J Trauma. 2001;51(2):395–7. PubMed PMID: 11493807 [r].

[85] Dunlap RH, Martinez R. Total colectomy for colon perforation after kayexalate administration: a case report and literature review of a rare complication. J Surg Case Rep. 2016;2016(10). http://dx.doi.org/10.1093/jscr/rjw167. PubMed PMID: 27765805; PMCID: PMC5055282 [A].

[86] Capitanini A, Bozzoli L, Rollo S, et al. The presence of crystals of sodium polystyrene sulfonate in the colonic wall: innocent bystander or pathogenic factor? G Ital Nefrol. 2016;33(2). PubMed PMID: 27067217 [A].

[87] Brown 2nd R, Samuel J, Parmar K, et al. Sodium polystyrene sulfonate-induced esophageal ulcer. Gastrointest Endosc. 2016;83(3):664. http://dx.doi.org/10.1016/j.gie.2015.09.022. discussion −5. PubMed PMID: 26422977 [A].

[88] Jacob SS, Parameswaran A, Parameswaran SA, et al. Colitis induced by sodium polystyrene sulfonate in sorbitol: a report of six cases. Indian J Gastroenterol. 2016;35(2):139–42. http://dx.doi.org/10.1007/s12664-016-0635-2. PubMed PMID: 27033844 [A].

[89] Kosiborod M, Rasmussen HS, Lavin P, et al. Effect of sodium zirconium cyclosilicate on potassium lowering for 28 days among

outpatients with hyperkalemia: the HARMONIZE randomized clinical trial. JAMA. 2014;312(21):2223–33. http://dx.doi.org/10.1001/jama.2014.15688. PubMed PMID: 25402495 [c].

[90] Linder KE, Krawczynski MA, Laskey D. Sodium zirconium cyclosilicate (ZS-9): a novel agent for the treatment of hyperkalemia. Pharmacotherapy. 2016;36(8):923–33. http://dx.doi.org/10.1002/phar.1797. PubMed PMID: 27393581 [r].

[91] Packham DK, Kosiborod M. Pharmacodynamics and pharmacokinetics of sodium zirconium cyclosilicate [ZS-9] in the treatment of hyperkalemia. Expert Opin Drug Metab Toxicol. 2016;12(5):567–73. http://dx.doi.org/10.1517/17425255.2016.1164691. PubMed PMID: 26998854 [R].

[92] Packham DK, Rasmussen HS, Lavin PT, et al. Sodium zirconium cyclosilicate in hyperkalemia. N Engl J Med. 2015;372(3):222–31. http://dx.doi.org/10.1056/NEJMoa1411487. PubMed PMID: 25415807 [c].

[93] Weiss KH, et al. Wilson Disease. In: Pagon RA, Adam MP, Ardinger HH, et al., editors. GeneReviews(R). Seattle (WA): University of Washington; 1993.

[94] Fung EB. The importance of nutrition for health in patients with transfusion-dependent thalassemia. Ann N Y Acad Sci. 2016;1368(1):40–8. http://dx.doi.org/10.1111/nyas.13003. PubMed PMID: 26824448 [r].

[95] Bhardwaj A, Swe KM, Sinha NK, et al. Treatment for osteoporosis in people with β-thalassaemia. Cochrane Database Syst Rev. 2016;3: CD010429. http://dx.doi.org/10.1002/14651858.CD010429.pub2. PubMed PMID: 26964506 [M].

[96] Oh E, Liu R, Nel A, et al. Meta-analysis of cellular toxicity for cadmium-containing quantum dots. Nat Nanotechnol. 2015;11:479–86. http://dx.doi.org/10.1038/nnano.2015.338 [M].

[97] Gray JP, Ray SD. Metal Antagonists. Side Effects of Drugs Annual. 2016;38:205–10 [M].

20

Antiseptic Drugs and Disinfectants

Dirk W. Lachenmeier[1]

Chemisches und Veterinäruntersuchungsamt (CVUA) Karlsruhe, Karlsruhe, Germany

[1]Corresponding author: lachenmeier@web.de

ALDEHYDES [SED-15, 1439, 1513; SEDA-31, 409; SEDA-32, 437; SEDA-33, 479; SEDA-34, 377; SEDA-36, 339; SEDA-37, 273; SEDA-38, 211]

Considering all disinfectants, aldehydes have a special status as they are able to pose occupational hazards even at very low concentrations in air (SEDA-36, 339; SEDA-37, 273). No new data on glutaraldehyde were identified this year.

Formaldehyde

The carcinogenicity classification of formaldehyde in the European Union was upgraded from category 2 (suspected human carcinogens) to category 1B (substances presumed to have carcinogenic potential for humans) and also to mutagen category 2 [1S]. The regulation entered into force as of 1 January 2016. For manufacturers of formaldehyde-containing disinfectants, new labelling and safety data sheet requirements are necessary as well as new registration requirements have to be applied. Legal changes also including remarks on requirements for occupational use of disinfectants were provided by Rühl [2r]. A survey from Sweden showed that formaldehyde releasers are widely used in skin care products (58 out of 247 tested products were positive with formaldehyde >2.5 mg/kg, from which 17 products were not declared to contain formaldehyde or formaldehyde-releasing preservatives) [3C]. A workplace exposure study from Australia showed that 2.5% of 4993 respondents were exposed to formaldehyde in the course of their work, most of them in the construction industry exposed through particle board or plywood [4C]. A study from Spain that evaluated 10 indoor air samples from homes found formaldehyde levels from 10 to 48 μg/m³ [5R].

Tumorigenicity

According to an updated assessment of the International Agency for Research on Cancer (IARC), formaldehyde was confirmed as carcinogenic to humans (Group 1). Formaldehyde causes cancer of the nasopharynx and leukemia [6S]. The IARC assessment and specifically the epidemiologic evidence on the association between formaldehyde exposure and risk of leukemia and other lymphohematopoietic malignancies have been previously discussed controversially [SEDA-36, 339; SEDA-37, 273]. A cohort mortality study of 11 043 US formaldehyde-exposed garment workers found that compared to the US population, myeloid leukemia mortality was elevated, but overall leukemia mortality was not. Overall leukemia mortality significantly increased with increasing exposure duration. The authors judged the data to provide limited evidence of an association between formaldehyde and leukemia [7C]. In vitro research in Hela cells detected that formaldehyde stimulation leads to downregulation of paxillin or p53 and its signaling complexes, while tyrosine phosphorylated paxillin and its signaling complexes are upregulated. The authors suggested that these alterations of normal signal transduction may finally lead to tumorigenesis [8E]. In vitro research showed that formaldehyde (10 μM) in simulated sweat is able to increase cell proliferation in malignant melanoma cells but not in normal keratinocytes [9E].

Immunologic

In a retrospective analysis of patch test data (1996–2012) in Northeastern Italy, the results from 23 774 patients showed a frequency of sensitization of 3.3%, without any significant time trend. Significant associations in health care, wood and textile industries and professional drivers were detected [10C]. In a trial with 15 formaldehyde-allergic individuals vs 12 controls in a repeated open application test during 4 weeks with

ISSN: 0378-6080

http://dx.doi.org/10.1016/bs.seda.2017.06.005

moisturizers releasing formaldehyde in concentrations of 2.5–40 mg/kg, 9 of the 15 allergic individuals, but none in the control group, developed reappearance or worsening of dermatitis in the treated areas. A significant dose–response effect between the reactions and different formaldehyde concentrations was detected. The results demonstrate the allergenic potential of formaldehyde even in the low concentrations found in skincare products containing formaldehyde-releasing preservatives [11c]. Two cases of patients developing allergic contact dermatitis and severe nail damage mimicking psoriasis were described following the use of nail hardeners containing formaldehyde (concentration in the products not stated) [12A]. A case of a 59-year-old man was presented who developed a grade 3 systemic anaphylaxis, 6 hours after receiving a tattoo. Symptoms included swelling and redness of the tattooed arm, as well as cheek, lips and tongue. The tattoo color contained 63 mg/kg total formaldehyde (11 mg/kg free formaldehyde) as well as several metal impurities. A combined effect of formaldehyde and metals (nickel and manganese) was suggested as triggers for the systemic anaphylaxis [13A].

Hematologic

The effects of inhalatory formaldehyde (3 mg/m^3) were studied experimentally in Balb/c mice in vivo for 2 weeks and in mouse spleens in vitro. Formaldehyde was shown to lead to reactive oxygen species and glutathione depletion in spleen cells. In combination with benzene, formaldehyde also leads to reduction of some immune cells in peripheral blood, and to decreased body weight and serum antibody levels [14E]. In another study by the same group with similar experimental design (probably the same experiment but other endpoints reported), formaldehyde was found toxic to the mouse hematopoietic system, including bone marrow stem/progenitor cells, and also in this case benzene-induced effects were enhanced [15E]. The interaction between formaldehyde and benzene was stressed in both studies as important because of the common co-exposure of both agents, e.g., as air pollutants [14E,15E].

Respiratory

A forensic investigation of commercial hair treatment lotions in Brazil detected extreme formaldehyde concentrations of 9%–19% (w/w) in three products, while two products were below the maximum concentration of 0.2% for preservative purposes [16A]. The products are mainly used by women to straighten hair and pose the risk of formaldehyde concentrations in air above occupational limits [17R]. This illegal practice has been known for several years, and anecdotally even led to fatal formaldehyde intoxication by inhalation (see Ref. [18E] and *SEDA-36, 339)* but products still appear regularly on the market. For example, the rapid alert system for dangerous non-food products (RAPEX) of the European Commission lists 34 illegal hair straightening product withdrawn or recalled from the market since 2010 [19S]. Another respiratory exposure to formaldehyde may be the use of electronic cigarettes. While formaldehyde is not directly contained in the liquids used for the electronic cigarettes (e.g. [20E]), it may be formed when the electronic cigarette devices were set at extremely high voltages (*SEDA-38, 211)*. New experimental research confirmed this potential, specifically when so-called direct drip atomizers may be involved or electronic cigarette devices are used off-label at extreme temperature. The formaldehyde exposure may then reach levels of conventional cigarettes (20–50 μg/mg nicotine) [21E]. In vitro research on lung epithelial cells exposed to an atmosphere of formaldehyde at 0.1 and 0.5 ppm for 3 days combined with genome-wide transcriptional analysis showed that metabolism, lipid biosynthesis and lung-associated functions are affected by the lower exposure level and processes affecting proliferation and apoptosis dominate the higher exposure level [22E].

Nervous System

The neurotoxicity of formaldehyde was studied in a cohort of formaldehyde-exposed workers ($n = 35$) compared to controls ($n = 32$) and acetylcholinesterase (AChE) as biomarker was analyzed. Significant induction of AChE activity was observed in the exposed workers with significant positive correlation between exposure levels and AChE activity. Susceptibility depended on ADH3 polymorphism [23c]. In an experimental in vivo study, 16 male mice were exposed to formaldehyde by inhalation (3 mg/m^3) for 7 days. Formaldehyde exposure impaired spatial memory associated with hippocampal neuronal death and elicited intensive oxidative stress by reducing systemic glutathione levels, in particular, decreasing brain melatonin concentrations [24E].

GUANIDINES

Chlorhexidine [SED-15, 714; SEDA-31, 410; SEDA-32, 439; SEDA-33, 480; SEDA-34, 378; SEDA-36, 340; SEDA-37, 273; SEDA-38, 212]

Drug Formulations

Chlorhexidine is used extensively in oral hygiene but can cause staining of the teeth and oral mucosa and adversely affect taste but rarely causes pain *[SEDA-30, 278; SEDA-31, 416; SEDA-34, 378; SEDA-36, 340; SEDA-37, 273; SEDA-38, 212]*. In a review about mouthwash ingredients, chlorhexidine was pointed out as an efficacious compound with both antiplaque and antibacterial activities; however, considering the adverse effects (discolorations, taste disturbances), chlorhexidine was suggested as best indicated for acute/short-term use [25R].

A further review reached the same conclusion that chlorhexidine is not indicated for long-term use as agent for post toothbrushing rinsing [26R]. In a clinical trial of different mouthwashes ($n = 50$ per group), side effects of 0.03% chlorhexidine were itching of the oral mucosa for 1 or 2 days in 2 patients, and one patient noted bitter taste in the oral cavity. For 0.12% chlorhexidine rinse, 3 patients reported itching sensation of the oral mucosa [27c]. Another clinical trial of 0.2% chlorhexidine gluconate mouthwash compared to some other mouthwash formulations found staining in 40%, taste disturbance in 25% and burning sensation in 2% of the subjects ($n = 90$) in the chlorhexidine group [28c].

Skin

A review regarding the use of chlorhexidine for skin antisepsis in preterm infants was critical about this practice, because the US Food and Drug Administration has not approved its use for this population. Skin toxicity such as skin irritation, skin burns and contact dermatitis has been described. Furthermore, absorption through the skin may potentially lead to systemic toxicity. Studies into the safety of chlorhexidine in preterm infants were suggested [29R]. A recent case of chlorhexidine-associated transient hyperchloremia in an infant confirmed the potential for systemic toxicity of chlorhexidine following topical application. The 58-day-old infant had her whole body cleansed with 2% chlorhexidine for 2 weeks on alternative days because of episodes of sepsis with various microorganisms. At the end of the second week the patient was hyperchloremic (125 mEq/L; normal range 98–107 mEq/L). When chlorhexidine cleaning was stopped, chloride levels had normalized 48 hours later [30A].

Immunologic

A Cochrane systematic review regarding the prevention of catheter-related infections in newborn infants with central venous catheters identified a single study reporting contact dermatitis as adverse effect: infants who received chlorhexidine dressing/alcohol cleansing were significantly more likely to develop contact dermatitis compared to infants who received polyurethane dressing/povidone-iodine cleansing (RR 43.06, 95% CI 2.61–710.44) [31M]. In a review of the literature between 1971 and 2012, increased reporting about hypersensitivity reactions to chlorhexidine was determined with complications ranging from mild irritant contact dermatitis to life-threatening anaphylaxis [32R]. A general review about chlorhexidine hypersensitivity reactions in dentistry concluded that this side effect is not well known in dentistry and must be considered if unexplained hypersensitivity reactions occur [33r]. A retrospective study of 8497 patients patch tested with chlorhexidine during 2003–2013 at Copenhagen University Hospital found

82 patients (1.0%) as positive. Most of the patients used chlorhexidine in a healthcare setting but for some cosmetic products were responsible [34C]. A case of allergic contact dermatitis following perioperative chlorhexidine skin disinfection was described of a 40-year-old woman needing laparoscopy for endometriosis. As instructed, she bathed with commercial 4% chlorhexidine solution the day before and the morning of her procedure. Intraoperatively, chlorhexidine was applied to her abdomen and groin. Two days later, a pruritic rash appeared on her abdomen and left upper thigh. The rash resolved with systemic steroids [35A].

Polyhexamethylene Guanidine [SEDA-36, 341; SEDA-37, 273; SEDA-38, 213]

Polyhexamethylene guanidine (PHMG) has been used as an antiseptic, especially for the suppression of hospital infection in the Russian Federation and as a disinfectant for sterilization of household humidifiers in Korea [SEDA-36, 341; SEDA-37, 273; SEDA-38, 213]. For a recent review, see Kim [36R].

Respiratory

Further evidence was gathered on the association of the disinfectants PHMG with lung disease (see SEDA-36, 341 and SEDA-37, 273 for description of cases). In a nationwide study of humidifier disinfectant lung injury in South Korea, 1994–2001, 374 possible cases were identified, from which 62 individuals died. PHMG exposure circumstances found to be significant in shortening survival included age < 4 at onset, use of disinfectant for 7 days per week, airborne density of $>800 \mu g/m^3$, and daily exposure >11 hours in duration [37C]. A community-based case–control study (28 cases, 60 matched controls) found a statistically significant exposure–response relationship between PHMG used as humidifier disinfectant and lung injury [38c]. In vivo animal research in mice (28 day study, intratracheal instillation of PHMG at 1.5 mg/kg) detected a gradually increasing lung inflammation and increases in collagen deposition and TGF-β production, which are indicators of pulmonary fibrosis [39E]. Using DNA microarray to identify gene expression changes in rats treated for 4 and 10 weeks with PHMG by inhalation, altered expression of genes involved in urea cycle, inflammation and oxidative stress was detected [40E].

Polyhexamethylene Biguanidine [SEDA-36, 341; SEDA-37, 273; SEDA-38, 213]

Immunologic

A review of the literature between 2009 and 2015 on safety and efficacy of PHMB identified only few reports of adverse effects, which included two cases of transient local skin erythema [41M].

Benzalkonium Compounds [SED-15, 421; SEDA-32, 440; SEDA-33, 481; SEDA-34, 379; SEDA-36, 341; SEDA-37, 273; SEDA-38, 213]

Sensory Systems

It is believed that eye drops containing benzalkonium chloride as preservative may contribute to ocular surface disease [see also SEDA-36, 341; SEDA-37, 273; *SEDA-38, 213*], see also the recent review [42R]. In a meta-analysis of clinical trials comparing benzalkonium chloride-preserved (0.02%) tafluprost vs preservative-free tafluprost eye drops, the incidences of irritation/burning/stinging, foreign body sensation, tearing, itching, and dry eye sensation significantly diminished to one-third of those reported for preserved latanoprost at baseline [43C]. Corneal toxicity (corneas damaged and exhibiting degenerated microvilli) was detected during an in vivo experiment in rabbits receiving benzalkonium chloride-preserved (0.02%) latanoprost, but not in benzalkonium-free latanoprost eye drops [44E].

Immunologic

In a retrospective analysis of patch test data (1998–2010) from a hospital in MN, USA, the rate of allergic patch test results increased in the period from 5.5% to 8.8% [45R]. In a study from OH, USA, 29 (20%) of 142 subjects patch tested positive for benzalkonium chloride and/or benzethonium chloride. The authors stressed the potential coreaction to benzethonium chloride if sensitization to benzalkonium chloride occurred [46C]. In a multicenter study in Korea, 584 patients were patch tested for preservative allergens with a positive test rate of 12.1% for benzalkonium chloride [47C].

Triclosan [SEDA-34, 379; SEDA-36, 342; SEDA-37, 276]

The exposure of triclosan to children was reviewed by Ginsberg and Balk [48R].

Fertility

In a study of 471 men recruited from a male reproductive health clinic, urinary triclosan concentrations were found to be associated with reduced semen quality (motility, morphology, concentration and count). The association was limited to the lowest tertile of triclosan levels, and further research was judged as necessary to confirm the association [49C]. In vitro research on human endometrial stromal cells determined that triclosan arrested the cell cycle at G2/M phase enhancing cell migration. Triclosan also increased gene expression and protein levels of some decidualization markers, such as insulin growth factor binding protein 1 and prolactin, amplifying the effect of progesterone alone. The data were interpreted that triclosan may alter human endometrium physiology, affecting fertility and pregnancy outcome [50E].

Immunologic

An unusual case of immunological contact urticaria including connubial/consort contact urticaria was presented. A 44-year-old woman showed pruritic reddish wheals on her skin/mucosa immediately after contact with triclosan-containing soaps and topical products. The use of a triclosan-containing toothpaste caused immediate swelling of lips and tongue, leading to breathing difficulties. Kissing her husband, having used the same toothpaste, or friends, having used triclosan-containing face products, caused wheals on the face/lips. Chamber tests with the cosmetic products as well as triclosan (2%) confirmed severe urticarial reactions within 10–15 min [51A]. In an experimental study in mice, triclosan was identified as a non-sensitizing compound capable of inducing stimulation of the immune system reflected by increases in numbers (B-cells, T-cells, NK cells and dendritic cells) and frequency (dendritic cells) in the draining lymph nodes, increased splenic IgM response to sheep red blood cells and increased liver weights and platelet counts following 28 days of dermal exposure. The need for additional long-term studies of triclosan was pointed out [52E].

Respiratory

In a large national representative sample of 639 asthmatic patients in the United States, triclosan exposure (as confirmed by urinary analysis) was significantly associated with a more than 70% increased risk of reporting an asthma exacerbation in the last year [53A].

Reproductive System

Through meta-analysis of data in animal experiments (rats), a 0.09% reduction in thyroxine concentration per mg triclosan/kg bodyweight in fetal and young rats was estimated for a prenatal exposure, and a 0.31% reduction for postnatal exposure. Sufficient non-human evidence but inadequate human evidence was concluded for the association between triclosan exposure and thyroxine concentrations. Consequently, triclosan was judged as being "possibly toxic" to reproductive and developmental health [54M].

HALOGENS

Sodium Hypochlorite [SED-15, 3157; SEDA-28, 262; SEDA-34, 380; SEDA-36, 342; SEDA-37, 273; SEDA-38, 214]

Teeth

Sodium hypochlorite is used to irrigate root canals in dentistry and can cause many adverse reactions [SEDA-34, 380; SEDA-36, 342; SEDA-37, 273; SEDA-38, 214]. While the adverse reactions are commonly fully reversible, a case of lasting sequelae was described. A 55-year-old woman underwent an endodontic procedure on a maxillary molar, whose roots were protruding into the maxillary sinus. After sodium hypochlorite root canal irrigation (undisclosed dosage and concentration), the patient immediately developed intense facial pain, facial edema, and periorbital cellulitis. Emergency department evaluation diagnosed an intense inflammatory disease of the maxillary sinus, with destruction of its bony walls, accompanied by midface paresthesia due to infraorbital nerve injury. Despite endoscopic endonasal opening of the maxillary sinus for profuse irrigation, the patient maintained a complete loss of function of the maxillary sinus, anesthesia–paresthesia of the midface, and inferior dystonia of the eye with an enophthalmos 2 years after the procedure [55A].

IODOPHORS [SED-15, 1896; SEDA-31, 411; SEDA-32, 440; SEDA-33, 485; SEDA-34, 380; SEDA-36, 342; SEDA-37, 273; SEDA-38, 215]

Polyvinylpyrrolidone (Povidone) and Povidone-Iodine

Immunologic

16 patients who developed burning and stinging sensation and swelling of the eyelids after intravitreal injection were patch tested. Five of the patients reacted to povidone-iodine [56A]. A case of an anaphylactic reaction to povidone-iodine following the use of skin antiseptics was described. The 56-year-old patient developed pruritus on the knee, spreading to the whole body and associated with general malaise, directly following the use of the wound disinfectant (concentration not provided). He then developed generalized erythema and diffuse sweating. Tachycardia and a drop in systolic blood pressure prompted emergency treatment. Allergy test performed 6 months later showed a positive prick test result with polyvinylpyrrolidone [57A].

PHENOLIC COMPOUNDS [SED-15, 2800; SEDA-32, 441; SEDA-33, 485; SEDA-34, 381; SEDA-36, 343]

Methyl Salicylate

Metabolism

A case of a 14-year-old male was described, who used an entire 60-g tube of a rubefacient containing 15% methylsalicylate to facilitate masturbation. Symptoms when presented to the emergency department included shortness of breath, chest pain, lightheadedness, vomiting and malaise. An arterial blood gas measurement revealed a pH of 7.44, pCO_2 of 18 mmHg, and a bicarbonate level of 12 mEq/L. The salicylate concentration was 68 mg/dL. Bicarbonate infusion was started to treat salicylate poisoning. The patient was discharged after 4 days in stable condition. The authors pointed out that methylsalicylate can be absorbed through the skin, and specifically through the scrotal skin which has a 40-fold greater absorption of certain substances. The dangerous misuse of the methylsalicylate-containing product was apparently caused by internet-based discussion forums suggesting the product's potential for enhancement of sensation during male masturbation. As rubefacients are available over the counter with up to 30% of methylsalicylate, the authors suggested warnings to avoid inadvertent scrotal contamination when using these products [58A].

Cresol

Metabolism

A case of a 61-year-old man was reported who was in the habit of soaking his feet in cresol-soap antiseptic solutions. Due to an inadvertently long exposure (5–6 hours), the patient was lethargic and developed a brownish discoloration of his feet. The detected presence of dark urine progressively cleared over an 8-hour period. Urine levels of p-cresol, m-cresol and phenol were 2608, 5391 and 156 mg/g creatine, respectively. Skin contact with cresol can result in chemical burns, while chronic exposure can cause dark skin discoloration. Following dermal absorption, cresols undergo metabolism to dark-colored substances, which are rapidly eliminated in the urine. The patient was discharged without any sequelae [59A].

References

[1] European Commission. Comission regulation (EU) No 605/2014 of 5 June 2014 amending, for the purposes of introducing hazard and precautionary statements in the Croatian language and its adaptation to technical and scientific progress, Regulation (EC) No 1272/2008 of the European Parliament and of the Council on classification, labelling and packaging of substances and mixtures. Off J Eur Union. 2014;L167:36–49 [S].

[2] Rühl R. Formaldehyd - ein krebserzeugender Stoff mit Wirkschwelle (in German). Analyticapro. 2016;2016:46–7 [r].

[3] Hauksson I, Pontén A, Isaksson M, et al. Formaldehyde in cosmetics in patch tested dermatitis patients with and without contact allergy to formaldehyde. Contact Dermatitis. 2016;74(3):145–51 [C].

[4] Driscoll TR, Carey RN, Peters S, et al. The Australian work exposures study: prevalence of occupational exposure to formaldehyde. Ann Occup Hyg. 2016;60(1):132–8 [C].

[5] Rovira J, Roig N, Nadal M, et al. Human health risks of formaldehyde indoor levels: an issue of concern. J Environ Sci Health A Tox Hazard Subst Environ Eng. 2016;51(4):357–63 [R].

[6] IARC Working Group on the Evaluation of Carcinogenic Risks to Humans. Formaldehyde. IARC Monogr Eval Carcinog Risks Hum. 2012;100F:401–35 [S].

[7] Meyers AR, Pinkerton LE, Hein MJ. Cohort mortality study of garment industry workers exposed to formaldehyde: update and internal comparisons. Am J Ind Med. 2013;56(9):1027–39 [C].

[8] Zhao Y, Wei C, Wu Y, et al. Formaldehyde-induced paxillin-tyrosine phosphorylation and paxillin and P53 downexpression in Hela cells. Toxicol Mech Methods. 2016;26(2):75–81 [E].

[9] Rizzi M, Cravello B, Tonello S, et al. Formaldehyde solutions in simulated sweat increase human melanoma but not normal human keratinocyte cells proliferation. Toxicol In Vitro. 2016;37:106–12 [E].

[10] Prodi A, Rui F, Belloni Fortina A, et al. Sensitization to formaldehyde in northeastern Italy, 1996 to 2012. Dermatitis. 2016;27(1):21–5 [C].

[11] Hauksson I, Pontén A, Gruvberger B, et al. Skincare products containing low concentrations of formaldehyde detected by the chromotropic acid method cannot be safely used in formaldehyde-allergic patients. Br J Dermatol. 2016;174(2):371–9 [c].

[12] Mestach L, Goossens A. Allergic contact dermatitis and nail damage mimicking psoriasis caused by nail hardeners. Contact Dermatitis. 2016;74(2):112–4 [A].

[13] Jungmann S, Laux P, Bauer TT, et al. From the tattoo studio to the emergency room. Dtsch Arztebl Int. 2016;113(40):672–5 [A].

[14] Wen H, Yuan L, Wei C, et al. Effects of combined exposure to formaldehyde and benzene on immune cells in the blood and spleen in Balb/c mice. Environ Toxicol Pharmacol. 2016;45:265–73 [E].

[15] Wei C, Wen H, Yuan L, et al. Formaldehyde induces toxicity in mouse bone marrow and hematopoietic stem/progenitor cells and enhances benzene-induced adverse effects. Arch Toxicol. 2017;91:921–33 [E].

[16] Oiye EN, Ribeiro MF, Okumura LL, et al. Forensic investigation of formaldehyde in illicit products for hair treatment by DAD-HPLC: a case study. J Forensic Sci. 2016;61(4):1122–5 [A].

[17] Weathersby C, McMichael A. Brazilian keratin hair treatment: a review. J Cosmet Dermatol. 2013;12(2):144–8 [R].

[18] Monakhova YB, Kuballa T, Mildau G, et al. Formaldehyde in hair straightening products: rapid ^{1}H NMR determination and risk assessment. Int J Cosmet Sci. 2013;35(2):201–6 [E].

[19] European Commission. Rapid alert system for dangerous non-food products (RAPEX). Brussels, Belgium: European Commission; [accessed on 2017-01-13]. https://ec.europa.eu/consumers/consumers_safety/safety_products/rapex/alerts/main/?event=main.search; 2017 [S].

[20] Hahn J, Monakhova YB, Hengen J, et al. Electronic cigarettes: overview of chemical composition and exposure estimation. Tob Induc Dis. 2014;12(1):23 [E].

[21] Talih S, Balhas Z, Salman R, et al. "Direct dripping": a high-temperature, high-formaldehyde emission electronic cigarette use method. Nicotine Tob Res. 2016;18(4):453–9 [E].

[22] Gostner JM, Zeisler J, Alam MT, et al. Cellular reactions to long-term volatile organic compound (VOC) exposures. Sci Rep. 2016;6:37842 [E].

[23] Zendehdel R, Fazli Z, Mazinani M. Neurotoxicity effect of formaldehyde on occupational exposure and influence of individual susceptibility to some metabolism parameters. Environ Monit Assess. 2016;188(11):648 [c].

[24] Mei Y, Duan C, Li X, et al. Reduction of endogenous melatonin accelerates cognitive decline in mice in a simulated occupational formaldehyde exposure environment. Int J Environ Res Public Health. 2016;13(3):258 [E].

[25] Tartaglia GM, Kumar S, Fornari CD, et al. Mouthwashes in the 21st century: a narrative review about active molecules and effectiveness on the periodontal outcomes. Expert Opin Drug Deliv. (in press). http://dx.doi.org/10.1080/17425247.2017.1260118 [R].

[26] Prasad M, Patthi B, Singla A, et al. The clinical effectiveness of post-brushing rinsing in reducing plaque and gingivitis: a systematic review. J Clin Diagn Res. 2016;10(5):ZE01–7 [R].

[27] Mor-Reinoso C, Pascual A, Nart J, et al. Inhibition of de novo plaque growth by a new 0.03% chlorhexidine mouth rinse formulation applying a non-brushing model: a randomized, double blind clinical trial. Clin Oral Investig. 2016;20(7):1459–67 [c].

[28] Chhina S, Singh A, Menon I, et al. A randomized clinical study for comparative evaluation of Aloe vera and 0.2% chlorhexidine gluconate mouthwash efficacy on de-novo plaque formation. J Int Soc Prev Community Dent. 2016;6(3):251 [c].

[29] Chapman AK, Aucott SW, Milstone AM. Safety of chlorhexidine gluconate used for skin antisepsis in the preterm infant. J Perinatol. 2012;32(1):4–9 [R].

[30] Celik IH, Oguz SS, Dilmen U. Chlorhexidine-associated transient hyperchloremia in an infant. Pediatr Dermatol. 2014;31(1):110–1 [A].

[31] Lai NM, Taylor JE, Tan K, et al. Antimicrobial dressings for the prevention of catheter-related infections in newborn infants with central venous catheters. Cochrane Database Syst Rev. 2016;3(3), CD011082 [M].

[32] Silvestri DL, McEnery-Stonelake M. Chlorhexidine: uses and adverse reactions. Dermatitis. 2013;24(3):112–8 [R].

[33] Pemberton MN, Gibson J. Chlorhexidine and hypersensitivity reactions in dentistry. Br Dent J. 2012;213(11):547–50 [r].

[34] Opstrup MS, Johansen JD, Zachariae C, et al. Contact allergy to chlorhexidine in a tertiary dermatology clinic in Denmark. Contact Dermatitis. 2016;74(1):29–36 [C].

[35] McEnery-Stonelake M, Silvestri DL. Allergic contact dermatitis to chlorhexidine after oral sensitization. Dermatitis. 2013;24(2):92–3 [A].

[36] Kim HR, Hwang GW, Naganuma A, et al. Adverse health effects of humidifier disinfectants in Korea: lung toxicity of polyhexamethylene guanidine phosphate. J Toxicol Sci. 2016;41(6):711–7 [R].

[37] Paek D, Koh Y, Park DU, et al. Nationwide study of humidifier disinfectant lung injury in South Korea, 1994–2011. Incidence and dose-response relationships. Ann Am Thorac Soc. 2015;12(12):1813–21 [C].

[38] Park JH, Kim HJ, Kwon GY, et al. Humidifier disinfectants are a cause of lung injury among adults in South Korea: a community-based case-control study. PLoS One. 2016;11(3). e0151849 [c].

[39] Lee SJ, Park JH, Lee JY, et al. Establishment of a mouse model for pulmonary inflammation and fibrosis by intratracheal instillation of polyhexamethyleneguanidine phosphate. J Toxicol Pathol. 2016;29(2):95–102 [E].

[40] Kim MS, Jeong SW, Choi SJ, et al. Analysis of genomic responses in a rat lung model treated with a humidifier sterilizer containing polyhexamethyleneguanidine phosphate. Toxicol Lett. 2017;268:36–43 [E].

[41] Fjeld H, Lingaas E. Polyhexanide—safety and efficacy as an antiseptic. Tidsskr Nor Laegeforen. 2016;136(8):707–11 [M].

[42] Aguayo Bonniard A, Yeung JY, Chan CC, et al. Ocular surface toxicity from glaucoma topical medications and associated preservatives such as benzalkonium chloride (BAK). Expert Opin Drug Metab Toxicol. 2016;12(11):1279–89 [R].

[43] Uusitalo H, Egorov E, Kaarniranta K, et al. Benefits of switching from latanoprost to preservative-free tafluprost eye drops: a meta-analysis of two Phase IIIb clinical trials. Clin Ophthalmol. 2016;10:445–54 [C].

[44] Uematsu M, Mohamed YH, Onizuka N, et al. Acute corneal toxicity of latanoprost with different preservatives. Cutan Ocul Toxicol. 2015;9527:1–6 [E].

[45] Wentworth AB, Yiannias JA, Davis MDP, et al. Benzalkonium chloride: a known irritant and novel allergen. Dermatitis. 2016;27(1):14–20 [R].

[46] Dao H, Fricker C, Nedorost ST. Sensitization prevalence for benzalkonium chloride and benzethonium chloride. Dermatitis. 2012;23(4):162–6 [C].

[47] Lee SS, Hong DK, Jeong NJ, et al. Multicenter study of preservative sensitivity in patients with suspected cosmetic contact dermatitis in Korea. J Dermatol. 2012;39(8):677–81 [C].

[48] Ginsberg GL, Balk SJ. Consumer products as sources of chemical exposures to children. Curr Opin Pediatr. 2016;28(2):235–42 [R].

[49] Zhu W, Zhang H, Tong C, et al. Environmental exposure to triclosan and semen quality. Int J Environ Res Public Health. 2016;13(2):224 [C].

[50] Forte M, Mita L, Cobellis L, et al. Triclosan and bisphenol A affect decidualization of human endometrial stromal cells. Mol Cell Endocrinol. 2016;422:74–83 [E].

[51] Özkaya E, Kavlak BP. An unusual case of triclosan-induced immunological contact urticaria. Contact Dermatitis. 2013;68(2):121–3 [A].

[52] Anderson SE, Meade BJ, Long CM, et al. Investigations of immunotoxicity and allergic potential induced by topical application of triclosan in mice. J Immunotoxicol. 2016;13(2):165–72 [E].

[53] Savage JH, Johns CB, Hauser R, et al. Urinary triclosan levels and recent asthma exacerbations. Ann Allergy Asthma Immunol. 2014;112(2):179–81 [A].

[54] Johnson PI, Koustas E, Vesterinen HM, et al. Application of the navigation guide systematic review methodology to the evidence for developmental and reproductive toxicity of triclosan. Environ Int. 2016;92–93:716–28 [M].

[55] Costa T, Ferreira E, Antunes L, et al. Antral bony wall erosion, trigeminal nerve injury, and enophthalmos after root canal surgery. Allergy Rhinol (Providence). 2016;7(2):99–101 [A].

[56] Veramme J, de Zaeytijd J, Lambert J, et al. Contact dermatitis in patients undergoing serial intravitreal injections. Contact Dermatitis. 2016;74(1):18–21 [A].

[57] Castelain F, Girardin P, Moumane L, et al. Anaphylactic reaction to povidone in a skin antiseptic. Contact Dermatitis. 2016;74(1):55–6 [A].

[58] Thompson T, Toerne T, Erickson T. Salicylate toxicity from genital exposure to a methylsalicylate-containing rubefacient. West J Emerg Med. 2016;17(2):181–3 [A].

[59] Liu LR, Huang MY, Huang ST. Black urine after medicinal foot baths. BMJ Case Rep. 2013;2013:bcr2013200771 [A].

21

Beta-Lactams and Tetracyclines

Rebecca A. Buckler[*,1], *Michelle M. Peahota*[†], *Jason C. Gallagher*[‡]

*Jefferson Health—Methodist Hospital Division, Philadelphia, PA, United States
†Thomas Jefferson University Hospital, Philadelphia, PA, United States
‡Temple University, Philadelphia, PA, United States
1Corresponding author: rebecca.buckler@jefferson.edu

CARBAPENEMS

Ertapenem

Organs and Systems

NERVOUS SYSTEM

Central nervous system toxicity is a well-known side effect of the carbapenems, including ertapenem. A 71-year-old man with multiple comorbidities, including morbid obesity, heart failure, chronic kidney disease, diabetes, hypertension, and hyperlipidemia was prescribed a 6 week course of intravenous daptomycin 1000 mg and ertapenem 1000 mg daily for osteomyelitis of the foot. After the fourth week of therapy, the patient presented to a hospital with weight gain, shortness of breath, hallucinations, and suicidal ideations. During this presentation, his mental status was noted to be dramatically changed from his baseline. Physical exam and laboratory testing were concerning for volume overload, attributed to heart failure. The patient was formally evaluated by Psychiatry and was prescribed haloperidol, which did not have an effect on his symptoms. On hospital day 4, ertapenem was discontinued and the patient's mental status returned to baseline after 72 hours. Given the negative psychiatric work up and resolution of symptoms following ertapenem discontinuation, it was felt that the patient's neurologic symptoms were attributed to ertapenem therapy. The authors hope to increase awareness of severe ertapenem-induced neurologic side effects, especially in the elderly patient population with underlying renal impairment [1A].

A 54-year-old man with end-stage renal disease, requiring continuous peritoneal dialysis, was hospitalized for pyelonephritis. On admission a urine culture was obtained and he was empirically initiated on ceftriaxone 1000 mg twice daily. His admission labs were notable for a serum creatinine of 9.91 mg/dL. His urine culture grew an extended spectrum beta-lactamase (ESBL) producing *Escherichia coli*. Based on his cultures, ceftriaxone was discontinued and ertapenem 1000 mg daily was initiated. On the fifth day of ertapenem therapy, the patient developed generalized tonic colonic seizures. Physical exam and imaging did not reveal abnormal central nervous system pathology. The authors did not report any further clinical course for this patient. Recommendations are available for ertapenem dose adjustment in patients with renal impairment, which were not followed in this patient. The authors highlight the importance of following carbapenem renal dose adjustment recommendations in patients with end-stage renal diseases [2A].

Imipenem/Cilastatin

Organs and Systems

RESPIRATORY

Acute eosinophilic pneumonia (AEP) is characterized by respiratory failure associated with pulmonary infiltrates, pulmonary eosinophilia, and fever. Antimicrobial-induced AEP has been described, with daptomycin and minocycline most frequently reported. A 60-year-old female, admitted to a hospital for colon resection and Hartmann's colostomy secondary to a perforated sigmoid colon, received imipenem/cilastatin 500 mg IV every 6 hours for treatment of an ESBL *Klebsiella pneumoniae* peritonitis. One day following imipenem/cilastatin initiation, she developed fever and required mechanical ventilation for hypoxic respiratory failure. Imaging of her chest revealed diffuse ground glass opacities.

Her white cell count was $15.6 \times 10/dL$ without esosino-philia. On the fourteenth day of antimicrobial therapy she developed peripheral eosinophilia (8%) and continued to be febrile. An extensive infectious workup was negative and her fevers resolved 3 days after imipenem/cilastatin cessation. On hospital day 23, the patient developed a fever and leukocytosis. A bronchoalveolar lavage (BAL) was performed which revealed 3120 nucleated cells/mm^3 without eosinophil and culture revealed an ESBL pathogen. Imipenem/cilastatin was restarted for pneumonia, but the patient continued to have fevers and developed a peripheral esosinophillia (18%). A subsequent BAL revealed 780 nucleated cells/mm^3 with an evaluated eosinophil percentage of 15%. The patient was diagnosed with imipenem/cilastatin-induced AEP and received a course of intravenous steroids followed by an oral steroid taper. Following imipenem/cilastatin cessation and steroid treatment, the patient had rapid resolution of fever, leukocytosis, eosinophilia and improvement of her chest X-ray. The authors report, to their knowledge, the first case of imipenem/cilastatin-induced AEP [3A].

NERVOUS SYSTEM

A 70-year-old woman with no significant neurologic past medical history was hospitalized for Macrophage Activation Syndrome. Imipenem/cilastatin was initiated for sepsis and, on day 6 of treatment, she developed confusion and an irregular multifocal myoclonus in her face, trunk, arms, and legs. An EEG showed a photoparoxysmal response (bilateral synchronous spike-and-wave discharges in posterior and anterior regions) during intermittent photic stimulation. Imipenem/cilastatin was discontinued and replaced with meropenem. A subsequent EEG, performed 3 days later, showed that the photoparoxysmal response had resolved. The authors demonstrate that photoparoxysmal response can be utilized as a marker for temporary brain dysfunction due to imipenem/cilastatin use, although the value of monitoring this is mostly academic [4A].

A 65-year-old man with no history of psychiatric diseases was prescribed imipenem/cilastatin and required mechanical ventilation for septic shock secondary to a urinary tract infection. Upon admission his serum creatinine was 2.4 mg/dL and his estimated glomerular filtration rate (eGFR) was 25 mL/min/1.73 m^2. He was extubated, sedatives were discontinued, and he demonstrated clinical improvement on day 2 of hospitalization. On day 3 his imipenem/cilastatin dose was increased as an adjustment to his improving renal function at the time (serum creatinine 0.9 mg/dL (eGFR, 65 mL/min/1.73 m^2). On day 4 the patient was agitated and developed violent visual and auditory hallucinations. Physical exam and laboratory testing were performed but did not reveal any abnormalities. His antibiotic was switched to ceftriaxone on day 5 and his mood returned to baseline and his hallucinations stopped within 24 hours. Similar symptoms, agitation and hallucination, developed 2 months later when treated with another course imipenem/cilastatin for urinary tract infection. Imipenem/cilastatin was again discontinued and his hallucination resolved within 48 hours. The authors highlight the importance of recognizing psychiatric side effects of antimicrobial therapy and stopping the offending medication when the side effect is recognized [5A].

PENICILLINS

Amoxicillin

Organs and Systems

NERVOUS SYSTEM

A 30-year-old female with no known drug allergy history was hospitalized with fever, headache, nuchal rigidity, myalgia, and photophobia which developed 2 days after starting treatment with amoxicillin/clavulanate for genital infection. Evaluation of her cerebral spinal fluid (CSF) revealed mononuclear pleocytosis, normal glucose, and elevated protein. CSF cultures were negative. Her symptoms resolved after amoxicillin/clavulanate cessation and symptomatic management. She was hospitalized 3 months later with similar symptoms that developed 48 hours after initiating amoxicillin for urinary tract infection. Again, her CSF demonstrated mononuclear pleocytosis with lymphocytic predominance, normal glucose, and elevated protein. An extensive infectious work up was negative. Other than amoxicillin, the patient did not admit to taking any other prescription or over-the-counter medications. Given her presentation and time course of amoxicillin exposure, she was diagnosed with drug-induced aseptic meningitis. The authors performed a literature review and found only 12 published cases of amoxicillin-induced aseptic meningitis. Onset of symptoms appears to occur several hours to 7 days following amoxicillin exposure and resolve within 72 hours of amoxicillin discontinuation. Notably, in all cases, aseptic meningitis occurred when the patient was re-challenged with amoxicillin. This report adds to the small body of literature that describes amoxicillin-induced aseptic meningitis, underscoring the importance of a thorough medication history in patients with suspected meningitis [6A].

SKIN

Acute generalized exanthematous pustulosis, a severe immune-mediated cutaneous reaction, is most commonly attributed to antimicrobials. An 85-year-old woman admitted to a hospital for heart failure exacerbation was prescribed amoxicillin/clavulanate for *E. coli* urinary tract infection. She developed a severe cutaneous reaction, disseminated edema, erythema, and non-follicular aseptic pustules localized at her thoracic region and the bilateral inferior limbs. She was diagnosed with acute generalized exanthematous pustulosis. Her symptoms resolved following amoxicillin/clavulanate cessation and initiation of systemic corticoids [7A].

Penicillin

Organs and Systems

NERVOUS SYSTEM

Neurotoxicity associated with penicillin use is a rare adverse effect which has primarily been documented in patients with renal failure who receive intravenous, high-dose, continuous infusion penicillin. Covelli and colleagues describe the first case, to their knowledge, of penicillin-induced encephalopathy associated with intermittent intravenous penicillin given in conjunction with probenecid. A 65-year-old female with a history of HIV was admitted for worsening headache, confusion, and lethargy. A neurologic exam on admission was normal and demonstrated intact cranial nerve function. CSF analysis revealed mononuclear pleocytosis (100), with an elevated protein (457 mg/dL), and a slightly elevated glucose (88 mg/dL). She was initiated on empiric ceftriaxone and vancomycin for presumed meningitis, although viral meningitis was suspected. Three days following lumbar puncture, her CSF VDRL results returned positive and her antimicrobial regimen was changed to 2.4 million units of intramuscular benzathine penicillin-G for one dose, followed by 4 million units of intravenous penicillin-G every 4 hours along with probenecid 500 mg four times daily. During the second day of penicillin therapy, the patient developed new-onset myoclonic jerking movements of her upper extremities, a severe depression of consciousness, and acute renal insufficiency. The patient was disoriented to place and time, with generalized rigidity and hyperflexia, which were not noted in her initial neurologic exam. Magnetic resonance imaging (MRI) of her brain found no acute pathology. Her new-onset symptoms were attributed to penicillin toxicity and penicillin and probenecid were discontinued. During the next 3 days, her mental status returned to baseline, myoclonus and rigidity resolved, and her renal function improved. Penicillin, without concomitant probenecid, was restarted and the patient did not demonstrate further recurrence of neurologic symptoms. Penicillin neurotoxicity, a rare adverse effect, should be considered in patients receiving high doses of intravenous penicillin and develop encephalopathy accompanied by myoclonic movements [8A].

MUSCULOSKELETAL

A 7-year-old boy, prescribed intramuscular benzathine penicillin-G four times weekly for rheumatic heart disease (diagnosed at age 4), presented with fever, left hip pain, and elevated inflammatory markers (C-reactive protein = 154 mg/L, erythrocyte sedimentation rate = 130 mm/hour) 46 days after his most recent penicillin injection. A scheduled dose of 900 mg of intramuscular benzathine penicillin-G was administered upon admission to the hospital. Two days following the injection, MRI of the left hip revealed extensive inflammatory changes within the right gluteus maximus, consistent with myositis. Given the correspondence with the injection site, his myositis was attributed to intramuscular benzathine penicillin-G injection. The boy continued to have significant injection-site pain for 5 days following his most recent benzathine penicillin-G dose. Intramuscular penicillin is a cornerstone in the management and secondary prevention of rheumatic heart disease; however, the injections are painful which may decrease adherence. The authors encourage the exploration of improved long-acting penicillin delivery systems for the prevention and management of rheumatic heart disease [9A].

CEPHALOSPORINS

Cefditoren

Organs and Systems

CARDIOVASCULAR

Kounis syndrome presents with acute coronary symptoms including coronary spasm, acute myocardial infarction and stent thrombosis triggered by allergic or anaphylactic insults, and has been previously reported in patients receiving cephalosporins [10r]. A 64-year-old male with a history of aortic valve replacement was hospitalized with community-acquired pneumonia after failing 2 weeks of amoxicillin–clavulanate therapy. He was initiated on intravenous ceftriaxone and clarithromycin and transitioned to oral cefditoren pivoxil after 3 days of therapy. Six hours after the first dose of cefditoren the patient developed epigastric pain radiating to the retrosternal, neck and interscapular regions. Emergent coronary angiography showed diffuse multivessel vasospasm, and cardiac enzymes were elevated (creatine kinase 133 U/L, creatine kinase-MB 8 ng/mL and troponin I 1.32 ng/mL). Three months later the patient was inadvertently administered intravenous ampicillin during a colonoscopy and complained of intense epigastric pain and nausea which terminated 10 minutes after the infusion was stopped. The patient had a negative skin-prick-test against cefditoren, and other allergy workup was also negative. The authors claim that despite negative allergy testing, a diagnosis of Kounis syndrome could not be excluded, as cephalosporin-induced Kounis syndrome without associated allergic symptoms has previously been reported [11A].

Cefepime

Organs and Systems

NERVOUS SYSTEM

Cefepime labeling includes a warning that renally impaired patients have an increased risk of seizures, encephalopathy, and myoclonus. These adverse events have not been extensively reported in patients with normal renal function. A 76-year-old African American female with a past medical history of adrenal insufficiency, noninsulin-dependent diabetes mellitus, hypertension and hyperlipidemia was hospitalized with generalized weakness and cough with sputum production. Chest X-ray showed moderate to large bilateral pleural effusions and minimal patchy infiltrate at the right base. Her serum creatinine was 0.58 mg/dL, heart rate 108 beats/min and white blood cell count 11.1 mg/dL on admission. She was started on vancomycin and cefepime 2 g IV every 8 hours for sepsis with a pulmonary source. Blood cultures on presentation grew coagulase negative *Staphylococcus* species in two of four bottles. On hospital day 5 the patient was found to be lethargic, non-conversational and unable to perform basic commands. The patient was afebrile and all labs were within normal limits with the exception of sodium (133 mmol/L). A head CT and MRI both showed no acute intracranial abnormalities, repeat chest X-ray showed no new consolidation, and repeat blood and urine cultures were negative. A lumbar puncture was performed which was also not remarkable. Electroencephalography showed diffuse slowing with triphasic waves and no electrographic seizures. The patient was switched from cefepime to piperacillin–tazobactam and gradual improvement in orientation and response to commands was noted. Three days following the switch to piperacillin–tazobactam the patient was back to baseline neurologically. The patient completed a 9-day course of antibiotics and was discharged to a subacute nursing facility with no further episodes of confusion or lethargy. The authors claim neurologic adverse events should be considered in patients receiving cefepime with normal renal function [12A].

Ceftaroline

General Adverse Drug Reactions

A meta-analysis of 3 phase III clinical trials comparing ceftaroline and ceftriaxone for the treatment of community-acquired pneumonia was conducted. The analysis included 1916 patients receiving ceftaroline 600 mg IV every 12 hours or ceftriaxone 1–2 g IV every 24 hours for 5–7 days. Adverse events were consistent across the trials evaluated, with 460 patients (46.3%) receiving ceftaroline and 444 patients (44.5%) receiving ceftriaxone experiencing at least one adverse event. Although the type of adverse events were not specified in the analysis, 34 patients (3.4%) and 32 patients (3.2%) discontinued ceftaroline and ceftriaxone, respectively, due to an adverse events [13M].

Safety and tolerability of ceftaroline has not been extensively evaluated in pediatric patients. A multicenter, randomized, observer-blinded, active-controlled study evaluated the safety and effectiveness of ceftaroline compared to ceftriaxone plus vancomycin in 40 pediatric patients age 2 months to 17 years with complicated community-acquired pneumonia. Ceftaroline 15 mg/kg IV every 8 hours (or 600 mg if weight >40 kg) was administered to patients ≥6 months and 10 mg/kg IV every 8 hours for patients <6 months. All patients received intravenous therapy for at least 3 days, and patients could be switched to an oral antibiotic on day 4 if they met study criteria. Twelve patients (40%) receiving ceftaroline experienced at least one treatment-emergent adverse event compared to 8 patients (80%) receiving ceftriaxone and vancomycin. One patient receiving ceftaroline experienced an increase in aspartate aminotransferase (AST) and alanine aminotransferase (ALT). The patient's AST returned to baseline 6 days after discontinuation of ceftaroline and ALT returned to baseline 10 days after discontinuation. One additional patient receiving ceftaroline discontinued therapy due to rash and pruritis, which resolved 6 days after discontinuation of the medication. The most common adverse events in the ceftaroline group were anemia (3 patients), pruritis (3) and vomiting (2) [14c].

Another multicenter, randomized, observer-blinded, active-controlled study evaluated the safety and efficacy of ceftaroline vs comparator (vancomycin or cefazolin, plus optional aztreonam) in 159 pediatric patients age 2 months to 17 years with acute bacterial skin and skin structure infections. Patients <6 months received ceftaroline 8 mg/kg IV every 8 hours and patients ≥6 months received 12 mg/kg IV every 8 hours (patients >33 kg received 400 mg IV every 8 hours). The proportion of patients experiencing at least one treatment-emergent adverse event was similar between groups (48% in the ceftaroline group and 43% in the comparator group). The most common adverse events in the ceftaroline group included diarrhea (8%), rash (8%), vomiting (7%) and pruritis (1%), and 48% of these events were mild to moderate in intensity. The most common adverse events related to study drug in the ceftatoline group were eosinophilia (5%) and rash (5%). Two patients receiving ceftaroline experienced a severe adverse event believed to be related to the study drug. One patient developed a hypersensitivity reaction on day 9 of treatment, which resolved 3 days after discontinuation of ceftaroline. Another patient developed *Clostridium difficile* colitis after 3 days of ceftaroline and 17 days of oral clindamycin. No deaths occurred during the study. Four patients discontinued ceftaroline due to adverse events. The authors concluded ceftaroline is safe in pediatric patients for the treatment of acute bacterial skin and skin structure infections [15c].

Organs and Systems

HEMATOLOGIC

Neutropenia is a known and uncommon adverse effect of cephalosporins as a class. There have been several reports of hematologic adverse drug reactions in patients treated with extended durations and with off-label dosing intervals of ceftaroline [16A,17c,18A]. A retrospective chart review of 67 patients aimed to determine the rate of neutropenia in patients treated with courses of ceftaroline ≥ 7 consecutive days. All patients were monitored with a complete blood count weekly over the course of therapy. Seven (10%) patients developed incident neutropenia a median of 29 days after initiation of ceftaroline therapy. Five of these patients required discontinuation of ceftaroline therapy. Among patients developing neutropenia, 5 were considered severe (ANC <500 cells/mm^3) and 2 were considered mild (ANC 1000–1800 cells/mm^3). Febrile neutropenia occurred in 2 patients with severe neutropenia, with one patient developing bacteremia with *Enterobacter cloacae*. The Naranjo score indicated a probable association with ceftaroline therapy in all of these cases. Of the 7 cases of neutropenia, 3 patients received ceftaroline 600 mg IV every 8 hours, 2 received 600 mg IV every 12 hours, 1 received 400 mg IV every 8 hours and 1 received 400 mg IV every 12 hours. The overall rate of incident neutropenia was 10%–14% for patients receiving ≥ 2 weeks of ceftaroline therapy and 21% for patients receiving ≥ 3 weeks of ceftaroline therapy. In all cases neutropenia resolved with discontinuation of ceftaroline therapy. The authors found no association between age, gender, prior antibiotic allergies, renal dysfunction or ceftaroline dose and incident neutropenia [19c].

Another retrospective chart review of 74 adult patients sought to evaluate the incidence of hematologic toxicities and rash in patients receiving ceftaroline over a 1 year period. The overall incidence of adverse drug reactions was 20%, with 15 patients developing 23 adverse events. Hematologic events occurred in 9 patients (17 events) and rash occurred in 6 patients. Anemia (hemoglobin <8 g/dL) occurred in 7 patients, leukopenia (WBC <3000 cells/μL) in 2 patients, neutropenia (ANC<1500 cells/μL) in 3 patients, and thrombocytopenia (platelets $<75\,000$ cells/μL) in 5 patients. Based on the Naranjo scale, 17 of these events were classified as having a possible association with ceftaroline therapy and 6 were considered a probable association. These events generally occurred after an extended duration of therapy (median onset 9 days). These events were not more likely to occur in patients receiving every 8 hour dosing compared to every 12 hour dosing (25% vs 17%, $P=0.4$). Rates of adverse events were similar in patients receiving ceftaroline as monotherapy compared to combination therapy with another agent (30% vs 33%, $P=0.5$). Ceftaroline was discontinued due to an adverse event in 7 patients. Patients receiving prolonged therapy with ceftaroline should be monitored for hematologic toxicities [20r].

Drug Administration

DRUG DOSAGE REGIMENS

Off-label doses of ceftaroline have been used to treat severe infections, but the safety of these regimens was not evaluated in clinical trials. A summary of studies evaluating the use of ceftaroline as salvage monotherapy for persistent *methicillin-resistant Staphylococcus aureus* bacteremia described adverse effects for 3 large case series [21R]. The first case series included 10 patients treated with ceftaroline 600 mg IV every 8 hours, or the renal dose equivalent, for a median of 26 days. Four of these patients experienced adverse events including *C. difficile* infection, eosinophilia, and rash. Discontinuation of ceftaroline occurred in both patients who developed rash [22c]. Another study reviewed 31 patients receiving ceftaroline who were followed for a median of 30 days to evaluate adverse events. Twelve patients (40%) received ceftaroline 600 mg IV every 8 hours; the rest received lower doses. Three patients (10%) required discontinuation of ceftaroline treatment for adverse events including diarrhea, rash and eosinophilic pneumonia. Two cases of peripheral eosinophilia resolved without discontinuation of ceftaroline [23c]. The last study was a large retrospective, observational, multi-center study including 527 patients treated with ceftaroline ≥ 72 hours. Forty-five patients received off-label, high-dose ceftaroline, principally 600 mg IV every 8 hours. Adverse events occurred in 8% of patients and no patients required discontinuation of therapy. Higher rates of adverse events occurred in patients who were bacteremic and those receiving off-label doses of ceftaroline. The most common adverse events included renal failure, diarrhea, nausea, rash, hypokalemia and *C. difficile* infection. Long-term follow-up for adverse events was not included in the study [24c].

Interactions

DRUG–DRUG INTERACTIONS

Ceftaroline has previously been reported to cause an increased risk of bleeding in patients taking warfarin [25A]. A 65-year-old African American male taking warfarin for a history of deep venous thrombosis and pulmonary embolism developed an increased international normalized ratio (INR) after treatment with ceftaroline 400 mg IV every 12 hours for cellulitis of the right lower extremity. The patient had a therapeutic INR for 2 years prior to initiation of ceftaroline and reported no recent changes in medications or diet. His INR was therapeutic (2.35) after 5 days of ceftaroline therapy. After 12 days of therapy his INR was >18 and prothrombin time (PT) >200. The patient had no signs or symptoms of bleeding and his INR was reduced to therapeutic range 48 hours after stopping ceftaroline and administration of phytonadione. The authors applied the Drug Interaction Probability Scale (DIPS), which indicated a probable likelihood of interaction between warfarin and ceftaroline. The authors hypothesize the interaction could be due to the effect of ceftaroline on gastrointestinal flora. This patient also experienced an increase in serum creatinine, and the authors suggest the relationship between acute kidney injury and the potentiation of the effects of ceftaroline and warfarin need to be examined further [26A].

Ceftazidime

Organs and Systems

NERVOUS SYSTEM

A 64-year-old male with a history of chronic lymphocytic leukemia receiving rituximab and alemtuzumab was hospitalized for catheter-associated bacteremia due to multidrug-resistant *Pseudomonas aeruginosa*. The patient's catheter was removed and he received 14 days of ceftazidime therapy. Repeat blood cultures were negative and on discharge the patient received oral sulfamethoxazole–trimethoprim and cefpodoxime for prophylaxis. Two days later the patient returned to the hospital with neutropenic fever. Upon presentation the patient was hypotensive, had a temperature of 38.5°C and a white blood count of $0.1 \times 10^3/mm^3$. The patient was initiated on intravenous fluids, ceftazidime 2 g IV and linezolid 600 mg IV. Chest imaging showed atelectasis and pneumonia in the lower lungs. On admission IV colistin was started while blood cultures were pending. On hospital day 2 ceftazidime 8 g/day via continuous IV infusion was added. Final blood cultures revealed multidrug-resistant *P. aeruginosa* susceptible to colistin (MIC 2 µg/mL) and resistant to ceftazidime (MIC

48 µg/mL). On hospital day 4 the patient developed septic shock and was transferred to the intensive care unit, where ceftazidime was increased to 16 g/day continuous IV infusion. Serum drug monitoring revealed a ceftazidime serum concentration of 80 to 100 µg/mL. On hospital day 8 ceftazidime was further increased to 19.2 g/day. One day later the patient became agitated and a CT scan showed a small subarachnoid hemorrhage in the right anterior frontal lobe and possible subdural hemorrhage. Two days later the patient experienced new-onset facial jerking, and electroencephalography revealed nonconvulsive status epilepticus. The patient also demonstrated myoclonus with arm and thigh twitching bilaterally. The patient was then administered anticonvulsive medication and intubated for airway protection. Ceftazidime was discontinued on hospital day 12, as follow-up blood cultures were negative. By hospital day 15 there was no further seizure activity. However, blood cultures from hospital day 14 and 15 again turned positive. On hospital day 18 the family decided to withdraw care. The authors state that although causality could not be determined, providers should be aware of the possibility of neurotoxicity with high-dose continuous infusion ceftazidime [27A].

Ceftazidime/Avibactam

General Adverse Drug Reactions

A large phase 3 randomized controlled trial evaluated the efficacy and safety of ceftazidime/avibactam plus metronidazole and meropenem for complicated intra-abdominal infections. Five hundred twenty-nine patients received at least one dose of ceftazidime/avibactam plus metronidazole and 529 received meropenem. Adverse events occurred at similar frequencies, with 243 (45.9%) patients receiving ceftazidime/avibactam plus metronidazole experiencing at least one adverse event compared to 227 (42.9%) patients who received meropenem. The most common adverse events were gastrointestinal disorders. Serious adverse events leading to study drug discontinuation occurred in 14 (2.6%) patients in the ceftazidime/avibactam plus metronidazole group compared to 7 (1.3%) patients receiving meropenem. The authors suggest the safety profile of ceftazidime/avibactam plus metronidazole was comparable to ceftazidime, metronidazole or meropenem alone [28MC].

The safety of ceftazidime/avibactam has not been extensively evaluated in pediatric patients. A phase I, open-label, pharmacokinetic study was conducted in 32 patients <18 years old who were hospitalized with infections. Patients were divided into 4 cohorts based on age (cohort 1: ≥12 to <18 years, cohort 2: ≥6 to

<12 years, cohort 3: ≥2 to <6 years, and cohort 4: ≥3 months to <2 years). Patients were given a single intravenous dose of ceftazidime/avibactam over 2 hours. Safety data were collected through day 3 after the dose was administered. Six patients (18.8%) reported 9 different adverse events. No adverse events occurred in cohorts 1 and 2. Four patients in cohort 3 and 2 patients in cohort 4 experienced an adverse event, all of which were mild to moderate in intensity. Gastrointestinal disorders (constipation, diarrhea, vomiting) occurred in 3 (9.4%) patients. One patient in cohort 4 with no history of cardiovascular conditions developed sinus tachycardia that occurred 1 hour after the infusion of ceftazidime/ avibactam and was considered to be related to the study drug [29c].

Organs and Systems

HEMATOLOGIC

Hemolytic anemia was not reported as an adverse event in phase III trials for ceftazidime/avibactam. A 67-year-old female was admitted to the hospital from a skilled nursing facility for surgical debridement of a left upper quadrant abdominal wall abscess secondary to prior chest tube placement. The patient was placed on ceftazidime/avibactam after cultures grew carbapenemase producing *K. pneumoniae*. Within 72 hours of initiation of the antibiotic the patient became tachycardic and hypotensive, and her hemoglobin dropped from 9.4 to 6.8 g/dL. The patient also had an undetectable haptoglobin, elevated lactate dehydrogenase and reticulocyte count, and a positive Coombs test. Ceftazidime/ avibactam was discontinued, the patient was treated with blood transfusions and had improvement of clinical symptoms within 3 days. Ceftazidime/avibactam should be considered as a causative agent if a patient develops hemolytic anemia [30A].

Ceftolozane/Tazobactam

General Adverse Drug Reactions

A phase I study assessed the pharmacokinetics, safety and tolerability of ceftolozane/tazobactam in healthy Japanese (10 subjects), Chinese (9) and white (10) subjects age 20 to 50 years. Subjects received a single 1.5 g intravenous dose (1 g ceftolozane and 0.5 g tazobactam), followed by a single 3 g intravenous dose (2 g ceftolozane and 1 g tazobactam) after a 48 hour washout period. Follow-up occurred 7 days after the second dose. Two Chinese subjects treated with 1.5 g ceftolozane/tazobactam experienced study drug-related adverse events including acute skin reactions, headache, and discolored feces. One Chinese subject and one white subject treated with 3 g ceftolozane/tazobactam experienced study drug-related adverse events including decreased appetite, dizziness and dry mouth. All adverse events were mild, and no serious events, deaths, or lab abnormalities were reported [31c].

Ceftriaxone

General Adverse Drug Reactions

The microbiological efficacy and tolerability of a single dose of ceftriaxone 1 g was evaluated in men with gonococcal urethritis. Adverse events were observed in 7 (3.2%) of the 220 patients who returned for follow-up. Diarrhea occurred in 4 patients, all classified as grade 1. Three men experienced urticaria during ceftriaxone administration. One of these events was classified as grade 1 and two events were classified as grade 3 [32C].

Organs and Systems

CARDIOPULMONARY

Ceftriaxone is not recommended to be administered to neonates ≤28 days old within 48 hours of receiving calcium-containing solutions due to the potential for an interaction resulting in crystalline materials in the pulmonary or renal vasculature. A systematic review conducted in 2016 included 3 older studies that reported adverse cardiopulmonary events in neonates receiving ceftriaxone [33M]. A prospective case series reported respiratory events for 51 of 86 patients aged 11 to 59 days who received IM ceftriaxone as outpatients. The authors state it is unclear which of these events could be attributed to ceftriaxone, as these events were not described in detail [34c]. Another study provided an assessment of eight cardiopulmonary events in neonates receiving concurrent ceftriaxone and calcium-containing products that were filed with the FDA Adverse Event Reporting System. Five patients were <3 weeks old, 2 patients were 4–8 weeks old and one patient was of unknown age. The ceftriaxone dosage varied and was not consistently reported among cases. Seven of 8 patients with reported events died and had autopsy findings consistent with the presence of crystalline material or white precipitate in the lungs [35c]. In a prospective case series, 3 neonates ≤3 days old receiving ceftriaxone died of cardiopulmonary events including asphyxia and persistent pulmonary hypertension. In addition, 11 patients experienced thrombocytosis [36c]. The authors of the review acknowledge that these studies had significant methodological limitations, but further support that concurrent administration of intravenous ceftriaxone and calcium-containing solutions should be avoided in neonates due to the risk of cardiopulmonary adverse events.

TETRACYCLINES AND GLYCYCLINES

Doxycycline

Organs and Systems

ENDOCRINE

An 80-year-old man with a history of insulin-dependent diabetes was enrolled into a clinical study of the treatment of bullous pemphigoid with tetracyclines. He had a 40-year history of well-controlled diabetes. The patient was randomized to receive doxycycline 200 mg daily, which was blinded at the time. Shortly after initiating doxycycline, the man experienced dizziness and lethargy in the evenings, for which he managed by eating an extra meal. After 3 weeks, he was advised to monitor his blood glucose levels during these episodes. At 4 weeks, the patient had a hypoglycemic episode, became unarousable, received oral glucose, and recovered without need for hospitalization. Doxycycline was discontinued and the patient's diabetic control normalized shortly after doxycyline cessation. The authors conclude that this patient's hypoglycemic episodes were a rare adverse effect of doxycyline. The case did not report the patient's diabetic medication regimen, concomitant medications, nor did they further define what criteria they used to consider his diabetes to be controlled. Without this additional information, it is difficult to draw a strong conclusion regarding the association between doxycyline use and hypoglycemia [37A].

PANCREAS

Drug-induced acute pancreatitis is relatively uncommon, accounting for about only 2% of acute pancreatitis cases. Moy and colleagues report a case of a 51-year-old man with a history of dyslipidemia and no significant social or family history who was prescribed doxycycline 100 mg orally twice daily for presumed Lyme disease. He presented with 1 week of fatigue, malaise, and confusion. The only medication he reported taking at the time was doxycyline. A physical exam revealed abdominal tenderness and no rash or lymphadenopathy. His laboratory results were notable for a serum bicarbonate of 15 meq/L, blood urea nitrogen of 80 mg/dL, serum creatinine of 4.6 mg/dL, serum glucose of 1161 mg/dL, serum lipase of 5410 units/L and serum amalyase of 1304 units/L. His serum triglyceride and ionized calcium concentrations were within normal limits. An infectious workup, including Lyme disease, influenza, hepatitis, HIV, and routine bacteria, was negative. Imaging revealed a normal right upper quadrant ultrasound and mild stranding in the fat near the pancreatic head on abdominal computed tomography scan. The patient was admitted to the intensive care unit and required ventilation, vasopressor support, aggressive fluid resuscitation, and hemodialysis. Doxycycline was discontinued and, along with supportive efforts, the patient's metabolic abnormalities improved. He required a 5 day stay in the intensive care unit and clinically improved. Following a review of the published literature, the authors found no association between Lyme disease and acute pancreatitis; although they debate that the patient likely did not have Lyme disease. The authors identified two case reports of doxycyline-induced acute pancreatitis. Given that other possible etiologies for acute pancreatitis was ruled out; such as alcohol use, gallstones, hypercalcemia, hyperlipidemia, and infection, the authors conclude the patient likely developed acute pancreatitis secondary to doxycycline use [38A].

SKIN

Phototoxicity is a well-known adverse effect associated with tetracyclines. Nguyen and colleagues report three cases of phototoxicity in adolescents receiving doxycyline 100 mg twice daily for inflammatory acne. A 14-year-old boy, 16-year-old boy, and 16-year-old girl developed rash that initiated on the dorsal thenar space before spreading to other areas of sun-exposed skin. One case noted that the patient received doxycyline for 3 months prior to phototoxicity, but the time from doxycyline initiation to rash development was not described in the other two cases. They note that all three patients received high doses of doxycyline and had frequent sun exposure. They suggest that common behaviors, which remove sunscreen from the hand, caused the rash to originate on the dorsal thenar spaces. The authors suggest that the "heart sign" can serve as an early indicator of doxycyline-induced phototoxicity [39A].

Bayhan and colleagues performed a case series to document the cutaneous side effects of doxycycline in pediatric brucellosis patients in Turkey. They retrospectively analyzed 189 brucellosis patients aged 1 month to 18 years treated between February 2014 and January 2016. Patients aged 8 years and older received doxycycline 200 mg per day plus rifampicin 15–20 mg/kg/day (those aged less than 8 years received trimethoprim–sulfamethoxazole in place of doxycycline, and thus were excluded). Of the 189 patients, 141 (74.6%) received doxycycline and rifampicin. Seven (5%) patients developed doxycycline-related cutaneous effects. The most common reaction described was nail hyperpigmentation; tooth discoloration, tongue hyperpigmentation, and photosensitivity were also described [40c].

Minocycline

Organs and Systems

RESPIRATORY

Reports of minocycline-induced hyperpigmentation of cartilage have been described [41A]. A 61-year-old female presented with blue-black discoloration of her skin, ears, and nails that had progressed over the last 3 years. She had been diagnosed with *Mycobacterium abscessus* pulmonary infection 5 years ago and had been receiving antimicrobial therapy, including minocycline 100 mg twice daily. A physical exam revealed blue-black hyperpigmentation of the nail beds, gingiva, teeth, and back portion of the pinna. A bronchoscopy also revealed a visible color change of her trachea cartilage to blue-black. Six months after minocycline discontinuation, her hyperpigmentation improved. The authors did not indicate how long the patient had been receiving minocycline prior to presentation. To the author's knowledge, this is the first case report describing minocycline-induced hyperpigmentation of trachea cartilage [42A].

SENSORY SYSTEMS

A 20-year-old woman underwent lacrimal gland biopsy for ocular swelling. Upon incision of the periosteum, olive-green bone in the region of the enlarged lacrimal gland was discovered. The bone biopsy, sent for pathology, was negative for neoplasia or significant inflammation, and the lacrimal gland biopsy results were unremarkable. The woman's physician, unaware that she had been treated with minocycline (doses ranging 100 to 200 mg per day) from ages 14–16, had ordered a number of different tests to find the cause of the discoloration. The authors recommend including minocycline-induced pigmentation in the differential diagnosis of bone pigmentation to avoid unnecessary testing [43A].

SKIN

Hanada and colleagues performed a retrospective cohort study to assess the incidence of minocycline-induced cutaneous hyperpigmentation as well as risk factors for its development in patients with orthopedic infections. Patients who received minocycline for orthopedic infection and long-term suppression were included in the study. 156 of 291 (54%) patients developed hyperpigmentation after a mean follow-up of 4.8 years (range 0.3 13.2 years). The mean duration of therapy prior to hyperpigmentation was 1.5 years (range 0.1–9 years). The risk of minocycline-induced hyperpigmentation was not significantly increased with high doses, as noted in previously published acne studies. Risk factors for hyperpigmentation included vitamin D deficiency, presence of shoulder prosthesis, and concomitant use of medications also known to cause hyperpigmentation. This study revealed that minocycline-induced hyperpigmentation in patients with orthopedic infections occurs frequently, with over half of patients developing symptoms. Prescribers should consider the risk associated with chronic minocycline use when selecting antimicrobial suppression therapy in patients with orthopedic infections [44C].

IMMUNOLOGIC

Drug reaction with eosinophilia and systemic symptoms (DRESS) is commonly associated with rash, hematologic abnormalities, and internal organ involvement. Although symptoms may resolve soon after the initial insult, autoimmune effects can develop long after the acute episode has subsided. A 13-year-old female developed DRESS 3 weeks after initiating minocycline for acne. Forty eight hours after presentation, she developed liver failure requiring liver transplantation. The patient was receiving tacrolimus, mycophenolate mofetil, and prednisone for immunosuppression. Five months after presentation, she was found to be hyperglycemic, which appeared to be chronic given her hemoglobin A_{1c} value of 9.4%. An autoimmune pathogenesis was suspected given the detection of glutamic acid decarboxylase antibodies. Additionally, antithyroid peroxidase and antithryroglobulin antibodies were detected, indicating thyroid involvement. The patient was placed on insulin therapy for management of diabetes. This case details a severe minocycline-induced DRESS reaction with long-term autoimmune sequelae involving the endocrine system. Providers should be aware of these complications in order to perform relevant laboratory testing in a timely manner [45A].

Tigecycline

Organs and Systems

PANCREAS

Tigecycline has been reported to cause pancreatitis, although studies have drawn mixed conclusions. Tigecycline's broad spectrum of activity has led to use in some cystic fibrosis (CF) patients for the management of chronic bronchitis and CF exacerbation. Patients with CF are at increased risk for pancreatitis due to a variety of genetic mutations. Hemphill and colleagues describe a case of tigecycline-induced pancreatitis in a CF patient. A 22-year-old male, with a history of CF, presented with cough and increased sputum production, necessitating an admission for CF-related bronchitis. He was initiated on tobramycin, meropenem, and vancomycin, and then tigecycline was added when sputum cultures yielded *Mycobacterium chelonae*. Ten days following initiation of tigecycline, he developed abdominal pain exacerbated by oral intake. His exam was notable for severe epigastric tenderness, his labs revealed a lipase of 732 U/L with normal transaminases, and abdominal imagining suggested pancreatitis. At this time, tigecycline was discontinued and the patient was managed with supportive care. Several months following his initial episode of pancreatitis, the patient was restarted on tigecycline, in addition to amikacin and clarithromycin, for persistent growth of *M. chelonae* in his sputum. Three days following initiation of tigecycline, the patient developed epigastric tenderness and nausea. Further workup revealed elevated amylase and lipase, but imaging was declined by the patient. The patient's symptoms and laboratory values improved 5 days following tigecycline discontinuation. This case was limited by several gaps in its reported information: triglyceride and alcohol use was not reported and his medication list was not consistent between both presentations. Despite the limitations, tigecycline-induced pancreatitis has been described in the literature and this patient's presentation appears to be consistent with drug-induced pancreatitis. Clinicians should be mindful for the risk of tigecycline-induced pancreatitis, especially in patient populations who are predisposed to develop pancreatitis [46A].

References

[1] Veillette JJ, Van Epps P. Ertapenem-induced hallucinations and delirium in an elderly patient. Consult Pharm. 2016;31:207–14 [A].

[2] Yılmaz F, Uslu H, Ersoy F. Ertapenem associated with seizures in treatment of pyelonephritis in a chronic peritoneal dialysis patient. Ther Apher Dial. 2016;20:89–90 [A].

[3] Foong KS, Lee A, Pekez M, et al. Imipenem/cilastatin-induced acute eosinophilic pneumonia. BMJ Case Rep. 2016;Published online (27 January 2017). http://dx.doi.org/10.1136/bcr-2016-214804 [A].

[4] Gschwind M, Simonetta F, Vulliemoz S. Reversible encephalopathy with photoparoxysmal response during imipenem/cilastatin treatment. J Neurol Sci. 2016;360:23–4 [A].

[5] Ninan J, George GM. Imipenem-cilastatin-induced psychosis: a case report. J Med Case Reports. 2016;10:107 [A].

[6] Turk VE, Šimić I, Makar-Aušperger K, et al. Amoxicillin-induced aseptic meningitis: case report and review of published cases. Int J Clin Pharmacol Ther. 2016;54:716–8 [A].

[7] Gaibino N, Bigotte Vieira M, Filipe P, et al. Acute generalised exanthematous pustulosis due to amoxicillin-clavulanate. BMJ Case Rep. 2016;Published online (25 January 2017). http://dx.doi.org/10.1136/bcr-2015-213839 [A].

[8] Covelli V, Khanapara DB, Naut ER. Penicillin encephalopathy: an unlikely adversary in the treatment of neurosyphilis—case report and review of the literature. Conn Med. 2016;80:143–5 [A].

[9] Francis JR, Wyber R, Remenyi B, et al. Myositis complicating benzathine penicillin-G injection in a case of rheumatic heart disease. IDCases. 2016;4:6–7 [A].

[10] Kounis NG. Coronary hypersensitivity disorder: the Kounis syndrome. Clin Ther. 2013;35:563–71 [r].

[11] Saleh AA. Kounis syndrome: acute inferior myocardial infarction with atroventricular node block due to ceftriaxone: a first reported case. Ann Saudi Med. 2014;34:250–3 [A].

[12] Meillier A, Rahimian D. Cefepime-induced encephalopathy with normal renal function. Oxf Med Case Reports. 2016;2016:118–20 [A].

[13] Taboada M, Melnick D, Iaconis JP, et al. Ceftaroline fosamil versus ceftriaxone for the treatment of community-acquired pneumonia: individual patient data meta-analysis of randomized controlled trials. J Antimicrob Chemother. 2016;71:862–70 [M].

[14] Blumer JL, Ghonghadze T, Cannavino C, et al. A multicenter, randomized, observer-blinded, active-controlled study evaluating the safety and effectiveness of ceftaroline compared with ceftriaxone plus vancomycin in pediatric patients with complicated community-acquired bacterial pneumonia. Pediatr Infect Dis J. 2016;35:760–6 [c].

[15] Korczowski B, Antadze T, Giorgobiani M, et al. A multicenter, randomized, observer-blinded, active-controlled study to evaluate the safety and efficacy of ceftaroline versus comparator in pediatric patients with acute bacterial skin and skin structure infection. Pediatr Infect Dis J. 2016;35:e239–47 [c].

[16] Rimawi RH, Frenkel A, Cook PP. Ceftaroline—a cause for neutropenia. J Clin Pharm Ther. 2013;38:330–2 [A].

[17] Jain R, Chan JD, Rogers L, et al. High incidence of discontinuations due to adverse events in patients treated with ceftaroline. Pharmacotherapy. 2014;34:758–63 [c].

[18] Yam FK, Kwan BK. A case of profound neutropenia and agranulocytosis associated with off-label use of ceftaroline. Am J Health-Syst Pharm. 2014;71:1457–61 [A].

[19] Furtek KJ, Kubiak DW, Barra M, et al. High incidence of neutropenia in patients with prolonged ceftaroline exposure. J Antimicrob Chemother. 2016;71:2010–3 [c].

[20] Dellabella A, Roshdy D, Martin KE. High incidence of adverse effects with extended use of ceftaroline. Ann Pharmacother. 2016;50:1068–9 [r].

[21] Burnett YJ, Echevarria K, Traugott KA. Ceftaroline as salvage monotherapy for persistent MRSA bacteremia. Ann Pharmacother. 2016;50:1051–9 [R].

[22] Lin JC, Aung G, Thomas A, et al. The use of ceftaroline fosamil in methicillin-resistant Staphylococcus aureus endocarditis and deep-seated MRSA infections: a retrospective case series of 10 patients. J Infect Chemother. 2013;19:42–9 [c].

[23] Polenakovik HM, Pleiman CM. Ceftaroline for meticillin-resistant Staphylococcus aureus bacteraemia: case series and review of the literature. Int J Antimicrob Agents. 2013;42:450–5 [c].

[24] Casapao AM, Davis SL, Barr VO, et al. Large retrospective evaluation of the effectiveness and safety of ceftaroline fosamil therapy. Antimicrob Agents Chemother. 2014;58:2541–6 [c].

[25] Bohm NM, Crosby B. Hemarthrosis in a patient on warfarin receiving ceftaroline: a case report and brief review of cephalosporin interactions with warfarin. Ann Pharmacother. 2012;46:e19 [A].

[26] Farhat NM, Hutchinson LS, Peters M. Elevated international normalized ratio values in a patient receiving warfarin and ceftaroline. Am J Health-Syst Pharm. 2016;73:56–9 [A].

[27] Collins RD, Tverdek FP, Bruno JJ, et al. Probable nonconvulsive status epilepticus with the use of high-dose continuous infusion ceftazidime. J Pharm Pract. 2016;29:564–8 [A].

[28] Mazuski JE, Gasink LB, Armstrong J, et al. Efficacy and safety of ceftazidime-avibactam plus metronidazole versus meropenem in the treatment of complicated intra-abdominal infection: results from a randomized, controlled, double-blind, phase 3 program. Clin Infect Dis. 2016;62:1380–9 [MC].

[29] Bradley JS, Armstrong J, Arrieta A, et al. Phase I study assessing the pharmacokinetic profile, safety, and tolerability of a single dose of ceftazidime-avibactam in hospitalized pediatric patients. Antimicrob Agents Chemother. 2016;60:6252–9 [c].

[30] Leuthner KD, Buechler K, Yousif A, et al. Drug-induced hemolytic anemia from ceftazidime/avibactam, a new old antimicrobial: a case report. Open Forum Infect Dis. 2016;3:1809 [A].

[31] Aiudi A, Miller B, Krishna G, et al. Pharmacokinetics, safety, and tolerability of ceftolozane/tazobactam in healthy Japanese, Chinese, and white subjects. Fundam Clin Pharmacol. 2016;30:625–33 [c].

[32] Ito S, Yasuda M, Hatazaki K, et al. Microbiological efficacy and tolerability of a single-dose regimen of 1 g of ceftriaxone in men with gonococcal urethritis. J Antimicrob Chemother. 2016;71:2559–62 [C].

[33] Donnelly PC, Sutich RM, Easton R, et al. Ceftriaxone-associated biliary and cardiopulmonary adverse events in neonates: a systematic review of the literature. Paediatr Drugs. 2017;19:21–34 [M].

[34] McCarthy CA, Powell KR, Jaskiewicz JA, et al. Outpatient management of selected infants younger than two months of age evaluated for possible sepsis. Pediatr Infect Dis J. 1990;9:385–9 [c].

[35] Bradley JS, Wassel RT, Lee L, et al. Intravenous ceftriaxone and calcium in the neonate: assessing the risk for cardiopulmonary adverse events. Pediatrics. 2009;123:e609–13 [c].

[36] Van Reempts PJ, Van Overmeire B, Mahieu LM, et al. Clinical experience with ceftriaxone treatment in the neonate. Chemotherapy. 1995;41:316–22 [c].

[37] Tan CH, Shelley C, Harman KE. Doxycycline-induced hypoglycaemia. Clin Exp Dermatol. 2016;41:43–4 [A].

[38] Moy BT, Kapila N. Probable doxycycline-induced acute pancreatitis. Am J Health Syst Pharm. 2016;73:286–91 [A].

[39] Nguyen TA, Krakowski AC. The "heart sign": an early indicator of dose-dependent doxycycline-induced phototoxicity. Pediatr Dermatol. 2016;33:e69–71 [A].

[40] Bayhan GI, Akbayram S, Ozaydin Yavuz G, et al. Cutaneous side effects of doxycycline: a pediatric case series. Cutan Ocul Toxicol. 2017;36:140–4 [c].

[41] Stichman JR, West SG. Minocycline-induced cartilage hyperpigmentation mimicking alkaptonuria in a patient with knee pain. J Rheumatol. 2016;43:825 [A].

[42] Asakura T, Nukaga S, Namkoong H, et al. Blue-black trachea as a result of minocycline-induced hyperpigmentation. Am J Respir Crit Care Med. 2016;193:e5–6 [A].

[43] Ballard TNS, Briceño CA. Minocycline-induced orbital rim discoloration. J AAPOS. 2016;20:182–4 [A].

[44] Hanada Y, Berbari EF, Steckelberg JM. Minocycline-induced cutaneous hyperpigmentation in an orthopedic patient population. Open Forum Infect Dis. 2016;3:ofv107. http://dx.doi.org/10.1093/ofid/ofv107 [C].

[45] Lan J, Lahoti A, Lew DB. A severe case of minocycline-induced DRESS resulting in liver transplantation and autoimmune sequelae. Ann Allergy Asthma Immunol. 2016;116:367–8 [A].

[46] Hemphill MT, Jones KR. Tigecycline-induced acute pancreatitis in a cystic fibrosis patient: a case report and literature review. J Cyst Fibros. 2016;15:e9–e11 [A].

22

Miscellaneous Antibacterial Drugs

Emily C. Tucker[1], *Matthew B. Roberts*, *David L. Gordon*

Flinders Medical Centre, Adelaide, South Australia, Australia
[1]Corresponding author: emily.tucker@sa.gov.au

AMINOGLYCOSIDES [SED-15, 118; SEDA-32, 461; SEDA-33, 509; SEDA-34, 399; SEDA-35, 463; SEDA-36, 363; SEDA-37, 293; SEDA-38, 229]

A meta-analysis examining the effect of gender on incidence of aminoglycoside-associated nephrotoxicity (AAN) included 24 studies from 1978 to 2015 including 5980 patients in univariate analysis and 2994 in multivariate analysis. The incidence of AAN was the same for males and females (odds ratio for females vs males 1.00 (0.81, 1.22), $P=0.97$, $n=5980$). No correlation was found between gender and risk of AAN (odds ratio 0.99 (0.58, 1.69), $P=0.96$, $n=2994$). Specifically, female gender was not an independent risk factor as previously believed [1M].

Amikacin [SED-15, 111; SEDA-32, 461; SEDA-33, 510; SEDA-34, 400; SEDA-35, 463; SEDA-36, 363; SEDA-37, 294; SEDA-38, 229]

Drug Studies

A systematic review of amikacin use and the influence of therapeutic drug monitoring on outcome and adverse events. Several outcomes were assessed. There were limited studies comparing clinical cure based on amikacin dosing regimen. However, amikacin was compared to other aminoglycosides in 4 studies (479 participants); the meta-analysis found no difference in clinical cure for amikacin vs other aminoglycosides. With regards to nephrotoxicity, 4 studies were found comparing amikacin dosing regimens. There was a non-significant trend favouring daily dosing with risk ratio 1.42 (95% CI 0.68–2.93). Nine studies (872 patients) comparing amikacin to another aminoglycoside found amikacin to be

favourable with an odds ratio of 0.48 (95% CI 0.23–0.72) compared to other aminoglycosides with regards to nephrotoxicity. With regards to ototoxicity, twice daily amikacin demonstrated a non-significant trend to being favourable (risk ratio 0.77 (95% CI 0.28–2.11)) based on combined results of 3 papers. However, compared to other aminoglycosides, amikacin had a non-significant less favourable risk ratio of 1.15 (95% CI 0.76–1.176) for ototoxicity and 1.61 (95% CI 0.39–6.68) for vestibular toxicity. Ultimately, the review was unable to find substantial evidence to support a dosing regimen or therapeutic drug monitoring target due to a paucity of suitable trials [2M].

Sensory Systems

A retrospective analysis of amikacin use for pulmonary non-tuberculous mycobacteria found 45 patients treated between 2002 and 2012. Eight (18%) experienced ototoxicity, only 3 of these were long-term. Only 1 patient experience transient vestibulo-ototoxicity based on clinical symptoms. Those with ototoxicity were more likely to have shorter durations of therapy, possibly owing to the onset of the ototoxicity [3c].

Urinary Tract

A retrospective cross-sectional study examined the incidence of nephrotoxicity across 2 intensive care units with relatively high rates of amikacin use, given a high prevalence of carbapenemase-resistant organisms. 313 patients between 2011 and 2015 received amikacin. 20.7% developed any kind of acute kidney injury. These individuals were compared to those that did not receive amikacin. The use of other nephrotoxic antimicrobials was an independent risk factor, including vancomycin, polymyxin and amphotericin B. Cases were not controlled for diagnosis, severity of illness or comorbidity. This highlights that in centres that use amikacin empirically, care should be taken to minimise concurrent use of other nephrotoxic agents where possible [4c].

Gentamicin [SED-15, 1500; SEDA-32, 461; SEDA-33, 510; SEDA-34, 400; SEDA-35, 463; SEDA-36, 364; SEDA-37, 294, SEDA-38, 229]

Drug Studies

A small clinical trial investigated the effects of single daily dosing (5 mg/kg) vs lower (1.7 mg/kg) three times daily dosing on nephrotoxicity and ototoxicity. 80 patients were randomised to each group who had presented with sepsis-syndrome. There are multiple deficiencies in the reporting of this study including clarity around how patients were selected, the appropriateness of gentamicin therapy and baseline characteristics of included patients. Outcomes on renal function were worse in the three times daily dosing, however, comparisons based on mean creatinine only. It is difficult to draw robust conclusions on the incidence of adverse effects from this trial [5c].

Prevention of surgical site infection utilising topical gel containing gentamicin (16.8 mg/mL) and vancomycin (18.8 mg/mL) was evaluated after colorectal surgery in a phase 2a double-blind, randomised trial for safety and tolerability. Topical doses of 10, 20 and 30 mL were used in 24 patients with 6 controls receiving placebo gel. The maximum serum gentamicin level for any patient was 2.36 μg/mL at 6 hours. Mean dose given was 149 mg of gentamicin, achieving a mean C_{max} of 0.642 mcg/mL and mean AUC of 14.2 h/mL. There were no reports of local tissue reaction or delayed wound healing. No serious adverse events were attributed to study drug. There was no change in serum creatinine from baseline to day 5 or 14. Ototoxicity was not evaluated [6c].

Urinary Tract

A retrospective analysis of a hip arthroplasty cohort ($n = 136$) found a lower incidence in post-operative acute kidney injury (AKI) when dicloxacillin was given alone compared to dicloxacillin plus gentamicin for perioperative prophylaxis. AKI was defined according to KDIGO classification. Mean maximum post-operative creatinine was higher in the dicloxacillin/gentamicin group vs the dicloxacillin alone group (126 μmol/L vs 93 μmol/L, $P = 0.04$). Mean doses of dicloxacillin were higher in the dicloxacillin/gentamicin group than the dicloxacillin alone group (4.92 g vs 4.49 g, $P = 0.01$). The mean gentamicin dose was 174 mg. Factors such as hypovolemia, bleeding, other medications were not evaluated and are likely to have changed given a clinical recognition of high rates of AKI post-operatively prior to the exclusion of gentamicin from prophylaxis regimens [7c].

Paediatric

Single vs multiple daily dosing of gentamicin was evaluated in a Cochrane review for both efficacy and safety in neonates with suspected or proven sepsis. Eleven studies were included for analysis ($n = 574$). Once daily dosing was associated with higher attainment of desired peak levels (>5 μg/mL) and greater clearance when measuring trough levels (<2 μg/mL) than multiple daily dosing regimens. However, there was significant heterogeneity of the results owing to differences in gestational age, birthweight of included subjects as well as differences in day of gentamicin therapy on which samples were taken. There was no difference in ototoxicity. Vestibular toxicity could not be assessed. Nephrotoxicity differences were not noted with either regimen, however, this is difficult to assess in this age-group owing to rapid changes in glomerular filtration rate. 1 study found once-daily dosing had smaller increases in N-acetyl-beta-D-glucosaminidase suggesting less nephrotoxicity. Based on pharmacokinetic properties once daily dosing appears superior, however, this has not yet been correlated with clinical outcomes of either efficacy or safety based on this Cochrane review [8M].

Tobramycin [SED-15, 3437; SEDA-32, 463; SEDA-33, 513; SEDA-35, 464; SEDA-36, 365; SEDA-37, 295; SEDA-38, 229]

Respiratory

An open-label, exploratory non-interventional trial of 41 cystic fibrosis patients with chronic Pseudomonas aeruginosa infection given 28 days of inhaled tobramycin followed by inhaled colistin with on-going monthly alternation over 6 months was undertaken. 18 adverse events were reported in 11 patients. Of the adverse events thought related to treatment, 4 events were cough, 3 were bronchial obstruction, 3 were dysphonia, and 2 were oropharyngeal pain, all were related to tobramycin inhalation. 1 patient experienced bronchial obstruction and severe haemoptysis following tobramycin [9c].

Long-term safety of tobramycin dry powder inhalation for cystic fibrosis patients chronically infected with P. aeruginosa was investigated over 48 weeks with a single-arm, open-label, multi-centre study. 157 participants were given up to 6 cycles of tobramycin via dry powder inhalation for 1 month, followed by 1 month off therapy. 96 completed the study. 134 experienced some form of adverse event. Most common events were post-inhalational cough, infective pulmonary exacerbation of cystic fibrosis, nasopharyngitis and haemoptysis. Cough and infective exacerbation were the most common reason for discontinuation, occurring in 9 patients. Cough was reported with less frequency with successive treatment cycles and was not associated with bronchospasm. 2 patients experienced bronchospasm by spirometric criteria. 9 of 36 cases of haemoptysis were thought treatment related. 5 patients experienced reduction in audiometric testing, 3 of which were noted to have baseline abnormal hearing. 1 patient discontinued study drug due to hearing loss at cycle 3 [10c].

Tolerability of a dry powder inhalation of tobramycin for non-cystic fibrosis bronchiectasis was assessed in 8 patients. FEV1 was measured following dosing and 2 of 32 measurements demonstrated $a \geq 10\%$ drop in FEV1 at some point post-inhalation. 2 participants experienced mild cough between 1 and 7 hours after administration. Bad taste after inhalation was alleviated by routine mouth rinsing [11c].

Urinary Tract

Once daily vs twice daily intravenous tobramycin dosing for treatment of pulmonary exacerbations of cystic fibrosis was evaluated retrospectively in paediatric patients at a single center. 59 patients were analysed in the once daily group and 44 in the twice daily group. Mean daily dose was similar between both groups (11.3 ± 1.9 vs 11.7 ± 2.4 mg/kg, $P = 0.32$). There was no renal failure or impairment documented in either group [12c].

Fluoroquinolones [SEDA-15, 1396; SEDA-32, 464; SEDA-33, 514; SEDA-34, 401; SEDA-36, 464; SEDA-36, 365; SEDA-37, 295; SEDA-38, 231]

Sensory Systems

The association between systemic fluoroquinolone use and retinal detachment was investigated in a meta-analysis involving 10 studies from 7 publications. There was no significant association found between fluoroquinolone use and retinal detachment with a risk ratio of 1.47 (95% CI 0.95–2.27, $P = 0.09$). The analysis was overall limited by heterogeneity of included studies, differences in reporting of retinal detachment and discrepancies between stated date of fluoroquinolone use and date of retinal detachment [13R].

A large retrospective cohort study found no association between fluoroquinolone use and uveitis when compared to a cohort of patients prescribed beta-lactams. However, fluoroquinolone use was associated with a subsequent diagnosis of an inflammatory disorder associated with uveitis, suggesting that fluoroquinolones are commonly prescribed to individuals earlier in the course of a yet to be diagnosed inflammatory disorder that predisposes to uveitis, rather than fluoroquinolones being associated with uveitis [14c]. These results should be interpreted with caution given the data was extracted from a medical claims database, however, they do shed some light on a complex issue.

Musculoskeletal

A review examined fluoroquinolone-associated musculoskeletal events in children and although the association was supported by animal studies, human trials comparing musculoskeletal adverse events in children taking fluoroquinolones vs those taking other antibiotics were less convincing, suggesting short courses may be suitable in low risk patients without an appropriate alternative [15r]. Clinical trials to definitively disprove this association remain lacking.

Ciprofloxacin [SED-15, 783; SEDA-32, 465; SEDA-33, 514; SEDA-34, 402; SEDA-35, 465; SEDA-36, 365; SEDA-37, 295; SEDA-38, 231]

Drug–Drug Interactions

Administration of quinine with ciprofloxacin to healthy volunteers was associated with reduced plasma clearance, greater total area under the concentration-time curve, and maximum plasma concentration of quinine, suggesting a downwards dose adjustment of quinine may be required when used concurrently with ciprofloxacin to reduce potential adverse effects [16E].

Skin

A 92-year-old female experienced drug-induced bullous pemphigoid after taking 8 days of ciprofloxacin for treatment of a urinary tract infection. Dermatological diagnosis was confirmed on biopsy. Temporally, ciprofloxacin was the only implicated drug. She had no personal history of dermatological disorder. Lesions resolved with ciprofloxacin cessation and topical corticosteroids. The authors highlight this as the second reported case of drug-induced bullous pemphigoid due to ciprofloxacin and the importance of drug history in patients with bullous pemphigoid [17A].

A 71-year-old woman experienced biopsy-proven cutaneous and gastro-intestinal leukocytoclastic vasculitis following a course of oral ciprofloxacin for a gastro-intestinal infection. The authors highlight that while there are several reports of ciprofloxacin associated systemic vasculitis, this is the first case reported with gastrointestinal involvement [18A].

Musculoskeletal

Rhabdomyolysis occurred in a 62-year-old woman on long-term simvastatin (40 mg daily) when given oral ciprofloxacin for a urinary tract infection for 4 days. Symptoms of rhabdomyolysis began 4 days into ciprofloxacin therapy. Muscle biopsy was not performed. Ciprofloxacin is a known weak inhibitor of CYP3A4; this interaction was thought to have increased simvastatin levels and thus precipitated rhabdomyolysis. The authors wish to highlight a potentially serious and rarely recognized drug interaction [19A].

A 72-year-old male with type 2 diabetes and end stage renal disease was treated for lumbar discitis and osteomyelitis with intravenous vancomycin and oral ciprofloxacin. 4 days into antibiotic therapy he developed acute right hip pain with MRI demonstrating partial tearing of the right gluteus medius tendon insertion and at the origin of the right hamstring tendons. This tendinopathy was thought related to fluoroquinonolone use and abated with cessation of ciprofloxacin. This case highlights that the Achilles is not the only area involved in tendinopathy [20A].

A 70-year-old man with chronic renal failure on corticosteroids and rituximab for minimal change disease developed spontaneous, atraumatic bilateral Achilles tendon rupture following 4 days of ciprofloxacin [21A].

Pediatric

A sustained-exposure formulation of ciprofloxacin microparticulates in a poloxamer named OTO-201 was administered during tympanostomy tube placement in children and compared to placebo and sham treatment for the prevention of tympanostomy otorrhoea. Adverse events were similar among all groups including audiometric outcomes [22c].

The combined analysis of 2 phase 3 trials utilising OTO-201 ciprofloxacin in randomised, sham-controlled clinical trials were reported in 2 publications. OTO-201 was examined to determine impact on otorrhoea post tympanostomy tube placement in 6 month to 17-year-olds. Reported adverse events were mild to moderate and not reported in detail but included pyrexia, post-operative pain, nasopharyngitis, cough and upper respiratory tract infection. There was no reported difference in otoscopic examination, audiometric analyses or tympanometry [23c,24c].

Levofloxacin [SED-15, 2047; SEDA-32, 467; SEDA-33, 516; SEDA-34, 403; SEDA-35, 465; SEDA-36, 366; SEDA-37, 296; SEDA-38, 232]

A comparison of 5 days of 750 mg daily intravenous levofloxacin to 10 days of 500 mg daily intravenous then oral levofloxacin for community acquired pneumonia found no significant difference in adverse events between groups. The most common adverse events overall were injection site reactions and gastrointestinal side effects [25c].

Nervous System

57 participants were randomised 1:1 in a controlled pilot study comparing standard tuberculosis therapy with standard therapy plus levofloxacin (10 mg/kg/day)

in patients with tuberculous meningitis. Those in the levofloxacin group were more likely to experience seizures (5/29 vs 0/28, $P = 0.02$). Other adverse events were experienced with equal frequency between groups [26c].

A 56-year-old female experienced transient muscle paralysis causing bilateral wrist drop and sensory deficit in the distribution of the radial nerve during levofloxacin infusion (within 30 minutes) that resolved spontaneously within 8 hours of symptom onset. There were no other contributing factors identified; levofloxacin was considered the cause of a transient bilateral peripheral neuropathy. The authors highlight this as the first reported case of large fiber neuropathy potentially due to levofloxacin [27A].

A 6-year-old girl with multi-drug resistant pulmonary tuberculosis experienced intra-cranial hypertension considered secondary to levofloxacin. Following diagnosis with isolated pulmonary tuberculosis she was commenced on ethambutol, isoniazid, ethionamide, pyrazinamide, amikacin, terizidone and pyridoxine in addition to levofloxacin at a dose of 15–20 mg/kg/day. After 12 weeks of treatment she underwent ophthalmic assessment as part of a research study and was noted to have isolated papilloedema. There were no other neurological symptoms or findings. CT brain and MRI were normal. Lumbar puncture opening pressure was >50 cm H_2O. There was no suggestion of intra-cranial tuberculosis on cerebrospinal fluid analysis or imaging. The most likely cause was thought to be levofloxacin prompting its cessation and institution of diuretics with subsequent normalisation of intracranial pressure on serial lumbar puncture. Her other anti-tuberculosis therapy was continued. No other contributory factors to intra-cranial hypertension were found. This represents the first case of probable levofloxacin-associated intracranial hypertension described in association with tuberculosis. The proposed mechanism is hypothesised to involve fluoroquinolone interaction with neurotransmitters and their receptors but is yet to be specifically linked to intracranial hypertension [28A].

Gastrointestinal

Helicobacter pylori eradication with levofloxacin, amoxicillin and omeprazole was compared to therapy with clarithromycin and omeprazole in a randomised trial involved 120 participants. The levofloxacin group had documented adverse effects of rash and nausea in 3.4% each and diarrhoea in 1.7% [29c].

Levofloxacin sequential therapy was compared to levofloxacin containing-triple therapy for eradication of H. pylori. Adverse events were overall more common in the sequential therapy group, with more dizziness, headache, nausea, taste distortion, bloating and vomiting. However, discontinuations were similar between groups. The triple therapy group also received metronidazole which may have contributed to a difference in adverse outcomes [30c].

Urinary Tract

The efficacy of levofloxacin peri-operative prophylaxis for ultrasound guided transrectal prostate biopsy was evaluated in a randomised multicentre trial involving 801 patients. Standard prophylaxis with physician determined intravenous antibiotics for 3 days was compared to 3 days of oral 500 mg levofloxacin. Patients were excluded if pre-operative urinary culture was positive. There was no difference in infective complications. No adverse events were reported in either group [31c].

Skin

Levofloxacin was associated with the development of toxic epidermal necrolysis in a 74-year-old female with chronic hepatitis C [32A].

Musculoskeletal

A literature review of levofloxacin-associated tendinopathy describes the risk as highest with longer courses and higher doses. Additional risk factors include older age, concomitant corticosteroids, renal dysfunction and solid organ transplantation. Levofloxacin appears to have a higher risk of tendinopathy than other fluoroquinolones [33R].

Systemic

The addition of levofloxacin to doxycycline and rifampicin for treatment of acute and subacute brucellosis was compared to doxycycline and rifampicin in a randomised trial involving 107 participants. Adverse effects appeared more frequently in the levofloxacin group (20.4% vs 11.3% ($P=0.059$) in doxycycline/rifampicin). The most common adverse events were epigastric pain, nausea and vomiting and diarrhoea [34c].

Moxifloxacin [SED-15, 2392; SEDA-32, 468; SEDA-33, 518; SEDA-34, 404; SEDA-35, 466; SEDA-36, 367; SEDA-37, 297; SEDA-38, 233]

Cardiac

Single-dose administration of 400 mg of moxifloxacin orally was shown to increase heart rate in healthy subjects; however, the maximum mean increase in heart rate at any time point after administration was small at 2.4 beats per minute. This observation could influence the analysis of QT evaluation studies [35c].

Respiratory

A meta-analysis of 9 studies compared standard tuberculosis therapy to moxifloxacin containing regimes. Safety analysis found no significant difference in adverse events between standard therapy and moxifloxacin containing-regimes [36M]. Similarly, the safety profile of moxifloxacin-containing tuberculosis treatment regimens was evaluated as being safe, particularly in the setting of liver dysfunction from standard tuberculosis regimes [37R].

A multi-centre, prospective randomised trial comparing moxifloxacin to levofloxacin for multi-drug resistant tuberculosis found musculoskeletal adverse events were more common in the levofloxacin group, but other adverse events were similar between both groups. The levofloxacin group had 29 of 77 experience musculoskeletal adverse events vs 11 of 74 in the moxifloxacin group ($P=0.001$) [38C].

Nervous System

A usually healthy 40-year-old male experienced acute onset of anxiety, hallucinations and insomnia while being treated with oral moxifloxacin for acute bronchitis. He had no known psychiatric disorder and there was complete resolution of symptoms within 12 hours of drug discontinuation. The authors report this as the first described case of moxifloxacin associated visual and auditory hallucinations [39A].

Sensory Systems

Use of intracameral moxifloxacin for endophthalmitis prophylaxis following ophthalmic surgery was not associated with any side effects in a single surgeon case-series of 4601 eyes [40c]. A smaller case series involving 91 eyes found one patient to develop iritis in both operated eyes after cataract surgery [41c].

Gastrointestinal

A comparison of 1 vs 2-week moxifloxacin containing therapy for *H. pylori* eradication found no difference in rate of adverse events. Common adverse events in both groups were nausea, dyspepsia and diarrhoea [42c]. The use of moxifloxacin as part of a sequential therapy regime for *H. pylori* eradication was compared to a moxifloxacin free regime. The moxifloxacin group had overall lower numbers of adverse effects reported [43c]. However, the differences in treatment regimens mean this difference in reported adverse effects cannot be attributed to the presence or absence of moxifloxacin alone.

Skin

A 25-year-old female being treated for tuberculosis with moxifloxacin, rifampicin, isoniazid, ethambutol and pyrazinamide experienced a drug reaction with eosinophilia and systemic symptoms (DRESS) prompting cessation of anti-tuberculosis therapy. Following reintroduction of alternative therapy she then had addition of moxifloxacin which was associated with onset of acute generalised exanthematous pustulosis (AGEP) [44A].

Ofloxacin [SED-15, 2597; SEDA-34, 405; SEDA-35, 466; SEDA-36, 368; SEDA-37, 297]

Allergic

A 24-year-old woman experienced angioedema after ingestion of ofloxacin for management of gastroenteritis. The authors highlight the importance of recognizing this rare side effect [45A].

KETOLIDES [SED-15, 1976; SEDA-33, 521; SEDA-34, 407; SEDA-35, 469; SEDA-36, 370; SEDA-37, 299; SEDA-38, 235]

Solithromycin

A review of the literature regarding solithromycin in the treatment of community acquired bacterial pneumonia was undertaken. Overall solithromycin has been well tolerated in clinical trials with no reported deaths. Gastrointestinal side effects were most commonly reported (10% patients). Approximately 5%–10% of patients developed transient transaminase elevations [46R].

A global double-blind, randomised, active-controlled, non-inferiority trial was undertaken comparing solithromycin ($n = 426$) to moxifloxacin ($n = 434$) for the treatment of community acquired bacterial pneumonia. The drugs had a similar safety profile. Gastrointestinal adverse events (diarrhea 4%, nausea 4% and vomiting 2% of patients on solithromycin) and nervous system disorders (headache 4% and dizziness 2% of patients on solithromycin) were the most commonly reported adverse events [47C].

GLYCOPEPTIDES [SEDA-33, 519; SEDA-34, 405; SEDA-35, 466; SEDA-36, 368; SEDA-37, 298; SEDA-38, 234]

Dalbavancin [SEDA-37, 297; SEDA-38, 234]

Drug Studies

A review of the safety profile of dalbavancin for treatment of skin and skin structure infections was undertaken. A pooled analysis of data on adverse events and laboratory assessments from seven late stage randomised controlled trials was undertaken. 1178 patients receiving dalbavancin were compared to 1124 receiving comparator antimicrobials (including vancomycin, linezolid, cefazolin, nafcillin, and oxacillin). Overall adverse event rates were similar or lower for patients receiving dalbavancin (799/1778; 44.9%) compared with those receiving comparator antimicrobials (573/1224; 46.8%, $P = 0.012$). The most frequently reported treatment-related adverse effects for dalbavancin were nausea, diarrhoea and pruritus [48R].

A double-blind, pharmacist-unblinded, randomised trial comparing the safety and efficacy of a single intravenous infusion of 1500 mg of dalbavancin to a two-dose regime (1000 mg on day 1 and 500 mg on day 8) for acute bacterial skin infection was performed. Doses were modified if the patient's creatinine clearance was <30 mL/min. The number of patients with adverse events was similar with each regimen. Nausea, headache and vomiting were the most frequently reported adverse events [49C].

Teicoplanin [SED-15, 3305; SEDA-32, 469; SEDA-33, 519; SEDA-34, 405; SEDA-35, 467; SEDA-36, 368; SEDA-37, 298; SEDA-38, 235]

Drug Studies

A retrospective review of records of patients receiving teicoplanin at a single centre was conducted to assess whether the systemic inflammatory response syndrome (SIRS) score could predict the pharmacodynamics of teicoplanin in sepsis. 133 patients were enrolled, 83 with SIRS and 50 without. The teicoplanin trough concentration (measured on day 4 or 5) was significantly lower in SIRS than non-SIRS patients (15.7 ± 7.1 vs 20.1 ± 8.6 μg/mL; $P < 0.01$). There was no significant difference in the loading doses administered. The findings suggest that the pharmacokinetics of teicoplanin are altered in SIRS patients, who may require a higher dose of teicoplanin to achieve a target trough concentration when compared with non-SIRS patients [50c].

Immunologic

A case of probable teicoplanin-induced DRESS syndrome following a cross-reaction with vancomycin has been reported. A 79-year-old man received vancomycin for a hospital acquired MRSA bacteraemia. After approximately 28 days of therapy the patient developed fever, extensive skin rash and eyelid oedema followed by a mild eosinophilia. A probable vancomycin-induced DRESS syndrome was suspected and as such vancomycin therapy was discontinued and teicoplanin therapy initiated. Six days later the patient developed diffuse pneumonic infiltrates. This initially improved with oral prednisolone. On cessation of prednisolone, on day 12 of teicoplanin therapy, the patient developed fever followed by recurrence of the rash and eosinophilia. A probable teicoplanin-induced DRESS syndrome was suspected. Teicoplanin was withdrawn after 16 days of therapy and the fever and rash resolved. Given the temporal relationship between administration of the antimicrobials and onset of symptoms it was thought that this most likely represented cross-reactivity between vancomycin and teicoplanin [51A].

Hematologic

A case of teicoplanin-induced pancytopenia has been reported. A 44-year-old man inadvertently received high-dose teicoplanin (400 mg twice daily) for 4 days. The patient developed pancytopenia on the fourth day of therapy which resolved after dose reduction of teicoplanin to 200 mg daily. The authors commented that teicoplanin-induced pancytopenia had not previously been demonstrated [52A].

Vancomycin [SED-15, 3593; SEDA-32, 470; SEDA-33, 520; SEDA-34, 406; SEDA-35, 467; SEDA-36, 369; SEDA-37, 298; SEDA-38, 235]

Urinary Tract

A meta-analysis of 9 clinical studies of the safety and efficacy of high (≥15 mg/L) vs low (≤15 mg/L) vancomycin trough levels in the treatment of patients with infections caused by MRSA found the variable of high vancomycin trough level was an independent factor for nephrotoxicity in MRSA infections (OR 2.14 95% CI 1.42–3.23; $P < 0.001$) [53M].

In a cohort of 94 critically ill paediatric oncology patients receiving intravenous vancomycin, a serum trough level of ≥20 μg/mL was an independent risk factor for toxicity ($P < 0.001$). Vancomycin-related nephrotoxicity was a predictor of death for up to 28 days ($P = 0.03$) [54c].

A meta-analysis was conducted to compare the efficacy and safety of continuous infusion of vancomycin (CIV) with intermittent infusion of vancomycin (IIV). Eleven studies were included. Patients receiving CIV had significantly lower incidence of nephrotoxicity compared with patients receiving IIV [risk ratio (RR) = 0.61, 95% confidence interval (CI) 0.47–0.80; $P < 0.001$] [55M].

3 cases of patients who received intravenous vancomycin and developed very high trough levels (>40 μg/mL) with associated severe acute kidney injury have been reported. In all cases the renal function improved with cessation of the vancomycin [56A].

Skin

A case of local skin necrosis was reported after extravasation of vancomycin administered via a peripheral cannula. An 84-year-old woman received intravenous vancomycin as treatment for hospital acquired pneumonia. Extravasation of vancomycin occurred during peripheral administration with severe painful blistering occurring at the site on the patient's wrist. The skin at the site became necrotic with ulcerated tissue under a black eschar. Venous duplex imaging showed evidence of thrombophlebitis. The wound healed slowly with topical management and surgical debridement was not required. Vancomycin is acidic (pH 2.5–4.0) and hyperosmolar (328 mOsm/L) and must be administered via a secure intravenous access or there is a risk of inadvertent extravasation and potential damage to local structures [57A].

Immunologic

A systematic case review of vancomycin hypersensitivity reactions (HSR) from 1982 to 2015 was undertaken. 57 articles were included describing 71 cases of vancomycin HSR; 7 immediate (anaphylaxis) and 64 nonimmediate. Non-immediate HSR included linear IgA bullous dermatosis (LABD, $n = 34$), drug rash eosinophilia and systemic symptoms (DRESS) syndrome ($n = 16$), acute interstitial nephritis (AIN, $n = 8$), and Stevens–Johnson syndrome/toxic epidermal necrolysis (SJS/TEN, $n = 6$). 16% of cases died with 6% being attributed to the HSR [58R].

A 73-year-old man with culture negative infective endocarditis developed fever, widespread maculopapular rash and severe progressive renal impairment. DRESS was considered the most likely diagnosis based on skin biopsy results and the clinical picture. Temporally, vancomycin was the most likely precipitant. The patient recovered following haemodialysis and systemic steroid therapy. The authors noted that this was the first case report of vancomycin-mediated DRESS leading to dialysis dependent renal failure in the literature [59A].

A case of vancomycin-induced immune thrombocytopenia has been reported. A 72-year-old woman received intravenous vancomycin for MRSA pneumonia. After 10 days of treatment she developed sudden, profound thrombocytopenia associated with a life-threatening gastrointestinal bleed. Vancomycin-dependant antiplatelet antibodies were detected by flow cytometry. The platelet count improved with drug cessation. The case highlighted the value of using flow cytometry to allow a definitive diagnosis of vancomycin-induced immune thrombocytopenia [60A].

A case of eosinophilic peritonitis has been reported in a 37-year-old female peritoneal dialysis patient. The patient received intra-peritoneal vancomycin for bacterial peritonitis with initial clinical improvement over the first 48 hours followed by rapid deterioration and development of eosinophilic peritonitis. Alternative causes were excluded and the patient quickly improved with cessation of the vancomycin. The authors noted that only one previous case of vancomycin-induced eosinophilic peritonitis had been reported in the literature [61A].

LINCOSAMIDES [SED-15, 2063; SEDA-33, 522; SEDA-34, 407; SEDA-35, 469; SEDA-36, 371; SEDA-37, 299; SEDA-38, 236]

Clindamycin [SEDA-38, 235]

Immunologic

A case of presumed anaphylaxis secondary to clindamycin has been reported. A 46-year-old woman received a 900 mg IV dose of clindamycin for a periodontal abscess. This was the only medication the patient received. 3 minutes post administration the patient became confused, dyspnoeic, tachycardic and hypotensive with decreased breath sounds bilaterally. There was no urticaria or other skin manifestations. She responded to a combination of methylprednisolone, epinephrine, diphenhydramine and albuterol. Confirmatory skin testing was not performed due to a lack of a standardised protocol. The authors noted that this was only the third documented case of clindamycin-induced anaphylaxis in the literature and emphasized the importance of being aware of the potential for drug-induced anaphylaxis with any medication [62A].

Liver

A case of presumed clindamycin-induced hepatotoxicity has been reported in a 62-year-old African American female who was prescribed clindamycin for a presumed dental infection. She had a background history of alcohol use. After 5 days of clindamycin treatment she was admitted to hospital with persisting gum pain, diagnosed as alveolar osteitis. On initial evaluation, she had an elevated alanine aminotransferase (ALT) at 423 IU/L, aspartate aminotransferase (AST) at 338 IU/L, gamma-glutamyl transpeptidase (GGT) at 179 IU/L and alkaline phosphatase (ALP) at 321 IU/L. INR and total bilirubin were within normal limits. She was initially managed for suspected acetaminophen toxicity with acetylcysteine. Her AST and ALT continued to rise and by day 9 of clindamycin therapy had peaked at 1812 IU/L and 1927 IU/L respectively. Clindamycin was ceased and the transaminases slowly improved. Screens for alternative causes of liver disease were unremarkable. A liver biopsy was not performed. The authors identified only 8 prior case reports of clindamycin-induced hepatotoxicity, the first reported in 1977 [63A].

Urinary Tract

A retrospective review of clindamycin-induced acute kidney injury (AKI) was undertaken in China between January 2009 and December 2013. 230 patients were identified with clindamycin-induced AKI in that period, 57 had a renal biopsy and of those 50 patients were selected to be included in the study. It was unclear why the 7 patients were excluded. Patients had no background history of renal disease, fulfilled the AKI network criteria of AKI within 72 hours of clindamycin infusion and had no obvious alternative causes of AKI. The most common doses of clindamycin were 0.75–1.25 g IV twice daily. The average onset of AKI was 1.5 days (range 0.7 hours to 3.5 days) after the first dose. Urine eosinophils were elevated in 93% of cases and blood eosinophils in 86%. In all cases, acute tubular necrosis (ATN) was seen and in 82% of patients there was renal tubulitis on renal biopsy. No immune complex deposition was seen. 72% of patients were diagnosed with acute interstitial nephritis and 20% with ATN. The average peak serum creatinine was $903.7 \pm 170.3 \, \mu mol/L$ and GFR was 6.43 mL/min on day 7. All patients required renal replacement therapy and 43% received oral prednisolone. On average, after approximately 14 days of treatment, 66% of patients had returned to normal serum creatinine levels and the other 34% had improved. The pathogenesis of the AKI was unclear [64c].

Gastrointestinal

A case of probable clindamycin-induced necrotising oesophagitis has been reported. A 43-year-old Caucasian woman was admitted with chest pain and dysphagia for solids and liquids. The symptoms began 24 hours after taking 300 mg orally of clindamycin as prophylaxis prior to a dental procedure. The patient had an unremarkable past medical history. She had been prescribed no other medications. Oesophagogastroduodenoscopy showed 8 cm of severe necrosis in the distal oesophagus. Clindamycin was discontinued and the patient was treated with a proton pump inhibitor. Follow-up endoscopy at 1 month showed mild gastro-oesophageal reflux disease only and the patient was free of symptoms. The authors note that clindamycin-induced necrotizing esophagitis has not been previously described [65A].

MACROLIDES [SED-15, 2183; SEDA-33, 522; SEDA-34, 408; SEDA-35, 469; SEDA-36, 371; SEDA-37, 299; SEDA-38, 236]

Azithromycin [SED-15, 389; SEDA-33, 522; SEDA-34, 408; SEDA-35, 469; SEDA-36, 371; SEDA-37, 299; SEDA-38, 236]

Cardiovascular

A retrospective cohort analysis was undertaken between November 2009 and January 2012 to evaluate the incidence of sustained ventricular tachycardia (VT) in patients with a prolonged QT interval (>450 ms) who were subsequently prescribed azithromycin therapy. 103 patients were included in the study with a median longest QTc of 485 ms. Only one patient (0.97%) developed sustained VT. The patient had multiple other cardiac co-morbidities and had one episode of self-terminating torsades de pointes and had a documented prolonged QT interval, prior to administration of azithromycin. 24 hours later he had recurrent VT followed by an asystolic cardiac arrest and died [66c].

Immunologic

A probable case of azithromycin-induced fixed drug eruption (FDE) has been described. A 35-year-old Indian man was prescribed azithromycin 500 mg for acne vulgaris. He was not receiving any concomitant drugs. The day after taking a single tablet he developed a bullous lesion over his left ankle, erosions over his genitalia and several non-bullous, pigmented lesions on his lower limbs. The year prior he had developed similar lesions over his genitalia and left ankle following use of azithromycin for a throat infection. A diagnosis of FDE was made based on the clinical picture. Azithromycin was ceased and he was treated with oral steroids and antihistamines. On follow-up, he had persisting post-inflammatory hyperpigmentation. Bullous FDE due to azithromycin has not been previously reported and the authors highlight the importance of prescribers being aware of this potential adverse event [67A].

A case of Stevens–Johnson syndrome (SJS) secondary to azithromycin has been described. A 58-year-old man presented with a 7-day history of painful, itchy rash, fever, malaise and oral discomfort and swelling which started and progressed a day after completing 5 days of oral azithromycin. The clinical findings were consistent with SJS. The azithromycin had been prescribed for symptoms that were later attributed to the patient's usual seasonal allergies. The authors highlight the importance of awareness of the potential for azithromycin to cause SJS and they strongly encouraged discretion when prescribing antimicrobials [68A].

Clarithromycin [SED-15, 799; SEDA-33, 523; SEDA-34, 408; SEDA-35, 470; SEDA-36, 372; SEDA-37, 299; SEDA-38, 237]

Cardiovascular

A population-based study was undertaken to compare the cardiovascular outcomes in adults receiving either oral clarithromycin ($n=108\,988$) or amoxicillin ($n=217\,793$) during 2005 to 2009 in Hong Kong. The propensity score adjusted rate ratio of myocardial infarction 14 days after antibiotic treatment was commenced was 3.66 (95% confidence interval 2.82–4.76) when comparing clarithromycin (132 events, rate 44.4

per 1000 person-years) with amoxicillin (149 events, 19.2 per 1000 person-years). There was no long-term increased risk observed. In the self-controlled case analysis, there was an association between current use of H. pylori eradication treatment containing clarithromycin and cardiovascular events. This returned to baseline after treatment had finished. The adjusted absolute risk difference for current use of clarithromycin vs amoxicillin was 1.90 excess myocardial infarction events (95% confidence interval 1.30–2.68) per 1000 patients [69MC].

Nervous System

A self-controlled case series study was conducted to examine the association between H. pylori therapy containing clarithromycin and acute neuropsychiatric events. It found evidence of a short-term increased risk of neuropsychiatric events associated with H. pylori therapy containing clarithromycin. 66 559 patients were included in the study. A total of 1824 patients had their first recorded neuropsychiatric event during the study period. An increased incidence rate ratio (IRR) of 4.12 (35 composite neuropsychiatric events during 72 person-years; 95% CI, 2.94–5.76) was identified during current use of clarithromycin compared with baseline (1766 events during 16 665 person-years) [70MC].

A case of akathisia following clarithromycin ingestion has been described. 77-year-old woman presented with a 4-day history of rapidly progressive generalized restless leg movements. She was prescribed clarithromycin 500 mg twice a day, prednisolone 30 mg orally daily and carbocisteine 375 mg three times daily for a respiratory tract infection. She had prior exposure to prednisolone and carbocisteine but never a macrolide antibiotic. A day after commencing treatment she developed agitation and restlessness affecting her head and all four limbs. On distraction, the limb movements could be reduced. She additionally described insomnia and visual hallucinations. There were no abnormalities in tone, reflexes, sensation or muscle power. The symptoms resolved with cessation of clarithromycin. The authors note that akathisia is a rare side effect of clarithromycin and clinicians should be vigilant for its occurrence [71A].

Erythromycin [SED-15, 1237; SEDA-33, 523; SEDA-34, 409; SEDA-35, 470; SEDA-36, 373; SEDA-37, 300; SEDA-38, 237]

Gastrointestinal

A systematic review and meta-analysis of postnatal erythromycin administration and infantile hypertrophic pyloric stenosis (IHPS) was undertaken. Nine studies were included, 2 randomised control trials (RCT) and 7 retrospective cohort studies. The total number of infants included was 3 008 453. 16 431 had received erythromycin. The two RCT had small numbers with no cases of IHPS in either arm so could not be included. Overall there was a significant association between erythromycin exposure and subsequent development of pyloric stenosis [OR 2.45 (1.12–5.35), $P=0.02$]. There was significant heterogeneity between the studies ($I^2=84\%$, $P<0.0001$) with a suggestion of publication bias. A further analysis was performed to assess the relationship between exposure to erythromycin in the first 14 days of life and development of IHPS. In this analysis only 4 of the 9 selected studies had sufficient documentation and an even stronger association was found between erythromycin exposure and subsequent development of IHPS [OR 12.89 (7.67–21 670, $P<0.00001$]. The study was limited by a lack of high quality published studies evaluating the relationship between erythromycin and development of IHPS and differences between the included studies' design [72M].

Drug–Drug Interaction

An open-label, randomised, two period cross-over study in healthy subjects investigated the edoxaban (a novel factor Xa inhibitor) drug–drug interaction with erythromycin. Edoxaban is a substrate of cytochrome P450 3A4 (CYP3A4) and P-glycoprotein (P-gp). A total of 36 healthy subjects received a single oral dose of 60 mg edoxaban with or without erythromycin 500 mg four times daily for 8 days. Three subjects discontinued due to erythromycin-related adverse effects. Coadministration with erythromycin resulted in an increase in both peak and total exposure of edoxaban of 68% and 78% higher, respectively, compared to edoxaban alone. The effect was thought primarily to be due to erythromycin inhibition of P-gp [73c].

OXAZOLIDINONES [SEDA-15, 2645; SEDA-33, 525; SEDA-34, 409; SEDA-35, 471; SEDA-36, 373; SEDA-37, 300; SEDA-38, 237]

Linezolid [SEDA-35, 469; SEDA-36, 373; SEDA-37, 300; SEDA-38, 237]

Metabolic

A 74-year-old man developed severe lactic acidosis (pH 6.9) after recently commencing oral linezolid and levofloxacin for management of a prosthetic joint infection. Sepsis was excluded as an etiology and linezolid was considered the most likely cause and was ceased. The patient had persisting reduced conscious state despite normalization of his lactic acid levels. MRI and MRA of the brain demonstrated acute bilateral globus pallidus hyperintensities consistent with necrosis. A CSF study showed normal lactate levels but elevated pyruvate levels. The patient's mental status slowly improved but he had persisting proximal muscle weakness. A biopsy was taken from the right vastus lateralis muscle and showed widespread mitochondrial dysfunction. Further work-up was negative for metabolic disorders. Sanger sequencing of the patient's mitochondrial DNA showed he belonged to the mitochondrial J1 haplotype which has previously been previously described as associated with increased risk of linezolid toxicity. The prevalence of the J1 haplotype is 8%–9% of the United States and European population and the authors recommend screening for this mitochondrial haplogroup in patients considered for prolonged linezolid therapy [74A].

Sensory Systems

A 49-year-old woman developed bilateral photophobia after receiving linezolid for 7 months for persistent MRSA septic arthritis. She had bilateral reduced visual acuity, moderate disc edema and central scotomas bilaterally. A diagnosis of linezolid-induced optic neuritis was made after alternative diagnoses were excluded. The changes improved with withdrawal of linezolid. The authors recommend that the safety of linezolid treatment for longer than 28 days has not been adequately evaluated and if long-term linezolid is unavoidable then regular ophthalmic examinations should be conducted [75A].

Hematologic

A retrospective observational cohort study of 221 Japanese patients who received linezolid therapy was performed. Thrombocytopenia developed in 48.4% of patients and anemia in 10.4%. The median time to development of thrombocytopenia was 9 days. In multivariate analysis, creatinine clearance (adjusted odds ratio=0.94 [0.92–0.95], $P<0.001$), hemodialysis (3.32 [1.14–9.67], $P=0.011$), and the duration of linezolid therapy (1.14 [1.07–1.21], $P<0.001$) were found to be significant risk factors for linezolid-induced thrombocytopenia. The duration of linezolid therapy (1.04 [1.01–1.07], $P=0.011$) was shown to be the only significant risk factor for anemia. The median time to development of anemia was 14 days [76c].

POLYMYXINS [SED-15; SEDA-33, 527; SEDA-34, 412; SEDA-35, 473; SEDA-36, 374; SEDA-37, 301; SEDA-38, 237]

Urinary Tract

A prospective multi-center cohort study of 491 adult patients was undertaken to compare the incidences of renal failure in patients receiving colistin methate sodium (CMS) or polymyxin B (PMB) for >48 hours. CMS was associated with significantly higher rates of renal failure than PMB. The overall incidence of renal failure was 16.9% (83 patients); 38.3% and 12.7% in the CMS and PMB groups, respectively, $P < 0.001$). In multivariate analysis, CMS therapy was an independent risk factor for renal failure (hazard ratio, 3.35; 95% confidence interval, 2.05–5.48; $P < 0.001$). The incidence of renal failure was higher in the CMS group regardless of the patient baseline creatinine clearance [77C].

Polymyxin B

Skin

An observational cohort study of 60 patients in Brazil was undertaken to assess the incidence of skin hyperpigmentation after administration of intravenous polymyxin B. Skin hyperpigmentation was noted in 9 (15%) patients. The skin hyperpigmentation manifested as rapid darkening of the entire facial skin. On average the change was 3 tones on the Von Luschan's Chromatic Scale. Changes were first noticeable on average 3 days after commencement of treatment. On review of the literature it appears that people with baseline darker skin are more likely to develop this adverse event [78c].

Three cases of generalized hyperpigmentation have been reported in neonates in India after receiving intravenous polymyxin B. Reversal of the changes was seen in one infant at day 45. The other two were lost to follow-up. The exact mechanism of hyperpigmentation is not known [79A].

STRETOGRAMINS [SED-15, 3182; SEDA-32, 528; SEDA-34, 413; SEDA-35, 473; SEDA-36, 375; SEDA-37, 301; SEDA-38, 238]

Pristinamycin [SEDA-34, 413; SEDA-35, 469; SEDA-36, 375; SEDA-38, 238]

A retrospective cohort study identified 98 patients treated with pristinamycin for a MRSA bone or joint infection. Median daily dose of pristinamycin was 3 g or 47.6 mg/kg. Typically, dosage was divided into 3 equal doses per day. The median duration of treatment for those not receiving long-term suppressive therapy was 9.3 weeks (IQR 1.4–20.4). 15 adverse events occurred in 14 patients. Nausea, vomiting and diarrhoea accounted for 10 of these adverse events. Three adverse events were allergic in nature with 1 isolated blood eosinophilia, 1 maculopapular rash and 1 anaphylactic reaction. Adverse events occurred more frequently in females. Additionally, higher doses were associated with

greater risk of adverse events, odds ratio 2.733 for additional 10 mg/kg daily dose (95% CI 1.006–7.424) [80c].

TRIMETHOPRIM AND TRIMETHOPRIM–SULFAMETHOXAZOLE [SED-15, 3216, 3510; SEDA-32, 477; SEDA-33, 528; SEDA-34, 414; SEDA-35, 474; SEDA-36, 375; SEDA-37, 301; SEDA-38, 238]

Trimethoprim

Nutrition

A randomised, double-blind, placebo-controlled trial in healthy male subjects investigated the effect of a 7 day course of trimethoprim 200 mg twice daily vs placebo. 30 subjects were randomly allocated to each group. Serum folate levels were measured at baseline and at the end of treatment. Serum folate was significantly lower in the trimethoprim group ($P = 0.018$) with a mean decrease of 1.95 nmol/L [81c].

Trimethoprim–Sulfamethoxazole [SEDA-35, 474; SEDA-36, 375; SEDA-37, 301; SEDA-38, 238]

A single centre retrospective review of HIV-positive patients with their first episode *Pneumocystis jirovecii* pneumonia treated with trimethoprim–sulfamethoxazole (TMP-SXT) that had not been taking trimethoprim–sulfamethoxazole as prophylaxis was conducted. The study aimed to determine frequency and risk factors for adverse drug reactions (ADRs) to TMP-SXT. 52 patients collected over 6 years were included in the study; 21 of whom developed an ADR. The most common ADRs were rash in 47.6%, liver function test derangement in 42.9% and elevated creatinine in 38.1%. ADRs were more likely to occur in those that received higher doses of TMP-SXT. The mean daily dose of TMP-SXT was 16.5 mg/kg of trimethoprim component (11.21–21.33) in those with ADRs vs 14.7 mg/kg (7.36–19.2) in those without ADRs ($P = 0.036$). Age and TMP-SXT dose were demonstrated to be independent risk factors for ADRs in cox-proportional analysis. When comparing dosing of 15–16 mg/kg/day, those on 16 mg/kg/day were more likely to experience ADRs (Log-rank test $P = 0.031$) [82c].

Nervous System

A 66-year-old male with spinal cord injury secondary to large B cell lymphoma developed bilateral upper extremity myoclonic jerks, asterixis and postural tremor while on high dose trimethoprim–sulfamethoxazole (15.6 mg/kg/day of trimethoprim) for *P. jiroveci* pneumonia. His symptoms only partially improved with levetiracetam and fully resolved with cessation of trimethoprim–sulfamethoxazole therapy [83A].

OTHER ANTIMICROBIAL DRUGS

Daptomycin [SED-15, 1053; SEDA-33, 529; SEDA-34, 416; SEDA-35, 474; SEDA-36, 375; SEDA-37, 302; SEDA-38, 238]

Hematologic

An observational cohort study of 65 patients who received daptomycin for treatment of a Gram-positive infection after cardiac surgery was undertaken. One patient developed mild neutropenia and one moderate neutropenia which resolved with termination of therapy. No other adverse events were reported in the study [84c].

A single case of daptomycin-induced thrombocytopenia and neutropenia has been reported. A 75-year-old woman received a prolonged course of daptomycin and cefepime for culture negative infective endocarditis. Thrombocytopenia occurred on day 28 of treatment and persisted despite cefepime withdrawal. Daptomycin was ceased on day 38 of treatment. On the same day, the patient developed a significant neutropenia. Both the thrombocytopenia and neutropenia resolved within a week of daptomycin withdrawal. Alternative causes for the thrombocytopenia and neutropenia were excluded. Only two cases of daptomycin-induced thrombocytopenia and a single case of daptomycin-induced neutropenia have been reported previously [85A].

Immunologic

A prospective cohort study was undertaken to evaluate the safety of high-dose daptomycin when used for the treatment of infective endocarditis. 102 patients were included. The median daptomycin dose was 8.2 mg/kg/day for a median of 20 days. The most common adverse event was a rise in peripheral blood eosinophils which occurred in 16 patients (15.7%). There were 3 cases of eosinophilic pneumonia. Muscle toxicity occurred in 15 patients. It was predominantly mild and reversible. Mild renal toxicity occurred in 9 patients (8.8%). Four patients (3.9%) had mild allergic or idiosyncratic reactions [86c].

An observational cohort study of 43 patients who received daptomycin at a dose of ≥6 mg/kg for treatment of a complex bone and joint infections was performed. Six patients had a severe adverse event including 2 confirmed cases of eosinophilic pneumonia [87c].

A case of possible daptomycin-induced eosinophilic pneumonia has been reported in a 67-year-old patient who received daptomycin monotherapy for a diabetic foot infection. On day 23 of daptomycin therapy the patient developed a bilateral pneumonia with a marked peripheral eosinophilia. A bronchoalveolar lavage or lung biopsy was not performed. The patient recovered after cessation of daptomycin. The authors highlight the importance of being aware of this severe potential adverse effect of daptomycin [88A].

Liver

A single case of potential daptomycin-induced acute liver failure has been reported. A 43-year-old woman with multiple medical comorbidities received daptomycin at a dose of 7 mg/kg for MRSA infective endocarditis. After 3 weeks of therapy she developed severe acute liver failure. Her liver function slowly improved after cessation of daptomycin. There was not a concomitant rise in the patient's creatinine kinase (CK). Only a small number of cases of daptomycin-induced liver injury have been previously reported and in most cases there was a concurrent rise in CK. This case suggests possible severe liver failure in the absence of rhabdomyolysis in a patient on high-dose, longer term daptomycin [89A].

Fosfomycin [SED-15, 1448; SEDA-34, 417; SEDA-35, 476; SEDA-36, 376; SEDA-37, 302; SEDA-38, 239]

Two reviews of fosfomycin have been published. Fosfomycin is generally considered a safe therapy with infrequent significant adverse effects. Mild, self-limiting gastrointestinal disturbance including nausea, diarrhoea and abdominal pain are the most common adverse events. Headaches, dizziness, infusion site reactions and fungal superinfections have been reported. Sodium overload and hypokalaemia are reported as potential important adverse events. Every gram of intravenous fosfomycin contains 0.32 g of sodium. Fosfomycin is thought to increase potassium secretion in the distal renal tubules. Transient neutropenia, eosinophilia, anaemia, thrombocytopenia and increases in liver enzymes have been reported [90R,91R].

Fusidic Acid [SED-15, 1460; SEDA-33, 530; SEDA-34, 417 SEDA-35, 475; SEDA-36, 376; SEDA-37, 302; SEDA-38, 239]

Musculoskeletal

A case of severe rhabdomyolysis has been reported in a 75-year-old man who was taking long-term atorvastatin and then subsequently commenced on fusidic acid and moxifloxacin for an infected vascular graft. Plasma concentrations of HMG-CoA reductase inhibitors such as atorvastatin are significantly increased when fusidic acid is co-administered. The mechanism of the interaction is not known. The patient fully recovered following cessation of fusidic acid. The authors emphasize that

HMG-CoA reductase inhibitors and fusidic acid should not be administered concurrently [92A].

Immunologic

A case of toxic epidermal necrosis due to oral fusidic acid has been reported. An 82-year-old woman developed a generalized bullous skin eruption 12 days after commencing oral fusidic acid for a skin infection. The patient had not been prescribed any other new medications in the preceding 2 months. On clinical examination, the patient was febrile with oral and ocular ulcerations and epidermal detachment involving more than 70% of her body surface area. Nikolsky's sign was positive. Lyell's syndrome was diagnosed. Cutaneous histology showed total epidermal necrosis and a normal dermis. The patient died within 24 hours. Whilst rare, the authors highlight the importance of considering fusidic acid as a potential source of severe cutaneous reactions [93A].

References

[1] Neugarten J, Golestaneh L. The effect of gender on aminoglycoside-associated nephrotoxicity. Clin Nephrol. 2016;86(10):183–9 [M].

[2] Jenkins A, Thomson AH, Brown NM, et al. Amikacin use and therapeutic drug monitoring in adults: do dose regimens and drug exposures affect either outcome or adverse events? A systematic review. J Antimicrob Chemother. 2016;71(10):2754–9 [M].

[3] Ellender CM, Law DB, Thomson RM, et al. Safety of IV amikacin in the treatment of pulmonary non-tuberculous mycobacterial disease. Respirology. 2016;21(2):357–62 [c].

[4] Tuon FF, Aragao BZ, Santos TA, et al. Acute kidney injury in patients using amikacin in an era of carbapenem-resistant bacteria. Infect Dis (Lond). 2016;48(11−12):869–71 [c].

[5] Saleh P, Abbasalizadeh S, Rezaeian S, et al. Gentamicin-mediated ototoxicity and nephrotoxicity: a clinical trial study. Niger Med J. 2016;57(6):347–52 [c].

[6] Bennett-Guerrero E, Minkowitz HS, Segura-Vasi AM, et al. A randomized, double-blind, placebo controlled safety, tolerability, and pharmacokinetic dose escalation study of a gentamicin vancomycin gel in patients undergoing colorectal surgery. Perioper Med (Lond). 2016;5:17 [c].

[7] Johansson S, Christensen OM, Thorsmark AH. A retrospective study of acute kidney injury in hip arthroplasty patients receiving gentamicin and dicloxacillin. Acta Orthop. 2016;87(6):589–91 [c].

[8] Rao SC, Srinivasjois R, Moon K. One dose per day compared to multiple doses per day of gentamicin for treatment of suspected or proven sepsis in neonates. Cochrane Database Syst Rev. 2016;12: CD005091 [M].

[9] Riethmuller J, Herrmann G, Graepler-Mainka U, et al. Sequential inhalational tobramycin-colistin-combination in CF-patients with chronic *P. aeruginosa* colonization—an observational study. Cell Physiol Biochem. 2016;39(3):1141–51 [c].

[10] Sommerwerck U, Virella-Lowell I, Angyalosi G, et al. Long-term safety of tobramycin inhalation powder in patients with cystic fibrosis: phase IV (ETOILES) study. Curr Med Res Opin. 2016;32(11):1789–95 [c].

[11] Hoppentocht M, Akkerman OW, Hagedoorn P, et al. Tolerability and pharmacokinetic evaluation of inhaled dry powder tobramycin free base in non-cystic fibrosis bronchiectasis patients. PLoS One. 2016;11(3)e0149768 [c].

[12] Brigg Turner R, Elbarbry F, Biondo L. Pharmacokinetics of once and twice daily dosing of intravenous tobramycin in paediatric patients with cystic fibrosis. J Chemother. 2016;28(4):304–7 [c].

[13] Alves C, Penedones A, Mendes D, et al. A systematic review and meta-analysis of the association between systemic fluoroquinolones and retinal detachment. Acta Ophthalmol. 2016;94(5):e251–9 [R].

[14] Sandhu HS, Brucker AJ, Ma L, et al. Oral fluoroquinolones and the risk of uveitis. JAMA Ophthalmol. 2016;134(1):38–43 [c].

[15] Binz J, Adler CK, So TY. The risk of musculoskeletal adverse events with Fluoroquinolones in children: what is the verdict now? Clin Pediatr (Phila). 2016;55(2):107–10 [r].

[16] Adegbola AJ, Soyinka JO, Adeagbo BA, et al. Alteration of the disposition of quinine in healthy volunteers after concurrent ciprofloxacin administration. Am J Ther. 2016;23(2): e398–404 [E].

[17] Cozzani E, Chinazzo C, Burlando M, et al. Ciprofloxacin as a trigger for bullous pemphigoid: the second case in the literature. Am J Ther. 2016;23(5):e1202–4 [A].

[18] Morgado B, Madeira C, Pinto J, et al. Leukocytoclastic vasculitis with systemic involvement associated with ciprofloxacin therapy: case report and review of the literature. Cureus. 2016;8(11) e900 [A].

[19] Goldie FC, Brogan A, Boyle JG. Ciprofloxacin and statin interaction: a cautionary tale of rhabdomyolysis. BMJ Case Rep. 2016;2016 [A].

[20] Goyal H, Dennehy J, Barker J, et al. Achilles is not alone!!! Ciprofloxacin induced tendinopathy of gluteal tendons. QJM. 2016;109(4):275–6 [A].

[21] Kawtharani F, Masrouha KZ, Afeiche N. Bilateral achilles tendon ruptures associated with ciprofloxacin use in the setting of minimal change disease: case report and review of the literature. J Foot Ankle Surg. 2016;55(2):276–8 [A].

[22] Mair EA, Moss JR, Dohar JE, et al. Randomized clinical trial of a sustained-exposure ciprofloxacin for intratympanic injection during tympanostomy tube surgery. Ann Otol Rhinol Laryngol. 2016;125(2):105–14 [c].

[23] Mair EA, Park AH, Don D, et al. Safety and efficacy of intratympanic ciprofloxacin otic suspension in children with middle ear effusion undergoing tympanostomy tube placement: two randomized clinical trials. JAMA Otolaryngol Head Neck Surg. 2016;142(5):444–51 [c].

[24] Park AH, White DR, Moss JR, et al. Phase 3 trials of thermosensitive ciprofloxacin gel for middle ear effusion in children with tubes. Otolaryngol Head Neck Surg. 2016;155(2):324–31 [c].

[25] Zhao T, Chen LA, Wang P, et al. A randomized, open, multicenter clinical study on the short course of intravenous infusion of 750 mg of levofloxacin and the sequential standard course of intravenous infusion/oral administration of 500 mg of levofloxacin for treatment of community-acquired pneumonia. J Thorac Dis. 2016;8(9):2473–84 [c].

[26] Kalita J, Bhoi SK, Betai S, et al. Safety and efficacy of additional levofloxacin in tuberculous meningitis: a randomized controlled pilot study. Tuberculosis (Edinb). 2016;98:1–6 [c].

[27] Pan L, Wang Z, Xu Y. Levofloxacin-induced transient musculospiral paralysis. Am J Emerg Med. 2017;35(2): 375 e1–e2 [A].

[28] van der Laan LE, Schaaf HS, Solomons R, et al. Probable levofloxacin-associated secondary intracranial hypertension in a child with multidrug-resistant tuberculosis. Pediatr Infect Dis J. 2016;35(6):706–8 [A].

[29] Haji-Aghamohammadi AA, Bastani A, Miroliaee A, et al. Comparison of levofloxacin versus clarithromycin efficacy in the eradication of Helicobacter pylori infection. Caspian J Intern Med. 2016;7(4):267–71 [c].

[30] Liou JM, Bair MJ, Chen CC, et al. Levofloxacin sequential therapy vs levofloxacin triple therapy in the second-line treatment of

helicobacter pylori: a randomized trial. Am J Gastroenterol. 2016;111(3):381–7 [c].

[31] Qiao LD, Chen S, Wang XF, et al. A multi-center, controlled, randomized, open-label clinical study of levofloxacin for preventing infection during the perioperative period of ultrasound-guided transrectal prostate biopsy. Eur J Clin Microbiol Infect Dis. 2016;35(11):1877–81 [c].

[32] Uzun R, Yalcin AD, Celik B, et al. Levofloxacin induced toxic epidermal necrolysis: successful therapy with omalizumab (Anti-IgE) and pulse prednisolone. Am J Case Rep. 2016;17:666–71 [A].

[33] Bidell MR, Lodise TP. Fluoroquinolone-associated tendinopathy: does levofloxacin pose the greatest risk? Pharmacotherapy. 2016;36(6):679–93 [R].

[34] Hasanain A, Mahdy R, Mohamed A, et al. A randomized, comparative study of dual therapy (doxycycline-rifampin) versus triple therapy (doxycycline-rifampin-levofloxacin) for treating acute/subacute brucellosis. Braz J Infect Dis. 2016;20(3):250–4 [c].

[35] Mason JW, Moon TE. Moxifloxacin increases heart rate in humans. Antibiotics (Basel). 2017;6(1):5 [c].

[36] Ruan Q, Liu Q, Sun F, et al. Moxifloxacin and gatifloxacin for initial therapy of tuberculosis: a meta-analysis of randomized clinical trials. Emerg Microbes Infect. 2016;5:e12 [M].

[37] Gillespie SH. The role of moxifloxacin in tuberculosis therapy. Eur Respir Rev. 2016;25(139):19–28 [R].

[38] Kang YA, Shim TS, Koh WJ, et al. Choice between levofloxacin and moxifloxacin and multidrug-resistant tuberculosis treatment outcomes. Ann Am Thorac Soc. 2016;13(3):364–70 [C].

[39] Mazhar F, Akram S, Haider N. Moxifloxacin-induced acute psychosis: a case report with literature review. J Res Pharm Pract. 2016;5(4):294–6 [A].

[40] Arshinoff SA, Modabber M. Dose and administration of intracameral moxifloxacin for prophylaxis of postoperative endophthalmitis. J Cataract Refract Surg. 2016;42(12):1730–41 [c].

[41] Zhou AX, Messenger WB, Sargent S, et al. Safety of undiluted intracameral moxifloxacin without postoperative topical antibiotics in cataract surgery. Int Ophthalmol. 2016;36(4):493–8 [c].

[42] Lim JH, Lee DH, Lee ST, et al. Moxifloxacin-containing triple therapy after non-bismuth quadruple therapy failure for Helicobacter pylori infection. World J Gastroenterol. 2015;21(46):13124–31 [c].

[43] Hwang JJ, Lee DH, Yoon H, et al. Efficacy of moxifloxacin-based sequential and hybrid therapy for first-line Helicobacter pylori eradication. World J Gastroenterol. 2015;21(35):10234–41 [c].

[44] Kim H, Bang ES, Lim SK, et al. DRESS syndrome and acute generalized exanthematous pustulosis induced by antituberculosis medications and moxifloxacin: case report. Int J Clin Pharmacol Ther. 2016;54(10):808–15 [A].

[45] Rawal G, Yadav S, Kumar R, et al. Ofloxacin induced angioedema: a rare adverse drug reaction. J Clin Diagn Res. 2016;10(11): FD03-FD4. [A].

[46] Zhanel GG, Hartel E, Adam H, et al. Solithromycin: a novel fluoroketolide for the treatment of community-acquired bacterial pneumonia. Drugs. 2016;76(18):1737–57 [R].

[47] Barrera CM, Mykietiuk A, Metev H, et al. Efficacy and safety of oral solithromycin versus oral moxifloxacin for treatment of community-acquired bacterial pneumonia: a global, double-blind, multicentre, randomised, active-controlled, non-inferiority trial (SOLITAIRE-ORAL). Lancet Infect Dis. 2016;16(4):421–30 [C].

[48] Dunne MW, Talbot GH, Boucher HW, et al. Safety of dalbavancin in the treatment of skin and skin structure infections: a pooled analysis of randomized, comparative studies. Drug safety. 2016;39(2):147–57 [R].

[49] Dunne MW, Puttagunta S, Giordano P, et al. A randomized clinical trial of single-dose versus weekly dalbavancin for treatment of acute bacterial skin and skin structure infection. Clin Infect Dis. 2016;62(5):545–51 [C].

[50] Nakano T, Nakamura Y, Takata T, et al. Change of teicoplanin loading dose requirement for incremental increases of systemic inflammatory response syndrome score in the setting of sepsis. Int J Clin Pharmacol. 2016;38(4):908–14 [c].

[51] Miyazu D, Kodama N, Yamashita D, et al. DRESS syndrome caused by cross-reactivity between vancomycin and subsequent teicoplanin administration: a case report. Am J Case Rep. 2016;17:625–31 [A].

[52] Choi HM, Choi MH, Yang YW. A case of teicoplanin-induced pancytopenia caused by excessive dosing. Am J Ther. 2016;23(1): e307–10 [A].

[53] Tongsai S, Koomanachai P. The safety and efficacy of high versus low vancomycin trough levels in the treatment of patients with infections caused by methicillin-resistant *Staphylococcus aureus*: a meta-analysis. BMC Res Notes. 2016;9(1):455 [M].

[54] Seixas GT, Araujo OR, Silva DC, et al. Vancomycin therapeutic targets and nephrotoxicity in critically ill children with cancer. J Pediatr Hematol Oncol. 2016;38(2):e56–62 [c].

[55] Hao JJ, Chen H, Zhou JX. Continuous versus intermittent infusion of vancomycin in adult patients: a systematic review and meta-analysis. Int J Antimicrob Agents. 2016;47(1):28–35 [M].

[56] Katikaneni M, Lwin L, Villanueva H, et al. Acute kidney injury associated with vancomycin when laxity leads to injury and findings on kidney biopsy. Am J Ther. 2016;23(4):e1064–7 [A].

[57] Peyko V, Sasson E. Vancomycin extravasation: evaluation, treatment, and avoidance of this adverse drug event. Case Rep Int Med. 2016;3(3):40 [A].

[58] Minhas JS, Wickner PG, Long AA, et al. Immune-mediated reactions to vancomycin: a systematic case review and analysis. Ann Allergy Asthma Immunol. 2016;116(6):544–53 [R].

[59] Webb PS, Al-Mohammad A. Enigma: infection or allergy? Vancomycin-induced DRESS syndrome with dialysis-dependent renal failure and cardiac arrest. BMJ Case Rep. 2016;2016 [A].

[60] Yamanouchi J, Hato T, Shiraishi S, et al. Vancomycin-induced immune thrombocytopenia proven by the detection of vancomycin-dependent anti-platelet antibody with flow cytometry. Intern Med (Tokyo, Japan). 2016;55(20):3035–8 [A].

[61] Deweese R, Slavens J, Barua A, et al. Vancomycin-induced eosinophilic peritonitis. Am J Health Syst Pharm. 2016;73(9):e243–6 [A].

[62] Bulloch MN, Baccas JT, Arnold S. Clindamycin-induced hypersensitivity reaction. Infection. 2016;44(3):357–9 [A].

[63] Okudo J, Anusim N. Hepatotoxicity due to clindamycin in combination with acetaminophen in a 62-year-old african american female: a case report and review of the literature. Case Rep Hepatol. 2016;2016:2724738 [A].

[64] Wan H, Hu Z, Wang J, et al. Clindamycin-induced kidney diseases: a retrospective analysis of 50 patients. Intern Med (Tokyo, Japan). 2016;55(11):1433–7 [c].

[65] Stanic Benic M, Karlovic K, Cubranic A. Clindamycin-induced necrotising oesophagitis. Postgrad Med J. 2016;92(1094):741 [A].

[66] Sears SP, Getz TW, Austin CO, et al. Incidence of sustained ventricular tachycardia in patients with prolonged QTc after the administration of azithromycin: a retrospective study. Drugs - Real World Outcomes. 2016;3:99–105 [c].

[67] Das A, Sancheti K, Podder I, et al. Azithromycin induced bullous fixed drug eruption. Indian J Pharm. 2016;48(1):83–5 [A].

[68] Nappe TM, Goren-Garcia SL, Jacoby JL. Stevens–Johnson syndrome after treatment with azithromycin: an uncommon culprit. Am J Emerg Med. 2016;34(3): 676.e1–3. [A].

[69] Wong AY, Root A, Douglas IJ, et al. Cardiovascular outcomes associated with use of clarithromycin: population based study. BMJ. 2016;352:h6926 [MC].

[70] Wong AY, Wong IC, Chui CS, et al. Association between acute neuropsychiatric events and helicobacter pylori therapy containing clarithromycin. JAMA Intern Med. 2016;176(6):828–34 [MC].

[71] Gbinigie II, Lasserson D. Clarithromycin-induced akathisia: a class effect of macrolides? BMJ Case Rep. 2016;2016 [A].

[72] Murchison L, De Coppi P, Eaton S. Post-natal erythromycin exposure and risk of infantile hypertrophic pyloric stenosis: a systematic review and meta-analysis. Pediatr Surg Int. 2016;32(12):1147–52 [M].

[73] Parasrampuria DA, Mendell J, Shi M, et al. Edoxaban drug-drug interactions with ketoconazole, erythromycin, and cyclosporine. Br J Clin Pharmacol. 2016;82(6):1591–600 [c].

[74] Abou Hassan OK, Karnib M, El-Khoury R, et al. Linezolid toxicity and mitochondrial susceptibility: a novel neurological complication in a lebanese patient. Front pharmacol. 2016;7:325 [A].

[75] Ishii N, Kinouchi R, Inoue M, et al. Linezolid-induced optic neuropathy with a rare pathological change in the inner retina. Int ophthalmol. 2016;36(6):761–6 [A].

[76] Hanai Y, Matsuo K, Ogawa M, et al. A retrospective study of the risk factors for linezolid-induced thrombocytopenia and anemia. J Infect Chemother. 2016;22(8):536–42 [c].

[77] Rigatto MH, Oliveira MS, Perdigao-Neto LV, et al. Multicenter prospective cohort study of renal failure in patients treated with colistin versus Polymyxin B. Antimicrob Agents Chemother. 2016;60(4):2443–9 [C].

[78] Mattos KP, Lloret GR, Cintra ML, et al. Acquired skin hyperpigmentation following intravenous polymyxin B treatment: a cohort study. Pigment Cell Melanoma Res. 2016;29(3): 388–90 [c].

[79] Gothwal S, Meena K, Sharma SD. Polymyxin B induced generalized hyperpigmentation in neonates. Indian J Pediatr. 2016;83(2):179–80 [A].

[80] Valour F, Boibieux A, Karsenty J, et al. Pristinamycin in the treatment of MSSA bone and joint infection. J Antimicrob Chemother. 2016;71(4):1063–70 [c].

[81] Meidahl Petersen K, Eplov K, Kjaer Nielsen T, et al. The effect of trimethoprim on serum folate levels in humans: a randomized, double-blind, placebo-controlled trial. Am J Ther. 2016;23(2): e382–7 [c].

[82] Chang HM, Tsai HC, Lee SS, et al. High daily doses of trimethoprim/sulfamethoxazole are an independent risk factor for adverse reactions in patients with pneumocystis pneumonia and AIDS. J Chin Med Assoc. 2016;79(6):314–9 [c].

[83] Gray DA, Foo D. Reversible myoclonus, asterixis, and tremor associated with high dose trimethoprim-sulfamethoxazole: a case report. J Spinal Cord Med. 2016;39(1):115–7 [A].

[84] Kornberger A, Luchting B, Kur F, et al. Daptomycin for the treatment of major gram-positive infections after cardiac surgery. J Cardiothorac Surg. 2016;11(1):120 [c].

[85] Leyra F, Perez-Chulia N, Jofre C, et al. Thrombocytopaenia and neutropaenia associated with daptomycin USE. J Chem (Florence, Italy). 2016;28(5):425–7 [A].

[86] Durante-Mangoni E, Andini R, Parrella A, et al. Safety of treatment with high-dose daptomycin in 102 patients with infective endocarditis. Int J Antimicrob Agents. 2016;48(1):61–8 [c].

[87] Roux S, Valour F, Karsenty J, et al. Daptomycin >6 mg/kg/day as salvage therapy in patients with complex bone and joint infection: cohort study in a regional reference center. BMC Infect Dis. 2016;16:83 [c].

[88] Hatipoglu M, Memis A, Turhan V, et al. Possible daptomycin-induced acute eosinophilic pneumonia in a patient with diabetic foot infection. Int J Antimicrob Agents. 2016;47(5):414–5 [A].

[89] Mo Y, Nehring F, Jung AH, et al. Possible hepatotoxicity associated with daptomycin: a case report and literature review. J Pharm Pract. 2016;29(3):253–6 [A].

[90] Falagas ME, Vouloumanou EK, Samonis G, et al. Fosfomycin. Clin Microbiol Rev. 2016;29(2):321–47 [R].

[91] Sastry S, Doi Y. Fosfomycin: resurgence of an old companion. J Infect Chemother. 2016;22(5):273–80 [R].

[92] Nandy A, Gaini S. Severe rhabdomyolysis as complication of interaction between atorvastatin and fusidic acid in a patient in lifelong antibiotic prophylaxis: a dangerous combination. Case Rep Med. 2016;2016:4705492 [A].

[93] Cluzel C, Pralong P, Logerot S, et al. Lethal Lyell's syndrome induced by fusidic acid. Ann Dermatol Venereol. 2016;143(3): 215–8 [A].

23

Antifungal Drugs

Dayna S. McManus[1]

Yale-New Haven Hospital, Yale University, New Haven, CT, United States
[1]Corresponding author: dayna.mcmanus@ynhh.org

COMPARATIVE HEPATOTOXICITY RISK AMONG ANTIFUNGAL AGENTS

Antifungal agents have a significant number of side effects with hepatotoxicity being one of the most common among all the classes of antifungals. Therefore, the start of this chapter looks at a review of the published literature on drug-induced hepatotoxicity from antifungal agents that are used to treated invasive fungal disease.

Amphotericin B deoxycholate (DAMB) is the first antifungal reviewed in the chapter. Overall amphotericin B deoxycholate is not typically associated with hepatotoxicity; however, there have been some reports of hepatotoxicity associated with this medications use. In one randomized controlled trial DAMB was administered to 68 cancer patients and none of which had to discontinue therapy due to abnormalities in liver function tests or concerns for hepatic toxicity. Another randomized controlled trial compared patients who received liposomal amphotericin B vs DAMB in adult and pediatric cancer patients. Increases in Alkaline phosphatase (ALP), Alanine Aminotransferase (ALT), Aspartate Aminotransferase (AST), and bilirubin were seen in 19.2, 14.0, 12.8, 19.2 of patients receiving DAMB compared to 22.2%, 14.6%, 12.8%, and 18.1% of patients receiving liposomal amphotericin (LAMB), respectively. In addition, a meta-analysis of the hepatotoxicity of antifungals was reviewed. A reported a risk of liver enzyme elevations that did not require cessation of treatment was found to be 13.3% (95% CI: 6.8–19.9) in subjects treated empirically with DAMB. The pooled risk was estimated to be only 0.2% (95% CI: 0–0.4) regarding liver biochemistries that require discontinuation. In this review, DAMB was found to be safer than the corresponding lipid formulations in terms of hepatotoxicity. There was a total of 300 cases of non-acetaminophen Drug-Induced Liver

Injury (DILI) that were reviewed and only 8 (2.7%) were attributed to antifungal agents, with no cases linked to amphotericin B products.

Liposomal amphotericin, like DAMB, is associated with a very low incidence of hepatotoxicity. The first study that was reviewed, in the chapter, was a retrospective single-center autopsy-controlled study that reviewed hepatotoxicity in 64 patients with hematologic malignancies who had received LAMB or Amphotericin B Lipid Complex (ABLC) for ≥7 days in a time period. Abnormal results of liver function tests [>fivefold of upper limit of normal (ULN) increase in serum bilirubin or ALT/AST in patients with normal baseline liver function; twofold increase in the aforementioned biochemistries in patients with abnormal baseline tests] were found in 12/32 (37.5%) and 10/32 (31.3%) of patients who received ABLC and LAMB, respectively. Of these cases one patient in the ALBC group and three in the LAMB group were attributed to other hepatotoxic agents such as triazoles. Nonspecific histopathological abnormalities were present in 94% of all patients and none of the patients with acquired liver dysfunction displayed the histopathologic findings that have been reported in animal studies with LAMB and ABLC and therefore was no signal for direct histopathologic evidence of toxicity associated with lipid formulations of AMB in this study. Another retrospectively review looked at the frequency of LAMB-induced laboratory adverse effects in 22 adult patients and saw an increase over the ULN of the total bilirubin, AST and ALT in 6 (27.3%), 8 (36.4%), and 8 patients (36.4%), respectively. Majority of the cases were mild elevations with only one case showing a sevenfold ULN increase. There was no association with dose and these lab abnormalities. Another study that looked at 201 patients with IFD who received LAMB at different doses found a lack of association with dose of LAMB and abnormal liver function

245

tests. In the study, abnormal liver function tests (>five times the ULN) were found in 15.7% of patients assigned to the 3-mg/kg group and in 14.4% in the 10-mg/kg group.

Finally, a case–control study of bone marrow transplant patients who experienced hepatotoxicity in association with antifungal agents reported an unadjusted incidence of hepatotoxicity of 0.78 cases per 100 patient-days of exposure to DAMB, 0.98 for fluconazole, and 1.50 for LAMB. LAMB and, to a lesser extent fluconazole were associated with a substantial increase in the risk of hepatotoxicity (OR 3.33; 95% CI: 1.61–6.88, and OR 1.99; 95% CI: 1.21–3.26, respectively). Among patients who were exposed to a single antifungal agent, the most significant association was recorded for LAMB (OR 3.78; 95% CI: 1.42–10; $P < 0.05$). Increased values of liver function tests were associated with increased exposure to LAMB; however, this correlation was not seen with patients that received DAMB. A follow-up analysis of this study was done to look at patients who developed hepatotoxicity but continued on antifungal medication. In the follow-up analysis, 32% of those receiving LAMB had increased bilirubin levels above 10 mg/dL, as opposed to 8% of patients treated with fluconazole. The authors, therefore, concluded that administration of both LAMB and fluconazole were associated with increased risk of hepatotoxicity, independently of other treatments received or patient characteristics.

The last study that was reviewed was a retrospective review of 100 consecutive patients receiving LAMB at doses of 1, 3, and 5 mg/kg. Hepatotoxicity, defined as an increase of bilirubin to >1.5 mg/dL or AST and ALT >three times the ULN, occurred in 16/75 patients (21%) with an unadjusted incidence of 2.2 cases per 100 patient-days. Cumulative dose was not associated with the occurrence of liver toxicity.

These reviews suggest that there is an overall low risk for serious hepatic toxicity with any amphotericin products; however, the risk may be slightly higher with the lipid formulations in comparison to the conventional formulation, DAMB.

Among the triazole antifungals ketoconazole has been shown to have the highest association with hepatic toxicity. In many countries ketoconazole has been removed from the market due to the high association with hepatic toxicity. Studies have shown the risk of liver toxicity from this agent occur at a rate of approximately 3.6%–4.3% without a clear correlation with dosing. In children rates have been found to be around 1.4%, which is much lower than that of adults. In one study of 90 847 Taiwanese users of oral antifungal agents, 52 patients presented DILI, 28 of which were attributed to ketoconazole (54%; incidence rate: 4.9 per 10 000 persons; rate increasing with cumulative dose). 12 cases were attributed to fluconazole (incidence ratio of 31.6 per 10 000 persons), and all

6 patients with fatal DILI in this study were attributed to fluconazole.

In terms of fluconazole, pilot exploratory study on safety and overall outcome, 41 neutropenic patients received either fluconazole or DAMB for febrile neutropenia. One patient in each arm developed drug-related hepatic disease, but only the patient from the amphotericin B arm had to discontinue its therapy. Fluconazole was compared to amphotericin B in another study of febrile neutropenic patients. 106 cancer patients were randomized to receive either fluconazole or DAMB. Overall adverse events occurred more frequently in the DAMB group ($P < 0.01$). Hyperbilirubinemia was found in 5 patients receiving fluconazole vs 9 patients receiving amphotericin. Another study of 206 patients with invasive candidiasis were randomly assigned to receive either DAMB or fluconazole. Elevation of liver enzymes occurred in 14% and 10% of patients receiving fluconazole and amphotericin B, respectively, which was a statistically significant difference. 2 out of 103 patients in the fluconazole arm (1.9%) had to stop treatment due to hepatotoxicity.

Another study performed a prospective, randomized, multicenter study comparing fluconazole and DAMB in the treatment of documented or presumed invasive candidiasis in 164 patients with and without neutropenia. Not surprisingly, adverse effects were more frequent with amphotericin B (35%) than with fluconazole (5%; $P < 0.0001$). Hepatic toxicity occurred in 3 vs 2 patients receiving DAMB and fluconazole, respectively. The patient who was receiving fluconazole had to discontinue treatment due to the hepatotoxicity. A meta-analysis estimated the pooled risk for mild elevation of liver enzyme levels under empirical treatment with fluconazole at 8.6% (95% CI: 1–16.1) and at 9.8% (95% CI: 2.5–17) when used for culture-documented therapy. Estimated pooled risk of discontinuing the empirical treatment with fluconazole due to DILI was 0.3% (95% CI: 0–0.9) vs 1.3% (95% CI: 0–2.8) that was calculated for culture-documented therapy. Overall this shows a relatively low risk for toxicity with fluconazole treatment.

Itraconazole was the next triazole antifungal that was reviewed in the chapter. The first study presented compared the efficacy and safety of itraconazole compared with DAMB in a randomized controlled trial of neutropenic patients being treated for proven or probable systemic fungal infections. There was no difference found in terms of hepatotoxicity between the two groups. Elevations in AST and ALP (more than 30% increase in pre-treatment values) were found in 40% and 10% for vs 55% and 25% of patients, respectively. In a different randomized, controlled, multicenter trial the efficacy and safety of intravenous and oral itraconazole were compared with DAMB as empirical antifungal therapy. There were fewer drug-related adverse events in the itraconazole group

(5% vs 54% of patients; $P = 0.001$), and the rate of withdrawal because of toxicity was significantly lower with itraconazole (19% vs 38%; $P = 0.001$). Specifically with DILI, none of the patients who received DAMB required discontinuation of treatment, while 3 patients in itraconazole's group were discontinued due to liver toxicity. Elevation in liver function tests occurred in 11 vs 8 patients who received itraconazole and DAMB, respectively. A study of 162 hematologic malignancy patients with persistent febrile neutropenia who received either intravenous followed by oral itraconazole suspension or intravenous DAMB showed significantly fewer itraconazole patients discontinued treatment due to any adverse events (22.2% vs 56.8% for; $P < 0.0001$). The main reason for discontinuation was a rise in serum creatinine (1.2% vs 23.5%). Elevated bilirubin levels were recorded in seven patients receiving itraconazole (8.6%) and in six patients (7.4%) in the DAMB group. A recent systematic review estimated the pooled risk of DILI was 17.4% (95% CI: 3.9–31) among itraconazole recipients, while the respective risk for DILI-attributed discontinuation of itraconazole was 1.5% (95% CI: 0–4).

Voriconazole was studied in a randomized controlled trial compared to DAMB in patients with possible or definite aspergillosis. Voriconazole-treated patients were found to have significantly fewer severe drug-related adverse events ($P = 0.008$), despite median therapy duration for voriconazole being much longer. Seven patients in the voriconazole arm (3.6%) presented with severe, potentially drug-related hepatic abnormalities vs four in the DAMB arm (2.2%; $P = 0.54$).

Another multicentered, randomized, noninferiority study compared voriconazole with DAMB followed by oral fluconazole for the treatment of candidemia in 370 nonneutropenic patients. There were significantly fewer serious adverse events ($P = 0.048$) and cases of renal toxicity ($P = 0.0002$) in the voriconazole group. Hepatic events, including increases in concentration of ALP, ALT, AST or bilirubin were comparable between groups (23%–24%) and they did not correlate with treatment discontinuation.

The toxicity of voriconazole and its correlation with CYP450 genotypes was investigated in a study of 95 patients. Visual disturbances and hallucinations were the most common adverse events, while hepatotoxicity was evident in 6 patients (6.3%) and to drug discontinuation in all cases. Notably, there was no correlation between DILI and other side effects, CYP2C19 genotype, CYP2C9 genotype, levels of voriconazole metabolites, or drug serum levels.

However, a large meta-analysis including 24 studies showed that patients with supratherapeutic Voriconazole serum concentrations (>4.0 mg/L) were at increased risk of toxicity (OR 4.17; 95% CI 2.08–8.36). The pooled incidence rate of hepatotoxicity was 5.7% and patients with supratherapeutic serum concentrations had almost fourfold the risk of hepatotoxicity as those with lower serum concentrations (12.4% vs 4.2%, $P = 0.001$; OR 3.70; 95% CI: 2.08–6.59; $I^2 = 37\%$). These findings support the idea that hepatotoxicity with voriconazole is a dose-dependent phenomena in most cases. In a study that investigated 6595 cases of hepatic adverse drug reactions in children from a worldwide pharmacovigilance database, voriconazole ranked 21st among all drugs with 52 cases (adjusted odds ratio 10.7; 95% CI: 7.9–14.6) and fluconazole was 30th (adjusted odds ratio 8.6; 95% CI: 6.2–12), while no other antifungal agent reached the frequency of 0.4%. A systematic review of randomized controlled trials estimated pooled risk of elevated liver enzyme levels for voriconazole at 19.7% (95% CI: 16.8–22.6). The rationale behind the higher incidence of hepatotoxicity with voriconazole compared with other triazoles is not completely understood, however, the fact that voriconazole is a substrate for several CYP450 enzymes could provide the explanation behind these findings.

Posaconazole, another triazole antifungal was compared to itraconazole or fluconazole in a randomized, multicenter study of prophylaxis in a total of 602 patients with prolonged neutropenia. Serious adverse events possibly or probably related to treatment were reported by 19 patients (6%) in the posaconazole group and 6 patients (2%) in the fluconazole and itraconazole group ($P = 0.01$). Three patients in the posaconazole arm had increased hepatic enzymes (1%) vs only one case recorded in the comparator group (0.3%; NS). Elevated bilirubin levels were found in 5 patients receiving posaconazole (1.6%) compared with 3 cases in the fluconazole/itraconazole group (1%). One patient (0.3%) in the posaconazole arm developed hepatic failure. In a nonrandomized comparison of posaconazole vs fluconazole and/or itraconazole in pediatric patients with hematological malignancies, the frequency of drug-related events did not differ significantly between groups and increase in ALT (>250% of ULN) ranged from 12.5% to 16.7% across groups. In a large randomized, double-blind trial in 600 patients, oral posaconazole was compared to oral fluconazole for prophylaxis against IFDs. The rates of treatment-related serious adverse events were 13% for posazonazole and 10% for fluconazole. There was no difference found in the frequency of individual liver and biliary disorders. There is no data to date that shows differences in toxicity risk among the different posaconazole formulations despite their different bioavailabilities.

Isavuconazole is a newly approved triazole antifungal with antifungal coverage similar to that of posaconazole. In a large phase III, randomized, double-blind study for treatment of probable and proven invasive aspergillosis treatment-emergent adverse events by system organ class was similar overall between people who received isavuconazole compared with voriconazole. However, isavuconazole-treated patients had a lower frequency of hepatobiliary disorders (23 [9%] vs 42 [16%]; $P = 0.016$). Based on the small amount of data available since the approval of isavuconazole it appears to have less potential for hepatic toxicity relative to voriconazole, however, this may change once more post-marketing data becomes available.

A systematic review of randomized controlled trials estimated risk of DILI that does not lead to treatment withdrawal at 8.7% when echinocandins were used for empirical therapy (95% CI: 6.4–11) and at 3.8% for definite therapy (95% CI: 2–5.5). The pooled risk for discontinuation of treatment with echinocandins due to DILI was also substantially lower than for other antifungal agents: 4.8% (95% CI: 3–6.5) in empirical and 3.7% (95% CI: 2.5–4.9) in definite therapy regimens. Among the individual echinocandins, DILI that did require cessation of treatment was more prevalent in patients under micafungin (pooled risk estimate at 2.7%; 95% CI: 0.7–4.6) than in those under anidulafungin (0.8%; 95% CI: 0–2.3) or caspofungin (0.2%; 95% CI: 0.1–0.4). Interestingly in this study, caspofungin and not micafungin was the echinocandin that had correlated stronger with elevation of liver enzymes. The corresponding pooled risk estimates for DILI that did not lead to discontinuation of administration were 7% (95% CI: 4.1–9.9) for caspofungin, 3% (95% CI: 1–5.1) for micafungin, and 2% (95% CI: 0.3–3.7) for anidulafungin.

In a randomized controlled trial that compared anidulafungin and fluconazole 11 patients in the anidulafungin arm had discontinuation of treatment due to adverse events (one due to elevation of transaminase levels), while in the fluconazole arm, 16 subjects were discontinued (two due to elevated transaminases). Drug-related elevation of hepatic enzymes was more frequent in the fluconazole arm (7.2% vs 1.5% in the anidulafungin group; $P = 0.03$). The overall frequency of elevated hepatic enzymes was observed in 11.2% of the fluconazole users vs 5.3% of patients under anidulafungin treatment. In an analysis of anidulafungin safety in 86 solid organ transplant patients none of the patients discontinued anidulafungin because of severe adverse effects. One patient developed mild liver toxicity that did not require discontinuation.

Caspofungin was compared with DAMB in a large double-blind trial for the primary treatment of invasive candidiasis in 239 subjects. Not surprisingly, there were significantly fewer drug-related adverse events and laboratory abnormalities in the caspofungin group than in the DAMB group ($P = 0.002$). Only 3 patients treated with caspofungin had therapy discontinued due to adverse events relative to 29 of those who received DAMB. Elevation in serum ALP was more frequent than the elevation in ALT/AST in both groups and was observed in

9 (8.3%) of caspofungin patients vs 19 patients (15.6%). At doses of three times the standard dosing regimen (i.e. 150 mg/day) for caspofungin there was significant drug-related adverse events occurred in 2/104 of patients receiving the standard regimen and in 3/100 of patients receiving the high-dose regimen. The most common drug-related adverse event in both groups was increased ALP (6.9% vs 2.0% in the high-dose group), followed by increased AST levels (4.0% vs 2.0% in the high-dose group), while the rates of drug-related discontinuations were similar between groups. Premature study discontinuation because of toxicity occurred less often in the caspofungin group than in the LAMB cohort ($P = 0.03$) in a study of patients receiving LAMB or caspofungin for treatment of fungal infections. Fewer patients who received caspofungin sustained a drug-related adverse event (54.4% vs 69.3%; $P < 0.001$) or discontinued therapy because of drug-related adverse events (5% vs 8%; $P = 0.04$). Regarding hepatotoxicity, 9% of patients in the caspofungin arm group had elevated liver function tests vs 12% of patients in the L-AMB arm group. In a prospective, multicenter, trial to evaluate caspofungin for prophylaxis in liver transplant patients six patients were discontinued prematurely due to potentially drug-related altered liver function. Grade IV elevations (>10 times ULN) of one or more liver function test enzyme were observed in 30% of patients on day +3 and in 27.7% of patients at the end of prophylaxis. All liver function tests, except ALP and GGT, improved during treatment with caspofungin.

Micafungin was compared for efficacy and safety with LAMB in a double-blind, randomized non-inferiority study in treatment of invasive candidiasis. Fewer treatment-related adverse events ($P = 0.082$) including those that were serious ($P = 0.138$) or led to treatment discontinuation ($P = 0.087$) were observed in the micafungin cohort. Increased liver enzymes attributed to the study drug were observed in eight patients receiving micafungin (3%) vs three patients receiving LAMB (1.1%; $P = 0.14$). Hepatic adverse events resulting in treatment discontinuation occurred in seven vs three patients. Thus, while hepatic adverse events seemed to be more prominent in micafungin recipients, this difference was not statistically significant. A second large randomized, double-blind trial compared micafungin (100 mg daily) and micafungin (150 mg daily) with a standard dosage of caspofungin (70 mg followed by 50 mg daily) in adults with invasive candidiasis. Abnormal results of liver function tests were among the most commonly observed treatment-emergent adverse events (≥2% of patients in all treatment arms). Drug-related events leading to withdrawal were evident in 5 patients who received micafungin 100 mg (2.5%), 6 with micafungin 150 mg (3%), and 7 with caspofungin (3.6%), and in one-third of these cases the reason was DILI. A randomized, double-blind, phase III trial involving 882 patients assessed the use of micafungin vs fluconazole as antifungal prophylaxis fewer micafungin-treated patients discontinued use of the study drug because of an adverse event (4.2% vs 7.2% in the fluconazole arm; $P = 0.058$). There were no differences between study groups in the occurrence of all hepatic-related adverse events and those considered to be related to study treatment (28% vs 28.7% and 5.2% vs 6.8%, respectively). In addition, an open-label, randomized trial of micafungin for the prevention of IFD in high-risk liver transplant recipients, micafungin was non-inferior to standard care (i.e. fluconazole, LAMB, or caspofungin). Adverse event profiles in the 344 subjects and liver function at the end of the prophylaxis period were similar. The rates of acute liver failure were comparable between groups (16.9% vs 19.2% of the standard care patients), but treatment-related hepatic adverse events were more frequent in the micafungin group (7 patients i.e. 4% vs 0.6% of standard care) and in 4 cases (2.3%), led to discontinuation. A black boxed warning can be found in the package insert for micafungin based on rat models have that showed development of foci of altered hepatocytes and hepatocellular tumors in treatment regimens lasting more than 3 months, however, there has been no signal of hepatocellular tumors during post-marketing.

Hepatotoxicity related to flucytosine usage typically causes elevation of hepatic transaminases. There is wide variation in the incidence of hepatotoxicity depending on the study and it can vary anywhere from 0% to 41% due to different definitions for hepatotoxicity. The increase in liver function tests is usually mild to moderate and reversible after discontinuation of flucytosine therapy. Two cases of severe liver necrosis have been reported in patients who received flucytosine for Candida endocarditis.

Hepatotoxicity is a well-known adverse event of terbinafine but the exact mechanisms remain to be identified. Toxicity to the liver seems to be both idiosyncratic and immune, as a metabolite of terbinafine was found to bind to hepatobiliary proteins and to induce an immune reaction; the primary pattern of DILI can either be hepatocellular or cholestatic, but typically evolves into a usually prolonged cholestatic pattern and may progress to the vanishing bile duct syndrome.

A prospective multicenter study concluded that DILI was an uncommon cause of acute liver failure with a preference to the female gender (71% women). Among 1198 acute liver failure subjects, 133 cases were attributed to DILI (11.1%) with 3 of them being associated with terbinafine use. A meta-analysis of the safety of oral antifungals in the treatment of superficial dermatophytosis and onychomycosis estimated that the probability of discontinuing terbinafine because of DILI was 0.34% (95% CI: 0.09–0.6); 0.70 (95% CI: 0.33–1.06) for itraconazole and

1.22 (95% CI: 0.00–5.30) for fluconazole. In a recent pharmacovigilance study 1964 cases of DILI most cases of DILI were attributed to terbinafine ($n = 422$; 27 with LF); the corresponding reporting odds ratio for liver failure among terbinafine recipients was 3.39 (95% CI: 2.32–4.96) [1R].

ALLYLAMINES [SEDA-36, 381; SEDA-37, 307; SEDA-38, 243]

Terbinafine [SEDA-36, 381; SEDA-37, 307; SEDA-38, 243]

Drug–Drug Interactions

A number of elegant review articles published in the past few years describe terbinafine's significant drug–drug interactions, particularly focusing on its strong inhibitory potential on CYP2D6. This enzyme is responsible for the metabolism of many beta-blockers and antidepressants which can lead to supratherapeutic levels of these medications when they are combined with terbinafine. Terbinafine can also lead to sub-therapeutic levels of tamoxifen, when combined with it because it inhibits the metabolism to the active metabolite of tamoxifen. Therefore, care should be taken whenever prescribing terbinafine to ensure these significant interactions are avoided [2r].

Amphotericin [SEDA-35, 483; SEDA-36, 382; SEDA-37, 307; SEDA-38, 244]

The safety of liposomal amphotericin was evaluated in a pharmacokinetics study of 40 pediatric patients who required antifungal therapy due to neutropenia. Doses administered included 2.5, 5, 7.5, and 10 mg/kg. A total of nine patients discontinued therapy due to adverse events and four of them were related to infusion-related reactions (11% of patients). There was a significant increase in serum creatinine levels. This increase in creatinine was more significant in patients that received doses >5 mg/kg/day. In addition, there was more hypokalemia and vomiting seen in doses of 10 mg/kg. Therefore, when using liposomal amphotericin doses >5 mg/kg in pediatric patients may be associated with a higher rate of side effects [3c].

A retrospective review of 33 Japanese patients, 65 years or older, with a hematologic malignancy who were being treated with liposomal amphotericin were compared to a group of 21 patients less than 65 years of age. No patients in the study discontinued therapy due to side effects, however, there was a two-time increase from baseline in creatinine, AST and ALT values in 21%, 39%, and 45.5%, respectively, compared to 38%, 62% and 52% in the younger cohort. Not surprisingly concomitant use of other nephrotoxic agents was a risk fact for the significant increases in creatinine. Based on these results liposomal amphotericin appears to have a similar safety profile whether patients are greater or less than 65 years of age [4c].

A retrospective review of 846 patients from South Africa who were treated with amphotericin B deoxycholate for HIV-associated cyptococcal meningitis were reviewed to establish the prevalence and monitoring of toxicities related to this antifungal therapy. Of the 846 patients 524 patients received amphotericin B deoxycholate and had complete record for review. In this patient population toxicity was seen commonly with the following rates anemia, 16% (86/524); hypokalemia, 43% (226/524) and nephrotoxicity, 32% (169/524). In the study monitoring occurred frequently with 64% ($n=333$) baseline labs, 40% ($n=211$) with pre-emptive hydration and 14% ($n=72$) with IV potassium and 19% ($n=101$) with oral. While on therapy 88% ($n=452$) of patients had fluid monitoring; 27% ($n=142$), 45% ($n=235$) and 44% ($n=232$) had hemoglobin, potassium and creatinine. Although toxicity with amphotericin B is common pre-emptive supportive care and close monitoring can help prevent serious side effects [5C].

Hepatic

The rate of hepatotoxicity in mice was evaluated when treatment doses of flucytosine and amphotericin B were combined. This combination is often used for treatment of Candida endocarditis in addition to Cryptococcal meningitis. There were three different dosing groups for the combination which included 50 mg/kg flucytosine and 300 μg/kg amphotericin B; 100 mg/kg flucytosine and 600 μg/kg amphotericin B; 150 mg/kg flucytosine and 900 μg/kg amphotericin B. The results of the study showed that this drug combination had a synergistic effect in increasing inflammation leading to hepatic toxicity also in a dose-dependent fashion. Therefore, when this combination has to be utilized to treat serious fungal infections the lowest possible dose should be utilized to decrease the risk for hepatic injury [6E].

A case of hepatotoxicity in an immunocompetent patient who was receiving Amphotericin B deoxycholate for bilateral renal fungal mycetomas due to Candida glabrata was reported. Typically amphotericin is associated with renal toxicity; however, there are some reports of hepatotoxicity. Many of the cases of hepatotoxicity are also in patients receiving chemotherapy and therefore it is difficult to discern if the hepatotoxicity is due to amphotericin or if it is due to the chemotherapy that the patients have received. In this case the patient was not on any other hepatotoxic medications along with the amphotericin. Early in the admission the patient had developed hepatic injury due to his multiple comorbidities and poor nutrition. The hepatic injury was improving until the patient received a dose of amphotericin when the patient suddenly developed worsening hepatotoxicity leading to discontinuation of the amphotericin. Although there may have been other causes for this hepatotoxicity caution should be utilized when administering this medication to patients with already existing hepatotoxicity [7A].

Antifungal Azoles [SEDA-33, 545; SEDA-34, 428; SEDA-35, 484; SEDA-36, 382; SEDA-37, 307; SEDA-38, 245]

For metronidazole see Chapter "Drugs Used in TB and Leprosy" by Meenakshi R. Ramanathan, James M. Sanders.

A major retrospective cohort study of 195 334 patients started on azole antifungal therapy was conducted to evaluate the incidence rate of acute liver injury in patients who received azole therapy. Of the 195 334 patients, 178 879 received fluconazole, 14 296 ketoconazole, 1653 itraconazole; 478 voriconazole, and 28 posaconazole. Overall fluconazole, ketoconazole and itraconazole were associated with the lowest incidence rates (events/1000 person-years [95% confidence intervals (CIs)]) of liver aminotransferases >200 U/L with (13.0 [11.4–14.6]), (19.3 [13.8–26.3]), and (24.5 [10.6–48.2]), respectively. Incident rates were much higher with voriconazole and posaconazole at (181.9 [112.6–278.0]) and (191.1 [23.1–690.4]). Similarly, severe acute liver injury was found to be relatively uncommon for patients on fluconazole (2.0 [1.4–2.7]), ketoconazole (2.9 [1.1–6.3]), and itraconazole (0.0 [0.0–11.2]); however, they were more frequently associated with voriconazole (16.7 [2.0–60.2]) and posaconazole (93.4 [2.4–520.6]). There was one patient in the study that developed acute liver failure due to ketoconazole. Not surprisingly, having pre-existing chronic liver disease was found to increase the risks of aminotransferases >200 U/L (hazard ratio 4.68 [95% CI, 3.68–5.94]) and severe acute liver injury (hazard ratio 5.62 [95% CI, 2.56–12.35]) [8MC].

Fluconazole [SEDA-33, 551; SEDA-34, 430; SEDA-35, 485; SEDA-36, 382; SEDA-37, 307; SEDA-38, 245]

Skin

A case of generalized exanthem trigged by fluconazole was reported in a 44-year-old women. The patient began taking clotrimazole 1% cream for anogenital itch and developed severe itching and redness in her groin area. The cream was discontinued and her physician changed to fluconazole 150 mg orally once. 48 hours after taking the fluconazole she broke out with widespread exanthem requiring the patient to be admission to the hospital and put on a 3 week steroid taper. After the event allergy patch testing was done which showed the patient was allergic to clotrimazole, methylisothiazolinone and methylchloroisothiazoline. The latter two items were in her baby wipes that she was using during the time of the allergic reaction. The patient was not tested for fluconazole allergy. Given the reaction worsened after administration of the clotrimazole there may be cross reactivity among topical and systemic azole antifungals [9A].

A case of a 23-year-old man who presented with erythematous and edematous plaques around his right axilla and above his right eyebrow. The patient noticed these skin lesions about 24 hours after taking a 300 mg dose of fluconazole for the treatment of tinea versicolor. He was taking no other medications at the time. His antifungal treatment was changed to itraconazole and his fixed drug eruption resolved [10A].

A randomized controlled trial was conducted of 240 patients who were treated with two doses of clotrimazole vaginal tablet 500 mg or two doses of oral fluconazole 150 mg for severe vulvovaginal candidiasis (SVVC) was conducted. The study looked at both safety and efficacy of the different treatment regiments. Clinical and mycological cure rates were similar for both regimens at both 7–14 days as well as 30–35 days. There were no differences in adverse events between the two agents and clotrimazole had mostly topical related side effects. Therefore, it appears either regimen is safe and effective for treatment of SVVC [11C].

Pregnancy

A retrospective review of 1 405 663 pregnancies from a Denmark registry were reviewed to assess for the risk of still birth. All pregnant patients were exposed to oral fluconazole during their pregnancy. These patients were matched with up to 4 pregnancies in which no exposure to fluconazole occurred. Among the 3315 women exposed to oral fluconazole ranging from 7 through 22 weeks' gestation, 147 experienced a spontaneous abortion. This result is compared with 563 among 13 246 unexposed matched women. This shows was a significantly increased risk of spontaneous abortion associated with fluconazole exposure (HR, 1.48; 95% CI, 1.23–1.77). In addition, among 5382 women exposed to fluconazole from gestational week 7 to birth, 21 experienced a stillbirth, compared with 77 among 21 506 unexposed matched women. Therefore, there was no association between fluconazole exposure and stillbirth (HR, 1.32 [95% CI, 0.82–2.14]). Based on the results of this study, providers should proceed with caution when prescribing fluconazole in pregnancy given the increase risk of spontaneous abortion seen in this study [12MC].

Itraconazole [SED-15, 1969; SEDA-33, 552; SEDA-34, 430; SEDA-35, 485; SEDA-36, 38; SEDA-37, 307]

A randomized controlled trial of 153 patients was conducted to assess the safety and efficacy of IV itraconazole in comparison to micafungin for empiric antifungal therapy in neutropenic patients with hematologic malignancies. The primary endpoint of treatment success, which was a composite of breakthrough invasive fungal infection, survival, premature discontinuation, defervescence and time to baseline fungal infection. There was a 7% point higher success rate in the micafungin group (64.4% vs 57.3%, $P = 0.404$), which met the criteria for non-inferiority. Serious grade 3 adverse events included hyperbilirubinemia (2 vs 7), elevation of transaminase levels (2 vs 4), electrolyte imbalance (1 vs 2), atrial fibrillation (1 vs 0), and anaphylaxis (1 vs 0) which occurred in 7 and 13 patients in the micafungin (10.4%) and itraconazole (18.8%) groups, respectively. Therefore, the authors of the study concluded that micafungin had favorable success rates with lower toxicity profile when compared to itraconazole, for febrile neutropenia in patients with hematological malignancies [13C].

Hepatotoxicity

A case of severe hepatotoxicity leading to hepatic failure, likely due to itraconazole, was reported in the literature. The patient had been receiving itraconazole for about 6 months for treatment of histoplasmosis. The patient's itraconazole levels were within therapeutic range (5 mg/mL). Typically, hepatotoxicity seen with intraconazole is in patients with elevated levels; however, this was not the case with this patient. The patient's aspartate transaminase levels were >20 times the upper limit of normal with their alanine transaminase reaching >15 times upper limit normal. The Naranjo probability scale and the Roussel Uclaf causality assessment method were used to assess the likelihood of itraconazole causing this toxicity. The Naranjo score found the relationship to be "probable" and "highly probable" in the case of the Roussel Uclaf assessment [14A].

Isavuconazole [SEDA-37, 307; SEDA-38, 246]

See Section Drug–Drug Interactions. There are no new studies or reports of side effects related to isavuconazole at this time.

Ketoconazole [SEDA-34, 430; SEDA-35, 486; SEDA-36, 383; SEDA-37, 307; SEDA-38, 246]

A retrospective review of all published literature related to ketoconazole drug interaction studies was conducted to evaluate the risks of ketoconazole-induced hepatotoxicity in these studies given the new warnings by the U.S. Food and Drug Administration (FDA) and the European Medicines Agency (EMA). Recently these agencies recommend against the use of these agents for drug interaction studies, which it has been the main stay of doing for some time now. In the drug interaction studies reviewed there were a total of 2355 participants who were treated for a median of 6 days. Of these patients only 40 participants were reported to have increased liver transaminase activity (1.7%), and no deaths were reported or associated with ketoconazole. In studies investigating ketoconazole treatment, patients were treated for 276 days (median), and 5.6% of patients had elevated liver enzyme activity. Likely because patients are treated for a much shorter duration in the drug interaction studies that is why the risk of drug-induced hepatic injury was shown to be very low. Based on this review ketoconazole could still be used as a CYP3A inhibitor for drug interaction studies without the risk of compromising the safety of the volunteers [15M].

One of the remaining uses of ketoconazole therapy is treatment of Cushing's disease. Given one of the side effects associated with ketoconazole use is QTc prolongation which can increased the risk for torsade de pointes. Patients with Cushing's may be at a higher risk for prolonged QTc given these patients often have hypokalemia and left ventricular hypertrophy. This study sought to review whether utilizing ketoconazole in this patient population puts them at an increased risk for QTc prolongation. The electrocardiograms of 15 patients with Cushing's disease receiving ketoconazole for treatment were reviewed. QTc values were done before and during ketoconazole treatment and other medications the patients were receiving were reviewed. On average, QTc was not significantly changed from before and after ketoconazole treatment (393.2 ± 7.17 vs 403.3 ± 6.05 ms in women; 424.3 ± 23.54 vs 398.0 ± 14.93 ms in men, N.S.) even in the context of other QT-prolonging drugs. Based on this review long-term use of ketoconazole in patients with Cushing's disease does not appear to be associated with significant prolongation of QT interval [16c].

Posaconazole [SEDA-33, 553; SEDA-34, 430; SEDA-35, 486; SEDA-36, 383; SEDA-37, 307; SEDA-38, 247]

There was a case of severe QT prolongation reported in a patient receiving posaconazole. The patient was a 26-year-old female who underwent surgery to remove calcifications on her left hip joint. After the procedure there was concern for post-surgical wound infection as the patient's clinical status worsened. The patient was started on broad spectrum antibiotics and when the clinical status did not improve amphotericin was added for concern of possible fungal etiology. After 9 days of treatment the patient was having persistant hypokalemia which prompted the switch from amphotericin to voriconazole. After 9 days of voriconazole therapy was changed to posaconazole, for reasons not documented in the case. Thirty-six hours after the dose of posaconazole was given the patient developed bradycardia and QT prolongation with normal electrolytes. The patient developed a cardiac arrest and had to be transferred to the cardiac ICU for continued episodes of cardiac arrest due to torsad des pointes that degenerated to lethal ventricular fibrillation. The posaconazole was discontinued and a temporary pacemaker was placed. QT prolongation has been associated with the azole class of antifungals; however, cases of torsad des pointes (TdP) remain limited in the literature. The most common agent to cause this per literature reports is voriconazole, which this patient did receive prior to the posaconazole. However, it seems likely that posaconazole was the cause for the QT interval prolongation and episodes of TdP either by itself or combined with voriconazole. The authors conclude this because the patient was treated with voriconazole for 9 days without an issue and the bradycardia and cardiac arrest occurred 36 hours after the first dose of posaconazole and approximately 48 hours after the last voriconazole dose. Based on half-lives posaconazole which is 20–35 hours and voriconazole which is about 9 hours it is unlikely there would be significant voriconazole present 48 hours later. Based on this case it is important to monitor for QT changes while on posaconazole and try to avoid combining it with other QT prolonging agents [17A].

Voriconazole [SEDA-33, 554; SEDA-34, 431; SEDA-35, 486; SEDA-36, 384; SEDA-37, 307; SEDA-38, 247]

A prospective study was done on AML patients undergoing chemotherapy who received voriconazole for antifungal prophylaxis to assess the safety and efficacy. A total of 75 patients with AML were included in the study for receiving voriconazole as prophylaxis. The overall incidence of proven/probable/possible (ppp) invasive fungal infection was found to be 6.6% (5/75). Voriconazole in comparison to fluconazole reduced the incidence of ppp invasive fungal infection (5/75, 6.6% vs 19/66, 29%; $P < 0.001$) and reduced mortality due to invasive fungal infection (1/75, 1.3% vs 6/66, 9%; $P = 0.0507$), but this was not significant. Only 3 patients discontinued voriconazole due to side effects.

Therefore, this study adds to the existing data that voriconazole is a safe and effective medication for prevention of invasive fungal infection in patients receiving chemotherapy [18c].

Voriconazole's use since its approval in 2002 has continued to increase due to its ability to treat a host of fungal infections without significant toxicity. With the significant amount of data now available we have seen the emergence of additional side effects that are related to the voriconazole use. To summarize this data a review was conducted which searched all available literature and voriconazole-related adverse effects. Many of the common adverse events such as cutaneous malignancies, arrhythmias, periostitis, neurologic effects, alopecia and nail changes were reported with their associated cases in the literature. It is important to continue to be aware of the side effects related to voriconazole so that patients can be monitored closely when they are receiving prolonged courses like many of the immunocompromised patients [19M].

The intravenous (IV) formulation of voriconazole is formulated with a product called cyclodextrin which may be related to nephrotoxicity particularly with patients with CrCl <50 mL/min. However, more recent reports show that a derivative of cyclodextrin, sulfobutylether β-cyclodextrin (SBECD), does not lead to nephrotoxicity in humans. Therefore, this prospective observational study was conducted on 25 hematologic malignancy patients who received IV voriconazole for treatment of invasive aspergillosis to assess the risk of nephrotoxicity. The frequency of severe adverse events in cases (3/7) was comparable to that of controls (4/18; $P = 0.355$). No patients had significant deterioration in renal function after the voriconazole therapy even in those patients with existing renal impairment. Although CrCl <50 mL/min was associated with higher voriconazole concentrations, its clinical impact remains unclear. Based on this study the SBECD-formulated intravenous voriconazole did not lead to a higher incidence of severe adverse events including nephrotoxicity in hematological patients with CrCl <50 mL/min [20c].

Sensory System

Two pediatric patients who developed neurologic side effects on voriconazole were presented. One patient was 9 years old and the other was 17 years old. The 9-year-old boy was a patient with cystic fibrosis who was being treated for invasive aspergillosis. While receiving the voriconazole the patient developed photophobia, altered color sensation, and fearful visual hallucination. The second patient also had cystic fibrosis and was being treated with voriconazole for allergic bronchopulmonary aspergillosis. Her neurologic side effects included photophobia, fatigue, impaired concentration, and insomnia. These side effects occurred when the dose of voriconazole therapy was increased from 12 to 16 mg/kg/day. After the voriconazole was discontinued the side effects resolved. In these two cases serum voriconazole concentration were not measured and that could have been helpful to prevent these toxicities as they are often seen with supratherapeutic levels of voriconazole [21A].

Skin

Voriconazole use has been associated with an increased risk of developing cutaneous squamous cell carcinoma (SCC). There is not clear guidance on how often this side effect occurs and when voriconazole should not be utilized to avoid this risk. Therefore, this retrospective cohort study of 455 lung transplant patients who received voriconazole for prophylaxis was conducted to evaluate the risk of developing SCC. Overall in this study voriconazole exposure was associated with a 73% increased risk of developing SCC (hazard ratio [HR] 1.73; 95% confidence interval [CI]: 1.04–2.88; $P = 0.03$). This risk was increased by 3.0% (HR 1.03; 95% CI: 1.02–1.04; $P < 0.001$) with each additional 30-day exposure. Voriconazole exposure reduced risk of Aspergillus colonization by 50% (HR 0.50; 95% CI: 0.34–0.72; $P < 0.001$). Cases of invasive aspergillosis infection were not measured given the small sample size. Voriconazole exposure significantly reduced all-cause mortality among subjects who developed Aspergillus colonization (HR 0.34; 95% CI: 0.13–0.91; $P = 0.03$) but had no significant impact on those without colonization. Voriconazole is effective in decreasing mortality in lung transplant patients who are colonized with Aspergillus, however, those benefits should be weighed with the increased risk of developing SCC when utilizing voriconazole long-term [22C].

Periostitis

Cases of voriconazole-induced periostitis continue to be reported. Voriconazole preparations contain fluoride and the mechanism of this adverse effect has been linked to the accumulation of fluoride which usually results in elevated levels in patients on therapy for at least 6 months. In most cases, the periostitis and fluoride accumulation ceases once voriconazole is stopped.

Fluoride integrates as fluorapatite into the bone crystal structure and promotes bone formation by stimulating osteoblasts. The integration of fluorapatite into bone causes alterations in bone crystal size and structure, making these more resistant to resorption. Ultimately this increases bone density and leads to osteosclerosis associated with brittleness, exostoses, pain, decreased mechanical competence of bone and increased susceptibility to fractures [23C].

Fluoride intoxication resembles hypertrophic osteoarthropathy and periostitis deformans, and several common features have been observed in skeletal imaging. Symmetric diffuse periosteal reactions including osteosclerosis and hyperostotic periostitis have been described together with osteoporosis, ligamentous calcification and periarticular changes; these have been located in various parts of the skeleton. Contrary to hypertrophic osteoarthropathy, voriconazole-induced periostitis is strongly associated with an elevated alkaline phosphatase and shows characteristically no digital clubbing [23C,24H].

Several etiological explanations may be considered for voriconazole-associated fluorosis. Fluorine is organically bound in voriconazole and hepatic oxidative metabolism may increase unbound fluoride levels after extensive voriconazole administration. Pharmacogenomic variations, especially polymorphisms in CYP2C19 enzyme may further alleviate this phenomena. Secondly, renal insufficiency or failure may increase the risk for toxicity during fluorine exposure, since its renal clearance is dependent on the patient's renal function [24H].

Periostitis Cases

Many of the cases of periostitis are in immunosuppressed patients including transplant and oncology patients. There are limited reports of periostitis in non-immunosuppressed patients. A case was presented of a 62-year-old male who presented with 3 months of increasingly painful nodules on his forearms and right hand. The patient had been receiving suppressive voriconazole for suppressive therapy of a *Candida glabrata* infection of the abdominal aortic stent-graft infection secondary to aortoduodenal fistula. The patient had been on voriconazole for 3 years prior to presenting with the bone pain and soft tissue nodules. Radiographic images were obtained which showed multifocal fluffy and nodular periostitis. A whole-body bone scan was also obtained, which revealed a multifocal increased radiotracer uptake throughout the axial and appendicular skeleton. This case demonstrates that periostitis can occur with anyone taking voriconazole and not just immunosuppressed patients [25A].

A case of voriconazole-induced periostitis in a allogenic hematopoietic stem cell transplant recipient was recently reported. The patient was receiving a low dose of voriconazole relative to what is typically presented in the literature. The patient was a 24-year-old male with paroxysmal nocturnal hemoglobinuria (PNH) who underwent a matched sibling allogeneic HSCT at our center, in May 2014. On day +47 post-transplant, the patient presented with gradually progressive, painful swellings over right ring finger. On physical examination, there were bony swellings in over the right ring finger which were mildly tender, but with no associated erythema. CT scan was done which showed bony swellings in areas corresponding to the clinical presentation and diffuse osteopenia along with multiple medullary transverse lines suggestive of healed stress fractures. Tc-99 MDP

bone scan showed increased tracer uptake in the right ring finger, proximal one-third of right tibia, mid shaft of left tibia, and left lateral malleolus. A urinary fluoride level was done which came out to be 1.76 ppm (normal <1 ppm). The patient had been on a very low dose of only 100 mg daily of voriconazole with for a total of 132 days prior to presentation. The cumulative dose of 26.4 g of voriconazole, whereas the lowest cumulative dosage described in literature is 55 g. Given voriconazole as the possible cause the patient was changed to itraconazole and had a complete resolution of his bony swellings in a period of 4 months. In India, where the patient lived, there is excess amounts of fluoride in the ground which was thought to have put the patient at an increased risk of developing periostitis. This should be taken into account and monitored closely in patients receiving long-term voriconazole [26A].

A retrospective observational study was done to characterize the frequency and clinical presentation of patients presenting with pain and fluoride excess in allogenic hematopoietic stem cell transplant (HSCT) recipient on voriconazole. With this information the authors hoped to identify when a plasma fluoride concentration was measured with respect to voriconazole initiation and onset of pain, and to describe the outcomes of patients with fluoride excess in the setting of HSCT. Of the 31 patients with fluoride measurement while on voriconazole, 29 (93.5%) had elevated fluoride levels. The median time to fluoride measurement was 128 days after voriconazole initiation (range, 28–692). At 1 year after the start of voriconazole, 15.3% of patients had developed pain associated with voriconazole use and 35.7% developed pain while on voriconazole after 2 years. Of the patients with an elevated fluoride level, 22 discontinued voriconazole. Pain resolved or improved in 15 of the patients, stabilized in 3, and worsened in 4 patients. Serum creatinine, estimated glomerular filtration rate, alkaline phosphatase, and voriconazole concentration did not predict for fluoride excess and associated pain. This review helps characterize the risk of periostitis in HSCT patients and helps providers better monitor for this side effect so that alternative antifungal agents with a lower risk for fluoride excess can be considered in patients receiving voriconazole who develop fluoride excess and pain [27c].

℞ Special Review

Drug–Drug Interactions and Pharmacogenomics of the Azoles Antifungal

Since many of the azole antifungals affect the hepatic cytochrome P450 system there are a large number of drug–drug interactions with many of these agents. Because of the large number of drug–drug interactions associated with the azole antifungals it is important to always review all medications, both prescription and over-the-counter, whenever starting a patient on an azole antifungal. The chart later shows the extent of the interactions with cytochrome P450 system that are commonly associated with drug interactions and the different azole antifungals effect on those cytochromes.

The other important factor that affects the potential severity with these drug–drug interactions involved pharmacogenomics. As discussed briefly in Section "Terbinafine", some individuals are classified as poor metabolizers or rapid metabolizers of certain cytochrome P450 enzyme systems. Depending on the patient's pharmacogenomics and therefore ability to metabolize certain medications through the CYP 450 system they may be at risk of being undertreated by a certain medication or potentially being over treated and therefore at risk for developing more side effects [28H,29R].

Voriconazole, in particular, has been one of the most difficult azoles to utilize effective dosing strategies because of the significant intra-patient variability in plasma concentrations due to nonlinear pharmacokinetics and patient characteristics such as age, sex, weight, liver disease, and genetic polymorphisms in the cytochrome P450 2C19 gene (CYP2C19) encoding for the CYP2C19 enzyme. The largest portion in variability in voriconazole dosing is the CYP2C19 polymorphisms and therefore it may be important, especially from an efficacy standpoint, to test CYP2C19 genotypes to help optimize the efficacy of voriconazole while decreasing the toxicity [29R].

A study done in pediatric patients in Japan highlight that there is a value to identifying these polymorphisms because they found there is an association between voriconazole plasma concentrations and the CYP2C19 phenotype. In this study 37 pediatric patients who had voriconazole plasma concentrations measured and were categorized as normal metabolizers, intermediate metabolizers, poor metabolizers, or hypermetabolizers based on genotype testing were retrospectively reviewed. Trough plasma concentrations of voriconazole were statistically significantly higher in the poor metabolizer and intermediate metabolizer groups compared with the normal metabolizer and hypermetabolizer groups

($P = 0.004$). Syndromes of inappropriate antidiuretic hormone secretion and cardiac toxicities were experienced by two patients in the high voriconazole concentration group. Dose adjustment based on CYP2C19 phenotype therefore may be useful during voriconazole therapy to improve efficacy and avoid toxicity. Japanese children, in particular, may benefit from this since they have a higher incidence of the poor metabolizer and intermediate metabolizer phenotypes as a group [30c].

Buprenorphine

A randomized, placebo-controlled crossover study with 12 healthy volunteers was conducted to evaluate the risk of developing toxicity from the drug–drug interaction between buprenorphine and either voriconazole or posaconazole. Patients in the study were given a dose of 0.4 mg (0.6 mg during placebo phase) sublingual buprenorphine after 5 days of oral placebo, voriconazole 400 mg twice daily on the first day and 200 mg twice daily, thereafter, or posaconazole 400 mg twice daily. Concentrations of buprenorphine and its primary active metabolite norbuprenorphine were monitored in the plasma and urine over 18 hours. In addition, the pharmacological effects were also measured. Voriconazole increased the mean area under the plasma concentration-time curve of buprenorphine 1.80-fold (90% confidence interval 1.45–2.24; $P < 0.001$), the peak concentration 1.37-fold ($P < 0.013$) and half-life 1.37-fold ($P < 0.001$) compared to placebo. Posaconazole increased the mean area under the plasma concentration-time curve of buprenorphine 1.25-fold ($P < 0.001$). Voriconazole, unlike posaconazole, increased the urinary excretion of norbuprenorphine 1.58-fold (90% confidence interval 1.18–2.12; $P < 0.001$) but there was no quantifiable parent buprenorphine in urine. Voriconazole, and to a lesser extent posaconazole, increase plasma exposure to sublingual buprenorphine, likely via the inhibition of cytochrome P450 and possibly via P-glycoprotein. Providers should use caution when using azole antifungals specifically voriconazole

This figure highlights some of the most common cytochrome P450 enzymes that are affected by antifungals and therefore are important to be aware of for pharmacogenomics differences as well as drug–drug interactions [28H,29R].

	CYP3A4		CYP2C9		CYP2C19	
	Substrate	Inhibitor	Substrate	Inhibitor	Substrate	Inhibitor
Fluconazole		Moderate		Moderate		Strong
Itraconazole	Major	Strong				
Voriconazole	Minor	Strong	Major	Moderate	Major	Moderate
Posaconazole		Strong				
Ketoconazole	Major	Strong		Moderate		Moderate
Miconazole						
Isavuconazole	Major	Moderate				Weak

in patients on buprenorphine given the interactions that can lead to adverse effects [31c].

Edoxaban

A drug interaction study was performed with edoxaban, a new factor Xa inhibitor, and ketoconazole. Because edoxaban is a substrate of cytochrome P450 3A4 and the efflux transporter P-glycoprotein (P-gp) there is concern with significant drug–drug interactions. In this study, healthy subjects received a single oral dose of 60 mg edoxaban with ketoconazole 400 mg once daily for 7 days and edoxaban on day 4. Co-administration of ketoconazole increased edoxaban total exposure by 87% and the peak concentration by 89% compared with edoxaban alone. The half-life remained unchanged. No clinically significant adverse events were observed. Administration of ketoconazole increased edoxaban exposure; however, no side effects were seen in this short pharmacokinetic study [32E].

ISAVUCONAZOLE

Isavuconazole, a new azole antifungal, was evaluated in a drug–drug interaction study with rifampin, ketoconazole, midazolam, and ethinyl estradiol/norethindrone in healthy adults. Because isavuconazole is metabolized by CYP3A4 this study sough to evaluate the interactions with this antifungal and other medications that are metabolized through the CYP system. In the study, isavuconazole oral (100 mg once daily) was administered with oral rifampin (600 mg once daily). Not surprisingly, given rifampin is a CYP3A4 inducer this combination resulted in a decreased isavuconazole area under the concentration-time curve by 90% and maximum concentration (C_{max}) by 75%. Whereas the coadministration of isavuconazole (200 mg single dose) with oral ketoconazole, a known CYP3A4 inhibitor, (200 mg twice daily) increased isavuconazole AUC and C_{max} by 422% and 9%, respectively. Next isavuconazole was coadministered (200 mg three times daily for 2 days, then 200 mg once daily) with single doses of oral midazolam, a known CYP3A4 substrate, (3 mg) or another 3A4 substrate ethinyl estradiol/norethindrone (35 µg/1 mg). Following coadministration, AUC increased 103% for midazolam, 8% for ethinyl estradiol, and 16% for norethindrone. The C_{max} increased by 72%, 14%, and 6%, respectively. No serious adverse effects leading to study discontinuation or deaths were reported. Some mild to moderate in intensity side effects were reported. Based on this study isavuconazole is a substrate and moderate inhibitor of CYP3A4 and should be used with caution when co-administered with inhibitors, inducers and substrates of 3A4 [33E].

Statins

Statins such as atorvastatin, simvastatin and other HMG-CoA reductase inhibitors and azole antifungals have known drug–drug interactions. Reports of these interactions continue to be published in the literature.

One particular case was a 47-year-old woman who had been treated with high-dose simvastatin for several years. After starting itraconazole for treatment of a fungal infection she developed muscle pain, elevated creatinine kinase and myoglobin. A muscle biopsy was compatible with statin-associated rhabdomyolysis. Once the itraconazole was stopped the patient's symptoms resolved. Simvastatin in addition to other statins such as atorvastatin and lovastatin are metabolized by the liver enzyme CYP3A4. This drug interaction was likely the cause of this patient's reaction given itraconazole is a known inhibitor of CYP3A4. It is not recommended to use these antifungals systemically if the patient is on a statin. It is recommended that another statin agent is utilized or temporarily discontinued until the antifungal treatment is complete [34A].

Another case of rhabdomyolysis in a patient on fluconazole and atorvastatin was presented. A case of a 70-year-old woman who was receiving atorvastatin for hyperlipidaemia without any problem for 4 years was presented. The patient was started on intravenous fluconazole for treatment of a fungal infection. After 2 weeks of the fluconazole and atorvastatin the patient developed rhabdomyolysis. At that time atorvastatin was stopped which resolved the patient's rhabdomyolysis. This is another case of why these statin agents should be separated from azole antifungals [35A].

Voriconazole has been associated with cases of cholestatic hepatitis. A case of a 44-year-old man who was on voriconazole for a year for treatment of pulmonary aspergillosis was started on 30 mg lansoprazole for gastroesophageal reflux symptoms. Five days after starting the lansoprazole, the patient developed fatigue, jaundice, and cholestatic hepatitis. The lansoprazole was stopped and soon after the hepatitis promptly resolved. Sixteen months after this event occurred the patient was started on simvastatin therapy. Two weeks after taking simvastatin the patient developed new onset fatigue, jaundice, and cholestatic hepatitis. As discussed previously voriconazole is metabolized by both CYP2C19 and CYP3A4. Lansoprazole is an inhibitor of the CYP2C19. The competition between voriconazole and lansoprazole likely led to increased voriconazole serum concentration and acute cholestatic hepatitis in this patient. Simvastatin a known inhibitor of CYP3A4 likely inhibited voriconazole metabolism which is represented by the voriconazole concentration remaining elevated (4.1 µg/mL) when measured 15 days after stopping simvastatin. Based on the Naranjo Adverse Drug Reaction Probability Scale score of 7 revealed that the cholestatic hepatitis was probably precipitated by lansoprazole. In terms of the simvastatin the patient's Naranjo score of 9 also revealed that cholestatic hepatitis was likely due to simvastatin being added to voriconazole [36A].

Pyrimadine Analogues [SEDA-36, 383; SEDA-37, 307; SEDA-38, 251]

Flucytosine

There are no new studies or reports of side effects related to flucytosine at this time.

ECHINOCANDINS [SEDA-33, 556; SEDA-34, 434; SEDA-35, 489; SEDA-36, 388; SEDA-37, 307; SEDA-38, 251]

Micafungin [SEDA-35, 489; SEDA-36, 388; SEDA-37, 307; SEDA-38, 251]

A case of a patient who was on micafungin for oesophageal candidiasis presented with polymorphic ventricular tachycardia. This is the first known case of polymorphic ventricular tachycardia with micafungin as the possible cause. There have been other cases of arrhythmias related to echinocandin use reported in the literature, however, no cases of polymorphic ventricular tachycardia. Providers should be aware of this potential adverse event and monitor patients receiving concomitant drugs that can prolong QT interval [37A].

Overall echinocandins are well tolerated; however, there have been reports of renal and hepatic adverse effects with micafungin. This study was a retrospective cohort study to evaluate the risk of developing hepatic or renal injury while on therapy. A total of 2970 micafungin recipients were matched to 6726 recipients of comparator parenteral antifungal agents. Baseline characteristics were similar between the two groups. There were similar rates of hepatic injury (micafungin, 13 events per 100 patients compared to 12 per 100 for other parenteral antifungals; HR = 0.99; 95% CI 0.86–1.14). There were lower rates of renal injury with micafungin, 63 events per 100 patients compared to other parenteral antimicrobial agents, 65 per 100; HR = 0.93; 95% CI 0.87–0.99) [38C].

Anidulafungin [SEDA-35, 489; SEDA-36, 388; SEDA-37, 307; SEDA-38, 252]

There are no new studies or reports of side effects related to anidulafungin at this time.

Caspofungin [SEDA-33, 556; SEDA-34, 434; SEDA-35, 490; SEDA-36, 389; SEDA-37, 307; SEDA-38, 252]

There are no new studies or reports of side effects related to caspofungin at this time.

References

[1] Kyriakidis I, Tragiannidis A, Munchen S, et al. Clinical hepatotoxicity associated with antifungal agents. Expert Opin Drug Saf. 2017;16:149–65 [R].

[2] Dürrbeck A, Nenoff P. Terbinafine: relevant drug interactions and their management. Hautarzt. 2016;67(9):718–23 [r].

[3] Seibel NL, Shad AT, et al. Safety, tolerability, and pharmacokinetics of liposomal amphotericin B in immunocompromised pediatric patients. Antimicrob Agents Chemother. 2017;61:e01477-16 [c].

[4] Ueda S, Miyamoto S, et al. Safety and efficacy of treatment with liposomal amphotericin B in elderly patients at least 65 years old with hematological diseases. J Infect Chemother. 2016;22(5):287–91 [c].

[5] Meiring S, Fortuin-de Smidt M, et al. Prevalence and hospital management of amphotericin B deoxycholate-related toxicities during treatment of HIV associated cryptococcal meningitis in South Africa. PLoS Negl Trop Dis. 2016;10(7): e0004865 [C].

[6] Folk A, Cotoraci C, et al. Evaluation of hepatotoxicity with treatment doses of flucytosine and amphotericin B for invasive fungal infections. Biomed Res Int. 2016;2016:5398730 [E].

[7] Wagner JL, Bell AM. Acute hepatic injury with amphotericin B deoxycholate in an immunocompetent patient. J Pharmacol Pharmacother. 2016;7(2):112–4 [A].

[8] Lo Re 3rd V, Carbonari DM, et al. Oral azole antifungal medications and risk of acute liver injury, overall and by chronic liver disease status. Am J Med. 2016;129(3): 283-91.e5 [MC].

[9] Nasir S, Goldsmith P. Anogenital allergic contact dermatitis caused by methylchloroisothiazolinone, methylisothiazolinone and topical clotrimazole with subsequent generalized exanthem triggered by oral fluconazole. Contact Dermatitis. 2016;74(5):296–7 [A].

[10] Lai O, Hsu S. Fixed drug eruption related to fluconazole. Dermatol Online J. 2016;22(4):18 [A].

[11] Zhou X, Li T, et al. The efficacy and safety of clotrimazole vaginal tablet vs. oral fluconazole in treating severe vulvovaginal candidiasis. Mycoses. 2016;59(7):419–28 [C].

[12] Mølgaard-Nielsen D, Svanström H, et al. Association between use of oral fluconazole during pregnancy and risk of spontaneous abortion and stillbirth. JAMA. 2016;315(1):58–67 [MC].

[13] Jeong SH, Kim DY, et al. Efficacy and safety of micafungin versus intravenous itraconazole as empirical antifungal therapy for febrile neutropenic patients with hematological malignancies: a randomized, controlled, prospective, cmulticenter study. Ann Hematol. 2016;95(2):337–44 [C].

[14] Pettit NN, Pisano J, Weber S, et al. Hepatic failure in a patient receiving itraconazole for pulmonary histoplasmosis-case report and literature review. Am J Ther. 2016;23(5):e1215–21 [A].

[15] Outeiro N, Hohmann N, Mikus G. No increased risk of ketoconazole toxicity in drug-drug interaction studies. J Clin Pharmacol. 2016;56(10):1203–11 [M].

[16] De Martin M, Toja PM, Goulene K, et al. No untoward effect of long-term ketoconazole administration on electrocardiographic QT interval in patients with Cushing's disease. Basic Clin Pharmacol Toxicol. 2016;118(4):279–83 [c].

[17] Panos G, Velissaris D, Karamouzos V, et al. Long QT syndrome leading to multiple cardiac arrests after posaconazole administration in an immune-compromised patient with sepsis: an unusual case report. Am J Case Rep. 2016;17:295–300 [A].

[18] Shah A, Ganesan P, Radhakrishnan V, et al. Voriconazole is a safe and effective anti-fungal prophylactic agent during induction therapy of acute myeloid leukemia. Indian J Med Paediatr Oncol. 2016;37(1):53–8 [c].

[19] Levine MT, Chandrasekar PH. Adverse effects of voriconazole: over a decade of use. Clin Transplant. 2016;30(11):1377–86 [M].

[20] Kim SH, Kwon JC, Park C, et al. Therapeutic drug monitoring and safety of intravenous voriconazole formulated with sulfobutylether β-cyclodextrin in haematological patients with renal impairment. Mycoses. 2016;59(10):644–51 [c].

[21] Demir SÖ, Atici S, Akkoç G, et al. Neurologic adverse events associated with voriconazole therapy: report of two pediatric cases. Case Rep Infect Dis. 2016;2016:3989070 [A].

[22] Mansh M, Binstock M, Williams K, et al. Voriconazole exposure and risk of cutaneous squamous cell carcinoma, aspergillus colonization, invasive aspergillosis and death in lung transplant recipients. Am J Transplant. 2016;16(1): 262–70 [C].

[23] Lindsay R. Fluoride and bone—quantity versus quality. N Engl J Med. 1990;322(12):845–6 [C].

[24] Whitford GM. Intake and metabolism of fluoride. Adv Dent Res. 1994;8(1):5–14 [H].

[25] Reber JD, McKenzie GA, Broski SM. Voriconazole-induced periostitis: beyond post-transplant patients. Skeletal Radiol. 2016;45(6):839–42 [A].

[26] Thekkudan SF, Kumar P, Nityanand S. Voriconazole-induced skeletal fluorosis in an allogenic hematopoietic stem cell transplant recipient. Ann Hematol. 2016;95(4):669–70 [A].

[27] Barajas MR, McCullough KB, Merten JA, et al. Correlation of pain and fluoride concentration in allogeneic hematopoietic stem cell transplant recipients on voriconazole. Biol Blood Marrow Transplant. 2016;22(3):579–83 [c].

[28] Ashbee HR, Gilleece MH. Has the era of individualized medicine arrived for antifungals? A review of antifungal pharmacogenomics. Bone Marrow Transplant. 2012;47(7):881–94 [H].

[29] Owusu Obeng A, Egelund EF, Alsultan A, et al. CYP2C19 polymorphisms and therapeutic drug monitoring of voriconazole: are we ready for the clinical implication of pharmacogenomics? Pharmacotherapy. 2014;34(7):703–18 [R].

[30] Narita A, Muramatsu H, Sakaguchi H. Correlation of CYP2C19 phenotype with voriconazole plasma concentration in children. J Pediatr Hematol Oncol. 2013;35(5):e219–23 [c].

[31] Fihlman M, Hemmilä T, Hagelberg NM, et al. Voriconazole more likely than posaconazole increases plasma exposure to sublingual buprenorphine causing a risk of a clinically important interaction. Eur J Clin Pharmacol. 2016;72(11):1363–71 [c].

[32] Parasrampuria DA, Mendell J, Shi M, et al. Edoxaban drug-drug interactions with ketoconazole, erythromycin, and cyclosporine. Br J Clin Pharmacol. 2016;82(6):1591–600 [E].

[33] Townsend R, Dietz A, Hale C, et al. Pharmacokinetic evaluation of CYP3A4-mediated drug-drug interactions of isavuconazole with rifampin, ketoconazole, midazolam, and ethinyl estradiol/ norethindrone in healthy adults. Clin Pharmacol Drug Dev. 2017;6(1):44–53 [E].

[34] Dybro AM, Damkier P, Rasmussen TB, et al. Statin-associated rhabdomyolysis triggered by drug-drug interaction with itraconazole. BMJ Case Rep. 2016;2016, http://dx.doi.org/10.1136/bcr-2016-216457 [A].

[35] Hsiao SH, Chang HJ, Hsieh TH, et al. Rhabdomyolysis caused by the moderate CYP3A4 inhibitor fluconazole in a patient on stable atorvastatin therapy: a case report and literature review. J Clin Pharm Ther. 2016;41(5):575–8 [A].

[36] Lopez JL, Tayek JA. Voriconazole-induced hepatitis via simvastatin- and lansoprazole-mediated drug interactions: a case report and review of the literature. Drug Metab Dispos. 2016;44(1):124–6 [A].

[37] Shah PJ, Sundareshan V, Miller B, et al. Micafungin and a case of polymorphic ventricular tachycardia. J Clin Pharm Ther. 2016;41(3):362–4 [A].

[38] Schneeweiss S, Carver PL, Datta K, et al. Short-term risk of liver and renal injury in hospitalized patients using micafungin: a multicentre cohort study. J Antimicrob Chemother. 2016;71(10):2938–44 [C].

24

Antiprotozoal Drugs

Dayna S. McManus*,1, Sidhartha D. Ray†

*Yale-New Haven Hospital, Yale University, New Haven, CT, United States
†Manchester University College of Pharmacy, Natural and Health Sciences, Fort Wayne, IN, United States
1Corresponding author: dayna.mcmanus@ynhh.org

ALBENDAZOLE

Treatments for lymphatic filariasis (LF) are limited due to the inability to clear the microfilaria from the blood. Therefore, a study was conducted to evaluate the safety and efficacy of two different drug-therapy regimens for treatment. Wuchereria bancrofti-infected Papua New Guineans adults were randomized to one of two regimens consisting of diethylcarbamazine (DEC) 6 mg/kg +albendazole (ALB) 400 mg (N=12) or DEC 6 mg/kg +ALB 400 mg+ivermectin (IVM) 200 μg/kg (N=12). The triple drug regimen induced >2-log reductions in microfilaria levels at 36 and 168 hours after treatment compared with approximately 1-log reduction with 2 drugs. All 12 individuals who received 3 drugs were microfilaria negative 1 year after treatment, whereas 11 of 12 individuals in the 2-drug regimen were microfilaria positive. In 6 participants followed 2 years after treatment, those who received 3 drugs remained microfilaria negative. The most common adverse effects in the study included fever, myalgias, pruritus, and proteinuria/hematuria. These side effects occurred in 83% of patients in the triple drug therapy arm compared with 50% of those receiving 2-drug treatment (P=0.021). All of the side effects resolved within 7 days after treatment and there were no serious adverse events that were reported in either group [1c].

A study was conducted to evaluate whether or not albendazole could be utilized for treatment of loiasis was conducted. Loiasis is a parasitic infection endemic in Africa. Typically, ivermectin is utilized for treatment, however, there is concerns with using it because it can induce serious adverse reactions in patients with high L loa microfilaraemia (LLM). Sixty men and women were randomized after stratification by screening LLM (≤30 000, 30 001–50 000, >50 000) to three treatment arms.

Patient received either two doses albendazole followed by 4 doses matching placebo (n = 20), six doses albendazole (n = 20) or 6 doses matching placebo (n = 20) administered every 2 months. During the study there were no adverse events recorded that were considered treatment related. The 6 dose group had the best response in terms of 50% decrease in LLM for ≥4 months at 53%. In addition, the 6 dose group also had 21%, the best response in LLM <8100 mf/mL for ≥4 months. The difference between the 6-dose and the placebo arm was statisticaly significant (P=0.01). Based on this the authors concluded that the 6-dose regimen reduced LLM significantly, but the reduction was insufficient to completely eliminate the risk of serious adverse reactions during ivermectin mass drug administration in loiasis co-endemic areas [2c].

ARTEMETHER–LUMEFANTRINE

A multicenter, randomized, open-label trial in four African countries was conducted to evaluate the safety and efficacy of artemisinin combination treatments for malaria in pregnant women. 3428 pregnant women in the second or third trimester who had falciparum malaria were treated with artemether–lumefantrine, amodiaquine–artesunate, mefloquine–artesunate, or dihydroartemisinin–piperaquine. The primary endpoint of the study was adjusted cure rates, which included cure of the original infection based on PCR, at day 63 and safety outcomes. The PCR-based cure rates were 94.8% in the artemether–lumefantrine group, 98.5% in the amodiaquine–artesunate group, 99.2% in the dihydroartemisinin–piperaquine group, and 96.8% in the mefloquine–artesunate group. There were no significant difference in the rate of serious adverse events and in birth outcomes was found among the treatment

Side Effects of Drugs Annual, Volume 39
ISSN: 0378-6080
http://dx.doi.org/10.1016/bs.seda.2017.06.034

groups. The most common adverse events of asthenia, poor appetite, dizziness, nausea, and vomiting occurred significantly more frequently in the mefloquine–artesunate group (50.6%) and the amodiaquine–artesunate group (48.5%) compared to the dihydroartemisinin–piperaquine group (20.6%) and the artemether–lumefantrine group (11.5%) (P < 0.001). Based on these results the authors concluded that artemether–lumefantrine was associated with the fewest adverse effects and with good cure rates but provided the shortest post-treatment prophylaxis, whereas dihydroartemisinin–piperaquine had the best efficacy and an acceptable safety profile [3C].

A multicentre, phase 4, open-label, non-inferiority trial in Burkina Faso, Kenya, and Tanzania was conducted in children ages 6–59 months to compare the efficacy and safety of fixed-dose artesunate–mefloquine to artemether–lumefantrine for treatment of uncomplicated Plasmodium falciparum malaria. This study was conducted because artemether–lumefantrine is typically used, however, the world health organization (WHO) recommends reconsidering the use of artesunate–mefloquine. Children in the study were randomly assigned using a computer-generated randomisation list, to receive 3 days' treatment with either one or two artesunate–mefloquine tablets (25 mg artesunate and 55 mg mefloquine) once a day or one or two artemether–lumefantrine tablets (20 mg artemether and 120 mg lumefantrine) twice a day. A total of 945 children were enrolled and randomized. 473 children were randomized to artesunate–mefloquine and 472 to artemether–lumefantrine. The per-protocol population had a total of 407 children in each group. The primary outcome of PCR-corrected adequate clinical and parasitological response (ACPR) at day 63 was 90.9% (370 patients) in the artesunate–mefloquine group and 89.7% (365 patients) in the artemether–lumefantrine group (treatment difference 1.23%, 95% CI −2.84% to 5.29%). Overall, the safety profiles of the two agents were comparable. There were low rates of early vomiting, 71 [15.3%] of 463 patients in the artesunate–mefloquine group vs 79 [16.8%] of 471 patients in the artemether–lumefantrine group, and few neurological adverse events, 10 [2.1%] of 468 vs 5 [1.1%] of 465, and there were no detectable psychiatric adverse events. Based on this study the authors concluded that artesunate–mefloquine is an effective and safe treatment option for treatment of uncomplicated P. falciparum malaria in African children younger than 5 years [4C].

Recently, the WHO updated their recommendations for treatment of acute uncomplicated P. falciparum malaria in Tanzania to include adding a single low-dose of primaquine (PQ) to standard artemisinin-based combination therapy (ACT), regardless of individual glucose-6-phosphate dehydrogenase (G6PD) status. This study aimed to evaluate the saftey and efficacy of these recommendations. Men and non-pregnant, non-lactating women aged ≥1 year with uncomplicated P. falciparum malaria were randomized to recieve either standard artemether–lumefantrine (AL) regimen alone or with a 0.25 mg/kg single-dose of PQ. The primary endpoint was mean percentage reduction in haemoglobin (Hb) concentration (g/dL) between days 0 and 7 by genotypic G6PD status and treatment arm. A total of 220 patients, 110 in each treatment arm, were enrolled. A total of 33/217 (15.2%) were phenotypically G6PD deficient, whereas 15/110 (13.6%) were genotypically hemizygous males, 5/110 (4.5%) homozygous females and 22/110 (20%) heterozygous females. Compared to genotypically G6PD wild-type/normal [6.8, 95% confidence interval (CI) 4.67–8.96], only heterozygous patients in AL arm had significant reduction in day-7 mean relative Hb concentration (14.3, 95% CI 7.02–21.55, P = 0.045), however, none fulfilled the pre-defined haemolytic threshold value of ≥25% Hb reduction. In the study, the majority of the adverse effects were mild and unrelated to the study drugs. There were, however, a total of 6 (4.4%) episodes, 3 in each treatment arm, of acute hemolytic anemia that all resolved without medical intervention. Of the events, 3 occurred in phenotypically G6PD-deficient patients, two in AL and one in AL + PQ arm. These findings show the recent WHO recommendations are safe and effective in the treatment of acute uncomplicated P. falciparum malaria regardless of G6PD status in Tanzania [5C].

Also in addition to these recent recommendations by the WHO a study was conducted to create a pharmacovigilance safety monitoring tool to assess the roll of the low-dose primaquine (PQ). The Primaquine Roll Out Monitoring Pharmacovigilance Tool (PROMPT) was comprised of the following: a standardized form to support the surveillance of possible adverse events following PQ treatment, a patient information card to enhance awareness of known adverse drug reactions of SLD PQ use and a database compiling recorded information. Patient characteristics, malaria diagnosis and treatment were collected. Hemoglobin (Hb) and G6PD deficiency were tested. After 13 months of follow-up PROMPT was considered to be well recieved and easy to use. Of the 102 patients enrolled who recieved PQ none were found to be G6PD deficent. A total of 4 (4.6%) patients had falls in Hb ≥25% from baseline, however, none of them presented with signs or symptoms of anaemia. No patient's had falls in Hb below 7 g/dL or that required a blood transfusion. A total of 11 (11%) patients reported an adverse event over the study period, however, only 3 were considered serious with 2 resulting in death and 1 in hospitalization. These effects were not concerned to be causally related to PQ. Of the non-serious adverse events, 4 were considered to be definitely, probably, or possibly related to PQ. Based on this study it is recommended to use PROMPT to improve pharmacovigilance to monitor and promote the safety of the WHO recommendations [6c].

The WHO recommends continued monitoring of efficacy of artemisinin combination therapies (ACTs) againsted *P. falciparum* every 2 years to ensure resistance is not developing. In order to follow these recommendations this study was conducted to assess the efficacy of artemether–lumefantrine (AL) (Coartem®) in treating the uncomplicated falciparum malaria in Eastern Ethiopia. A standard six-dose regimen of AL was administered over 3 days and followed up for measuring therapeutic responses over 28 days. There were a total of 91 patients enrolled and at the the the day-28 analysis 83 patients had adequate clinical and parasitological responses (ACPRs). Based on a per protocol analysis, PCR-uncorrected and corrected cure rates of AL among the study participants were 97.6% (95% CI: 93.6–99.5) and 98.8% (CI: 93.5%–100%), respectively. From day 3 and onward there were no parasites detected. Mean hemoglobin levels were significantly increased ($P < 0.000$) from 12.39 g/dL at day 0 to 13.45 g/dL on day 28. There were no serious adverse drug reactions observed among the study participants. Based on the results of this study there is still a high efficacy of AL in the treatment of uncomplicated *P. falciparum* malaria in the Eastern Ethiopia. Although there were no major side effects there was a high incidence of repeated cough and oral ulceration which warrents futher investigation [7c].

A multicenter, randomized, double-blind, comparative, parallel-group trial was conducted to evaluate a fixed-dose combination of arterolane maleate (AM), a new synthetic trioxolane, with piperaquine phosphate (PQP), a long half-life bisquinoline, compared to artemether–lumefantrine in patients with an uncomplicated *P. falciparum* malaria. A total of 1072 patients aged 12–65 years with *P. falciparum* infection received either AM-PQP (714 patients) once daily or artemether–lumefantrine (AL; 358 patients) twice daily for 3 days. A total of 638 (89.4%) of the 714 patients in the AM-PQP group completed the study and 301 (84.1%) of the 358 patients in the AL group. In both groups, the PCR was used to evaluate adequate clinical and parasitological response (PCR-corrected ACPR) on day 28 in intent-to-treat (ITT) and per-protocol (PP) populations was 92.86% and 92.46% and 99.25% and 99.07%, respectively and on day 42 in the ITT and PP populations were 90.48% and 91.34%, respectively. After adjusting for survival ITT, the PCR-corrected ACPR on day 42 was >98% in both groups. The incidence of adverse events was comparable between the two treatment arms. Therefore, the authors concluded that AM-PQP is a comparible option to AL in terms of safety adn efficiacy in the treatment of uncomplicated *P. falciparum* malaria [8C].

Large scale safety studies have not been conducted on artemisinin combination therapies such as artemether–lumefantrine (AL) despite the face they are typically first line options for treatment of uncomplicated acute *P. falciparum* malaria. Therefore, this study was conducted to evaluate the safety of AL in public health facilities in Tanzania using the Cohort Event Monitoring (CEM) method. A prospective, observational cohort study included patients who presented to public health facilities in four regions of Tanzania who were prescribed AL. Pre- and post-treatment forms were used to record baseline information and new health events before and 7 days after treatment. 8040 patients were enrolled in the study with 6147 being able to be included in the analysis. After starting treatment, a total of 530 adverse events were reported in 6% (383) of the patients. The most frequent post-treatment adverse events that were reported included vomiting, nausea, diarrhea, abdominal pain and anorexia and 25% of patients had a side effect related to the neurological system. After a causality assessment of the events it was determined that 51.9% (275/530) were possibly related to AL. There was a significant difference in the frequency of adverse events by age-group as the incidence of side effects increased as age increased ($P < 0.001$). There was no significant difference in the frequency of the events between males and females ($P = 0.504$). There were no new adverse effects identified as all were consistent with the adverse effects reported in the product information and in other studies. This study shows that based on a large scale analysis AL continues to be a safe option for treatment of malaria [9C].

Commonly in Ghana unsweetened natural cocoa is consumed has antimalarial properties. Cocoa powder contains about 1.9% theobromine and 0.21% caffeine. It is suspected that concomitant consumption of cocoa and artemether/lumefantrine (AL) may have protective effect on the heart and kidney despite (AL) administration. To evaluate this effect, 30 male guinea pigs were divided into 5 groups of 6 animals each. One group recieved 75 mg/kg body weight of AL, the other group received 300, 900 and 1500 mg/kg body weight cocoa powder for 14 days orally and AL for the last 3 days and the control group recieved distilled water. After euthanisation of the animals, an analysis revealed increases in HDL levels ($P > 0.05$) while there were decreases in LDL levels ($P > 0.05$), creatine kinase and AST levels ($P < 0.05$) in animals that received cocoa powder compared to AL only administered group. Urea levels reduced significantly by 53% ($P < 0.05$) in group that received 1500 mg/kg cocoa powder. The results of this study showed that natural cocoa powder proved to possess cardioprotective and renoprotective effects during artemether–lumefantrine administration [10E].

A prospective audit of pediatric outpatients in four general hospitals in Nigeria over a 3-month period was conducted to assess for adverse drug events and drug–drug interactions. A total of 1233 patients were eligible and of them 208 (16.9%) received prescriptions with at least one potential drug–drug interaction. Of the possible interactions, there were a total of 7 drug classes and antimalarial combination therapies were the most commonly reported. The most common exposure to a single drug–drug interaction involved promethazine, artemether/lumefantrine, ciprofloxacin and artemether/lumefantrine. This study shows the importance of close monitoring for drug–drug interactions when prescribing antimalaria medications [11c].

Artemether and lumefantrine (AL), commonly used for treatment of malaria, are metabolized via CYP3A4. Lopinavir/ritonavir, which inhibits CYP3A4, is used for treatment of HIV which could possibly result in significant drug–drug interactions. In order to assess these interactions a pharmacokinetic study was conducted in HIV-infected patients without malaria who were either antiretroviral-naïve or stable on lopinavir/ritonavir-based antiretrovirals. Both groups received the recommended six-dose artemether–lumefantrine treatment. A total of 34 patients were enrolled and at day-7 lumefantrine concentrations were about 10-fold higher in the lopinavir group than the antiretroviral-naïve group [3170 vs 336 ng/mL; $P=0.0001$], with AUC(0-inf) and Cmax increased fivefold [2478 vs 445 μg h/mL; $P=0.0001$], and threefold [28.2 vs 8.8 μg/mL; $P<0.0001$], respectively. Artemether exposure, however, was similar between groups, however, the Cmax and AUC(0–8 hours) of its active metabolite dihydroartemisinin were initially twofold higher in the lopinavir group [$P=0.004$ and $P=0.0013$, respectively]. After 21 days of starting AL there were similar numbers of treatment emergent side effects (42 vs 35) and adverse reactions (12 vs 15, $P=0.21$) in the lopinavir and antiretroviral-naïve groups, respectively. There were no serious adverse events and no difference in electrocardiographic QTcF- and PR-intervals. This study shows there is a significant drug–drug interaction that occurs between AL which results in higher lumefantrine levels, however, it did not result in any sifnificant side effects. Patients who are recieving this combination should be monitored for side effects closely [12c].

ARTESUNATE

Artesunate is throught to possibly attenuate the progression of atherosclerosis lesion formation alone or combined with rosuvastatin. To test this hypothesis, a study in Western-type diet (WD) fed mice was conducted. The results of the study show that artesunate could attenuate the progression of atherosclerosis lesion formation alone or combined with rosuvastatin in WD fed mice.

The mechanism is suspected to be due to reduction in pro-inflammatory cytokine, such as TNF-α and IL-6 in addition to down-regulation of the pro-inflammatory chemokines such as IL-8 and MCP-1 in aorta of mice. Rosuvastatin combined with artesunate could more effectively attenuate the progression of atherosclerosis lesions than when treated by one of them, demonstrating that lipid-lowering agents combined with anti-inflammatory agents could provide the greater benefit for cardiovascular disease patients. Based on this study more investigation of artesunate as a treatment alone or in combination of atherosclerosis is warrented [13E].

WHO recommends utilizing artemisinin-based combination therapy (ACT) as first line treatment of malaria. Ghana adopted these recommendations in 2004 and therefore a study was conducted to evaluate reporting of adverse events prior to and after the change to ACT for treatment of malaria. The study consisted of 60 in-depth interviews with health workers, chemical shop owners and patients with malaria who were given ACT at the health facilities. Body weakness and dizziness were most commonly reported as side effects from the used of ACT by study participants. Additional side effects reported included swollen testes, abdominal pain and shivering. Side effects were mostly associated with the use of artesunate–amodiaquine compared to other artemisinin-based combinations. Factors found to effect reporting included patients not being provided information about the side effects of the drugs, long queues at health facilities and unfriendly health worker attitude, wrong use of ACT at home, farming and commercial activities also affected effective adverse events reporting in the study area. These causes for poor reporting should be taken into account as it may negatively affect patient's reporting [14c].

Recently, artesunate (ART) has started to be used for add-on therapy in patients with breast cancer. When used for treatment of malaria the drug has been considered to be safe, however, the safety when used for treatment of breast cancer is not as well known. Therefore, a phase I study aimed to determine the daily dose of ART that is well tolerated as add-on therapy in patients with breast cancer for 4 weeks of therapy specifically monitoring for ototoxicity which could occur when used for this indication. This study was a prospective, open, uncontrolled, phase I dose-escalation study to evaluate the safety and tolerability of ART in patients with advanced breast cancer. Patients received either 100, 150 or 200 mg oral ART daily for 4 weeks in addition to their additional oncology treatment. A total of 23 female patients were included in the study of which 4 patients had auditory related adverse events which may be related to ART. Another 4 patients had an vertigo as a result of treatment and of of the reactions was considered to be severe, however, it resolved after the treatment was stopped. Audiological results after 4 weeks of therapy with ART did not show any dose-limiting auditory toxicity. However, audiological monitoring is still recommended when utilizing higher doses that were not evaluated in this study [15c].

A study was conducted to assess the safety and efficacy of pyronaridine–artesunate after inital treatment vs repeated treatment of malaria given the lack of data available in this area. The study was a randomized, open-label done at six health facilities in patients (aged ≥6 months and bodyweight ≥5 kg) with uncomplicated microscopically confirmed Plasmodium spp. malaria. In the study the primary safety endpoint was incidence of hepatotoxicity which was defined as alanine aminotransferase of greater than five times the upper limit of normal (ULN) or Hy's criteria (alanine aminotransferase or aspartate aminotransferase greater than three times the ULN and total bilirubin more than twice the ULN) after treatment of the first episode of malaria and re-treatment (≥28 days after first treatment) with pyronaridine–artesunate. After inital treatment, 13 (1%) of 996 patients had hepatotoxicity (including one [<1%] possible Hy's law case) vs two (1%) of 311 patients on re-treatment (neither a Hy's law case). Based on this study, there is no evidence that pyronaridine–artesunate re-treatment increased safety risk based on laboratory values, reported adverse event frequencies, or electrocardiograph findings. In terms of efficacy, all first treatment or re-treatment episodes, pyronaridine–artesunate ($n=673$) day 28 crude ACPR was 92.7% (95% CI 91.0–94.3) vs 80.4% (77.8–83.0) for artemether–lumefantrine ($n=671$). This study shows that pyronaridine–artesunate is safe and efficacious on first malaria treatment vs re-treatment [16C].

A study was conducted to evaluate the interaction between lopinavir/ritonavir (LR) and artesunate (AS), amodiaquine (AQ) or a fixed dose of AS/AQ in a mouse model of chloroquine-resistant Plasmodium berghei. To evaluate these interaction, LR with graded doses of AS or AQ resulted in a significant reduced the median effective dose. At day 3 till day 21 everything cleared completely in the animals infected. All the animals survived till day 21 post-infection. In contrast, survival on day 21 in animals treated with AQ alone or AQ with LR was 20% and 60%, respectively. Based on this analysis in mice, LR appears to enhance the antimalarial drugs AS and AQ likely through the CYP enzyme system [17E].

DIHYDROARTEMISININ–PIPERAQUINE

Piperaquine, a commonly used antimalarial medication, has been associated with delayed ventricular depolarization resulting in prolonged QT interval. Overall the safety data regarding dihydroartemisinin/piperaquine (DHA/PPQ) for the treatment of uncomplicated malaria is lacking. Therefore, electrocardiograms (ECG) were performed to evaluate the safety of DHA/PPQ, at baseline before the use of DHA/PPQ and on day 3, before the final dose and at day 7 post-administration. 1315 patients gave consent and were enrolled and 1147 (87%) had complete information for analyses. Median age was 8 (5–14) years and 25% of the patients were children under 5 years of age ($n=287$). There were no clinical significant changes in blood counts. Mean QTcF values were higher on day 3 before and after administration of the treatment as well as on day 7 (post-treatment) compared with day 1 (12, 22 and 4 times higher, $P<0.001$). The QTcF and QTcB were highest on day 3 after drug intake in all age groups. There were 79 (7%) events of significantly prolonged mean QTcF, however, these were not clinically significant. This study demonstrates that DHA/PPQ at therapeutic doses in patients with uncomplicated malaria and no predisposing cardiac conditions in Africa was associated QTc prolongation and therefore this should be monitored in patients receiving this treatment [18C].

A double-blind, randomized, controlled trial involving 300 pregnant adolescents or women in Uganda was conducted to assess safety of different malaria treatment options. Patients were randomly assigned to a sulfadoxine–pyrimethamine regimen (106 participants), a three-dose dihydroartemisinin–piperaquine regimen (94 participants), or a monthly dihydroartemisinin–piperaquine regimen (100 participants). The prevalence of histopathologically confirmed placental malaria, the primary outcome of the study, was significantly higher in the sulfadoxine–pyrimethamine group (50.0%) than in the three-dose dihydroartemisinin–piperaquine group (34.1%, $P=0.03$) or the monthly dihydroartemisinin–piperaquine group (27.1%, $P=0.001$). The prevalence of adverse birth effects was lowest in the monthly dihydroartemisinin–piperaquine group (9.2%) than in the sulfadoxine–pyrimethamine group (18.6%, $P=0.05$) or the three-dose dihydroartemisinin–piperaquine group (21.3%, $P=0.02$). During pregnancy, the incidence of symptomatic malaria was significantly higher in the sulfadoxine–pyrimethamine group (41 episodes over 43.0 person-years at risk) than in the three-dose dihydroartemisinin–piperaquine group (12 episodes over 38.2 person-years at risk, $P=0.001$) or the monthly dihydroartemisinin–piperaquine group (0 episodes over 42.3 person-years at risk, $P<0.001$). The risk of vomiting after administration of any dose of the study agents was less than 0.4% and there were no significant differences among any of the groups in terms of adverse effects. Based on this study dihydroartemisinin–piperaquine appears to be superior with limited side effects. In addition, monthly treatment with dihydroartemisinin–piperaquine was found to be superior to three-dose dihydroartemisinin–piperaquine [19C].

OXANTEL PAMOATE–ALBENDAZOLE

Recent studies have shown oxantel pamoate to be effective against *Trichuris trichiura*. Therefore, this study was done to assess the optimum dose for oxantel pamoate in treatment of this infection. A randomized, placebo-controlled, single-blind trial with oxantel pamoate in school-aged children (aged 6–14 years) infected with *T. trichiura* was evaluated. Children were excluded if they suffered from any systematic illness. Children were randomly assigned to 6 different oxantel pamoate doses (5–30 mg/kg) or a placebo. A total of 480 participants were enrolled and 350 children were randomly assigned to the different oxantel pamoate doses or the placebo. The dose of 5 mg/kg was shown to be the minimum effective dose (10 of 46 children cured [cure rate 22%, 95% CI 11–36]; egg-reduction rate 85%, 64.5–92.9). As doses increased the probability of being cured increased as well. At a dose of 25 mg/kg oxantel pamoate 27 of 45 children were cured (cure rate 60%, 95% CI 44–65) and at 30 mg/kg 27 of 46 children were cured (59%, 43–73). Overall it was well tolerated at all doses with only mild adverse events. This study shows a oxantel pamoate if well tolerated and effective in children with *T. trichiura*. The optimal dose range was found to be 15–30 mg/kg oxantel pamoate [20C].

PRIMAQUINE

As mentioned previously in this chapter, a single low dose of 0.25 mg/kg of primaquine is recommended by the WHO to be added to Artemisinin-based Combination Therapies (ACTs) without testing G6PD. This study sought to evaluate the adverse events and haemoglobin variations after implimentation of this low dose primaquine in both G6PD normal and deficient patients. The single dose primaquine was combined with dihydroartemisinin–piperaquine (DHA-PPQ) given three times at monthly intervals in 819 patients. There were no adverse events related to primaquine that were observed throughout the study. The mean fractional hemaoglobin changes after each primaquine treatment were greater in G6PD-deficient subjects (−5.0%, −4.2% and −4.7%) compared to G6PD normal subjects (0.3%, −0.8% and −1.7%) but these changes were not clinically significant. This study does support that the low dose (0.25 mg/kg) of primaquine can utilized safely in patients regardless of G6PD testing [21C].

A case of a 57-year-old male whose death was thought to be due to primaquine (PQ)-triggered hemolysis was reported. The article discusses how in 2012, 2 deaths were related to primaquine (PQ)-triggered hemolysis that had occurred in glucose-6-phosphate dehydrogenase (G6PD)-deficient patients who were being treated for

Plasmodium vivax infection. Both of these patients were receiving chloroquine (25 mg/kg in 3 days) and PQ (0.5 mg/kg/d for 7 days). The hemolysis developed after the third day of the recommended PQ dose. Only one patient was available for postmortem analysis which was the 57-year-old man. On autopsy it was found the man also had mild alcoholic steatohepatitis. He was found to have had a severe hemolytic crisis including acute renal failure, respiratory distress, and severe anemia. Based on PCR analysis he was found to have *G6PD* mutations associated with the A(−) allele (202 G/A and 376 A/G), which is the most common in people of African descent. The article also reports that in total there have been 14 deaths due to PQ that have been reported. Of these 14 cases 12 of them were in confirmed G6PD-deficient individuals, however, only one of the genotypes was known. Based on this information it is important to identify patients with *G6PD* A(−), because of the possibly life-threatening hemolysis that can occur when these patients are treated with PQ therapy [22A].

Primaquine is a major CYP2D6 substrate and therefore it can be effected by being co-administration with drugs that induce or inhibit CYP2D6 which may effect the concentrations of primaquine. To assess this interaction a study was conducted to assess the inhibition potential of the selective serotonin reuptake inhibitor (SSRI) and serotonin norepinephrine reuptake inhibitor (SNRI) classes on primaquine metabolism using a pharmacological assay. The different drugs within the SSRI and SNRI classes varied in their ability to primaquine metabolism. Fluoxetine and paroxetine were the most potent inhibitors primaquine metabolism and desvenlafaxine was the least potent. Fluoxetine and primaquine were given together in a mouse malaria model to assess the clinical effect of this interaction. This interaction showed that co-administration reduced the anti-malarial efficacy of primaquine when it was given with fluoxetine. Therefore, it is recommeneded that potent CYP2D6 medications, like fluoxetine, be avoided in combination with primaquine [23E].

A review article discussed the pharmacology of primaquine and how pharmacogenomics may play an important role in the safety and efficacy of this agent. As discussed previously, primaquine is a substrate of CYP2D6 and therefore is effected by inhibitors and inducers of CYP2D6. In addition, it has been shown that metabolism via CYP2D6 may be necessary in order for primaquine to exert its activity. If this is the case then patients who are poor CYP2D6 metabolizers may experience treatment failures when primaquine is used for treatment of their malaria. The article goes on to discuss that primaquine may be an important drug for CYP genotype testing prior to administering or if a patient fails therapy. If they are a poor metabolizer this may be the result of the failure rather than non-compliance or another issue. The article also goes on to discuss the possible interactions between inhibitors and inducers of CYP2D6 and primaquine. This article highlights why pharmacogenomics may be very important with the administration of some medications and how drug interactions can also play a big part in safety and efficacy [24R].

QUINACRINE

Historically, quinacrine has been used for its activity against malaria; however, this agent may have an additional role in the treatment of ulcerative colitis (UC). UC remains a very difficult to treat chronic IBD as treatment often results in symptom management without an ability to cure the disease. Quinacrine has been used to treat other inflammatory related diseases such as rheumatoid arthritis and lupus erythematosus. Therefore, this study of two doses of quinacrine was conducted in mouse models of UC. The results of this study showed that quinacrine was able to suppress colitis without any toxicity or side effects in a mouse models. Further investigation in humans is warranted [25E].

MEFLOQUINE

Mefloquine is often reported to cause different acute and chronic neurological side effects despite the underlying mechanism remaining relatively unclear. Recently, a case of a 30-year-old man, from Pakistan, presented with new compliants of dizziness and diplopia after taking mefloquine. He started to develop macular changes and was subsequently diagnosed as acute central serous chorioretinopathy by angiography and optical coherence tomography. The visual changes seen in this case and are similar to those seen after recieving other quinoline derivative. Providers should be aware of chorioretinopathy as a potential ophthalmological sign of mefloquine CNS toxicity. This should be monitored closely in patients recieving mefloquine therapy [26A].

As mentioned with the first case, mefloquine (MQ) is often associated with neurologic and/or psychiatric adverse events which can range from mild to severe. In the United States the package information for MQ recommends to discontinue the medication if there is any neurologic or psychatric side effects that develop. This systematic review was conducted of drug labeling in different countries to identify possible prodromal reactions for which there is complete or partial agreement in prescribing and patient recommendations. A total of 6 primarily English-speaking countries' packaging were reviewed. Recommendations were available for 22 neuropsychiatric reactions. Complete or partial international agreement was found for reactions in 11 (50%) of the 22 reactions. A detailed table with these reactions and recommendations is available within the article. Based on this review there is opportunity to optimize and standardize the recommendations and wording in the labeling of mefloquine throughout the countries reviewed [27r].

A review article was published which aimed to summarize any published studies which document evidence of the neuropsychiatric effects that may be caused by antimalarial drugs. Of all the published data reviewed in this study over the last few decades only mefloquine was identified as having clear documentation of serious neurological and/or psychiatric side effects. Continued monitoring and caution prior to prescribing of mefloquine is warrented given the documented association with these side effects in patients recieving therapy for malaria [28r].

A case report of possible rhabdomyolysis related to mefloquine use has been reported. There are no previously reported cases of rhabdomyolysis possible related to mefloquine that have been reported in the literature. The case that was reported was a 36-years-old man who presented to the hospital with complaints of malaise, fatigue, and difficulty functioning in his daily activities. The symptoms had been ongoing over several weeks and he noted that they after receiving mefloquine for prophylaxis against malaria during a recent trip to Nigeria. No fevers were reported by the patient so a extensive work-up was performed which included blood tests. The results of the blood test was concerning for rhabdomyolysis with a CK 2978 U/L, sodium 133 mmol/L, and of creatinine 1.24 mg/dL. All other tests that were sent were negative which ruled out other possible causes including malaria, hepatitis, dengue fever and chikungunya. The patient was given symptomatic treatment with intravenous and after 12 hours of fluids the CK value decreased to 641 U/L, and creatinine and sodium were within normal limits. Within 2 days all blood tests were normal and he was back to his normal state of health. Based on the lab values and time course the most likely explanation was rhabdomyolysis related to mefloquine, which has not been reported previously and therefore providers should be aware of this as a potential side effect [29A].

A review on use of mefloquine in military personnel was published. In the report the evidence suggests that mefloquine may be the least safe antimalarial agent yet it continues to be used routinely in military personnel. The report suggests better strategies for educating providers on alternatives to mefloquine and ways to monitor for side effects more effectively [30r].

Mefloquine is being considered as a safer alternative to sulfadoxine/pyrimethamine for treatment of malaria in pregnant patients. However, there is not much known about the interaction of mefloquine and sulfamethoxazole and trimethoprim in pregnant patients since they may be recieving this for an HIV infection. To evaluate this interaction a double-blinded, placebo-controlled study was conducted in 124 HIV-infected, pregnant women who were receiving sulfamethoxazole/trimethoprim as part of their prophylaxis. Of the 124 women 72 of them received 3 doses of mefloquine (15 mg/kg) at monthly intervals. There was not any noticable changes in mefloquine pharmacokinetics in patinets that were also on sulfamethoxazole/trimethoprim prophylaxis. There was no difference with trimethoprim steady-state levels either, however, sulfamethoxazole levels showed a significant 53% decrease after mefloquine administration compared to the placebo. Although there was a decrease in sulfamethoxazole levels, there was no changes in clinical effects as there was no increase in hospital admissions due to secondary bacterial infections. Therefore, these agents should be able to be used together without major clinical effect [31c].

A study was conducted to evaluate for any pharmacokinetic interaction between the artesunate–mefloquine and lopinavir boosted with ritonavir (LPV/r) since many patients receive both of these medication together. The study was an open-label, three-way, cross-over, study in 16 healthy adults. Patients were given the following treatment regiments standard 3-day artesunate–mefloquine combination followed by a 2 months washout followed by oral LPV/r 400 mg/100 mg twice a day for 14 days and finally artesunate–mefloquine and LPV/r twice a day for 3 days. When artesunate was combined with LPV/r the Cmax and systemic exposure of artesunate were significantly increased by 45%–80%. Mefloquine Cmax and systemic exposure were significantly reduced by 19%–37%. Artesunate–mefloquine and lopinavir resulted in a significantly reduced lopinavir by 22%, however, there was no significant change in systemic drug exposure. Overall the drug treatments were generally well tolerated with no serious adverse events. The most common side effects that were reported were vertigo, nausea and vomiting. Based on this data caution should be advised when these medications are used together to monitor for possible treatment failure. Additional studies are warrented to furthur investigate this potential interaction [32c].

References

[1] Thomsen EK, et al. Efficacy, safety, and pharmacokinetics of coadministered diethylcarbamazine, albendazole, and ivermectin for treatment of bancroftian filariasis. Clin Infect Dis. 2016;62(3):334–41 [c].

[2] Kamgno J, et al. Effect of two or six doses 800 mg of albendazole every two months on loa loa microfilaraemia: a double blind, randomized placebo-controlled trial. PLoS Negl Trop Dis. 2016;10(3):e0004492 [c].

[3] PREGACT Study Group, Pekyi D, Ampromfi AA, et al. Four artemisinin-based treatments in African pregnant women with malaria. Malawi Med J. 2016;28(3):139–49 [C].

[4] Sirima SB, et al. Comparison of artesunate-mefloquine and artemether-lumefantrine fixed-dose combinations for treatment of uncomplicated plasmodium falciparum malaria in children younger than 5 years in sub-Saharan Africa: a randomised, multicentre, phase 4 trial. Lancet Infect Dis. 2016;16(10):1123–33 [C].

[5] Mwaiswelo R, et al. Safety of a single low-dose of primaquine in addition to standard artemether-lumefantrine regimen for treatment of acute uncomplicated Plasmodium falciparum malaria in Tanzania. Malar J. 2016;15:316 [C].

[6] Poirot E, et al. Development of a pharmacovigilance safety monitoring tool for the rollout of single low-dose primaquine and artemether-lumefantrine to treat Plasmodium falciparum infections in Swaziland: a pilot study. Malar J. 2016;15(1):384 [c].

[7] Nega D, et al. Therapeutic efficacy of artemether-lumefantrine (Coartem®) in treating uncomplicated P. falciparum malaria in metehara, eastern ethiopia: regulatory clinical study. PLoS One. 2016;11(4)e0154618 [c].

[8] Toure OA, et al. A phase 3, double-blind, randomized study of arterolane maleate-piperaquine phosphate vs artemether-lumefantrine for falciparum malaria in adolescent and adult patients in Asia and Africa. Clin Infect Dis. 2016;62(8):964–71 [C].

[9] Mssusa AK, et al. Safety profile of artemether-lumefantrine: a cohort event monitoring study in public health facilities in Tanzania. Clin Drug Investig. 2016;36(5):401–11 [C].

[10] Asiedu-Gyekye IJ, et al. A dietary strategy for the management of artemether-lumefantrine-induced cardiovascular and renal toxicity. BMC Complement Altern Med. 2016;16:348 [E].

[11] Oshikoya KA, et al. Potential drug-drug interactions in pediatric outpatient prescriptions in Nigeria and implications for the future. Expert Rev Clin Pharmacol. 2016;9(11):1505–15 [c].

[12] Kredo T, et al. The interaction between artemether-lumefantrine and lopinavir/ritonavir-based antiretroviral therapy in HIV-1 infected patients. BMC Infect Dis. 2016;16:30 [c].

[13] Jiang W, et al. Artesunate attenuated progression of atherosclerosis lesion formation alone or combined with rosuvastatin through inhibition of pro-inflammatory cytokines and pro-inflammatory chemokines. Phytomedicine. 2016;23(11):1259–66 [E].

[14] Chatio S, et al. Factors influencing adverse events reporting within the health care system: the case of artemisinin-based combination treatments in northern Ghana. Malar J. 2016;15:125 [c].

[15] König M, et al. Investigation of ototoxicity of artesunate as add-on therapy in patients with metastatic or locally advanced breast cancer: new audiological results from a prospective, open, uncontrolled, monocentric phase I study. Cancer Chemother Pharmacol. 2016;77(2):413–27 [c].

[16] Sagara I, et al. Safety and efficacy of re-treatments with pyronaridine-artesunate in African patients with malaria: a substudy of the WANECAM randomised trial. Lancet Infect Dis. 2016;16(2):189–98 [C].

[17] Abiodun OO, Gbimadee N, Gbotosho GO. Lopinavir/ritonavir enhanced the antimalarial activity of amodiaquine and artesunate in a mouse model of Plasmodium berghei. J Chemother. 2016;28(6):482–6 [E].

[18] Kabanywanyi AM, et al. Multi-country evaluation of safety of dihydroartemisinin/piperaquine post-licensure in African public hospitals with electrocardiograms. PLoS One. 2016;11(10) e0164851 [C].

[19] Kakuru A, et al. Dihydroartemisinin-piperaquine for the prevention of malaria in pregnancy. N Engl J Med. 2016;374(10):928–39 [C].

[20] Moser W, et al. Efficacy and safety of oxantel pamoate in school-aged children infected with *Trichuris trichiura* on Pemba Island, Tanzania: a parallel, randomised, controlled, dose-ranging study. Lancet Infect Dis. 2016;16(1):53–60. http://dx.doi.org/10.1016/S1473-3099(15)00271-6. Epub 2015 Sep 18, [C].

[21] Bancone G, et al. Single low dose primaquine (0.25 mg/kg) does not cause clinically significant haemolysis in G6PD deficient subjects. PLoS One. 2016;11(3):e0151898 [C].

[22] Monteiro WM, et al. Fatal primaquine-induced hemolysis in a patient with plasmodium vivax malaria and G6PD A(-) variant in the Brazilian Amazon. Clin Infect Dis. 2016;62(9): 1188 [A].

[23] Jin X, et al. Pre-clinical evaluation of CYP 2D6 dependent drug-drug interactions between primaquine and SSRI/SNRI antidepressants. Malar J. 2016;15(1):280 [E].

[24] Marcsisin SR, et al. Primaquine pharmacology in the context of CYP 2D6 pharmacogenomics: current state of the art. Pharmacol Ther. 2016;161:1–10 [R].

[25] Chumanevich AA, et al. Repurposing the anti-malarial drug, quinacrine: new anti-colitis properties. Oncotarget. 2016;7(33):52928–39 [E].

[26] Jain M, Nevin RL, Ahmed I. Mefloquine-associated dizziness, diplopia, and central serous chorioretinopathy: a case report. J Med Case Rep. 2016;10(1):305 [A].

[27] Nevin RL, Byrd AM. Neuropsychiatric adverse reactions to mefloquine: a systematic comparison of prescribing and patient safety guidance in the US, UK, Ireland, Australia, New Zealand, and Canada. Neurol Ther. 2016;5(1):69–83 [r].

[28] Grabias B, Kumar S. Adverse neuropsychiatric effects of antimalarial drugs. Expert Opin Drug Saf. 2016;15(7):903–10 [r].

[29] Comelli I, et al. Mefloquine-associated rhabdomyolysis. Am J Emerg Med. 2016;34(11). 2250.e5–2250.e6, [A].

[30] Quinn JC. Better approach needed to detect and treat military personnel with adverse effects from mefloquine. BMJ. 2016;352:i838 [r].

[31] Green M, et al. Pharmacokinetics of mefloquine and its effect on sulfamethoxazole and trimethoprim steady-state blood levels in intermittent preventive treatment (IPTp) of pregnant HIV-infected women in Kenya. Malar J. 2016;15:7 [c].

[32] Rattanapunya S, et al. Pharmacokinetic interactions between artesunate-mefloquine and ritonavir-boosted lopinavir in healthy Thai adults. Malar J. 2015;14:400 [c].

25

Antiviral Drugs

Sreekumar Othumpangat[*],[1], Sidhartha D. Ray[†], John D. Noti[*]

[*]National Institute for Occupational Safety and Health, Centers for Disease Control and Prevention, Morgantown, WV, United States

[†]Manchester University College of Pharmacy, Natural & Health Sciences, Fort Wayne, IN, United States

[1]Corresponding author: seo8@cdc.gov

Abbreviations

3TC	lamivudine (dideoxythiacytidine)
AZT	zidovudine (azidothymidine)
D4T	stavudine (didehydrodideoxythymidine)
DDI	didanosine (dideoxyinosine)
ETV	etravirine
FTC	emtricitabine
RPV	rilpivirine
SIM	simeprevir
SOF	sofosbuvir

DRUGS ACTIVE AGAINST CYTOMEGALOVIRUS

Human cytomegalovirus (CMV) is a major cause of morbidity and mortality among immunocompromised individuals, especially those who have undergone allogeneic hematopoietic cell transplantation (HCT). Several available drugs induce significant side effects which deter their use for CMV; specifically, Ganciclovir (GCV), CDV, and Foscarnet (FOS). There are novel promising drugs without myelosuppressive properties or renal toxic effects, such as Maribavir (MBV), Letermovir (LMV) and Brincidofovir (BCV), which are very promising anti-CMV drugs that are in randomized phase II and III trials [1R].

Cidofovir [SED-15, 771; SEDA-32, 529; SEDA-33, 577; SEDA-34, 447; SEDA-35, 503; SEDA-36, 401; SEDA-37, 329; SEDA-38, 261]

See also Section Brincidofovir.

Cidofovir (CDV) was FDA approved in 1996 as an IV formulation for the treatment of a broad-range of DNA virus infections. CDV is a phosphonate (monophosphate analogue) and does not require initial viral phosphorylation. Cellular kinases add additional phosphates to produce CDV diphosphate, which could incorporate into the viral DNA by pUL54 leading to the termination of viral DNA replication. CDV has a very long intracellular half-life and is effective in the treatment of CMV retinitis in AIDS patients. CDV is also considered as a second-line antiviral drug for the treatment of CMV infection due to some concerns regarding its poor oral bioavailability, dose-related nephrotoxicity, and myelosuppression [2R].

Letermovir [SEDA-38, 261]

Letermovir (LMV) is a direct-acting antiviral that could lead to the emergence of LMV-resistant virus variants in CMV patients treated with LMV. Monitoring the emergence of resistant strains has been an integral part of the clinical studies. So far, only a small number of amino acid substitutions conferring LMV resistance have been identified. A suboptimal use of LMV leads to the emergence of LMV-resistant strains. The efficacy of different LMV (AIC246, MK8228) doses (60, 120, and 240 mg/day) against CMV was evaluated in a phase 2 dose-range-finding prophylaxis study in HSCT patients infected with CMV. The LMV resistance mutation emerged when a suboptimal prophylactic dose (60 mg/day) was used, but a higher dose of 240 mg/day achieved complete suppression of viremia [3c].

Three antiviral agents, GCV, FOS and CDV, are currently approved by Food and Drug Administration (USA) for the treatment of CMV infections. They all target the viral DNA polymerase and are associated with significant side effects. Combinations of novel antiviral compounds acting on different targets such as artesunate (ART) with currently approved drugs or eventually LMV or MBV may result in synergistic effects. The concentrations of GCV, FOS, CDV and ART that reduced the GLuc activity by 50% were 3.92 ± 1.64, 62.45 ± 8.39, 0.68 ± 0.19 and 3.86 ± 1.25 μM, respectively, whereas those of MBV and LMV were 64 ± 22 and 2.50 ± 0.83 nM, respectively. The combination of ART with GCV, CDV or MBV was associated with synergism, whereas combination of ART with FOS or LMV resulted in moderate synergism. These results suggest that the combination of ART with the antiviral agents could be an effective strategy for the treatment CMV [4c].

Brincidofovir

Brincidofovir (BCV), part of a new class of anti-viral drugs, is an oral nucleotide analog that has been a promising candidate against CMV. BCV is less nephrotoxic than CDV and could prevent CMV infection in HSCT patients. In a phase 2 clinical trials, BCV showed a dose–response relationship for the prevention of CMV infection in adult allogeneic HSCT recipients [5c].

A case study reported, a 68-year-old woman with stage III follicular lymphoma who underwent chemotherapy, showed complete remission. She developed CMV antigenemia during chemotherapy. The patient received IV of FOS for 19 days and was on valganciclovir (900 mg/day) for another 117 days. Later (249 days) she developed CMV reactivation and continued to receive FOS (60 mg/day). Although these treatments cleared the CMV, the patient developed acute kidney injury (AKI). FOS was discontinued and BCV was started (150 mg, twice weekly). In 4 days, the patient developed nausea and diarrhea. BCV was discontinued for next 5 days and on sixth onwards a mixture of BCV and FOS were given, in 2 weeks the CMV was cleared. However, the patient developed leukemia and sepsis that led to her death [6A].

A 59-year-old man underwent donor cell transplantation for acute lymphoblastic leukemia. The patient developed CMV infection and was on oral valganciclovir for a week. Side effects resulting from the treatment were vomiting, loose stools, and increase in CMV count. The patient's medication was changed to GCV for the next 44 days. CMV resistance to GCV was developed and the medication was replaced with FOS (90 mg/kg/day). The patient developed diarrhea and to overcome the side effect, BCV (100 mg twice daily) was added to FOS, and CMV became undetectable in 33 days. The patient died on day 419 due to other complications but not from CMV [6A].

Foscarnet [SED-15, 1447; SEDA-34, 448; SEDA-35, 504; SEDA-36, 403; SEDA-37, 329; SEDA-38, 262]

Observational Study

A 50-year-old woman who received double cord blood HSCT as part of her leukemia treatment showed CMV infection and treated with FOS. CMV was cleared in 2 weeks and the patient was subsequently kept on valaciclovir (900 mg/day). In about 152 days, the CMV count was elevated and valaciclovir was replaced with GCV. Resistant strains were again detected with a mutation in UL97, and FOS was given at 60 mg/kg/dose. CMV further increased and BDF 200 mg/kg/dose was started; this caused considerable decrease in CMV count within 2 weeks. Meanwhile, the patient developed abdominal discomfort and gastrointestinal disease involving stomach, duodenum and colon. Even after increasing the concentration of BCV, the side effects persisted. The patient died of gastrointestinal bleeding, septic shock and ongoing gastrointestinal CMV on the 342nd day of treatment [6A].

Ganciclovir and Valganciclovir [SED-15, 1480; SEDA-34, 449; SEDA-35, 504; SEDA-36, 404; SEDA-37, 330; SEDA-38, 262]

Observational Study

GCV is a myelosuppressive drug, which is intracellularly phosphorylated to GCV monophosphate by a viral kinase encoded by CMV gene UL97. The most relevant side effect of GCV is bone marrow depression, particularly neutropenia, which has been associated with risk factors such as impaired renal function, high baseline viral load, and low-level neutrophil counts.

Combination Study

A comparative study in tissue transplant patients on the effect of GCV has been reported. In this study 22 solid organ transplant (SOT) and 17 HSCT patients were included. Of the 39 patients, 15 showed GCV resistance mutations and 11 had tissue-invasive CMV. Virological failure occurred in 33% and 31% showed relapses of viremia. HSCT patients showed higher mortality (31%). GCV resistance was higher in SOT patients compared to HSCT. The most common adverse event (AE) reported was renal dysfunction in 20 patients by the end of treatment and 7 patients after 6 months of treatments [7c].

CMV infection was studied using a murine model to understand the role of CMV in birth defects, mental retardation and non-genetic sensorineural hearing loss. The pharmacokinetics of GCV was assessed in adult mice and pups after 5 days of IP injection of GCV.

In adult rats, the intra-cochlear diffusion of GCV reached the same concentration as in blood. GCV was also capable of crossing the transplacenta in gestating mice and diffused into the brain and the perilymphatic space of the inner ear. High dose of GCV resulted in significant hematotoxicity in different blood cell populations of the mice [8E].

Valaciclovir

A study was conducted in 68 heart transplant patients, who were given 1000 mg/day valaciclovir to prevent CMV infection. The results from this study confirm that the daily use of low-dose valaciclovir (1000 mg/day) is sufficient for CMV prophylaxis without any significant AEs reported [9C].

Similarly, an open-label, phase II study showed that a high dosage of valaciclovir could prevent CMV in transplant patients. Oral administration of high-dosage valaciclovir to mothers significantly reduced the viral load and produced therapeutic concentrations in the blood of infected fetuses [10c].

Monoclonal Antibodies

The in vitro activities of two human monoclonal antibodies, LJP538 and LJP539, has been evaluated for CMV treatment in a study using a combination of these monoclonal antibodies (known as CSJ148) that is currently evaluated for safety and efficacy in clinical trials of CMV infection in HSCT patients. The antibodies target glycoproteins gB and the pentameric (gH/gL/UL128/UL130/UL131) complex. In vitro, LJP538 and LJP539 inhibited CMV infection in five epithelial and three endothelial cell lines; LJP538 also blocked the infection of fibroblasts. No loss of susceptibility to the combination of antibodies was observed for more than 400 days in culture and the binding regions of LJP538 and LJP539 are conserved among clinical isolates. These data provide a hope for the use of these monoclonal antibodies for clinical trials in CMV patients [11E].

DRUGS ACTIVE AGAINST HERPES VIRUSES [SEDA-32, 530; SEDA-33, 577; SEDA-34, 450; SEDA-35, 507; SEDA-36, 407; SEDA-37, 332; SEDA-38, 263]

Acyclovir

The most frequent AEs reported for acyclovir (ACV) are nausea, diarrhea, and headache. Another uncommon but serious side effect of ACV treatment is neurotoxicity that may lead to confusion, hallucinations, and seizures.

Observational Studies

Valacyclovir and ACV were used for the treatment of herpes zoster ophthalmicus in immunocompetent patients. Herpes zoster ophthalmicus affects the eye and vision and is caused by the varicella zoster virus. Patients treated with ACV and Valacyclovir showed side effects such as vomiting, eyelid or facial edema, and disseminated zoster [12R].

Herpes simplex virus-1 (HSV-1) and HSV-2 are closely related human herpesviruses. HSV-1 typically causes common cold sores, encephalitis, and over 400 000 cases of sight-threatening corneal disease annually. ACV is used to treat acute infections and reduces viral shedding and disease associated with HSV reactivations. The authors screened 26 synthetic α-hydroxytropolones, of which compound 118 showed significant inhibition of HSV. ACV resistant virus also failed to replicate in the presence of compound 118. The authors are of the opinion that troponoid drugs administered alone or in combination with existing nucleos(t)ide analogs could suppress the HSV replication without any significant side effects [13E].

Studies have been reported in predicting the risk factors for varicella zoster virus (VZV) infection and postherpetic neuralgia (PHN) after HSCT. This retrospective review was conducted in 163 patients who underwent HSCT between November 2004 and July 2014. Overall, the male/female (M/F) ratio was 80/83, median age at HSCT was 54 (range 15–69) years, and the autologous/allogeneic HCT (auto/allo-HCT) ratio was 71/92. Forty-four patients developed VZV infection after HSCT. All cases were successfully treated with ACV or valacyclovir, and there was no VZV-related death. Nine (20%) of the 44 patients developed PHN after resolution of zoster. The authors indicate that receiving immunosuppressive therapy at the cessation of ACV is a significant risk factor for allo-HSCT recipients [14C].

Famciclovir

The most common adverse experiences with the use of famciclovir were headache, nausea, and diarrhea.

Neurlogical

A 67-year-old man, who was on botulinum toxin A injections to control trigeminal neuralgia was infected with herpes labialis and herpes zoster. The patient was treated with famciclovir and showed significant improvement in pain and subsequent control of trigeminal neuralgia. No significant side effects of famciclovir was reported [15A].

Valacyclovir

Valacyclovir is an antiviral drug also used for the treatment of HSV. The most frequent ADRs reported for valacyclovir were headache, nausea, and abdominal pain.

Renal Toxicity

A female patient 35 years of age was hospitalized due to complaints of a hip blister, fever and kidney dysfunction. The patient was diagnosed with herpes simplex due to the hip blister with unknown causes accompanied by slight erythema. The patient was orally administered with valacyclovir hydrochloride tablets to treat herpes simplex. Subsequently, the patient experienced a significant reduction in quantity of urine produced, and an apparent elevation in serum creatinine levels. The patient was given the anti-inflammatory oral liquid combined with the iodophor solution. The patient's lumbar discomfort was not improved and the patient experienced dysuria and hypourocrinia. Serum creatinine was increased to 592.7 µmol/L and uric acid increased to 624 µmol/L. Renal tubular epithelial cell granule and vacuolar degeneration were also observed in the patient. The patient was given glutathione to alleviate renal tubular injury and sodium bicarbonate was given to induce the alkalized urine that could prevent the tubular formation. Compound polymyxin and topical use of iodophor were able to control HSV infection in this patient [16A].

Observational Studies

HSV-2 infection may increase HIV-1 replication leading to greater infectivity and disease progression. A randomized clinical trial of valacyclovir for HSV-2 suppression in HIV co-infected patients was conducted between March and December 2005 in Peru. Women who were 18 years of age or older, HIV-1 and HIV-2 seropositive and not using antiretroviral or anti-HSV medications were selected for the study. Twenty HSV-2/HIV-1 co-infected women were enrolled in the study. The median age was 28 years and the median CD4 count was 372 cells/µL. The results from their study confirm that HSV-2 suppressive therapy with valacyclovir has little effect in reducing inflammation in the mucosal environment in HSV-2/HIV-1 coinfected women [17c].

A 52-year-old man with hypertension, diastolic congestive heart failure, end-stage renal disease and a remote history of a hemorrhagic stroke was admitted to the emergency department with a vesicular rash on his left arm. Diagnosis revealed that he had herpes zoster infection. The patient was discharged home on valacyclovir 1 g, three times a day for 7 days. The patient took two doses of valacyclovir, but reported with irritability and hallucinations. Over the next several days, the patient's neurologic status declined and he became disoriented and increasingly somnolent. Acyclovir was initiated intravenously at 600 mg (10 mg/kg) for every 12 hours. The patient subsequently had a seizure during dialysis and was felt to have status epilepticus due to ACV and valacyclovir neurotoxicity. The patient underwent daily hemodialysis for removal of the drug and eventually made a full neurologic recovery. ACV side effects resulted in status epilepticus, hallucinations, and altered consciousness [18A].

A case study of a 51-year-old woman was reported with recurrent, dusky and erythematous macules at fixed sites after taking valacyclovir for HSV infection. The patient had already reported similar adverse drug reactions (ADRs) after ACV. Patch and prick tests were performed for ACV, valacyclovir, and famciclovir at a concentration of 1% in petrolatum base, on normal and previous lesional skin. However, the patch and prick tests showed a negative response. The oral challenge test was done with valacyclovir 2 weeks after the patch test. Skin biopsy was performed on an erythematous patch on the lateral thigh, and histopathological findings were consistent with fixed drug eruption, an uncommon adverse drug reaction caused by delayed cell-mediated hypersensitivity. Famciclovir provoked the same ADR at previous lesion sites within 2 hours after administration. This study demonstrates concomitant sensitization to ACV, valacyclovir and famciclovir. Cross-reactions between ACV, valacyclovir and famciclovir in allergic contact dermatitis could be due to their close chemical structures, including a 2-aminopurine nucleus. This case study suggests that ACV, valacyclovir, and famciclovir could have cross-reactions and that could cause the macular drug eruptions, along with exanthematous drug eruptions [19A].

Vaccines

Herpes zoster (HZ), which is commonly referred to as shingles, is caused by reactivation of varicella zoster virus (VZV). The virus is reactivated when immunity to VZV declines mostly with aged or in immune compromised persons. Post-herpetic neuralgia, defined as pain persisting more than 3 months after the skin rash has healed, is a serious consequence of HZ. HZ vaccine reduces the incidence of HZ by 50%. The most common side effects of the vaccine are minor local injection site reactions and headache [20R].

DRUGS ACTIVE AGAINST HEPATITIS VIRUSES

Adefovir [SED-15, 35; SEDA-32, 530; SEDA-33, 578; SEDA-34, 452; SEDA-35, 507; SEDA-36, 409; SEDA-37, 333; SEDA-38, 264]

Urinary Tract

ADV has side effects in osteomalacia patients and could induce Fanconis's syndrome. A case report from

Japan showed altered urinary β-2 microglobulin (β2MG) levels in a patient receiving ADV therapy for HBV infection. A 66-year-old woman reported to have hypophosphatemia and a slightly elevated serum alkaline phosphatase (ALP) level was admitted to the hospital. She had a normal physical condition including normal muscle strength. She was previously diagnosed with chronic HBV infection and was on 3TC (100 mg/day) for 13 years and later on ADV (10 mg/day). Laboratory data showed she had elevated levels of urinary β2MG and N-acetyl-β-D-glucosaminidase levels. The ADV treatment induced temporary pain in her right ankle and hypophosphatemic osteomalacia was reported. ADV levels were reduced by prescribing ADV 10 mg on alternative days that resulted in reduced the β2MG levels. The authors suggest that β2MG could be used as a sensitive marker for drug-induced renal damage [21c].

Direct-Acting Antiviral Protease Inhibitors [SEDA-35, 508; SEDA-36, 409; SEDA-37, 334]

Entecavir [SEDA-33, 578; SEDA-34, 452; SEDA-35, 512; SEDA-36, 411; SEDA-37, 335]

Observational study: Entecavir (ETV) is a nucleoside analogue of 2-deoxyguanosine that inhibits the replication of the HBV. The role of ETV has been reviewed, where the authors shows the advantages of ETV in a combination therapy against HBV infections. A continuous therapy with ETV improves liver histology and reduces the risk of liver failure and hepatocellular carcinoma. Patients with 3TC/ADV resistance or baseline 3TC-resistant mutants should use the combination therapy with ETV in order to overcome the 3TC/ADV resistant HBV mutants [22R].

Another similar study conducted in 30 patients reported the efficacy of ETV in combination with ADV to eliminate the HBV mutants [23c].

Ribavirin [SEDA-33, 578; SEDA-34, 452; SEDA-35, 512; SEDA-36, 412; SEDA-37, 335; SEDA-38, 267]

Neurological

Ribavirin (RBV) is useful in cases like HCV genotype 1, treatment-experienced, cirrhotic patients, or patients with decompensated cirrhosis, and in HCV genotype 3, cirrhotic patients. In these cases RBV shorten the treatment period to 12 weeks. The need of RBV remains to be determined in cirrhotic patients with SOF plus SIM regimen. Generally, the addition of RBV to different combinations of direct-acting antivirals increases the risk of anemia [24R].

Sofosbuvir (SEDA-37, 335; SEDA-38, 268)

Observational Study

A case study reported, a 72-year-old man infected with HCV genotype 1b admitted with cirrhosis and no prior history of inflammatory bowel disease. He developed drug-induced bloody diarrhea within 3 weeks of HCV antiviral therapy with SOF (400 mg/day), SIM (150 mg/day) and RBV (800 mg/day). During the third week of treatment, the patient complained of nausea, vomiting, abdominal pain and constipation [25A].

The use of direct-acting agents for HCV kidney transplant and kidney transplant recipient patients has been reviewed and was suggested to be safe in these particular patients [26R].

A prospective, open-label multicenter pilot study was reported in which adults with recent HCV infection received SOF, 400 mg daily and, weight-based RBV (<75 kg, 1000 mg/day; ≥75 kg, 1200 mg/day) for 6 weeks. Nineteen participants were enrolled between October 2014 and May 2015 through a network of tertiary hospitals in Australia and New Zealand. HCV RNA was below the limit of detection in 47%, 74%, and 79% of patients at weeks 1, 2, and 4 of treatment, respectively. At posttreatment week 12, 13 of 19 patients had treatment failure. One patient discontinued after 2 weeks of treatment. The remaining 12 participants demonstrated virological failure: 2 nonresponse, 9 posttreatment relapse, and 1 reinfection. Both participants with virological nonresponse had high HCV RNA. Another clinical ADRs were reported by 14 participants (74%), with most ADRs being of mild (68%) or moderate (29%) severity. In this, two serious ADRs were reported, one AKI requiring hospitalization and another *Escherichia coli* bloodstream infection; however, both were considered as unrelated to the study drug [27c].

Lung injury was reported in a liver transplant patients treated with SOF. Twenty-four liver transplant recipients with recurrent chronic HCV were treated: 8 received the SOF along with SIM, 6 with ledipasvir, 5 with daclatasvir, and 5 with RBV. At 8 weeks of direct-acting antiviral therapy all patients had achieved undetectable serum HCV-RNA. Moreover, all but one had reached serum virus recovery (SVR). Overall, SOF treatment was well tolerated in the study population with only mild degree of ADRs in 42% of patients. The most common ADRs were fatigue (25%), headache (13%), gastrointestinal disturbances (8%), and anemia (55%) in the RBV group. However, one patient who developed a serious ADE was a 52-year-old woman who had undergone a liver transplant 10 years ago. The patient was in the SOF-daclatasvir treatment group. Ten days after she was admitted in the hospital complaining of severe fatigue, nonproductive cough, dyspnea, and fever. She also developed respiratory failure. The patient was treated with high-dose corticosteroids (60 mg methylprednisolone every 8 hours), and SOF was replaced with SIM. Patient was recoverd from the ADRs and in 24 weeks she achieved SVR. The authors concluded that the respiratory failure and SOF-associated lung injury are rare but potentially life-threatening conditions in patients that develop respiratory symptoms soon after beginning HCV therapy [28c].

A phase 2, multicenter, open-label study was conducted in 44 HCV genotype 4 patients in France from March to November 2014. Participants took a fixed-dose combination tablet of 90 mg of ledipasvir and 400 mg of SOF orally once daily for 12 weeks. The majority of the patients were white and male (64%). Of the 44 patients who were treated with ledipasvir/SOF, 41 (93%) reached the primary endpoint of SVR12. The most common AEs reported were asthenia, headache, and fatigue. All ADRs were mild or moderate in severity, and no patients experienced a serious AE or discontinued treatment because of an ADR. Authors conclude that the treatment with once-daily oral regimen of ledipasvir/SOF for 12 weeks resulted in a high rate of SVR among treatment-naïve and -experienced patients with HCV genotype 4 [29C].

A retrospective cohort study included 260 patients who were treated with a SOF-containing therapy between January 2014 and December 2015 in Germany. Patients were treated with SOF/DCV or SOF/LDV. Of the 256 patients, 240 patients achieved SVR12; 4 out of 256 lost follow-up and 12 patients suffered from relapse. One hundred and forty-seven patients reported side effects during treatment. In general, side effects were mild in intensity, thus, just one patient discontinued treatment prematurely due to back-pain. Overall, fatigue, headache, bone pain or joint pain, and myalgia were the most frequently reported side effects. Hospital admissions were required during treatment with SOF-based regimens in 22 (8.6%) patients. The reasons for hospitalization were infections ($n=8$); hepatic decompensation ($n=3$); cardiovascular disease ($n=3$); cholestatic hepatitis after liver transplantation ($n=2$); treatment of hepatocellular carcinoma ($n=2$); and lumbago, vomitus, diabetes insipidus and right upper quadrant pain ($n=1$, each). Of those hospitalized, two patients died from infectious complications (right-heart failure), and two patients died from cardiovascular disease (intracerebral bleeding) [30C].

A retrospective analysis with prospective follow-up was performed of post-kidney transplant patients with chronic HCV treated with DAAs in three academic centers in Boston, MA. Twenty-four kidney transplant recipients with chronic HCV infection received DAA during the study period. Patients were included irrespective of their liver fibrosis stage, genotype, or prior HCV treatment status. SOF was prescribed at 400 mg/day orally; SIM was prescribed at 150 mg/day orally; ledipasvir

was prescribed at 90 mg/day administered orally in co-formulation with SOF 400 mg; RBV was prescribed according to body weight (1000 mg daily in patients who were <75 kg and 1200 mg daily in patients who were >75 kg). The treatment duration varied between 12 and 24 weeks based on HCV genotype, the stage of underlying liver fibrosis and prior treatment history. Twenty-three patients had SVR12 assessment; one patient had SVR4 assessment. Eleven patients (46%) reported AEs. Overall, there were three serious AEs. Of the seven patients that received RBV, two discontinued RBV due to side effects (fatigue, shortness of breath and gout flare), but they continued combined DAA treatment. Two of the seven patients developed anemia. The serious ADRs were gastrointestinal bleeding, portal vein thrombosis, and sinus bradycardia, and the common ADRs were shortness of breath, fatigue, headache, dizziness, diarrhea, pain in the lower extremity, photosensitivity, insomnia, and rashes [31C].

Antiviral treatment with a combination of SOF/LDV is highly effective, safe, and well tolerated in HCV patients who had orthotropic liver transplantation. The addition of RBV along with SOF often results in severe anemia and required dose reduction or discontinuation to avoid the side effects [32c].

Early treatment of HCV infection with IF-α is highly effective. A prospective, open-label, multicenter, single-arm pilot study in adults having acute HCV genotype 1 monoinfection was reported from 10 centers in Germany. Patients were administered ledipasvir (90 mg) plus SOF (400 mg) as a fixed-dose combination tablet once daily for 6 weeks. The primary efficacy outcome was the proportion of patients with SVR 12 weeks after the end of treatment. All patients achieved a SVR 12 weeks after the end of treatment (20 out of 20 patients). Treatment was well tolerated, and up to 12 weeks after treatment, 22 possible drug-related adverse drug events (ADRs) were reported but none of them was a serious ADRs. There was one serious ADE, which was judged as unrelated to the study drug [33C].

Simeprevir [SEDA-38, 269]

A SIM plus SOF regimen was recommended for certain patients with HCV genotype 1 infection. A multicenter observational study reported included 583 patients with HCV genotype 4 infection were treated with SIM plus SOF for 12 weeks. The overall SVR rate was 95.7% (558 out of 583 patients). Side effects included rash in 21 patients, photosensitivity in 18 patients, pruritus in 44 patients and hyperbilirubinemia in 42 patients [34C].

Dermatological reactions caused by SIM+SOF treatment in HCV patients has been reported [35c].

SOF and SIM combination therapy early after allo-HSCT was also reported to clear the HCV without any significant ADRs [36c].

Sixty-two patients with HCV cirrhosis underwent organ liver transplant (OLT) at a transplant center. Five patients developed recurrence HCV in the form of severe FCH and were treated with SOF and SIM for 24 weeks. All patients achieved significant improvement in HCV viral load. One patient developed refractory pruritus and acute pancreatitis. The third patient showed hepatic artery thrombosis and developed sepsis and renal failure [37C].

DRUGS ACTIVE AGAINST HUMAN IMMUNODEFICIENCY VIRUS: COMBINATIONS

Abacavir/Lamivudine/DTG

Dolutegravir (DTG) in combination with abacavir (ABC)/3TC is one of the preferred regimens in multiple clinical scenarios, including treatment-naive and treatment-experienced patients. Triple combination therapy with ABC/3TC/DTG should be considered among the initial options for treatment-naïve HIV patients, being effective, well tolerated, with a high genetic barrier to resistance along with a convenient once-daily administration. DTG inhibits HIV integrase by binding to the integrase active site and blocking the strand transfer step of retroviral DNA integration into host cell DNA. ABC and 3TC are both metabolized sequentially by intracellular kinases to the respective 5'-triphosphates, which are the active moieties with extended intracellular half-lives. The main antiviral activity of ABC and 3TC is through the incorporation of the monophosphate form into the viral DNA chain, resulting in chain termination.

DTG has relatively fewer side effects and is generally better tolerated than most other available ARVs. Common AEs reported for DTG included headache, insomnia, nausea, and diarrhea, but the proportion of patients reporting severe reactions never exceeded 1%. Hypersensitivity reactions were reported in <1% of trial participants, despite the fact that ABC has been associated with serious and sometimes fatal multiple-organ hypersensitivity reactions. Creatinine elevation is the most frequently observed biochemical alteration due to DTG use. Transaminase elevation might occur in 5% of subjects receiving DTG but were mild [38M].

Elvitegravir/Cobicistat/FTC/Tenofovir

Observational Studies

An open-label, non-comparative switch study evaluated the efficacy and safety of ETV/COB/FTC/TAF in HIV/HBV-coinfected adults. At 48 weeks, 91.7% of the 72 participants maintained or achieved virologic suppression. ETV/COB/FTC/TAF was associated with improved renal function and reduced bone turnover. These data support the use of ETV/COB/FTC/TAF in treating HIV/HBV coinfection without significant AEs [39c].

Acute kidney injury (AKI) was reported in children treated with highly active antiretroviral therapy (HRRT). Sixty-three children were included in the study with a mean age of 5.3 ± 4.27 years (range 1–14 years); 44 (69.8%) were younger than 7 years; and 35 (55.6%) were females. Forty-three (68.3%) patients were using HRRT prior to admission, but 20 were not on HRRT. Among all patients using HRRT, 37 were using 3TC; 31 on AZT; 16 on LPV; and 5 were treated with TDF. One patient needed hemodialysis and one patient died. One patient showed microscopic hematuria and three had proteinuria. Among all patients, the most frequent opportunistic infections (OIs) were pneumonia (44.4%), pulmonary tuberculosis (9.5%), and varicella zoster/chickenpox (6.3%). AKI was observed in 33 children, of which 19 children were classified as risk, 13 children were classified as injury, and 1 child considered as failure. Prevalence of AKI was lower in those on HRRT than those not on HRRT [40c].

A 47-year-old black man with a solitary kidney who was infected with HIV was treated with EFV 600 mg/ETV 200 mg/TDF 300 mg, daily for 19 months. The patient showed no evidence of nephrotoxicity over the course of 19 months on ART. He maintained adequate renal function, comparable to his baseline renal function. The authors suggest that, for patients with solitary kidneys, ART containing TDF maybe a better choice [41c].

An open-label, non-comparative switch study evaluated the efficacy and safety of coformulated ETV, COB, FTC, and tenofovir alafenamide (TAF) in HIV/HBV-coinfected adults. Of the 100 adults screened, 74 received at least one dose of ETV/COB/FTC/TAF. The participants were predominantly male. At 48 weeks, 72 participants maintained or achieved virologic suppression. ETV/COB/FTC/TAF was associated with improved renal function and reduced bone turnover. There was no proximal tubulopathy or drug discontinuation because of renal AEs. The most frequently reported study drug-related AEs were diarrhea (4.1%) and increased appetite (2.7%). One participant (1.4%) discontinued ETV/COB/FTC/TAF because of AEs of increased weight and appetite. Serious AEs were infrequent (8.1%) and there was no death reported by the treatment. There were small increases in total cholesterol, direct LDL cholesterol and HDL cholesterol, but not affecting the total cholesterol-to-HDL ratio [39c].

DRUGS ACTIVE AGAINST HUMAN IMMUNODEFICIENCY VIRUS: NUCLEOSIDE ANALOGUE REVERSE TRANSCRIPTASE INHIBITORS (NRTI) [SEDA-15, 2586; SEDA-32, 534; SEDA-33, 585; SEDA-34, 456; SEDA-35, 516; SEDA-36, 415; SEDA-37, 337; SEDA-38, 270]

Abacavir [SEDA-15, 3; SEDA-32, 534; SEDA-33, 585; SEDA-34, 456; SEDA-35, 516; SEDA-36, 415; SEDA-37, 337; SEDA-38, 270]

Observational Studies

The efficacy and safety data from phase 2 and 3 clinical study on a combination of ABC/3TC/DTG, particularly on the results of both SPRING (1 and 2) and SINGLE studies suggest that the use of these combination compounds reduced the side effects. The authors are of the opinion that the triple combination therapy with ABC/3TC/DTG should be considered among the initial options for treatment-naive HIV patients, being effective, well tolerated, with a high genetic barrier to resistance along with a convenient once-daily administration [38c].

Lamivudine [SED-15, 1989; SEDA-32, 531; SEDA-33, 587; SEDA-34, 456; SEDA-35, 517; SEDA-36, 416; SEDA-37, 338]

Observational Studies

An observational study was conducted in the antiretroviral treatment center in North India from February 2009 to December 2013 to record the effects of 3TC-induced rashes. 3TC-induced skin rash occurred in 23 HIV-infected individuals out of 3213 HIV-infected patients who were on ZDV/TDF+3TC+NVP/EFV during the study period. 3TC-induced rash was more common in women than men [42c].

A 54-year-old white woman diagnosed with HIV infection started treatment with FTC/TDF in combination with NVP. An itchy rash on the neckline, abdomen and limbs appeared 8 hours after the first dose. The symptoms improved with antihistamine treatment. However, 24 hours after this reaction, the patient took another dose and a new rash with extensive skin scaling appeared, accompanied by oral and genital ulceration, fever, hepatitis, diarrhea, and loss of consciousness. Nine months later, the patient resumed HAART, and subsequently suffered from three milder episodes after FTC/TDF with etravirine, ABC/3TC with RAL, and FTC/TDF

with RAL. However, the patient continued to have the rashes. The patient started an alternative treatment plan with TDF, RAL and ritonavir/lopinavir for a year without having any episode of rashes [43A].

Zidovudine [SED-15, 3713; SEDA-32, 536; SEDA-33, 588; SEDA-34, 458; SEDA-35, 517; SEDA-36, 417; SEDA-37, 338]

HIV-infected pediatric patients, aged <18 years from 14 cohorts participating in EPPICC's pharmacovigilance program who were on AZT/3TC tablets between 2008 and 2012, were included in this study. Data from 541 patients on AZT/3TC were taken for the study. Five patients aged <10 years and six ≥10 years at start of AZT/3TC tablets had grade ≥3 neutropenia. Two patients aged <10 years had a grade ≥3 ALT event. One patient aged <10 years had a grade ≥3 AST event 12–24 months after starting AZT/3TC. Five patients aged <10 years had grade ≥3 hyperbilirubinemia. Five patients aged <10 years had grade ≥3 anemia. Two patients aged <10 years had grade ≥3 platelet results (both <12 months after starting AZT/3TC). There was only 1 grade ≥3 WBC event among patients aged ≥10 years [44C].

DRUGS ACTIVE AGAINST HUMAN IMMUNODEFICIENCY VIRUS: NUCLEOTIDE ANALOGUE REVERSE TRANSCRIPTASE INHIBITORS

Tenofovir [SED-15, 3314; SEDA-32, 537; SEDA-33, 588; SEDA-34, 458; SEDA-35, 518; SEDA-36, 418; SEDA-37, 338; SEDA-38, 272]

Renal Toxicity

Combination therapy including nucleoside and nucleotide analogues for the treatment of chronic HBV with multidrug resistance has been recommended as an effective treatment, but it has shown side effects. A study was conducted from December 2012 to June 2014 in patients exhibiting antiviral drug resistance who were treated with TDF for more than 6 months. The patients were categorized into three groups: 3TC-resistance (LAM-R) group (n=290), and LAM-R+ADV-resistance (ADV-R) group (n=43), and LAM-R+ETV-resistance (ETV-R) group (n=113). TDF mono-rescue therapy in the entire cohort was well tolerated, and no clinically significant side effects were reported. Thirteen patients had a low eGFR

($\leq$50 mL/min/1.73 m^2) at the onset of TDF initiation and were treated with a reduced dose of TDF, which normalized the eGFR level [45C].

Bone Density

When treated with TDF, HIV-infected patients showed a decrease in the bone mineral density (BMD). This study compared the effects of EFV/FTC/TDF with the effects of RAL/DRV/r on BMD on antiretroviral treatment-naïve African American subjects. Thirty-five HIV patients were randomized to receive either EFV/FTC/TDF or RAL/DRV/r. All of the subjects received supplemental vitamin D-3 and calcium. CD4 counts, HIV RNA, parathyroid hormone, osteocalcin, N-telopeptide, and 25-hydroxyvitamin D levels were obtained at baseline and at 8, 24, 36, and 48 weeks, but the 25-hydroxyvitamin D levels were decreased in both groups. By week 48, the levels of 25-hydroxyvitamin D in the RAL/DRV/r group increased but not in the EFV/FTC/TDF group [46c].

A review article also discusses the bone safety of TDF in HIV patients [47R].

A phase 1, single-dose, pharmacokinetic (PK) investigation of TDF and FTC treatment in 49 healthy female volunteers participated in the clinical trial between April 2012 and August 2013 included in the study. A mathematical modeling was also used to determine the number of doses required for effective HIV pre-exposure prophylaxis (PrEP). A PK/pharmacodynamic (PD) model was developed by measuring mucosal tissue concentrations of TAF, FTC, and their active metabolites (tenofovir diphosphate and FTC triphosphate, respectively), and competing endogenous nucleotides (dATP and dCTP) in all participants. This model is predictive of PrEP trial results in which 2–3 doses/week were 75%–90% effective in men but not effective in women [48C].

A single-arm, open-label study recruited 242 patients with mean age of 58 years. Tenofovir alafenamide (TAF) is a novel tenofovir pro-drug with improved renal and bone safety. A 48-week safety and efficacy study on a once-daily single tablet regimen of ETV 150 mg, COB 150 mg, FTC 200 mg, and TAF 10 mg (ETV/COB/FTC/TAF) was conducted in HIV-1-infected patients. The primary endpoint was the change from baseline in eGFR. Through week 48, no significant change in estimated CrCl was observed. Two patients (0.8%) discontinued the study drug due to decreased creatinine clearance. Subjects had significant improvements in proteinuria, albuminuria, and tubular proteinuria. Hip and spine bone mineral density significantly increased from baseline to week 48. Ninety-two percent of the patients maintained less than 50 copies of HIV-1 RNA at week 48 [49C].

DRUGS ACTIVE AGAINST HUMAN IMMUNODEFICIENCY VIRUS: NON-NUCLEOSIDE REVERSE TRANSCRIPTASE INHIBITORS (NNRTI) [SEDA-15, 2553; SEDA-31, 486; SEDA-32, 537; SEDA-33, 590; SED-34, 459; SEDA-35, 519; SEDA-36, 420; SEDA-37, 339; SEDA-38, 273]

Efavirenz [SEDA-15, 1204; SEDA-32, 537; SEDA-33, 590; SEDA-34, 459; SEDA-35, 519; SEDA-36, 420; SEDA-37, 339; SEDA-38, 273]

The impact of Efavirenz (EFV), Etravirine, RPV and NVP on the integrity of the blood–brain barrier, and their impact on severity of stroke, was studied in an animal model. EFV altered claudin-5 expression, increased endothelial permeability, and disrupted the blood–brain barrier integrity and also increased the severity of stroke in the middle cerebral artery occlusion in mice [50E].

Observational Studies

The efficacy, safety, and anti-inflammatory effects of cenicriviroc (CVC) with EFV in treatment-naive, HIV-1-infected adults were studied. In this study, a randomized, double-blind, double-dummy phase 2b trial at 43 institutions (USA and Puerto Rico) was conducted in 143 HIV-1-infected adults for 48 weeks. Study participants were randomized to receive CVC 100 mg (59 patients), CVC 200 mg (56 patients), or EFV 600 mg (28 patients), each administered with FTC/TDF. Virologic success was obtained at week 24 and at week 48. Resistance mutations emerged in five CVC-treated participants. Treatment-related AEs of at least grade 2 and discontinuations due to AEs were less frequent in CVC-treated study participants. Total and low-density lipoprotein cholesterol decreased with CVC, but increased with EFV. The authors suggest that CVC showed better efficacy and favorable safety in treatment-naive HIV-1-infected patients and that the drug could go on to phase 3 trials [51C].

Neurological

The first case of complex partial seizures arising due to EFV treatment in HIV patient was reported. A 33-year-old Nigerian man was treated with an EFV-based antiretroviral regimen for HIV infection. He reported with seizures soon after starting the antiretroviral drugs. His blood levels of sodium, glucose, urea, and creatinine were within normal limits. His electroencephalogram showed intermittent bursts of sharp waves and spikes bilaterally over front temporoparietal regions. His seizures stopped following a switch to a non-EFV-based regimen [52A].

Four black African children, between the ages of 4 and 8 years and between 1 and 20 months post-EFV initiation, developed cerebellar dysfunction and generalized seizures. Plasma EFV levels ranged from 20 to 60 mg/L, 5–15 times the upper limit. All abnormal central nervous system manifestations abated after EFV discontinuation. This study suggests that CYP2B6 single-nucleotide polymorphisms should be analyzed before starting the antiviral treatment to avoid the neurological side effects [53A].

Nevirapine [SEDA-33, 593; SEDA-34, 460; SEDA-35, 521; SEDA-36, 421; SEDA-37, 339; SEDA-38, 274]

See also Section Efavirenz.

Rilpivirine [SEDA-35, 521; SEDA-36, 423; SEDA-37, 340; SEDA-38, 274]

PAINT is a phase II, open-label, single-arm, 2-part study, with an 8-week screening period, an initial 48-week treatment period and an ongoing post-week 48-treatment extension period. The study was conducted between December 2010 and June 2014 for 48 weeks. Thirty-six patients were enrolled and treated in the study, and at the end of 48 weeks, 8 patients (22%) discontinued for various reasons. In Cohort 1 of the study, the PK, safety, efficacy and virology of RPV taken in combination with an investigator-selected dual NTRTI background regimen was evaluated. The median time to virologic response was 11.4 weeks. Study demonstrated that RPV 25 mg combined with two NTRTI was effective and generally well tolerated over 48 weeks in HIV-1-infected patients. AEs considered to be at least related to RPV were somnolence (14%), nausea (6%), dizziness, headache, abdominal pain, blurred vision, pyrexia, drug hypersensitivity, skin papilloma, and rash in 3% of the patients [54C].

DRUGS ACTIVE AGAINST HUMAN IMMUNODEFICIENCY VIRUS: PROTEASE INHIBITORS [SED-15, 2586; SEDA-32, 541; SEDA-33, 593; SEDA-34, 461; SEDA-35, 522; SEDA-36, 423; SEDA-37, 340; SEDA-38, 274]

Atazanavir

Observational Study

Ritonavir-boosted atazanavir (ATV/r) is the preferred treatment for HIV patients in resource-limited settings and with ADRs for other drugs. Data analyzed on the ATV/r-associated ADRs in Southern India. In this prospective study, 111 HIV patients treated with ATV/r for at least 2 years who followed a follow-up visits for the emergence of hyperbilirubinemia, hypertransaminasemia, and serum creatinine elevation were included in the study. The incidence of severe hyperbilirubinemia, hypertransaminasemia, and creatinine elevation was 28.6, 0.76, and 1.62 cases/100 person years, respectively. 3TC/FTC + TDF were found to be significantly associated with hypertransaminasemia and creatinine elevation [55C].

Cardiovascular risk among HIV-infected patients treated with ATV has been reviewed [56R]. In this systematic review of cardiovascular disease in HIV-infected patients receiving ATV, there was no increase in the risk or occurrence of adverse clinical outcome with boosted and unboosted ATV compared to other antiviral agents.

DRUGS ACTIVE AGAINST HUMAN IMMUNODEFICIENCY VIRUS: INHIBITORS OF HIV FUSION [SEDA-33, 598; SEDA-34, 464; SEDA-35, 525; SEDA-36, 428; SEDA-37, 341; SEDA-38, 275]

Enfuvirtide

Fusion inhibitors are a class of molecules designed to disrupts the HIV-1 fusion protein equipment at the final stage of fusion with the host cell. HIV binds to the host CD4+ cell receptor via the viral protein gp120 and gp41, and then undergoes a conformational change that assists in the fusion of the viral membrane with the host cell membrane. Enfuvirtide binds to gp41 and thus preventing the formation of an entry pore for the capsid of the HIV-virus. Enfuvirtide has side effects include diarrhea, fatigue, nausea, and reactions at the site injection [57R].

DRUGS ACTIVE AGAINST HUMAN IMMUNODEFICIENCY VIRUS: INTEGRASE INHIBITORS [SEDA-33, 599; SEDA-34, 465; SEDA-35, 525; SEDA-36, 428; SEDA-37, 342; SEDA-38, 275; SEDA-38, 276]

Dolutegravir

Observational studies: DTG is one of the preferred antiretroviral agents in cART. A cohort study including all patients who started DTG in two HIV treatment centers in the Netherlands. All cART-naïve and cART-experienced patients who had started DTG were identified from the institutional HIV databases. In total, 556 patients were included, of whom 102 (18.4%) were cART-naïve at initiation of DTG. Median follow-up time was 225 days. Overall, in 85 patients (15.3%), DTG was stopped. In 76 patients (13.7%), this was due to intolerability. Insomnia and sleep disturbance (5.6%), gastrointestinal complaints (4.3%) and neuropsychiatric symptoms such as anxiety, psychosis and depression (4.3%) were the predominant reasons for switching from DTG. In regimens that included ABV, DTG was switched more frequently. In particular, DTG was stopped more frequently if the regimen included ABV [58c].

Raltegravir

The use of RAL in clinical practice raised new hopes in the achievement of HIV eradication, since its mechanism of action based on the inhibition of HIV integration in uninfected cells.

Observational Study

A prospective cohort study was conducted of HIV-1-infected adult patients from January 2011 through December 2012 receiving a stable antiretroviral regimen for at least 12 months including a ritonavir-boosted PI plus two NRTIs for at least 6 months. All patients who switched to a dual antiretroviral regimen constituting RAL (400 mg twice daily) and darunavir/ritonavir (800/100 mg daily) were enrolled in the study and followed for 48 weeks. This study enrolled 82 patients with a mean age of 45.2 years, of which 60 patients were male. The reasons for switch to RAL plus darunavir/ritonavir were renal toxicity (increased creatinine, hypophosphoremia, or tubular proteinuria), reduced BMD, hyperlipidemia, gastrointestinal symptoms, or resistance to nucleoside/nucleotide analogues. After 48 weeks from the switch to RAL plus darunavir/ritonavir, 6 discontinued, 2 due to virological failure and 4 due to non-serious AEs. The four discontinuations for non-serious AEs were due to diarrhea with abdominal discomfort in three cases and nausea with lack of appetite in one. The authors concluded that the dual therapy containing RAL and darunavir/ritonavir was well tolerated after a 48-week follow-up as a strategy in persistently suppressed HIV-infected patients [59c].

DRUGS ACTIVE AGAINST HUMAN IMMUNODEFICIENCY VIRUS: CHEMOKINE RECEPTOR CCR5 ANTAGONISTS [SEDA-33, 600; SEDA-34, 465; SEDA-35, 528; SEDA-36, 430; SEDA-37, 343; SEDA-38, 276]

Maraviroc

Observational study: Maraviroc is an entry inhibitor registered for the treatment of HIV. Binding of MVC to CCR5 prevents interaction with the third hypervariable loop (V3 loop) of the viral envelope protein gp120 and thereby prevents HIV entry into the cell. A retrospective cohort study was reported in patients with an HIV-1 diagnosis who were ≥18 years of age. Sixty-two patients were included in the study. In 40 patients, plasma HIV-RNA was detectable (≥50 copies/mL) at the start of MVC, whereas in 22 patients MVC was started when plasma HIV-RNA was undetectable. Thirty-four patients (54.8%) started MVC because of virological failure of their previous regimen, whereas 15 patients (24.2%) switched to MVC-containing regimen because of toxicity problems. MVC-containing regimens were well tolerated. Twelve patients (19.4%) discontinued MVC therapy. Of these patients, three re-started MVC treatment after 6 months. Three patients discontinued MVC due to side effects. Out the remaining patients, four developed increased ALT levels, but was not related to MVC therapy. Increased plasma creatinine level was found in five patients. However, all five patients were known to have renal insufficiency before the start of MVC. Five patients (8.1%) died during follow-up. Causes of death were pneumonia (two cases), B-cell lymphoma, squamous cell carcinoma, and cardiomyopathy in combination with pulmonary hypertension (3 cases). There appeared to be no direct correlation between MVC therapy and any of the deaths [60C].

A multicenter, randomized, open-label, 96-week noninferiority switch study of MVC was reported. Participants were included if they were HIV-1-infected adults aged ≥18 years. Seven hundred ninety-five participants were screened from sites in 13 countries (Argentina, Australia, Canada, Chile, France, Germany, Ireland, Japan, Mexico, Poland, Spain, Thailand, and United Kingdom). Twenty-three percent of participants were women. Sixty-eight percent were on tenofovir-based N(t)RTI backbones; 35%, 28%, and 17% were on ritonavir-boosted ATV, lopinavir (LPV/r), or darunavir, respectively. Eight hundred and eighty-four AEs were reported; 86% were determined as not related or probably not related to study drugs. During the 48 weeks of follow-up, 1 patient died, 1 patient in the MVC+PI/r arm developed an AIDS-defining illness, and 9 had serious non-AIDS-defining events (2 and 7 in the control and MVC arms, respectively). One myocardial infarction event was reported as a safety alert in a patient on MVC [61c].

DRUGS ACTIVE AGAINST INFLUENZA VIRUSES: NEURAMINIDASE INHIBITORS [SED-15, 2436; SEDA-32, 544; SEDA-33, 601; SEDA-34, 466; SEDA-35, 528; SEDA-36, 431; SEDA-37, 344; SEDA-38, 277]

Oseltamivir (Tamiflu)

Oseltamivir is well tolerated in influenza patients and the most commonly reported side effect is associated with the gastrointestinal system [62R].

A survey was conducted in a cross-sectional, multiple-choice, adult patients and adult caregivers of pediatric patients who were admitted to the emergency department with flu-like symptoms. The survey asked about the use of oseltamivir in flu-like symptoms. The survey responders were of the opinion that they were not willing to take the medication since it may have adverse effects on kidney and liver [63c].

A novel cyclopentane neuraminidase inhibitor of influenza virus, Peramivir, was active against both A and B strains of influenza virus, and was approved by the Food and Drug Administration in December 2014. Common side effects of peramivir were gastrointestinal disorders and decreased neutrophil counts [64R].

OTHER DRUGS

Imiquimod [SED-15, 1718; SEDA-35, 530; SEDA-36, 431; SEDA-37, 344; SEDA-38, 277]

Imiquimod is an immune response modifier. The mechanism of action of imiquimod has been detailed [65R].

Cervical intraepithelial neoplasia (CIN) is the premalignant condition of cervical cancer and is caused by cervical human papillomavirus (HPV) infection. Imiquimod has been employed to treat CIN [66C].

A 67-year-old male patient presenting with infiltrating basal cell carcinoma above the left eyebrow was treated with Imiquimod. The reported side effects of imiquimod were multiple eruptive milia, erythema, irritation and crusting [67c].

Dermatological studies: Periocular melanoma was treated with 5% Imiquimod cream and showed no systemic side effects [68c].

A recent survey of case studies pertaining to antivirals was published in 2015 [69].

Disclaimer

The findings and the conclusions in this report are those of the authors and do not necessarily represent the views of the National Institute for Occupational Safety and Health.

References

[1] Maffini E, Giaccone L, Festuccia M, et al. Treatment of CMV infection after allogeneic hematopoietic stem cell transplantation. Expert Rev Hematol. 2016;9(6):585–96 [R].

[2] Campos AB, Ribeiro J, Boutolleau D, et al. Human cytomegalovirus antiviral drug resistance in hematopoietic stem cell transplantation: current state of the art. Rev Med Virol. 2016;26(3):161–82 [R].

[3] Lischka P, Michel D, Zimmermann H. Characterization of cytomegalovirus breakthrough events in a phase 2 prophylaxis trial of letermovir (AIC246, MK 8228). J Infect Dis. 2016;213(1):23–30 [c].

[4] Drouot E, Piret J, Boivin G. Artesunate demonstrates in vitro synergism with several antiviral agents against human cytomegalovirus. Antivir Ther. 2016;21(6):535–9 [c].

[5] Randall Lanier E, Foster S, Brundage T, et al. Analysis of mutations in the gene encoding cytomegalovirus DNA polymerase in a phase 2 clinical trial of brincidofovir prophylaxis. J Infect Dis. 2016;214(1):32–5 [c].

[6] El-Haddad D, El Chaer F, Vanichanan J, et al. Brincidofovir (CMX-001) for refractory and resistant CMV and HSV infections in immunocompromised cancer patients: a single-center experience. Antiviral Res. 2016;134:58–62 [A].

[7] Avery RK, Arav-Boger R, Marr KA, et al. Outcomes in transplant recipients treated with foscarnet for ganciclovir-resistant or refractory cytomegalovirus infection. Transplantation. 2016;100(10):e74–80 [c].

[8] Boujemla I, Fakhoury M, Nassar M, et al. Pharmacokinetics and tissue diffusion of ganciclovir in mice and rats. Antiviral Res. 2016;132:111–5 [E].

[9] Kervan U, Kucuker SA, Kocabeyoglu SS, et al. Low-dose valacyclovir for cytomegalovirus infection prophylaxis after a heart transplant. Exp Clin Transplant. 2016;14(5):551–4 [C].

[10] Leruez-Ville M, Ghout I, Bussières L, et al. In utero treatment of congenital cytomegalovirus infection with valacyclovir in a multicenter, open-label, phase II study. Am J Obstet Gynecol. 2016;215(4): 462.e1–462.e10 [c].

[11] Patel HD, Nikitin P, Gesner T, et al. In vitro characterization of human cytomegalovirus-targeting therapeutic monoclonal antibodies LJP538 and LJP539. Antimicrob Agents Chemother. 2016;60(8):4961–71 [E].

[12] Schuster AK, Harder BC, Schlichtenbrede FC, et al. Valacyclovir versus acyclovir for the treatment of herpes zoster ophthalmicus in immunocompetent patients. Cochrane Database Syst Rev. 2016;2016(11) Article number CD011503, [R].

[13] Ireland PJ, Tavis JE, D'Erasmo MP, et al. Synthetic α-hydroxytropolones inhibit replication of wild-type and acyclovir-resistant herpes simplex viruses. Antimicrob Agents Chemother. 2016;60(4):2140–9 [E].

[14] Kanbayashi Y, Matsumoto Y, Kuroda J, et al. Predicting risk factors for varicella zoster virus infection and postherpetic neuralgia after hematopoietic cell transplantation using ordered logistic regression analysis. Ann Hematol. 2017;96:311–5 [C].

[15] Emeriewen K, Macgregor C, Athanasiadis Y, et al. Neuropathic pain in multiple sclerosis improved with oral famciclovir: a case report. Ophthal Plast Reconstr Surg. 2016;32(5): e119–21 [A].

[16] Zhang Y, Cong Y, Teng Y. Acute renal injury induced by valacyclovir hydrochloride: a case report. Exp Ther Med. 2016;12(6):4025–8 [A].

[17] Andersen-Nissen E, Chang JT, Thomas KK, et al. Herpes simplex virus suppressive therapy in herpes simplex virus-2/human immunodeficiency virus-1 coinfected women is associated with reduced systemic CXCL10 but not genital cytokines. Sex Transm Dis. 2016;43(12):761–4 [c].

[18] Hoskote SS, Annapureddy N, Ramesh AK, et al. Valacyclovir and acyclovir neurotoxicity with status epilepticus. Am J Ther. 2016;23(1):e304–6 [A].

[19] Lee HJ, Kim JM, Kim GW, et al. Fixed drug eruption due to acyclovir, valacyclovir and famciclovir. J Eur Acad Dermatol Venereol. 2016;30(8):1417–9 [A].

[20] Sampathkumar P. Herpes zoster and post-herpetic neuralgia. Current Geriatrics Rep. 2016;5(1):9–15 [R].

[21] Takagi J, Morita H, Ito K, et al. Urinary β-2 microglobulin levels sensitively altered in an osteomalacia patient receiving add-on adefovir dipivoxil therapy for hepatitis B virus infection. Intern Med. 2016;55(12):1599–603 [c].

[22] Lee HW, Park JY, Ahn SH. An evaluation of entecavir for the treatment of chronic hepatitis B infection in adults. Expert Rev Gastroenterol Hepatol. 2016;10(2):177–86 [R].

[23] Oh M, Lee H. Antiviral efficacy of entecavir versus entecavir plus adefovir for hepatitis B virus rtA181V/T mutants alone. Saudi J Gastroenterol. 2016;22(1):37–42 [c].

[24] Hézode C, Bronowicki JP. Ideal oral combinations to eradicate HCV: the role of ribavirin. J Hepatol. 2016;64(1):215–25 [R].

[25] Izzo I, Zanotti P, Chirico C, et al. Colitis during new direct-acting antiviral agents (DAAs) therapy with sofosbuvir, simeprevir and ribavirin for genotype 1b hepatitis C. Infection. 2016;44(6):811–2 [A].

[26] Rostaing L, Alric L, Kamar N. Use of direct-acting agents for hepatitis C virus-positive kidney transplant candidates and kidney transplant recipients. Transpl Int. 2016;29(12):1257–65 [R].

[27] Martinello M, Gane E, Hellard M, et al. Sofosbuvir and ribavirin for 6 weeks is not effective among people with recent hepatitis C virus infection: the DARE-C II study. Hepatology. 2016;64(6):1911–21 [c].

[28] Benítez-Gutiérrez L, de Mendoza C, Baños I, et al. Drug-induced lung injury in a liver transplant patient treated with sofosbuvir. Transplant Proc. 2016;48(7):2515–8 [c].

[29] Abergel A, Metivier S, Samuel D, et al. Ledipasvir plus sofosbuvir for 12 weeks in patients with hepatitis C genotype 4 infection. Hepatology. 2016;64(4):1049–56 [c].

[30] Werner CR, Schwarz JM, Egetemeyr DP, et al. Second-generation direct-acting-antiviral hepatitis C virus treatment: efficacy, safety, and predictors of SVR12. World J Gastroenterol. 2016;22(35):8050–9 [C].

[31] Lin MV, Sise ME, Pavlakis M, et al. Efficacy and safety of direct acting antivirals in kidney transplant recipients with chronic hepatitis C virus infection. PLoS One. 2016;11(7)e0158431 [C].

[32] Ciesek S, Proske V, Otto B, et al. Efficacy and safety of sofosbuvir/ledipasvir for the treatment of patients with hepatitis C virus re-infection after liver transplantation. Transpl Infect Dis. 2016;18(3):326–32 [c].

[33] Deterding K, Spinner CD, Schott E, et al. Ledipasvir plus sofosbuvir fixed-dose combination for 6 weeks in patients with acute hepatitis C virus genotype 1 monoinfection (HepNet Acute HCV IV): an open-label, single-arm, phase 2 study. Lancet Infect Dis. 2017;17:215–22 [C].

[34] El-Khayat HR, Fouad YM, Maher M, et al. Efficacy and safety of sofosbuvir plus simeprevir therapy in Egyptian patients with chronic hepatitis C: a real-world experience. Gut. 2016; (in press) [C].

[35] Lacaita MV, Carpentieri A, Buongiorno S, et al. Dermatologic reactions in patients with hepatitis C receiving direct-acting antiviral (DAAs). Giornale Italiano di Farmacia Clinica. 2016;30(3):158–63 [c].

[36] Piñana JL, Serra MÁ, Hernández-Boluda JC, et al. Successful treatment of hepatitis C virus infection with sofosbuvir and simeprevir in the early phase of an allogeneic stem cell transplant. Transpl Infect Dis. 2016;18(1):89–92 [c].

[37] Issa D, Eghtesad B, Zein NN, et al. Sofosbuvir and simeprevir for the treatment of recurrent hepatitis C with fibrosing cholestatic hepatitis after liver transplantation. Int J Organ Transplant Med. 2016;7(1):38–45 [C].

[38] Comi L, Maggiolo F. Abacavir+dolutegravir+lamivudine for the treatment of HIV. Expert Opin Pharmacother. 2016;17(15):2097–106 [M].

[39] Gallant J, Brunetta J, Crofoot G, et al. Brief report: efficacy and safety of switching to a single-tablet regimen of elvitegravir/cobicistat/emtricitabine/tenofovir alafenamide in HIV-1/hepatitis B-coinfected adults. J Acquir Immune Defic Syndr. 2016;73(3):294–8 [c].

[40] Soares DDS, Cavalcante MG, Ribeiro SMV, et al. Acute kidney injury in HIV-infected children: comparison of patients according to the use of highly active antiretroviral therapy. J Pediatr (Rio J). 2016;92(6):631–7 [c].

[41] Biagi M, Badowski M, Chiampas T, et al. Administration of tenofovir disoproxil fumarate-based antiretroviral therapy in an HIV-infected patient following unilateral nephrectomy. Int J STD AIDS. 2016;27(9):808–11 [C].

[42] Sachdeva RK, Sharma A, De D, et al. Lamivudine-induced skin rash remains an underdiagnosed entity in HIV. J Int Assoc Provid AIDS Care. 2016;15(2):153–8 [c].

[43] Suárez-Lorenzo I, Castillo-Sainz R, Cárden-Santana MA, et al. Severe reaction to emtricitabine and lamiduvine: evidence of cross-reactivity. Contact Dermatitis. 2016;74(4):253–4 [A].

[44] Bailey H, Thompson L, Childs T, et al. Safety of zidovudine/lamivudine scored tablets in children with HIV infection in Europe and Thailand. Eur J Clin Pharmacol. 2016;1–6 (in press) [C].

[45] Lee S, Park JY, Kim DY, et al. Prediction of virologic response to tenofovir mono-rescue therapy for multidrug resistant chronic hepatitis B. J Med Virol. 2016;88(6):1027–34 [C].

[46] Cook PP, Stang AT, Walker LR, et al. Bone mineral density and vitamin D levels in HIV treatment-naïve African American individuals randomized to receive HIV drug regimens. South Med J. 2016;109(11):712–7 [c].

[47] Bedimo R, Rosenblatt L, Myers J. Systematic review of renal and bone safety of the antiretroviral regimen efavirenz, emtricitabine, and tenofovir disoproxil fumarate in patients with HIV infection. HIV Clin Trials. 2016;17(6):246–66 [R].

[48] Cottrell ML, Yang KH, Prince HMA, et al. A translational pharmacology approach to predicting outcomes of preexposure prophylaxis against HIV in men and women using tenofovir disoproxil fumarate with or without emtricitabine. J Infect Dis. 2016;214(1):55–64 [C].

[49] Pozniak A, Arribas JR, Gathe J, et al. Switching to tenofovir alafenamide, coformulated with elvitegravir, cobicistat, and emtricitabine, in HIV-infected patients with renal impairment: 48-week results from a single-arm, multicenter, open-label phase 3 study. J Acquir Immune Defic Syndr. 2016;71(5):530–7 [C].

[50] Bertrand L, Dygert L, Toborek M. Antiretroviral treatment with efavirenz disrupts the blood–brain barrier integrity and increases stroke severity. Sci Rep. 2016;6 Article number 39738, (in press) [E].

[51] Thompson M, Saag M, Dejesus E, et al. A 48-week randomized phase 2b study evaluating cenicriviroc versus efavirenz in treatment-naive HIV-infected adults with C-C chemokine receptor type 5-tropic virus. AIDS. 2016;30(6):869–78 [C].

[52] Shehu NY, Ojeh V, Osaigbovo G, et al. A 33-year-old patient with human immunodeficiency virus on antiretroviral therapy with efavirenz-induced complex partial seizures: a case report. J Med Case Reports. 2016;10(1):93 [A].

[53] Pinillos F, Dandara C, Swart M, et al. Case report: Severe central nervous system manifestations associated with aberrant efavirenz metabolism in children: the role of CYP2B6 genetic variation. BMC Infect Dis. 2016;16(1):56 [A].

[54] Lombaard J, Bunupuradah T, Flynn PM, et al. Rilpivirine as a treatment for HIV-infected antiretroviral-naïve adolescents: week 48 safety, efficacy, virology and pharmacokinetics. Pediatr Infect Dis J. 2016;35(11):1215–21 [C].

[55] Subashini D, Dinesha T, Boobalan J, et al. Incidence of atazanavir-associated adverse drug reactions in second -line drugs treated south Indian HIV-1 infected patients. Indian J Pharmacol. 2016;48(5):582–5 [C].

[56] Chow D, Shikuma C, Ritchings C, et al. Atazanavir and cardiovascular risk among human immunodeficiency virus-infected patients: a systematic review. Infect Dis Ther. 2016;5(4):473–89 [R].

[57] Berretta M, Caraglia M, Martellotta F, et al. Drug-drug interactions based on pharmacogenetic profile between highly active antiretroviral therapy and antiblastic chemotherapy in cancer patients with HIV infection. Front Pharmacol. 2016;7: Article number 71, [R].

[58] De Boer MGJ, Van Den Berk GEL, Van Holten N, et al. Intolerance of dolutegravir-containing combination antiretroviral therapy regimens in real-life clinical practice. AIDS. 2016;30(18):2831–4 [c].

[59] Calza L, Danese I, Magistrelli E, et al. Dual raltegravir–darunavir/ritonavir combination in virologically suppressed HIV-1-infected patients on antiretroviral therapy including a ritonavir-boosted protease inhibitor plus Two nucleoside/nucleotide reverse transcriptase inhibitors. HIV Clin Trials. 2016;17(1):38–47 [c].

[60] Van Lelyveld SFL, Symons J, Van Ham P, et al. Clinical outcome of maraviroc-containing therapy in heavily pre-treated HIV-1-infected patients. Int J Antimicrob Agents. 2016;47(1):84–90 [C].

[61] Pett SL, Amin J, Horban A, et al. Maraviroc, as a switch option, in HIV-1-infected individuals with stable, well-controlled HIV replication and R5-tropic virus on their first nucleoside/nucleotide reverse transcriptase inhibitor plus ritonavir-boosted protease inhibitor regimen: week 48 results of the randomized, multicenter March study. Clin Infect Dis. 2016;63(1):122–32 [c].

[62] Çiftçi E, Karbuz A, Kendirli T. Influenza and the use of oseltamivir in children. Turk Pediatri Ars. 2016;51(2):63–71 [R].

[63] Schauer SG, Varney SM, Aden JK, et al. Patient perceptions of oseltamivir for the treatment of influenza. South Med J. 2016;109(8):477–80 [c].

[64] Alame MM, Massaad E, Zaraket H. Peramivir: a novel intravenous neuraminidase inhibitor for treatment of acute influenza infections. Front Microbiol. 2016;7: Article number 450, [R].

[65] Hanna E, Abadi R, Abbas O. Imiquimod in dermatology: an overview. Int J Dermatol. 2016;55(8):831–44 [R].

[66] Koeneman MM, Kruse AJ, Kooreman LFS, et al. TOPical imiquimod treatment of high-grade cervical intraepithelial neoplasia (TOPIC trial): study protocol for a randomized controlled trial. BMC Cancer. 2016;16(1) Article number 132, [C].

[67] Dillies AS, Gras-Champel V, Fraitag-Spinner S, et al. Eruptive epidermoid cysts during topical imiquimod treatment. Ann Dermatol Venereol. 2016;144:212–5 [c].

[68] Elia MD, Lally SE, Hanlon AM, et al. Periocular melanoma in situ treated with imiquimod. Ophthal Plast Reconstr Surg. 2016;32(5):371–3 [c].

[69] Othumpanagat S, Noti J, Ray SD. Antiviral drugs. Side Effects of Drugs Annual. 2016;38:261–81 [R].

26

Drugs Used in TB and Leprosy

Meenakshi R. Ramanathan[*,1], *James M. Sanders*[*,†]

*The University of North Texas Health Science Center System College of Pharmacy, Fort Worth, TX, United States
†JPS Health Network, Fort Worth, TX, United States
1Corresponding author: meenakshi.ramanathan@unthsc.edu

AMINOGLYCOSIDES AND CAPREOMYCIN

The aminoglycosides are second-line injectable agents used in tuberculosis (TB), with amikacin, kanamycin, and streptomycin (STR) being the most common. Amikacin and kanamycin are considered the preferable agents given increased resistance patterns against STR. Capreomycin, although structurally different, is often linked to aminoglycosides as it is thought to have a similar mechanism of action. Capreomycin is generally reserved in the situation that the strain is resistant to amikacin and kanamycin. Commonly cited side effects of the aminoglycosides include nephrotoxicity, ototoxicity, neuromuscular blockade, and respiratory tract paralysis [1S,2S,3S].

Electrolyte Disturbances

Amalia and colleagues performed a retrospective and concurrent cohort study to determine the effects of kanamycin and capreomycin on serum potassium levels in multidrug-resistant TB (MDR-TB) patients. A total of 72 patients were reviewed: 53 patients on kanamycin and 19 patients on capreomycin. On a monthly basis for a total of 5 months, patients were evaluated on serum potassium levels, incidence of hypokalemia, and severity level. Capreomycin was found to have a stronger hypokalemic effect compared to kanamycin, where serum potassium levels were 2.95 mEq/L vs 3.82 mEq/L in the first month ($P < 0.001$) and 2.85 mEq/L vs 3.81 mEq/L in the second month ($P < 0.001$), respectively. There was a higher incidence of hypokalemia in the capreomycin group compared to the kanamycin group in the first month (89.5% vs 28.3%, $P < 0.001$) and second month (81.8% vs 29.2%, $P < 0.001$). The mechanism of hypokalemia is thought to be due to stimulation of the calcium-sensing receptor (CaSR), which disrupts the electrolyte transport via inhibition of various pathways. Capreomycin is thought to have a stronger hypokalemic effect, as it has more amino groups compared to kanamycin, allowing for its potency [4c].

Santra and colleagues report Gitelman-like syndrome with the use of kanamycin for MDR-TB in a 22-year-old female. The patient was started on kanamycin, cycloserine (CS), ethionamide, pyrazinamide (PZA), and moxifloxacin (MXF). After 2 months of therapy, the patient presented with muscle cramps and carpopedal spasm. Laboratory findings included hypokalemia with metabolic alkalosis, hypomagnesemia, hypochloremia, and hypocalciuria. The patient's potassium was replaced both orally and intravenously and kanamycin discontinued. The hypokalemia and metabolic alkalosis slowly resolved 1 month after discontinuation [5A].

Ototoxicity

Sogebi and colleagues performed a prospective analytical study looking at the incidence of aminoglycoside-induced ototoxicity during the intensive phase of drug-resistant TB therapy in 70 patients. At admission and 4-week intervals until 4 months after discharge, patients underwent serial pure tone audiometries (PTAs). Incidence of aminoglycoside-induced ototoxicity was found in 16 patients (22.9%). In their evaluation of clinical predictors for ototoxicity, age, body mass index (BMI) on admission, and co-existing retroviral infection were found to be the primary predictors [6c].

BEDAQUILINE

Bedaquiline (BDQ), a novel entity for the treatment of MDR-TB, has limited available evidence regarding safety and efficacy [7R]. The utilization of this agent remains selective due to previous trials demonstrating enhanced mortality and a propensity to prolong the QTc-interval [8R,9R]. A recent study of 197 patients aimed to determine the experience of patients in Belarus receiving BDQ for treatment of MDR-TB. Upon interim analysis, the most common (those occurring >30%) reported side effects were metabolism and nutrition disorders (68%), hepatobiliary disorders (64%), electrolyte disorders (47%), cardiac disorders, including abnormal electrocardiogram and arrhythmia (41%), and gastrointestinal disorders (35%). Two deaths were reported with one purported to be related to therapy [10c]. In 2016, the first case regarding prolonged BDQ treatment (i.e., 18 months) of extensively drug-resistant TB (XDR-TB) was published [11A].

A 20-year-old, otherwise healthy female from Romania presented with XDR-TB with resistance to first-line agents—fluoroquinolones (FQs), prothionamide, and other intravenous agents. Her modified treatment regimen, based on resistance testing, consisted of BDQ, linezolid (LNZ), PZA, CS, azithromycin and para-aminosalicylic acid. Treatment initiation occurred at week 8. Initially, the patient received the recommended 24 weeks of BDQ and restarted the agent at week 38 due to intolerability to LNZ and CS. The patient experienced an initial QTc-interval increase of 54 milliseconds (ms) that plateaued at 14 ms above her baseline of 411 ms. Two weeks after reinitiating BDQ, she experienced a peak QTc-interval of 495 ms; thus, azithromycin therapy was discontinued resulting in a median QTc-interval of 472 ms for the remainder of therapy. Electrolytes remained within normal limits and no arrhythmias were documented. Per report, no other significant adverse events were documented and treatment resulted in cure [11A].

Future evidence for the safety and efficacy of BDQ will be guided by the Evaluation of a Standardised Treatment Regimen of Anti-TB Drugs for Patients with MDR-TB2 (STREAM2). This multicenter randomized controlled trial focuses on the efficacy of an all enteral, 9-month BDQ-based regimen. In addition to efficacy, the trial will collect the percentage of patients with severe adverse events [12c].

Drug–Drug Interactions

BDQ and the M2 metabolite metabolism occur via cytochrome P450 3A4 (CYP3A4) [13R]. The antiretrovirals nevirapine (NVP) and lopinavir/ritonavir (LPV/r) induce and inhibit the CYP3A4 enzyme, respectively. A pharmacokinetic study conducted in patients from South Africa on BDQ compared human immunodeficiency virus (HIV) seronegative patients, patients on NVP-based HIV regimens and patients on LPV/r-based regimens. Patients receiving concomitant LPV/r demonstrated significantly increased area under the curve (AUC_{0-48}), time to maximum concentration (T_{max}), and half-life for BDQ, but not the M2 metabolite. Independent predictors of BDQ exposure included male sex, duration of BDQ therapy, and concomitant LPV/r [14c]. Further studies are needed to confirm the relevance of these interactions on potential safety and to guide dose adjustments.

Pharmacokinetics

Toxicity may result from altered drug pharmacokinetics including alterations in metabolite disposition. A population pharmacokinetic modeling study based on the Phase IIb studies demonstrated that weight and albumin significantly alter the kinetics of BDQ and M2 along with age [15c]. The understanding of these parameters carries the potential to guide appropriate dosing to achieve desired drug exposure while balancing safety parameters.

CLOFAZIMINE

Clofazimine (CFZ) as part of combination therapy represents a treatment modality for non-tubercular mycobacterium, MDR-TB, and more commonly, leprosy [16R]. CFZ, a dye-based product, results in discoloration of tissues and pigmentation of the eye [16R]. A case study demonstrated the development of CFZ-induced premaculopathy in a patient with vitiligo that resolved upon discontinuation [17A]. Enteropathy represents a rare side effect of CFZ. A recent case study demonstrated this adverse event during the treatment of *Mycobacterium abscessus* [18A].

Special populations, such as pregnancy, breastfeeding and children, must be considered when treating leprosy and MDR-TB due to toxicity and limited evidence in these populations. A case demonstrated an uncomplicated pregnancy following treatment of a mother with CFZ; however, the baby experienced skin discoloration while the mother was breastfeeding. Resolution occurred following discontinuation of breastfeeding [19c]. A recent observational trial of children with XDR-TB and pre-XDR-TB demonstrated CFZ tolerability in 20 children. Adverse events reported were red discoloration of the skin, ichthyosis with spontaneous resolution, and gastritis [20c].

CYCLOSERINE

Cycloserine (CS) due to its propensity to cause profound neuropsychiatric side effects and limited efficacy data against TB remains a last-line treatment option [9R]. However, the emergence of MDR-TB and XDR-TB necessitates its use in select cases. A recent case series from India demonstrated the treatment of genital MDR-TB in six females. All six received CS as part of the combination therapy. Reported side effects included depression among the entire cohort and half of the patients described suicidal thoughts [21c]. CS utilization has expanded to the treatment of neuropsychiatric and pain disorders. Side effects demonstrated in trials for panic disorder and obsessive–compulsive disorder, at a low dose (i.e., 50 and 125 mg once), include fatigue, headache, nausea/vomiting, dizziness, and sedation [22c,23c]. For treatment of chronic back pain, patients received 100, 200 and 400 mg/day each for 2 weeks. Headache, numbness and/or tingling, and lower extremity edema were commonly reported side effects [24c].

DAPSONE

Dapsone is a mainstay for the combination treatment of leprosy due to its activity against *Mycobacterium leprae* [25R]. Dapsone provides an alternative to sulfamethoxazole–trimethoprim for the prophylaxis of *Pneumocystis jiroveci*. A report of 19 patients with HIV and concomitant sulfa allergy demonstrated that 13 patients tolerated dapsone with those not tolerating the agent experiencing rash [26c].

Cardiovascular

Dapsone may result in dapsone hypersensitivity syndrome (DHS). The syndrome presents across a spectrum from mild to severe life-threatening reactions [25R].

A 35-year-old female presented with epigastric pain with vomiting, cutaneous pain, myalgia, and dark urine. Prior to admission, she received 7 weeks of triple drug therapy, including dapsone, for leprosy. Her assessment was positive for a skin rash and lymphadenopathy. Also, the patient was found to have hemolytic anemia and fulminant hepatitis. The diagnosis of DHS was made, and the patient was successfully treated with corticosteroid therapy. A month and a half post discharge, the patient succumbed to myocarditis purported to have resulted from DHS [27A].

A review of dapsone overdose cases revealed that approximately 30% had some presentation of an adverse cardiovascular event. Patients who experienced an adverse cardiovascular event were approximately six times more likely to die [28c].

Hematologic Disorders

In 2016, the two hematologic disorders reported were methemoglobinemia and red cell aplasia [29c,30c,31A, 32A,33A]. Dapsone-induced methemoglobinemia, primarily due to overdose, resulted in prolonged methemoglobin levels necessitating higher doses of methylene blue relative to methemoglobinemia resulting from other toxic agents [29c]. Following dapsone overdose, hemolytic anemia occurred in approximately 70% of patients lasting upwards of 6 days and resulting in prolonged admission and ICU length of stay [30c]. A case study from India presented a rare case of red cell aplasia with associated cholestatic jaundice [33A].

DELAMANID

Delamanid demonstrates activity against MDR-TB and XDR-TB while demonstrating limited side effects in the approval trials [34R]. XDR-TB often necessitates the utilization of agents demonstrating potential additive toxicities. Cardiotoxicity may result from BDQ and delamanid hindering the use of the combination. A recent case study demonstrated the utilization of delamanid and BDQ for treatment of XDR-TB [35A].

A 39-year-old Tibetan woman presented in India with a second relapse of TB with ongoing treatment failure with four past treatment regimens. Drug susceptibility testing demonstrated resistance to first- and second-line treatment options including intravenous agents. Testing demonstrated susceptibility to CFZ. The patient was initiated on delamanid, BDQ, CFZ, terizidone, meropenem, and amoxicillin/clavulanate. After 8 doses the patient's QTc-interval increased to 486 ms (baseline < 450 ms) and BDQ was stopped. Consultation with the TB Consilium resulted in restarting BDQ with recommendations to stop CFZ if QTc-interval increased to > 500 ms and to add verapamil. At restart of BDQ, the QTc-interval was 489 ms and remained stable on day 27 at 491 ms [35A].

A paucity of data exists for the utilization of delamanid in children, especially for prolonged courses. A recent report demonstrated safety and efficacy in a 12-year old with XDR-TB requiring the addition of delamanid due to intolerability and resistance to other available agents. The child's QTc-interval remained in 410–444 ms range throughout treatment with no other untoward effects reported after a successful 24-month treatment course [36A].

Drug–Drug Interactions

Delamanid previously was shown to have relatively few drug–drug interactions related to its non-cytochrome

P450 mediated metabolism. New in vitro data demonstrates no significant interaction with drug transporters affecting drug absorption, distribution, and excretion [37E]. Delamanid showed no significant interactions with first-line anti-TB medications, rifampin, isoniazid (INH), PZA, and ethambutol (EMB), and antiretroviral agents, ritonavir, tenofovir, efavirenz (EFV), and LPV/r, thus limiting the possibility for reducing safety or efficacy when used concomitantly [38c].

ETHAMBUTOL

Ethambutol (EMB) remains a component of first-line quadruple therapy for the treatment of drug-susceptible TB [39R]. Of the four first-line agents, rifampin, INH, PZA and EMB (RIPE), EMB demonstrates the lowest potential to cause hepatotoxicity. A review of 2070 patients with drug-induced hepatitis while on traditional RIPE therapy demonstrated zero percent of the cases having EMB as the presumed cause [40C]. Paradoxical worsening of TB may result upon anti-TB therapy (ATT) initiation. Of 67 patients with an identified paradoxical reaction almost a quarter were able to reinitiate EMB safely [41c].

Hematologic

A case report reported a rare incidence of EMB-induced hemolytic anemia [42A].

A 71-year-old male was on treatment with rifampin, INH, and EMB for TB. On day 5, the patient had acute elevation in total and direct bilirubin with resulting jaundice. Subsequently, a diagnosis of acute hemolysis syndrome was made and treated with methylprednisolone. Clinical course and laboratory parameters continued to decline with the patient dying on day 8. Diagnosis of drug-induced autoimmune hemolytic anemia was made with EMB-positive eluate testing (negative in absence of all drugs and in presence of rifampin and INH) [42A].

Hypersensitivity

A report of patch-testing confirmed EMB-induced hypersensitivity syndrome resulted in pruritic erythema, oral erosions, lymphadenopathy, and fever. Successful treatment included corticosteroid and intravenous immunoglobulin (IVIG) therapy [43A]. In HIV patients, patch testing for diagnostic purposes in patients with prior cutaneous reaction to ATT results in systemic reactions (e.g., eosinophilia, transaminitis and fever), specifically EMB caused two reactions [44c].

Pharmacokinetics/Pharmacogenomics

A novel urine metabolite of EMB, 2-aminobutyric acid, was discovered in a small cohort of patients from India [45c]. The role the metabolite plays in safety of EMB remains to be determined. Pharmacogenomic analysis revealed that single-nucleotide polymorphisms affect the pharmacokinetics of EMB [46c]. Due to the renal excretion of EMB, renal adjustment and renal replacement therapy play a key role in drug exposure. Adjustment of doses based on EMB levels during extended daily dialysis resulted in titration of dose without any associated side effects. Concomitant extracorporeal membrane oxygenation (ECMO) had no clear effect on EMB levels [47A].

Visual Effects

The incidence of toxic optic neuropathy in a Korean cohort was found to be 0.7% with a reduced incidence, 0.3%, in patients receiving low dose EMB (≤15 mg/kg/day) [48c]. Concomitant therapy of EMB and LNZ resulted in a case of toxic optic neuropathy with improvement following discontinuation of both agents [49A]. Visual function tests demonstrated the ability to detect early, subclinical changes of ocular toxicity to EMB preceding demonstrative visual changes [50c]. Macular thickness determined via optic coherence neuropathy may provide a potential for predicting EMB ocular toxicity [51c]. Retreatment with a prolonged course of EMB (14 months) was tolerated after a 10-year hiatus following previous EMB optic neuropathy [52A].

FLUOROQUINOLONES

The most commonly used fluoroquinolones (FQs) for TB include moxifloxacin (MXF), levofloxacin (LVX), and ofloxacin [1S,2S,3S]. Ciprofloxacin is no longer considered a valid therapeutic option for TB due to poor microbial kill and rapid emergence of resistance [53E]. According to the WHO Treatment of TB guidelines (2010) and the WHO Treatment guidelines for Drug-Resistant-TB (2016 update), the FQs are considered group 3 drugs for MDR-TB and should be used if susceptible and considered efficacious [2S, 3S]. Per the American Thoracic Society/CDC/IDSA guidelines for the treatment of drug-susceptible TB, MXF and LVX are considered second-line agents [39R]. Gatifloxacin has also been used in the past and in third world countries for treatment of TB, but with increasing reports of dysglycemia and decreased market availability, it is no longer recommended [54H]. Many studies have looked into using the FQs upfront in the place of INH where INH resistance may be an issue. In May 2016, the FDA released reports stating that FQs should be avoided in less severe infections (e.g., uncomplicated urinary tract infections, acute sinusitis, and acute bronchitis) where the risks outweigh the benefits due to undue side effects associated with them [55S]. Common adverse effects associated with the FQs include photosensitivity, antibiotic associated diarrhea, *C. difficile* infections, neurotoxicity, and tendon rupture [1S].

Conde et al. performed a phase 2 randomized trial looking at the bactericidal activity, safety, and tolerability of rifapentine (RPT) plus MXF-based regimens (along with PZA and EMB) for treatment of pulmonary TB in adults. The proportion of grade 3 or higher adverse events were similar between the low-dose RPT and MXF group vs standard therapy (5/62 (8%) vs 6/59 (10%), $P=0.76$) [56C].

Kalita et al. performed an open label randomized controlled trial reviewing the safety and efficacy of adding LVX to standardized RIPE therapy in TB meningitis. The primary outcomes of the study were death and secondary outcomes included disability and adverse events. Adverse events were found to be similar between the groups, with an increased incidence of seizures found in the group with the added LVX [57C].

A meta-analysis by Ruan et al. reviewed the safety and efficacy of MXF and gatifloxacin for initial therapy in TB. Although these regimens may result in an increased incidence of relapse when used upfront in short-course regimens in lieu of INH or EMB, the review found no significant difference in adverse events between the MXF and gatifloxacin regimens compared to standard therapy [58M].

Kang et al. presented a continuation of a randomized study reviewing the use of LVX vs MXF in MDR-TB outcomes. More adverse events were present in the LVX group vs the MXF group (79.2% vs 63.5%, $P=0.03$), with a higher prevalence of musculoskeletal adverse events in the LVX group (37.7% vs 14.9%, $P=0.001$) [59C].

van der Lann and colleagues report a case of a 6-year-old pulmonary MDR-TB patient with secondary intracranial hypertension due to LVX. The patient had been started on INH, EMB, ethionamide, LVX, terizidone, PZA, amikacin, and pyridoxine administered once daily. After 12 weeks of therapy, bilateral papilledema was noted on the ophthalmologic assessment. LVX was found to be the culprit and was discontinued. *Para*-aminosalicylic acid was added to the regimen, and in order to decrease the intracranial pressure, the patient received acetazolamide 30 mg/kg every 8 hours [60A].

ISONIAZID

Considered a first-line agent in the treatment of active TB and latent TB infections (LTBI), isoniazid (INH) was first approved by the US FDA in 1953. Although the exact mechanism of action is unknown, it is thought that it inhibits mycolic acid synthesis and causes disruption of the cell wall. Hepatotoxicity accounts for the most

common adverse effect of INH, followed by neuropathy and neurotoxicity. Other more serious side effects include dermatologic, hematologic, immunologic, and musculoskeletal toxicities. Increasing resistance has been noted in the literature; thus, making providers choose second-line agents that may not be as effective, safe, and cost-effective [1S,2S].

Dermatologic

Catano et al. looked into the use of INH chemoprophylaxis for TB reactivation in patients who were on biological therapy for psoriasis. Patients were started on INH 5 mg/kg for LTBI, with a maximum dose of 300 mg/day. Anti-TNF therapy was started 2–9 months after initiation of chemoprophylaxis. In the case patients developed intolerance or toxicity to INH, patients were given rifampin as a second-line agent for 4 months total. Active TB developed in 3 out of the 101 patients (2.9%) and 17 patients (16.8%) were found to have INH intolerance or toxicity. The primary toxicities noted included allergic reactions, gastric intolerance, and hepatotoxicity [61C].

Hepatotoxicity

Gray et al. performed a retrospective chart review of 100 consecutive patients between 2010 and 2014 who were given preventive therapy for LTBI. The primary endpoints of the study looked at demographics, compliance, completion rates, and adverse events. The secondary endpoints reviewed the rates of INH hepatotoxicity and any contributory factors. The study found that 33% of patients on INH and 23% of patients on rifampin experienced liver function test (LFT) abnormality. INH therapy was stopped in 3% of patients due to asymptomatic hepatic dysfunction. The contributory factors for liver dysfunction were found to be risk factors for liver disease and abnormal pre-therapy LFT [62c].

Ben Fredj et al. reviewed the risk factors associated with INH-induced hepatotoxicity (IIH) in 71 Tunisian TB patients. Major risk factors for IIH included a serum concentration of INH over 3.69 mg/L and a combined genotype of cytochrome P450 2E1 (CYP2E1) slow acetylation. Because of this, therapeutic drug monitoring and the determination of polymorphisms in the N-acetyltransferase-2 (NAT2) and CYP2E1 are necessary in predicting and preventing IIH [63c].

Immunologic

Shah et al. presented a case report of a 21-year-old female with INH-induced lupus being retreated for tuberculous synovitis. The patient had received INH, rifampicin (RMP), PZA, EMB, and STR (HRZES) for 2 months, followed by INH, RMP, PZA, and EMB (HREZ) for 1 month, and INH, RMP, and EMB (HRE) for 26 days. Three days prior to presentation, RMP was removed from the regimen due to thrombocytopenia and oral ulcers; however, the lesions persisted and worsened in severity. The patient was found to have rashes over her face and palms, extensive oral mucosal ulcers with anemia with pancytopenia, and a low-grade fever for 7 days. Her auto-immune profile revealed elevated anti-nuclear antibody (ANA), anti-ds DNA, and anti-histone antibody titers. After discontinuation of ATT, improvement in oral ulcers, total leukocyte count, and platelets were seen. The patient was re-initiated on ATT excluding INH, where the patient was given STR for 1 month in addition to RMP, EMB, and LVX. The patient tolerated the regimen well without recurrence of symptoms [64A].

Neurologic

Chaitanya et al. present a case report of a 53-year-old male patient with INH-induced cerebellitis on peritoneal dialysis. This patient was started on ATT with INH (5 mg/kg/day) and pyridoxine (40 mg/day). After 15 days of starting treatment, the patient experienced many neurologic clinical features, his MRI was positive for bilateral T2-weighted hyperintensities in dentate nuclei of cerebellar hemispheres, and the trough plasma pyridoxal-5-phospahte (PLP) levels were low at <5 mcg/L. The INH was discontinued and pyridoxine dose increased to 120 mg/day, with clinical symptoms resolved in a week [65A].

LINEZOLID

Linezolid (LNZ) was the first oxazolidinone approved by the US FDA in 2000, which works by inhibiting bacterial protein synthesis by binding to the 23S ribosomal subunit of the 50S subunit; thus, preventing the formation of the 70S initiation complex. Its primary uses include vancomycin-resistant *Enterococcus faecium* infections, nosocomial pneumonia, community-acquired pneumonia, and complicated and uncomplicated skin and structure infections. The WHO Treatment of TB guidelines (2010) consider LNZ as a group 5 drug, an agent with an unclear role in the treatment of drug-resistant TB. According to the CDC's Treatment of TB guidelines (2003), LNZ was considered an alternative agent that required more data to support its use. With increasing resistance, LNZ has more commonly been used in MDR-TB and XDR-TB. Common side effects noted include thrombocytopenia and neurotoxicity/neuropathy generally seen around 2 weeks of therapy. As LNZ is a weak monoamine oxidase inhibitor (MAOI), caution

is advised with other MAOIs and serotonergic agents. LNZ use has become more prevalent in the treatment of pediatric TB [1S,3S].

Ramirez-Lapausa et al. performed a retrospective chart review looking into the tolerability and efficacy of LNZ in MDR-TB in 21 patients receiving a LNZ-containing regimen vs 34 patients receiving a non-LNZ-containing regimen from 1998 to 2014. In general, LNZ was added to therapy when no other sensitive drugs could be added and an additional agent was needed to complete ATT. Most patients received LNZ 600 mg by mouth daily, except for two patients who received LNZ 600 mg by mouth twice daily. Patients also received vitamin B6 to help prevent hematologic toxicity and peripheral neuropathy. They assessed the frequency of myelosuppression, peripheral neuropathy, and optic neuropathy. A majority of the LNZ patients did not have any adverse events at all (81%). Four patients developed toxicity to LNZ, which included anemia in two patients and moderate paresthesia in another. After lowering the dose from 1200 to 600 mg/day, the adverse effects improved. None of the patients discontinued LNZ due to side effects [66c].

Yi et al. presented a single-center retrospective chart review of 26 Japanese patients assigned to LNZ for treatment of MDR-TB or XDR-TB between 2009 and 2015. Patients were started on either oral or intravenous LNZ at a dose of 600–1200 mg daily with other TB medications. Side effects for LNZ were monitored carefully, and in the case that the patient experienced side effects, LNZ dosage was decreased or LNZ withdrawn altogether. Of the 26 patients evaluated, 7 patients were considered MDR-TB susceptible to kanamycin and LVX, 12 patients were considered MDR-TB with resistance to either injectable drugs or FQs (pre-XDR-TB), and 7 patients were considered XDR-TB. Eleven (42%) patients either withdrew or had a reduced dose of LNZ due to the adverse effects associated with the drug. The primary adverse effects noted were myelosuppression (e.g., anemia, leukopenia, thrombocytopenia) in 10 patients, severe anorexia in 2 patients, and suspected liver toxicity in 2 patients. Dose reductions from 1200 mg daily to 600 mg daily or 1200 mg every other day was observed in 6 patients, whereas dosage adjustments from 600 mg daily to 300 mg daily or 600 mg every other day was observed in 5 patients. Neuropathy was not observed in the study [67c].

Arbex et al. performed a retrospective observational study looking into the safety and effectiveness of imipenem/clavulanate (IC) and LNZ for the treatment of MDR-TB and XDR-TB in Brazilian patients. All 12 patients were started on IC 1000 mg daily plus amoxicillin/clavulanic acid 500 mg/125 mg three times a day in addition to LNZ 600 mg daily, except for 1 patient who did not receive LNZ because of co-administration with ethionamide to avoid peripheral neuropathy due to a prior history. No adverse effects were reported for IC, although two patients (17%) experienced minor, yet reversible adverse effects to LNZ. The first patient experienced peripheral neuropathy, which when restarted resulted in no further problems. The second reported diarrhea, which was managed symptomatically, without discontinuation of ATT [68c].

Zeng and colleagues studied the clinical results of using LNZ for MDR-TB. LNZ was administered at 600 mg/day for 6 months followed by 300 mg/day for at least 3 months, in addition to ATT. The study included a total of 12 patients aged 21–58 years. Only three patients were considered cured at the end of therapy, while the other nine patients showed improvement in clinical symptoms, cavity narrowing, and sputum conversion. Of the latter group, three patients failed treatment, two patients discontinued therapy due to adverse effects (including acroanesthesia, insomnia, and palpitations), and another patient relapsed after 4 months [69c].

A systematic review and meta-analysis by Agyeman and Ofori-Asenso analyzed the safety and efficacy of LNZ in MDR-TB. The outcomes assessed included culture conversion, treatment success, and incidence of adverse events. A total of 23 studies were included across 14 countries with 507 patients. LNZ was given at a minimum dose of 300 mg to a maximum dose of 1200 mg daily, ranging from 1 to 36 months in duration. Common adverse effects noted in these studies included myelosuppresion, neuropathy, nausea, vomiting, hyperpigmentation of the oral cavity, and transient visual impairment. Pooled proportion data showed the following percentages of incidence: (1) major adverse events leading to LNZ discontinuation, 15.81% (95% confidence interval (CI) = 9.68%–23.11%, $P < 0.0001$); (2) myelosuppression, 32.93% (95% CI = 23.13%–43.54%, $P < 0.0001$); (3) neuropathy, 29.92% (95% CI = 20.53%–40.25%); (4) other adverse effects, 33.60% (95% CI = 20.41%–48.23%, $P < 0.0001$). Upon comparing LNZ daily doses ≤ 600 mg and >600 mg, there was no difference in culture conversion or treatment success, but myelosuppression was more prevalent in the latter group (19.58% vs 50%, respectively, 95% CI = 15.77%–44.94%, $P < 0.0001$). Neuropathy (34.17% vs 41.67%, respectively, 95% CI = 6.84% to 22.79%, $P = 0.3213$) and other side effects leading to permanent LNZ discontinuation (18.02% vs 18.75%, respectively, 95% CI = 9.44% to 14.72%, $P = 0.9050$) were similar between the groups [70M].

PYRAZINAMIDE

Pyrazinamide (PZA), a pyrazine analogue of nicotinamide, is considered a first-line agent in the treatment of TB. Originally approved in 1971 by the US FDA for treatment of TB, the exact mechanism of action is unknown. Common side effects attributed to PZA include nausea, vomiting, hyperuricemia, arthralgia, anemia, and hepatotoxicity. This drug is contraindicated in individuals with hypersensitivity reactions, severe liver damage, and/or acute gout [1S,2S].

RIFAMYCIN

The rifamycins continue to be the backbone for the first-line TB medications along with INH, with RMP/rifampin being the most common agents being used. Other agents in the rifamycin class used for TB include rifabutin (RBT) and RPT. RMP/rifampin and RPT are also commonly used in LTBI. The rifamycins work by blocking RNA transcription by binding the beta subunit of the DNA-dependent RNA polymerase. As the rifamycins, especially RMP/rifampin, are potent CYP3A4 inducers, one must take into account the multiple drug–drug interactions at play, especially in HIV co-infected patients, as many of the protease inhibitors (PIs) and non-nucleoside reverse transcriptase inhibitors (NNRTIs) are dependent on this cytochrome P450 system for metabolism. RMP/rifampin has also remained a mainstay in the treatment of leprosy. More and more regimens are trying to shorten the duration of therapy or use high-dose rifamycin protocols for the treatment of TB [1S,2S].

Adrenal Insufficiency

Denny and colleagues report a case of a 55-year-old Indian man who presented with RMP-induced adrenal crisis, with tuberculous infiltration of the adrenal glands. The patient was started on standard ATT for drug-susceptible pulmonary TB. Patient presented to the hospital with drowsiness and dehydration after 1 week of initiation of ATT. The patient was transferred to the critical care unit for treatment of severe septic shock secondary to hospital-acquired pneumonia. The patient was started on intravenous crystalloids, antibiotics, followed by norepinephrine. Intravenous hydrocortisone was added, leading to an improvement in vasopressor requirements. RMP was deemed the culprit for the Addisonian crisis and was discontinued. The patient made a full recovery after the initiation of hydrocortisone and discontinuation of RMP. The patient also showed progressive mixed cholestatic and hepatic compromise, with elevations over fivefold the upper limit of normal in alanine aminotransferase (ALT), alkaline phosphatase (ALP), and gamma-glutamyl transferase (GGT). Thus, INH and PZA were replaced with STR and MXF, although MXF also caused an acute transaminitis and was withdrawn. INH was reintroduced with monitoring of LFTs. The patient received 2 months of STR, INH, and EMB, followed by 16 months of INH and EMB. The mechanism of RMP-induced adrenal insufficiency appears to be linked to its potent induction of CYP3A4. RMP increases the metabolism of cortisol to 6β-hydroxycortisol by selectively upregulating liver microsomal CYP3A4, which can occur over the course of 5 days of oral therapy. Although this adverse effect is rare, it can be life-threatening [71A].

Hepatotoxicity/Renal Toxicity

A randomized Phase II trial by Jindani and colleagues studied the toxicities associated with high-dose RMP to treat pulmonary TB. Doses of RMP 10, 15, and 20 mg/kg were used. The primary objective reviewed whether these high doses increased the incidence of grade 3 or 4 hepatic adverse events. Three hundred patients were randomized to one of three groups: (1) control group (R10) of EMB, INH, RMP 10 mg/kg, and PZA daily for 8 weeks followed by INH and RMP daily for 18 weeks; (2) similar to R10 with the RMP dose increased to 15 mg/kg to be given over the first 16 weeks of therapy (R15 group); (3) similar to R10 with the RMP dose increased to 20 mg/kg to be given over the first 16 weeks of therapy (R20 group). As far as hepatotoxicity, seven grade 3 increases in ALT (1% of R10 group, 2% of R15 group, and 4% of R20 group) were demonstrated. One patient in the R15 group experienced jaundice, which required a treatment modification. No grade 4 ALT increases were seen. No significant difference in adverse events was found amongst the groups [72C].

Chogtu et al. report a case of a 28-year-old male patient with pulmonary TB relapse who presented in rifampin-induced renal failure and hepatitis. He was started on directly observed therapy (DOT) with a five drug regimen of INH, RMP, PZA, EMB, and STR. Patient presented with complaints of vomiting, abdominal pain, fever, and decreased urine output; all of which began 7 days after starting ATT. Other positive findings on physical examination included icterus, elevated heart rate (103 beats per minute), and hepatomegaly. Pertinent laboratory findings include the following: WBC 33 200/μL, neutrophils 77%, urea 62 mg/dL, creatinine 2.3 mg/dL (increasing up to 10.2 mg/dL on serial testing), total bilirubin 8.6 mg/dL, direct bilirubin 2.6 mg/dL, and aspartate aminotransferase (AST) 285 IU/L. Drug-specific antibody to RMP was present upon serological testing. The treatment plan for this patient was to stop the patient's ATT, initiate intravenous fluids, followed by hemodialysis. After the patient's renal and LFTs came back to normal, ATT was restarted in a step wise fashion. However, upon re-introduction of RMP, abnormalities in

renal function and liver function were seen again. RMP was discontinued, and the patient continued the other four medications for a total of 2 months, followed by a 10-month regimen of INH, EMB, and LVX. Patient's renal function normalized, and the patient was deemed cured at the end of 12 months [73A].

A similar report by Gopi and Seshadri showed RMP-induced hepatitis in a 24-year-old female patient diagnosed with bilateral pulmonary TB, with primary effects on the patient's bilirubin. Although the exact mechanism of RMP-induced hepatotoxicity is unknown, it is thought to be due to an idiosyncratic reaction to RMP metabolites, which may induce liver injury. Upon 3 days of starting her category 1 TB regimen under directly observed treatment, short course (DOTS), the patient noticed a yellow discoloration of sclera but continued to take her medications. The patient later experienced nausea and vomiting, which prompted her visit to the hospital. Upon presentation, the patient was found to be deeply icteric with tender hepatomegaly. The patient's LFTs showed normal transaminases, LDH, and ALP, but a direct bilirubin of 3.5 mg/dL and indirect bilirubin of 10 mg/dL. Patient's current ATT was discontinued and restarted with INH, EMB, and ofloxacin. Patient showed gradual improvement with the bilirubin dropping to 1.3 mg/dL after 1 week. The patient was restarted on RMP. After 1 week of RMP therapy, the bilirubin had dropped to 1 mg/dL, but the patient continued to spike fevers and have a persistent neutrophilic leukocytosis. A repeat sputum culture grew out *Staphylococcus aureus*, which was treated with amoxicillin/clavulanate. An ultrasound then revealed miliary TB of the liver. After LFTs normalized, PZA was added. Patient continued to spike fevers after 1 week of completion of amoxicillin/clavulanate; thus, leading to the addition of STR. The patient became afebrile within 2 weeks of the addition of STR [74A]. A similar biphasic effect of RMP on bilirubin was reported by McColl et al. [75A].

Ji and colleagues report a case of a 42-year-old female patient with RMP-induced antineutrophil cytoplasmic antibody (ANCA)-positive vasculitis, who was started on ATT for pulmonary TB with INH, RMP, EMB, and PZA. After 5 days of initiation, she developed renal dysfunction with elevated serum creatinine (420.2 μmol/L) and blood urea nitrogen (16.9 μmol/L). The ATT was discontinued, and a protective renal strategy was started. The patient developed oliguria after re-challenge with RMP, which was then discontinued. She was then restarted on INH, EMB, PZA, and MXF. The mechanism of RMP-induced vasculitis is thought to be due to RMP–anti-RMP antibody complex, which acts on renal tubular epithelial cells; thus, activating the complement system resulting in renal injury. After 4 months of treatment with prednisone and ATT, the patient's renal function and ANCA tests normalized [76A].

Immunologic

Syrigou et al. reported anaphylaxis in a 72-year-old male patient being treated with RMP, INH, PZA, and EMB for miliary TB. The patient had an extensive history of reactions to both RMP and RBT. Because of this, the patient underwent a de-sensitization protocol for RMP using the skin prick test and intradermal skin testing. Within 30 minutes of administration of the RMP 50 mg dose, the patient experienced signs of anaphylaxis [77A].

SPECIAL POPULATIONS

The utilization of ATT often requires the consideration of special populations regarding the tolerability of the various agents. For example, patients on renal replacement therapy and underlying diabetes mellitus (DM) are more prone to developing side effects [78c,79c]. In particular, 83% of patients on hemodialysis with concomitant ATT reported adverse side effects, including syncope, peripheral neuropathy, and elevated LFTs [78c]. The presence of DM carried an over threefold higher chance of experiencing an adverse drug event. A statistically higher portion of patients reported restlessness, hypoglycemia, foot pain, and back pain with TB and DM [79c]. ATT with the novel agents BDQ and delamanid requires special consideration in patients with DM including pharmacokinetic and pharmacodynamics alterations, efficacy, and safety [80R]. Many gaps remain in understanding the novel therapeutic and repurposed drugs regarding the treatment of MDR-TB in the pediatric population, necessitating further study to understand the safety [81R].

Acknowledgements

The authors are grateful to Brook Amen, the research and education librarian at UNTHSC, for her continued support throughout the project.

References

[1] U.S. Food and Drug Administration [Internet]. Silver Spring, MD: U.S. Food and Drug Administration; 2017. Available from: http://www.fda.gov/ [7 March 2017], [S].

[2] Treatment of tuberculosis: guidelines. WHO guidelines approved by the guidelines review committee. 4th ed. Geneva: World Health Organization; 2010 [S].

[3] WHO treatment guidelines for drug-resistant tuberculosis, 2016 update. WHO guidelines approved by the guidelines review committee. Geneva: World Health Organization; 2016 [S].

[4] Amalia L, Zulfa IM, Soeroto AY. Comparative study of kanamycin and capreomycin on serum potassium level of multidrug resistance tuberculosis patients at a hospital in Bandung, Indonesia. Int J Pharm Pharm Sci. 2016;8(1):307–3010 [c].

[5] Santra G, Paul R, Karak A, et al. Gitelman-like syndrome with kanamycin toxicity. J Assoc Physicians India. 2016;64(5): 90–2 [A].

[6] Sogebi OA, Adefuye BO, Adebola SO, et al. Clinical predictors of aminoglycoside-induced ototoxicity in drug-resistant tuberculosis patients on intensive therapy, Auris Nasus Larynx. 2017;44(4): 404–10. http://dx.doi.org/10.1016/j.anl.2016.10.005 [c].

[7] Yadav S, Rawal G, Baxi M. Bedaquiline: a novel antitubercular agent for the treatment of multidrug-resistant tuberculosis. J Clin Diagn Res. 2016;10(8):FM01–2 [R].

[8] Sloan DJ, Lewis JM. Management of multidrug-resistant TB: novel treatments and their expansion to low resource settings. Trans R Soc Trop Med Hyg. 2016;110(3):163–72 [R].

[9] Tiberi S, Scardigli A, Centis R, et al. Classifying new anti-tuberculosis drugs: rationale and future perspectives. Int J Infect Dis. 2017;56:181–4 [c].

[10] Skrahina A, Hurevich H, Falzon D, et al. Bedaquiline in the multidrug-resistant tuberculosis treatment: Belarus experience. Int J Mycobacteriol. 2016;5(Suppl 1):S62–3 [c].

[11] Lewis JM, Hine P, Walker J, et al. First experience of effectiveness and safety of bedaquiline for 18 months within an optimised regimen for XDR-TB. Eur Respir J. 2016;47(5): 1581–4 [A].

[12] Moodley R, Godec TR, Team ST. Short-course treatment for multidrug-resistant tuberculosis: the STREAM trials. Eur Respir Rev. 2016;25(139):29–35 [c].

[13] Chahine EB, Karaoui LR, Mansour H. Bedaquiline: a novel diarylquinoline for multidrug-resistant tuberculosis. Ann Pharmacother. 2014;48(1):107–15 [R].

[14] Pandie M, Wiesner L, McIlleron H, et al. Drug-drug interactions between bedaquiline and the antiretrovirals LPV/r and nevirapine in HIV-infected patients with drug-resistant TB. J Antimicrob Chemother. 2016;71(4):1037–40 [c].

[15] Svensson EM, Dosne AG, Karlsson MO. Population pharmacokinetics of bedaquiline and metabolite M2 in patients with drug-resistant tuberculosis: the effect of time-varying weight and albumin. CPT Pharmacometrics Syst Pharmacol. 2016;5(12):682–91 [c].

[16] Cholo MC, Steel HC, Fourie PB, et al. Clofazimine: current status and future prospects. J Antimicrob Chemother. 2012;67(2): 290–8 [R].

[17] Kasturi N, Srinivasan R. Clofazimine-induced premaculopathy in a vitiliginous patient. J Pharmacol Pharmacother. 2016;7(3):149–51 [A].

[18] Szeto W, Garcia-Buitrago MT, Abbo L, et al. Clofazimine enteropathy: a rare and underrecognized complication of mycobacterial therapy. Open Forum Infect Dis. 2016;3(3): ofw004 [A].

[19] Ozturk Z, Tatliparmak A. Leprosy treatment during pregnancy and breastfeeding: a case report and brief review of literature. Dermatol Ther. 2016;30(1):e12414. http://dx.doi.org/10.1111/dth.12414 [c].

[20] Swaminathan A, du Cros P, Seddon JA, et al. Treating children for drug-resistant tuberculosis in Tajikistan with Group 5 medications. Int J Tuberc Lung Dis. 2016;20(4):474–8 [c].

[21] Sharma JB, Kriplani A, Sharma E, et al. Multi drug resistant female genital tuberculosis: a preliminary report. Eur J Obstet Gynecol Reprod Biol. 2016;210:108–15 [c].

[22] Otto MW, Pollack MH, Dowd SM, et al. Randomized trial of D-cycloserine enhancement of cognitive-behavioral therapy for panic disorder. Depress Anxiety. 2016;33(8):737–45 [c].

[23] de Leeuw AS, van Megen HJ, Kahn RS, et al. D-Cycloserine addition to exposure sessions in the treatment of patients with obsessive-compulsive disorder. Eur Psychiatry. 2016;40:38–44 [c].

[24] Schnitzer TJ, Torbey S, Herrmann K, et al. A randomized placebo-controlled pilot study of the efficacy and safety of D-cycloserine in people with chronic back pain. Mol Pain. 2016;12:1–8 [c].

[25] Kar HK, Gupta R. Treatment of leprosy. Clin Dermatol. 2015;33(1):55–65 [R].

[26] May SM, Motosue MS, Park MA. Dapsone is often tolerated in HIV-infected patients with history of sulfonamide antibiotic intolerance. J Allergy Clin Immunol Pract. 2017;5(3):831–3 [c].

[27] Hoogeveen RM, van der Bom T, de Boer HH, et al. A lethal case of the dapsone hypersensitivity syndrome involving the myocardium. Neth J Med. 2016;74(2):89–92 [A].

[28] Kang KS, Kim HI, Kim OH, et al. Clinical outcomes of adverse cardiovascular events in patients with acute dapsone poisoning. Clin Exp Emerg Med. 2016;3(1):41–5 [c].

[29] Kim YJ, Sohn CH, Ryoo SM, et al. Difference of the clinical course and outcome between dapsone-induced methemoglobinemia and other toxic-agent-induced methemoglobinemia. Clin Toxicol (Phila). 2016;54(7):581–4 [c].

[30] Cha YS, Kim H, Kim J, et al. Incidence and patterns of hemolytic anemia in acute dapsone overdose. Am J Emerg Med. 2016;34(3):366–9 [c].

[31] Toker I, Yesilaras M, Tur FC, et al. Methemoglobinemia caused by dapsone overdose: which treatment is best? Turk J Emerg Med. 2015;15(4):182–4 [A].

[32] Graff DM, Bosse GM, Sullivan J. Case report of methemoglobinemia in a toddler secondary to topical dapsone exposure. Pediatrics. 2016;138(2). http://dx.doi.org/10.1542/peds.2015-3186 [A].

[33] Sawlani KK, Chaudhary SC, Singh J, et al. Dapsone-induced pure red cell aplasia and cholestatic jaundice: a new experience for diagnosis and management. J Res Pharm Pract. 2016;5(3):215–8 [A].

[34] Podany AT, Swindells S. Current strategies to treat tuberculosis. F1000Res. 2016;5. 2579 [version 1; referees: 2 approved], http://dx.doi.org/f1000research.7403/f1000research.7403.1 [R].

[35] Tadolini M, Lingtsang RD, Tiberi S, et al. First case of extensively drug-resistant tuberculosis treated with both delamanid and bedaquiline. Eur Respir J. 2016;48(3):935–8 [A].

[36] Esposito S, Bosis S, Tadolini M, et al. Efficacy, safety, and tolerability of a 24-month treatment regimen including delamanid in a child with extensively drug-resistant tuberculosis: a case report and review of the literature. Medicine (Baltimore). 2016;95(46): e5347 [A].

[37] Sasabe H, Shimokawa Y, Shibata M, et al. Antitubercular agent delamanid and metabolites as substrates and inhibitors of ABC and solute carrier transporters. Antimicrob Agents Chemother. 2016;60(6):3497–508 [E].

[38] Mallikaarjun S, Wells C, Petersen C, et al. Delamanid coadministered with antiretroviral drugs or antituberculosis drugs shows no clinically relevant drug-drug interactions in healthy subjects. Antimicrob Agents Chemother. 2016;60(10): 5976–85 [c].

[39] Nahid P, Dorman SE, Alipanah N, et al. Official American thoracic society/centers for disease control and prevention/infectious diseases society of America clinical practice guidelines: treatment of drug-susceptible tuberculosis. Clin Infect Dis. 2016;63(7): e147–95 [R].

[40] Bright-Thomas RJ, Gondker AR, Morris J, et al. Drug-related hepatitis in patients treated with standard anti-tuberculosis chemotherapy over a 30-year period. Int J Tuberc Lung Dis. 2016;20(12):1621–4 [C].

[41] Chahed H, Hachicha H, Berriche A, et al. Paradoxical reaction associated with cervical lymph node tuberculosis: predictive factors and therapeutic management. Int J Infect Dis. 2017;54:4–7 [c].

[42] Nicolini A, Perazzo A, Gatto P, et al. A rare adverse reaction to ethambutol: drug-induced haemolytic anaemia. Int J Tuberc Lung Dis. 2016;20(5):704–5 [A].

[43] Yoshioka Y, Hanafusa T, Namiki T, et al. Drug-induced hypersensitivity syndrome by ethambutol: a case report. J Dermatol. 2016;43(8):971–2 [A].

[44] Lehloenya RJ, Todd G, Wallace J, et al. Diagnostic patch testing following tuberculosis-associated cutaneous adverse drug reactions induces systemic reactions in HIV-infected persons. Br J Dermatol. 2016;175(1):150–6 [c].

[45] Das MK, Arya R, Debnath S, et al. Global urine metabolomics in patients treated with first-line tuberculosis drugs and identification of a novel metabolite of ethambutol. Antimicrob Agents Chemother. 2016;60(4):2257–64 [c].

[46] Fatiguso G, Allegra S, Calcagno A, et al. Ethambutol plasma and intracellular pharmacokinetics: a pharmacogenetic study. Int J Pharm. 2016;497(1–2):287–92 [c].

[47] Strunk AK, Ciesek S, Schmidt JJ, et al. Single- and multiple-dose pharmacokinetics of ethambutol and rifampicin in a tuberculosis patient with acute respiratory distress syndrome undergoing extended daily dialysis and ECMO treatment. Int J Infect Dis. 2016;42:1–3 [A].

[48] Yang HK, Park MJ, Lee JH, et al. Incidence of toxic optic neuropathy with low-dose ethambutol. Int J Tuberc Lung Dis. 2016;20(2):261–4 [c].

[49] Libershteyn Y. Ethambutol/linezolid toxic optic neuropathy. Optom Vis Sci. 2016;93(2):211–7 [A].

[50] Kim KL, Park SP. Visual function test for early detection of ethambutol induced ocular toxicity at the subclinical level. Cutan Ocul Toxicol. 2016;35(3):228–32 [c].

[51] Peng CX, Zhang AD, Chen B, et al. Macular thickness as a predictor of loss of visual sensitivity in ethambutol-induced optic neuropathy. Neural Regen Res. 2016;11(3):469–75 [c].

[52] Bouffard MA, Nathavitharana RR, Yassa DS, et al. Re-treatment with ethambutol after toxic optic neuropathy. J Neuroophthalmol. 2017;37(1):40–2 [A].

[53] Gumbo T, Louie A, Deziel MR, et al. Pharmacodynamic evidence that ciprofloxacin failure against tuberculosis is not due to poor microbial kill but to rapid emergence of resistance. Antimicrob Agents Chemother. 2005;49(8):3178–81 [E].

[54] Chiang CY, Van Deun A, Rieder HL. Gatifloxacin for short, effective treatment of multidrug-resistant tuberculosis. Int J Tuberc Lung Dis. 2016;20(9):1143–7 [H].

[55] Fluoroquinolone antibacterial drugs: drug safety communication—FDA advises restricting use for certain uncomplicated infections, 2016, Silver Spring, MD: U.S. Food and Drug Administration; 2016. [cited 2017 Feb 20]. Available from: https://www.fda.gov/Drugs/DrugSafety/ucm500143.htm [S].

[56] Conde MB, Mello FC, Duarte RS, et al. A phase 2 randomized trial of a rifapentine plus MXF-based regimen for treatment of pulmonary tuberculosis. PLoS One. 2016;11(5)e0154778 [C].

[57] Kalita J, Bhoi SK, Betai S, et al. Safety and efficacy of additional LVX in tuberculous meningitis: a randomized controlled pilot study. Tuberculosis (Edinb). 2016;98:1–6 [C].

[58] Ruan Q, Liu Q, Sun F, et al. MXF and gatifloxacin for initial therapy of tuberculosis: a meta-analysis of randomized clinical trials. Emerg Microbes Infect. 2016;5:e12 [M].

[59] Kang YA, Shim TS, Koh WJ, et al. Choice between LVX and MXF and multidrug-resistant tuberculosis treatment outcomes. Ann Am Thorac Soc. 2016;13(3):364–70 [C].

[60] van der Laan LE, Schaaf HS, Solomons R, et al. Probable LVX-associated secondary intracranial hypertension in a child with multidrug-resistant tuberculosis. Pediatr Infect Dis J. 2016;35(6):706–8 [A].

[61] Catano J, Morales M. Isoniazid toxicity and TB development during biological therapy of patients with psoriasis in Colombia. J Dermatolog Treat. 2016;27(5):414–7 [C].

[62] Gray EL, Goldberg HF. Baseline abnormal liver function tests are more important than age in the development of isoniazid-induced hepatoxicity for patients receiving preventive therapy for latent tuberculosis infection. Intern Med J. 2016;46(3):281–7 [c].

[63] Ben Fredj N, Gam R, Kerkni E, et al. Risk factors of isoniazid-induced hepatotoxicity in Tunisian tuberculosis patients. Pharmacogenomics J. 2016; http://dx.doi.org/10.1038/tpj.2016.26 [c].

[64] Shah R, Ankale P, Sinha K, et al. Isoniazid induced lupus presenting as oral mucosal ulcers with pancytopenia. J Clin Diagn Res. 2016;10(10):OD03–5 [A].

[65] Chaitanya V, Sangeetha B, Reddy MH, et al. Isoniazid cerebellitis in a peritoneal dialysis patient. Nephrology (Carlton). 2016;21(5):442 [A].

[66] Ramirez-Lapausa M, Pascual Pareja JF, Carrillo Gomez R, et al. Retrospective study of tolerability and efficacy of linezolid in patients with multidrug-resistant tuberculosis (1998–2014). Enferm Infecc Microbiol Clin. 2016;34(2):85–90 [c].

[67] Yi L, Yoshiyama T, Okumura M, et al. Linezolid as a potentially effective drug for the treatment of multidrug-resistant tuberculosis in Japan. Jpn J Infect Dis. 2017;70(1):96–9 [c].

[68] Arbex MA, Bonini EH, Kawakame Pirolla G, et al. Effectiveness and safety of imipenem/clavulanate and linezolid to treat multidrug and extensively drug-resistant tuberculosis at a referral hospital in Brazil. Rev Port Pneumol. 2016;22(6):337–41 [c].

[69] Zeng Q, LIang J, Wang J, et al. Clinical results of linezolid treatment for multidrug-resistant tuberculosis in China: cases report and literature review. Int J Clin Exp Med. 2016;9(9):18554–8 [c].

[70] Agyeman AA, Ofori-Asenso R. Efficacy and safety profile of linezolid in the treatment of multidrug-resistant (MDR) and extensively drug-resistant (XDR) tuberculosis: a systematic review and meta-analysis. Ann Clin Microbiol Antimicrob. 2016;15(1):41 [M].

[71] Denny N, Raghunath S, Bhatia P, et al. Rifampicin-induced adrenal crisis in a patient with tuberculosis: a therapeutic challenge. BMJ Case Rep. 2016; http://dx.doi.org/10.1136/bcr-2016-216302 [A].

[72] Jindani A, Borgulya G, de Patino IW, et al. A randomised Phase II trial to evaluate the toxicity of high-dose rifampicin to treat pulmonary tuberculosis. Int J Tuberc Lung Dis. 2016;20(6):832–8 [C].

[73] Chogtu B, Surendra VU, Magazine R, et al. Rifampicin-induced concomitant renal injury and hepatitis. J Clin Diagn Res. 2016;10(9):OD18–9 [A].

[74] Gopi M, Seshadri MS. Biphasic effect of rifampicin on bilirubin—a case report. J Clin Diagn Res. 2016;10(4):OD14–5 [A].

[75] McColl KE, Thompson GG, el Omar E, et al. Effect of rifampicin on haem and bilirubin metabolism in man. Br J Clin Pharmacol. 1987;23(5):553–9 [A].

[76] Ji G, Zeng X, Sandford AJ, et al. Rifampicin-induced antineutrophil cytoplasmic antibody-positive vasculitis: a case report and review of the literature. Int J Clin Pharmacol Ther. 2016;54(10):804–7 [A].

[77] Syrigou E, Grapsa D, Nanou E, et al. Anaphylaxis during rapid oral desensitization to rifampicin. J Allergy Clin Immunol Pract. 2016;4(1):173–4 [A].

[78] Hamadah AM, Beaulieu LM, Wilson JW, et al. Tolerability and healthcare utilization in maintenance hemodialysis patients undergoing treatment for tuberculosis-related conditions. Nephron. 2016;132(3):198–206 [c].

[79] Siddiqui AN, Khayyam KU, Sharma M. Effect of diabetes mellitus on tuberculosis treatment outcome and adverse reactions in patients receiving directly observed treatment strategy in India: a prospective study. Biomed Res Int. 2016;2016:7273935 [c].

[80] Hu M, Zheng C, Gao F. Use of bedaquiline and delamanid in diabetes patients: clinical and pharmacological considerations. Drug Des Devel Ther. 2016;10:3983–94 [R].

[81] Harausz EP, Garcia-Prats AJ, Seddon JA, et al. New/repurposed drugs for pediatric multidrug-resistant tuberculosis: practice-based recommendations. Am J Respir Crit Care Med. 2017;195(10):1300–10 [R].

27

Antihelminthic Drugs

Igho J. Onakpoya[1]

University of Oxford, Oxford, United Kingdom

[1]Corresponding author: igho.onakpoya@phc.ox.ac.uk

ALBENDAZOLE

Observational Study

In a non-randomized comparative study ($n=60$), the clinical effectiveness of liposomal albendazole and albendazole tablet in the treatment of hepatic cystic echinococcosis were compared [1c]. The most common adverse events observed were abdominal discomfort, diarrhea and dizziness. There was no statistically significant difference in the frequency of adverse events between groups ($P>0.05$).

Placebo-Controlled Trial

In a randomized, double-blind, placebo-controlled trial ($n=60$), the safety and efficacy of two or six doses of 800 mg albendazole every 2 months for treatment of Loa loa microfilariae were evaluated [2c]. No treatment related adverse events were observed.

Meta-Analysis

See Section Ivermectin.

Liver

Albendazole-induced hepatic failure in a 38-year-old woman has been described [3A].

- A 38-year-old Iraqi woman with known hydatid cysts presented to the emergency department with a 2-week history of worsening malaise, nausea, fatigue, and jaundice. *Echinococcus* was established 3 months prior, while during work-up for abdominal pain, and ultrasound revealed 2 hydatid cysts measuring 7.4 cm × 6.7 cm and 6.7 cm × 5.2 cm. Laboratory studies indicated positive echinococcus IgG enzyme-linked immunosorbent assay with confirmatory Western

blot. The patient was initiated on albendazole 400 mg twice daily and remained well for a month before her presentation to our facility. On presentation, she was found to have abnormal chemistries with elevated aspartate aminotransferase (AST) 1705 IU/L, alanine aminotransferase (ALT) 2118 IU/L, total bilirubin 5.0 mg/dL, and international normalized ratio 1.3. An examination revealed jaundice and scleral icterus, with no asterixis and normal mentation. She was admitted for expedited work-up of acute liver injury and albendazole was discontinued. Over the next 48 hours, her liver function worsened with laboratory results showing AST 2438 IU/L, ALT 2748 IU/L, total bilirubin 12.6 mg/dL, and an international normalized ratio of 1.7. Work-up results for the cause of liver failure including anti-hepatitis A virus IgM, hepatitis B core antibody, anti-hepatitis B core IgM, anti-hepatitis C virus, anti-hepatitis E virus IgM, anti-cytomegalovirus IgM, anti-Epstein–Barr virus IgM, and anti-herpes simplex virus IgM were nonreactive. Antinuclear, anti-mitochondrial, and anti-smooth muscle antibodies were negative, and ceruloplasmin was within normal limits. Duplex sonography showed no abnormality of hepatic vascular inflow and outflow. A trans-jugular liver biopsy was performed on day 3 revealing severe acute hepatitis with areas of confluent necrosis, scattered eosinophils, and no plasma cell infiltrates. The patient was initiated on *N*-acetylcysteine for presumed severe drug-induced liver injury; however, she grew increasingly encephalopathic and required admission to the intensive care unit for intubation and airway protection. Coagulopathy and mentation did not improve on *N*-acetylcysteine, and the patient was listed Status IA for liver transplant. A suitable donor organ was identified, and she received an orthotopic liver transplant on day 10 of hospitalization. Explant pathology demonstrated massive hepatic necrosis and hydatid cysts with necrotic lamellated membranes. Her post-transplant course was uneventful, and the patient remains in good health with normal liver allograft and neurologic function 1.5 years post-transplant.

IVERMECTIN

Systematic Review

The safety and efficacy of doxycycline plus ivermectin vs ivermectin alone have been evaluated in a systematic review of three randomized controlled trials ($n=466$) [4M]. Adverse events reported included itching, headaches, body pains, vertigo and diarrhea. None of the studies reported significant differences between intervention groups.

Meta-Analysis

The safety and efficacy of ivermectin compared with albendazole or thiabendazole in the treatment of *Strongyloides stercoralis* infection have been assessed in a meta-analysis of seven randomized clinical trials including 1147 participants [5M]. Four trials were conducted in endemic communities in low- to middle-income settings, while three trials recruited participants from endemic areas in high-income settings. The most common adverse events were nausea, dizziness and disorientation. No serious adverse events were reported. In four trials that compared ivermectin vs albendazole ($n=518$), there was no significant difference in the frequency of adverse events: RR 0.80, 95% CI 0.59–1.09; however, the quality of the evidence was low. In three trials that compared ivermectin vs thiabendazole ($n=507$), the frequency of adverse events was significantly reduced with ivermectin: RR 0.31, 95% CI 0.20–0.50; the quality of the evidence was moderate.

LEVAMISOLE

Levamisole-Contaminated Cocaine

Abuse of levamisole-contaminated cocaine continues to pose a public health challenge. Majority of abusers are females, and the average age of abusers is 43 years [6A]. Recent reports of abuse in the scientific literature are here presented.

Respiratory System

The first case of laryngeal involvement in levamisole-induced vasculitis has been reported [7A].

- *An adult patient with a history of crack cocaine abuse presented with several days of malaise, painful violacious purpura, and necrosis of bilateral cheek and ear skin. Lesions were non-blanching centrally, with a rim of erythema. Similar lesions were present on the thighs and hard palate. The patient's voice was rough and breathy. Endoscopy revealed normal hypopharyngeal and supraglottic mucosa, but bilateral ulcerative lesions of the true vocal folds with surrounding edema were detected. There were no mucosal stigmata to suggest burn injury. Complete blood cell count findings were normal, while results of antinuclear antibody (ANA) and antineutrophil cytoplasmic antibody (ANCA) testing were positive. Result of urine toxicology testing was positive for cocaine metabolites, which was in concordance with the presumed diagnosis of levamisole-induced vasculitis. The facial lesions were treated with oral steroids and petroleum jelly ointment, and the patient was counseled to cease cocaine use. When seen at follow-up visits at 1, 8, and 16 weeks, the patient's facial lesions had healed with minimal scaring. The patient's voice remained rough and breathy, with stiffening of the bilateral vocal folds observed on videostroboscopy.*

Renal System

Renal manifestation of vasculitis caused by levamisole-adulterated cocaine has again been described [8A].

- *A 44-year-old black woman presented to the hospital with right flank pain associated with fever, fatigue, and nausea. Review of systems was significant for dark urine, rash over arms and legs, discoloration of ears with burning, and intermittent bilateral shoulder and knee arthralgias. She reported tobacco and marijuana use and denied use of other illicit substances. Four weeks prior, she had been evaluated in the emergency department for abdominal pain, nausea, vomiting, and urinary urgency and frequency. A diagnosis of focal enteritis then was managed with ciprofloxacin and metronidazole. During that visit, she was also found to have a small right pelvic hematoma thought to be secondary to a hysterectomy 2 months prior. Physical examination revealed blood pressure of 191/106 mmHg, heart rate of 106 beats/min, boggy and erythematous nasal turbinates, right upper quadrant tenderness, chronic interphalangeal hyperextension of bilateral thumbs, and necrotic-appearing rash over the earlobes, nose, left upper arm, and posterior thighs. Cardiopulmonary examination was unremarkable. Laboratory investigations revealed hemoglobin of 8 mg/dL (12–16 mg/dL) and leukopenia 4000/μL (4.5–11/μL), with normal platelet count. Creatinine was elevated from baseline of 0.5–1.23 mg/dL (0.6–1.6 mg/dL); albumin 3.5 g/dL (3.2–4.8 g/dL); erythrocyte sedimentation rate 85 mm/h (0–19 mm/h); C-reactive protein 21 mg/dL (0–0.5 mg/dL). Urinalysis revealed proteinuria of 300 mg/dL, large amount of blood, and no casts. Immune screening tests were positive for anti-nuclear antibody > 1:640 (<1:40), homogeneous pattern of staining, anti-dsDNA > 1000 IU/mL*

(<30 IU/mL), cryoglobulin, perinuclear ANCA, myeloperoxidase 2.9 U (<0.4 U), proteinase 3 (PR3) 3.2 U (<0.4 U) and rheumatoid factor 20 IU/mL (0–14 IU/mL). Negative immune studies included anti-Smith antibody, cytoplasmic ANCA, human immunodeficiency virus, and hepatitis B and C viruses. C3 and C4 were normal. Blood and urine cultures grew Escherichia coli. Urine drug screen positive for cocaine and urinary detection of levamisole by gas chromatography/mass spectroscopy confirmed cocaine adulteration. Computed tomographic scan revealed a large right perinephric hematoma; renal arteriogram uncovered dye extravasation and multiple intrarenal micro aneurysms suggestive of polyarteritis nodosa. Spontaneous renal artery bleed was attributed to blood vessel wall compromise. Renal artery bleeding completely resolved after coli embolization of the affected renal vasculature with return of creatinine to baseline. Skin manifestations resolved rapidly after starting short prednisolone taper, but primarily, the patient was managed conservatively and counselled to stop cocaine use and seek substance abuse treatment. Escherichia coli bacteremia was managed accordingly. After this admission, the patient had recurring emergency room visits for cocaine intoxication with mild cutaneous lesions managed conservatively, and no further serological tests were done.

Skin

The clinical, serologic, and histopathologic findings in pyoderma gangrenosum (PG) caused by levamisole-adulterated cocaine have been described in a cohort of eight patients [9A].

• The primary lesions were similar to those observed in patients with conventional PG with tender, ulcerated serpiginous plaques with necrotic ulcer beds. In the entire cohort, vesicopustular, bullous, ulcerative, and vegetative types of lesions were also observed. Importantly, no petechiae, palpable purpura, or other physical examination findings suggestive of the more typical vasculitis was seen in most of the patients who presented with early lesions. None of the patients were found to have any of the medical comorbidities classically associated with PG, including inflammatory bowel disease, arthritides, or hematologic disease. Only 3 patients with the ulcerative lesions of PG also presented with concomitant retiform purpura more commonly associated with thrombotic levamisole toxicity. The PG lesions in these patients had no surrounding retiform purpura or petechiae to suggest an ulcer taking origin in vasculitis. Lesions appeared primarily on the upper (6 of 8 patients) and lower (all 8 patients) extremities. Most patients demonstrated elevated titers for p-ANCA and antiphospholipid antibodies, and a diffuse dermal infiltrate dominated by neutrophils was seen in all biopsy specimens. Lesions improved or remained stable with conservative management or short courses of steroids, and recurrence was only noted on re-exposure to adulterated cocaine.

Extensive necrotic purpura in an intoxicated female has also been described [10A].

• A 40-year-old woman presented with painful skin lesions on her right upper extremity without medical examination. According to the patient, the lesions healed spontaneously in 2 weeks. A recurrence of the lesions was observed 1 month later in the same location and without medical consultation. A third episode was again observed 2 months after the first episode with painful skin lesions of the nose, cheeks, ears, back of the hands, and lower extremities. Five days after hospitalization, the patient admitted to using heroin and cocaine immediately before the skin lesions appeared in both episodes. For the recent episode, she reported only smoking cocaine and heroin that was supplied to her by her regular supplier. The patient had a past medical history of heroin (intravenous) and cocaine (intravenous and sniff) abuse, hepatitis C virus, and septic shock with staphylococcus aureus and streptococcus infections in 2009. No previous documented history of any type of autoimmune disorder was reported prior to the described episode. Neither documented allergy nor allergy manifestation was reported too. In the emergency department and during hospitalization, she presented with necrotic evolution of the skin lesions with enlargement. Skin grafts on the lower extremities and wound healing of the rest of the skin lesion were performed. The addiction medicine unit of the hospital proposed treatment for her cocaine and heroin addiction, but she declined this medical follow-up and did not attend all of her dermatologic consultations. The laboratory investigations did not show signs of infection in the blood sample cultures or in the cerebrospinal fluid. The laboratory analyses showed acute kidney failure (serum creatinine 15 mg/L) without additional anomalies such as anemia (12.2 g/dL of hemoglobin; 227 000/mm^3 blood platelets; 12 000/mm^3 leukocytes; and 8300/mm^3 neutrophils) or thrombocytopenia (increased activated partial thromboplastin time [APTT] measured at 57 s and normal prothrombin time [PT]). Antibodies anti-beta2 glycoprotein 1 or anticardiolipin were negative. Lupus anticoagulant screening was positive, with a Rosner Index of 40.7. Antinuclear antibodies (ANA) were weakly positive with a titer of 1:80 (positivity threshold 1/80), cytoplasmic antimyeloperoxydase antibodies (anti-MPO) were positive but not significant (16.99 U/mL, normal range < 20 U/mL), and specific searching for pANCA specificity anti-human neutrophil elastase (anti-HNE) was positive with high titer (>100 U/mL). A positive type III cryoglobulinemia was observed (0.56 g/L) with a HVC serology positive for the 3a genotype (viral load at 332 557 IU/mL). HIV and HVB serology were negative. C protein and its complement were normal. Microscopic observations of the sample showed a superficial perivascular neutrophilic infiltration with fibrinoïd degeneration of the vessel wall and erythrocyte extravasations with several micro thrombi, which were compatible with leukocytoclastic vasculitis. The direct *immunofluorescence study revealed positive C3 and IgG depositions. Blood samples for toxicology were negative. Urine toxicology was positive for cocaine and methadone. Hairs analysis found a positive result for levamisole in all 6 cm of hair length, including chronic and repeated levamisole intoxication with 1 ng/mg in the first proximal fraction of hair (48 mg, 2 cm), 1.24 ng/mg in the second fraction of hair (85 mg, 2 cm), and 1.78 ng/mg in the third fraction of hair (68 mg, 2 cm).*

MEBENDAZOLE

Observational Study

The safety of mebendazole for treating nematode infections in nursing mothers has been evaluated in a case series involving 45 breastfeeding women who had all suffered from pinworm infection associated with rectal itching [11c]. Single- or repeat-dose mebendazole regimens were administered as treatment. Irrespective of the treatment protocol used, mebendazole was well tolerated and was not associated with any adverse events in infants of lactating mothers. Mild GI irritability was observed in two women.

Placebo-Controlled Trials

The safety of mebendazole has been assessed in a randomized multi-arm, placebo-controlled trial of 1760 children aged 12 months with soil-transmitted helminth infections [12C]. The children were followed up for 24 months. A total of 18 serious adverse events (11 deaths and 7 hospitalisations) and 31 minor adverse events were reported. There was no significant difference in the frequency of serious adverse events between the mebendazole and placebo groups: (odds ratio [OR] = 1.21; 95% confidence interval [CI] = 0.47–3.09); there was also no significant difference in the frequency of minor adverse events between the groups: OR = 0.84; 95% CI = 0.41–1.72.

Congenital Malformations

The effect of mebendazole and pyrvinium administration during pregnancy on birth outcomes has been investigated in a large Danish cohort study including 713 667 births [13C]. A total of 2567 mothers received a prescription for mebendazole; 1588 for pyrvinium. Logistic regression analysis was used to adjust for potential confounders. There was no association between exposure to mebendazole and major congenital malformations (OR = 0.7 (CI 95% 0.5–1.1)) or other negative birth outcomes. There was no association between exposure to pyrvinium and major congenital malformations (OR = 0.8 (CI 95% 0.4–1.5)) or other negative birth outcomes. There was also no increased risk of having negative birth outcomes after exposure at any trimester during pregnancy.

Immune System

Angioedema after administration of mebendazole, cotrimoxazole and leaf extracts has been reported in a child [14A].

- A 12-year-old boy presented to the Paediatric Nephrology Clinic with a day history of periorbital swelling, skin rash, pruritus and low grade fever. A day prior to the onset of these symptoms, he had been given mebendazole tablets as anti-helminthic—300 mg in the morning and in the evening. The following morning, he was noticed to have peri-orbital swelling and subsequently facial swelling. He was also noticed to have pruritic rash about the same time. This involved the face, trunk and upper limbs. The upper part of the child's body was also noticed to have been bigger than normal. There was no preceding insect bite, ingestion of a new type of food or contact with latex. There was also no family history of such ailment. This was the first episode of body swelling and first episode of mebendazole intake. He had been given oral cotrimoxazole, vitamin C and bitter leaf extracts before presentation in the hospital. Physical examination revealed that he had peri-orbital oedema with submental fullness and papular skin rash involving the face, trunk and upper limbs. He was not dyspnoeic and had respiratory rate of 16/min. His pulses were of normal volume, and his heart rate and blood pressure were 80/min and 100/60 mmHg, respectively. The heart sounds were heart sounds 1 and 2, and were normal. He did not have any other significant abnormalities in other systems. Investigations including urinalysis, blood electrolytes and urea, full blood count, and fasting lipids profile were within normal ranges. A diagnosis of angioneurotic edema was made. Other differential diagnoses considered were acute glomerulonephritis and nephrotic syndrome. He was placed on steroids—oral prednisolone 60 mg daily for 3 days. By the second day on admission, oedema was regressing and by the third day it had resolved completely as well as the rash. The parents pressed for discharge and were allowed home on the fourth day on admission. He was lost to follow-up.

OXANTEL PAMOATE

Dose-Comparison Study

The efficacy and safety of six different disease of oxantel pamoate (5–30 mg/kg) in the treatment of *Trichuris trichiura* in school-aged children have been evaluated in a single-blind trial including 350 children [15C]. The most common adverse events reported were abdominal cramps (2%). There were no significant differences in the frequency of adverse events across groups based on doses. No serious adverse events were reported.

PRAZIQUANTEL

Placebo-Controlled Trials

The safety of praziquantel therapy in the treatment of schistosomiasis during pregnancy has been assessed in a double-blind randomized trial including 370 participants [16C]. Severe adverse events observed included headache, fever and malaise. There were no significant differences in the rates of abortion, fetal demise in-utero, or congenital anomalies.

The safety and efficacy of praziquantel for treating light infections of *Opisthorchis viverrini* have been evaluated in a randomised parallel, single blind, dose-ranging, phase 2 trial including 217 adults [17c]. The daily dosages of praziquantel were 30, 40, 50, 3×25 mg/kg. The most common adverse events observed were nausea, headache and vertigo. No serious adverse events were observed.

PYRVINIUM

Congenital Malformations

See Section Mebendazole.

THIABENDAZOLE

Meta-Analysis

See Section Ivermectin.

TRIBENDIMIDINE

Randomized Clinical Trial

The safety and efficacy of tribendimidine in the treatment of *Opisthorchis viverrini* have been evaluated in two randomized, parallel-group-single-blind, dose-ranging phase 2 trials of children ($n = 39$) and adults ($n = 318$) [18c]. The doses of tribendimidine were 25, 50, 100, 200, 400, or 600 mg in adolescents and adults; in children the doses were 50, 100, 200, or 400 mg. The adverse events were generally mild. The most common adverse events observed in adolescents and adults occurring 3-hour post-treatment included vertigo (11%), headache (3%), nausea (2%), and fatigue (1%). Common adverse events reported in children included headache (2%), vertigo (1%), and fatigue (1%). No moderate or serious adverse events were observed.

References

[1] Li H, Song T, Shao Y, et al. Comparative evaluation of liposomal albendazole and tablet-albendazole against hepatic cystic echinococcosis: a non-randomized clinical trial. Medicine (Baltimore). 2016;95(4):e2237 [c].

[2] Kamgno J, Nguipdop-Djomo P, Gounoue R, et al. Effect of two or six doses 800 mg of albendazole every two months on Loa loa microfilaraemia: a double blind, randomized, placebo-controlled trial. PLoS Negl Trop Dis. 2016;10(3):e0004492 [c].

[3] Aasen TD, Nasrollah L, Seetharam A. Drug-induced liver failure requiring liver transplant: report and review of the role of albendazole in managing echinococcal infection. Exp Clin Transplant. 2016. http://dx.doi.org/10.6002/ect.2015.0313 [A].

[4] Abegunde AT, Ahuja RM, Okafor NJ. Doxycycline plus ivermectin versus ivermectin alone for treatment of patients with onchocerciasis. Cochrane Database Syst Rev. 2016;(1):CD011146 [M].

[5] Henriquez-Camacho C, Gotuzzo E, Echevarria J, et al. Ivermectin versus albendazole or thiabendazole for strongyloides stercoralis infection. Cochrane Database Syst Rev. 2016;(1):CD007745 [M].

[6] Larocque A, Hoffman RS. Levamisole in cocaine: unexpected news from an old acquaintance. Clin Toxicol (Phila). 2012;50(4):231–41 [A].

[7] Alemi AS, Faden DL. Otolaryngologic manifestations of levamisole-induced vasculitis. JAMA Otolaryngol Head Neck Surg. 2016;142(3):299–300 [A].

[8] Machua W, Oliver AM. Another vasculitis red herring: spontaneous renal artery bleed associated with levamisole-adulterated cocaine. J Clin Rheumatol. 2016;22(1):47–8 [A].

[9] Jeong HS, Layher H, Cao L, et al. Pyoderma gangrenosum (PG) associated with levamisole-adulterated cocaine: clinical, serologic, and histopathologic findings in a cohort of patients. J Am Acad Dermatol. 2016;74(5):892–8 [A].

[10] Le Garff E, Tournel G, Becquart C, et al. Extensive necrotic purpura in levamisole-adulterated cocaine abuse—a case report. J Forensic Sci. 2016;61(6):1681–5 [A].

[11] Karra N, Cohen R, Berlin M, et al. Safety of mebendazole use during lactation: a case series report. Drugs R&D. 2016;16(3):251–4 [c].

[12] Joseph SA, Montresor A, Casapía M, et al. Adverse events from a randomized, multi-arm, placebo-controlled trial of mebendazole in children 12–24 months of age. Am J Trop Med Hyg. 2016;95(1):83–7 [C].

[13] Torp-Pedersen A, Jimenez-Solem E, Cejvanovic V, et al. Birth outcomes after exposure to mebendazole and pyrvinium during pregnancy—a Danish nationwide cohort study. J Obstet Gynaecol. 2016;36(8):1020–5 [C].

[14] Ashubu OF, Ademola AD, Asinobi AO. A case report of suspected angioedema in a child after administration of mebendazole, cotrimoxazole and leaf extracts. Ann Ib Postgrad Med. 2016;14(1):41–3 [A].

[15] Moser W, Ali SM, Ame SM, et al. Efficacy and safety of oxantel pamoate in school-aged children infected with Trichuris trichiura on Pemba Island, Tanzania: a parallel, randomised, controlled, dose-ranging study. Lancet Infect Dis. 2016;16(1):53–60 [C].

[16] Olveda RM, Acosta LP, Tallo V, et al. Efficacy and safety of praziquantel for the treatment of human schistosomiasis during pregnancy: a phase 2, randomised, double-blind, placebo-controlled trial. Lancet Infect Dis. 2016;16(2):199–208 [C].

[17] Sayasone S, Meister I, Andrews JR, et al. Efficacy and safety of praziquantel against light infections of Opisthorchis viverrini: a randomised parallel single blind dose-ranging trial. Clin Infect Dis. 2016;64(4):451–8 [c].

[18] Sayasone S, Odermatt P, Vonghachack Y, et al. Efficacy and safety of tribendimidine against Opisthorchis viverrini: two randomised, parallel-group, single-blind, dose-ranging, phase 2 trials. Lancet Infect Dis. 2016;16(10):1145–53 [c].

28

Vaccines

Kendra M. Damer*,[1], Carrie M. Maffeo*, Deborah Zeitlin*,[†],
Carrie M. Jung*,[‡], Medhane G. Cumbay[§]

*Butler University College of Pharmacy and Health Sciences, Indianapolis, IN, United States
[†]Indiana University Health, Indianapolis, IN, United States
[‡]Butler University, Eskenazi Health, Indianapolis, IN, United States
[§]Marian University College of Osteopathic Medicine, Indianapolis, IN, United States
[1]Corresponding author: kmdamer@butler.edu

Abbreviations

AVA	anthrax vaccine adsorbed
BCG	bacillus Calmette–Guérin
DTaP	diphtheria + tetanus toxoids + acellular pertussis vaccine
HAV	hepatitis A virus
HBV	hepatitis B virus
Hib	haemophilus influenzae type b
HPV	human papillomavirus
HPV4	quadrivalent human papillomavirus vaccine
HZ/su	herpes zoster subunit vaccine
HZV	herpes zoster virus
IIV	inactivated influenza vaccine
IPV	inactivated poliovirus vaccine
JE	Japanese encephalitis
JE-CV	Japanese encephalitis chimeric vaccine
LAIV	live attenuated influenza vaccine
MenB	neisseria meningitidis serogroup B
MenC	neisseria meningitidis serogroup C
MMR	measles + mumps + rubella
OPV	oral poliovirus vaccine
PCV13	13-valent pneumococcal conjugate vaccine
PCV7	7-valent pneumococcal conjugate vaccine
PPSV23	23-valent pneumococcal polysaccharide vaccine
RV	rotavirus
Tdap	tetanus toxoid + diphtheria toxoid + acellular pertussis vaccine
VZV	varicella zoster virus
YF	yellow fever

℞ Mucosal Vaccines: Combining Adjuvants With Ideal Delivery Systems

Many human pathogens gain entry through mucosal membranes. The protective mucosal immune system stands as first line of defense and provides an ideal target for vaccine application. In contrast to parenteral administration, engaging the mucosal immune system can produce robust localized (targeted mucosal membrane) and systemic protective immunity [1R,2R,3R]. Ease of application (which could facilitate mass vaccination and curb costs) and less invasive administration are some of the advantages of targeting vaccines to mucosal surfaces. Although the first oral vaccine was introduced in 1961, currently mucosal vaccines licensed for human immunization only target five infective agents: poliovirus, rotavirus, influenza virus, vibrio cholera, and Salmonella typhi. Elements that limit the development of mucosal vaccines include poor stability and inefficient uptake of immunogenic factor introduced to various mucosal environments, and the resulting low immunogenicity. Advances in nanotechnology and development of adjuvants have provided new avenues to address these limitations of mucosal immunizations [2R].

Immunological adjuvants modify immunogenic effects of antigens. Elucidations of mechanisms that underlie immunogenicity have identified multiple selective adjuvants that can potentiate immune responses. Of particular interest are agents that act on toll-like receptors (TLRs) [4R,5R]. TLRs are one class of Pattern Recognition Receptors (PRR) that function as a link between innate and adaptive immunity. TLRs contribute to adaptive immunity by enhancing the cell surface presentation on antigen-presenting cells (APCs), in particular dendritic cells, by promoting the release of specific cytokines. Subsequent activation of CD4+ T-helper cells, CD8+ cytotoxic cells, and B-cells in the mucosal areas results in the migration of differentiated T-lymphocytes and B-cells into systemic circulation. Synthetic and naturally (e.g. lipopolysaccharide) occurring agonist of various subtypes (TLR 1-10) of TLRs have been shown to be effective adjuvants [6R]. In a mouse model of melanoma, TLR agonist gardiquimod and a related compound, imiquimod, *significantly improved immune response-dependent anti-tumor effects of dendritic cells loaded with tumor lysate [7E]. Although in this study gardiquimod and the tumor lysate carrying dendritic cells were administered intravenously, subsequent studies have shown that the addition of gardiquimod to intranasally delivered Norwalk virus-like particles can enhance systemic IgG responses, and other systemic immunological responses, comparable to an established and well-characterized immunomodulator, cholera toxin [8E]. The ability to potentiate mucosal immune response has been observed with multiple combinations of TLRs agonists and various antigenic factors, and there is preclinical and clinical data to support their role as effective adjuvants [6R]. Another PRR with promising potential as an adjuvant for mucosal vaccinations are the nucleotide-binding oligomerization domain-like receptors (NLRs) [9R]. Similar to TLRs, NLRs receptors respond to various components (i.e. components of bacterial peptidoglycans) of pathogens and behave as immunomodulators. Unlike TLRs, NLRs seem to produce their effects through a transactivation pathway that impacts dendritic cells indirectly, which raises the possibility that a combination of TLRs and NLRs adjuvants may provide more effective immunogenic response [9R]. Although the combination of TLRs and other adjuvants (e.g. aluminum salts) has been clinically evaluated, the combination of agonists that target TLRs and NLRs is yet to be explored. Because these adjuvants can significantly improve antigenic response, they help to address one of the factors that limits efficacy of mucosal vaccines, low immunogenicity. Furthermore, the applicability of adjuvants to the prophylactic and therapeutic use of vaccines makes them useful for a wide array of therapeutic goals.*

In addition to enhanced immunogenicity, the antigenic factor used for mucosal vaccination (and potentially the adjuvant) must be protected from degradation, readily traverse the mucus layer, and be efficiently taken up by microfold (M) cells [2R]. Addressing these factors involves careful design of the delivery system used to reach different mucosal membranes, accounting for the size as well as the physical and chemical properties of the final product. In a novel study in which the contribution of nanoparticle surface charge and its effect on efficacy of a pulmonary vaccine was selectively measured, different surface charges accounted for nearly a 100-fold difference in potency as assessed by the, in part, antigen-specific T-cell proliferation [10E]. Size and shape differences in nanoparticles can also dictate the extent and nature of immune response [11R]. Identifying the most effective mixture of properties will likely be facilitated by the myriad of building tools available to develop nanoparticles. Nanoparticles that carry both an antigenic factor and an adjuvant are likely to show the greatest promise for the delivery of effective mucosal vaccines. An illustration of this concept comes from studies in which adjuvants combined with antigenic factors where incorporated into nanoparticle vehicles and administered parenterally or by mucosal route [12E]. In contrast to parenteral administration, mucosal administration resulted in enhanced antigen presentation, increased T-cell activation and expansion, and prolonged mucosal and systemic

immunity. The utilization of mucosal surfaces as targets for vaccine delivery, along with the appropriate packaging, adjuvant, and antigen, produces robust immunogenic effects.

GENERAL [SEDA-36, 465]

An adverse event following immunization (AEFI) is defined by the World Health Organization (WHO) as any untoward medical occurrence that follows immunization and does not necessarily have a causal relationship with the use of the vaccine. The event could consist of any unfavorable sign, abnormal laboratory result, symptom and/or disease. Specific causes associated with AEFI may include the vaccine product, the quality of the vaccine product, an error related to immunization, and/or immunization-related anxiety.

A causality assessment is the systematic review of data surrounding an AEFI that is conducted to determine the likelihood of a causal association between the event and the vaccine(s) administered. The WHO established the Global Advisory Committee for Vaccine Safety (GACVS) which commissioned a group of experts from GACVS, Advisory Committee on Causality Assessment (ACCA), Vaccine Adverse Event Surveillance & Communication of the European Union (EU/VAESCO), Clinical Immunization Safety Assessment (CISA) and the Council for International Organizations of Medical Sciences (CIOMS) to update and publish a manual to assist healthcare personnel in the investigation of and causality assessment of AEFI. The manual presents background information, checklists, algorithms, classification schemes, and examples that can be utilized in various settings. The classifications of AEFI cases with adequate information for causality conclusions include (1) consistent causal association to immunization, (2) indeterminate (e.g. temporal relationship), (3) inconsistent causal association to immunization (coincidental). A case that lacks adequate information for causality conclusion is categorized as "unclassifiable" and requires further investigation. The association between immunization and AEFI is of vital importance to further enhance knowledge of vaccine safety and for continued patient education and healthcare professional advocacy of immunization practices as a major public health initiative to prevent vaccine-preventable illness worldwide [13H,14S].

VIRAL VACCINES

Dengue Vaccine

General

The WHO issued the first position paper focusing on the dengue vaccine in July 2016. One dengue vaccine has been registered in a number of countries. The vaccine is a recombinant, yellow fever-17D-dengue virus, live attenuated, tetravalent dengue vaccine (CYD-TDV, or Dengvaxia). The vaccine is administered in a three-dose series at 0, 6, and 12 months and is indicated for individuals aged 9–45 years living in dengue endemic areas. Pooled safety data were described for subjects aged 9–60 years. Local and systemic adverse events (AE) were comparable following receipt of CYD-TDV compared to other live attenuated vaccines. Fever was reported in 5% in subjects aged 18–60 years and 16% of recipients aged 9–17 years. The most common solicited systemic reactions were headache (>50%), malaise (>40%), and myalgia (>40%). Injection site reactions were reported in 49.6% of CYD-TDV recipients compared to 38.5% in placebo subjects. The most common reaction was pain, reported in 45.2% in subjects aged 18–60 and 49.2% in those aged 9–17 years. The vaccine's yellow fever (YF) 17D backbone presents a theoretical risk of acute viscerotropic or neurotropic disease; however, no cases have been detected to date [15S]. A safety signal emerged from the youngest age group studied. The relative risk (RR) of hospitalized dengue illness was increased among participants aged 2–5 years during the third year following dose one (RR of 7.5 [95% CI 1.2–313.8]). This increased risk was not observed for older age group [16R]. Therefore, at this time, the dengue vaccine is not recommended for children aged less than 9 years. The position of the WHO states a consideration to introduce dengue vaccine only in geographical settings with a high burden of disease based on epidemiological data (~70% or great seroprevalence) in order to achieve optimal public health impact [15S].

Susceptibility Factors

AGE AND ETHNICITY

Significant study of the CYD-TDV vaccine conducted in five Asian and five Latin American countries demonstrated comparable efficacy and safety data. Recently, a multi-center, observer-blinded, randomized, placebo-controlled phase 2 trial was completed in India. Included subjects were aged 18–45 years and were in good health. Participants received a three-dose series of the CYD-TDV vaccine at 0, 6, and 12 months via the subcutaneous route. Solicited injection site and systemic reactions were reported more frequently in the CYD-TDV group (9.5% and 19%, respectively) compared to placebo (4.9% and 6.6%, respectively). The authors did not describe systemic reaction results in this publication. Of the 188 subjects included in the safety analysis, one subject in each group experienced at least one serious adverse event (SAE). One subject in the CYD-TDV group experienced megaloblastic anemia and one subject in the placebo group experience a viral upper respiratory tract infection. Neither event was considered associated with the study vaccine. No deaths were reported during the study and zero

virologically confirmed cases of dengue illness occurred. The safety profile of CYD-TDV vaccine in this adult population was deemed acceptable and comparable to previously reported studies in Asian and Latin American children [17C].

Drug Interactions

DRUG–DRUG INTERACTIONS

The safe and effective co-administration of childhood vaccines remains a key focus of vaccine research given the numerous vaccines recommended for children for prevention of diseases. The dengue vaccine CYD-TDV was studied in children aged 12–15 months to assess safety and immunogenicity when administered concomitantly with measles–mumps–rubella (MMR) vaccine. The enrolled children were randomized to one of four groups and received three doses of CYD-TDV or control vaccines (varicella or hepatitis A) according to vaccine schedule recommendations. One group received concomitant CYD-TDV and MMR vaccine and the final group received CYD-TDV and placebo. Pain and erythema were the most commonly reported local reactions. The frequency did not increase with subsequent doses of CYD-TDV vaccine. Fever, abnormal crying, and irritability were reported in 20%–26.7% of children after CYD-TDV vaccination. The co-administration of CYD-TDV and MMR vaccine did appear to slightly more reactogenic compared to the CYD-TDV/placebo group with higher rates of reported fever following co-administration. Overall, SAEs were reported in 10 children (4.8%). Three children reported febrile convulsions following co-administration of CTD-TDV and MMR vaccine. While all three cases were assessed as unrelated to the study vaccines by the study investigator, the study sponsor considered one case possibly related to the co-administered vaccines. Ultimately, the safety profile of the CYD-TDV vaccine was deemed satisfactory and comparable to other vaccines routinely administered to children aged 12–15 months. The co-administration of CYD-TDV and MMR vaccine tended to be more reactogenic compared to CYD-TDV vaccine alone. The authors concluded that the study results support further examination of the dengue vaccine in larger phase 3 trials to assess co-administration with other vaccines recommended for children [18C].

Ebolavirus Vaccine

General

The world's worst Ebola Virus Disease (EVD) outbreak has resulted in greater than 28 000 cases of EVD and more than 11 000 deaths in western Africa. The WHO has declared the outbreak as an international public health emergency. The development of an effective and safe vaccine to prevent EVD represents a significant public health initiative [19c,20C].

Drug Administration

DRUG FORMULATIONS

A number of phase 1 clinical trials have been initiated to determine the safety and immunogenicity of ebola-virus vaccine candidates. The replication-competent recombinant vesicular stomatitis virus (rVSV)-vectored Zaire ebolavirus (rVSV-ZEBOV) candidate vaccine was studied in phase 1 trials in Gabon, Kenya, Germany, and Switzerland. A single dose (range 300 000 plaque-forming units [PFUs] to 50 million PFUs) was administered intramuscularly to 150 healthy adults aged 18–65 years, 8 subjects received placebo for a total of 158 participants. No SAEs were associated with the study vaccine. Ninety-two percent of participants reported at least one AE. The majority of events were mild or moderate in severity. Fever was reported in 25% of the Germany and Switzerland subjects, 30% of Kenya subjects, and 13% of subjects in Gabon. Hematologic changes were noted soon after the study vaccine was administered. In Gabon, transient leukopenia was observed in 60% of subjects receiving the 300 000 PFU dose and in 42% of those receiving the 3 million PFU dose. These results were also observed in 71% of the subjects in Switzerland and all participants in Germany. Additionally, lymphocyto-penia was noted in 11% of subjects in the 3 million PFU dose group in Gabon. Other notable AEs included arthri-tis and skin lesions. In Switzerland, 11 (22%) of the sub-jects reported arthralgia and arthritis was confirmed in 9 of the 11 subjects. At the 6-month follow-up, 10 of the 11 subjects were free of symptoms. Of the 11 subjects who reported arthralgia, three developed mild maculo-papular rashes with few tender vesicles on fingers or toes (characterized as subepidermal dermatitis with necrotic keratinocytes). Given the seemingly self-limiting nature of skin and joint involvement following vaccination, administration of the vaccine appears to present a favor-able risk–benefit relationship, and the results support the continued study of this candidate vaccine in phase 2 and 3 trials [21C].

A phase 2/2a randomized, double-blinded, placebo-controlled trial examined the safety and immunogenicity of the monovalent, recombinant, chimpanzee adenovirus type 3 vector-based Ebola Zaire (ChAd3-EBO-Z) vaccine candidate in healthy adults aged 18–65 years in Switzer-land. Subjects received either high dose or low dose study vaccine or placebo. At least one AE was reported in 87% of subjects receiving study vaccine compared to 50% of subjects in the placebo group ($P = 0.0015$). No vaccine-related SAEs occurred during the study period. The majority of AEs were mild in severity and self-limiting.

The most common systemic AEs were fatigue or malaise and headache. Musculo-articular pain was commonly reported as well. Two AEs were deemed possibly related to the study vaccine. The first was an episode of macro-scopic hematuria with pain and dysuria and mild left costovertebral angle tenderness observed within 24 hours of vaccination. The second was herpetiform dermatitis that occurred 15 days after the vaccination and lasted for 2 weeks. Other notable AEs observed included mild, transient lymphocytopenia ($n = 51$), anemia ($n = 6$), and neutropenia ($n = 6$). Seven Grade 3 AEs were reported and included one case of local erythema of 11 cm, two sudden onset and strong headaches, two fevers with tem-peratures >39°C, and two cases of severe neutropenia. All Grade 3 AEs resolved. Both cases of Grade 3 neutro-penia resolved within 3 days. At the 3-month follow-up, three mild to moderate AEs were reported and deemed possibly related to the study vaccine. The AEs included one case of axillary lymph node enlargement at day 63 post vaccination lasting 2 days, one case of mild fatigue at day 34 lasting 1 week, and one case of moderate fatigue at day 34 lasting 3 weeks. At the 6-month follow-up, one AE was reported as possibly related to the study vaccine; the AE was described as a case of mild arthralgia that lasted 1 month. Overall, the frequencies and severity of AEs were similarly reported between the two vaccines groups; however, fevers with higher temperatures were reported in the high dose group and three of the seven Grade 3 AEs occurred in the high dose group. The study results appear to support further examination of the safety and efficacy of this vaccine candidate [20C].

Hepatitis A Vaccines [SED-16, 255–293, 696–706; SEDA-38, 308]

Organs and Systems

CARDIOVASCULAR

A 20-month-old female was diagnosed with Kawasaki disease 6 days following vaccination against hepatitis A and rotavirus. The vaccines given were a second dose of Lanzhou lamb rotavirus (LLR) vaccine, the only licensed rotavirus vaccine in China, and the first dose of freeze-dried live attenuated hepatitis A vaccine. The child initially presented 5 hours after vaccination with fever and runny nose attributed to a cold and began treat-ment for acute tonsillitis. Five days later, the patient had persistent fever with a rash and itching. Additional find-ings during physical examination included superficial lymph nodes, strawberry tongue, conjunctival and pha-ryngeal congestion, rough breath sounds, chapped lips, and enlarged adenoids. Cardiac echo revealed mildly dilated left and right coronary arteries. She was diag-nosed with Kawasaki disease and sepsis and given intra-venous immunoglobulin, aspirin and dipyridamole, and imipenem–cilastatin. The patient recovered 10 days post-vaccination. While this case does not demonstrate a definitive causal relationship between the vaccination and development of Kawasaki disease, the authors felt it prudent to report given the closely associated timeframe of vaccination and onset of symptoms [22A].

SENSORY SYSTEMS: EYES

A 51-year-old male presented to the emergency department with complaints of bilateral periorbital pain, ocular pain and decreased visual acuity. His past medical history was significant only for vitamin B12 deficiency and remote pulmonary and cutaneous sarcoidosis. The patient was only receiving vitamin B12 supplementation. He had received hepatitis A and typhoid vaccines 2 weeks prior to presentation. Assessment of the patient, including multiple laboratories and a biopsy, was negative with the exception of an MRI showing optic nerve enhancement. A diagnosis of acute bilateral optic neuritis was made. The patient received treatment with intravenous thiamine, benzylpenicillin, and methylprednisolone, oral steroids, and intravenous immunoglobulin without improvement. An MRI obtained 6 weeks after presentation showed resolved optic nerve enhancement. Two years after presentation, the patient's vision was not restored. Given the timing of vaccination and the lack of other identifiable causes, including the lack of diagnosis of any other neurological disorders, the patient was suspected to have had a rare reaction to vaccination against hepatitis A and typhoid vaccines [23A].

Susceptibility Factors
AGE AND ETHNICITY

Three hepatitis A vaccines were studied in an adolescent Korean population for comparative immunogenicity and safety. The three studied vaccines were adult and pediatric doses of two formaldehyde-inactivated liquid hepatitis A adsorbed onto aluminum hydroxide (Avaxim™ and Havrix®) and a formalin-inactivated liquid vaccine attached to virosomes (Epaxal®). Adverse events after vaccination were minimal amongst all groups. The most common adverse events were local site reactions including pain, redness, and swelling. Systemic reactions occurred similarly between groups and most commonly included headache, myalgia, and gastrointestinal disorders. The vaccines were deemed safe in an adolescent population [24C].

A combined hepatitis A and typhoid vaccine is approved for use in Australia for individuals 16 years and older. Due to the ease of use, it has been used off-label for children 2–16 years of age. A study by Lau and colleagues evaluated the tolerability of the combined vaccine compared to the individual vaccines in children 2–16 years old. Children received either the combined

vaccine intramuscularly, hepatitis A vaccine and typhoid vaccine intramuscularly, or hepatitis A vaccine intramuscularly with oral typhoid vaccine. The third option was available only for children 6 years and older. Parents and children were allowed to choose the vaccine option. A total of 425 children received the combined vaccine. Of these, 236 had no other vaccines on the same day and were assessed for systemic reactions. There were an additional 89 patients who did have vaccines on the same day, but not in the same arm as the combined vaccine. This totaled 325 patients who were assessed for local reactions. Follow-up occurred 3 days after vaccination. A total of 114 participants did not experience any local or systemic AEFIs and no SAEs were reported. Soreness (70.5%), redness (16%), and swelling (11.1%) were the most common reactions in participants who did not receive other injections in the same arm. Redness and swelling tended to occur more commonly in younger children, but this was not significant. The percentage of participants reporting local AEs was significantly more than reported for the individual vaccines within age groups. Tiredness/lethargy/malaise (5.9%), headache (4.2%), fever (3.4%), sore muscles/joints (3.4%), and nausea (2.5%) were the most common systemic AEs in the combined vaccine group. Fever occurred significantly more often in younger participants (<6 years of age). Overall, the combination of hepatitis A and typhoid vaccine was considered well tolerated in children 2–16 years of age [25C].

Drug Administration
DRUG DOSAGE REGIMEN

Petrecz and colleagues investigated the efficacy and safety of concomitantly administered hepatitis A vaccine with diphtheria–tetanus–acellular pertussis (DTaP) and Haemophilus influenzae type b (Hib) vaccines. Subjects were divided into five groups: (1) Hepatitis A + DTaP + Hib concomitantly on day 1 and hepatitis A again at week 24; (2) DTaP + Hib on day 1 and hepatitis A at weeks 4 and 28; (3) Hepatitis A + Hib on day 1 and hepatitis A again at week 24; (4) Hib on day 1 and hepatitis A at weeks 4 and 28; (5) hepatitis A vaccine only on day 1 and at week 24. Stage I of the study included groups 1–4. Subjects in this stage were healthy children 15 months of age without a history of hepatitis A, immune deficiency, neoplasm, drug-induced immunodeficiency, or allergy to vaccine components. Stage II (group 5) subjects were similar, although could be 12–17 months of age upon receipt of the first vaccine. A 14-day follow-up period occurred for all subjects after visits 1, 2, and 3, including for those groups who did not receive vaccination at visit 2. A total of 1271 subjects were randomized. A total of 260 subjects completed the study in groups 1 and 3, 237 completed in groups 2 and 4, and 597 completed the study in group 5. Immunity was comparable for between concomitantly administered and non-concomitantly administered vaccine groups. Safety was also comparable between groups. Subjects receiving the vaccines separately reported less clinical adverse effects, but the difference was not significant. The most common systemic adverse effects were pyrexia (21.5% in the concomitant group vs 23.4% in the non-concomitant group), irritability (10.6% vs 16.2%, respectively), and diarrhea (9.9% vs 9.6%, respectively). Serious adverse events occurred in two patients in the non-concomitant group and four patients in the safety cohort (group 5), but none of these were deemed related to the vaccine. No subjects died or discontinued the study due to adverse events. Concomitant administration of DTaP + Hib + hepatitis A is considered favorable with regard to both immunogenicity and safety in a young pediatric population [26C].

Hepatitis B Vaccines [SED-16, 255–293, 696–706; SEDA-36, 466; SEDA-37, 384; SEDA-38, 307–308]

Organs and Systems

SKIN

A 2-month-old girl presented 2 days after vaccination with diphtheria–tetanus–pertussis and hepatitis B vaccines with tense vesicles and bullae. The lesions affected her face, limbs, palms, soles with fewer found on the abdomen, scalp, and mucosae. Hematological work-up was unrevealing and histologic work-up confirmed a diagnosis of infantile bullous pemphigoid. The patient was treated with prednisolone 1 mg/kg daily for 2 weeks and then slowly tapered. The lesions resolved during this period, and the patient remained without occurrence 6 months after initial presentation. She received subsequent vaccinations according to schedule with no recurrence. Given the timeframe of onset and lack of other potential causes, the presentation of bullous pemphigoid in this patient was possibly due to vaccination [27A].

Human Papillomavirus Vaccines (HPV) [SED-16, 255–293, 861; SEDA-36, 466; SEDA-37, 384; SEDA-38, 308–309]

General

The GACVS has previously released numerous reports on the safety of the human papillomavirus (HPV) vaccines and found no safety issues to revise the current recommendations for vaccination. Another review of the safety of the HPV vaccines was completed by GACVS and released in December 2015. A retrospective cohort study of autoimmune conditions post-HPV vaccination, including >2 million girls, found a slightly increased risk

of Guillain–Barré syndrome (GBS) during the first 3 months post-vaccination compared to unvaccinated individuals. Other autoimmune conditions occurred similarly between vaccinated and unvaccinated groups. The GACVS recommended additional studies to investigate the true risk of GBS, since this has not been reported in smaller studies. Additionally, the GACVS reviewed data on complex regional pain syndrome (CRPS) and postural orthostatic tachycardia syndrome (POTS). Upon review, they concluded these syndromes are not associated with HPV vaccination. The GACVS continues to recommend ongoing pharmacovigilance regarding HPV vaccines and increased awareness of the health benefits of HPV vaccination [28S].

Three additional studies evaluating the adverse events of HPV vaccination have also provided information on the safety of the vaccines. The first study evaluated hospital admissions data in Scotland to evaluate the incidence of 59 diagnoses after introduction of the HPV vaccine. Bell's Palsy, celiac disease, ovarian dysfunction, type 1 diabetes, demyelinating disease and juvenile rheumatoid arthritis all had slightly increased incidences, but none were significant [29c]. The second study reviewed AEFI documented in a national registry in Slovenia from 2009 to 2013. There was a higher reporting rate of AEFIs compared to documented rates in other countries. It was suspected that this was related to the mandatory reporting by physicians in Slovenia. Five serious adverse events occurred during the reporting period, but only one, migraine headache, was previously undocumented as a potential adverse event following HPV vaccination [30c]. The final study also utilized a national AEFI registry in Alberta, Canada from 2006 to 2014. This study found low rates of AEFI and the AEFIs documented were consistent with previous reports following HPV vaccination [31c]. All three of these studies were completed in females receiving the vaccine and add to the body of evidence supporting the safety of the HPV vaccines in females.

Organs and Systems

CARDIOVASCULAR: VENOUS THROMBOEMBOLISM

Post-licensure studies of the quadrivalent HPV (HPV4) vaccine have suggested an increased risk of venous thromboembolism (VTE) following vaccination. Previous editions of SEDA have reviewed small studies concerning the risk of VTE. Two large studies have since been completed to evaluate the risk of VTE in individuals receiving the HPV4 vaccine. The first study reviewed claims data for females 9–26 years of age who received the HPV4 vaccine. VTE risk factors were also assessed in this study. Over 1.4 million doses of HPV4 vaccine were given. No increased risk for VTE was found in this study population, even when stratifying by post-vaccination timeframe and controlling for additional risk factors, particularly contraceptive use [32c]. The second study reviewed claims data in the Vaccine Safety Datalink (VSD) for males and females aged 9–26 years who received the HPV4 vaccine. VTE risk factors were controlled for in this study. Over 1.2 million doses of vaccine were given to this study group. Of the 313 people who were identified with a diagnosis of VTE, only three were male. Similar to the Yih study, there was no increased risk of VTE in the study population in any post-vaccination timeframe or amongst patients with additional risk factors for VTE [33c].

NERVOUS SYSTEM

Acute disseminated encephalomyelitis (ADEM) is a rare, but documented, adverse event following immunization against HPV. Two cases have been documented in Japanese females. The first female was a 16-year-old who received the bivalent HPV vaccine. Symptoms of ADEM began 14 days after her second dose of the vaccine. Other causes were ruled out, and MRI was consistent with a diagnosis of ADEM. She was treated with methylprednisolone 1 g daily intravenously for 3 days and had resolution of her symptoms. She had no residual effects during a 2-year follow-up period. She did not receive the third dose of the vaccine. The second case was a 15-year-old female who received the HPV4 vaccine. Symptoms began 16 days after vaccination and MRI results 3 weeks after vaccination were consistent with ADEM. The patient's symptoms spontaneously resolved by 40 days post-vaccination and the MRI returned to normal. She did not have a relapse in symptoms during a 2-year follow-up period. The third dose of vaccine was not administered to this patient either. Both cases were deemed likely related to vaccination against HPV [34A].

SENSORY SYSTEMS: EYES

A 30-year-old female presented with decreased visual acuity in her right eye 3 days after vaccination with HPV vaccine. MRI showed enhancement of the right optic nerve and no other abnormalities. She had left eye optic neuritis 2 months earlier, which had begun 7 days following the first dose of HPV vaccine. The patient had no prior history of autoimmune disease and had given birth just days before her first dose of vaccine. She had not taken any other medications. Neuromyelitis optica-immunoglobulin G was discovered in this patient. She was treated with high-dose methylprednisolone for 5 days and a month-long taper of oral prednisolone. She had mild improvement in her visual acuity, which still persisted at 12 months following the second episode. She did not receive any additional doses of HPV vaccine. It was concluded that both episodes of optic neuritis were possibly due to HPV vaccination [35A].

URINARY TRACT: KIDNEYS

Two cases of tubulointerstitial nephritis and uveitis (TINU) syndrome were described following HPV vaccination. The first case occurred in a 14-year-old female 4 days following the third dose of HPV vaccine. Laboratory evaluation was consistent with interstitial nephritis and renal biopsy confirmed the diagnosis. Oral corticosteroids relieved her symptoms. However, 1 week after discontinuation of the steroids, she presented with bloodshot eyes and photophobia. Physical examination by an ophthalmologist led to diagnosis of anterior uveitis and subsequently TINU syndrome. Oral and topical corticosteroids were used to treat her symptoms. Topical steroids were still necessary 3 years after diagnosis for uveitis. The second case was in a 14-year-old girl also following her third dose of HPV vaccine. She presented with bloodshot eyes and photophobia 10 weeks after HPV vaccination. Laboratory evaluation was consistent with renal damage and abdominal ultrasound showed mild bilateral renal swelling. Eye examination by an ophthalmologist confirmed a diagnosis of anterior uveitis. Subsequently, the diagnosis of TINU syndrome was made. Oral and topical corticosteroids were utilized and resolved this patient's symptoms. The two cases were likely due to HPV vaccination [36A].

Susceptibility Factors

AGE

The VIVIANE study investigated the efficacy, safety, and immunogenicity of a bivalent HPV vaccine in women older than 25 years of age. A 7-year follow-up study evaluating the end-of-analysis of the efficacy, safety, and immunogenicity data was recently completed. Safety endpoints were published after the 48-month follow-up period. However, serious AEFIs continued to be documented during the 7-year follow-up period. Five women had serious events possibly related to the vaccine (0.2%) in the vaccine group vs eight women (0.3%) in the control group. Of the 13 deaths in the vaccine group and 5 deaths in the control group, none were attributed to the vaccine. Ongoing analysis suggests the safety of the bivalent HPV vaccine in women older than 25 years of age [37MC].

Influenza Vaccines [SEDA-16, 98–106, 263–265, 269, 276, 277, 280, 281; SEDA-36, 467; SEDA-37, 385; SEDA-38, 309]

Organs and Systems

NERVOUS SYSTEM: NARCOLEPSY

Narcolepsy is a chronic sleep disorder associated with unintended sleep episodes, excessive daytime sleepiness (EDS), and typically hypothalamic hypocretin deficiency.

It is suspected to have an autoimmune etiology. Narcolepsy is rare, with an estimated incidence of 0.74–1.37 cases per 100 000 person/years. The association of the monovalent influenza A (H1N1)pdm09 adjuvanted with Adjuvanted System containing alpha-Tocopherol and squalene in an oil-in-water emulsion (AS03) vaccine (Pandemrix™) and narcolepsy continues to undergo extensive study. Cases of narcolepsy surfaced in 2010 and by January 2015, a total of 1379 reports of narcolepsy following Pandemrix™ vaccination have been received by the EMA Eudravigilance database. Increased risk of narcolepsy has been noted in children and adolescent who received the AS03-adjuvanted vaccine and studies continue to be conducted to assess the association between the vaccine and narcolepsy. Study results are under much examination to determine the impact of any potential for biases (e.g. ascertainment bias, recall bias, selection bias, and confounding) that could influence the results. It is noted that an association between narcolepsy and the AS03-adjuvanted vaccine persists, but the true risk may be lower than reported due to the presence of biases [38H,39H]. Further study and strict consideration of potential biases is warranted to determine the true risk of narcolepsy following vaccination with AS03-adjuvanted influenza vaccine (Pandemrix™) [38H,39H,40H].

RESPIRATORY SYSTEM

Two patient cases of interstitial pneumonia are described following receipt of a seasonal influenza vaccine containing the influenza A (H1N1)pdm09 antigen. The patients include a 71-year-old female and 67-year-old male presented with worsening dry cough 36 and 41 days following vaccination, respectively. Chest imaging was suggestive of organizing pneumonia in both cases, and a diagnosis was made of drug-induced interstitial lung disease based upon diagnostic criteria. Prednisolone was initiated for treatment given negative results for tested pathogens. Both patients responded well to therapy. The authors were unable to conclude that the influenza A (H1N1)pdm09 antigen was specifically associated with the development of interstitial pneumonia in the two patient cases. The results of this study suggest the need for providers to be aware of the interstitial pneumonia as a potential complication following influenza vaccination and ensure a thorough evaluation of patients with similar complaints presenting after vaccination [41A].

SKIN

Local injection site reactions are common following influenza vaccination. A report of a severe, local cutaneous reaction following vaccination with the influenza A (H1N1)pdm09 vaccine was recently described. A 20-year-old Indian female presented 2 weeks following vaccination with erythematous, edematous, tender induration over the left arm. The reaction began 1 day after vaccination with redness and swelling at the injection site that progressed to intense itching and peeling of the skin over a few days followed by oozing and crusting. A 4-cm plaque with small erythematous papules was visualized at the periphery of the plaque. The patient did not express any systemic symptoms. She was treated with oral antibiotics, antihistamines, analgesics, and topical steroid with good response in 1 week. The report does not include the specific influenza vaccine received by the patient. The case does emphasize the importance of remaining vigilant during the assessment and reporting of AEFI [42r].

Second-Generation Effects

PREGNANCY

The administration of vaccines during pregnancy has been associated with significant reductions in infections pertussis and influenza in young infants. The safety of providing vaccines during pregnancy remains an important area of study to further support this public health intervention and increase the uptake of vaccination in this patient population. A recent study was conducted in Western Australia to assess the reactogenicity of seasonal trivalent-inactivated influenza vaccine (IIV3) and/or diphtheria–tetanus–acellular pertussis (Tdap) vaccine in a cohort of pregnant women. Pregnant women who received IIV3 exclusively, Tdap exclusively, or concomitant IIV3/Tdap vaccine(s) during pregnancy were contacted on their mobile phone via short message service (SMS) 7 days after vaccination. A total of 4347 pregnant women completed the AEFI information request(s) sent via SMS of which 468 (10.8%) reported an AEFI. Local reactions of pain or swelling at the injection site were reported in 5.1% of women. Local reactions were more common in women who received Tdap exclusively compared to IIV3 exclusively (7.1% and 3.2%, respectively; OR, 2.29; 95% CI, 1.61–3.26). Women who received concomitant IIV3/Tdap vaccines reported higher rates of local reactions compared to IIV3 exclusively (5.4% and 3.2%, respectively; OR, 1.73; 95% CI, 1.21–2.47). The receipt of Tdap vaccine in the third trimester was more than twice as often associated with local reaction compared to receiving IIV3 in the third trimester (OR, 2.5; 95% CI, 1.32–4.74). Seventy women in the study had previously received Tdap vaccine ∼3 years prior to the present study. Results indicated that AEFI was reported more frequently in women who had record of a previous dose of Tdap ($P=0.04$) compared to those with no previous dose. Pain or swelling at the injection site was more common in women with a previous dose of Tdap compared to those who did not receive a previous dose (OR, 2; 95% CI, 0.94–4.25, $P=0.06$). There was no difference between the vaccine groups in regards to the frequency of seeking medical care for AEFI ($P>0.05$). All women who sought medical care experienced a resolution of symptoms and all infants delivered at the time of follow-up were healthy. Results of reported AEFI with IIV3 and/or Tdap vaccine are consistent with previously reported data. Future study is warranted to assess the impact of closely spaced doses of Tdap vaccine to evaluate the potential for increased local reactogenicity. Overall, the study results support the safety of continued vaccination of this population with IIV3 and/or Tdap vaccine [43MC].

Susceptibility Factors

AGE

An Institute for Vaccine Safety white paper was recently published with the objective to summarize available published English-language literature on the safety of influenza vaccination in children. The publication consisted of a systematic review of the literature focused on available influenza vaccines, manufacturing and development progress of influenza vaccines over time, and published literature assessing causality between vaccination and reported AEs. Overall, most influenza vaccines were found to be generally safe, but rare SAEs may occur. Continued study of influenza vaccines in children is recommended to increase the quantity and value of evidence related to AEs associated with influenza vaccine in this population. The authors concluded that vaccination with influenza vaccine far outweighs the risk of complications or AEs following vaccination [44M].

AGE AND PHYSIOLOGICAL FACTORS: OVERWEIGHT AND OBESE CHILDREN

The number of overweight and obese children has increased worldwide. In 2010, the Advisory Committee on Immunization Practices (ACIP) in the United States (US) added obesity (specifically, adults with a body mass index [BMI] ≥ 40) to the list of conditions for which influenza vaccination is strongly recommended based on observed morbidity and mortality data in obese patients during the 2009 influenza pandemic. A small ($n=51$) prospective cohort study was conducted in Italy to assess the immunogenicity and safety of trivalent-inactivated influenza vaccine (IIV3) in already primed children aged 3–14 years with documented overweight or obesity compared to health controls. The frequency of local and systemic reactions was similar between the two groups 14 days after vaccination. The most commonly reported local AE was pain, reported in 29.6% and 8.7% of overweight/obese subjects and normal weight subjects, respectively ($P=0.09$). The most frequently reported systemic reactions were sleepiness and vomiting/diarrhea, reported in 14.8%, 4.3% and 14.8%, 4.3% of overweight/obese subjects and normal weight subjects,

respectively ($P=0.36$ and $P=0.36$). No SAEs were reported. The results of the study indicated a satisfactory immunologic response to influenza vaccine in overweight and obese children and an acceptable safety profile. Further study in the overweight and obese populations is recommended to assess immunogenicity and safety of the influenza vaccine [45c].

DISEASE: SYSTEMIC LUPUS ERYTHEMATOSUS

Systemic lupus erythematosus (SLE) is an autoimmune disease associated with dysregulation of the immune system and autoantibody production. The disease can affect several organs and is thought to impair immunity, which is associated with increased susceptibility to infection. The efficacy and safety of influenza vaccination in patients with SLE continue to be disputed in the literature. A meta-analysis was performed to evaluate the published literature with regard to the immunogenicity and safety of influenza vaccines administered to patients with SLE compared to healthy individuals. Included studies were published between 1978 and 2013 in 8 countries and included 1966 SLE patients and 1112 health controls. All SLE patients were treated with drug therapy that affects the immune system and may affect immune response to vaccination. Influenza vaccines utilized in the studies included antigens of influenza A (H1N1), (H3N2) and/or influenza B viruses administered as monovalent, bivalent, or trivalent vaccines. The authors reports all "side effects" were mild, manageable, and transient. The rate was not significantly greater than in the healthy individuals (OR, 3.24; 95% CI, 0.62–16.76). However, it was noted that 32 SLE subjects experienced mild SLE exacerbations and 5 had "serious side effects". No specific details were reported for any reported AEs from the studies included in the meta-analysis. The five "serious side effects" included one death, two hospitalizations, and two severe SLE exacerbations. The authors stated that "most" of the SAEs could not be attributed to the influenza vaccine; however, no details were provided to discuss any causality evaluation between vaccination and the reported SAEs. It was noted that there was a lack of evidence to verify an association between influenza vaccine and SLE disease exacerbation or SAEs. Future questions also include the need for assessment of SLE drug therapy on immune response following vaccination. Based upon the results of the meta-analysis, the authors conclude that influenza vaccine is an option to protect SLE patients during pandemic periods. Further study is necessary in the SLE patient population to assess safety and immunogenicity of influenza vaccine [46M].

OTHER: HOSPITALIZED SURGICAL PATIENTS

Current ACIP recommendations for influenza vaccine in the US include eligible hospitalized patients before hospital discharge. Patient admitted for surgical procedures are often not targeted for influenza vaccination prior to discharge. Potential reasons may include concerns for AEs in the perioperative period, which may lead to unnecessary evaluations or reflect poorly on surgical performance by increasing post-surgical complication rates following vaccination. A retrospective cohort study was conducted including patients enrolled in the Kaiser Permanente Southern California (KPSC) health care system to assess for outcomes related to outpatient visits, readmission, emergency department visits, or fever 7 days following vaccination with influenza vaccine. Included patients ranged from 6 months to 106 years of age (mean, 56.5 years). The most common surgery types were general surgery (28%), orthopedic (26%) and obstetrics/gynecology (11%). Among the patients vaccinated between hospital admission and discharge, most (78%) received the vaccination on the day of discharge. Of the patients that did not receive a vaccine prior to discharge, 53% were aged 6–17 years and 16% were 85 years or greater. Patients who underwent vascular surgery (18.4%) were most likely to receive vaccination during admission, followed by cardiac surgery (17.4%), and orthopedic surgery (17%). Patients admitted for ear/nose/throat surgery (8.3%) and neurosurgery (9.2%) were least likely to receive influenza vaccine. In general, vaccination rates increased during the study period. Patients who received influenza vaccine during hospital admission did have a slightly higher risk for outpatient visits following discharge (RR, 1.05; 95% CI, 1–1.1). Non-statistically significant increased in adjusted absolute risk for inpatient visits, emergency department visits, and clinical work-ups for infection were noted in the study results. The clinical significance of the study results requires further examination. The authors concluded that the results suggest that administration of influenza vaccine in hospitalized surgical patients is safe as strong evidence of increased risk of post surgical emergency department or inpatient visits or infection work-up were not detected. The increased risk of outpatient visits among surgical patients warrants further evaluation and should be weighed against the known benefits of influenza vaccination [47MC].

OTHER: SOLID ORGAN TRANSPLANT RECIPIENTS

Solid organ transplant rejection is associated with significant graft failure among transplanted patients. A number of factors and conditions may contribute to solid organ transplant rejection, including infection with influenza. Therefore, transplant recipients are at increased risk for complications of influenza and are a high-risk group recommended to receive the influenza vaccine. Reports of solid organ transplant rejection surfaced following vaccination with the monovalent influenza A (H1N1)pdm09 split-virion-inactivated vaccine

adjuvanted with AS03 (Pandemrix™). A study of solid organ transplant recipients was conducted in the United Kingdom (UK) based upon data extracted from the Clinical Practice Research Datalink (CPRD) and Hospital Episodes Statics (HES) systems. The objective of the study was to assess the risk of solid organ transplant rejection 30 and 60 days following vaccination with Pandemrix™ vaccine. Of the 254 rejection events reported, 79 occurred in patients exposed to Pandemrix™. Relative incidence estimates for rejection were 1.05 (95% CI, 0.52–2.14) and 0.8 (95% CI, 0.42–1.5) within 30 and 60 days following vaccination, respectively. Analyses were conducted to assess for covariates (vaccination with IIV3, opportunistic infections, malignancies, etc.) without significant change to the relative incidence estimates. None of the statistical analyses demonstrated a statistically significant increased risk of rejection following vaccination with Pandemrix™ vaccine. The authors noted that results might have been confounded by the inability to assess for the presence of other risk factors that may impact the development of rejection. Overall, the results do not suggest an increased risk of rejection following vaccination with Pandemrix™ vaccine in solid organ transplant recipients [48C].

Drug Administration

DRUG ADDITIVES

As described earlier, the high risk of morbidity and mortality related to influenza infection in solid organ transplant recipients necessitates the protection from infection with safe and effective vaccination practices. This population has also been noted to have a decreased immunologic response to influenza vaccine compared to immunocompetent patients. The addition of adjuvants to vaccines has been studied in various populations and typically results in increased immunogenicity. The MF59 adjuvant is an oil-in-water emulsion that contains squalene and polysorbate-80 and acts to attract inflammatory cells to the site of injection. Kumar and colleagues conducted a randomized controlled trial in adult kidney transplant recipients to assess the safety and immunogenicity of MF59-adjuvanted (Fluad®) vs non-adjuvanted (Agriflu®) influenza vaccine. In terms of safety, local tenderness was the reported in a significantly greater percentage of subjects who received MF59-adjuvanted vaccine compared to non-adjuvanted vaccine (77.4% vs 51.6%; $P = 0.034$). No other significant differences were noted for either local or systemic AEs between the two groups. In addition, no evidence of de novo or nonspecific HLA alloantibody formation was noted following adjuvanted vaccination. Six hospitalizations occurred during the study period, none were associated with the study vaccines. One death due to progressive small cell lung cancer occurred in the adjuvanted vaccine group.

This population consisted of stable long-term kidney transplant recipients. Further study regarding the safety of adjuvanted vaccines soon after transplant is warranted. In this stable population, no evidence of safety concerns was noted following MF59-adjuvanted influenza vaccine. This study supports the safe use of the adjuvanted vaccine in transplant recipients [49c].

Anaphylaxis following influenza vaccination is a rare event but remains of significant concern given the potentially fatal outcome associated with the condition. Historically, a concern for hypersensitivity reactions following influenza vaccination has focused on the potential for egg albumin exposure in patients with egg allergy. Published studies and the US ACIP support the administration of egg-based influenza vaccines even in patients with severe egg allergy, suggesting that some other vaccine component may be attributing to reactions. A study conducted in Japan investigated an increased incidence of anaphylaxis following influenza vaccine associated with one specific manufactured product during the 2011–2012 season. The one difference in this product compared to other vaccines during that season was the inclusion of the preservative 2-phenoxyethanol (2-PE). The other influenza vaccines utilized thimerosal. Nineteen subjects diagnosed with anaphylaxis according to the Brighton Collaboration case definition were studied against two age-matched control groups. Only 21% of the subjects diagnosed with anaphylaxis reported egg allergy and none were severe reactions. Levels of influenza antigen-specific IgE and vaccine-induced expression of CD203c were significantly higher in the anaphylaxis group compared to controls. There was no demonstrable binding to the excipients used in the vaccines. At higher vaccine dilutions, 2-PE demonstrated significantly enhanced CD203c expression, but thimerosal showed no effect on basophil activation. Three subjects were vaccinated with influenza vaccine containing thimerosal the following season without evidence of anaphylaxis occurrence. Two subjects did experience extensive local swelling and one had a mild cough. The study findings support a thorough investigation of anaphylactic reactions and suggest that hypersensitivity reactions to influenza vaccine may be associated with another component of the vaccine rather than the low concentrations of egg albumin [50c].

DRUG DOSAGE REGIMENS

Influenza is a significant cause of morbidity and mortality among patients with a history of hematopoietic cell transplantation (HCT). The immunologic response to influenza vaccination has been lower compared to healthy controls in published trials, potentially related to the impaired humoral response in HCT patients [51c]. Increasing the dose of antigen delivered in the influenza vaccine has demonstrated positive immunogenic

results in the elderly (≥65 years) patient population, another group commonly associated with poor response to influenza vaccine. This strategy has also been studied in adults aged 50–64 years and has demonstrated enhanced immune response following high-dose influenza vaccine [52C]. In an effort to evaluate this strategy in HCT patients, a prospective, randomized, double-blinded, phase 1 study was conducted to assess the safety and immunogenicity of trivalent high-dose-inactivated influenza vaccine (IIV3-HD) compared to standard-dose vaccine (IIV3-SD) in adult allogeneic HCT recipients. Forty-four subjects were enrolled in the study. The median age was 50.1 years (range, 19.6–72.8 years) and the median time from HCT was 7.9 months (range, 5.7–105.6 months). A higher rate of injection site reactions was noted in the IIV3-HD group (67%) compared to the IIV3-SD group (31%, $P=0.33$). No differences were reported between the groups with regard to systemic reactions. The majority of local and systemic reactions were mild to moderate in intensity and resolved within 3 days following vaccination. Three SAEs were reported during the study, none were associated with the study vaccines. The utilization of IIV3-HD was safe and well tolerated in HCT patients in this phase 1 study. Further study is necessary to assess the immune response to IIV3-HD in HCT patients [51c].

DRUG FORMULATIONS

The majority of available influenza vaccines are manufactured with the process of propagated influenza virus in embryonated hen's eggs. This method has noted limitations that may impact vaccine supply. Cell-culture vaccine manufacturing methods may represent an opportunity to improve vaccine production and limit potential contamination. Two trivalent-inactivated cell-culture-derived subunit influenza vaccines (ccIIV3) have been produced utilizing Madin-Darby Canine Kidney (MDCK) cells. One vaccine is licensed in the US (Flucelvax®) and the other in Europe (Optaflu®). The vaccines are approved for use in persons aged 18 years or older. The Flucelvax® vaccine was first administered to patients in the US during the 2013–2014 influenza season. A review of the Vaccine Adverse Event Reporting System (VAERS) was conducted to assess reported AEs following the initiation of Flucelvax® vaccine for routine influenza vaccination during the first two seasons (2013–2015) of use. Of the 629 reports following vaccination with ccIIV3, 309 (49.1%) described an AE. The most frequent AE category was "general disorders and administration site conditions" (49.2%). Nineteen of the reports were reported as SAEs (6.1%). Two reports of anaphylaxis were included, both fully recovered, and four reports of GBS were also included. Hypersensitivity and GBS events were not disproportionately reported compared to previously published data for influenza vaccines.

One death was reported in a patient with significant comorbidities who died of cardiovascular disease due to diabetes. The only signal identified in the assessment of reported AEs included the term "drug administered to patient of inappropriate age", which indicated administration to a patient <18 years of age. Only 10 (3%) reports described an AE, none of these AEs were serious and included arm pain/injection site reaction (3), nausea and/or vomiting (2), non-anaphylaxis allergic reaction (2), and one report each of asthma attack, syncope, and fever with nasal congestion. While data extracted from the VAERS database is valuable, caution must be noted due to the limitations of such data collection. Limitations include the potential for over and under-reporting of events, inconsistency in quality and completeness of reports, and the general inability to assess causality. Overall, the authors did not identify any new or unexpected safety concerns during the first two seasons of ccIIV3 utilization in the US. The only finding that was disproportionate involved the vaccination of persons <18 years with Flucelvax® vaccine. Continued examination of the safety of Flucelvax® is recommended to enhance the knowledge of AEs associated with this cell-culture-derived vaccine product [53C].

Evaluation of the safety and tolerability of the Flucevax® vaccine continues as a research focus. A phase 3 observer-blinded, randomized, multicenter study was conducted in 5 countries to assess the safety of the ccIIV3 vaccines in children <18 years of age. Healthy children aged 4–17 years were randomized to receive either ccIIV3 or IIV3. Children who have not been previously vaccinated received 2 doses of vaccine 28 days apart. Safety data were analyzed for 2052 subjects. Most AEs were mild to moderate in intensity and resolved within 7 days of vaccination. The most commonly reported local reaction was pain, and the rates were similar across all groups; however, children aged 9–17 years reported less pain in the IIV3 group (42%) compared to the ccIIV3 subjects (52%). A higher percentage of subjects in the ccIIV3 groups reported systemic reactions compared to children in the IIV3 groups. The most commonly reported reaction in 4–8 year olds was malaise with a rate of 16% in the ccIIV3 group and 13% in the IIV3 group. The most common reaction among 9–17 year olds was headache with a frequency of 19% in the ccIIV3 group and 17% in the IIV3 group. No deaths or vaccine-related SAEs occurred during the study period. Medically attended AEs were similar between the ccIIV3 (33%) and IIV3 (36%) groups. Most were deemed not related to the study vaccines. One case of psoriasis in the IIV3 group was considered possibly related to the vaccine due to the temporal relationship and lack of clear alternative cause. Overall, the results indicated that both vaccines were well tolerated in this age group. Furthermore, the ccIIV3 vaccine was safe in children aged 4–17 years and tolerability is similar to IIV3. The results support further study and

consideration of utilizing ccIIV3 vaccine in patients younger than 18 years [54MC].

A second phase 3 randomized, observer-blinded, multicenter trial was conducted in Spain to assess the safety of ccIIV3 compared to IIV3 in children aged 3 to <18 years with underlying medical conditions that place them at high risk for complications related to influenza infection. Of the 426 enrolled subjects who received at least one vaccination, 73% reported at least one AE. In general, rates of AE were lower after the second vaccine dose compared to the first dose in subjects who had not been vaccinated previously. The majority of AEs were mild to moderate in intensity. In subjects less than 6 years of age, the most commonly reported local reaction was site tenderness (44% in the ccIIV3 groups and 56% in IIV3 groups). The most commonly reported systemic reaction was irritability (22% in the ccIIV3 groups and 24% in the IIV3 groups). The most commonly reported local reaction in subject greater than 6 years of age was pain (57% in the ccIIV3 groups and 60% in the IIV3 groups) and the most common systemic reaction was headache (21% in ccIIV3 subjects and 22% in IIV3 subjects). A total of 22 SAEs in 16 subjects were reported during the study period (4% in the ccIIV3 groups and 3% in the IIV3 groups). No SAEs were considered vaccine related. Medically attended AEs were similar between the ccIIV3 and IIV3 groups. The most common medically attended AEs were categorized at "infections and infestations" followed by respiratory, thoracic, and mediastinal disorders and gastrointestinal disorders. No AEs lead to study withdrawal and no deaths were reported during the study period. Overall, the study results indicate an acceptable safety profile for ccIIV3 in this age group of children with risk factors for influenza-related complications. The rates of AE were higher than in the study conducted by Nolan and colleagues described earlier; however, this may be due to the inclusion of children with comorbidities, which may increase their susceptibility to reactions. No safety signals were identified during the study or 6-month follow-up, and results were comparable to AEs observed following vaccination with egg-based influenza vaccines. These results support further study and potential utilization of ccIIV3 vaccines in children with comorbidities associated with increased risk of influenza complications [55C].

An additional new influenza vaccine formulation utilizing recombinant DNA technology to produce influenza hemagglutinin in cell culture continues to undergo study in expanding patient populations to assess safety and immunogenicity of this new technology. The recombinant-inactivated influenza vaccine (RIV3) is approved for use in adults aged ≥18 years in the US. A new study was conducted to assess the safety of RIV3 (Flublok®) in adults aged ≥50 years to support this indication. Among subject-reported possible hypersensitivity reactions, rash was the most common event reported. Rash was reported at a higher frequency among RIV3 recipients compared to IIV3 subjects. The majority of rashes were mild and transient in nature. The adjudicated possible hypersensitivity events were similar between the two vaccine groups. The most common local reaction was tenderness, and total local reactions were more frequently reported in the RIV3 group compared to IIV3 group ($P = 0.042$). No deaths were reported during the duration of the study. Thirty-seven SAEs were reported, but none were considered related to the study vaccines. The RIV3 vaccine appeared well tolerated and continued study and expansion of utilization in older patients is supported by the study results [56MC].

The utilization of live attenuated influenza vaccine (LAIV) continues to undergo study to assess safety and efficacy in various patient populations. A recent study examining a quadrivalent LAIV (Fluenza Tetra®) was conducted in the UK to evaluate safety of the vaccine in children aged 2–17 years (median age 4 years). Of the 385 participants, a significant number reported having pre-existing medical conditions including asthma (85), diabetes mellitus (2), heart disease (2), chronic kidney disease (1), and immunosuppression (1). A total of 237 participants reported at least one AE during the study period. The most frequently reported AE was nasal congestion (43.4%) followed by malaise (22.6%) and cough (20.8%). Less than 5% of subjects reported wheezing (2.3%). Five reports of hypersensitivity were reported; however, no "true" hypersensitivity reactions based on the description of the symptoms by participants (i.e. "feeling dizzy" or "lightheaded"). Rates of wheezing were ~30 times higher in the group of subjects with pre-existing asthma (50.1 per 1000 patient-weeks; 95% CI, 25.1–100.2) compared to those without a history of asthma (1.7 per 1000 patient-weeks; 95% CI, 0.2–11.9). It was noted by the authors that information related to the current level of control for the asthma subjects was largely unknown; therefore, the etiology of the wheezing was undetermined. No SAEs were described during the course of the study. The authors concluded that no significant safety signals were identified during the study and continued study of LAIV in this population will enhance surveillance of safety of influenza vaccines [57C].

Severe human diseases associated with influenza A (H7N9) virus continue to occur in China. Over 630 cases of human laboratory-confirmed infections have been documented in China, with a mortality rate greater than 30%. Candidate vaccines for influenza A (H7N9) continued to undergo study to assess safety and immunogenicity given the concerning characteristics of H7N9 viruses to perpetuate a pandemic. Two recent studies assessed the safety of pandemic live attenuated influenza vaccines (pLAIVs) in adult patients [58c,59c]. The most commonly reported AEs included nasal congestion, runny nose, and headache. Results from one study indicated reports of fever in six (20%) of pLAIV subjects compared to one (10%) of placebo subjects [58c]. All AEs were mild in nature and self-limiting. No SAEs were noted in either study. Overall, the pLAIVs were well tolerated in study subjects. The authors have concluded that further study is warranted to continue to assess safety of pLAIVs in larger studies to determine the safety and efficacy of pLAIVs in preparation for any potential H7N9 pandemic [58c,59c].

Japanese Encephalitis Vaccines [SED-16, 393–396; SEDA-36, 475; SEDA-37, 393; SEDA-38, 319]

General

Infection with the Japanese encephalitis (JE) virus is the most common cause of viral encephalitis in children that live in South and East Asian countries and the Western Pacific. In a phase 3, open-label study in the Republic of Korea, the live attenuated Japanese encephalitis chimeric vaccine (JE-CV), Imojev®, was studied in 119 children 12–24 months of age who were previously vaccinated with JE-CV at 12–24 months of age received a JE-CV booster at 12–24 months after primary vaccination. Safety was assessed 28 days post-vaccination, and SAEs were monitored 6 months post-vaccination. No immediate (30 minutes after vaccination) AEs were observed. Predefined injection site reactions (pain, erythema and swelling) were recorded 7 days post-vaccination, and the most common systemic reactions (fever, headache, malaise and myalgia) were recorded for 14 days post-vaccination (also considered by definition to be related to the vaccination). Overall, 37.8% of participants experienced an injection site reaction and 47.1% of participants experienced a systemic reaction, with very few being Grade 3 (<1% for individual injection site reactions and ≤7% for individual systemic reactions). The most common injection site reaction was pain (28.6%), and the most common systemic reaction was malaise (40.3%). No deaths or SAEs were reported. This study demonstrates the safety and tolerability of a JE-CV booster dose at 12–24 months in Korean children. Additional studies with a larger sample size are needed to confirm these findings [60C].

Measles–Mumps–Rubella (MMR) Vaccine [SED-16, 257, 259, 264, 269, 278, 756–775; SEDA-36, 473; SEDA-37, 391; SEDA-38, 319]

Organs and Systems

ENDOCRINE

The increasing incidence of type 1 diabetes mellitus has been observed in most regions around the worldwide. A number of studies continue to investigate any potential risk associated with the development of type

1 diabetes in children. A systematic review and meta-analysis were conducted to assess the association between routine vaccination practices and the risk of type 1 diabetes development in childhood. The studies included in the review evaluated a number of routine vaccines, and the measles, mumps, and rubella-containing vaccines were most commonly studied. The meta-analysis found no significant association between any of the 11 vaccines studied and the risk of type 1 diabetes. Of the 15 studies that examined a measles vaccine, a non-statistically significant decrease in the risk of developing type 1 diabetes was noted (OR, 0.75; 95% CI, 0.54–1.05; $P=0.09$). The limitations of this systematic review and meta-analysis include heterogeneity of the study design among the studies included. Analyzed results indicate no evidence to support an association between routine childhood vaccination and the development of type 1 diabetes [61M].

NERVOUS SYSTEM

Aseptic meningitis is a complication of natural mumps infection. It occurs in roughly 10% of patients following infection with the mumps virus and typically resolves within a week without any further sequelae. Aseptic meningitis has been linked to vaccination with the measles–mumps–rubella (MMR) vaccine as well. A retrospective study was conducted to determine any association between MMR vaccination with the Leningrad–Zagreb attenuated mumps viral strain and the development of aseptic meningitis in Iranian children. Hospitalized children were included in the study if the diagnosis of aseptic meningitis was identified within 6 weeks of receipt of MMR vaccine. Researchers assessed the cerebral spinal fluid (CSF) for presence of the mumps virus via polymerase chain reaction (PCR) analysis. The mumps virus was present in 49 (39%) of patient CSF samples. Most patients were male (70%) and between the ages of 1 and 5 years (50%). Aseptic meningitis cases were observed within 10–33 days of MMR vaccination (average 19 days). The authors concluded that there is a risk of aseptic meningitis following MMR vaccination with a vaccine containing the Leningrad–Zagreb mumps virus strain. Previously published reports indicate that this strain of mumps virus may be more reactogenic compared to the Urabe and Jeryl Lynn strains [62C]. In addition to the Leningrad–Zagreb, Urabe, and Jeryl Lynn strains, three additional strains (Torii, Miyahara, and Hoshino) have been studied in monovalent mumps vaccines in Japan. Findings indicated a higher incidence of seizure as opposed to aseptic meningitis in children less than 3 years of age. Aseptic meningitis was still observed following vaccination with the Torii, Miyahara, and Hoshino strains [63MC]. Results reported here further support the importance of performing a thorough assessment of AEFI to determine any and all

potential associations between vaccine products and observed/reported AEs [62C].

SKIN

Acute hemorrhagic edema of infancy (AHEI) is characterized as a rare leuckocytoclastic vasculitis condition of the skin that typically affects children less than 2 years of age. Identified triggers for AHEI include infection, drugs, and vaccination. A report of a 2-year-old male with a 5-day history of progressive dusky red indurated plaques with a targetoid appearance over the face and extremities is described. The subject received the MMR vaccine 2 weeks prior to symptom onset. No history of preceding infection or medication was reported. The subject was labeled with AHEI based upon clinical presentation and skin biopsy. He was treated with prednisolone 1 mg/kg over 3 weeks that resulted in a complete recovery determined at a 1-month follow-up assessment. One other case of AHEI following MMR vaccine was reported in the literature in 2007. This report of AHEI 2-weeks following MMR vaccination was described as "apparently triggered" by the vaccine. No formal causality assessment for the present case was discussed, but a temporal relationship between vaccination and the event did exist [64A].

Susceptibility Factors

AGE

Vaccination with MMR vaccine is recommended in children aged 14 months and at 9 years of age in the Netherlands. During a measles outbreak in 2013 and 2014, the MMR vaccine was offered to all infants aged 6–14 months living in municipalities with MMR vaccine coverage <90% to protect younger infants from measles infection. An observational study utilizing an online questionnaire was conducted to assess the tolerability of early MMR vaccination. The median age of early vaccination was 7 months (range, 5.7–14.9 months). Parents of 59 infants (6.1%) reported at least one AE following vaccination. A trend of increasing frequency of local AEs with increasing age was noted, but was not statistically significant ($P=0.08$). Redness was the most commonly reported local AE (5.5%) followed by pain (4.2%) and swelling (3.4%). Parents of 8 infants reported pronounced redness, pain, or swelling. At least one systemic AE was reported for 350 (36.4%) infants following vaccination. Parents of the youngest infants (aged 6–8 months) reported AEs less frequently than those of the older infants. Systemic AEs were reported in 31.7%, 45.5%, and 42.5% of infants aged 6–8 months, 9–11 months, and 12–14 months, respectively. Listlessness was reported most commonly (28%) followed by fever (19%), crying (19%), rash (12%), and sleeping problems (10%). The frequencies of AEs in this study were lower than previous reports. The study design may have impacted the results as the parents may have experienced a time lag between vaccination and completing the questionnaire; therefore, potential underestimation of AEs may have occurred. The study results may have limited generalizability beyond countries similar to the Netherlands. Overall, the study appears to support the utilization of the MMR vaccine in younger infants during the time of an outbreak in terms of safety to protect infants from measles infection [65C].

In the US, two doses of the MMR vaccine are recommended routinely during childhood and one or two doses of MMR vaccine may be recommended in adulthood based up age and risk factors. A number of measles (and mumps) outbreaks continue to occur in the US and in countries in the European Union. Control of outbreaks may involve the recommendation for adults to receive additional MMR vaccination(s). An assessment of the AEs in adult (≥19 years) was conducted utilizing the US VAERS database. The database reports were reviewed over a 10-year period (2003–2013). Over 3000 reports were received in adults following MMR vaccination. Nearly half of the patients had also received a concomitant vaccine. The median interval from vaccination to the onset of symptoms was 2 days (range, 0–954 days). The median age was 37 years (range, 19–101 years) and females represented 77.1% of the patients. The most common AEs included fever (19.3%), rash (16.5%), and pain (13%). Serious reports were present for 5.3% of patients including 7 deaths. Four of the 7 deaths were associated with cardiac or cardiovascular conditions. Serious reports included encephalitis (8), seizures (5), GBS (17), anaphylaxis (13), and myocarditis (4). Pregnancy reports were identified for 131 patients. No AEs were reported in 61.9% of the pregnancy reports. The most common pregnancy-related AE was spontaneous abortion (12.7%). Overall, the authors did not detect any new, concerning, or unexpected AEs in adults following MMR vaccination. Limitations to this study include the inability to perform a causality assessment related the reported AEs given the passive nature of the surveillance system. Further investigation of AEs following MMR vaccination in adults appears warranted given the current state of continued outbreaks of vaccine-containing viruses [66R].

Poliovirus Vaccines [SED-16, 257, 847–853; SEDA-38, 320]

General

Based on an endorsement by the WHO Strategic Advisory Group of Experts (SAGE) on Immunization, trivalent oral poliovirus vaccine (OPV) was replaced globally in April 2016 with bivalent OPV. An additional recommendation states at least one dose of inactivated poliovirus vaccine (IPV) should be administered in countries exclusively using OPV as a strategy to prevent the re-emergence of type 2 poliovirus. The action further supports recommendations from the Polio Eradication and Endgame Strategic Plan 2013–2018 created in 2012 [67S].

Susceptibility Factors

IMMUNOCOMPROMISED: SEVERE COMBINED IMMUNODEFICIENCY AND MAJOR HISTOCOMPATIBILITY COMPLEX CLASS II DEFICIENCY

Two infants, from Libya and Saudi Arabia, who received OPV, were treated in Germany for their underlying immunodeficiencies diagnosed as severe combined immunodeficiency and major histocompatibility complex class II deficiency. Due to the immunodeficiencies, the infants received bone marrow transplantation 19 weeks after hospitalization. During hospitalization, stool samples identified type 2 poliovirus in both infants. The infection in one patient was identified after 3 months of hospitalization by an Enterovirus reverse transcriptase polymerase chain reaction (PCR) assay and in the second patient after 1 month through a virus culture using a routine protocol. Because these cases are vaccine-derived polioviruses (VDPV), all personnel in contact with these patients or their feces were tested; no cases of VDPV transmission were detected. After transplant, both infants cleared the VDPV infection at 5 and 4 weeks, respectively. The authors concluded rare cases of prolonged poliovirus exist in immunodeficient people, but unrecognized VDPV excretion is a concern, and potential patients should be screened [68c].

Drug Administration

DRUG FORMULATIONS

Safety and immunogenicity of a novel monovalent high-dose-inactivated poliovirus type 2 vaccine (mIPV2HD) were evaluated in 233 healthy infants from Panama. The regimen was two doses of bivalent OPV at weeks 6 and 10. At week 14 subjects were randomly assigned (1:1) for vaccination with one intramuscular dose of either mIPV2HD or IPV along with a third dose of OPV. At week 18, all infants received one dose of monovalent OPV2. Serial neutralizing antibody titers for poliovirus types 1, 2 and 3 were obtained at weeks 6, 14, 15, 18, and 19. Eighty-seven percent (201 infants) completed the trial. All infants were seroprotected against poliovirus types 1 and 3; however, 1 week after receiving OPV2, 98.2% of the mIPV2HD group and 91.2% of the IPV group were seroconverted to poliovirus type 2. Serious adverse events occurred in 8 (7%) infants in the mIPV2HD group and 15 (13%) infants in the IPV group with 6 and 7 infants, respectively during the 8-week period following vaccination. Per the authors, none of the SAEs were judged as related to the vaccination, and mIPV2HD can be considered an option for primary prevention or for an outbreak of poliovirus type 2 infection [69C].

Rotavirus Vaccines [SED-16, 252–256; SEDA-36, 473; SEDA-37, 391]

Organs and Systems

GASTROINTESTINAL

The risk of intussusception (IS) following rotavirus (RV) vaccination was identified after the first RV vaccine, Rotashield® (RRV-TV), was licensed in 1998 and subsequently withdrawn from the market in 1999. The occurrence of IS remains a central component of post-licensure safety surveillance worldwide for the second generation of available RV vaccines, Rotateq® (RV5), Rotarix® (RV1), and Rotavac®. In recent years, studies have identified a small increased risk of IS with both RV1 and RV5 vaccines predominantly after the first dose within 7 days after administration [70C].

A retrospective surveillance study from 2000 to 2013 was conducted assessing hospitalization IS rates before (2000–2005) and after (2007–2013) the introduction of RV1 and RV5 vaccines administered in the US. Hospitalizations in children <12 months of age for IS were identified through the State Inpatient Databases (SID) which is sponsored by the Agency for Healthcare Research and Quality. In the pre-vaccine years, before RV1 and RV5 introduction, IS hospitalization rates remained constant, averaging 35.9 per 100 000 children. In the post-vaccine years, significantly elevated IS rates per 100 000 children <12 months were observed in years 2007 (40.7; RR: 1.13, 95% CI: 1.07–1.20) and 2010 (40.3; RR: 1.12, 95% CI 1.06–1.20). However, no differences in IS rates were observed in all other post-vaccine years. A subset analysis of age groups identified a significant increase rate of IS hospitalizations in children 8–11 weeks in all post-vaccine years (range 16.7–22.9 per 100 000), when compared to pre-vaccine baseline years (11.4 per 100 000), except years 2011 (15.0 per 100 000) and 2013 (14.7 per 100 000). These results are consistent with other recent studies that have identified a small increased risk of IS, predominantly after administration of the first dose of RV vaccine [70C].

A surveillance study in Finland used a self-controlled case-series method to assess the risk of IS during days 1–21 (days after first dose) compared to the control period (days 22–42 days post-vaccination). The incidence of IS risk during the days after first dose compared to the control period was 2.0 (95% CI 0.5–8.4; $P=0.34$). The number of excess IS cases after the first dose was estimated to be 1.04 per 100 000 vaccine doses (95% CI 0.0–2.5). No excess risk after the second and third dose was identified [71c].

An observational study conducted in Brazil compared the incidence of IS before and after the RV1 Rotarix® vaccine was introduced into the National Immunization Program in 2006. Retrospective data collected from 21 hospital discharge diagnoses codes from 2001 to 2005 established a pre-vaccine IS baseline average of 31 cases per year (range 24–42). Using a prospective reporting system developed post-vaccine, the same 21 hospitals reported an average of 26 IS cases in 2007 and 19 IS cases in 2008; both annual averages are lower than the identified annual pre-vaccine IS cases [72c].

Drug Administration

DRUG DOSAGE REGIMENS

In the US, the ACIP recommends the use of the same RV vaccine to complete the vaccination series; however, in practice using same vaccine formulation (RV1 vs RV5) is not always possible. A randomized, multi-centered, open-label study of 1393 children was conducted designed to examine the non-inferiority of immune responses of mixed RV schedules (RV1 and RV5) compared to singe RV vaccine (RV1 or RV5) schedules. Gastrointestinal and systemic side effects were monitored 8 days after each RV vaccine administered. No statistically significant differences in solicited symptoms after each RV dose (fever, diarrhea or vomiting) were found between the mixed RV schedules and single RV schedules groups. However, the overall proportion of children with solicited symptoms was significantly higher in the mixed RV1–RV5–RV5 group ($n=94$), 0.20 (95% CI 0.15–0.24) vs the single RV1–RV1 group ($n=64$), 0.29 (95% CI 0.24–0.34). One case of IS was reported 91 days after the last RV dose, but researchers determined the case was unrelated to the RV vaccine. The study concluded that mixed schedules are equally safe and tolerated and result in comparable immune responses [73C].

Varicella Vaccine and Herpes Zoster Vaccines [SED-16, 360–365; SEDA-36, 474; SEDA-37, 391; SEDA-38, 320]

Organs and Systems

INFECTION RISK

A 76-year-old Caucasian male developed herpes zoster 7 days after receiving the varicella zoster virus (VZV) vaccine (Varixax®). His past medical history was significant for a recent episode of poison ivy with completion of a 7-day taper of methylprednisolone. Within a couple of days after completing the methylprednisolone taper the patient received the VZV vaccine and subsequently 7 days later developed a erythematous, vesicular eruption in a dermatomal distribution. No specimens were collected to confirm if the rash was caused by the

VZV or the wild type-strain. This case report identifies the need for further research to determine the incidence of zoster-like rashes after VZV vaccination [74A].

Susceptibility Factors

GENETICS

Studies regarding herpes zoster virus (HZV) vaccination in Asian adults are lacking. An open-label, multi-center, single-arm study was conducted in 180 Korean adults 50 years of age and older to investigate the safety and immunogenicity of the live attenuated herpes zoster virus (HZV) vaccine (Zostavax®). Individuals were vaccinated on day 1 and monitored for herpes zoster (HZ) development as well as safety and tolerability of the vaccine for 42 days post-vaccination. 62.8% developed at least one AE with 53.3% reporting injection site AEs, with erythema most frequently reported at 45%. No SAEs or VZV-like rashes were reported. This study demonstrated that the HZV vaccine is well tolerated in healthy Korean adults 50 years of age and older. Additional studies with a larger sample size are needed to confirm these findings [75c].

DISEASE AND AGE: DIABETES MELLITUS AND ELDERLY

A double-blinded, randomized, placebo-controlled single-center study of patients with diabetes 60–70 years of age examined the safety and immunogenicity after administration of one dose of the live attenuated herpes zoster virus (HZV) vaccine (Zostavax®). Pneumococcal polysaccharide vaccine (PPSV23) was simultaneously administered. Using an intention-to-treat analysis, primary endpoints of safety outcomes and cellular-mediated immunity measured by the varicella skin test reaction and were assessed at 3 months. Local and systemic AEs were monitored 42 days post vaccination; SAEs and development of HZ were monitored for 1 year. Twenty-seven patients were randomized into each group. No changes were observed in the varicella skin test reaction scores, 0.41 ± 0.80 and 0.11 ± 0.93 in the vaccine and placebo groups, respectively ($P = 0.2155$). Vaccine-related AEs (local and systemic) were similar between groups, 3 (11.1%) and 4 (14.8%) in the vaccine and placebo groups, respectively ($P = 0.6419$). No SAEs or VZV-like rashes were reported. The study concluded that HZV vaccine can safely be used in elderly patients with diabetes but may not boost VZV immunity [76c].

IMMUNOCOMPROMISED: TRANSPLANT PATIENTS

Hematopoietic stem cell transplantation (HSCT) recipients are at high risk for VZV infections, and data regarding the safety and efficacy of VZV vaccination and especially HZV vaccination in HSCT patients are limited. A retrospective review of 47 patients with a median age

of 5.6 years who all underwent allogeneic HSCT was conducted. Of the 47 HSCT patients, 31 received the live attenuated herpes zoster virus (HZV) vaccine (Zostavax®). The interval from HSCT to HZV vaccination varied; recipients had to be free of graft-vs-host disease, immunosuppressive treatments, and no longer receiving transfusions and intravenous immunoglobulin for greater than 3 months. Seventeen patients were vaccinated within 24 months of HSCT; however, the seropositivity of these patients did not differ from the patients vaccinated greater than 24 months after HSCT. Of the HZV vaccine recipients, 18 (58.1%) were seropositive with a median interval from HSCT to vaccination of 21.0 months vs 13 (41.9%) were seronegative with a median interval from HSCT to vaccination of 20.6 months ($P = 0.52$). One patient developed wild-type VZV infection 13 days after vaccination confirmed by DNA sequence analysis. During the median follow-up period of 4.8 years no VZV or HZV cases were observed. This study suggests HZV vaccination may be safe in pediatric HSCT patients and a beneficial approach to prevent VZV infection [77c].

Drug Administration

DRUG FORMULATION

A new investigational formulation of a herpes zoster subunit vaccine (HZ/su, GSK Vaccines) containing VZV glycoprotein E and the $AS01_8$ adjuvant system has been developed. A randomized, placebo-controlled phase 3 trial conducted in 18 countries studied the efficacy and safety of the HZ/su vaccine in adults 70 years of age or older. 13 900 patients with a mean age of 75.6 years were randomized to receive two doses of HZ/su or a placebo (saline) intramuscularly, 2 months apart. Efficacy against HZ and post-herpetic neuralgia (PHN) was evaluated over an average of 3.7 years. Efficacy of the HZ/su vaccine for preventing HZ was 89.8% (95% CI: 84.2–93.7; $P < 0.001$). When compared between age groups, similar efficacy rates were observed, 90.0% for individuals 70–79 years of age vs 89.1% for individuals 80 years of age and older. HZ/su vaccine efficacy for preventing PHN was 88.8% (95% CI: 68.7–97.1; $P < 0.001$). Vaccine safety was assessed by a randomly selected subgroup of 1025 patients stratified by age through solicited reports for injection site reactions and systemic reactions for 7 days after both injections. Solicited reactions were more common in the HZ/su group than placebo (79.0% vs 29.5%); with injection site reactions occurring most frequently, 74.1% in the HZ/su group vs 9.9% in the placebo group. SAEs were similar in the two groups, 16.6% of HZ/su recipients and in 17.5% of placebo recipients. However, SAEs considered by the investigators to be related to the trial intervention occurred in 12 HZ/su recipients (0.2%) and in 8 placebo participants (0.1%). Potential immune-mediated diseases occurred in 1.3% of HZ/su recipients vs 1.4% of placebo recipients. Death occurred in 426 (6.1%) participants in the HZ/su group and 459 (6.6%) participants in the placebo group. One death was considered related to the HZ/su vaccine; a 90-year old with pre-existing thrombocytopenia and acute myeloid leukemia was diagnosed 75 days post HZ/su first vaccination and died from neutropenic sepsis 97 days after vaccination. The new HZ/su vaccine is safe and effective in preventing HZ and PHN in patient 70 years of age and older. Additional investigational studies are required for approval of this new VZV vaccine formulation [78MC].

DRUG ADDITIVES

Two monovalent varicella vaccines are currently available in Europe, Varilrix® (GSK Vaccines) and Varivax® (Merck & Co., Inc.), both of which are derived from the Japanese Oka strain. Human serum albumin (HSA) is incorporated in live attenuated vaccines as a stabilizer to prevent immunogens from adhering to vial walls. The European Medicine Agency has recommended the elimination of all blood-derived product of human origin from vaccine manufacturing. Therefore, the manufacturing process removed the addition of HSA. Therefore, the existing HSA containing varicella vaccine, Varilrix®, underwent a non-inferiority clinical trial to compare the newly formulated non-HSA containing varicella vaccine, Varilrix® to compare the immunogenicity and safety. A phase 2, double-blinded, randomized, non-inferiority study was conducted at 14 centers in the Czech Republic and Hungary in healthy children aged 11–21 months. Children received two doses 42–65 days apart of the varicella vaccine without HSA (group A) or with HSA (group B). The rate of solicited and unsolicited symptoms was similar after both vaccines; 43 days after dose one the rate was 76% in group A and 69.7% in group B; after dose two the rate was 71.9% and 68.6%, respectively. After both doses in both groups, redness was the most common solicited local symptom with no statistical difference observed. Seven SAEs were reported; none were fatal or considered to be vaccine related. The new varicella vaccine without HSA has a comparable safety profile to the current varicella vaccine with HSA [79MC].

DRUG DOSAGE REGIMENS

A prospective study in 200 patients 50 years of age and older was conducted to evaluate the effect of a live attenuated herpes zoster virus (HZV) vaccine (Zostavax®) booster dose 10 years after receipt of the first dose. Participants were randomized into 4 groups; group 1 were individuals 70 years of age or older who received the HZV vaccine more than 10 years ago and groups 2, 3, and 4 were individuals who never received the HZV vaccine that were aged 70 and older, 60–69 years of age, and

50–59 years of age, respectively. Participants received a single dose of HZV and were monitored for local and systemic side effects through week 6. SAEs were followed up at weeks 12 and 26 over the phone and in person at week 52. In groups 1 and 2, 57% of participants reported at least 1 or more AE, while in groups 3 and 4, 75% of participants reported at least 1 or more AE. Injection site reactions were the most common AE reported among all groups, occurring most frequently during days 1–5 post vaccination and included pain and erythema. There were no vaccine-related SAEs reported in all groups for the 52-week study duration [80C].

Yellow Fever Vaccines [SEDA-16, 537–540; SEDA-36, 475; SEDA-37, 392; SEDA-38, 321]

General

Serious adverse events associated with the yellow fever (YF) vaccination include viscerotropic disease (YEL-AVD), neurologic disease (YEL-AND), and anaphylaxis. Post marketing surveillance is needed to continue to describe and understand risk factor associated with these SAE. In the US the only YF vaccine licensed for use is YF-VAXVR®, a live attenuated vaccine manufactured by Sanofi Pasteur. A retrospective review of adverse effects reported to the US. VAERS database from 2007 through 2013 following yellow fever vaccination was conducted. AEs reported more than 60 days post vaccination were excluded as well as dosing errors and YF vaccines administered by military organizations. The Brighton Collaboration Viscerotropic Disease Work Group guidelines for case definitions for YEL-AVD was used in this study. A total of 938 AE reports following YF vaccination were reviewed, 854 (91%) were classified as non-serious and 84 (9%) were classified as SAE. A total of 75 (89%) of the reported SAEs patients were hospitalized. Of the YF vaccine AE cases reported, 618 (66%) were administered with other vaccines, these included typhoid ($n=36$), hepatitis A ($n=7$), inactivated poliovirus ($n=16$), tetanus/diphtheria/pertussis ($n=12$) and combined recombinant hepatitis A and B ($n=11$) vaccines. Reported rates of YEL-AND and YEL-AVD were 0.8 and 0.3 per 100 000 doses distributed, respectively; with both rates increased with increasing age. The highest relative risk of YEL-AND was 2.5 in the 60–69 years age group and the highest relative risk of YEL-AVD was 4.0 in the greater than 70 years age group, all cases occurred in men. Overall, 12 (71%) YEL-AND cases occurred in males with a median age of 61 years. Five deaths (0.2 per 100000 doses distributed) were reported following YF vaccination, which included two cases of YEL-AVD, and one case each of stroke, cardiac arrest and drug overdose. This retrospective review is consistent with previously identified increased risks of

YEL-AND and YEL-AVD occurring in older patients, in particular men [81c].

Organs and Systems

SKIN

Cold contact urticarial (CCU) is primarily idiopathic but rare cases can be secondary to infectious disease, with or without cryoproteins. A 29-year-old man with no past medical history was referred for evaluation and treatment of cold contact urticaria (CCU) 3 years after onset due to persistence of his symptoms. His initial symptoms appeared 3 weeks after receiving YF vaccine (Stamarile®) and hepatitis A vaccines (Havrix®). The patient was treated with 80 mg of desloratadine per day, with partial improvement of his symptoms. An epinephrine auto-injector was prescribed for subsequent exposure to environmental triggers. The authors recognize this case does not prove a causal relationship between CCU and YF or hepatitis A vaccines; however, it is noteworthy to keep in mind that CCU may occur post-vaccination, in rare cases [82r].

Susceptibility Factors

INFECTION RISK

A case report of YEL-AVD presenting with fever and jaundice was reported in a 65-year-old man 5 days after receiving a primary dose of YF vaccine 17D-204 (YF-VAXVR®), in Hong Kong prior to his scheduled travel to South America. The patient developed fever, loss of appetite, headache and mild myalgia. At 10 days post-vaccination, he became confused, lethargic, jaundiced and was admitted to the hospital. Two days after admission (day 11 post-vaccination) both blood and cerebral spinal fluid (CSF) samples were obtained for a real-time PCR test for YF virus. Both samples were positive and confirmed to be the vaccine strain. Blood tests for yellow fever PCR became negative on day 14 post-vaccination; however, his fever did not resolve until day 12 after admission. The patient was discharged from the hospital after 14 days. The development of YEL-AVD within 10 days of YF vaccination is a known risk as demonstrated with this case report. Patients should be advised of the rare but serious risks of YF vaccination and balance this with the preventative benefits when traveling to endemic areas [83r].

OTHER: HEMODIALYSIS

A cross-sectional study assessing the YF vaccination safety in adult patients with chronic kidney disease receiving regular dialysis therapy was conducted in São Carlos, Brazil. Patients at the São Carlos Dialysis Service were screened for YF vaccination status. Patients that had not received any YF vaccine or a booster within the last 10 years were referred to receive the YF vaccine. Of the patients 181 screened, 130 were included in the study. Previous YF vaccination was verified in 44 patients within the last 10 years, 26 patients received YF vaccination more than 10 years ago (with no mention of adverse effects), 36 patients had never been vaccinated and 24 had an unknown YF vaccination status. As a result, 86 patients met the criteria for YF vaccination and received a referral for the vaccine of which 45 patients (52%) received the YF vaccine. 24.4% reported mild local adverse effects and 4.4% reported a fever. No SAEs related to YF vaccination were observed; patients were followed for 2 months post-vaccination and monitored for reports of anaphylaxis, YEL-AND or YEL-AVD. Due to the small sample size, conclusions regarding the safety of YF vaccination in dialysis are limited and suggest the need of further studies to evaluate the risk vs benefit [84c].

BACTERIAL VACCINES

Anthrax Vaccines [SED-16, 270, 527]

General

Anthrax is an acute infectious disease that is secondary to exposure to *Bacillus anthracis*, a non-motile spore forming bacteria. Anthrax infection is potentially fatal and may be associated with the skin (cutaneous), gastrointestinal tract, and/or the lungs (inhalation). Vaccination against anthrax is primarily directed towards individuals with increased risk of exposure (pre-exposure prophylaxis) or those exposed to the anthrax (post-exposure prophylaxis) [85C].

Organs and Systems

IMMUNOLOGIC

Military personnel are among the three groups of individuals the Centers for Disease Control and Prevention (CDC) recommends pre-exposure prevention with the anthrax vaccine adsorbed (AVA) in the US. A recent study was conducted to determine any identifiable demographic predictors of AEs and assess serologic markers in persons reporting large local reactions (LLRs) and systemic reactions (SRs) following AVA vaccination. The LLRs were defined as local redness or swelling >2 in. in diameter, a nodule, or numbness or burning at the site for >24 hours. A SR was defined as >24 hours of headache, muscle or joint pain, fatigue or other systemic response that interred with work or recreation. One hundred fifty three subjects (6.3%) reported LLRs (67.3%) or SRs (32.7%). Results indicated that sex, ethnicity, and age are associated with AEs following AVA vaccination. Women were more likely to report AEs compared to men (22.5% vs 4.6%; $P < 0.0001$) [86C]. An increase in AEs reported by women following AVA vaccine has been previously reported [87C]. Hispanic persons were less likely to report AEs compared to non-Hispanic subjects ($P = 0.03$; OR = 0.27 [95% CI = 0.09–0.86]) and Asian subjects were more likely to report AEs ($P = 0.03$; OR = 3.39 [95% CI = 1.26–9.1]). In addition, AEs were reported at a significantly increased rate in subjects greater than the age of 30 years compared to those between 18 and 29 years ($P < 0.0001$; OR = 0.31 [95% CI = 0.22–0.43]). Immunologic data indicated that subjects reporting a LLR had higher levels of protective antigen (PA)-specific IgE levels compared to matched controls (88.3 vs 60.5 ng/mL; $P < 0.01$). The PA-specific IgE levels did not differ among the subjects reporting SRs. Additionally; PA-specific IgG levels did not differ in either the LLR vs control or the SR vs control populations [86C]. Whereas, elevated PA-specific IgG levels among subjects with tenderness and swelling following AVA vaccination has been previously reported [87C]. Plasma interferon-gamma inducible protein 10 (IP-10) levels were increased in the LLR group compared to matched controls as well ($P = 0.03$). In the SR population, C-reactive protein (CRP) levels were elevated compared to controls (6.88 vs 1.86 mg/L; $P = 0.02$). The levels of CRP did not differ between the LLR and control groups of subjects. The immunologic results of this study provide insight into the mechanisms behind AEs and data to support possible adjustments in future study design regarding the administration of AVA vaccine based upon the subject demographic data and potential immunologic responses [86C].

Drug Administration

DRUG ADDITIVES AND DRUG DOSAGE REGIMENS

The CPG 7909 adjuvant, a synthetic immune-stimulatory oligonucleotide, is currently under investigation in combination with the BioThrax® anthrax vaccine adsorbed (AVA) product in the post-exposure setting. A phase 2 multi-center, double-blind, randomized, parallel-group, active-control study was conducted to assess the safety and immunogenicity of the AV7909 formulation in healthy, unexposed adults aged 18–50 years in the US. Subjects were randomized to one of five groups comprising three immunization schedules (days 0/14, 0/28, or 0/14/28) and two dosage regimens (full dose AV7909 or half dose AV7909) or BioThrax® on days 0/14/28 intramuscularly (IM). Overall, the study vaccine was well tolerated; however, the incidence of AEs was lower in the BioThrax® group (65.2%) compared to the four AV7909 groups (73.9%–81.8%). Six of nine AEs that lead to discontinuation of vaccination were deemed related to the study vaccine (AV7909). Four subjects reported generalized rash and pruritus, one subject with rash, one subject with elevated transaminase enzymes, and one with injection site erythema >13 cm. Greater

than 50% of subjects across the study reported tenderness, injection site pain, arm motion limitation, and muscle ache after the first vaccination. Of the reports of injections site and systemic reactogenicity, 93.5% and 83.3% of subjects reported a mild or moderate severity, respectively. Five subjects in the AV7909 population reported Grade 3 systemic reactions (fever [1], fatigue/tiredness, muscle ache, and headache [1], headache and fever [1], fatigue/tiredness [1]). Four SAEs were reported, none of which were related to the study vaccines. The study results demonstrate that further study is warranted and appropriate given the immunogenicity and safety data reported, particularly with the full dose AV7909 vaccine provided at days 0 and 14 [88C].

Bacillus Calmette–Guérin Vaccines [SED-16, 267, 797-806]

Organ and Systems

CARDIOVASCULAR

The Bacillus Calmette–Guérin (BCG) vaccine is a live, attenuated organism of the Calmette–Guérin strain of *Mycobacterium bovis* administered to stimulate active immunity to prevent and control tuberculosis. The BCG vaccine may also be administered as an intravesical instillation for local superficial bladder cancer treatment. The mechanism of action is thought to work through inflammatory effects and an immune response to slough the bladder wall epithelium and destroy superficial cancer cells [89]. An 85-year-old male, who was in remission for bladder cancer after 4 months of intravesical BCG vaccine treatment, developed hemoptysis 11 months after the intravesical installation. The results from the sputum culture showed growth of *Mycobacterium bovis*. Initial *M. bovis* treatment was rifampin, isoniazid, ethambutol and pyrazinamide, but ethambutol was discontinued after 8 weeks, and pyrazinamide was stopped after 4 weeks due to resistance. Five months later, this patient presented with a rapid onset aortobronchial fistula and massive hemoptysis that was diagnosed as a thoracic aortic mycotic aneurysm in the descending thoracic aorta. Due to the patient's age and poor baseline status, the family elected to withdraw care. This is thought to be the first report of a BCG-related mycotic aneurysm in the descending thoracic aorta in a patient receiving treatment for *M. bovis*. [90A].

HEMATOLOGIC

A randomized trial evaluated Danish infants, minimal gestational age of 32 weeks, to receive ($n = 2118$) or not receive ($n = 2133$) the BCG SSI (Danish strain 1331) vaccine at birth or up to 7 days. Two children diagnosed with regional lymphadenitis and suppurative lymphadenitis, which were hospitalized and received ultrasonic examination, were categorized as developing severe adverse reactions related to BCG vaccine. There were 10 total episodes of suppurative lymphadenitis and 13 cases of regional lymphadenitis. Suppurative lymphadenitis occurred in the left axilla, the same arm that the vaccine was administered, and median onset was 87 days (range 25–200 days). All perforated spontaneously and healed with a median scar time of 198 days (range 63–328 days). No deaths were considered related to the BCG vaccine [91C].

SKIN

An infant Japanese girl developed erythema induratum of Bazin (EIB) in her lower extremities 1 month after receiving a BCG vaccination in her upper arm at 6 months. It produced multiple, indurated 3–4 cm, subcutaneous nodules with dark-reddish or violaceous erythema. These subcutaneous nodules regressed spontaneously without treatment within 1 month without recurrence. Macrophages assist in the initiation and maintenance of the immune response to *Mycobacterium tuberculosis*. The M1 macrophages, which are characterized by their pro-inflammatory response and microbicidal capacity, and monocyte chemotactic protein (MCP)-1, which assists in the recruitment of macrophages and memory T cells to inflammatory sites, may have had a role, due to the M1 macrophage infiltration and MCP-1 expression. Previously published reports have identified cutaneous manifestations following BCG vaccination; therefore, the development of EIB in this child was likely associated with BCG vaccine [92A].

MUSCULOSKELETAL

The BCG vaccine rarely causes osteitis, but this complication is severe and the current mean incidence is 6.4 per 100 000 vaccinated newborns. A cohort study conducted in Finland looked at the presence and severity of orthopedic effects through a questionnaire sent to 203 former BCG osteitis patients. There were 160 responses. The median age was 31 years (range 19–47 years) and 85 were females. Their responses reported "long-term ailments" and if they had been treated or followed regarding these adverse events. Twenty-two patients reported orthopedic complications in infancy, but classified them as mild, and 5 required surgery for the orthopedic complications. Leg length discrepancy within 2–3 cm was reported in 11 patients, chronic pain in four patients, abnormal gait in two patients, and one patient each reported tibial fracture, hip joint problems and restricted upper limb movements. There was no causality noted; however, this population is of interest since Finland has a much higher prevalence than other countries [93C].

INFECTION RISK

Two case reports described the development of tuberculosis in patients receiving intravesical instillation of BCG vaccine for bladder cancer treatment. One patient was 66 years old and after 5 years of treatment developed spinal tuberculosis with tubercle bacilli and tubercular granulation tissue. Symptomatic back pain encircling the chest occurred along with progressive paralysis of the lower limbs, which caused destruction of the intervertebral disc and vertebral endplates. The second patient was 35 years old and also received 18 months of intravesical installation of BCG vaccine therapy. However, after another intravesical dose, girdle chest pain occurred and spondylitis was diagnosed most likely caused by tuberculosis. The positive Babinski reflex resolved after anti-mycobacterial treatment and 3 weeks of bed rest. Extra-bladder complications after intravesical BCG vaccine administration are rare, but intravesical administration may cause BCG spreading through microdamages of the bladder and spread to surrounding tissue through the circulatory system [94A].

Susceptibility Factors

AGE

In countries that are endemic for tuberculosis, the BCG vaccine is typically administered to newborns. An infant, who received the BCG vaccine at 2 months, was hospitalized at 8 months with a disseminated mycobacterial infection and noted to have a novel nuclear factor xB essential modulator gene (NEMO), which led to elevated ferritin levels of 1160 µg/dL. He was diagnosed with disseminated BCG disease (BCG-osis) and a suspected defect of interferon-gamma. By age 2, he had failed to thrive due to multiple complications including continued elevated ferritin levels that increased to 14 300 µg/dL. The assumed cause of high ferritin levels was the high inflammatory response from BCG-osis. The authors concluded that a combination of immunologic factors might have lead to the development of BCG-osis in this child [95A].

Drug Administration

DRUG FORMULATIONS

A phase 1 1-year trial performed in the United Kingdom enrolled 30 healthy volunteers, aged 18–55 years, who had received a BCG vaccine at least 6 months prior to the study. The study assessed the safety and immunogenicity of a tuberculosis vaccine. The immunogenicity-enhancing protein called IMX313 was studied and is used to increase a vaccine's immunogenicity and effectiveness. This small protein, IMX313, was combined with a Modified Vaccinia virus Ankara expressing the immunodominant *M. tuberculosis* antigen 85A, MVA85A-IMX313. Patients were randomized to three groups to received low dose MVA85A-IMX313, standard dose MVA85A-IMX313, or standard dose MVA85A. All volunteers completed the study and were included in the analysis. All groups experienced scaling and mild to moderate local symptoms, but one patient administered standard dose MVA85A developed severe swelling. Mild to moderate systemic symptoms of fever, arthralgia, myalgia, fatigue, headache, nausea and malaise were noted in all groups. Only one patient developed severe symptoms of nausea, malaise, and fatigue in the standard dose MVA85A-IMX313 that may have been attributed to a diarrheal illness that the entire family experienced. The authors concluded that further research optimizing molecular proteins should be conducted in recombinant viral vectors [96c].

Meningococcal Vaccines [SED-16, 269, 825–829; SEDA-36, 476; SEDA-37, 393; SEDA-38, 322]

Organs and Systems

SKIN

A 4-year-old boy developed severe cold contact urticaria for 3 months beginning 5 days after his first vaccination with Meningitec® (anti-*Neisseria meningitidis* serogroup C conjugate vaccine). He also experienced generalized hives with malaise and pharyngeal discomfort when drinking cold beverages. After a 3-minute ice-cube test on the volar aspect of his forearm, a large wheal formed within 10 minutes of removal. Management of cold contact urticaria included avoidance of cold-water swimming, cold liquids, foods, and weather, and treatment with desloratidine 5 mg daily, montelukast 4 mg daily and an epinephrine auto-injector. Partial remission occurred 6 months later. The authors concluded this allergic reaction may be associated with the vaccine [82r].

MUSCULOSKELETAL

A 5-month-old girl presented with upper extremity dysfunction, myositis, periostitis and (peri-) vasculitis of the left arm and hand after receiving a second dose of a 4-component meningococcal serogroup B (4CMenB) vaccination (Bexero®) administered to the left deltoid muscle. This vaccine was given concomitantly with a 6-in-1 pediatric vaccine containing diphtheria, tetanus, pertussis, hepatitis B, poliomyelitis and invasive infections caused by *Haemophilus influenza* type b (Hexyon™) and pneumococcal 13-valent Conjugate Vaccine [Diphtheria CRM197 Protein] (Prevnar 13®) in her right and left legs. This reaction did not occur after the first 4CMenB vaccine in the same deltoid muscle. Symptoms completely resolved after 2 months; however, ibuprofen twice daily for 5 days and ceftriaxone and clindamycin intravenously for 7 days were administered. The authors concluded the reaction may be caused by an increased specific local immune response, and 4CMenB vaccination administration is preferred in the thigh [97c].

Drug Administration

DRUG FORMULATIONS

Safety of Tumenba®, a *Neisseria meningitidis* serogroup B (MenB) vaccine (bivalent rLP2086), was studied in this phase 3, randomized, active-controlled study. Participants, aged 10–25 years, in Australia, Europe and the United States were assigned (2:1) to receive bivalent rLP2086 at months 0, 2, and 6 or hepatitis A virus (HAV) vaccine (Havrix®) at months 0 and 6 and saline at month 2. Of the 5712 randomized, 4986 subjects completed the series (84.5% bivalent rLP2086; 87.2% HAV vaccine/saline) with 1% of participants withdrawing due to adverse events. More serious events were noted in HAV vaccine/saline (2.5%) compared to bivalent rLP2086 (1.6%). However, two events in each group were considered vaccine related, neutropenia and an anaphylactic reaction (bivalent rLP2086) and demyelination and spontaneous abortion (HAV vaccine/saline). Medically attended adverse events were 14.4% and 14.6% in bivalent rLP2086 and HAV vaccine/saline groups respectively, but vaccine-related events occurred in 0.2% of the bivalent rLP2086 group for pyrexia, injection site pain and swelling, and headaches compared to only headaches (0.2%) for HAV/saline. Newly diagnosed chronic medical conditions related to the study vaccination were rare. One case of alopecia areata was identified in the bivalent rLP2086 group, and one subject in the HAV vaccine/saline group reported multiple sclerosis. More subjects receiving bivalent rLP2086 reported any adverse event within 30 days of vaccination including reactogenicity events considered mild to moderate in severity. When comparing the treatment groups, the rates of serious adverse events were similar and rare, and the reactogenicity that occurred in the bivalent rLP2086 group did not interfere with completion of the vaccination schedule [98C].

Three hundred healthy Koreans, aged 11–55 years, were vaccinated with a quadrivalent meningococcal (serogroups A, C, Y and W-135) polysaccharide diphtheria toxoid conjugate (MenACYW-D, Menactra®) in a 2:1 ratio with Tdap vaccine, and serum titers were evaluated on days 0 and 28. At 28 days, seroconversion was higher for all MenACYW-D serogroups compared to Tdap with serogroups C and W-135 having the highest rates. No participants experienced serious adverse events or withdrew due to side effects. The authors concluded MenACYW-D is well tolerated and elicits a robust immune response [99C].

DRUG DOSAGE REGIMENS

Infants, who previously received a studied 4CMenB schedule, were enrolled in a phase 2b randomized, controlled trial to evaluate the rate of bactericidal antibody waning. These infants were assessed for maintenance of vaccine-induced bactericidal antibodies at ≥12 months and immunogenicity of a 4CMenB booster dose given at 12, 18 or 24 months. There were 1481 infants enrolled in this follow-up study within six European countries. The human serum bactericidal antibody (hBSA) titers of ≥1:5 were met in all infants, who received the 4CMenB booster at 12 months, but decreased when boosters were administered at 18 and 24 months. Seventy serious adverse events occurred in 58 participants. Three events were classified as possibly related to the vaccine. One child from the United Kingdom in the control 12, 14-month group was diagnosed with autism at 3 years after presenting with speech delay and learning difficulties at 18 months and had received 4CMenB at 15 and 17 months. The investigators determined, due to the temporal association, that it is not possible to exclude an association with the vaccine. Another child, who was vaccinated with 4CMenB along with routine vaccines at 2, 4, and 6 months, developed convulsions at 27 months, which was 106 days after a booster dose of 4CMenB at 24 months. The child experienced 6 seizures (febrile and afebrile) by the age of 3.5 years, but none after 38 months. The last child in the control 12, 14-month group developed 2 febrile convulsions, who also had atypical pneumonia at the time, when vaccinated at 12 months. The 4CMenB booster vaccine given at 12 months may help infants overcome waning hBSA titers, but this vaccine appears to be more reactogenic, and further studies are recommended to assess its usage [100C].

One dose of a quadrivalent meningococcal CRM-conjugate vaccine (MenACWY-CRM, Menveo®) (ACWY1) was compared to two doses (ACWY2) in healthy children 2–10 years of age in a 1:1 ratio in this phase 3b randomized, placebo-controlled trial. The two doses of ACWY2 or one placebo dose followed by a dose of MenACWY-CRM (ACWY1) were given 2 months apart, and patients were monitored for a year after the second vaccination. Results showed ACWY2 participants had a higher seroresponse; however, overall seroresponse demonstrated non-inferiority between the regimens at 1 year. One SAE of idiopathic thrombocytopenia was considered possibly related to the MenACWY-CRM vaccine. This occurred in a 6-year old, who was randomized to the ACWY1, about 10 weeks after receiving the MenACWY-CRM vaccine. Based on the subject's inadequate history, even though a previous episode of bruising and scleral hemorrhage had occurred with another bicycle accident, the possible effect from the vaccine could not be ruled out [101C].

Interactions

DRUG–DRUG INTERACTIONS

Bivalent rLP2086 (Trumenba®), administered in 2:2:1 ratio with or without quadrivalent human papillomavirus vaccine (HPV4) (bivalent rLP2086 + HPV-4, bivalent rLP2086 + saline, or saline + HPV-4), was evaluated in this phase 2, randomized, active-control, multi-center study completed in the United States. Subjects, aged 11–17 years, received vaccines at months 0, 2, and 6. Of the initial 2499 subjects, 2127 completed the study with similar rates. Non-inferiority criteria were met for the 2 MenB strains and all HPV antigens except HPV-18. No serious vaccine-related adverse events occurred, and the authors support usage of these vaccines together [102C].

Block et al. studied the administration of a 3 (2/4/12 months)—and 4 (2/4/6/12 months)—dose vaccination series of MenACWY-CRM with concomitant administration of a 13-valent pneumococcal conjugate vaccine (PCV13), Prenvar®, at months 7 and 13 and other routine vaccinations compared to PCV13 administered only with routine vaccines. This phase 3b trial evaluated 751 infants in Canada and the United States. Five hundred seventy-one infants (75%) finished the study, and withdrawal of consent and loss to follow-up were most common reasons for discontinuation. Non-inferiority criteria for an immune response were met for both the 3- and 4-dose MenACWY-CRM vaccine and PCV13 at 13 months. The primary solicited AEs were local reactions and irritability. No serious adverse events were considered vaccine related, but more infants in the MenACWY-CRM group experienced them. Four infants withdrew early due to adverse events; 1 (3-dose MenACWY-CRM series) developed Krabbe disease on day 117 after the third vaccination, 1 in the routine group developed bronchiolitis on day 14 after the first vaccine, and 2 (4-dose MenACWY-CRM series) experienced convulsions; the first had a severe seizure on day 38 after the fourth vaccination, and the second had a potential mild seizure on day 2 after the third vaccination. The authors concluded that the safety and reactogenicity for the groups that received MenACWY-CRM were similar to those who received routine vaccinations, and no relationship was seen between the vaccine and the AEs [103C].

Pertussis Vaccines (Including Diphtheria–Tetanus–Acellular/Whole-Cell Pertussis-Containing Vaccines) [SEDA-16, 257, 258, 261, 269, 645–654, 764-767, 1011–1014; SEDA-36, 478; SEDA-37, 396; SEDA-38, 325]

Organs and Systems

SKIN

A healthy 2-year-old girl developed localized urticaria on cold air-exposed areas 7 days after receiving PCV13 (Prevnar®) and Pentavac® (diphtheria, tetanus, pertussis, poliomyelitis/Haemophilus influenzae type b vaccine). Her clinical exam and all blood tests were normal or within normal limits. She was treated with dexchlorpheniramine and hydroxyzine, which provided partial effectiveness 5 months later. The cause of the urticaria may be an immune allergic reaction to the vaccine or associated with infectious diseases, but at this time, the mechanism has not been identified [82r].

Second-Generation Effects

PREGNANCY

Pregnant women or their infants were followed to determine the incidence of adverse events using the US. VAERS database after Tdap was administered during pregnancy according to the 2011 and 2012 ACIP recommendations. These subjects were then compared for incidence of events in a similar patient population prior to the ACIP Tdap pregnancy recommendations. From October 2011 until June 2015, a total of 8795 reports were obtained after Tdap vaccination, but only 392 events were included. Recorded administration of Tdap in 333 pregnant patients primarily occurred during the third trimester (79.2%), and brands of Tdap included Adacel® (59.7%), Boostrix® (33.2%) or unknown (7.1%). Twenty-seven events (6.9%) were classified as serious meaning death, hospitalization, prolonged hospitalization, life-threatening illness, or persistent or significant disability. Only one neonatal death occurred and was classified as umbilical cord occlusion with fetal vascular thrombus formation. The incidence of the other events included stillbirth 11 (2.8%), preterm birth 11 (2.8%), spontaneous abortion 4 (1%), major birth defect 4 (1%), and injection site reactions or arm pain 47 (11.9%). When compared to the events reported from January 2005 until June 2010, the majority of the 132 reported Tdap vaccinations administered during pregnancy were administered during the first trimester (77%) and only 6 (4.5%) experienced serious adverse events. The incidence of stillbirth, preterm birth, major birth defects, and injection site reactions and arm pain was less compared to vaccination administered from October 2011; however, the rate of spontaneous abortion was greater with 22 occurrences (16.7%). Data on Tdap vaccination during pregnancy are limited, and this makes it difficult to estimate reporting rate for pregnancy conditions when using VAERS, since this system has many inherent limitations the authors discuss including underreporting, reporting biases and inconsistency in the quality of the data. With the new Tdap pregnancy recommendation, more studies are being conducted regarding the safety of Tdap administration during pregnancy, and current data show that Tdap is safe [104M].

A similar cohort trial assessed 631 256 pregnancies between 2007 and 2013 in the United States. The study goal was to assess the acute safety of a population of 14–49 year olds, who received (53 885 patients) or did not receive (109 253 patients) Tdap during pregnancy. Vaccination rates did improve significantly in 2010 from 12.7% of pregnancies to 41.7% by 2013. Results showed that women who received Tdap were less likely to be hospitalized (8.3% compared to 9.1%) and more likely to have appropriate prenatal care (78.8% compared to 74.6%). Only 43 women receiving Tdap required medical attention within 3 days of vaccination, and episodes consisted of allergic reactions, fever and malaise, seizure, altered mental status, or local or other reaction (8.1 per 10 000). When compared to the unvaccinated group within 3 days of the matched index date, their event rate was 6.8 per 10 000. There was an increased rate of fever within 3 days post Tdap vaccination (2.8 per 10 000) compared to the unmatched cohort (<1 per 10 000). The authors concluded that there was no observed increased risk for any pre-specified maternal safety outcomes within 42 day of Tdap vaccination [105C].

Another study assessing Tdap safety during pregnancy was conducted in New Zealand to monitor pregnant women up to 4 weeks post vaccination who were administered Tdap between 28 and 38 weeks gestation. Boostrix® was administered and differs from the United States formulation, since it contains 0.5 mg of aluminum as aluminum hydroxide and phosphate. The United States formulation is comprised of no more than 0.39 mg aluminum as aluminum hydroxide. Participants were recruited differently based on where they lived, Northern arm or Canterbury arm, but were assessed the same. A total of 793 pregnant women participated. A majority of participants were of New Zealand European ethnicity (73.5%) with a mean age of 32 and 61.4% were between the ages of 25 and 35 years. Concomitant administration of an influenza vaccine occurred in 27.9%, and preexisting conditions in 18% included preeclamptic toxemia, symphysis pubis dysfunction, low lying placenta, shortening cervix and poor fetal growth. Mild to moderate pain was the most common reaction (79%) with 2.6% reporting severe pain, and 83.9% reported the pain onset within 24 hours of vaccination. Swelling (7.6%) and erythema (5.8%) occurred within 48 hours and few episodes were greater than 5 cm. Systemic events included fever, headache, dizziness, nausea and vomiting, fatigue, and myalgias or arthralgias with an incidence of less than 4% in all women, but fatigue occurred in 8.4%. There were 31 (3.9%) SAEs reported including 23 hospitalizations for obstetric bleeding (4), hypertension (2), infection (4), tachycardia (1), preterm labor (9), exacerbation of pre-existing condition (2), and pre-eclampsia (1). Eight events occurred during labor and delivery and included perinatal deaths (2), a cyanotic episode (1) and concern of fetal well-being (5). One of the perinatal deaths was due to a congenital abnormality. The authors concluded that none of the SAEs were caused by exposure to the Tdap vaccine [106C].

TERATOGENICITY

A cohort of 403 infants from New Zealand were followed between 6 and 12 months after birth to determine if any adverse outcomes occurred due to exposure of Tdap during pregnancy. The average gestational age when Tdap was administered was 33.9 weeks and the average gestational age at delivery was 39.2 weeks (range 33–42 weeks). The results of this study did not find an increased risk of adverse events when being exposed to the Tdap vaccine in utero compared to the incidence of the baseline population [107C].

Drug Administration

DRUG DOSAGE REGIMENS

Timing of DTaP vaccination was assessed in Australian children in this cohort study to determine if there was a correlation with vaccination timing and the risk of food allergies and eczema at the age of one. Of the 4487 infants who received the first dose of DTaP, 109 (2.5%) were vaccinated at least 1 month later than recommended with a median time frame of 103 days compared to 3 days in the on-time group. Factors associated with delayed vaccination included older age at recruitment, not attending childcare, having siblings, smokers at home, and not receiving artificial formula. Food allergy risk was associated with having siblings ($P = 0.04$ for 1–2 siblings and $P = 0.001$ for ≥ 3 siblings), and having smokers at home was associated with eczema ($P = 0.02$), both were inverse associations. Overall results found no significant association between delayed DTaP and the development of food allergies or atopic sensitization, and there was a reduced risk of developing eczema (aOR (adjusted odds ratio): 0.57; 0.34–0.97, $P = 0.04$) or using eczema medications (aOR: 0.45; 0.24–0.83, $P = 0.01$) compared to children vaccinated on time. There was also no difference in the incidence of bronchiolitis admissions or wheezing [108C].

Pneumococcal Vaccines [SEDA-16, 836–840; SEDA-36, 477; SEDA-37, 395; SEDA-38, 327]

Organs and Systems

INFECTION RISK

In the US, parapneumonic empyema started increased before the introduction of the 7-valent pneumococcal conjugate vaccine (PCV7) in children under 18 years of age. In 2000 PCV7 was introduced in the US; however, serotypes commonly associated with parapneumonic empyema (1, 3, 7F and 19A) were not included in the vaccine. The introduction of PCV7 has been cited as a reason for the ongoing increase in cases of parapneumonic empyema due to the higher representation of serotypes associated with condition. In 2010, PCV13 was introduced and the included serotypes associated with parapneumonic empyema (1, 3, 7F and 19A). A retrospective study using Nationwide Inpatient Sample and Consensus data (1997–2013) calculated annual empyema hospitalization rates during four periods based on PCV7 and PCV13 introductions; excluding years of PCV introduction: pre-PCV7 (1997–1999), early-PCV7 (2001–2005), late-PCV7 (2006–2009) and post-PCV13 (2011–2013), and pre-specified age groups (<2, 2–4 and 5–17 years). Among all children, the annualized rate of parapneumonic empyema hospitalizations per 100 000 persons was 2.1 (95% CI, 1.7–2.4) in the pre-PCV7 period and increased to 3.6 per 100 000 in the late-PCV7 period [RR: 1.70 (95% CI, 1.11–2.60)]. Rates in the post-PCV13 period decreased to 1.7 per 100 000 (95% CI, 1.4–2.0). Rates in the post-PCV13 period were similar to the pre-PCV7 period rates [RR: 0.95 (95% CI, 0.76–1.18)]. This study demonstrates that empyema hospitalization rates in US children have decreased after the introduction of PCV13. Ongoing surveillance is needed to demonstrate the persistence of this data [109c].

Susceptibility Factors

AGE

A randomized, double-blinded, multi-center phase 3 trial conducted in the US to assess the safety and immunogenicity of a second PCV13 dose 5 years after the initial dose in adults 50 years of age and older. Participants 50–59 years of age received one dose of PCV13 and IIV during the 2007/2008 season simultaneously (group 1) or 1 month apart (group 2); both groups received a second PCV13 dose 5 years later. Local injection site reactions and systemic AEs were monitored 14 days post-vaccination, and SAEs or any newly diagnoses chronic medical conditions were monitored for 6 months after each vaccination. 1116 subjects were enrolled, 727 were revaccinated with PCV13 at year 5, and 712 completed the 6-month follow-up. Of the 727 participants, 678 (93.3%) were Caucasian, 428 (58.9%) were female, and the average age was 59.8 (±2.8) years. Local reactions were mostly mild (redness, swelling, and injection site pain) and lasted an average of 3 days. The most common systemic AEs included new muscle pain, headache, and fatigue. The mean duration of any systemic event was less than 6 days. Within 1 and 6 months of revaccination with PCV13, AEs reported by subjects were 4.7% and 0.7%, respectively. When AEs were compared from initial PCV13 vaccination to PCV13 revaccination, a statistically significantly higher proportion of subjects reported increased redness and swelling after PCV13 revaccination; 12.8% vs 19.4% (95% CI, 1.2–11.9) and 14.2% vs 20.4% (95% CI, 1.1–11.2), respectively. However, a statistically significantly lower proportion of subjects reported pain and limitation of arm movement after PCV13 revaccination compared with initial PCV13 vaccination; pain 85.8% vs 81.5% (95% CI, −7.9 to −0.7) and limitation of arm movement 38.4% vs 27.6% (95% CI, −16.3 to −5.1). No SAEs were vaccine related, no deaths occurred, and no participant withdrew from the study because of AE post-vaccination. This study suggests that revaccination with PCV13 5 years apart in adults over the age of 50 is safe with no increase in SAE [110C].

Drug Administration

DRUG FORMULATIONS

To date, pneumococcal conjugate vaccines (PCV) available worldwide contain 7–13 different serotypes that cover greater than 80% of invasive pneumococcal disease (IPD) in most counties. In Africa, however, coverage of IPD is less, about 60%. Costs of PCV vaccines and limitations of serotype replacement to cover global control of IPD is a limitation of available PCV in developing countries. To overcome these barriers new pneumococcal vaccines are being developed. One of these investigational vaccines contains 2 proteins; pneumococcal histidine triad protein D (PhtD) and pneumolysin toxid (dPly, defined as detoxified pneumolysin). This new vaccine contains 30 micrograms each of dPly and PHtD and was combined with a 10-valent pneumococcal conjugate vaccine: PHid-CV/dPly/PhtD-30. The new PHid-CV/dPly/PhtD-30 pneumococcal vaccine was studied in phase 2 randomized trial in children aged 2–4 years of age. The trial enrolled 120 pneumococcal naïve children and assessed the immunogenicity and safety of the new PHid-CV/dPly/PhtD-30 pneumococcal vaccine compared to the PCV13 vaccine. Seventeen children were excluded from analysis (8 receiving PHid-CV/dPly/PhtD-30 and 9 receiving PCV13) due to concomitant receipt of OPV. Local and systemic AEs were monitored 4 days post-vaccination, and SAEs were reported for 6 months post-vaccination. The mean age of children was 2.8 years in the PHid-CV/dPly/PhtD-3030 group and 2.9 years in the PCV13 group. One Grade 3 injection site reaction was reported in the PHid-CV/dPly/PhtD-30 group and systemic reactions between both groups were similar with fever being the most common, 4 (6.7%) in the PHid-CV/dPly/PhtD-30 group and 2 (3.3%) in the PCV13 group. One child receiving PHid-CV/dPly/PhtD-30 reported loss of appetite during the 4-day post-vaccination period. No other local or systemic AEs were reported and no SAEs were reported during the study period. This study demonstrated the new PHid-CV/dPly/PhtD-30 vaccine was well tolerated in pneumococcal naïve vaccine children 2–4 years of age. Studies in a larger patient population are ongoing by the investigators [111c].

PARASITIC VACCINES

Malaria Vaccine [SED-16, 733, 734]

General

It has been estimated that 438 000 people died from malaria in 2015. The majority (>90%) of the deaths occurred in sub-Saharan Africa followed by South-East Asia and South America. Nearly all deaths related to malaria result from infection with the *Plasmodium falciparum* species of the parasite. Malaria control activities have significantly impacted the malaria mortality rates. The activities include long-lasting insecticidal nets (LLINs), indoor residual spraying (IRS) of insecticides, prompt diagnosis using rapid diagnostic tests (RDTs), and treatment with highly effective artemisinin-combination therapies (ACTs). In addition to malaria control activities, vaccine development efforts have focused on the *P. falciparum* species given the associated mortality [112S].

The WHO issued the first position paper on malaria vaccine in January 2016. Of the greater than 30 malaria vaccine candidates undergoing preclinical or clinical evaluation, the paper focused on the one vaccine candidate with results from phase 3 studies with a positive regulatory assessment [112S]. The RTS,S/AS01 malaria vaccine is a hybrid recombinant protein vaccine that targets the pre-erythrocytic state of *P. falciparum* to induce cell-mediated and humoral immune response to the circumsporozoite protein present on the surface of sporozoites and liver stage schizonts [112S,113MC]. The vaccine is formulated with the $AS01_E$ adjuvant system. Vaccine safety data for 5- to 17-month-old children indicated similar rates of reported AEs within 30 days of each vaccine dose (95% CI, 84.1–89.2). Pain, drowsiness, irritability, loss of appetite, and fever were reported more frequently among subjects in the study vaccine groups compared to the control groups. Fever was the most common systemic reaction, occurring in 31.1% of RTS,S/AS01 subjects compared to 13.4% of subjects in the control group (95% CI, 12–14.9). Fever was more common with subsequent doses of the study vaccine. Reported SAEs were less common in this age group receiving the study vaccine compared to control group subjects. Children in the 6- to 12-week age category who received study vaccine reported similar AEs when compared to the control subjects (79.4% and 81.3%, respectively). The rates of systemic reactions (fever, drowsiness, and irritably) were greater in the RTS,S/AS01 subjects compared to controls. Fever occurred in 30.6% of RTS,S/AS01 subjects compared to 21.1% of control subjects (95% CI, 19.4–22.8). The reported SAEs were comparable between the study and control subject groups.

According to the position paper, phase 3 studies have indicated a risk of febrile convulsions within 7 days of vaccination and two safety signals for meningitis and cerebral malaria have emerged. The cause for these reactions remains unknown. In children aged 5–17 months, the incidence of febrile convulsions following any of the first three vaccinations was 1 per 1000 doses compared to 0.5 per 1000 doses of the control vaccine (RR = 1.8, 95% CI, 0.6–4.9). The rates of febrile convulsion were lower in the children aged 6–12 weeks groups

(0.16 per 1000 doses and 0.47 per 1000 doses, respectively). The incidence of febrile convulsions did increase following receipt of a fourth dose of RTS,S/AS01 vaccine in both age groups. Meningitis was reported as a SAE in 16 children in the 5- to 17-month age group who received the RTS,S/AS01 vaccine compared to one child in the control group (RR = 8, CI, 1.1–60.3). There was no temporal association with any dose of the study vaccine; these findings may be due to chance [112S]. The authors of the study concluded that a causal relationship could not be confirmed or excluded at this point in time given the lack of a temporal relationship and low biological plausibility [113MC]. A greater number of cerebral malaria cases were reported in this age group receiving RTS,S/AS01 vaccine compared to controls (22 and 6 cases, respectively). It was concluded that these findings could be due to chance as well. Further investigation of the RTS, S/AS01 vaccine is recommended by the WHO to determine any potential causal relationship between the vaccine candidate and cases of meningitis and cerebral malaria, in addition to additional surveillance for AEFI [112S].

The data from phase 3 trials also indicated a great number of deaths from all causes among girls vaccinated with RTS,S/AS01 compared to girls in the control groups (mortality ratio was 1.91; 95% CI, 1.3–2.79; $P = 0.0006$). These results were not observed in boys vaccinated with the study vaccine (mortality ratio 0.84; 95% CI, 0.61–1.17; $P = 0.3343$). The WHO concluded that the results could be due to chance; however, further investigation and additional surveillance regarding the sex differences related to all-cause mortality may be warranted in order to identify any potential causal relationship as well as strategies to reduce mortality in girls [112S,114r].

Drug Administration

DRUG FORMULATIONS

The majority of effort in malaria vaccine development has focused on *P. falciparum* followed by *P. vivax*. Outside of sub-Saharan Africa, *P. vivax* is the most prevalent cause of malaria cases. The *P. vivax* species is associated with significant morbidity and mortality; therefore, studies of vaccines to prevent infection are underway. A phase 1 non-randomized, open-label, dose-escalation study was conducted in 36 adult volunteers. Subjects were divided into three groups and received one of three doses of the vivax malaria protein 001 (VMP001) adjuvanted with AS01$_B$ (VMP001/AS01$_B$) study vaccine. Overall, the study vaccine was well tolerated. No subject withdrawals occurred as a result of an AE. One SAE occurred that was not related to the study vaccine. Mild to moderate pain was the most common local AE reported, which was reported in 100% of subjects. Fatigue and headache were the most common systemic AEs reported. The frequency of occurrence increased with additional vaccine doses. Fatigue reports increased from 17% to 21% of subjects and headache from 17% to 45% from vaccination one to three, respectively. Myalgia and arthralgia were reported in 41% and 21% of subjects, respectively, and was greatest following vaccination three. Fever was reported in 10% of subjects and was also more frequently reported following vaccination three. A trend was noted for increased numbers of AE with each subsequent dose of the study vaccine. The study results support continued investigation of the VMP001/AS01$_B$ vaccine candidate [115c].

References

[1] Azegami T, Yuki Y, Kiyono H. Challenges in mucosal vaccines for the control of infectious diseases. Int Immunol. 2014;26(9):517–28 [R].

[2] Srivastava A, Gowda DV, Madhunapantula SV, et al. Mucosal vaccines: a paradigm shift in the development of mucosal adjuvants and delivery vehicles. APMIS. 2015;123(4):275–88 [R].

[3] Kim S-H, Jang Y-S. The development of mucosal vaccines for both mucosal and systemic immune induction and the roles played by adjuvants. Clin Exp Vaccine Res. 2017;6(1):15–21 [R].

[4] Dowling JK, Mansell A. Toll-like receptors: the Swiss army knife of immunity and vaccine development. Clin Transl Immunology. 2016;5:e85 [R].

[5] Gutjahr A, Tiraby G, Perouzel E, et al. Triggering intracellular receptors for vaccine adjuvantation. Trends Immunol. 2016;37(9):573–87 [R].

[6] Mifsud E, Tan A, Jackson D. TLR agonists as modulators of the innate immune response and their potential as agents against infectious disease. Front Immunol. 2014;5:79 [R].

[7] Ma F, Zhang J, Zhang J, et al. The TLR7 agonists imiquimod and gardiquimod improve DC-based immunotherapy for melanoma in mice. Cell Mol Immunol. 2010;7(5):381–8 [E].

[8] Velasquez LS, Hjelm BE, Arntzen CJ, et al. An intranasally delivered toll-like receptor 7 agonist elicits robust systemic and mucosal responses to norwalk virus-like particles. Clin Vaccine Immunol. 2010;17(12):1850–8 [E].

[9] Maisonneuve C, Bertholet S, Philpott DJ, et al. Unleashing the potential of NOD- and toll-like agonists as vaccine adjuvants. Proc Natl Acad Sci. 2014;111(34):12294–9 [R].

[10] Fromen CA, Robbins GR, Shen TW, et al. Controlled analysis of nanoparticle charge on mucosal and systemic antibody responses following pulmonary immunization. Proc Natl Acad Sci. 2015;112(2):488–93 [E].

[11] Kumar S, Anselmo AC, Banerjee A, et al. Shape and size-dependent immune response to antigen-carrying nanoparticles. J Control Release. 2015;220(Pt A):141–8 [R].

[12] Li AV, Moon JJ, Abraham W, et al. Generation of effector memory T cell-based mucosal and systemic immunity with pulmonary nanoparticle vaccination. Sci Transl Med. 2013;5(204):204ra130 [E].

[13] Halsey NA, Edwards KM, Dekker CL, et al. Algorithm to assess causality after individual adverse events following immunization. Vaccine. 2012;30(39):5791–8 [H].

[14] World Health Organization. Causality assessment of an adverse event following immunization (AEFI), WHO Press, World Health Organization, Geneva, Switzerland; 2017. Published March 2013. Accessed April 29 [S]. http://www.who.int/vaccine_safety/publications/gvs_aefi/en/.

[15] Dengue vaccine: WHO position paper. Wkly Epidemiol Rec. 2016;91(30):349–64 [S].

[16] Hadinegoro SR, Arredondo-García JL, Capeding MR, et al. Efficacy and long-term safety of dengue vaccine in regions of endemic disease. N Engl J Med. 2015;373:1195–206 [R].

[17] Dubey AP, Agarkhedkar S, Chhatwal J, et al. Immunogenicity and safety of a tetravalent dengue vaccine in healthy adults in India: a randomized, observers-blind, placebo-controlled phase II trial. Hum Vaccin Immunother. 2016;12(2):512–8 [C].

[18] Crevat D, Brion JB, Gailhardou S, et al. First experience of concomitant vaccination against dengue and MMR in toddlers. Pediatr Infect Dis J. 2015;34(8):884–92 [C].

[19] Regules JA, Beigel JH, Paolino KM, et al. A recombinant vesicular stomatitis virus Ebola vaccine. N Engl J Med. 2017;376: 330–41 [c].

[20] De Santis O, Audran R, Pothin E, et al. Safety and immunogenicity of a chimpanzee adenovirus-vectored Ebola vaccine in health adults: a randomized, double-blind, placebo-controlled, dose-finding, phase 1/2a study. Lancet Infect Dis. 2016;16:311–20 [C].

[21] Agnandji ST, Huttner A, Zinser ME, et al. Phase I trials of rVSV Ebola vaccine in Africa and Europe. N Engl J Med. 2016;374(17):1647–60 [C].

[22] Yin S, Liubao P, Chongqing T, et al. The first case of Kawasaki disease in a 20-month old baby following immunization with rotavirus vaccine and hepatitis A vaccine in China: a case report. Hum Vaccin Immunother. 2015;11(11):2740–3 [A].

[23] O'Dowd S, Bafiq R, Ryan A, et al. Severe bilateral optic neuritis post hepatitis A virus (HAV) and typhoid fever vaccination. J Neurol Sci. 2015;357(1–2):300–1 [A].

[24] Yoon SH, Kim HW, Ahn JG, et al. Reappraisal of the immunogenicity and safety of three hepatitis A vaccines in adolescents. J Korean Med Sci. 2016;31:73–9 [C].

[25] Lau CL, Streeton CL, David MC, et al. The tolerability of a combined hepatitis A and typhoid vaccine in children aged 2-16 years: an observational study. J Travel Med. 2016;23(2):1–8 [C].

[26] Petrecz M, Ramsey KP, Stek JE, et al. Concomitant use of VAQTA with PedvaxHIB and Infanrix in 12 to 17 month old children. Hum Vaccin Immunother. 2016;12(2):503–11 [C].

[27] Bisherwal K, Pandhi D, Singal A, et al. Infantile bullous pemphigoid following vaccination. Indian Pediatr. 2016;53:425–6 [A].

[28] Global advisory committee on vaccine safety, 2–3 December 2015. Wkly Epidemiol Rec. 2016;91(3):21–32 [S].

[29] Cameron RL, Ahmed S, Pollock KGJ. Adverse event monitoring of the human papillomavirus vaccines in Scotland. Intern Med J. 2016;46(4):452–7 [c].

[30] Šubelj M, Učakar V, Kraigher A, et al. Adverse events following school-based vaccination of girls with quadrivalent human papillomavirus vaccine in Slovenia, 2009 to 2013. Euro Surveill. 2016;21(14):1–6 [c].

[31] Liu XC, Bell CA, Simmonds KA, et al. Adverse events following HPV vaccination, Alberta 2006–2014. Vaccine. 2016;34(15):1800–15 [c].

[32] Yih WK, Greene SK, Zichittella L, et al. Evaluation of the risk of venous thromboembolism after quadrivalent human papillomavirus vaccination among US females. Vaccine. 2016;34(1):172–8 [c].

[33] Naleway AL, Crane B, Smith N, et al. Absence of venous thromboembolism risk following quadrivalent human papillomavirus vaccination, Vaccine Safety Datalink, 2008–2011. Vaccine. 2016;32(1):167–71 [c].

[34] Sekiguchi K, Yasui N, Kowa H, et al. Two cases of acute disseminated encephalomyelitis following vaccination against human papilloma virus. Intern Med. 2016;55(21): 3181–4 [A].

[35] Chang H, Lee HL, Yeo M, et al. Recurrent optic neuritis and neuromyelitis optica-IgG following first and second human papillomavirus vaccinations. Clin Neurol Neurosurg. 2016;144:126–8 [A].

[36] Sawai T, Shimizu M, Sakai T, et al. Tubulointerstitial nephritis and uveitis syndrome associated with human papillomavirus vaccine. J Pediatr Ophthalmol Strabismus. 2016;53(3):190–1 [A].

[37] Wheeler CM, Skinner SR, Del Rosario-Raymundo MR, et al. Efficacy, safety, and immunogenicity of the human papillomavirus 16/18 AS04-adjuvanted vaccine in women older than 25 years: 7-year follow-up of the phase 3, double-blind, randomised controlled VIVIANE study. Lancet Infect Dis. 2016;16:1154–68 [MC].

[38] Johansen K, Brasseur D, MacDonaald N, et al. Where are we in our understanding of the association between narcolepsy and one of the 2009 adjuvanted influenza A (H1N1) vaccines? Biologicals. 2016;44:276–80 [H].

[39] Verstraeten T, Cohet C, Santos GD, et al. Pandemrix™ and narcolepsy: a critical appraisal of the observational studies. Hum Vaccin Immunother. 2016;12(1):187–93 [H].

[40] Bollaerts K, Shinde V, Dos Santos G, et al. Applications of probabilistic multiple-bias analyses to a cohort-and a case-control study on the association between Pandemrix™ and narcolepsy. PLoS One. 2016;11(2):1–14 [H].

[41] Hibino M, Kondo T. Interstitial pneumonia associated with the influenza vaccine: a report of two cases. Intern Med. 2017;56:197–201 [A].

[42] Narasimhan M, Ahmed PB, Venugopal V, et al. Severe allergic eczematous skin reaction to 2009 (H1N1) influenza vaccine injection. Int J Dermatol. 2015;54:1338–41 [r].

[43] Regan AK, Tracey LE, Blyth CC, et al. A prospective cohort study assessing the reactogenicity of pertussis and influenza vaccines administered during pregnancy. Vaccine. 2016;34:2299–304 [MC].

[44] Halsey NA, Talaat KR, Greenbaum A, et al. The safety of influenza vaccines in children: an Institute for Vaccine Safety white paper. Vaccine. 2015;33:F1–F67 [M].

[45] Esposito S, Giavoli C, Trombetta C, et al. Immunogenicity, safety and tolerability of inactivated trivalent influenza vaccine in overweight and obese children. Vaccine. 2016;34:56–60 [c].

[46] Liao Z, Tang H, Xu X, et al. Immunogenicity and safety of influenza vaccination in systemic lupus erythematosus patients compared with healthy controls: a meta-analysis. PLoS One. 2016;11(2):1–13 [M].

[47] Tartof SY, Qian L, Rieg GK, et al. Safety of seasonal influenza vaccination in hospitalized surgical patients. Ann Intern Med. 2016;164:593–9 [MC].

[48] Cohet C, Haguinet F, Dos Santos G, et al. Effect of the adjuvanted (AS03) A/H1N1 2009 pandemic influenza vaccine on the risk of rejection in solid organ transplant recipients in England: a self-controlled case series. BMJ Open. 2016;6(1):1–10 [C].

[49] Kumar D, Campbell P, Hoschler K, et al. Randomized controlled trial of adjuvanted versus nonadjuvanted influenza vaccine in kidney transplant recipients. Transplantation. 2016;100:662–9 [c].

[50] Nagao M, Fujisawa T, Ihara T, et al. Highly increased levels of IgE antibodies to vaccine components in children with influenza vaccine-associated anaphylaxis. J Allergy Clin Immunol. 2016;137:861–7 [c].

[51] Halasa NB, Savani BN, Asokan I, et al. Randomized double-blind study of the safety and immunogenicity of standard-dose trivalent inactivated influenza vaccine versus high-dose trivalent inactivated influenza vaccine in adult hematopoietic stem cell transplantation patients. Biol Blood Marrow Transplant. 2016;22:528–35 [c].

[52] DiazGranados CA, Saway W, Gouaux J, et al. Safety and immunogenicity of high-dose trivalent inactivated influenza vaccine in adults 50–64 years of age. Vaccine. 2015;33:7188–93 [C].

[53] Moro PL, Winiecki S, Lewis P, et al. Surveillance of adverse events after the first trivalent inactivated influenza vaccine produced in mammalian cell culture (Flucelvax®) reported to the Vaccine Adverse Event Reporting System (VAERS), United States, 2013–2015. Vaccine. 2015;33:6684–8 [C].

[54] Nolan T, Chotpitayasunondh T, Rosario Capeding M, et al. Safety and tolerability of a cell culture derived trivalent subunit inactivated influenza vaccine administered to healthy children and adolescents: a phase II, randomized, multicenter, observer-blind study. Vaccine. 2016;34:230–6 [MC].

[55] Diez-Domingo J, de Martino M, Garcia-Sicilia Lopez J, et al. Safety and tolerability of cell culture-derived trivalent influenza vaccines in 3 to <18 year-old children and adolescents at risk of influenza-related complications. Int J Infect Dis. 2016;49:171–8 [C].

[56] Izikson R, Leffell DJ, Bock SA, et al. Randomized comparison of the safety of Flublok® versus licensed inactivated influenza vaccine in healthy, medically stable adults ≥50 years of age. Vaccine. 2015;33:6622–8 [MC].

[57] McNaughton R, Lynn E, Osborne V, et al. Safety of intranasal quadrivalent live attenuated influenza vaccine (QLAIV) in children and adolescents: a pilot prospective cohort study in England. Drug Saf. 2016;39:323–33 [C].

[58] Rudenko L, Isakova-Sivak I, Naykhin A, et al. H7N9 live attenuated influenza vaccine in healthy adults: a randomized, double-blind, placebo-controlled, phase I trial. Lancet Infect Dis. 2016;16:303–10 [c].

[59] Sobhanie M, Matsuoka Y, Jegaskanda S, et al. Evaluation of the safety and immunogenicity of a candidate pandemic live attenuated influenza vaccine (pLAIV) against influenza A (H7N9). J Infect Dis. 2016;213:922–9 [c].

[60] Kim D, Jang G, Houillon G, et al. Immunogenicity and safety of a booster dose of a live attenuated Japanese encephalitis chimeric vaccine given 1 year after primary immunization in healthy children in the Republic of Korea. Pediatr Infect Dis. 2016;35(2): e60–4 [C].

[61] Morgan E, Halliday SR, Campbell GR, et al. Vaccinations and childhood type I diabetes mellitus: a meta-analysis of observation studies. Diabetologia. 2016;59:237–43 [M].

[62] Mamishi S, Sarkardeh M, Pourakbari B, et al. Aseptic meningitis after measles-mumps-rubella (MMR) vaccination. Br J Biomed Sci. 2016;73(2):84–6 [C].

[63] Muta H, Nagai T, Ito Y, et al. Effect of age on the incidence of aseptic meningitis following immunization with monovalent mumps vaccine. Vaccine. 2015;33:6049–53 [MC].

[64] Binamer Y. Acute hemorrhagic edema of infancy after MMR vaccine. Ann Saudi Med. 2015;35(3):245–6 [A].

[65] van der Maas NAT, Woudenberg T, Hahné SJM, et al. Tolerability of early measles-mumps-rubella vaccination in infants aged 6–14 month during a measles outbreak in The Netherlands in 2013–2014. J Infect Dis. 2016;213:1466–71 [C].

[66] Sukamaran L, McNeil MM, Moro PL, et al. Adverse events following measles, mumps, and rubella vaccine in adults reported to the Vaccine Adverse Event Reporting System (VAERS), 2003–2013. Clin Infect Dis. 2015;60(10):e58–65 [R].

[67] Polio vaccine: WHO position paper. Wkly Epidemiol Rec. 2016;91(12):145–68 [S].

[68] Schubert A, Böttcher S, Eis-Hübinger AM. Two cases of vaccine-derived poliovirus infection in an oncology ward. N Eng J Med. 2016;374(13):1296–8 [c].

[69] Sáez-Llorens X, Clemens R, Leroux-Roels G, et al. Immunogenicity and safety of a novel monovalent high-dose inactivated poliovirus type 2 vaccine in infants: a comparative, observer-blind, randomized, control trial. Lancet Infect Dis. 2016;16:321–30 [C].

[70] Tate J, Yen C, Steiner C, et al. Intussusception rates before and after the introduction of rotavirus vaccine. Pediatrics. 2016;138(3):1–7 [C].

[71] Leino T, Ollgren J, Strömberg N, et al. Evaluation of the intussusception risk after pentavalent rotavirus vaccination in finnish infants. PLoS One. 2016;11(3): e0144812 [c].

[72] Fernandes E, Leshem E, Sato H, et al. Hospital-based surveillance of intussusception among infants. J Pediatr (Rio J). 2016;92(2):181–7 [c].

[73] Libster R, McNeal M, Edwards K, et al. Safety and immunogenicity of sequential rotavirus vaccine schedules. Pediatrics. 2016;137(2)e20152603 [C].

[74] Gustafson C, Woodard M, Hanke C. A unique case of herpes zoster within one week of varicella zoster vaccination. J Drugs Dermatol. 2016;15(2):241–3 [A].

[75] Choi WS, Choi JH, Choi JY, et al. Immunogenicity and safety of a live attenuated zoster vaccine (Zostavax™) in Korean adults. J Korean Med Sci. 2016;31:13–7 [c].

[76] Hata A, Inoue F, Ohkubo T, et al. Efficacy and safety of live varicella zoster vaccine in diabetes: a randomized, double-blind, placebo-controlled trial. Diabet Med. 2016;33(8):1094–101 [c].

[77] Aoki T, Koh K, Hanada R, et al. Safety of live attenuated high-titer varicella-zoster virus vaccine in pediatric allogeneic hematopoietic stem cell transplantation recipients. Biol Blood Marrow Transplant. 2016;22(4):771–5 [c].

[78] Cunningham A, Lai H, Downey H, et al. Efficacy of the herpes zoster subunit vaccine in adults 70 years of age or older. N Engl J Med. 2016;375(11):1019–32 [MC].

[79] Prymula R, Simko R, Povey M, et al. Varicella vaccine without human serum albumin versus licensed varicella vaccine in children during the second year of life: a randomized, double-blind, non-inferiority trial. BMC Pediatr. 2016;16:7 [MC].

[80] Levin MJ, Schmader KE, Williams-Diaz A, et al. Cellular and humoral responses to a second dose of herpes zoster vaccine administered 10 years after the first dose among older adults. J Infect Dis. 2016;213(1):14–22 [C].

[81] Lindsey NP, Rabe IB, Miller ER, et al. Adverse event reports following yellow fever vaccination, 2007–13. J Travel Med. 2016;23(5):1–6 [c].

[82] Raison-Peyron N, Philibert C, Bernard N, et al. Cold contact urticaria following vaccination: four cases. Acta Derm Venereol. 2016;96:852–3 [r].

[83] Leung WS, Chan MC, Chik SH, et al. First case of yellow fever vaccine-associated viscerotropic disease (YEL-AVD) in Hong Kong. J Travel Med. 2016;23(4):1–3 [r].

[84] Facincani T, Guimarães MNC, De Sousa dos Santos S. Yellow fever vaccination status and safety in hemodialysis patients. Int J Infect Dis. 2016;48:91–5 [c].

[85] Bernstein DI, Jackson L, Patel SM, et al. Immunogenicity and safety of four different dosing regimens of anthrax vaccine adsorbed for post-exposure prophylaxis for anthrax in adults. Vaccine. 2014;32:6284–93 [C].

[86] Garman L, Smith K, Muns EE, et al. Unique inflammatory mediators and specific IgE levels distinguish local from systemic reactions after anthrax vaccine adsorbed vaccination. Clin Vaccine Immunol. 2016;23(8):664–71 [C].

[87] Pondo T, Rose Jr. CE, Martin SW, et al. Evaluation of sex, race, body mass index, and pre-vaccination serum progesterone levels and post-vaccination serum anti-0anthrax protective immunoglobulin G on injection site adverse events following anthrax vaccine adsorbed (AVA) in the CDC AVA human clinical trial. Vaccine. 2014;32:3548–54 [C].

[88] Hopkins RJ, Kalsi G, Montalvo-Lugo VM, et al. Randomized, double-blind, active-controlled study evaluating the safety and immunogenicity of three vaccination schedules and two dose levels of AV7909 vaccine for anthrax post-exposure prophylaxis in health adults. Vaccine. 2016;34:2096–105 [C].

[89] Bacillus Calmette-Guérin Vaccine. Lexi-Comp Online®, AHFS DI (Adult and Pediatric), Hudson, Ohio: Lexi-Comp, Inc. Accessed: April 12, 2017.

[90] Hui D, Stoeckel DA, Kaufman EE, et al. Massive hemoptysis from an aortobronchial fistula secondary to BCG-related mycotic thoracic aorta aneurysm. Ann Thorac Surg. 2016;101:350–2 [A].

[91] Nissen TN, Birk NM, Kjaergaard J, et al. Adverse reactions to the Bacillus Calmette-Guérin vaccine in new-born infants-an

evaluation of the Danish strain 1331 SSI in a randomized clinical trial. Vaccine. 2016;34:2477–82 [C].

[92] Sekiguchi A, Motegi S, Ishikawa O. Erythema induratum of Bazin associated with bacillus Calmette-Guérin vaccination: implication of M1 macrophage infiltration and monocyte chemotactic protein-1 expression. J Dermatol. 2016;43(1):111–3 [A].

[93] Pöyhönen L, Pauniaho S, Kröger L, et al. Orthopedic complications in former Bacillus Calmette-Guérin osteitis patients. Pediatr Infect Dis J. 2016;35(5):579–80 [C].

[94] Bialecki J, Nowak-Misiak N, Rapala K, et al. Spinal tuberculosis with severe neurological symptoms as a complication of intravesical BCG therapy for carcinoma of the bladder. Neurol Neurochir Pol. 2016;50:131–8 [A].

[95] Karaca NE, Aksu G, Ulusoy E, et al. Disseminated BCG infectious disease and hyperferritinemia in a patient with a novel NEMO mutation. J Investig Allergol Clin Immunol. 2016;26(4):268–71 [A].

[96] Minhinnick A, Satti I, Harris S, et al. A first-in-human phase 1 trial to evaluate the safety and immunogenicity of the candidate tuberculosis vaccine MVA85A-IMX313, administered to BCG-vaccinated adults. Vaccine. 2016;34:1412–21 [c].

[97] Tenenbaum T, Niessen J, Schroten H. Severe upper extremity dysfunction after 4CMen B vaccination in a young infant. Pediatr Infect Dis J. 2016;35:94–6 [c].

[98] Ostergaard L, Lucksinger GH, Absalon J, et al. A phase 3, randomized, active-controlled study to assess the safety and tolerability of meningococcal serogroup B vaccine bivalent rLP2086 in healthy adolescents and young adults. Vaccine. 2016;34:1465–71 [C].

[99] Kim DS, Kim MJ, Cha S, et al. Safety and immunogenicity of a single dose of a quadrivalent meningococcal conjugate vaccine (MenACYW-D): a multicenter, blind-observer, randomized, phase III clinical trial in the Republic of Korea. Int J Infect Dis. 2016;45:59–64 [C].

[100] Snape MD, Voysey M, Finn A, et al. Persistence of bactericidal antibodies after infant serogroup B meningococcal immunization and booster dose response at 12, 18 or 24 months of age. Pediatr Infect Dis J. 2016;35:e113–23 [C].

[101] Johnston W, Essink B, Kirstein J, et al. Comparative assessment of a single dose and 2-dose vaccination series of a quadrivalent meningococcal CRM-conjugate vaccine (MenACWY-CRM) in children 2-10 years of age. Pediatr Infect Dis J. 2016;35:e19–27 [C].

[102] Senders S, Bhuyan P, Jiang Q, et al. Immunogenicity, tolerability and safety in adolescents of bivalent rLP2086, a meningococcal serogroup B vaccine, coadministered with quadrivalent human papilloma virus vaccine. Pediatr Infect Dis J. 2016;35:548–54 [C].

[103] Block SL, Shepard J, Garfield H, et al. Immunogenicity and safety of a 3- and 4-dose vaccination series of a meningococcal ACWY conjugate vaccine in infants. Pediatr Infect Dis J. 2016;35:e48–59 [C].

[104] Moro P, Cragan J, Tepper N, et al. Enhanced surveillance of tetanus toxoid, reduced diphtheria toxoid, and acellular pertussis (Tdap) vaccines in pregnancy in the Vaccine Adverse Event Reporting System (VAERS), 2011–2015. Vaccine. 2016;34:2349–53 [M].

[105] Kharbanda EO, Vazquez-Benitez G, Lipkind HS, et al. Maternal Tdap vaccination: coverage and acute safety outcomes in the Vaccine Safety Datalink, 2007–2013. Vaccine. 2016;34:968–73 [C].

[106] Petousis-Harris H, Walls T, Watson D, et al. Safety of Tdap vaccine in pregnant women: an observational study. BMJ Open. 2016;6:e010911. http://dx.doi.org/10.1136/bmjopen-2015-010911 [C].

[107] Walls T, Graham P, Petousis-Harris H, et al. Infant outcomes after exposure to Tdap vaccine in pregnancy: an observational study. BMJ Open. 2016;6:e009536. http://dx.doi.org/10.1136/bmjopen-2015-009536 [C].

[108] Kiraly N, Koplin JJ, Crawford MW, et al. Timing of routine infant vaccinations and risk of food allergy and eczema at one year of age. Allergy. 2016;71:541–9 [C].

[109] Wiese AD, Griffin MR, Zhu Y, et al. Changes in empyema among U.S. children in the pneumococcal conjugate vaccine era. Vaccine. 2016;34:6243–9 [c].

[110] Frenck Jr. RW, Fiquet A, Gurtman A, et al. Immunogenicity and safety of a second administration of 13-valent pneumococcal conjugate vaccine 5 years after initial vaccination in adults 50 years and older. Vaccine. 2016;34:3454–62 [C].

[111] Odutola A, Ota MO, Ogundare EO, et al. Reactogenicity, safety and immunogenicity of a protein-based pneumococcal vaccine in Gambian children aged 2–4 years: a phase II randomized study. Hum Vaccin Immunother. 2016;12(2):393–402 [c].

[112] World Health Organization. Malaria vaccine: WHO position paper, January 2016. Wkly Epidemiol Rec. 2016;91(4):33–52 [S].

[113] The RTS, S Clinical Trials Partnership. Efficacy and safety of the RTS, S/AS01 malaria vaccine during 18 months after vaccination: a phase 3 randomized, controlled trial in children and young infants at 11 African sites. PLoS One. 2014;11(7):1–24 [MC].

[114] Sl Klein, Shann F, Moss WJ, et al. RTS, S malaria vaccine and increased mortality in girls. MBio. 2016;7(2):1–2 [r].

[115] Bennett JW, Yadava A, Tosh D, et al. Phase 1/2a trial of *Plasmodium vivax* malaria vaccine candidate VMP001/AS01$_B$ in malaria-naïve adults: safety, immunogenicity, and efficacy. PLoS Negl Trop Dis. 2016;10(2):1–16 [c].

29

Blood, Blood Components, Plasma, and Plasma Products

Maria Cardinale[*,†,1], *Kent Owusu*[‡], *Tamara Malm*[‡,§]

[*]Ernest Mario School of Pharmacy, Rutgers, The State University of New Jersey, Piscataway, NJ, United States
[†]Saint Peter's University Hospital, New Brunswick, NJ, United States
[‡]Yale-New Haven Hospital, New Haven, CT, United States
[§]University of Saint Joseph School of Pharmacy, University of Saint Joseph, West Hartford, CT, United States
[1]Corresponding author: maria.cardinale@pharmacy.rutgers.edu

ALBUMIN AND DERIVATIVES
[SEDA-15, 54; SEDA-36, 483; SEDA-37, 403; SEDA-38, 335]

Albumin [SEDA-15, 54; SEDA-36, 483; SEDA-37, 403; SEDA-38, 335]

Albumin plays a major role in volume expansion in critically ill patients requiring fluid resuscitation. There is also a role for albumin in cirrhosis, spontaneous bacterial peritonitis (SBP), and hepatorenal syndrome [1R]. Current guidelines recommend administering albumin after large volume paracentesis to prevent hematologic abnormalities [2M]. However, regular use of albumin may be less practical when compared to crystalloids, due to cost and availability [3R].

Hematologic

A decrease in fibrinogen and coagulation proteins is seen after plasma exchange using albumin. These changes in clotting proteins cause a delay in clot firmness and a reduction in clot firmness [4c]. A randomized control trial of 40 patients undergoing radical cystectomy examined the effects of 5% human albumin (HA) compared to lactated ringers (LR) on coagulation. At the end of anesthesia, and in the recovery room, albumin administration was associated with decreased platelets, elevated aPPT, and increased INR [5c].

Renal

A meta-analysis assessing the impact of timely albumin administration on renal impairment in patients diagnosed with SBP found that albumin administered within 6 hours of SBP detection improved both mortality and renal impairment, with a number needed to treat of 6 and 4, respectively [6M]. Large volume paracentesis is often conducted under concomitant albumin infusion [7c]. A retrospective review of patients requiring continuous large volume paracentesis and concomitant albumin infusion, found an improvement in serum creatinine, with no increase in bacterial infections [8c]. A randomized, single-center study of patients undergoing off-pump coronary artery bypass surgery, found that administering 20% albumin immediately before surgery, in patients with baseline albumin <4 g/dL, increased urine output and decreased risk of acute kidney injury, with few adverse effects [9C].

BLOOD TRANSFUSION [SEDA-15, 529; SEDA-36, 483; SEDA-37, 404; SEDA-38, 336]

Erythrocytes

Anemia is common among hospitalized patients and transfusion of erythrocytes to prevent related hypoxia is not uncommon in this setting [10c,11M]. A retrospective cohort study assessed the incidence of further bleeding and mortality in patients with nonvariceal upper gastrointestinal bleeding who received red blood cell (RBC) transfusions. Of 2128 adult patients who met inclusion criteria, transfusion of 4 or more units of RBCs was associated with higher odds of further bleeding in patients with a hemoglobin level >9 g/dL (OR, 11.9; 95% CI, 3.2–45.7;

$P \leq 0.001$), without an increase in mortality. However, when patients were administered 5 or more units of fresh frozen plasma, there was an increased rate of 30-day mortality (HR, 2.8; 95% CI, 1.3–5.9; $P = 0.008$) as well as an increase in 1-year mortality (HR, 2.6; 95% CI, 1.3–5.0; $P = 0.005$). This increase in mortality observed here was dose dependent and independent of administration of RBCs [10c].

Cardiovascular: A recent meta-analysis was performed to review the impact of red blood cell transfusions on acute coronary syndrome. It included a total of 17 studies with 2 525 550 patients from 2001 through 2015. Included were 4 secondary analysis of randomized control trials, 12 cohort studies, and 1 case–control study. Here, erythrocyte transfusions were found to be associated with higher short- and long-term all-cause mortality as well as reinfarction rates (adjusted RR 2.23; 95% CI 1.47–3.39; HR 1.93; 95% CI 1.12–3.34; RR 2.61; 95% CI 2.17–3.14, respectively) in comparison to no transfusion. When stratified by hemoglobin, transfusion and risk of all-cause mortality was significant at hemoglobin levels below 8.0 g/dL (RR 0.52; 95% CI 0.25–1.06) and was associated with an increased risk of mortality at a hemoglobin above 10 g/dL (RR 3.34; 95% CI 2.25–4.97) [11M].

Granulocytes

Systemic Review: In a Cochrane review of 10 studies of 587 neutropenic patients with infection, there was insufficient evidence to observe a difference in all-cause mortality between patients receiving therapeutic granulocyte transfusions and those that did not (six studies; 321 participants; RR 0.75, 95% CI 0.54–1.04). Serious adverse effects were reported in three studies. There was insufficient evidence to observe a difference in pulmonary serious adverse events between patients receiving therapeutic granulocyte transfusions and those that did not (one study; 24 participants; RR 0.85, 95% CI 0.38–1.88) [12M].

Pulmonary: Pulmonary reactions are an important short-term consequence occurring within 48 hours of granulocyte transfusion and are reported at a rate of 0%–53%. Possible mechanisms include the flare-up of existing pneumonia because of neutrophil trafficking to the infection site. Transfusion-related acute lung injury may also be due to alloimmunization, virus transmission, volume overload, or allergic reactions [13R].

Platelets: The British Blood Transfusion Society (BBTS) published highlights from a special interest group meeting held in November 2015 that touched on controversies in platelet components and medical and surgical uses of platelet transfusions [14H]. In addition, the British Committee for Standards in Haematology (BCSH) published guidelines in 2016 on the appropriate use and indications for prophylactic and therapeutic indications for platelet transfusion [15H].

Cardiovascular: Platelet transfusions are associated with thrombosis and negative outcomes, including increased mortality. Specifically, increased mortality has been reported in patients with consumptive platelet disorders, cancer patients, and patients who recently underwent coronary stent placement. Some of the factors that may contribute to thrombotic potential include platelet dysfunction in trauma patients, the prevalence of microparticles in platelet concentrates, nongroup-O blood, and storage at 4°C compared to 22°C [16H]. The PATCH study was a multi-center, randomized, open-label study in which 190 patients with a supratentorial intracerebral hemorrhage were randomized within 6 hours of presentation to standard care or standard care plus platelet transfusion. To be enrolled, patients must have used antiplatelet therapy for at least 7 days prior and have a Glasgow Coma Scale of at least eight. The odds of death or dependence at 3 months were higher in the platelet transfusion group compared with the standard care group (OR 2.05; $P = 0.0114$). Although the mechanism of increased mortality is unknown, the authors speculate that impaired collateral perfusion may have led to cerebral ischemia, and thrombosis could result in lesion expansion [17C].

In a retrospective, non-randomized study of adult patients with dengue fever and platelet count less than 20 000/mm^3, 486 patients received prophylactic platelet transfusion. There was no difference in clinical bleeding, but the patients that received platelets experienced slower platelet recovery (3 days vs 2 days, $P < 0.0001$) and longer hospital length of stay (6 days vs 5 days, $P < 0.0001$) compared to those that did not [18c].

Immunologic: Transfusion reactions can occur following transfusions of platelet concentrates. Removal of leukocytes from cellular blood components (leukoreduction) reduces the risk of febrile non-hemolytic transfusion reactions. In a retrospective study of pediatric patients who received transfusions at a single institution, total transfusion reactions, including febrile non-hemolytic and allergic transfusion reactions, were significantly reduced when the institution transitioned to leukocyte-reduced platelets. In this study, 7.6% of patients who received leukoreduced platelet concentrate experienced transfusion reactions, of which 90.5% were allergic reactions. On univariate analysis, allergic reactions were significantly associated with older age, male gender, hematological and malignant disease, number of transfusions and history of transfusion with other products [19C]. The BCSH guidelines recommend that patients with a history of allergic transfusion reactions should receive platelets suspended in Platelet Additive Solution (PAS) [20H].

Infection risk: Sepsis has also been reported following platelet transfusions. Despite aseptic collection techniques, bacterial contamination can still occur during phlebotomy [21r]. Hong and colleagues reported the results of active and passive surveillance of platelet transfusions over a 7-year span by platelet aliquot. In this study, 20 of 51 440 platelet units transfused (0.004%; 389 per million) were bacterially contaminated and resulted in 5 reported septic transfusion reactions, which occurred between 9 and 24 hours following transfusion. All of the septic reactions occurred in patients with neutropenia, and there was one fatality. The authors highlight that none of these septic reactions were detected by passive surveillance strategies, highlighting the limitations of passive surveillance for determining the rate of septic transfusion reactions [22MC]. Rapid diagnostic tests are available to detect bacterial contamination on the day of transfusion, but are not routinely performed in transfusion centers [21r].

In recent years, worldwide outbreaks of the zika virus, a mosquito-borne virus, were increasingly a major public health concern. An editorial published in the New England Journal of Medicine describes two patients that tested positive for the zika virus on PCR assay following receipt of platelet transfusion from a donor found to have the virus. Patient 1 was a 54-year-old woman with primary myelofibrosis syndrome and patient 2 was a 14-year-old girl with acute myeloid leukemia who was receiving immunosuppressive therapy following a bone marrow transplant. Fortunately, neither patient experienced any symptoms of zika virus during the investigation [23r].

Regarding other viral infections, the British Committee for Standards in Haematology guidelines of 2016 list the risk of HIV infection from platelet transfusion as 1 in 7 million, the risk of hepatitis C as 1 in 30 million, and the risk of hepatitis B as 1 in 1 million [24H].

BLOOD SUBSTITUTES [SEDA-36, 485; SEDA-37, 406; SEDA-38, 339]

Hemoglobin-Based Oxygen Carriers [SEDA-36, 485; SEDA-37, 406; SEDA-38, 339]

Hemoglobin-based oxygen carriers (HBOC) have the potential to increase blood oxygen content in patients with life-threatening anemia in whom red blood cell transfusion is not an option. Weiskopf and colleagues analyzed data from a large randomized trial of Hemopure (HBOC-201) in orthopedic patients to assess the impact of HBOC treatment on mortality. Although adverse effects were not reported in this study, when compared to comparable, untransfused surgical patients, patients that received HBOC had a higher survival rate ($P < 0.014$; HR, 0.42) [25r]. Similar mortality benefits were seen in patients included in compassionate-use programs when compared to similar hospitalized, untransfused patients. However, concerns of adverse effects due to oxidative damage nitric oxide scavenging have previously

limited the development of an acceptable HBOC product. Modifications to the molecular structure of future HBOC products are currently being researched to reduce the oxidative potential [26E].

PLASMA AND PLASMA PRODUCTS [SEDA-15, 84; SEDA-36, 486; SEDA-37, 407; SEDA-38, 340]

Alpha 1-Antitrypsin

Alpha 1-antitrypsin (AAT), a serine protease inhibitor produced by the hepatocytes in response to inflammation, has been used for inflammatory conditions in the setting of AAT deficiency. More recently, an open-label, prospective, observational, phase I/II clinical trial, aimed to assess the safety of administration of AAT in pediatric patients with a diagnosis of type I diabetes mellitus. Twenty four included patients were assigned to treatment with AAT at escalating doses of 40, 60, and 80 mg per kg actual body weight ($n = 8$, in each dosage group) infused over a period of 28 weeks, with a 9-week follow-up period. Safety endpoints included any reported adverse events, diabetic ketoacidosis (DKA) (defined as a serum pH < 7.31 and requirement of an insulin infusion), episodes of severe hypoglycemia (blood glucose < 70 mg/dL associated with coma and/or seizures or the need for glucagon administration), infusion-site reactions, weight changes, daily insulin requirements, electrocardiogram, physical examination, and laboratory assessments. Nineteen of the 24 patients reported 158 adverse events of which only 45 adverse events among 11 patients (45.6%) were classified to be related to AAT administration. Notable adverse events included headache, abdominal pain, and cough. Infusion-related adverse events included hypotension in one patient who received a high dose (80 mg per kg per dose) and an infusion site related blister formation [27c].

C1 Esterase Inhibitor Concentrate

Human complement component-1 esterase inhibitors (C1INH) are utilized in the treatment of Hereditary angioedema (HAE) in patients deficient in endogenous or functional C1INH which leads to an overproduction of bradykinin. Manifestations of HAE include episodes of skin inflammation, abdominal pain, and laryngeal edema. Available C1INH products in the United States (US) include *Berinert*, *Cinryze*, and *Ruconest*. While previous safety data published in a total of 236 subjects who received *Ruconest* reported no safety concerns related to hemodynamics or cardiotoxicity, hematology, or urinalysis, recent reports have highlighted serious hypersensitivity reactions. Additionally, Ruconest should be avoided in patients with a history of allergic reactions to rabbits or rabbit-derived products due to risk of serious hypersensitivity reactions [28c].

Cryoprecipitate

Cryoprecipitate a derivative of fresh frozen plasma thawed at 4°C, contains fibrinogen (200 mg/unit), Factor VIII, fibronectin, factor XIII, and von Willebrand Factor (vWF). Cryoprecipitate has been widely used for a variety of indications surrounding hypofibrinogenemia. Most recently, cryoprecipitate has been recommended for hypofibrinogenemia following administration of alteplase due to the increased risk of parenchymal hematoma following alteplase administration for acute ischemic stroke (AIS). It has been noted that approximately 10 units of cryoprecipitate will raise fibrinogen levels by about 70 mg/dL in an average 70-kilogram (kg) patient [29S]. Adverse events associated with the administration of cryoprecipitate include transmission of infectious diseases, transfusion-associated circulatory overload (TACO), and transfusion-related acute lung injury (TRALI).

Fresh Frozen Plasma [SEDA-36, 486; SEDA-37, 408; SEDA-38, 341]

Fresh frozen plasma (FFP) contains all coagulation factors including varying levels of vitamin K+-dependent factors II, VII, IX, and X. Due to variation of coagulation factor concentration, effects on hemostasis are unpredictable and concerning in the setting of a life-threatening bleeding event. FFP is commonly used in the setting of coagulopathy including coagulation factor deficiencies and in the setting of intracranial or extracranial bleeding events. One mL of FFP per kg of body weight generally increases the levels of coagulation factors by approximately 1 IU/dL.

Neurology: Hematoma expansion is an established cause of mortality in the setting of intracranial hemorrhage (ICH). A 2016 multicenter, prospective, randomized, open-label, blinded trial aimed to assess the safety and efficacy of administration of FFP in comparison to PCC in patients with vitamin K antagonist-related ICH. Outcomes were assessed in 50 patients with an INR of at least 2.0 within 12 hours after onset of VKA-associated ICH. Individuals were randomized to receive either 4-factor PCC or 20 mL per kg body weight of FFP [30c]. In assessing the primary outcome of INR reduction to 1.2 or lower within 3 hours of initiation of treatment, only 9% of patients in the FFP arm achieved this endpoint when compared to 67% of patients in the 4-factor PCC arm (adjusted OR 30.6, 95% CI 4.7–197.9; $P = 0.0003$). There was a smaller change in hematoma volume in the PCC group in comparison to the FFP group when assessed per head computer tomography (CT) scan at 24 hours [30c]. Despite the aforementioned differences, there were no differences in clinical outcomes.

PLASMA SUBSTITUTES [SEDA-36, 487; SEDA-37, 408; SEDA-38, 341]

Dextrans [SEDA-36, 487; SEDA-37, 408; SEDA-38, 341]

Systematic Reviews: In a meta-analysis of 31 randomized controlled trials of patients undergoing major elective surgery over 5 years, coagulation competence (measured by thromboelastography (TEG) maximum amplitude), hemorrhage rates, and outcomes were compared between patients receiving various colloids and crystalloids during surgery. In the two trials that compared dextran to crystalloid fluids, there were no differences between groups in terms of blood loss (mean difference: −120.44, 95% CI: −319.38 to 78.5, $I^2 = 50\%$) or reoperation (OR: 1.40; 95% CI: 0.53 – 3.70; $I^2 = 0\%$) [31M].

Etherified Starches [SEDA-15, 1237; SEDA-36, 487; SEDA-37, 408; SEDA-38, 341]

Hematologic: In the meta-analysis of surgical patients by Rasmussen and colleagues, hydroxyethyl starch (HES) was compared to crystalloids in 20 randomized trials. In 17 trials comparing blood loss volume, 12 (70%) reported an increased blood loss in patients receiving HES compared to crystalloids (Mean difference: 21.8 mL, $P < 0.003$). When restricted to noncardiovascular surgery, the difference was still significant ($P < 0.0009$). Perioperative hemorrhage increased by 20% with HES compared to crystalloids. Coagulation competence using thromboelastography-maximum amplitude (TEG-MA) was also assessed in nine studies comparing HES to crystalloids and four studies comparing HES to albumin. In all but one these studies, HES administration led to an increased reduction in TEG-MA following HES administration; however, there was significant heterogeneity (69%) [32M]. When restricting the analysis to low molecular weight HES compared to crystalloids, the results are similar ($P < 0.004$ for blood volume $P < 0.0001$ for coagulation competence) [32M].

Urinary Tract: Acute kidney injury (AKI) is an important concern of HES therapy in critically ill septic patients, but this adverse effect is less well described in surgical patients. In addition, it is unknown whether newer-generation HES pose the same risks as older generations. A retrospective study evaluated 1641 living donors who underwent a donor right hepatectomy and received either crystalloids or 6% HES 130/0.4, a third-generation

HES. After a 1:3 propensity score matching was performed, 206 donors were analyzed for post-operative AKI, defined by the RIFLE or AKIN criteria. In this study, the risk of AKI did not differ between patients receiving HES or crystalloids. The authors state that large trials are needed to settle the controversy of intraoperative HES use and nephrotoxicity [33c].

Gelatin [SEDA-36, 487; SEDA-37, 409; SEDA-38, 342]

Gelatins exhibit similar adverse effects as other synthetic colloids [34r]. A meta-analysis of 30 randomized trials included 3629 hypovolemic patients that were administered gelatin or crystalloids or albumin for resuscitation. Surgical, critically ill, and pediatric patients were included in the analysis. Administration of gelatin increased the risk of anaphylaxis (RR: 3.01, 95% CI: 1.27 – 7.14) and may have led to an increased risk of mortality, with a difference that trended toward significance (RR: 1.15, 95% CI: 0.96 – 1.38). In addition, the relative risk for requirement for allogeneic blood transfusion was 1.10 (95% CI: 0.86 – 1.41), and the relative risk for acute kidney injury was 1.35 (95% CI: 0.58 – 3.14) [35MC].

GLOBULINS

Immunoglobulins [SEDA-15, 1719; SEDA-36, 488; SEDA-37, 409; SEDA-38, 342]

Intravenous Immunoglobulin

IVIG therapy is considered very safe, although systemic adverse effects occur in 20%–40% of patients. Typical adverse effects associated with IVIG include headaches, flushing, fever, nausea, diarrhea, urticaria, blood pressure change, and tachycardia, and are more likely to occur with a large infusion dose. Serious and potentially fatal side effects include anaphylactic reactions, aseptic meningitis, acute renal failure, and other thrombotic complications [36c]. A retrospective review of 13 studies including 70 patients with mucous membrane pemphigoid (MMP) treated with IVIG found that majority of studies reported mild adverse effects, while 2 studies did not report any side effects [37M]. An open-label study using Gammaplex in children aged 3–16 to treat primary immunodeficiency diseases found that mild adverse events occurred in 56% of patients, 26% of which were determined to be temporally related (≤72 hours after infusion) [38c].

Cardiovascular: Thromboembolic events are reported in 0.5%–15% of patients that receive IVIG. In a retrospective cohort study of 10 759 Medicare patients treated for chronic lymphocytic leukemia or multiple myeloma with

IVIG demonstrated a transient increased risk of arterial thrombosis during the day of IVIG infusion and the following day (HR: 3.40, 95% CI: 1.25–9.25). The arterial thrombosis risk declined over the remainder of the 30-day treatment period, and the 1-year period attributable risk was estimated as 0.7% (95% CI: −0.2% to 2%) [39MC].

A case report describing two patients diagnosed with common variable immunodeficiency (CVID) in their childhood received IVIG therapy and subsequently experienced a stroke 3–6 days afterward. Both patients were young (≤37 years old) and had minimal vascular risk factors. Neither patient experienced further stroke occurrence after treatment [40A].

Nervous System: A retrospective observational study in 70 patients with West Syndrome used IVIG to promote seizure cessation. Two patients experienced adverse effects (0.8%): the first patient became hypertensive and the second developed aseptic meningitis. Both adverse effects resolved after cessation of IVIG [41c].

Hematologic: Clinically significant hemolysis secondary to IVIG occurs in 1.6%–6.7% of infusions. A case report of a 63-year-old patient with chronic inflammatory demyelinating polyneuropathy was treated with IVIG for 3 days, when he experienced progressive jaundice. Hemolysis was confirmed through elevated reticulocytes, elevated bilirubin, elevated lactate dehydrogenase, and decreased haptoglobin. The patient was diagnosed with severe intravenous immune globulin induced hemolysis and pigment nephropathy, which was subsequently treated with partial red cell exchange with group O blood, which stabilized renal function and reduced hemoglobinuria [42A].

Hemolytic anemia following high dose IVIG has also been reported in association with the treatment of Kawasaki disease. A case report of a 2-month-old boy presented with symptoms and signs suggestive of incomplete Kawasaki disease. Treatment with high dose (2 g/kg) IVIG was used for 5 days; however, the child's hemoglobin and hematocrit began to drop. A direct Coombs' test was positive and indirect Coombs' test was negative, which led to the suspected development of hemolytic anemia. IVIG therapy was discontinued, and the patient recovered over the next 30 days [43A]. Another case report of a 10-month-old child with Kawasaki disease was also treated with high dose IVIG and developed severe hemolytic anemia [44A].

A post-hoc analysis of 102 pregnant women with fetal and neonatal alloimmune thrombocytopenia (FNAIT) examined the rate of anemia in different blood groups after administration of either high dose IVIG (2 g/kg/week) or low dose IVIG (1 g/kg/week)+0.5 mg/kg/day of prednisone. Women receiving 2 g/kg/week IVIG were more likely to have anemia (hemoglobin <10 g/dL) if they were blood group A and/or

B ($P = 0.0005$), compared to blood group O. Women receiving 1 g/kg/week+0.5 mg/kg/day of prednisone had the same rate of anemia, regardless of blood group. The mean decrease in hemoglobin was greater in blood group A and/or B (1.9 g/dL) compared to blood group O (1.1 g/dL, $P = 0.004$). Maternal blood groups may play a role in selecting the appropriate treatment for FNAIT [45C].

Drug Formulation: All immunoglobulins employed in IVIG formulations are derived from human blood donors and differ only in their purification methods. A retrospective study compared the different brands of IVIG (Flebogamma, IgVena, Gammagard, Kiovig) for the treatment of chronic inflammatory demyelinating polyradiculoneuropathy (CIDP) and multifocal motor neuropathy (MMN). There were no differences seen in the rate of adverse effects, and all adverse effects were transient [46c].

A case report described an incident in China, where 6 patients died after receiving IVIG products from a specific lot. An unusually high level of aggregates and microparticles contained in this particular lot led to a blockage of the pulmonary circulation and contributed to the fatalities [47c].

Nephrotoxicity associated with IVIG has been attributed to sucrose stabilizers added to some formulations. Sucrose-free IVIG is an option for patients being treated with IVIG that have unstable renal function. In a retrospective, matched cohort study, kidney transplant recipients receiving high-dose, sucrose-free IVIG were compared to recipients that did not receive any IVIG. Sucrose-free IVIG was not associated with any acute kidney injury episode at 3 months, but an increased frequency of tubular macrovacuoles (28% vs 2.8%, $P < 0.001$). Among the different sucrose-free IVIG formulations, patients treated with amino-acid-stabilized formulations developed fewer macrovacuoles at 3 months (12% vs 60%; $P < 0.001$) than those treated with carbohydrate-stabilized IVIG [48C]. In patients ≥60 years of age, sucrose-free IVIG administration is an independent risk factor for adverse effects, including renal failure [49C].

Subcutaneous Immunoglobulin

Subcutaneous immunoglobulin (SCIG) provides an alternative delivery method for patients that cannot tolerate the intravenous route, or require a formulation that can be administered at home. IVIG is administered every 34 weeks for replacement therapy, while SCIG is typically administered weekly. A novel formulation of SCIG uses hyaluronidase to facilitate absorption and allows for less frequent administration. Adverse effects with this novel formulation are milder compared to IVIG, but more severe compared with non-hyaluronidase SCIG. Adverse effects seen in a review study include flu-like symptoms, and transient, local inflammatory symptoms [50R]. An observational study with retrospective control group showed that there were changes in reported adverse effects between the 20% and 16% concentrations of SCIG [51C]. A retrospective case series of 19 patients treated with SCIG for polymyositis, dermatomyositis, and inclusion body myositis found patients experienced mild adverse effects including headache and local skin reactions [52c]. A meta-analysis of 8 studies examining the safety of SCIG as treatment for multifocal motor neuropathy, and chronic inflammatory demyelinating polyneuropathy, found that SCIG had similar efficacy to IVIG for treatment of these conditions. SCIG had a 28% reduction in relative risk of moderate and/or systemic adverse effects [53M]. An observational study of patients receiving SCIG for idiopathic inflammatory myopathies examined the quality of life and tolerance of patients who switched from IVIG to SCIG. Quality of life was determined to be unaffected by a difference in route, and most common adverse effects included injection site reactions (50%), cutaneous tissue disorders (18.2%), and nervous system disorders (13.6%) [54c].

Anti-D Immunoglobulin

The Serious Hazards of Transfusion (SHOT) conference highlighted the role of human error in transfusion-related incidents. There were 3288 incidents reported in the SHOT report published in *Transfusion Medicine*. Of these, 350 were associated with anti-D immunoglobulin, and 77% of these were related to late administration or omission. As a consequence, three women developed anti-D in the current pregnancy [55H].

COAGULATION PROTEINS [SEDA-36, 493; SEDA-37, 411; SEDA-38, 344]

Factor I

Plasma-derived or recombinant fibrinogen (factor I) is the final protein in the common pathway of the coagulation cascade, and rare adverse events have been reported with its administration. A meta-analysis of randomized control trials (RCTs) in adult and pediatric surgical patients identified 14 RCTs comprising of a total of 1035 patients between 2009 and 2016 [56M]. Of included trials, two trials were conducted in 2016. One evaluated the impact of factor I administration on transfusion requirements in liver transplantation and the other assessed effects of preoperative supplementation with fibrinogen concentrate on postoperative blood loss in cardiac surgery [57C,58C]. There was a lower non-statistically significant rate of any adverse events in comparison to placebo (68% vs 75%; $P = 0.644$). These included infectious, neurological, cardiac, and respiratory complications. There was a lower rate of thrombotic events in comparison to placebo (2.2% vs 11.4%, $P = 0.102$) [57C].

Factor II

A wide variety of topical agents are approved as potential therapies in the maintenance of hemostasis during surgical procedures. Topical thrombin may be either from a bovine or recombinant source. Thrombin plays a central role in coagulation, both activating platelets and cleaving fibrinogen. In a retrospective study of children with post-tonsillectomy bleeding, an absorbable gelatin-thrombin hemostatic matrix sealant demonstrated efficacy in preventing bleeding complications and was not associated with any adverse effects [59c].

Factor VIIa [SEDA-15, 1318; SEDA-36, 493; SEDA-37, 412; SEDA-38, 345]

Recombinant factor VIIa (rFVIIa) has a diverse range of labelled indications including use in congenital hemophilia A or B with inhibitors, congenital factor VII deficiency, acquired hemophilia, Glanzmann's thrombasthenia, and for the treatment of refractory bleeding after cardiac surgery in nonhemophiliac patients. Safety of rFVIIa was recently assessed in 30 patients under extracorporeal membrane oxygenation (ECMO) who received rFVIIa in comparison to a matched control [60c]. An efficacy rate of 93.3% was reported, while there were no statistically significant differences observed among groups with respect to thromboembolic events ($P = 0.00$), circuit change, ventilation time ($P = 0.71$), and infectious complications ($P = 0.61$), as well as survival at ECMO explantation [60c].

Factor VIII [SEDA-15, 1319; SEDA-36, 494; SEDA-37, 412; SEDA-38, 345]

Afstyla® is a recombinant antihemophilic factor indicated in pediatric and adult patients with congenital Factor VIII deficiency to control bleeding episodes and the management of perioperative bleeding as well as routine prophylaxis in reducing the frequency of bleeding episodes. Safety of Afstyla® was evaluated in 258 pediatric and adult patients with severe hemophilia A who received at least one dose of agent either as routine prophylaxis, for the treatment of active bleeding episodes or during the perioperative management of bleeding complications. Of the 28 492 injections of Afstyla®, the most common (>0.5%) adverse reactions reported were dizziness and hypersensitivity reactions. No events of anaphylaxis, thrombosis, or development of neutralizing antibodies to FVIII or antibodies to host cell proteins were reported [61S].

Kovaltry® is an unmodified, full-length recombinant human FVIII product with improved manufacturing technologies that have resulted in a rFVIII product with a consistent purity. In three clinical trials, Kovaltry® was used in patients with Hemophilia A either as prophylaxis and during surgery (LEOPOLD I/LEOPOLD II), and for the treatment of bleeds and surgical management (LEOPOLD kids). A total of 41 patients were assessed ($n = 25$, LEOPOLD I), ($n = 15$, LEOPOLD II), ($n = 1$, LEOPOLD kids) [16c]. In all 3 trials, there were no hemostasis-related complications and none of the patients developed FVIII inhibitors [62c].

Factor IX [SEDA-15, 1319; SEDA-36, 494; SEDA-37, 412; SEDA-38, 345]

Continuous intravenous infusion of recombinant factor IX (rFIX) was administered to a patient with hemophilia B during a coronary artery bypass grafting with cardiopulmonary bypass. Continuous infusion of rFIX appears to be more desirable in lieu of intermittent bolus dosing due to the decreased variability of serum factor concentrations as well as the decreased requirement of extrinsic factor administration in the perioperative setting. Authors reported no clinically significant complications during the infusion period [63A].

A recent development of a recombinant fusion protein that links rFIX with recombinant albumin (rIX-FP; Idelvion®) provides an extended half-life of factor IX with the inclusion of albumin (mean terminal half-life of 102 hours), while capitalizing on the function of the coagulation factor. Results of a recent phase III trial assessing the pharmacokinetic profile, efficacy, and safety of rIX-FP in 63 previously treated male patients with hemophilia B, demonstrated a 100% reduction in median annualized spontaneous bleeding rates and 100% resolution of target joints when patients were transitioned from an on-demand regimen and received prophylactic doses. There was a 98.6% success rate with respect to the treatment of bleeding episodes, no development of inhibitors was observed, and no additional safety concerns were noted [64c].

Prothrombin Complex Concentrate [SEDA-36, 494; SEDA-37, 412; SEDA-38, 345]

Cardiac surgery: A retrospective analysis aimed to assess the efficacy and safety of prothrombin complex concentrate (PCC) in comparison to FFP in patients undergoing cardiac surgery found no significant differences in the amount of bleeding within the first 12 hours from the end of the procedure [65c]. In patients who received PCC, there was a significantly higher volume of total blood loss at 24 hours when compared to patients who received FFP (median CI, 1213 mL [1244–1641]), $P = 0.0034$. Additionally, there were no differences in thrombotic events, acute kidney injury, or 30-day mortality reported between groups following surgery [65c].

The safety and efficacy of PCC when administered as a first-line agent in treatment of cardiac surgery associated bleeding were assessed in a recent Critical Care publication. After one-to-one propensity score-matching, this observational study included 225 patient pairs who received PCC. While PCC was associated with a lower risk of RBC transfusions (OR 0.50; 95% CI 0.31–0.80), patients who received PCC had an increased risk of post-operative acute kidney injury (OR 1.70, 95% CI 1.20–2.43, $P = 0.003$) as well as increased risk of renal replacement therapy (OR 3.35, 95% CI 1.13–9.90). This effect was not found to be dose dependent and may have been due to a hypovolemic balance with exclusive PCC administration in the setting of blood loss. FFP may have conversely provided a renal protective effect on the kidney with the administration of excess volume [66C].

von Willebrand Factor (vWF)/Factor VIII Concentrates [SEDA-36, 494; SEDA-37, 413; SEDA-38, 346]

The administration of sole recombinant human FVIII (rFVIII) may be associated with increased rates of inhibitor production. Administration of FVIII concentrate concomitantly with von Willebrand factor (VWF) aims to protect FVIII from phagocytosis by dendritic cells and perhaps lead to lower rates of inhibitor production against FVIII [67M,68c]. The association of thrombotic events and repeat administration of VWF/FVIII containing concentrates has also been suggested to be due to high concentrations of FVIII in combination products [67M].

Vocento® is a low-volume, high active, plasma-derived VWF (pdVWF)/FVIII concentrate indicated for the prophylaxis and treatment of bleeding events in subjects with haemophilia. A phase III, multi-center, double-blind, randomized, cross over trial evaluated the efficacy and safety of Vocento® in patients 12 years or older with haemophilia A who required treatment of non-surgical bleeds, treatment during surgical events, or who received Vocento for prophylaxis. In 81 patients assessed for efficacy and safety during exposure to Vocento®, 39 patients (48.1%) reported a total of 143 treatment emergent adverse events of which 18 events in 8 patients were considered to be possibly related to the administration of Vocento®. These included palpitations, constipation, oral paresthesia, asthenia, increased alanine aminotransferase (ALT), back pain, dysgeusia, anxiety, and skin burning sensation. Serious adverse events reported included hepatic echinococcosis, aggravation of pre-existing hypertension, and aggravation of pre-existing FVIII inhibitor production in one patient [68c].

Wilate®, is a double virus-inactivated, plasma-derived concentrate with native VWF and FVIII complex in a physiological 1:1 activity ratio. Its safety was prospectively assessed in the prevention and treatment of surgical bleeding in 28 patients with inherited VWD who underwent 30 surgical procedures. Eight non-serious adverse events in five patients reported included hypersensitivity reactions (including one with moderate severity leading to discontinuation of drug), chest discomfort, feeling hot, dizziness, and decrease in blood pressure. Hematoma formation was noted in the postoperative setting in three patients although none required intervention. No thromboembolic events or formation of factors to either VWF or FVIII were noted [69c].

Antithrombin III

Although no longer recommended in international guidelines, antithrombin supplementation is used to treat sepsis-induced disseminated intravascular coagulation (DIC) in Japan. In a retrospective study (J-SEPTIC DIC), patients in Japan with severe sepsis or septic shock who developed DIC in 42 intensive care units were evaluated. There were 461 propensity-matched pairs analyzed. The average antithrombin level prior to enrollment was 60% in the control group and 51% in the antithrombin group. When evaluating survival, the early in-hospital mortality rate for patients receiving antithrombin was lower compared to the control group ($P = 0.007$); however, the mortality rate was similar when comparing late in-hospital mortality. Importantly, the frequency of bleeding events requiring transfusion was higher in the antithrombin group compared to the control group, but severe bleeding complications were similar between the groups [70MC].

Similarly, in a Cochrane review of antithrombin III supplementation in critically ill patients, antithrombin was associated with an increased risk of bleeding, with a relative risk of 1.58 (95% CI 1.35–1.84, I^2 statistic = 0%, 11 trials, 3019 participants). In a subgroup analysis of patients receiving concomitant heparin, there was no statistical increase in bleeding seen in patients receiving antithrombin (RR: 0.95) [71M]. In another multicenter study of septic DIC patients with a reduced antithrombin level who received antithrombin, the rate of bleeding was heparins: 9.09% in patients receiving concomitant heparin and 3.03% in patients not receiving heparin, but this difference was not significant ($P = 0.224$) [72C].

ERYTHROPOIETIN AND DERIVATIVES [SEDA-36, 494; SEDA-37, 413; SEDA-38, 346]

Anemia is a common complication of chronic kidney disease (CKD) as well as cancer. In the setting of end stage renal disease (ESRD), erythropoietin-stimulating agents (ESAs) have an established role. In the setting of cancer, myelosuppressive chemotherapy complicates therapy and may induce anemia leading to need for blood transfusions, decreased quality of life, among other complications. Administration of ESAs including epoetin alfa and darbepoetin alfa (DA) increase hemoglobin levels and may decrease the need for transfusions.

Pediatrics: Adverse events were reported from a recent prospective observational registry study in pediatric patients 16 years of age or younger with CKD-related anemia who received DA. Of the 319 patients who were included, a total of 434 serious adverse events were reported. Among them, the most common were peritonitis, gastroenteritis, and hypertension. While six deaths occurred, authors concluded that they were unrelated to DA administration [73C].

THROMBOPOIETIN AND RECEPTOR AGONISTS [SEDA-15, 3409; SEDA-36-495; SEDA-37, 414; SEDA-38, 347]

The use of recombinant human thrombopoietin for immune thrombocytopenia (ITP) is limited by antibody production. Thrombopoietin receptor agonists (TPO-RAs), or thrombopoietin mimetics, bind directly to the thrombopoietin receptor, leading to increased platelet production and reduced bleeding risk. There are two agents currently available: romiplostim and eltrombopag. Both agents appear to be well tolerated. In clinical trials, romiplostim was rarely associated with headache, fever, and arthralgia, while nasopharyngitis, elevated alanine amino-transferase levels, and headaches were reported with eltrombopag [74H]. Both are very rarely associated with thrombosis, including pulmonary embolism, but mainly in patients with other risk factors. Although not yet proven, these agents are also associated with concerns of myelofibrosis and reversible reticulin deposition in bone marrow, leading to the possibility of malignancy [75H].

Cardiovascular: One potential safety concern with thrombopoeitin receptor agonists (TPO-RAs) is thrombosis. In a Cochrane review of patients with hematological malignancies undergoing intensive chemotherapy or stem cell transplantation, rates of thromboembolism ranged from 0% to 9.1% for patients treated with TPO-RAs compared to 5.9%–15.8% for patients treated with control, suggesting TPO-RAs did not increase thrombosis rates in these patients [76M]. However, in a retrospective study of 31 patients with refractory ITP who received TPO-RAs to improve platelet count prior to therapeutic splenectomy, 75% of patients achieved platelet count

increase, but two patients developed thrombosis. Due to the limited study design, an association between TPO-RAs and thrombosis cannot be ruled out [77c]. In addition, LaMoreaux and colleagues reported two cases of patients with antiphospholipid antibodies who received romiplostim for presumed ITP and developed catastrophic antiphospholipid syndrome. Both patients, one pediatric and one adult, were hospitalized for severe thrombotic complications. The authors recommend administering TPO-RAs cautiously to patients with positive antiphospholipid antibodies [78A].

Observational studies: In a phase-2, single-arm study of adults with newly diagnosed ITP treated with romiplostim for less than 12 months, the most common adverse events were headache (16%), arthralgia (15%), nasopharyngitis (12%), haematoma (11%), petechiae (9%) and epistaxis (8%). Serious adverse effects included gastritis, increased transaminases and reversible ischaemic neurological deficit, and occurred in one patient each [79c]. In a multicenter, retrospective study of 124 patients treated with TPO-RAs for ITP, the most frequent reason for discontinuation was failure of treatment. Thrombotic events occurred in 2% of patients treated with romiplostim and 3% with eltrombopag [80c].

Tarantino and colleagues described a phase-3, placebo-controlled, double-blind study of 62 pediatric patients with chronic ITP receiving weekly romiplostim injection for 24 weeks. Serious adverse effects occurred in 24% of patients receiving romiplostim, and included epistaxis, contusion, and headache, bronchiolitis, nausea, petechiae, epilepsy, fever, thrombocytosis, urinary tract infection, and vomiting [81c]. In another retrospective study of 79 pediatric patients treated with TPO-RAs for ITP (ICON2 study), there were two pulmonary emboli reported, but neither patient experienced thrombocytosis [82c].

Major review: In a meta-analysis of 13 studies including 1126 ITP patients, there were no differences in serious adverse events in those receiving TPO-RAs or control therapy. Specifically, there was no signal of thrombosis, bone marrow reticulin increases, or the generation of neutralizing antibodies to TPO-RAs [83R].

Pregnancy: There is limited data supporting the safety of TPO-RAs in pregnancy. Purushothaman and colleagues described a case of a 27-year-old multigravida with known ITP who presented at 26 weeks gestation with muscosal bleeding and reduced platelet count. She was started on eltrombopag, which maintained her platelet count between 30–50 000/μL, and she delivered at 36 weeks gestation. The authors state that the mother and baby were in good health at the time of hospital discharge, and there were no adverse effects associated with eltrombopag administration in the third trimester of pregnancy [84A].

Transmission of Infectious Agents Through Blood Donation [SEDA-36, 495; SEDA-37, 414; SEDA-38, 347]

A database was created from the voluntary records of the major blood donation centers in the United States. In an analysis of 14.8 million blood donations over a 2-year period, the overall frequency of surveillance-positive donations of hepatitis B virus was 0.757 per 10 000; hepatitis C virus was 2.007 per 10 000; and human immunodeficiency virus was 0.282 per 10 000 [85MC]. Strategies to reduce infectious complications of transfusions are currently under investigation. For example, the Mirasol Pathogen Reduction Technology system has been in use in Poland in 2009. In a report on hemovigilance data, there appear to be no difference in adverse reaction rates, including infectious complications, between transfusions taking place during the Mirasol time period or the period prior to institution of the technology [86MC]. Randomized controlled trials are underway (PREPAReS trial) to test the safety and efficacy of pathogen-reduced platelet concentrates treated with the Mirasol system [87S].

Virus: In 2016, the Center for Disease Control reported that there have been no reported cases of Zika virus transmission via blood transfusion in Puerto Rico or the US mainland, but during periods of outbreak, Zika virus nucleic acid was detected retrospectively in 2.8% of asymptomatic blood donors in French Polynesia, and transfusion-related Zika virus infection was reported in Brazil [88S].

STEM CELLS [SEDA-36, 496; SEDA-37, 415; SEDA-38, 348]

Hematopoietic stem cell transplant (HSCT) is a well-established treatment for many malignant and nonmalignant conditions. Research in the field has led to increased understanding of the effects of donor selection, graft-vs-host disease (GVHD), and conditioning regimens, which has contributed to decreased long-term adverse effects [89M]. Advances in transplantation techniques have led to improved survival rates and reduced incidence of complications like GVHD, thus lowering the rates of transplant-related morbidity and mortality [90M]. Despite these advances in stem cell therapy, adverse reactions (ADRs) during the infusion of cellular products still occurs, and late effects of infusion include GVHD, infections, secondary malignancies, respiratory disease and cardiovascular disease [91R]. A retrospective observational study in children determined that an independent risk factor for a serious ADR included stem cell source, while the use of manipulated cellular therapy products was protective. White blood cell count and granulocyte content were not found to be risk factors [92C].

GVHD: GVHD is a major complication of hematopoietic stem cell transplants (HSCT), associated with increased morbidity and mortality [93R]. A retrospective study compared patients with early acute GHVD to patients with late acute GVHD who all underwent allogeneic HSCT between 2007 and 2012. Overall 2-year survival was 59% in late acute GVHD, vs 50% in those with early acute GVHD. Only the development of grade III or IV early onset acute GVHD was associated with higher high of developing late acute GVHD; age, graft source, and conditioning intensity had no independent effect on the risk of late acute GVHD. 100-day mortality was no different between groups (HR 0.96; 95% CI: 0.59–1.55; $P = 0.85$); however, the risk of chronic GVHD was doubled in patients with late acute GVHD (HR 1.81; 95% CI: 1.16–2.82; $P = 0.01$) [94C]. This mortality rate is comparable to other studies of similar populations [95C]. A different study found that late acute GVHD and bronchiolitis obliterans had particularly high 2-year mortality rates [96C].

Endocrine: It is known that the endocrine system is damaged by HSCT preparative regimens using high dose chemotherapy and irradiation. Metabolic syndrome is prevalent, occurring in 31%–49% of HSCT recipients [97R]. A retrospective study examining 114 children and adults that received reduced intensity conditioning found that despite the reduced regimen, children and adults still had significant deficits in height, vitamin D levels, and thyroid function [98C]. Bone mineral density loss occurs early after HSCT and is affected by steroids, vitamin D, and chronic GVHD. Younger age and higher pre-transplant body mass index are protective against osteopenia/osteoporosis and play an influential role in recovery [99C].

Hematopoietic stem cell transplant-associated thrombotic microangiopathy (TA-TMA) is a complex disorder that occurs in ~30% of HSCT recipients [100R]. Presentation of TA-TMA can include thrombocytopenia, hemolysis, acute renal failure, and involvement of other organs. Due to suboptimal treatment options, mortality rate is high [101R]. Complement modifying therapy (i.e. eculizumab) is the most promising treatment option at this time [101R].

Cardiopulmonary: Venous thromboembolism (VTE) is becoming an increasingly more recognized problem in patients receiving HSCT. Risk factors for VTE in HSCT patients include history of VTE, GVHD, infections and indwelling catheters [102R]. Arrhythmias also occur within the first 100 days of HSCT, as well as long-term. A retrospective study examining the cardiovascular health outcomes of patients undergoing HSCT found that patients experiencing an arrhythmia after HSCT had longer hospital stays (32 days vs 23 days, $P < 0.001$) and had a greater chance of being admitted to the medical intensive care unit (52% vs 7%, $P < 0.001$), compared to those patients that did not experience an arrhythmia. Patients with arrhythmia had greater probability of death within 1 year of transplant (41% vs 15%, $P < 0.001$) [103C].

Pleural effusion is a rare complication of HSCT recipients. A retrospective review of 618 patients receiving allogeneic HSCT between 2008 and 2013, found 71 patients experienced pleural effusion (cumulative incidence 9.9% at 1 year). Pleural effusion was most commonly associated with infections, volume overload, and chronic GVHD. Higher comorbidity index ($P = 0.03$) and active GVHD ($P = 0.018$) were both independent risk factors for pleural effusion development [104C]. A case report of pulmonary hypertension as a complication of HSCT also suggests high mortality rates [105c].

References

[1] Italian Association for the Study of the Liver (AISF), Italian Society of Transfusion Medicine and Immunohaematology (SIMTI). AISF-SIMTI position paper: the appropriate use of albumin in patients with liver cirrhosis. Dig Liver Dis. 2016;48(1):4–15 [R].

[2] Kutting F, Schubert J, Franklin J, et al. Insufficient evidence of benefit regarding mortality due to albumin substitution in HCC-free cirrhotic patients undergoing large volume paracentesis. J Gastroenterol Hepatol. 2016;32(2):327–38 [M].

[3] Zazzeron L, Gattinoni L, Caironi P. Role of albumin, starches and gelatins versus crystalloids in volume resuscitation of critically ill patients. Curr Opin Crit Care. 2016;22(5):428–36 [R].

[4] Blasi A, Cid J, Beltran J, et al. Coagulation profile after plasma exchange using albumin as a replacement solution measured by thromboelastometry. Vox Sang. 2016;110(2):159–65 [c].

[5] Rasmussen KC, Hojskov M, Johansson PI, et al. Impact of albumin on coagulation competence and hemorrhage during major surgery: a randomized controlled trial. Medicine. 2016;95(9):e2720 [c].

[6] Jamtgaard L, Manning SL, Cohn B. Does albumin infusion reduce renal impairment and mortality in patients with spontaneous bacterial peritonitis? Ann Emerg Med. 2016;67(4):458–9 [M].

[7] Tan HK, James PD, Wong F. Albumin may prevent the morbidity of paracentesis-induced circulatory dysfunction in cirrhosis and refractory ascites: a pilot study. Dig Dis Sci. 2016;61(10):3084–92 [c].

[8] Martin DK, Walayat S, Jinma R, et al. Large-volume paracentesis with indwelling peritoneal catheter and albumin infusion: a community hospital study. J Community Hosp Intern Med Perspect. 2016;6(5):32421 [c].

[9] Lee EH, Kim WJ, Kim JY, et al. Effect of exogenous albumin on the incidence of postoperative acute kidney injury in patients undergoing off-pump coronary artery bypass surgery with a preoperative albumin level of less than 4.0 g/dl. Anesthesiology. 2016;124(5):1001–11 [C].

[10] Subramaniam K, Spilsbury K, Ayonrinde OT, et al. Red blood cell transfusion is associated with further bleeding and fresh-frozen plasma with mortality in nonvariceal upper gastrointestinal bleeding. Transfusion. 2016;56(4):816–26 [c].

[11] Wang Y, Shi X, Du R, et al. Impact of red blood cell transfusion on acute coronary syndrome: a meta-analysis. Intern Emerg Med. 2016. http://dx.doi.org/10.1007/s11739-016-1594-4 [Epub ahead of print] [M].

[12] Estcourt LJ, Stanworth SJ, Hopewell S, et al. Granulocyte transfusions for treating infections in people with neutropenia or neutrophil dysfunction. Cochrane Database Syst Rev. 2016;4: CD005339 [M].

[13] Yoshihara S, Ikemoto J, Fujimori Y. Update on granulocyte transfusions: accumulation of promising data, but still lack of decisive evidence. Curr Opin Hematol. 2016;23:55–60 [R].

[14] Murphy MF, Gill R, Moss R, et al. Spotlight on platelets: summary of BBTS combined special interest group autumn meeting, November 2015. Transfus Med. 2016;26(1):8–14 [H].

[15] Estcourt LJ, Birchall J, Allard S, et al. Guidelines for the use of platelet transfusions. Br J Haematol. 2016;176:365–94 [H].

[16] Schmidt AE, Refaai MA, Blumberg N. Platelet transfusion and thrombosis: more questions than answers. Semin Thromb Hemost. 2016;42:118–24 [H].

[17] Baharoglu MI, Cordonnier C, Salman RA, et al. Platelet transfusion versus standard care after acute stroke due to spontaneous cerebral haemorrhage associated with antiplatelet therapy (PATCH): a randomised, open-label, phase 3 trial. Lancet. 2016;387:2605–13 [C].

[18] Lee TH, Wong JGX, Leo YS, et al. Potential harm of prophylactic platelet transfusion in adult dengue patients. PLoS Negl Trop Dis. 2016;10(3), e0004576 [c].

[19] Yanagisawa R, Shimodaira S, Sakashita K, et al. Factors related to allergic transfusion reactions and febrile non-haemolytic transfusion reactions in children. Vox Sang. 2016;110:376–84 [C].

[20] Estcourt LJ, Birchall J, Allard S, et al. Guidelines for the use of platelet transfusions. Br J Haematol. 2016;176:365–94 [H].

[21] Benjamin RJ. Transfusion-related sepsis: a silent epidemic. 2016; 127:380–1 [r].

[22] Hong H, Xiao W, Lazarus HM, et al. Detection of septic transfusion reactions to platelet transfusions by active and passive surveillance. Blood. 2016;127(4):496–502 [MC].

[23] Motta IJF, Spencer BR, Cordeiro da Silva SG, et al. Evidence for transmission of Zika virus by platelet transfusion. N Engl J Med. 2016;375:1101–3 [r].

[24] Estcourt LJ, Birchall J, Allard S, et al. Guidelines for the use of platelet transfusions. Br J Haematol. 2016;176:365–94 [H].

[25] Weiskopf RB, Beliaev AM, Shander A, et al. Addressing the unmet need of life-threatening anemia with hemoglobin-based oxygen carriers. Transfusion. 2017;57(1):207–14 [r].

[26] Silkstone GGA, Silkstone RS, Wilson MT, et al. Engineering tyrosine electron transfer pathways decreases oxidative toxicity in hemoglobin: implications for blood substitute design. Biochem J. 2016;473:3371–83 [E].

[27] Strauss RM, Benzaquen DN, Horesh O. Alpha-1 antitrypsin therapy is safe and well tolerated in children and adolescents with recent onset type 1 diabetes mellitus. Pediatr Diabetes. 2016;17:351–9 [c].

[28] No authors. A recombinant C1 esterase inhibitor (Ruconest) for hereditary angioedema. Med Lett Drugs Ther. 2016;58(1491): e44–5 [c].

[29] Frontera J, Lewin III JJ, Rabinstein AA, et al. Guideline for reversal of antithrombotics in intracranial hemorrhage. Neurocrit Care. 2016;24:6–46.

[30] Steiner T, Poli S, Griebe M. Fresh frozen plasma versus prothrombin complex concentrate in patients with intracranial haemorrhage related to vitamin K antagonists (INCH): a randomised trial. Lancet Neurol. 2016;15:566–73 [c].

[31] Rasmussen KC, Secher NH, Pedersen T. Effect of perioperative crystalloid or colloid fluid therapy on hemorrhage, coagulation competence, and outcome: a systematic review and stratified meta-analysis. Medicine. 2016;95(31):e4498 [M].

[32] Rasmussen KC, Secher NH, Pedersen T. Effect of perioperative crystalloid or colloid fluid therapy on hemorrhage, coagulation competence, and outcome A systematic review and stratified meta-analysis. Medicine. 2016;95(31):e4498 [M].

[33] Kim SK, Choi SS, Sim JH, et al. Effect of hydroxyethyl starch on acute kidney injury after living donor hepatectomy. Transplant Proc. 2016;48:102–6 [c].

[34] Pisano A, Landoni G, Bellomo R. The risk of infusing gelatin? Die-hard misconceptions and forgotten (or ignored) truths. Minerva Anestesiol. 2016;82(10):1107–14 [r].

[35] Moeller C, Fleischmann C, Thomas-Rueddel D, et al. How safe is gelatin? A systematic review and meta-analysis of gelatin-containing plasma expanders vs. crystalloids and albumin. J Crit Care. 2016;35:75–83 [MC].

[36] Moon KP, Kim BJ, Lee KJ, et al. Prediction of nonresponsiveness to medium-dose intravenous immunoglobulin (1 g/kg) treatment: an effective and safe schedule of acute treatment for Kawasaki disease. Korean J Pediatr. 2016;59(4):178–82 [c].

[37] Tavakolpour S. The role of intravenous immunoglobulin in treatment of mucous membrane pemphigoid: a review of literature. J Res Med Sci. 2016;21:37 [M].

[38] Melamed IR, Gupta S, Stratford Bobbitt M, et al. Efficacy and safety of Gammaplex(®) 5% in children and adolescents with primary immunodeficiency diseases. Clin Exp Immunol. 2016;184(2):228–36 [c].

[39] Ammann EM, Jones MP, Link BK, et al. Intravenous immune globulin and thromboembolic adverse events in patients with hematologic malignancy. Blood. 2016;127(2):200–7 [MC].

[40] Nakano Y, Hayashi T, Deguchi K, et al. Two young stroke patients associated with regular intravenous immunoglobulin (IVIg) therapy. J Neurol Sci. 2016;361(15):9–12 [A].

[41] Matsuura R, Hamano S, Hirata Y, et al. Intravenous immunoglobulin therapy is rarely effective as the initial treatment in West syndrome: A retrospective study of 70 patients. J Neurol Sci. 2016;368(15):140–4 [c].

[42] Lasica M, Zantomio D. Severe intravenous immunoglobulin-induced hemolysis with pigment nephropathy managed with red cell exchange. J Clin Apher. 2016;31(5):464–6 [A].

[43] Kim NY, Kim JH, Park JS, et al. A 2-month-old boy with hemolytic anemia and reticulocytopenia following intravenous immunoglobulin therapy for Kawasaki disease: a case report and literature review. Korean J Pediatr. 2016;59(Suppl 1):S60–3 [A].

[44] Tocan V, Inaba A, Kurano T, et al. Severe hemolytic anemia following intravenous immunoglobulin in an infant with kawasaki disease. J Pediatr Hematol Oncol. 2017;39(2):e100–2 [A].

[45] Lakkaraja M, Jin JC, Manotas KC, et al. Blood group A mothers are more likely to develop anemia during antenatal intravenous immunoglobulin treatment of fetal and neonatal alloimmune thrombocytopenia. Transfusion. 2016;56(10):2449–54 [C].

[46] Gallia F, Balducci C, Nobile-Orazio E. Efficacy and tolerability of different brands of intravenous immunoglobulin in the maintenance treatment of chronic immune-mediated neuropathies. J Peripher Nerv Syst. 2016;21(2):82–4 [c].

[47] Yu CF, Hou JF, Shen LZ, et al. Acute pulmonary embolism caused by highly aggregated intravenous immunoglobulin. Vox Sang. 2016;110(1):27–35 [c].

[48] Luque Y, Anglicheau D, Rabant M, et al. Renal safety of high-dose, sucrose-free intravenous immunoglobulin in kidney transplant recipients: an observational study. Transpl Int. 2016;29(11):1205–15 [C].

[49] Lozeron P, Not A, Theaudin M, et al. Safety of intravenous immunoglobulin in the elderly treated for a dysimmune neuromuscular disease. Muscle Nerve. 2016;53(5):683–9 [C].

[50] Bonilla FA. Intravenous and subcutaneous immunoglobulin G replacement therapy. Allergy Asthma Proc. 2016;37(6):426–31 [R].

[51] Canessa C, Iacopelli J, Pecoraro A, et al. Shift from intravenous or 16% subcutaneous replacement therapy to 20% subcutaneous immunoglobulin in patients with primary antibody deficiencies. Int J Immunopathol Pharmacol. 2017;30:73–82. pii: 0394632016681577, [C].

[52] Cherin P, Belizna C, Cartry O, et al. Long-term subcutaneous immunoglobulin use in inflammatory myopathies: a retrospective review of 19 cases. Autoimmun Rev. 2016;15(3):281–6 [c].

[53] Racosta JM, Sposato LA, Kimpinski K. Subcutaneous vs. intravenous immunoglobulin for chronic autoimmune neuropathies: a meta-analysis. Muscle Nerve. 2017;55(6):802–9. http://dx.doi.org/10.1002/mus.25409 [M].

[54] Hachulla E, Benveniste O, Hamidou M, et al. High dose subcutaneous immunoglobulin for idiopathic inflammatory myopathies and dysimmune peripheral chronic neuropathies treatment: observational study of quality of life and tolerance. Int J Neurosci. 2016;14:1–8 [c].

[55] Bolton-Maggs PHB. SHOT conference report 2016: serious hazards of transfusion—human factors continue to cause most transfusion-related incidents. Transfus Med. 2016;26:401–5 [H].

[56] Fominskiy E, Nepomniashchikh VA, Lomivorotov VV, et al. Efficacy and safety of fibrinogen concentrate in surgical patients: a meta-analysis of randomized controlled trials. J Cardiothorac Vasc Anesth. 2016;30(5):1196–204 [M].

[57] Sabate A, Gutierrez R, Beltran PM, et al. Impact of preemptive fibrinogen concentrate on transfusion requirements in liver transplantation: a multicenter, randomized, double-blind, placebo-controlled trial. Am J Transplant. 2016;16:2421–9 [C].

[58] Jeppsson A, Walden K, Roman-Emmanuel C, et al. Preoperative supplementation with fibrinogen concentrate in cardiac surgery: a randomized controlled study. Br J Anaesth. 2016;116:208–14 [C].

[59] Binnetoglu A, Demir B, Yumusakhuylu AC, et al. Use of a gelatin-thrombin hemostatic matrix for secondary bleeding after pediatric tonsillectomy. JAMA Otolaryngol Head Neck Surg. 2016;142(10):954–8 [c].

[60] Anselmi A, Guinet P, Ruggieri VG, et al. Safety of recombinant factor VIIa in patients under extracorporeal membrane oxygenation. Eur J Cardiothorac Surg. 2016;49(1):78–84 [c].

[61] Afstyla® [package insert]. Kankakee, IL. CSL Behring LLC; 2016, [S].

[62] Oldenburg J, Windyga J, Hampton K. Safety and efficacy of BAY 81–8973 for surgery in previously treated patients with haemophilia A: results of LEOPOLD clinical trial programme. Haemophilia. 2016;22:349–53 [c].

[63] Suzuki T, Kawamoto S, Kumagai K. Coronary artery bypass grafting in a patient with hemophilia B: continuous recombinant factor IX infusion as per the Japanese guidelines for replacement therapy. Gen Thorac Cardiovasc Surg. 2016;64:481–3 [A].

[64] Santagostino E, Martinowitz U, Lissitchkov L. Long-acting recombinant coagulation factor IX albumin fusion protein (rIX-FP) in hemophilia B: results of a phase 3 trial. Blood. 2016;127(14):1761–9 [c].

[65] Arachchillage DJ, Deplano S, Dunnett E, et al. Efficacy and safety of prothrombin complex concentrate in patients undergoing major cardiac surgery. Blood. 2016;128:3852 [c].

[66] Cappabianca G, Mariscalco G, Biancari F, et al. Safety and efficacy of prothrombin complex concentrate as first-line treatment in bleeding after cardiac surgery. Crit Care. 2016;20:5 [C].

[67] Harper P, Favaloro EJ, Curtin J, et al. Human plasma-derived FVIII/VWD concentrate (Biostate): a review of experimental and clinical pharmacokinetic, efficacy and safety data. Drugs Context. 2016;5:212292 [M].

[68] Skotnicki A, Lissitchkov T, Manonov V, et al. Efficacy, safety, and pharmacokinetic profiles of a plasma-derived VWFFVIII concentrate (VONCENTO®) in subjects with haemophilia A (SWIFT-HA study). Thromb Res. 2016;137:119–25. http://dx.doi.org/10.1016/j.thromres.2015.10.014 [c].

[69] Srivastava A, Serban M, Werner S, et al. Efficacy and safety of a VWF/FVIII concentrate (Wilate®) in inherited von Willebrand disease patients undergoing surgical procedures. Haemophilia. 2017;23:264–72 [c].

[70] Hayakawa M, Kudo D, Saito S, et al. Antithrombin supplementation and mortality in sepsis-induced disseminated intravascular coagulation: a multicenter retrospective observational study. Shock. 2016;46(6):623–31 [MC].

[71] Allingstrup M, Wetterslev J, Ravn FB, et al. Antithrombin III for critically ill patients. Cochrane Database Syst Rev. 2016;2: CD005370 [M].

[72] Iba T, Gando S, Saitoh D, et al. Efficacy and bleeding risk of antithrombin supplementation in patients with septic

disseminated intravascular coagulation: a third survey. Clin Appl Thromb Hemost. 2017;23:422–8. http://dx.doi.org/10.1177/1076029616648405 [C].

[73] Schaefer F, Hoppe B, Jungraithmayr T, et al. Safety and usage of darbepoetin alfa in children with chronic kidney disease: prospective registry study. Pediatr Nephrol. 2016;31:443–53 [C].

[74] Nomura S. Advances in diagnosis and treatments for immune thrombocytopenia. Clin Med Insights Blood Disord. 2016;9:15–22 [H].

[75] Gutti U, Pasupuleti SR, Sahu I, et al. Erythropoietin and thrombopoietin mimetics: natural alternatives to erythrocyte and platelet disorders. Crit Rev Oncol Hematol. 2016;108:175–86 [H].

[76] Desborough M, Estcourt LJ, Doree C, et al. Alternatives, and adjuncts, to prophylactic platelet transfusion for people with haematological malignancies undergoing intensive chemotherapy or stem cell transplantation. Cochrane Database Syst Rev. 2016;(8). Article No. CD010982 [M].

[77] Zaja F, Barcellini W, Cantoni S, et al. Thrombopoietin receptor agonists for preparing adult patients with immune thrombocytopenia to splenectomy: results of a retrospective, observational GIMEMA study. Am J Hematol. 2016;91:E293–5 [c].

[78] LaMoreaux B, Barbar-Smiley F, Ardoin S, et al. Two cases of thrombosis in patients with antiphospholipid antibodies during treatment of immune thrombocytopenia with romiplostim, a thrombopoietin receptor agonist. Semin Arthritis Rheum. 2016;45:e10–2 [A].

[79] Newland A, Godeau B, Priego V, et al. Remission and platelet responses with romiplostim in primary immune thrombocytopenia: final results from a phase 2 study. Br J Haematol. 2016;172:262–73 [c].

[80] Mazza O, Minoia C, Melpignano A, et al. The use of thrombopoietin-receptor agonists (TPO-RAs) in immune thrombocytopenia (ITP): a "real life" retrospective multicenter experience of the Rete Ematologica Pugliese (REP). Ann Hematol. 2016;95:239–44 [c].

[81] Tarantino MD, Bussel JB, Blanchette VS, et al. Romiplostim in children with immune thrombocytopenia: a phase 3, randomized, double-blind, placebo-controlled study. Lancet. 2016;388:45–54 [c].

[82] Neunert C, Despotovic J, Haley K, et al. Thrombopoietin receptor agonist use in children: data from the Pediatric ITP Consortium of North America ICON2 Study. Pediatr Blood Cancer. 2016;63:1407–13 [c].

[83] Wang L, Gao Z, Chen X, et al. Efficacy and safety of thrombopoietin receptor agonists in patients with primary immune thrombocytopenia: A systematic review and meta-analysis. Sci Rep. 2016;6:39003. http://dx.doi.org/10.1038/srep39003 [R].

[84] Purushothaman J, Puthumana KJ, Kumar A, et al. A case of refractory immune thrombocytopenia in pregnancy managed with elthrombopag. Asian J Transfus Sci. 2016;10(2):155–8 [A].

[85] Dodd RY, Notari EP, Nelson D, et al. Development of a multisystem surveillance database for transfusion-transmitted infections among blood donors in the United States. Transfusion. 2016;56:2781–9 [MC].

[86] LeRtowska M, Przybylska Z, Piotrowski D, et al. Hemovigilance survey of pathogen-reduced blood components in the Warsaw Region in the 2009 to 2013 period. Transfusion. 2016;56:S39–44 [MC].

[87] Ypma PF, van der Meer PF, Heddle NM, et al. A study protocol for a randomised controlled trial evaluating clinical effects of platelet transfusion products: the Pathogen Reduction Evaluation and Predictive Analytical Rating Score (PREPAReS) trial. BMJ Open. 2016;6:e010156. http://dx.doi.org/10.1136/bmjopen-2015-010156 [S].

[88] Vasquez AM, Sapiano MRP, Basavaraju SV, et al. Survey of blood collection centers and implementation of guidance for prevention of transfusion-transmitted Zika virus infection—Puerto Rico, 2016. MMR Weekly. 2016;65(14):375–8 [S].

[89] Singh AK, McGuirk JP. Allogenic stem cell transplantation: a historical and scientific overview. Cancer Res. 2016;76(22):6445–51 [M].

[90] Parmesar K, Raj K. Haploidentical stem cell transplantation in adult haematological malignancies. Adv Hematol. 2016;2016:3905907 [M].

[91] Mosesso K. Adverse late and long-term treatment effects in adult allogeneic hematopoietic stem cell transplant survivors. Am J Nurs. 2015;115(11):22–34 [R].

[92] Truong TH, Moorjani R, Dewey D, et al. Adverse reactions during stem cell infusion in children treated with autologous and allogeneic stem cell transplantation. Bone Marrow Transplant. 2016;51:680–6 [C].

[93] Villarreal CD, Alanis JC, Perez JC, et al. Cutaneous graft-versus-host disease after hematopoietic stem cell transplant—a review. An Bras Dermatol. 2016;91(3):336–43 [R].

[94] Omer AK, Weisdorf DJ, Lazaryan A, et al. Late acute graft-versus-host disease after allogeneic hematopoietic stem cell transplantation. Biol Blood Marrow Transplant. 2016;22(5):879–83 [C].

[95] Holtan SG, Khera N, Levine JE, et al. Late acute graft versus host disease: a prospective analysis of clinical outcomes and circulating angiogenic factors. Blood. 2016;128(19):2350–8 [C].

[96] Arora M, Cutler CS, Jagasia MH, et al. Late acute and chronic graft-versus-host disease after allogeneic hematopoietic cell transplantation. Biol Blood Marrow Transplant. 2016;22(3):449–55 [C].

[97] DeFilipp Z, Duarte RF, Snowden JA, et al. Metabolic syndrome and cardiovascular disease following hematopoietic cell transplantation: screening and preventive practice recommendations from CIBMTR and EBMT. Bone Marrow Transplant. 2016;22:1493–503. http://dx.doi.org/10.1038/bmt.2016.203 [R].

[98] Myers KC, Howell JC, Wallace G, et al. Poor growth, thyroid dysfunction and vitamin D deficiency remain prevalent despite reduced intensity chemotherapy for hematopoietic stem cell transplantation in children and young adults. Bone Marrow Transplant. 2016;51(7):980–4 [C].

[99] Anandi P, Jain NA, Tian X, et al. Factors influencing the late phase of recovery after bone mineral density loss in allogeneic stem cell transplantation survivors. Bone Marrow Transplant. 2016;51:1101–6 [C].

[100] Jodele S, Dandoy CE, Myers KC, et al. New approaches in the diagnosis, pathophysiology, and treatment of pediatric hematopoietic stem cell transplantation-associated thrombotic microangiopathy. Transfus Apher Sci. 2016;54(2):181–90 [R].

[101] Elsallabi O, Bhatt VR, Dhakal P, et al. Hematopoietic stem cell transplant-associated thrombotic microangiopathy. Clin Appl Thromb Hemost. 2016;22(1):12–20 [R].

[102] Chaturvedi S, Neff A, Nagler A, et al. Venous thromboembolism in hematopoietic stem cell transplant recipients. Bone Marrow Transplant. 2016;51(4):473–8 [C].

[103] Blaes A, Konety S, Hurley P. Cardiovascular complications of hematopoietic stem cell transplantation. Curr Treat Options Cardiovasc Med. 2016;18(4):25 [C].

[104] Modi D, Jang H, Kim S, et al. Incidence, etiology, and outcome of pleural effusions in allogeneic hematopoietic stem cell transplantation. Am J Hematol. 2016;91(9):E341–7 [C].

[105] Pate A, Rotz S, Warren M, et al. Pulmonary hypertension associated with bronchiolitis obliterans after hematopoietic stem cell transplantation. Bone Marrow Transplant. 2016;51:310–2 [c].

30

Vitamins, Amino Acids and Drugs and Formulations Used in Nutrition

Sara Al-Dahir, Nisha Vithlani†, Anna Smith†, Jon F. Davis‡,
Sunil Sirohi†,1*

*College of Pharmacy, Xavier University of Louisiana, New Orleans, LA, United States
†Laboratory of Endocrine and Neuropsychiatric Disorders, College of Pharmacy, Xavier University of Louisiana,
New Orleans, LA, United States
‡Washington State University, Pullman, WA, United States
1Corresponding author: ssirohi@xula.edu; sirohilab@outlook.com

VITAMIN A [SEDA-35, 607, SEDA-36, 503; SEDA-38, 355]

A review of randomized controlled clinical trial studies published from 1993 to 2015 concluded that contrary to the popular belief, intake of vitamin A, E, D, C and folic acid in high-dose could actually be detrimental to the health [1M].

A 20-year-old female (52 kg) was presented to a Psychiatric clinic with symptoms of decreased appetite, irritability, grandiosity and sleep disturbance. Physical examination revealed acne on the forehead. She was receiving isotretinoin 20 mg/day for acne vulgaris, 45 days before admission and admitted taking isotretinoin three times a day without prior authorization for the last 15 days. Based on the International Classification of Diseases (ICD-10), the patient was diagnosed with isotretinoin-induced psychosis manic [2A].

This study investigated macular degeneration as a result of daily intake of vitamins and minerals using a 198-item food frequency questionnaire in 848 subjects (30–60 years). The study reported a heightened risk of macular drusen (>63 μm; odd ratio = 1.82, CL_{95} = 1.02–3.24, $P = 0.042$) as a result of an increase in intake of vitamin A, when adjusted for age, group and gender. A significant interaction with CFHY402H (age-related macular degeneration-related polymorphisms in complement factor H gene; $P = 0.038$) was also reported. Authors concluded that higher vitamin A intake increases macular drusen risk in subjects with CFHY402H [3C].

An article summarizing several clinical cases of ocular side effects following Isotretinoin (vitamin A derivative) therapy has been presented [4A].

- A 39-year-old female patient reported blurred vision, dry eyes, transient loss of some parts of the visual field, facial and lips erythema. She was taking 20 mg/kg of Isotretinoin daily for 7.5 weeks. Several abnormalities were recorded, which included punctate corneal staining, conjunctival hyperemia, Meibomian gland dysfunction and changes in the shape of cornea. These symptoms disappeared after seven and half weeks of Isotretinoin discontinuation.

- A 19-year-old female patient was presented with painless and sudden vision loss in her left eye. She was taking oral 30 mg/kg of Isotretinoin daily for 4 months. Further investigation revealed premacular hemorrhage, which disappeared following discontinuation of Isotretinoin treatment, indicating that the adverse reaction was linked to Isotretinoin treatment.

- A 19-year-old male patient reported a sudden and multiple episodes of right eye ptosis which were later accompanied by double vision. The patient was taking oral 1 mg/kg Isotretinoin daily for 6 months. Testing revealed antibodies against thyroid-stimulating hormone (TSH) receptors, thyroiditis and ocular myasthenia gravis, which indicated a relationship with Isotretinoin therapy as other causal or predisposing factors were absent in this case.

Side Effects of Drugs Annual, Volume 39
ISSN: 0378-6080
http://dx.doi.org/10.1016/bs.seda.2017.06.012

An in vitro study shedding light on the mechanism by which retinoic acid-induced side effects (skin dryness) demonstrated increased expression of aquaporin channel (AQP3) protein in keratinocyte cell culture models [5E].

A study provided evidence of vitamin A-induced inhibition of UGT2B7 (enzymes that carry out the glucuronidation reaction during phase II drug-metabolizing reactions) and shed light on the mechanism by which vitamin A may induce adverse effects [6E].

All-trans retinoic acid (ATRA) was orally administered to a 34-year-old patient who was diagnosed with acute promyelocytic leukemia (APL). The patient developed differentiation syndrome (DS) on the 25th day of treatment and an improvement of symptoms was observed following administration of methylprednisolone and suspending ATRA therapy. However, the patient reported severe abdominal pain on day 48 and multiple ulcers and perforations were identified following resected ileocecal intestines examination. It was concluded that these adverse effects could be due to DS or ATRA [7A].

A recent review reported dietary supplement-induced liver injury. A total of 18 reports were highlighted in which 58 cases of hepatotoxicity were due to vitamin A containing dietary supplements [8R].

A 12-week, single-center, clinical trial examined the efficacy of a 0.5% retinol and 30% vitamin C combined formulation treatment in 44 women with hyperpigmented and photodamaged facial skin. Although clinical improvement was observed in all parameters assessed; facial dryness was significantly increased at 4 and 8 weeks [9c].

A 24-week, single-center study evaluated effectiveness of 4.0% hydroquinone and 0.02% tretinoin cream in 39 females with mild to moderate melisma and photodamage. Although the treatment was generally well-tolerated and significantly improved clinical outcomes, severe cutaneous erythema was observed in one patient at 4 weeks [10c].

A study evaluated rheumatic side effects (i.e., low back pain, musculoskeletal pain, Sacroiliitis) in 73 patients treated with Isotretinoin for acne vulgaris. Patients received 0.4–0.8 mg/kg/day Isotretinoin for 6–8 months. Mechanical and inflammatory lower back pain was reported by 20 and 16 patients, respectively. Further diagnostic evaluation revealed acute Sacroiliitis (an inflammation of sacroiliac joints) in 5 females and 1 male patient. Study concluded high incidence of Sacroiliitis in patients receiving Isotretinoin [11c].

A female (9-year-old) with medulloblastoma, treated with a multimodal regimen, which included cis-retinoic acid, developed premature epiphyseal closure and later diagnosed with growth hormone deficiency and hypothyroidism. Following 7 months of growth hormones therapy, radiographical evaluation revealed bilateral premature closure of the proximal tibia growth plates and distal femur. Authors concluded increased risk of premature closure of the lower-extremity growth plates as a result of high doses of vitamin A and its analogues in animals and children [12A].

A recent study reported that Cisplatin (cis-diammine dichloroplatinum (II), CDDP; a widely used anticancer drug) when combined with all-trans retinoic acid induce nephrotoxicity [13E].

Two cases of ATRA-associated genital vasculitis were reported. Both patients were receiving arsenic trioxide (ATO), ATRA and prophylactic steroid therapy [14A].

An in vitro study reported enhanced tumor size and tumor invasiveness following combination of all-trans-retinoic-acid (ATRA) with 5-aza-2′deoxycytidine (5-AZA), DNA-methyltransferase inhibitor and a similar trend when combined with the histone deacetylase (HDAC) inhibitor suberoylanilide hydroxamic acid (SAHA). Authors concluded that combining ATRA and epigenetic drug therapy may trigger undersized adverse effects [15E].

A study evaluated the impact of dietary vitamin supplement prior to and/or during pregnancy on child behavior. During third trimester of pregnancy and after 3 years of birth, 1271 pairs of Japanese pregnant women received a self-administered questionnaire and Japanese Child Behavior Checklist (ages 2–3 years), respectively. Even after adjusting for several variables (age, parent's income and no of deliveries, etc.), vitamin A/β-carotene supplements intake in pregnancy was linked with aberrant child behavior at 3 years of age [16C].

VITAMINS OF THE B GROUP
[SEDA-34, 531; SEDA-35, 607; SEDA-38, 355]

Cobalamins (Vitamin B12)

A study evaluated benefits of dietary supplements, including vitamin B12 for the treatment of tinnitus. A total of 1788 subjects from 53 different countries completed the survey of which 413 (23.1%) were taking dietary supplements. Data suggested marginal benefits in sleep; however, in general dietary supplements were not effective and produced many adverse effects, including bleeding, headache and diarrhea [17MC].

A study examined the impact of various drugs and vitamins on homocysteine and dimethylglycine levels in 117 middle-age men drinking white wine. The subjects were randomly divided in five groups. Group 1 received only wine and other groups received one of the supplements (vitamin B12 or B6, betaine or folic acid) along with wine. Data suggested that betaine and folic acid supplementation as beneficial in lowering the homocysteine concentration following drinking period and attenuating the adverse effects of moderate alcohol drinking. However, supplementation with vitamin B12 or B6 was ineffective in regulating homocysteine levels [18C].

A phase II study evaluated oral vitamin B12 supplementation in lung cancer patients receiving pemetrexed treatment. 25 subjects received vitamin B12 and folic acid orally for more than a week before pemetrexed therapy. However, the study could not meet the end point and failed to assess safety and efficacy of the vitamin B12 oral treatment [19c].

A 23-year-old male was reported to have recurrent paraparesis due to nitrous oxide abuse, which resulted in more severe paraparesis attack. His symptoms improved after stopping nitrous oxide use and were treated with vitamin B12 supplement. Death occurred eventually due to abusive substances intoxication [20A].

Folic Acid and Folinic Acid

A review article summarized various peer-reviewed publications questioning the 2015 World Health Organization's guidelines and showed that an excessive intake of folic acid could be detrimental to the health. Worsening of anemia, cognitive impairments and adverse clinical and biochemical outcomes because of high folate intake in elderly patients were highlighted. Furthermore, women who took excessive amount of folic acid had low activity of the natural killer cells. Authors concluded that in certain population a high intake of folic acid could be a significant concern [21R]. Another review supporting this conclusion also summarized studies linking high folic acid intake and adverse effects [22R].

An expert panel from the Office of Dietary Supplements of the National Institutes of Health and the United States National Toxicology Program (NTP) highlighted the current research requirements regarding the safe use of high folic acid consumption. A clinical summary reported increased colorectal cancer risk in humans due to insufficient dietary folate intake; however, supplementation in case of adequate baseline folate was not beneficial for caner reduction. However, in light of human studies suggesting negative effects of folic acid supplements on cancer growth, further research is warranted. In addition, observational studies suggest exacerbation of neurological problems as a result of low vitamin B12 status and high folic acid intake; however, the mechanisms underlying this effect are unclear. Due to limited data, the effects of high folate status or high folic acid consumption on glucose/insulin metabolism or diabetes risk are inconclusive. It is also unclear if high folic acid intake has any adverse effects on thyroid disease. Future studies are needed to examine the impact of high folic acid intake on insulin resistance and fat mass based on evidence from observational studies [23S].

The effect of B-vitamins on endothelial function and inflammation was investigated within an interventional study on 2919 hyperhomocysteinemic elderly subjects receiving vitamin B12 (500 µg) and folic acid (400 µg) for 2 years. The study concluded that vitamin B12 and folic acid intake did not influence systemic inflammation or endothelial function [24MC].

A case of ventricular septal rupture was reported in a 64-year-old male patient 25 days following alcohol septal ablation treatment for hypertrophic cardiomyopathy. The patient was receiving FOLFOX (folinic acid, 5 FU, oxaliplatin) chemotherapy for stage II colon cancer [25A].

To assess the safety and efficacy of any vitamin supplementation on the risk of miscarriage, a study examined all randomized and quasi-randomized trials (a total of 40) evaluating any vitamin supplementation use before 20 weeks' gestation. Overall, authors concluded ineffectiveness of any supplement usage prior to or during pregnancy in preventing miscarriage. However, risk of still birth was reduced in women taking multivitamins along with iron and folic acid [26M].

A mega-cohort study, evaluated the effects of periconceptional folic acid intake on pregnancy outcomes in 1 535 066 women (aged 20–49) in 220 selected counties in China. The data demonstrated that if taken early before conception, periconceptional folic acid intake had protective effects against birth defects and adverse pregnancy outcomes [27MC].

A study examined the interaction between folic acid supplementation and passive smoking during pregnancy on children autism spectrum disorder (ASD) behaviors. The primary caregivers completed the self-administered questionnaires and an Autism Behavior Checklist (ABC) assessed the children ASD behaviors. The study reported a significant association of passive smoking with children ASD behaviors, whereas no such association was found in case of folic acid supplements. Furthermore, a negative association was reported with children ASD behaviors and folic acid supplements in children in the absence of passive smoking by mothers during pregnancy. A positive association was detected between ASD behaviors and passive smoking even when mothers were taking folic acid supplementation during pregnancy. Authors concluded a significant interaction effect between folic acid intake and passive smoking on children ASD behavior during pregnancy [28C].

A retrospective study examined the association of menstruation-related changes with preconceptional folic acid use in 219 in Chinese women. A total of 32 women reported menstruation-related changes (change in cycle length, bleeding between cycle, less blood loss and algomenorrhea). These symptoms were recovered following discontinuation of folic acid supplementation in 15 out of 17 women, indicating that folic acid or multivitamins containing folic acid contributed to these changes [29C].

Authors reported a placebo-controlled, double-blind trial, which examined the impact of folic acid in children with sickle cell anemia. Authors did not find any such trial in adults. Authors concluded that effects of folic acid supplementation on sickle cell disease are inconclusive and further studies are warranted [30c].

A phase II study evaluated the safety and efficacy of a treatment regimen of 5-fluorouracil (5-FU), folinic acid and oxaliplatin (mFOLFOX6) with bevacizumab, and 5-FU, folinic acid and irinotecan (FOLFIRI) with bevacizumab on 52 metastatic colorectal cancer patients. The study concluded that the alternating treatment regimen was well-tolerated and was an effective chemotherapy combination for patients with metastatic colorectal cancer [31c].

A multicenter, cross-section observational study evaluated the impact of 5 and 30 mg weekly folic acid supplementation on the tolerability of methotrexate. There was no between regimes difference in the methotrexate tolerability. However, lower disease activity score was reported in the 5 mg of folic acid weekly supplement group [32C].

A phase III, open-label trial, which evaluated the impact of nanoliposomal irinotecan alone or combined with folinic acid and fluorouracil in 417 patients with metastatic pancreatic ductal adenocarcinoma who had earlier received gemcitabine-based treatment. The trial was conducted in 14 counties at 76 sites with survival as primary endpoint after 35 events along with the safety assessment. Authors reported extended survival with reasonable safety level following Nanoliposomal irinotecan in combination with folinic acid and fluorouracil treatment [33MC].

Hopantenic Acid

A study evaluated the tolerability and efficacy of rac-hopantenic acid (pantogam activ) for treating anxiety and depressive disorders in 50 patients with chronic cerebral ischemia. A total of 30 patients received 1200 mg of Rac-hopantenic acid daily for 21 days in addition to the standard SSRI antidepressant therapy. Authors concluded rapid decrease in anxiety, depression and cognitive impairments in the treatment group in addition to less adverse events [34c].

Pantothenic Acid

An experimental study demonstrated beneficial effects of pantothenic acid (vitamin B5, a precursor of CoA) supplementation on high sugar diet-induced hyperglycemia and fatty acid accumulation [35E].

Pyridoxine

A 3-year study reported pyridoxine-related convulsions in children with refractory epilepsy. Authors concluded pyridoxine-dependent convulsions are rare (3.5%) and respond well to the appropriate treatment within 2 weeks [36c].

Tetrahydrobiopterin and Sapropterin

Two randomized, placebo-controlled, double-blinded crossover studies examined the impact of an acute treatment (single dose of BH4; 400 mg; $n = 18$) and short-term treatment (BH4; 400 mg daily for 1 week; $n = 15$) on endothelial function. Data suggested improvement in endothelial function following both regimens. However, no change in aortic pulse wave velocity was evident following either treatment [37c].

A study evaluated the long-term effects of Tetrahydrobiopterin (BH4; sapropterin) treatment in 9 hyperphenylalaninemia (HPA) children at least following 2 years. Authors concluded that BH4-treated patients could tolerate very high intake of dietary phenylalanine without any adverse effects. No change in median zinc, vitamin B12, selenium, levels or anthropometric assessment was evident following BH4 therapy. However phenylalanine/tyrosine ratio declined in the treatment group [38c].

Thiamine

A study tested the hypothesis that adjuvant thiamine treatment would improve treatment outcomes in patients with major depressive disorders. A total of 51 patients received standard SSRI treatment and were randomly assigned to placebo or thiamine and symptoms of depression were evaluated following 3, 6 and 12 weeks of treatment. Authors reported improvement in depression symptoms following 6 weeks of treatment without any adverse effects. However, no difference in treatment vs placebo groups was evident towards the end of the study [39c].

A randomized, multicenter, blinded study evaluated the efficacy/safety of gabapentin (GBP) when combined with thiamine (B1) and cyanocobalamine (B12) compared to pregabalin (PGB) in 270 patients with painful diabetic neuropathy for a duration of 12 weeks. The GBP/B1 (100 mg)/B12 (20 mg) group of patients received 300–3600 mg, whereas the PGB group received 75–600 mg/day from day 1 to the end of the treatment duration. The study concluded both treatments were equally effective. However, the GBP+B1+B12 group experienced less dizziness and vertigo [40MC].

A review focused on evaluating the safety and efficacy of vitamin supplements treatment for the genetic defects (SLC19A2, SLC19A3, SLC25A19 and TPK1) of thiamine transport and metabolism. Authors concluded that improvement was observed following thiamine treatment in case of patients with SLC19A3-, SLC19A-2 and

TPK1 defects. However, different doses were needed in each case, i.e., 25–200 mg/day for SLC19A2, 10–40 mg/kg per day for SLC19A3, and 30 mg/kg per day for TPK1 [41R].

VITAMIN C (ASCORBIC ACID) [SEDA-34, 531; SEDA-35, 609; SEDA-38, 355]

A systematic analysis of the safety and efficacy of vitamin C in preventing atrial fibrillation (AF) following cardiac surgery was conducted and included 8 randomized controlled trials with a total 1060 patients. The study concluded that vitamin C is safe and effective in decreasing the occurrence of postoperative atrial fibrillation [42MC].

A prospective, uncontrolled study examined the impact of polyethylene glycol plus vitamin C administered before colonoscopy. Study concluded that hypovolemia caused by polyethylene glycol plus vitamin C could be related to the serum albumin concentration in the elderly patients [43c].

A double-blind, randomized, placebo controlled study reported failure of intravenous vitamin C administration in reducing intraoperative blood loss in 50 women during laparoscopic myomectomy [44c].

A randomized prospective trial evaluated the safety and efficacy of vitamin C as adjuvant therapy to deferoxamine, DFO; deferiprone, DFP; and deferasirox, DFX in vitamin C deficient patients with b-thalassemia. Authors concluded that DFO efficacy was greatly enhanced by vitamin C adjuvant therapy compared to DFP and DFX, without any adverse events [45c].

The effect of oral, low-dose (250 mg daily for 3 months) vitamin C on erythropoietin dose needed for stable hemodialysis patients with functional iron deficiency was evaluated. Study concluded that daily vitamin C dose decreased erythropoietin dose requirements in the patient population without adverse effects [46c].

A prospective pilot study evaluated the clinical benefit of combining cranberries, Lactobacillus rhamnosus, and vitamin C in recurrent urinary tract infections in women (rUTI). Following 3 and 6 months of combined supplement intake 42 women with rUTI were evaluated. Authors concluded that combined administration of above supplement is safe and effective for the management of rUTI [47c].

A study evaluated the impact of vitamin C intake (both dietary and supplementation) on occurrence of kidney stone. This prospective (11.3–11.7 years) cohort study analyzed 156735 women and 40536 men, and reported a significant association of total and supplemental intake of vitamin C with the incidence of kidney stones in men, but not in women [48MC].

A study documented clinical response associated with administering high doses of intravenous vitamin C (25–100 g/day) in 9 cancer patients. Authors concluded improvement in the survival and clinical outcomes. However, discontinuation of vitamin C therapy negatively impacted the clinical condition and transient Jarisch-Herxheimer reaction was experienced by some patients [49A].

The impact of an intravenous high dose of vitamin C on pain and morphine use in patients undergoing laparoscopic colectomy was investigated in 97 patients. Authors reported significantly decreased pain scores and morphine consumption at 2 h following surgery in the vitamin C treated patient group [50c].

Two cases were reported in which a high-dose of vitamin C was given to patients with burn resuscitation. Death occurred in both cases following acute kidney injury and autopsy identified calcium oxalate crystals were found in the renal tubules [51A].

- A 31-year-old Caucasian woman was presented in a treatment facility following 65% TBSA thermal injury. Initial diagnosis showed grade I inhalation injury and the patient was given Lactated Ringers and later escharotomies were performed on her upper and lower extremities. She received albumin (0.4 mL/kg/%TBSA/24 h) and vitamin C (66 mg/kg/hr) following 8- and 11-h following burn, respectively. A total of 101 g of vitamin C was administered in 18 h and acute kidney injury was registered followed by hypotension and heart block. Eventually, death occurred on 2nd day. The autopsy identified calcium oxalate crystals in intratubular spaces in both kidneys and mild cerebral edema.

- A 20-year-old man was admitted with 67% TBSA thermal but no inhalation injuries and was intubated upon arrival. Vitamin C (66 mg/kg/hr) infusion was administered 8 h following burning. He received a total of 224 g vitamin C infusion during 20 h and 200 mg as a parental nutrition. Escharotomies were performed on his upper and lower extremities. The patient developed metabolic acidosis, shock, acute kidney injury and underwent left above-the-knee amputation followed by lactic acidosis and fever. Pupil fixation and dilation showed cerebral edema and tonsillar herniation on the 3rd day. In addition to the calcium oxalate crystals in the intratubular space in the both kidneys, the autopsy identified cerebellar herniation with necrosis of cerebellum, brain stem and cervical spinal cord.

VITAMIN D ANALOGUES [SEDA-34, 532; SEDA-35, 609; SEDA-38, 355]

A case of vascular calcifications related to hypervitaminosis D was reported in which a 64-year-old man was presented in the clinic reporting weakness, stupor and renal colic. The patient was diagnosed with hypertension, polyuria and small masses in the glutei. Laboratory and imaging tests further identified elevated serum calcium, creatinine and phosphate levels, extremely high Vit-D and reduced parathyroid hormone levels with widespread vascular calcifications, pelvic ectasia and gluteal calcification. The patient received saline and furosemide intravenous infusion with prednisone and omeprazole, which improved kidney function and consciousness. It was identified that the patient received exceptionally high slow released intramuscular preparation of cholecalciferol and had a recent history of urinary stones. The patient was discharged following discontinuation of intravenous treatment. Following discharge patient received prednisone, oral hydration, omeprazole and furosemide for approximately 6 months. The patient was readmitted due to microhematuria 12 years later and testing revealed minor vascular calcification [52A].

The safety and efficacy of Vit-D supplementation (200 000 IU loading dose and 25 000 IU every 2 weeks for 4 months) was evaluated in 80 young (15–21 years) girls. This Vit-D therapy was found to be safe and effective in improving premenstrual syndrome-induced mood disorders in women with severe hypovitaminosis D [53c].

A single center, double-blind and randomized pilot study characterized the immunological effects and safety profile of daily high (10 400 IU) vs low (800 IU) cholecalciferol dose for 6 months in 40 multiple sclerosis (MS) patients. It was reported that high cholecalciferol dose was safe, tolerable and had immunomodulatory effects in MS patients [54c].

A study reported safety and efficacy of a single high dose (300 000 IU) of vitamin D in 28 vitamin D deficient young subjects [55c].

A 60-day pilot study examined the safety and efficacy of a sustained release tablet (containing extracts of green coffee bean, banaba leaf, *Moringa oleifera* leaf and vitamin D3) in 30 subjects. The study reported improvement in the quality of life and changes in the body composition (decrease in fat mass and increase in fat free mass) in the treatment group [56c].

A randomized, double-blind, placebo-controlled study assessed the safety and efficacy of a forced high dose ($\leq$3 loading doses, 100 000 IU) and a maintenance dose (3420 IU/day) of vitamin D (Vit-D) in 50 patients with vitamin D deficiency who were undergoing an omega-loop gastric bypass (OLGB). The study concluded that the intervention was not only safe and effective in OLGB patients but also was more effective in patients with liver fibrosis [57c].

A study evaluated the impact of Vit-D supplement in 28 patients with moderate-severe Crohn's disease receiving infliximab. The study concluded a negative correlation between vitamin D levels and infliximab-induced clinical remission following 14 weeks [58c].

A randomized controlled study assessed the safety/efficacy of Vit-D (20 000 IU/week) intervention in 511 pre-diabetic patients for 5 years. The study concluded that Vit-D therapy was safe, but ineffective in preventing progression of diabetes [59C].

Another similar study reported ineffectiveness of a very high dose (30 000 IU; once a week for 8 weeks) in prediabetes, diabetes, beta-cell function, glycemic control or insulin sensitivity [60c].

A meta-analysis of side effects (kidney stones, hypercalciuria and hypercalcemia) reported in randomized clinical trials related to Vit-D supplementation for $\geq$24 weeks was carried out. A total of 48 studies ($n = 19833$) were identified. The study concluded heightened risk of hypercalciuria and hypercalcemia but not kidney stones following long-term Vit-D supplementation [61MC].

A 69-year old woman was admitted with acute kidney injury, metabolic acidosis, hypercalcemia and symptoms of systemic vasculitis. The patient had ANCA-associated vasculitis for 4 years and received cytotoxic therapy. She was currently on immunosuppressant therapy and was in remission. A kidney biopsy identified interstitial inflammation, calcium phosphate crystals and acute tubular necrosis. The patient admitted taking Vit-D containing multivitamins and huge doses of over-the counter Ca^+ containing antacid. Discontinuation of drugs improved renal function [62A].

A study reported the largest series of 62 cases of malpractice-related Vit-D toxicity with hypercalcemia and acute kidney injury. 51 cases of de novo acute kidney injury and 11 cases of chronic kidney disease were presented with a mean age 60 ± 14 and 62 ± 13 and Vit-D injections ranging from 4 to 28 and 3 to 24 million units, respectively [63A].

A 1-year, randomized, double-blind controlled trial evaluated high Vit-D dose (2000 IU vs 400 IU for 1 year) on lumbar spine areal bone mineral density in adolescents and children with Osteogenesis imperfecta. Although Vit-D supplementation increased serum 25OHD levels, no effect on the desired outcome was evident [64c].

A review summarized current data related to the skeletal and extraskeletal effects of vitamin D, methods of assessing 25-hydroxyvitamin D and safety and efficacy of vitamin D replacement therapy [65R].

A placebo-controlled, double-blind 5 months study examined the safety/efficacy of 5 grass pollen sublingual 300 IR immunotherapy with 1000 IU Vit-D daily supplementation in 50 children (5–12 years old) with allergic rhinitis. The study concluded that the supplementation was well-tolerated and more effective in treating allergic rhinitis in children [66c].

Efficacy and safety of vitamin D3 (4000 IU/day) compared to the usual dose (600 IU) was evaluated in a single site, double-blind, randomized, phase 3 clinical trial in patients displaying aromatase inhibitor-associated musculoskeletal (AIMS) symptoms. The study reported no benefits of the higher dose in improving AIMS symptoms. In addition, no adverse effects on reproductive hormones, anastrozole or letrozole pharmacokinetics, were reported following 4000 IU administration [67c].

A controlled, randomized, double-blind trial evaluating the impact of 2 cholecalciferol doses (400 and 2000 IU/day) in 57 pregnant women concluded that a dose of 2000 IU was effective not only in improving Vit-D status but also in preventing adverse events due to inflammation during pregnancy [68c].

A study evaluating data from 15 trials reported significantly higher 25(OH)D levels in pregnant women supplementing with Vit-D and that such an intake was beneficial in reducing risk of preeclampsia. However, further studies were warranted [69M].

A randomized, placebo-controlled and double-blind vitamin D Antenatal Asthma Reduction Trial was conducted at 3 centers across the United States to evaluate the safety and efficacy of prenatal Vit-D supplement in the prevention of recurrent wheezing and asthma in early childhood. An insignificant decrease (6.1%) in the occurrence of recurrent wheeze and asthma in children was reported [70MC].

A review study evaluated several randomized and quasi-randomized trials assessing the safety and efficacy of Vit-D supplementation alone or in combination with vitamins, calcium and minerals in pregnancy. Authors concluded that Vit-D supplementation during pregnancy could be beneficial in reducing risk of pre-eclampsia, low birth weight and preterm birth; however, rigorous randomized trails are needed to draw any conclusion. No significant between group differences in adverse effects were reported [71M].

VITAMIN E (TOCOPHEROL) [SEDA-35, 610; SEDA-36, 515; SEDA-38, 355]

A review evaluating the efficacy and safety of medical interventions for anthracycline-induced cardiotoxicity showed no difference in overall survival, mortality due to heart failure, echocardiographic function or adverse events. The interventions studied were enalapril, phosphocreatine and a control treatment of vitamin C, vitamin E, adenosine triphosphate and oral coenzyme Q10 [72R].

In November 2016, a case–control study, 32 patients (mean age 68.6) undergoing endoscopic sinus surgery were randomized to receive alpha-tocopherol acetate compared or gomenol oil. Increased mucosal healing was noted in the vitamin E acetate-treated group after 7-day, 15-day, and 1–3-month follow-up. No adverse events were noted with the topical vitamin E therapy [73c].

In a study of 32 healthy volunteers (16 smokers and 16 non-smokers), a significant decrease in the vitamin E levels were found in the smokers, suggesting that exposure to smoking decreases antioxidant biomarkers significantly [74c].

In a 2016 Cochrane review of antioxidant treatment for schizophrenic patients, a total of 22 randomized control trials were included for analysis. Included antioxidants were vitamin E and vitamin C. Adverse events were not well reported among the trials, and only three trials included "Serious adverse events." The results were equivocal across the trials (3 RCTs, $n = 234$, RR 0.65, 95% CI 0.19–2.27, low quality evidence) [75R].

In a Cochrane Review of the effects of vitamin E on mild cognitive impairment in dementia, there was no evidence that alpha-tocopherol prevented progression to dementia. There was no link between vitamin E and risk of adverse events or mortality [76R].

Participants in a randomized control trial (60 male patients) in Iran received combination of omega-3+vitamin E vs omega-3+placebo vs double placebo for 2 months. Serum glucose, lipid and insulin levels were monitored. Though Omega-3 supplementation was found to increase serum glucose levels, the addition of vitamin E decreased both insulin and insulin resistance with no observation on adverse events [77c].

A systematic review of the adverse effects of herbal dietary supplementation in G6PD deficiency patients showed that there was insufficient evidence to suggest that herbal supplements at therapeutic doses were associated with adverse events. Studied supplements included vitamin C, vitamin E, vitamin K, Gingko Biloba and alpha-lipoic acid [78R].

In an observational study on the efficacy of VeDrops (vitamin E oral solution) for treatment of vitamin E deficiency among 274 children in 7 European centers; vitamin E levels were noted to improve in 89% of children within 6 months. No serious adverse events were reported [79C].

In a placebo-controlled randomized trial, 300 patients with chronic kidney disease were randomized 1:1 to receive 0.9% saline infusion+vitamin E prior and post coronary angiography or to receive placebo. Prophylactic short-term high-dose vitamin E combined was superior to placebo to prevent acute kidney injury in these patients. No side effects related to the interventions were observed [80C].

In a randomized control trial of oral interdialytic oral protein supplementation, 92 hemodialysis patients were randomized to one of three groups (vitamin E 600 IU fortified whey vs fortified whey vs vitamin E 600 IU).

A short-term improvement was found in the Subjective Global Assessment (SGA) nutritional score. Few adverse events were reported in any group [81c].

In a study of therapies used for Restless Leg Syndrome among Chronic Kidney Disease patients, adverse events were reported with different pharmacologic and non-pharmacologic interventions. Among the vitamins studied (C, E and C plus E), an increase in nausea and dyspepsia was noted [82R].

In a case–control study, 31 patients received chemical peeling with glycolic acid, iontophoresis with ascorbyl 2-phosphate 6-palmitate and DL-alpha-tocopherol for the treatment of post-inflammatory hyperpigmentation (PIH). An improvement was seen in PIH cases. The only observed adverse event was mild redness and irritation in four patients [83c].

In a review of six studies on the effects of vitamin E in scar management, it was concluded that there are insufficient evidence that support topical vitamin E monotherapy for the treatment of scars. Two of these six studies reported an increase in contact dermatitis, rash and itching following vitamin E application [84R].

In a review of pharmacologic and non-pharmacologic treatments for Friedreich ataxia, a total of 12 studies were identified that used antioxidant therapy (idebenone, coQ10 and vitamin E). Though the quality of evidence was low, no significant differences in adverse events between the placebo and antioxidant groups were reported [85R].

Pro-apoptotic analogues of vitamin E are postulated to exert anticancer effects in animal models. Due to the low solubility of vitamin E in aqueous mediums, use of liposomal formulations has been developed. In this review article, the liposomal formulation was evaluated with regard to reducing the undesirable side effects of the drug and using pre-clinical models, anticancer effects of liposomal VE analogues were demonstrated [86R].

In a double-blind, randomized, controlled clinical trial at 21 clinical sites, older adults with Downs Syndrome were recruited to receive 1000 IU of vitamin E twice daily for 3 years or placebo. A total of 337 people were randomized. No significant difference in adverse events between the control group and the placebo occurred [87C].

A May 2016 Cochrane Review of the utility of vitamin supplementation to prevent miscarriage, found no difference in adverse events between vitamin supplementation (vitamin C and vitamin E) vs placebo (RR 1.16, 95% CI 0.39–3.41, one trial, 739 women; moderate-quality evidence) [88R].

A 2016 review of the use of dietary supplements in dysmenorrhea, only 4 of the 27 studies included adverse events. There was no evidence that there was a difference in adverse events between the groups. Among the vitamins studied was vitamin B1 and E [89R].

VITAMIN K ANALOGUES [SEDA-35, 610; SEDA-36, 515; SEDA-38, 355]

An 8-year-old female child with tubercular meningitis was initiated on antibiotics. After 12 days of antibiotics, the patient developed presumed antibiotic induced thrombocytopenia. A slow intravenous vitamin K (2 mg diluted in 2 mL normal saline) injection was given which led to respiratory arrest requiring CPR (cardiopulmonary resuscitation) [90A].

In a retrospective study of 46 pregnant women with mechanical heart valve in a West China Women and Children's Hospital, data was collected on pre-Cesarean section vitamin K1 administration for anticoagulation reversal. Increased warfarin resistance was noted in these patients during the bridging with warfarin phase after cesarean [91c].

In a prospective study on the use of 0.01% Vitamin K1 cream after the administration of Cetuximab for patients with metastatic colorectal cancer to reduce Cetuximab-induced acneiform skin rash, the appearance of skin rash was decreased in the 41 observed patients. In addition, the vitamin K1 cream was well tolerated with no significant side effects on coagulation [92c].

In an interim-analysis of a trial evaluating the administration of oral vitamin K2 alone or with sorafenib on 72 Hepatocellular Carcinoma patients who underwent liver resection or transplantation, reported no noticeable adverse effects in the patients receiving vitamin K2, except for skin rash in one patient. Furthermore, no adverse effects related to vitamin K2 were noticeable at the 6-month point. vitamin K with or without sorafenib was associated with the improvement in anti-tumor effects in a small proportion of patients [93c].

AMINO ACIDS [SEDA-36, 515; SEDA-38, 355]

Arginine

In a 2016 review from the American Society for Nutrition, the safety and effectiveness of Arginine at oral administration levels ~20 g/day has been found to be beneficial for lean tissue deposition and insulin resistance. At these doses, no serious adverse events were noted. The Society recommends additional study regarding the safety and efficacy of arginine supplementation [94R].

A 2016 systematic review of arginine supplementation among military personnel was conducted using 17 databases and 5 adverse event report portals. The study found that, though most studies had few participants with a risk of bias that could affect results, L-arginine did not offer improved performance effects. In addition, gastrointestinal and cardiovascular adverse events were reported. The authors recommend a computational model-based approach to assess the safety and efficacy of L-arginine [95r].

Ornithine

A systematic review of 41 trials involving 3881 participants of randomized and quasi-randomized trials of elderly patients with hip fractions revealed inconclusive evidence of the occurrence of nausea, vomiting, and diarrhea as a result of oral supplements, possible because of methodological limitations due to the risk of bias assessment [96MC].

In a review of cirrhotic patients with portosystemic encephalopathy, it was noted that L-ornithine-L-aspartate improved performance in Psychometric Tests for hepatic encephalopathy. L-ornithine-L-aspartate had few side effects and was well tolerated in both oral and parenteral form [97r].

PARENTERAL NUTRITION [SEDA-35, 610; SEDA-36, 515; SEDA-38, 355]

In a prospective exploratory study of 48 patients with end-stage cancer and advance chronic bowel disease, patients ≥18 years old with an indication for home parenteral nutrition therapy were followed for 2–24 months. By week 4, patients with tumors showed a deterioration in phase angle and patients with bowel disease improved extracellular mass:body cell mass ratio. The authors concluded that both groups benefitted from home parenteral nutrition therapy without harmful side effects [98c].

In a prospective, randomized double-blind trial, 97 patients received either partial parenteral nutrition or total parenteral nutrition in a hospital setting and were followed between days 7 and 14. The results indicated that both groups showed improvement in the nutritional status measured by protein, albumin, serum albumin and serum transferrin. Though not directly studied, the authors suggested that the use of parenteral nutrition and enteral nutrition may reduce side effects with parenteral nutrition, though no specific side effects were mentioned. Recommendation was made for precise studies in the future to evaluate which method is better as well as tolerable [99c].

In a retrospective study of surgical critically ill patients receiving parenteral nutrition, 69 patients were divided into the parenteral nutrition vs non-parenteral nutrition groups. A significant increase in the mean blood glucose concentration was reported in the PN group compared to the non-PN group ($P = 0.004$). Consequently, consumption of insulin was increased as well. The authors recommend close monitoring of blood glucose levels as mortality increases in critically ill patients as blood glucose exceeds 180 mg/dL [100c].

Electrolytes and Minerals

In a retrospective cohort study of the effects of calcium supplementation outside of the TPN due to calcium gluconate shortage, the adverse events of total parenteral nutrition–calcium interactions were recorded. A total of 259 ICU total parenteral nutrition patients were included in the study. For non-mechanically ventilated and non-vasopressor dependent when PN started, logistic regression revealed that calcium administration was associated with mortality, acute respiratory failure, new-onset shock, and the combined end point. Adverse outcomes odds increased as the calcium dose increased with total parenteral nutrition administration [101C].

Manganese levels were tracked in a retrospective review of 16 adult patients with short bowel syndrome on long-term Home Parenteral Nutrition (duration 4–96 months). The parenteral nutrition therapy contained a daily dose of manganese (80 and 470 microgram/day; 1.2–8.5 pg/kg/day). Whole blood manganese concentration was almost double in the patients under observation compared to the control group (16.2 microgram/L; 12.9–20.4 microgram/L vs 7.4 microgram/L; 6.4–8.4 microgram/L, respectively). Symptoms of cholestatic hepatopathy were also reported in five patients. The authors recommend close monitoring of manganese levels as well using single element trace element options in compounding parenteral nutrition as opposed to standard trace minerals [102c].

Though hypersensitivity reaction to parenteral nutrition is rare, it has been reported as an adverse event among children. In a 1-month-old breastfed baby with gastroenteritis, 60 min after the initiation of the infusion on day 2, the patient had an allergic reaction with an overall diffused rash. Similarly, in a 4-year-old girl with a background of stage III neuroblastoma, the patient showed sudden facial edema on day 3 of PN. Finally, a 3rd case is a 10-year-old boy with a diagnosis of an acute peritonitis showed a general wheal rash after initiation of parenteral nutrition. Each allergic reaction was modified by changing the amino acid formulation, lipid formulation or vitamin/trace mineral components in the TPN [103A].

A 47-year-old woman with a history of bulimia and gastroparesis was on 8 weeks of total parenteral nutrition therapy. The patient presented with a painful, perioral, perineal, and acral eruption of 7 weeks' duration. These symptoms were complicated by diarrhea, vomiting, and a 13.5-kg weight loss. Physical examination revealed perioral and perineal, erythematous, scaly plaques with yellow crusting requiring punch biopsies [104A].

Contamination and Infectious

A study reported an outbreak of *Candida albicans* in the neonatal pediatric ward as a result of TPN solution contamination [105c].

In a report of two cases, patients suffering from megacystis microcolon intestinal hypoperistalsis syndrome were receiving long-term parenteral nutrition therapy via a central venous catheter. Both patients developed infection-related glomerulonephritis presenting with proteinuria, hematuria, and hypocomplementemia. The infectious agent was Staphylococcus epidermidis in the central venous catheter. The cure was achieved with catheter removal with or without pulse prednisolone therapy [106A].

A 2016 review of 36 trials evaluating enteral vs parenteral therapy in cancer patients, reported no significant differences in the endpoints between two therapies. However, more infections incidents occurred in the case of parenteral nutrition ($P = 0.03$) [107M].

A 2016 review of 21 clinical trials compared positive nutrition markers as well as lipid markers following synthetic structured triglycerides (STGs) vs physical mixtures of medium and long chain triglycerides parenteral nutrition regimens in total surgical and critically ill patients. The meta-analysis reported a significantly higher pre-albumin, albumin, better cumulative nitrogen balance. The structured triglycerides group had significantly lower plasma triglycerides levels, total bilirubin and Liver function tests when compared to the medium chain/long chain group. No significant adverse events were reported [108M].

In a comprehensive review of 789 full-text articles, of which 114 were included (87 human studies), the rate of adverse effects associated with intravenous lipid emulsion (ILE) infusion was described. The adverse effects associated with acute ILE administration were multisystem and included cardiac arrest, acute lung injury, ventilation perfusion mismatch, acute kidney injury, hypersensitivity, fat embolism, venous thromboembolism, fat overload syndrome, extracorporeal circulation machine circuit obstruction, pancreatitis, increased susceptibility to infection and allergic reaction. Adverse reactions commensurate with the dose and rate of infusion [109R].

In a review of lipid emulsion formulas of soybean oil, olive oil, or several oils, safety and efficacy of different lipid emulsion formulas were collected. From March 2014, 15 studies were identified comparing two or multiple lipid emulsion components. The meta-analysis suggested that patients receiving mixed-based lipid (soybean, fish oil, olive oil) had higher plasma concentrations of plasma oleic acid, alpha-tocopherol, docosahexaenoic acid and ω-3 PUFAs eicosapentaenoic. A correlation between low plasma concentrations of long-chain ω-6 polyunsaturated fatty acids and olive oil- and mixed-based lipids was reported and their effects on the liver function were like soybean oil-based emulsions. Safety profiles were similar across the lipid emulsions [110M].

ENTERAL NUTRITION (NON-ORAL: GASTRIC AND JUJENAL) [SEDA-35, 610; SEDA-36, 515; SEDA-38, 355]

In one study, 341 patients receiving pancreaticoduodenectomy were randomized to receive parenteral nutrition + enteral nutrition (PN + EN) vs total parenteral nutrition (TPN) alone. A significant higher occurrence of pulmonary infection, delayed gastric emptying and probable intraperitoneal infection were reported in the PN + EN group. In addition, these patients also had longer nasogastric tube time, increased postoperative hospital stay and hospitalization cost [111C].

A randomized control trial of 161 acute pancreatitis patients assigned subjects to abdominal pancreatic drainage or no drainage and initiated on enteral therapy. The incidence of gastrointestinal events was similar in both groups, except for diarrhea. This trial demonstrated gastrointestinal complication with the initiation of enteral feeding, with or without surgery [112C].

In a 2016 published study, 120 patients on mechanical ventilation were randomized to receive fiber enriched or fiber free tube feedings. On days 4 and 5, the fiber-enriched group had higher volume ratios ($P < 0.05$). 59% of the patients had at least one gastrointestinal complication, 44 (73%) of them were controls and 27 (45%) of them study patients. Diarrhea was the most often reported gastrointestinal complication. With increased incidence in the fiber-free group ($P < 0.001$). No significant between-group differences in vomiting and regurgitation were observed [113C].

A clinical analysis of 47 children receiving enteral nutrition revealed abdominal pain and bloating ($n = 3$), vomiting ($n = 7$), secondary respiratory infections ($n = 5$) and diarrhea ($n = 12$) as the most common adverse events [114c].

A pilot study investigating the effects of peptide-based vs high-protein enteral formulas on tolerance and safety among 49 patients did not find between groups differences in the adverse events and undesired gastrointestinal events at baseline and post-baseline points. In addition, the peptide-based group had significantly fewer days with adverse events ($P = 0.0336$; $n = 24$/group) and undesired gastrointestinal events ($P = 0.0489$; $n = 24$/group). Thus, gastrointestinal side effects continue to be reported regardless of protein enteral formula used [115c].

A study reported an incidence of frequent vomiting (50.0%), nausea (14.8%), loss of appetite (45.2), nervous perspiration during feeding (7.5%), skin irritation

(1.9%) and local tissue granulation (5.2%) in 425 infants and children receiving enteral feeds [116C].

Aspiration and aspiration pneumonia remains a complication of initiation of enteral feeding. In one study comparing liquid vs semisolid percutaneous endoscopic gastrostomy (PEG) tube feedings, one hundred and seventeen patients were initiated on a hospital base protocol to one of the two groups. Fewer adverse events (i.e., feeding-related aspiration pneumonia and shorter postoperative hospital length of stay) were experienced in the semi-solid feed group. However, no significant difference in the frequency of peristomal infection, feeding-related diarrhea and 30-day mortality rates were reported. Thus, changing feeding formula bulk had a positive impact on pulmonary related complications of enteral feeding [117C].

A retrospective review of 114 pediatric patients with an abnormal videofluoroscopic swallow found patients fed with a g-tube vs orally had a median admission rate of 2 vs 1 ($P < 0.0001$) and increased hospital stay (median 24 vs 2, $P < 0.001$). There was no difference in total pulmonary admissions. The study concluded 2 times higher admission in patients receiving g-tube placement compared to the orally fed patients [118C].

In a 2016 Cochrane Review of the safety and efficacy of nutrition support therapy in critically ill children, studies were reviewed from 1992 until February 2016 and is an update to the 2009 review. All randomized controlled trials involving pediatric patients who received nutrition within the first 7 days of admission in a pediatric intensive care unit and had at least one pre-conceived outcome (e.g., the number of ventilator days, morbid complications or length of stay). Authors found only one trial relevant to the conditions, which involved 77 children with burns admitted to the intensive care who received enteral nutrition within 24 or 48 h. There were no differences in the sepsis, length of stay, ventilator days, resting energy expenditure, unexpected adverse events, albumin levels, nitrogen balance or mortality. Since it was only a small trial, results need to be interpreted with caution [119R].

A review of recommended advances in the nutrition therapy in inflammatory bowel disease found that enteral nutrition therapy remains a safe method of providing nutrition in this patient population [120R].

Acknowledgements

This publication was made possible by funding, in part, from the NIMHD-RCMI grant number 5G12MD007595 from the National Institute on Minority Health and Health Disparities and the NIGMS-BUILD grant number 8UL1GM118967 to S.S. This project was also supported, in part, by Alcohol and Drug Abuse Program (ADARP) at Washington State University grant # 2550–1324 to J.F.D. Authors declare no conflict of interest.

References

[1] Hamishehkar H, Ranjdoost F, Asgharian P, et al. Vitamins, are they safe? Adv Pharm Bull. 2016;6(4):467–77 [M].

[2] Lucca JM, Varghese NA, Ramesh M, et al. A case report of isotretinoin-induced manic psychosis. Indian J Dermatol. 2016;61(1):120 [A].

[3] Munch IC, Toft U, Linneberg A, et al. Precursors of age-related macular degeneration: associations with vitamin A and interaction with CFHY402H in the Inter99 Eye Study. Acta Ophthalmol. 2016;94(7):657–62 [C].

[4] Bergler-Czop B, Bilewicz-Stebel M, Stańkowska A, et al. Side effects of retinoid therapy on the quality of vision. Acta Pharm Zagreb Croat. 2016;66(4):471–8 [A].

[5] Xing F, Liao W, Jiang P, et al. Effect of retinoic acid on aquaporin 3 expression in keratinocytes. Genet Mol Res GMR. 2016;15(1):15016951 [E].

[6] Liu X, Cao Y-F, Dong P-P, et al. The inhibition of UDP-glucuronosyltransferases (UGTs) by vitamin A. Xenobiotica. 2017;47(5):376–81. 1–6 [E].

[7] Kimura K, Takeuchi M, Hasegawa N, et al. Severe stomatitis and ileocecal perforation developed after all-trans retinoic acid monotherapy in an HLA-B51-positive patient with acute promyelocytic leukemia. Rinsho Ketsueki. 2016;57(6):765–70 [A].

[8] García-Cortés M, Robles-Díaz M, Ortega-Alonso A, et al. Hepatotoxicity by dietary supplements: a tabular listing and clinical characteristics. Int J Mol Sci. 2016;17(4):537 [R].

[9] Herndon JH, Jiang LI, Kononov T, et al. An open label clinical trial to evaluate the efficacy and tolerance of a retinol and vitamin C facial regimen in women with mild-to-moderate hyperpigmentation and photodamaged facial skin. J Drugs Dermatol JDD. 2016;15(4):476–82 [c].

[10] Rendon M, Dryer L. Investigator-blinded, single-center study to evaluate the efficacy and tolerability of a 4% hydroquinone skin care system plus 0.02% tretinoin cream in mild-to-moderate melasma and photodamage. J Drugs Dermatol JDD. 2016;15(4):466–75 [c].

[11] Baykal Selçuk L, Aksu Arıca D, Baykal Şahin H, et al. The prevalence of sacroiliitis in patients with acne vulgaris using isotretinoin. Cutan Ocul Toxicol. 2017;36(2):176–9 [c].

[12] Noyes JJ, Levine MA, Belasco JB, et al. Premature epiphyseal closure of the lower extremities contributing to short stature after cis-retinoic acid therapy in medulloblastoma: a case report. Horm Res Paediatr. 2016;85(1):69–73 [A].

[13] Elsayed AM, Abdelghany TM, Akool el-S, et al. All-trans retinoic acid potentiates cisplatin-induced kidney injury in rats: impact of retinoic acid signaling pathway. Naunyn Schmiedebergs Arch Pharmacol. 2016;389(3):327–37 [E].

[14] Yanamandra U, Khadwal A, Saikia UN, et al. Genital vasculitis secondary to all-trans-retinoic-acid. BMJ Case Rep. 2016. pii: bcr2015212205. http://dx.doi.org/10.1136/bcr-2015-212205 [A].

[15] Schmoch T, Gal Z, Mock A, et al. Combined treatment of ATRA with epigenetic drugs increases aggressiveness of glioma xenografts. Anticancer Res. 2016;36(4):1489–96 [E].

[16] Ishikawa Y, Tanaka H, Akutsu T, et al. Prenatal vitamin A supplementation associated with adverse child behavior at 3 years in a prospective birth cohort in Japan. Pediatr Int Off J Jpn Pediatr Soc. 2016;58(9):855–61 [C].

[17] Coelho C, Tyler R, Ji H, et al. Survey on the effectiveness of dietary supplements to treat tinnitus. Am J Audiol. 2016;25(3):184–205 [MC].

[18] Rajdl D, Racek J, Trefil L, et al. Effect of folic acid, betaine, vitamin B_6, and vitamin B12 on homocysteine and dimethylglycine levels in middle-aged men drinking white wine. Nutrients. 2016;8(1). http://dx.doi.org/10.3390/nu8010034 [C].

[19] Takagi Y, Hosomi Y, Nagamata M, et al. Phase II study of oral vitamin B12 supplementation as an alternative to intramuscular injection for patients with non-small cell lung cancer undergoing pemetrexed therapy. Cancer Chemother Pharmacol. 2016;77(3):559–64 [c].

[20] Hirvioja J, Joutsa J, Wahlsten P, et al. Recurrent paraparesis and death of a patient with "whippet" abuse. Oxf Med Case Rep. 2016;2016(3):41–3 [A].

[21] Selhub J, Rosenberg IH. Excessive folic acid intake and relation to adverse health outcome. Biochimie. 2016;126:71–8 [R].

[22] Patel KR, Sobczyńska-Malefora A. The adverse effects of an excessive folic acid intake. Eur J Clin Nutr. 2017;71(2):159–63. http://dx.doi.org/10.1038/ejcn.2016.194 [R].

[23] Boyles AL, Yetley EA, Thayer KA, et al. Safe use of high intakes of folic acid: research challenges and paths forward. Nutr Rev. 2016;74(7):469–74 [S].

[24] van Dijk SC, Enneman AW, Swart KM, et al. Effect of vitamin B12 and folic acid supplementation on biomarkers of endothelial function and inflammation among elderly individuals with hyperhomocysteinemia. Vasc Med Lond Engl. 2016;21(2):91–8 [MC].

[25] Liebregts M, Bol GM, Groen J-W, et al. FOLFOX chemotherapy as a cause of ventricular septal rupture after alcohol septal ablation for obstructive hypertrophic cardiomyopathy? Int J Cardiol. 2016;207:208–10 [A].

[26] Balogun OO, da Silva Lopes K, Ota E, et al. Vitamin supplementation for preventing miscarriage. Cochrane Database Syst Rev. 2016;5:CD004073 [M].

[27] He Y, Pan A, Hu FB, et al. Folic acid supplementation, birth defects, and adverse pregnancy outcomes in Chinese women: a population-based mega-cohort study. Lancet Lond Engl. 2016;388(Suppl 1):S91 [MC].

[28] Jiang H, Liu L, Sun DL, et al. Interaction between passive smoking and folic acid supplement during pregnancy on autism spectrum disorder behaviors in children aged 3 years. Zhonghua Liu Xing Bing Xue Za Zhi. 2016;37(7):940–4 [C].

[29] Shen L, Chu Z, Yang J, et al. The risk of menstrual abnormalities after preconceptional use of folic acid or a folic acid-containing multivitamin in Chinese women. Ecol Food Nutr. 2016;55(2):111–8 [C].

[30] Dixit R, Nettem S, Madan SS, et al. Folate supplementation in people with sickle cell disease. Cochrane Database Syst Rev. 2016;2:CD011130 [c].

[31] Miwa K, Oki E, Emi Y, et al. Phase II trial of an alternating regimen consisting of first-line mFOLFOX6 plus bevacizumab and FOLFIRI plus bevacizumab for patients with metastatic colorectal cancer: FIREFOX plus bevacizumab trial (KSCC0801). Int J Clin Oncol. 2016;21(1):110–7 [c].

[32] Koh KT, Teh CL, Cheah CK, et al. Real-world experiences of folic acid supplementation (5 versus 30 mg/week) with methotrexate in rheumatoid arthritis patients: a comparison study. Reumatismo. 2016;68(2):90–6 [C].

[33] Wang-Gillam A, Li C-P, Bodoky G, et al. Nanoliposomal irinotecan with fluorouracil and folinic acid in metastatic pancreatic cancer after previous gemcitabine-based therapy (NAPOLI-1): a global, randomised, open-label, phase 3 trial. Lancet Lond Engl. 2016;387(10018): 545–57 [MC].

[34] Gekht AB, Kanaeva LS, Avedisova AS, et al. [Possible applications of rac-hopantenic acid in the treatment of anxiety and depressive disorders in patients with chronic cerebral ischemia]. Zh Nevrol Psikhiatr Im S S Korsakova. 2016;116(11):45–57 [c].

[35] Palanker Musselman L, Fink JL, Baranski TJ. CoA protects against the deleterious effects of caloric overload in Drosophila. J Lipid Res. 2016;57(3):380–7 [E].

[36] Chandra SR, Issac TG, Deepak S, et al. Pyridoxine-dependent convulsions among children with refractory seizures: a 3-year follow-up study. J Pediatr Neurosci. 2016;11(3):188–92 [c].

[37] Mäki-Petäjä KM, Day L, Cheriyan J, et al. Tetrahydrobiopterin supplementation improves endothelial function but does not alter aortic stiffness in patients with rheumatoid arthritis. J Am Heart Assoc. 2016;5(2). http://dx.doi.org/10.1161/JAHA.115.002762, pii: e002762 [c].

[38] Tansek MZ, Groselj U, Kelvisar M, et al. Long-term BH4 (sapropterin) treatment of children with hyperphenylalaninemia—effect on median Phe/Tyr ratios. J Pediatr Endocrinol Metab JPEM. 2016;29(5):561–6 [c].

[39] Ghaleiha A, Davari H, Jahangard L, et al. Adjuvant thiamine improved standard treatment in patients with major depressive disorder: results from a randomized, double-blind, and placebo-controlled clinical trial. Eur Arch Psychiatry Clin Neurosci. 2016;266(8):695–702 [c].

[40] Mimenza Alvarado A, Aguilar Navarro S. Clinical trial assessing the efficacy of gabapentin plus B complex (B1/B12) versus pregabalin for treating painful diabetic neuropathy. J Diabetes Res. 2016;2016:4078695 [MC].

[41] Ortigoza-Escobar JD, Molero-Luis M, Arias A, et al. Treatment of genetic defects of thiamine transport and metabolism. Expert Rev Neurother. 2016;16(7):755–63 [R].

[42] Hu X, Yuan L, Wang H, et al. Efficacy and safety of vitamin C for atrial fibrillation after cardiac surgery: a meta-analysis with trial sequential analysis of randomized controlled trials. Int J Surg Lond Engl. 2017;37:58–64 [MC].

[43] Ogino N, Aridome G, Oshima J, et al. Serum albumin concentrations predict hypovolaemia caused by polyethylene glycol plus ascorbic acid prior to colonoscopy in elderly patients. Drugs Aging. 2016;33(5):355–63 [c].

[44] Lee B, Kim K, Cho HY, et al. Effect of intravenous ascorbic acid infusion on blood loss during laparoscopic myomectomy: a randomized, double-blind, placebo-controlled trial. Eur J Obstet Gynecol Reprod Biol. 2016;199:187–91 [c].

[45] Elalfy MS, Saber MM, Adly AAM, et al. Role of vitamin C as an adjuvant therapy to different iron chelators in young β-thalassemia major patients: efficacy and safety in relation to tissue iron overload. Eur J Haematol. 2016;96(3):318–26 [c].

[46] Sultana T, DeVita MV, Michelis MF. Oral vitamin C supplementation reduces erythropoietin requirement in hemodialysis patients with functional iron deficiency. Int Urol Nephrol. 2016;48(9):1519–24 [c].

[47] Montorsi F, Gandaglia G, Salonia A, et al. Effectiveness of a combination of cranberries, lactobacillus rhamnosus, and vitamin C for the management of recurrent urinary tract infections in women: results of a pilot study. Eur Urol. 2016;70(6):912–5 [c].

[48] Ferraro PM, Curhan GC, Gambaro G, et al. Total, dietary, and supplemental vitamin C intake and risk of incident kidney stones. Am J Kidney Dis. 2016;67(3):400–7 [MC].

[49] Raymond YC, Glenda CS, Meng LK. Effects of high doses of vitamin C on cancer patients in Singapore: nine cases. Integr Cancer Ther. 2016;15(2):197–204 [A].

[50] Jeon Y, Park JS, Moon S, et al. Effect of intravenous high dose vitamin C on postoperative pain and morphine use after laparoscopic colectomy: a randomized controlled trial. Pain Res Manag. 2016;2016:9147279 [c].

[51] Buehner M, Pamplin J, Studer L, et al. Oxalate nephropathy after continuous infusion of high-dose vitamin C as an adjunct to burn resuscitation. J Burn Care Res. 2016;37(4):e374–9 [A].

[52] Cirillo M, Bilancio G, Cirillo C. Reversible vascular calcifications associated with hypervitaminosis D. J Nephrol. 2016;29(1):129–31 [A].

[53] Tartagni M, Cicinelli MV, Tartagni MV, et al. Vitamin D supplementation for premenstrual syndrome-related mood

disorders in adolescents with severe hypovitaminosis D. J Pediatr Adolesc Gynecol. 2016;29(4):357–61 [c].

[54] Sotirchos ES, Bhargava P, Eckstein C, et al. Safety and immunologic effects of high- vs low-dose cholecalciferol in multiple sclerosis. Neurology. 2016;86(4):382–90 [c].

[55] Chen P-Z, Li M, Duan X-H, et al. Pharmacokinetics and effects of demographic factors on blood 25(OH)D3 levels after a single orally administered high dose of vitamin D3. Acta Pharmacol Sin. 2016;37(11):1509–15 [c].

[56] Stohs SJ, Kaats GR, Preuss HG. Safety and efficacy of banaba-Moringa oleifera-green coffee bean extracts and vitamin D3 in a sustained release weight management supplement. Phytother Res PTR. 2016;30(4):681–8 [c].

[57] Luger M, Kruschitz R, Kienbacher C, et al. Vitamin D3 loading is superior to conventional supplementation after weight loss surgery in vitamin D-deficient morbidly obese patients: a double-blind randomized placebo-controlled trial. Obes Surg. 2017;27(5):1196–207. http://dx.doi.org/10.1007/s11695-016-2437-0 [c].

[58] Reich KM, Fedorak RN, Madsen K, Kroeker KI. Role of vitamin D in infliximab-induced remission in adult patients with Crohn's disease. Inflamm Bowel Dis. 2016;22(1):92–9 [c].

[59] Jorde R, Sollid ST, Svartberg J, et al. Vitamin D 20,000 IU per week for five years does not prevent progression from prediabetes to diabetes. J Clin Endocrinol Metab. 2016;101(4):1647–55 [C].

[60] Wagner H, Alvarsson M, Mannheimer B, et al. No effect of high-dose vitamin D treatment on β-cell function, insulin sensitivity, or glucose homeostasis in subjects with abnormal glucose tolerance: a randomized clinical trial. Diabetes Care. 2016;39(3):345–52 [c].

[61] Malihi Z, Wu Z, Stewart AW, et al. Hypercalcemia, hypercalciuria, and kidney stones in long-term studies of vitamin D supplementation: a systematic review and meta-analysis. Am J Clin Nutr. 2016;104(4):1039–51 [MC].

[62] Choudhry WM, Nori US, Nadasdy T, et al. An unexpected cause of acute kidney injury in a patient with ANCA associated vasculitis. Clin Nephrol. 2016;85(5):289–95 [A].

[63] Wani M, Wani I, Banday K, et al. The other side of vitamin D therapy: a case series of acute kidney injury due to malpractice-related vitamin D intoxication. Clin Nephrol. 2016;86(11):236–41 [A].

[64] Plante L, Veilleux L-N, Glorieux FH, et al. Effect of high-dose vitamin D supplementation on bone density in youth with osteogenesis imperfecta: a randomized controlled trial. Bone. 2016;86:36–42 [c].

[65] Glendenning P, Inderjeeth CA. Controversy and consensus regarding vitamin D: recent methodological changes and the risks and benefits of vitamin D supplementation. Crit Rev Clin Lab Sci. 2016;53(1):13–28 [R].

[66] Jerzynska J, Stelmach W, Rychlik B, et al. The clinical effect of vitamin D supplementation combined with grass-specific sublingual immunotherapy in children with allergic rhinitis. Allergy Asthma Proc. 2016;37(2):105–14 [c].

[67] Shapiro AC, Adlis SA, Robien K, et al. Randomized, blinded trial of vitamin D3 for treating aromatase inhibitor-associated musculoskeletal symptoms (AIMSS). Breast Cancer Res Treat. 2016;155(3):501–12 [c].

[68] Zerofsky MS, Jacoby BN, Pedersen TL, et al. Daily cholecalciferol supplementation during pregnancy alters markers of regulatory immunity, inflammation, and clinical outcomes in a randomized controlled trial. J Nutr. 2016;146(11):2388–97 [c].

[69] Palacios C, De-Regil LM, Lombardo LK, et al. Vitamin D supplementation during pregnancy: updated meta-analysis on maternal outcomes. J Steroid Biochem Mol Biol. 2016;164:148–55 [M].

[70] Litonjua AA, Carey VJ, Laranjo N, et al. Effect of prenatal supplementation with vitamin D on asthma or recurrent wheezing in offspring by age 3 years: the VDAART randomized clinical trial. JAMA. 2016;315(4):362–70 [MC].

[71] De-Regil LM, Palacios C, Lombardo LK, et al. Vitamin D supplementation for women during pregnancy. Cochrane Database Syst Rev. 2016;1:CD008873 [M].

[72] Cheuk DK, Sieswerda E, van Dalen EC, et al. Medical interventions for treating anthracycline-induced symptomatic and asymptomatic cardiotoxicity during and after treatment for childhood cancer. In: The Cochrane Collaboration ,editor. Cochrane Database of Systematic Reviews. Chichester, UK: John Wiley & Sons, Ltd; 2016. http://dx.doi.org/10.1002/14651858.CD008011.pub3 [R].

[73] Testa D, Marcuccio G, Panin G, et al. Nasal mucosa healing after endoscopic sinus surgery in chronic rhinosinusitis of elderly patients: role of topic alpha-tocopherol acetate. Aging Clin Exp Res. 2017;29:191–5 [c].

[74] Lymperaki E, Makedou K, Iliadis S, et al. Effects of acute cigarette smoking on total blood count and markers of oxidative stress in active and passive smokers. Hippokratia. 2015;19(4):293–7 [c].

[75] Magalhães PVS, Dean O, Andreazza AC, et al. Antioxidant treatments for schizophrenia. In: The Cochrane Collaboration, editor. Cochrane Database of Systematic Reviews. Chichester, UK: John Wiley & Sons, Ltd; 2016. http://dx.doi.org/10.1002/14651858.CD008919.pub2 [R].

[76] Farina N, Llewellyn D, Isaac MGEKN, et al. Vitamin E for Alzheimer's dementia and mild cognitive impairment. In: The Cochrane Collaboration ,editor. Cochrane Database of Systematic Reviews. Chichester, UK: John Wiley & Sons, Ltd; 2017. http://dx.doi.org/10.1002/14651858.CD002854.pub4 [R].

[77] Saboori S, Djalali M, Yousefi Rad E, et al. Various effects of omega 3 and omega 3 plus vitamin E supplementations on serum glucose level and insulin resistance in patients with coronary artery disease. Iran J Public Health. 2016;45(11):1465–72 [c].

[78] Lee SWH, Lai NM, Chaiyakunapruk N, et al. Adverse effects of herbal or dietary supplements in G6PD deficiency: a systematic review. Br J Clin Pharmacol. 2017;83(1):172–9 [R].

[79] Thébaut A, Nemeth A, Le Mouhaër J, et al. Oral tocofersolan corrects or prevents vitamin E deficiency in children with chronic cholestasis. J Pediatr Gastroenterol Nutr. 2016;63(6):610–5 [C].

[80] Rezaei Y, Khademvatani K, Rahimi B, et al. Short-term high-dose vitamin E to prevent contrast medium-induced acute kidney injury in patients with chronic kidney disease undergoing elective coronary angiography: a randomized placebo-controlled trial. J Am Heart Assoc. 2016;5(3)e002919 [C].

[81] Sohrabi Z, Eftekhari MH, Eskandari MH, et al. Intradialytic oral protein supplementation and nutritional and inflammation outcomes in hemodialysis: a randomized controlled trial. Am J Kidney Dis. 2016;68(1):122–30 [c].

[82] Gopaluni S, Sherif M, Ahmadouk NA. Interventions for chronic kidney disease-associated restless legs syndrome. Cochrane Database Syst Rev. 2016;11:CD010690 [R].

[83] Kurokawa I, Oiso N, Kawada A. Adjuvant alternative treatment with chemical peeling and subsequent iontophoresis for postinflammatory hyperpigmentation, erosion with inflamed red papules and non-inflamed atrophic scars in acne vulgaris. J Dermatol. 2017;44(4):401–5. http://dx.doi.org/10.1111/1346-8138.13634 [c].

[84] Tanaydin V, Conings J, Malyar M, et al. The role of topical vitamin E in scar management: a systematic review. Aesthet Surg J. 2016;36(8):959–65 [R].

[85] Kearney M, Orrell RW, Fahey M, et al. Pharmacological treatments for Friedreich ataxia. In: The Cochrane Collaboration , editor. Cochrane Database of Systematic Reviews. Chichester, UK: John Wiley & Sons, Ltd; 2016. http://dx.doi.org/10.1002/14651858.CD007791.pub4 [R].

[86] Koudelka S, Turanek Knotigova P, Masek J, et al. Liposomal delivery systems for anti-cancer analogues of vitamin E. J Control Release. 2015;207:59 [R].

[87] Sano M, Aisen PS, Andrews HF, et al. Vitamin E in aging persons with Down syndrome: a randomized, placebo-controlled clinical trial. Neurology. 2016;86(22):2071–6 [C].

[88] Balogun OO, da Silva Lopes K, Ota E, et al. Vitamin supplementation for preventing miscarriage. In: The Cochrane Collaboration ,editor. Cochrane Database of Systematic Reviews. Chichester, UK: John Wiley & Sons, Ltd; 2016. http://dx.doi.org/10.1002/14651858.CD004073.pub4 [R].

[89] Pattanittum P, Kunyanone N, Brown J, et al. Dietary supplements for dysmenorrhoea. In: The Cochrane Collaboration , editor. Cochrane Database of Systematic Reviews. Chichester, UK: John Wiley & Sons, Ltd; 2016. http://dx.doi.org/10.1002/14651858.CD002124.pub2 [R].

[90] Choudhary B, Kumari S, Dhingra B, et al. A clinically suspected case of anaphylactoid reaction to vitamin K injection in a child—a case report and review of literature. Indian J Pharmacol. 2016;48(4):45–75 [A].

[91] Bian C, Qi X, Li L, et al. Anticoagulant management of pregnant women with mechanical heart valve replacement during perioperative period. Arch Gynecol Obstet. 2016;293(1):69–74 [c].

[92] Pinta F, Ponzetti A, Spadi R, et al. Pilot clinical trial on the efficacy of prophylactic use of vitamin K1-based cream (vigorskin) to prevent cetuximab-induced skin rash in patients with metastatic colorectal cancer. Clin Colorectal Cancer. 2014;13(1):62–7 [c].

[93] Jung D-H, Hwang S, Song G-W, et al. An interim safety analysis of hepatocellular carcinoma patients administrating oral vitamin K with or without sorafenib. Korean J Hepato-Biliary-Pancreat Surg. 2015;19(1):1–5 [c].

[94] McNeal CJ, Meininger CJ, Reddy D, et al. Safety and effectiveness of arginine in adults. J Nutr. 2016;146(12) 2587S-93S [R].

[95] Brooks JR, Oketch-Rabah H, Low Dog T, et al. Safety and performance benefits of arginine supplements for military personnel: a systematic review. Nutr Rev. 2016;74(11):708–21 [r].

[96] Avenell A, Smith TO, Curtain JP, et al. Nutritional supplementation for hip fracture aftercare in older people. In: The Cochrane Collaboration ,editor. Cochrane Database of Systematic Reviews. Chichester, UK: John Wiley & Sons, Ltd; 2016. http://dx.doi.org/10.1002/14651858.CD001880.pub6 [MC].

[97] Kircheis G. Current state of knowledge of hepatic encephalopathy (Part V): clinical efficacy of L-ornithine-L-aspartate in the management of HE. Metab Brain Dis. 2016;31(6):1365–7 [r].

[98] Girke J, Seipt C, Markowski A, et al. Quality of life and nutrition condition of patients improve under home parenteral nutrition: an exploratory study. Nutr Clin Pract. 2016;31(5):659–65 [c].

[99] Radpay R. Poor zamany nejat kermany M, radpay B. Comparison between total parenteral nutrition vs. Partial parenteral nutrition on serum lipids among chronic ventilator dependent patients: a multicenter study. Tanaffos. 2016;15(1):31–6 [c].

[100] Yan C-L, Huang Y-B, Chen C-Y, et al. Hyperglycemia is associated with poor outcomes in surgical critically ill patients receiving parenteral nutrition. Acta Anaesthesiol Taiwan. 2013;51(2):67–72 [c].

[101] Dotson B, Larabell P, Patel JU, et al. Calcium administration is associated with adverse outcomes in critically ill patients receiving parenteral nutrition: results from a natural experiment created by a calcium gluconate shortage. Pharmacotherapy. 2016;36(11):1185–90 [C].

[102] Dastych M, Dastych Jr. M, Senkyrík M. Manganese in whole blood and hair in patients with long-term home parenteral nutrition. Clin Lab. 2016;62(1–2):173–7 [c].

[103] Hernández CR, Ponce EC, Busquets FB, et al. Hypersensitivity reaction to components of parenteral nutrition in pediatrics. Nutrition. 2016;32(11–12):1303–5 [A].

[104] Zhu LY, Broussard KC, Boyd AS, et al. An eruption while on total parenteral nutrition. Cutis. 2016;97(3):E3–5 [A].

[105] Guducuoglu H, Gultepe B, Otlu B, et al. Candida albicans outbreak associated with total parenteral nutrition in the neonatal unit. Indian J Med Microbiol. 2016;34(2):202–7 [c].

[106] Okada M, Sato M, Ogura M, et al. Central venous catheter infection-related glomerulonephritis under long-term parenteral nutrition: a report of two cases. BMC Res Notes. 2016;9:196. http://dx.doi.org/10.1186/s13104-016-1997-3 [A].

[107] Chow R, Bruera E, Chiu L, et al. Enteral and parenteral nutrition in cancer patients: a systematic review and meta-analysis. Ann Palliat Med. 2016;5(1):30–41 [M].

[108] Wu GH, Zaniolo O, Schuster H, et al. Structured triglycerides versus physical mixtures of medium- and long-chain triglycerides for parenteral nutrition in surgical or critically ill adult patients: systematic review and meta-analysis. Clin Nutr. 2017;36:150–61. http://dx.doi.org/10.1016/j.clnu.2016.01.004 [M].

[109] Hayes BD, Gosselin S, Calello DP, et al. Systematic review of clinical adverse events reported after acute intravenous lipid emulsion administration. Clin Toxicol. 2016;54(5): 365–404 [R].

[110] Dai Y-J, Sun L-L, Li M-Y, et al. Comparison of formulas based on lipid emulsions of olive oil, soybean oil, or several oils for parenteral nutrition: a systematic review and meta-analysis. Adv Nutr Int Rev J. 2016;7(2):279–86 [M].

[111] Lu J-W, Liu C, Du Z-Q, et al. Early enteral nutrition vs parenteral nutrition following pancreaticoduodenectomy: experience from a single center. World J Gastroenterol. 2016;22(14):3821–8 [C].

[112] Hongyin L, Zhu H, Tao W, et al. Abdominal paracentesis drainage improves tolerance of enteral nutrition in acute pancreatitis: a randomized controlled trial. Scand J Gastroenterol. 2017;52(4):389–95 [C].

[113] Yagmurdur H, Leblebici F. Enteral nutrition preference in critical care: fibre-enriched or fibre-free? Asia Pac J Clin Nutr. 2016;25(4):740–6 [C].

[114] Zhuang RD, Tang LJ, Fang YH, et al. Clinical analysis of enteral nutrition in 47 children. Zhonghua Er Ke Za Zhi. 2016;54(7): 500–3 [c].

[115] Seres DS, Ippolito PR. Pilot study evaluating the efficacy, tolerance and safety of a peptide-based enteral formula versus a high protein enteral formula in multiple ICU settings (medical, surgical, cardiothoracic). Clin Nutr. 2017;36(3):706–9. http://dx.doi.org/10.1016/j.clnu.2016.04.016 [c].

[116] Pahsini K, Marinschek S, Khan Z, et al. Unintended adverse effects of enteral nutrition support: parental perspective. J Pediatr Gastroenterol Nutr. 2016;62(1):169–73 [C].

[117] Toh Yoon E, Yoneda K, Nishihara K. Semi-solid feeds may reduce the risk of aspiration pneumonia and shorten postoperative length of stay after percutaneous endoscopic gastrostomy (PEG). Endosc Int Open. 2016;04(12):E1247–51 [C].

[118] McSweeney ME, Kerr J, Amirault J, et al. Oral feeding reduces hospitalizations compared with gastrostomy feeding in infants and children who aspirate. J Pediatr. 2016;170:79–84 [C].

[119] Joffe A, Anton N, Lequier L, et al. Nutritional support for critically ill children. In: The Cochrane Collaboration ,editor. Cochrane Database of Systematic Reviews. Chichester, UK: John Wiley & Sons, Ltd; 2016. http://dx.doi.org/10.1002/14651858.CD005144.pub3 [R].

[120] Wedrychowicz A, Zajac A, Tomasik P. Advances in nutritional therapy in inflammatory bowel diseases: review. World J Gastroenterol. 2016;22(3):1045–66 [R].

31

Drugs That Affect Blood Coagulation, Fibrinolysis and Hemostasis

Hanna Raber[*,1], *Jason Isch*[†], *Kirk Evoy*[‡]

*College of Pharmacy, University of Utah, Salt Lake City, UT, United States
[†]Graduate Medical Education, Saint Joseph Health System, Mishawaka, IN, United States
[‡]College of Pharmacy, University of Texas at Austin, Austin, TX, United States
[1]Corresponding author: hanna.raber@pharm.utah.edu

COUMARIN ANTICOAGULANTS
[SEDA-36, 529; SEDA-37, 419; SEDA-38, 365]

Warfarin [SEDA-36, 529; SEDA-37, 419; SEDA-38, 365]

Monitoring Therapy

The SAMe-TT$_2$R$_2$ score was recently developed to predict the likelihood of atrial fibrillation (AF) patients on warfarin to have a time in therapeutic range (TTR) above 70% (i.e., patient's international normalized ratio (INR) is within the target range ≥70% of the period studied), with a TTR of ≥70% the goal for patients managed on warfarin [1C]. A single-center retrospective study of 1428 Chinese patients was conducted to validate the SAMe-TT$_2$R$_2$ score. This study was the first to assess the validity of the SAMe-TT$_2$R$_2$ score in an Asian population, as previous studies validating the score were performed in primarily Caucasian populations. While overall TTR among patients included in this study was quite low (mean TTR was 38.2% ± 24.4% (interquartile range: 17.9%)), the SAMe-TT$_2$R$_2$ score did correlate well with TTR and ischemic stroke incidence. Using a SAMe-TT$_2$R$_2$ score of 2 as a cutoff, the sensitivity and specificity to predict a TTR ≥70% were 85.7% and 18.2%, respectively, while the positive and negative predictive values were 11.2% and 91.3%, respectively. Additionally, the SAMe-TT$_2$R$_2$ score displayed significant association with annual ischemic stroke risk. In patients with a SAMe-TT$_2$R$_2$ score ≤2, the annual risk of ischemic stroke was significantly lower (3.49%/year) than patients with a SAMe-TT$_2$R$_2$ score ≥4 (6.41%/year, $P < 0.001$). The study's authors concluded that the SAMe-TT$_2$R$_2$ score

correlates well with TTR in Chinese AF patients, with a score above 2 having a high sensitivity and negative predictive value for poor TTR. This may be useful in clinical practice, as patients with a SAMe-TT$_2$R$_2$ score >2 may benefit from closer follow-up, increased warfarin-related patient education, or alternative anticoagulation strategies.

A retrospective study of 258 patients on warfarin (with an INR ≤3 at the time of the procedure) was conducted at a single Japanese dental surgery center to assess whether the HAS-BLED score could successfully predict post-tooth-extraction bleeding (defined as a bleed requiring medical hemostatic procedures to terminate the bleed) [2C]. In this study, 21 of the 258 patients experienced a post-tooth-extraction bleed. The mean HAS-BLED score was not significantly different in those who experienced a bleed (1.3 ± 0.9) vs those who did not (1.2 ± 0.8, $P = 0.467$), and the HAS-BLED score was deemed insufficient to predict post-tooth-extraction bleeding risk.

Nephropathy

A case of warfarin-related nephropathy in a 56-year-old Chinese woman with atrial fibrillation and a mechanical mitral valve replacement was reported [3A]. The woman had been taking warfarin for multiple years, with no recent changes in her medications or diet. Her INR upon diagnosis was elevated (4.95), though this was detected during a routine follow-up, and she had no perceived signs or symptoms of bleeding. Further workup revealed a significantly elevated serum creatinine (317 micromol/L) and microscopic hematuria. Due to persistent acute kidney injury (AKI), a renal biopsy was performed 12 days later with findings suggestive of background IgA

Side Effects of Drugs Annual, Volume 39
ISSN: 0378-6080
http://dx.doi.org/10.1016/bs.seda.2017.06.013

nephropathy. However, the patient had normal renal function prior to this event, and the authors concluded that warfarin over-anticoagulation likely precipitated an AKI in this patient with probable background IgA nephropathy. After a 5-day discontinuation of all anticoagulation followed by temporary bridge-therapy with enoxaparin and treatment with oral acetylcysteine 1.2 g twice daily and oral prednisolone 30 mg daily, the serum creatinine improved to 274 micromol/L but did not return to baseline at 3-month follow-up.

Hematologic

A single-center retrospective evaluation compared 164 pediatric patients undergoing warfarin therapy, 93 of which were monitored with patient self-testing at home while 71 received INR assessments from a hospital or pathology service [4C]. Patients undergoing home self-testing achieved similar TTR with no difference in major bleeding events. No previously unreported adverse events (AE) emerged.

A single-center retrospective study of 646 patients anticoagulated with warfarin with a current INR >3 sought to evaluate the frequency of abdominal hemorrhagic complications through the use of abdominal computed tomography (CT) scans [5C]. The study identified hemorrhagic complications via abdominal CT in 11.5% of patients ($n = 74$). Investigators found that frequency of hemorrhagic complications was correlated with intensity of anticoagulation. 5.9% of those in the lowest studied INR range of 3.01–3.99 experienced hemorrhagic complications and this percentage increased with each 1 point increase in INR range. Among patients in the highest reported INR category (INR of 10 or greater), 28.9% of patients experienced a hemorrhagic event.

A meta-analysis of 8 cohort studies (7 retrospective and 1 prospective) including 9539 patients with AF undergoing hemodialysis sought to assess whether stroke risk differed based on whether or not they were taking warfarin [6M]. The study identified a greater risk of stroke among patients receiving warfarin (relative risk (RR) 1.50, 95% confidence interval (CI): 1.13–1.99). This was driven predominantly by an increase in the risk of hemorrhagic stroke (RR 2.30, 95% CI: 1.62–3.27) and not ischemic stroke (RR 1.01, 95% CI: 0.65–1.57).

A retrospective study of a large US administrative claims database compared outcomes of 20158 patients receiving novel anticoagulants (NOACs, specifically dabigatran, rivaroxaban, or apixaban) to warfarin among patients with AF with valvular heart disease (post-valve repair or bioprosthetic replacement, rheumatic mitral stenosis, non-rheumatic mitral stenosis, and either mitral regurgitation, aortic stenosis, or aortic insufficiency) [7C]. In this study, major bleeding events were lower with NOACs than warfarin (hazard ratio (HR) 0.84, 95% CI: 0.72–0.97) amongst patients with aortic stenosis

(AS) or insufficiency (AI) or mitral regurgitation (MR). However, while the purpose of the study was to assess the safety and efficacy of NOACs across the spectrum of valvular heart disease, the vast majority ($n = 19351$) had AS/AI/MR, and thus data from the study can only safely be generalized to the AS/AI/MR group. There was no statistical difference in bleeding event rates among patients with post-surgical valve disease treated with NOACs vs warfarin, though only 79 such patients were treated with NOACs for such conditions. Thus, there is insufficient evidence to make strong recommendations for the use of NOACs in such patients.

Cardiovascular

Following a recent study that identified increased arterial calcification in breasts of women taking warfarin, a single-center retrospective matched cohort study was conducted to assess whether warfarin was similarly associated with increased arterial calcification in the lower extremities and in men [8C]. Peripheral arterial calcification was identified via lower leg or foot radiograph in 30.2% of patients with current or past warfarin use vs 20.9% ($P = 0.0023$) among patients with no warfarin use. Use of warfarin for more than 5 years was significantly associated with increased calcification ($P = 0.001$), whereas patients with less than 5 years of warfarin therapy displayed similar calcification rates to the control group. Both genders displayed similar calcification rates. The authors note that this data is consistent with past animal and human studies and postulate the mechanism to be inhibition of matrix Gla protein.

Skin

A case of a 76-year-old woman who developed bilateral necrotic lesions on her lower legs 1 month after starting warfarin for AF was reported [9A]. After further workup, the patient was diagnosed with skin-biopsy-confirmed calciphylaxis. Despite stopping warfarin and receiving wound care and antibiotics, the ulcers worsened. After more than 6 months the ulcers had not healed, eventually culminating in death from severe sepsis with multi-organ failure. Her physicians concluded that the calciphylaxis was warfarin-induced.

HEPARINS [SEDA-36, 530; SEDA-37, 419; SEDA-38, 367]

Enoxaparin [SEDA-36, 530; SEDA-37, 419; SEDA-38, 367]

Skin

A case of a 71-year-old Caucasian man who developed asymptomatic, erythematous, blood-filled vesicles and bullae on his limbs 2 weeks after initiating subcutaneous enoxaparin 80 mg every 12 hours for deep vein thrombosis (DVT) was reported [10A]. These lesions were not present near the enoxaparin injection sites. Workup revealed normal blood counts, coagulation studies, and serum chemistry, while the lesions were found to contain predominantly red blood cells without signs of vasculitis or intravascular thrombus. The patient was diagnosed with enoxaparin-induced bullous hemorrhagic dermatosis. Despite symptoms, the patient remained on enoxaparin for 6 months, with lesions coming and going. Following enoxaparin discontinuation, the symptoms completely resolved. The study authors noted 18 other cases of bullous hemorrhagic dermatosis associated with low-molecular-weight heparins have been reported.

Hematologic

Pregnant and post-partum women are at increased risk of venous thromboembolism (VTE), particularly in obese patients and/or following post-cesarean delivery [11c]. However, little evidence exists to determine whether these patients should be anticoagulated and, if so, what the ideal anticoagulant dose is. Therefore, a single-center, randomized controlled trial (RCT) was conducted including 84 women with a body mass index $\geq$35 post-cesarean delivery, with half receiving a fixed dose of enoxaparin 40 mg once a day and half receiving enoxaparin 0.5 mg/kg every 12 hours. The weight-based dosing regimen led to significantly higher rates of patients achieving target prophylactic anti-Xa blood levels. Major AEs were similar among groups.

A single-center retrospective analysis assessed the persistence of prolonged activated partial thromboplastin time (aPTT) following various bolus doses of unfractionated heparin (UFH) in patients with chronic kidney disease (CKD, defined in this study as a creatinine clearance <60 mL/min) following a ST-segment elevation myocardial infarction (STEMI) to determine at which UFH bolus doses persistent prolongation of aPTT occurs [12C]. Of the 1071 patients included in the study, 195 had CKD. The investigators noted that 6 hours after primary percutaneous coronary intervention (PCI), patients with CKD had a higher aPTT ratio (5.1) vs patients without CKD (3.4, $P < 0.001$). They also found CKD patients were more likely to have a markedly high aPTT at least four times that of the control (OR 2.04, 95% CI: 1.27–3.27), and that the highest risk of markedly high aPTT occurred with UFH bolus doses $\geq$130 IU/kg (OR 3.69, 95% CI: 1.85–7.36). CKD was also associated with greater risk of bleeding complications (OR 2.78, $P < 0.001$) and major adverse cardiac events (OR 2.52, $P < 0.001$) in this study. The authors concluded that CKD presents risk for persistently prolonged aPTT in STEMI patients undergoing primary PCI and that reducing the dose of UFH in CKD patients may reduce bleeding complications.

DIRECT THROMBIN INHIBITORS
[SEDA-36, 531; SEDA-37, 422; SEDA-38, 368]

Bivalirudin [SEDA-32, 633; SEDA-35, 619; SEDA-38, 368]

Cardiovascular

A retrospective observational cohort study analyzed a database that includes clinical and economic information from more than 600 US hospitals [13C], in order to compare outcomes of congestive heart failure (CHF) patients undergoing PCI with either bivalirudin $\pm$ glycoprotein IIb/IIIa inhibitors (GPI) or UFH $\pm$ GPI. A total of 89 948 propensity-score-matched patients were included ($n =$ 42 474 for each group). Bivalirudin patients experienced lower risk of death (OR 0.851, $P < 0.0001$), bleeding (OR 0.885, $P < 0.0001$), bleeding requiring transfusion (OR 0.845, $P < 0.0001$), and transfusion (OR 0.857, $P < 0.0001$).

A meta-analysis of 18 observational studies and 12 RCT comparing bivalirudin to UFH during PCI was conducted [14M]. In total, 51 593 patients were included. The primary outcomes were major cardiovascular events (myocardial infarction (MI), death or urgent revascularization and stent thrombosis, major bleeding, and transfusion) within 30 days. Among bivalirudin-treated patients, major bleeding (OR 0.59, $P < 0.0001$) and transfusion (OR 0.79, $P = 0.01$) were significantly reduced, while major adverse cardiovascular events were similar (OR 0.98, $P = 0.80$), and stent thrombosis was higher (OR 1.52, $P = 0.009$).

A similar meta-analysis compared bivalirudin to UFH $\pm$ GPI in patients with acute STEMI undergoing primary PCI [15M]. The meta-analysis included six studies ($n = 14 095$ patients). With regards to 30-day outcomes, all-cause mortality (RR 0.81, $P = 0.041$), cardiac mortality (RR 0.68, $P = 0.009$), and major bleeding (RR 0.63, $P = 0.12$) were significantly lower in the bivalirudin group, while major cardiac AE (RR 1.02, $P = 0.800$), MI (RR 1.41, $P = 0.089$), target vessel revascularization (RR 1.37, $P = 0.122$) and net adverse clinical events (RR 0.81, $P = 0.069$) were not statistically significantly different from UFH. The risk of acute stent thrombosis (RR 3.31, $P < 0.001$) was significantly higher in the bivalirudin group.

A patient-level pooled analysis of three previously conducted RCT comparing bivalirudin ($n = 7413$ total; $n = 1870$ women) to UFH plus GPI ($n = 7371$ total; $n = 1910$ women) in patients undergoing PCI was conducted to assess the outcomes in female patients, specifically [16R]. Among the women included in these studies, bivalirudin-treated patients experienced lower 30-day major bleeding risk (HR 0.56, $P < 0.001$) and mortality (HR 0.66, $P = 0.02$) than UFH/GPI-treated patients. When comparing males to females, while 1-year mortality was higher among women than men, multivariate analyses identified female gender as an independent predictor of reduced 1-year mortality after adjusting for gender differences in 30-day major bleeding complications (which were higher in women, HR 1.80, $P < 0.001$ for major bleed). The authors concluded that bleeding complications are the strongest predictor of increased mortality in patients undergoing PCI, as opposed to female gender.

Dabigatran Etexilate [SEDA-36, 531; SEDA-37, 422; SEDA-38, 369]

Hematologic

A post-hoc subgroup analysis of the RE-LY randomized controlled trial, which compared dabigatran (110 or 150 mg twice daily) with warfarin for the treatment of AF, was conducted to assess perioperative outcomes associated with each drug among patients requiring a surgery/procedure [17C]. A total of 4168 patients (23.1% of the study population) underwent an elective surgery/procedure, while 353 patients (2% of study population) underwent an urgent surgery/procedure. For both urgent and elective surgeries, the rates of major bleed, life-threatening bleed, thromboembolism, and mortality were not statistically different based on anticoagulant received.

A retrospective study utilized national prescription and hospital records from New Zealand to compare bleeding risk of AF patients aged ≥65 and newly initiated on warfarin or dabigatran in a real-world setting [18C]. Two different propensity-matched cohorts were studied. In the first cohort, which included 4385 patients taking dabigatran at any dose and 4385 patients taking warfarin, dabigatran was associated with significantly lower total hemorrhage events (HR 0.45, 95% CI: 0.37–0.55) and intracerebral hemorrhages (HR 0.29, 95% CI: 0.09–0.86), while gastrointestinal bleeding risk was numerically higher without statistical significance (HR 1.16, 95% CI: 0.87–1.56). In the second cohort, which consisted of 3395 patients receiving dabigatran 110 mg twice daily, 2153 patients receiving dabigatran 150 mg twice daily and 2283 patients receiving warfarin, both dabigatran 110 mg (HR 0.40, 95% CI: 0.31–0.52) and 150 mg (HR 0.29, 95% CI: 0.19–0.41) were associated with lower risk of total hemorrhage events. Of note, hemorrhage events were defined as bleeding events requiring admission to the hospital. Finally, mortality was assessed using national mortality registry data to identify deaths within 7 days after the original bleeding event and patients receiving dabigatran at either dose displayed a lower 7-day mortality rate than those receiving warfarin (adjusted odds ratio 0.72, 95% CI: 0.59–0.87).

A population-based observational study comparing dabigatran (110 or 150 mg twice daily; $n = 15\,918$) and warfarin ($n = 47\,192$) in AF patients was also conducted in Canada [19C]. Notably, 67.3% of the study population

was ≥75 years old, and the authors compared outcomes of this cohort to the patients ≤75 years. Among patients ≥75 years, dabigatran ($n = 9548$) was associated with similar overall bleeding risk (HR 0.94, 95% CI: 0.86–1.01), less ICH (HR 0.60, 95% CI: 0.47–0.76) and more gastrointestinal bleeding (HR 1.30, 95% CI: 1.14–1.50) compared with warfarin ($n = 32\,930$).

Similarly, a single-center, retrospective, observational study compared dabigatran 110 mg twice daily ($n = 129$) to warfarin ($n = 442$) in Chinese patients aged ≥80 years with nonvalvular AF [20C]. At baseline, patients exhibited a mean CHA_2DS_2-VASc score of 4.8 ± 1.6 and HAS-BLED score of 2.4 ± 0.8. Over a mean follow-up duration of 2.6 years, 4 dabigatran patients (1.4%/year) experienced an ischemic stroke vs 83 warfarin patients (6.9%/year; HR 0.22, 95% CI: 0.23–0.67). One patient receiving dabigatran (0.35%/year) and seven patients receiving warfarin (0.59%/year) experienced an intracranial hemorrhage (ICH). The authors concluded that dabigatran reduced stroke risk with similar rates of ICH compared with warfarin in elderly Chinese AF patients.

A meta-analysis of 22 observational studies (including 26 817 patients taking dabigatran 110 mg twice daily, 43 298 patients taking dabigatran 150 mg twice daily, and 266 878 patients taking vitamin K antagonists (VKA)) compared the bleeding risk of dabigatran vs VKA for AF treatment [21M]. Studies were required to include at least 1000 AF patients, directly compare dabigatran and VKA, and report bleeding events to be included. Patients receiving 110 mg dabigatran displayed a significantly lower risk of any bleeding (HR 0.78, 95% CI: 0.69–0.89) and major bleeding (HR 0.84, 95% CI: 0.73–0.97) vs VKA. Patients taking 150 mg dabigatran exhibited lower bleeding risk (HR 0.83, 95% CI: 0.60–1.14) and lower major bleeding risk (HR 0.77, 95% CI: 0.55–1.07) than VKA but did not reach statistical significance.

A multicenter, retrospective, observational study was conducted in Turkey to compare outcomes of patients with nonvalvular AF newly initiated on dabigatran (110 or 150 mg twice daily) with a non-matched cohort of warfarin patients from the same study centers [22C]. Several significant limitations of this study exist that may reduce the validity of these results compared to those of other studies contained in this text. Limitations include the fact that the cohorts were unmatched and most baseline characteristics differed significantly among the treatment groups, the TTR in the warfarin group was only 32%, the median follow-up period was much longer for warfarin (15 months) than dabigatran (6 months), and the number of patients was small compared to many recent studies comparing these two drugs.

A small, prospective observational study displayed statistically similar rates of stroke and AEs among patients receiving the VKA acenocoumarol ($n = 74$) and dabigatran

110 mg twice daily ($n = 9$). However, this study was likely underpowered to show differences given the small number of dabigatran patients studied [23c].

A case report was published regarding a 71-year-old man taking dabigatran who reported to the emergency department with an acute gastrointestinal hemorrhage [24A]. Initial labs revealed an INR >10, aPTT of 93 seconds, hemoglobin of 12 g/dL, and an acute kidney injury (serum creatinine of 5.8 mg/dL compared to his baseline of 1.1 mg/dL 3 months prior). He was given 5 mg oral phytonadione, 2 units of fresh frozen plasma, 1 g calcium gluconate, 10 units of insulin and 25 g dextrose solution. An hour after admission the patient became hypotensive (77/39 mm Hg) and eventually was placed on norepinephrine infusion to stabilize blood pressure. Twelve hours after admission, the patient developed hemorrhagic shock and was administered 3500 units of 4-factor prothrombin complex concentrate (4F-PCC). He was also initiated on hemodialysis to increase dabigatran elimination. Four hours after 4F-PCC administration and hemodialysis initiation, the patient's coagulation levels were markedly reduced (INR 1.7, PT 17 seconds). No further dialysis or pro-coagulants were administered, and the patient discharged on hospital day 8. The authors note this to be the first case published regarding gastrointestinal hemorrhage and hypovolemic shock reversal in a patient with an AKI while taking dabigatran.

Cardiovascular

A report of an 83-year-old woman presenting with a type A aortic dissection thought to be induced by dabigatran 110 mg was published [25A]. Upon admission, the patient's prothrombin time (190 seconds; reference 10.5–13.5 seconds), aPTT (55 seconds; reference 25–37 seconds), and thrombin time (>150 seconds; reference 14–20 seconds) were all significantly elevated. The patient's dabigatran level was 240 ng/mL, and her renal function was impaired (eGFR 48 mL/min). Dialysis was initiated and lowered the dabigatran concentration to 140 ng/mL. However, the patient's plasma dabigatran concentration began to rise again 2 hours after dialysis (which the authors postulate was due to redistribution of protein-bound dabigatran). With the patient remaining anticoagulated, 20 units/kg factor VIII was administered to reduce the anticoagulant activity for surgery. A successful ascending aortic replacement was subsequently performed. Thus, the authors concluded that while hemodialysis may reduce dabigatran levels, dabigatran levels may subsequently rise shortly after due to redistribution.

Esophageal

A small, multi-center retrospective study was conducted in Japan to assess the frequency and endoscopic characteristics of dabigatran-induced esophagitis among the 91 patients identified who were taking dabigatran (110 or 150 mg twice daily) at the time they had undergone an upper gastrointestinal endoscopy [26c]. Dabigatran-induced esophagitis was identified in 20.9% ($n = 19$) of patients. Thirteen of these patients experienced associated symptoms including odynophagia, dysphagia, chest pain, heartburn, nausea, epigastric pain, melena, or abdominal fullness. Five patients had a follow-up endoscopy, three of whom had their dabigatran discontinued, while the other two were instructed to drink more water and maintain an upright position for at least 30 minutes after taking their dabigatran. In each of these patients the lesions were resolved on follow-up endoscopy. The study authors note this to be the first study to assess prevalence of dabigatran-induced esophagitis by endoscopy.

A case report of a 75-year-old Japanese man who developed an esophageal mucosal injury shortly after initiating dabigatran 110 mg twice daily was published [27A]. Asymptomatic whitish mucosal thickening in the upper esophagus was first observed on routine screening endoscopy 3 days after beginning dabigatran. One week later, the lesion had become diffuse throughout the upper and middle esophagus. Esophageal mucosal coagulation necrosis was established via biopsy. Dabigatran was discontinued, and the patient was initiated on warfarin therapy. The lesions were resolved upon follow-up 4 weeks later.

Ocular

A case report of a 79-year-old woman with hypertension, CHF, AF, and coronary artery disease presenting with painless, acute bilateral vision loss (visual acuity of 20/400 in the right eye and 20/500 in the left) was published [28A]. Patient workup revealed spontaneous hyphemia, fibrin accumulation, vitreous hemorrhage, and bilateral choroidal detachment believed to be induced by dabigatran, which she had started taking less than a year prior at a dose of 150 mg twice daily for AF. Despite discontinuation of dabigatran, neither topical nor oral steroids resolved the injury, and surgery was required. One month post-surgery the patient's vision was reportedly stable. Per report authors, this was the first such event reported related to dabigatran therapy.

DIRECT FACTOR XA INHIBITORS
[SEDA-36, 532; SEDA-37, 423; SEDA-38, 370]

Apixaban [SEDA-32, 635; SEDA-34, 546; SEDA-38, 370]

Death

An analysis of the AMPLIFY-EXT trial ($n = 2486$) studied the effects of extended anticoagulation over 12 months with apixaban on hospitalization rates for patients with VTE [29R]. Compared to placebo, both apixaban 2.5

and 5 mg twice daily significantly reduced the rate of all-cause hospitalization (HR 0.64, $P=0.026$ and HR 0.54, $P=0.004$). Both apixaban doses significantly reduced the time to first hospitalization (by 43 and 49 days, respectively). Median length of hospital stay was longer for placebo compared to both apixaban doses (by 2 and 2.5 days, respectively). The study promotes the use of extended anticoagulation for VTE vs standard length of therapy. Based on 2016 CHEST guidelines for VTE, extended therapy is now recommended in patients with unprovoked DVT or PE and at lower bleeding risk over 3 months of therapy [30].

Hematologic

Subgroup analysis from the AVERROES trial examined the safety of apixaban in the elderly population compared with aspirin [31R]. The trial of 5599 patients included 1898 patients ≥ 75 years and 366 patients ≥ 85 years. Compared to aspirin, apixaban was significantly more efficacious in preventing both pulmonary emboli and strokes in the elderly population. In regards to safety, apixaban and aspirin showed similar rates of major bleeding in the ≥ 85 year population (4.7%/year vs 4.9%/year). However, rates of intracranial bleeding were lower with apixaban vs aspirin in this age group (0.5%/year vs 2.9%/year; HR 0.17, $P=0.04$). The study authors concluded that apixaban is superior to aspirin in the elderly population due to increased efficacy and slightly less intracranial bleeding.

A meta-analysis of three studies ($n=1057$) analyzed the safety and efficacy of uninterrupted periprocedural apixaban in patients undergoing AF catheter ablation compared to VKA [32M]. No statistical differences were noted in overall bleeding (OR 0.94, 95% CI: 0.55–1.58), major bleeding (OR 1.37, 95% CI: 0.33–5.67) or minor bleeding (OR 0.89, 95% CI: 0.50–1.55). The authors concluded that apixaban is a safe and effective alternative to VKA in AF ablation.

A meta-analysis of four phase III RCT ($n > 70\,000$) compared the relative safety and efficacy of the NOACs to VKA for patients with non-valvular atrial fibrillation [33M]. The studies included were the ARISTOTLE trial (apixaban), the RE-LY trial (dabigatran 110 or 150 mg twice daily), the ENGAGE AF-TIMI trial (edoxaban 30 or 60 mg daily), and the ROCKET-AF trial (rivaroxaban). The study concluded that all of the NOACs have comparable safety and efficacy to warfarin with a few statistically significant differences among the NOACs. Efficacy data significantly favored apixaban (HR 0.70, 95% CI: 0.55–0.88), high-dose dabigatran (HR 0.57, 95% CI: 0.44–0.75), rivaroxaban (HR 0.77, 95% CI: 0.62–0.96), and high-dose edoxaban (HR 0.77, 95% CI: 0.66–0.90) compared to edoxaban 30 mg daily. High-dose dabigatran was favored over rivaroxaban (HR 0.74, 95% CI:

0.56–0.97), edoxaban 60 mg (HR 0.74, 95% CI: 0.57–0.97), and low-dose dabigatran (HR 0.72, 95% CI: 0.57–0.90), but not apixaban (HR 0.82, 95% CI: 0.61–1.08). In regards to safety data, patients given apixaban, and low-dose edoxaban had significantly less major bleeding, GI bleeding, and other major bleeding compared to rivaroxaban or dabigatran 150 mg. The authors of the study further conclude that apixaban has the best balance of safety, efficacy, and tolerability compared to the rest of the NOACs. However, there are several limitations that should be considered including the variability in CHADS2 score used as an exclusion criteria in each study. The mean TTR for warfarin was also significantly lower in the ROCKET-AF trial. Conclusions from this meta-analysis should be taken with caution as each trial was created with several differences in design.

A case of a 78-year-old man with a left ventricular assist device (LVAD) and history of recurrent gastrointestinal bleeding described successful anticoagulation with apixaban over the course of a year with no recurrent gastrointestinal bleeding [34A]. Further studies assessing the use of apixaban for prophylactic anticoagulation of patients with LVADs are warranted.

Liver

A 72-year-old woman experienced elevated liver transaminase levels and symptomatic hepatotoxicity after initiation of apixaban [35A]. Hepatocellular injury was already present before initiation of therapy but worsened when apixaban was started. Patient's status resolved after therapy discontinuation. Hepatotoxicity associated with apixaban has been published previously, but the mechanism has not yet been defined.

Edoxaban [SEDA-34, 546; SEDA-35, 620; SEDA-38, 370]

Hematologic

The ENSURE-AF trial, a multicenter, prospective, RCT ($n=2199$) analyzed the safety and efficacy of edoxaban 60 mg daily vs enoxaparin/warfarin in patients undergoing AF cardioversion [36MC]. The dose of edoxaban was reduced to 30 mg daily if any of the following factors were observed: creatinine clearance 15–50 mL/min, low bodyweight (≤ 60 kg), or concomitant use of P-glycoprotein inhibitors. The primary safety endpoint monitored both major and non-major bleeding which was similar between groups (1% vs 1%, OR 1.48, 95% CI: 0.64–3.55). Results were independent of anticoagulation status prior to treatment and cardioversion strategy. The study concluded that both edoxaban and enoxaparin/warfarin are safe and effective for patients undergoing cardioversion during AF. The X-VERT trial showed that rivaroxaban was a safe and effective alternative for warfarin in cardioversion [37]. ENSURE-AF provides a second study to corroborate this finding.

A review of the ENGAGE AF-TIMI 48 trial examined the impact of renal function on outcomes with edoxaban vs warfarin in 14 071 patients with AF at moderate-to-high stroke risk [38R]. In patients with moderate renal dysfunction (creatinine clearance (CrCl) 30–50 mL/min), patients on edoxaban displayed 4.0%/year incidence of major bleeding vs 5.3%/year with warfarin (HR 0.76, $P = 0.036$). Patients with mild renal dysfunction (CrCl >50–95 mL/min) showed a numerical decrease in major bleeding on edoxaban compared to warfarin, but this difference was not significant (HR 0.89, $P = 0.15$). In patients with CrCl >95 mL/min, major bleeding was lower with edoxaban (1.4%/year vs 2.3%/year, HR 0.6, $P = 0.004$). Intracranial hemorrhage incidence was also significantly reduced with edoxaban in patients with mild and moderate renal dysfunction. Interestingly, incidence of gastrointestinal bleeding was significantly lower with warfarin in patients with mild renal dysfunction (5.0%/year vs 4.5%/year, HR 0.90, $P = 0.002$). The authors concluded that edoxaban demonstrates superior safety and comparable efficacy to warfarin in patients with AF.

Another review of the ENGAGE AF-TIMI 48 trial analyzed concomitant use of single antiplatelet therapy (SAPT) with edoxaban compared to warfarin in patients with AF [39R]. Of the 14 977 patients enrolled, 4912 patients were selected to receive SAPT. A total of 92.5% of these patients received aspirin, while 92% of these patients on aspirin had doses <100 mg. This patient population was more frequently male, with higher incidence of coronary artery disease and diabetes, and also had higher baseline CHADS$_2$-VASc and HAS-BLED scores than those not receiving SAPT. Patients receiving SAPT exhibited significantly higher incidence of major bleeding vs those not receiving SAPT (HR$_{adj}$ 1.46, $P < 0.001$). Furthermore, edoxaban showed a decrease risk of major bleeding without SAPT (HR$_{adj}$ 0.80, 95% CI: 0.68–0.95) or with SAPT (HR$_{adj}$ 0.82, 95% CI: 0.65–1.03) compared to warfarin without and with SAPT, respectively. The authors conclude that edoxaban or other Xa inhibitors should be selected over warfarin if SAPT is required in addition to anticoagulation therapy.

A third review of the ENGAGE AF-TIMI 48 trial further studied the safety and efficacy of edoxaban in the East Asian population [40R]. This sub-analysis ($n = 1943$) identified significantly reduced major bleeding with edoxaban (2.86%) vs warfarin (4.80%) in the higher dose (60 mg daily) subgroup of edoxaban (HR 0.61, $P = 0.011$) and in the lower dose (30 mg daily) subgroup (1.59%; HR 0.34, $P < 0.001$). Like the ENGAGE AF-TIMI 48 study, this sub-analysis concluded that once-daily edoxaban provides similar efficacy to warfarin while reducing major bleeding risk in the East Asian population.

Rivaroxaban [SEDA-36, 532; SEDA-37, 423; SEDA-38, 371]

Hematologic

A subgroup analysis of the ROCKET-AF trial ($n = 14\,264$) studied the impact of the number of concomitant medications used on the safety and efficacy of rivaroxaban for patients with AF [41R]. The trial identified that patients taking ≥ 10 medications had significantly higher incidence of major or non-major, clinically relevant bleeding than the cohort with 0–4 medications (HR 1.47, 95% CI: 1.31–1.65). The study also assessed the impact of taking ≥ 1 cytochrome P450 3A4 and/or P-glycoprotein inhibitor. No evidence of differing outcomes in this patient population were identified. The authors conclude that increasing medication use was associated with higher risk of bleeding but not stroke while on rivaroxaban. There are a number of limitations that should be considered when evaluating these conclusions, most notably, the nature of the retrospective, exploratory design of the trial.

Post-hoc analysis of patients from the ROCKET-AF trial with worsening renal function (WRF; defined as a 20% CrCl decrease from baseline at any point in the study) sought to determine whether the primary efficacy and safety endpoints differed in WRF patients taking rivaroxaban vs warfarin [42C]. Among the 3320 patients with WRF included, patients randomized to rivaroxaban displayed a lower rate of stroke or systemic embolism (1.54/100 patient years) vs warfarin (3.25/100 patient years) which was not observed in patients with stable renal function ($P = 0.05$ for the interaction). There was no difference in major or nonmajor clinically relevant bleeding events in WRF patients based on treatment assignment (HR 1.06, 95% CI: 0.80–1.39).

Liver

A 71-year-old male patient developed severe jaundice due to intrahepatic cholestasis after initiation of rivaroxaban 15 mg for AF 1 month prior [43A]. On lab evaluation, the patient exhibited a pattern of elevated liver function tests (LFTs). Other possible causes were ruled out, and rivaroxaban was discontinued. The patient showed rapid biochemical and clinical recovery within 1 day of cessation. Two weeks post-discontinuation, the patient's LFTs returned to baseline and symptoms resolved. The proposed mechanism of liver injury is unknown but is hypothesized to involve complex interactions of several immune-mediated reactions.

Immunologic

A 65-year-old man developed a drug reaction with eosinophilia and systemic symptoms (DRESS) 10 days after rivaroxaban (10 mg daily) initiation [44A]. The patient began to experience chills with fever followed by skin erythema and pruritus requiring hospital admission. Several laboratory abnormalities were noted, including elevated white cell count with increased eosinophils, acute renal failure, and mild cholestasis. Rivaroxaban was identified as the probable cause and was discontinued. The patient received corticosteroids, and symptoms resolved over 3 months. Rivaroxaban has not been associated with DRESS in the past, but should now be considered as a possible cause of this condition.

Pregnancy

One cohort study ($n=63$) observed the outcomes of patients exposed to rivaroxaban during pregnancy [45c]. One case of major fetal malformation (a conotruncal cardiac defect leading to termination of pregnancy) was noted, and one case of major bleeding was observed. Due to the limited sample size, the authors could not make a conclusion on the safety of rivaroxaban during pregnancy. However, they did conclude that treatment with rivaroxaban during the first trimester should be reconsidered.

Drug–Drug Interactions

A large non-interventional, phase IV study, analyzed concomitant drug use and associated outcomes in patients ($n=17\,701$) receiving rivaroxaban for the prevention of VTE after major orthopedic surgery [46MC]. The observational trial specifically looked at cytochrome P450 3A4 inhibitors and P-glycoprotein inducers/inhibitors, platelet aggregation inhibitors (PAIs), and non-steroidal anti-inflammatory drugs (NSAIDs). The results showed minimal concomitant use of CYP3A4/P-glycoprotein inhibitors/inducers, but 52% and 7% used NSAIDs and PAIs, respectively. NSAID use had little effect on efficacy outcomes, but did significantly increase major bleeding risk [OR 1.70, 95% CI: 1.06–2.03]. Use of PAIs with rivaroxaban did not significantly alter efficacy or bleeding risk. The authors concluded that concomitant use of NSAIDs was common and associated with higher frequency of bleeding events in patients receiving rivaroxaban or other forms of anticoagulation.

INDIRECT FACTOR XA INHIBITORS
[SEDA-34, 547; SEDA-35, 621; SEDA-38, 371]

Fondaparinux [SEDA-34, 547; SEDA-35, 621; SEDA-38, 371]

Bleeding Risk

A clinical trial conducted at 2 Japanese hospitals compared a regimen of intravenous tranexamic acid (TXA) 1000 mg prior to initial skin incision and subcutaneous fondaparinux 1.5 mg on postoperative days 2–4 vs intermittent pneumatic compression (IPC) devices alone in 391 patients undergoing elective hip surgery [47C]. The rate of DVT was numerically lower in the TXA/fondaparinux group (3.1%) vs the IPC group (6.0%, $P=0.19$), though this was not statistically significant. None of the DVTs were considered symptomatic, and all resolved spontaneously within 6 months. No significant bleeding events were observed in either group.

A prospective RCT randomized 78 patients to either prophylactic post-operative fondaparinux (2.5 mg subcutaneously daily for 11 days or until hospital discharge) or placebo for the prevention of VTE following coronary artery bypass graft (CABG) surgery [48c]. The authors identified one asymptomatic DVT in the placebo group and one major and three minor post-operative hemorrhages in the fondaparinux group and concluded that the trial did not support prophylactic fondaparinux for this indication.

THROMBOLYTIC DRUGS [SEDA-36, 532; SEDA-37, 424; SEDA-38, 371]

Alteplase [SEDA-36, 532; SEDA-37, 424; SEDA-38, 371]

Cardiovascular

An 87-year-old man developed orolingual angioedema followed by transient bradycardia with subsequent hypotension, resulting in the deterioration of his neurological signs and expansion of the ischemic legion [49A]. The authors of this study warn that concomitant use of ACE inhibitors may increase the risk of recombinant tissue plasminogen activator (rt-PA)-associated orolingual angioedema. The authors also conclude that providers should monitor cardiac function for cardiovascular instability that may result in reduced blood supply to the penumbra following rt-PA-associated orolingual angioedema.

DRUGS THAT ALTER PLATELET FUNCTION [SEDA-34, 547; SEDA-35, 621; SEDA-38, 372]

Anagrelide [SEDA-32, 637; SEDA-33, 719; SEDA-38, 372]

Hematologic

Patients with essential thrombocytopenia on anagrelide therapy were analyzed to determine whether genetic mutations affected the development of AE [50c]. The mutations examined include JAK2V617F, CALR, and MPL. Of the 67 patients included in the retrospective analysis, anemia developed in 20.8% of patients after 2 years and 30.3% of patients after 5 years of treatment.

Patients who were positive for CALR mutations were more likely to develop anemia (46.15% vs 11.43%, $P = 0.015$ and 60% vs 11.43%, $P = 0.035$ at 2- and 5-year follow-up, respectively).

GLYCOPROTEIN IIb–IIIa INHIBITORS
[SEDA-35, 622; SEDA-37, 426; SEDA-38, 372]

Eptifibatide [SEDA-36, 533; SEDA-37, 426; SEDA-38, 372]

Hematologic

A 71-year-old female with inferior STEMI received eptifibatide infusion during PCI [51A]. During eptifibatide infusion, a severe drop in platelet count from 210 000/μL to 35 000/μL was observed and eptifibatide was discontinued. One hour later, acute stent thrombosis developed. Platelet function testing suggested eptifibatide induced thrombocytopenia mediated by activating autoantibodies.

Immunologic

A 71-year-old male was admitted to the hospital for expiratory wheezes in all lung fields [52A]. A diagnostic coronary angiography was planned, and the patient was administered eptifibatide infusion (bolus of 180 μg/kg followed by an infusion at 2 μg/kg/min). Two hours after infusion initiation, the patient developed chills, rigors, and hypoxemia followed by purpuric lesions on his face and arms the following morning. The eptifibatide infusion was discontinued and 8 hours later a complete blood count was performed, which revealed a platelet count of 6000 μL.

Tirofiban [SEDA-36, 533; SEDA-37, 426; SEDA-38, 372]

Hematologic

A 66-year-old male undergoing PCI was administered tirofiban infusion periprocedurally [53A]. Within 1 hour after the procedure, the patient developed sudden shortness of breath, hemoptysis, and hypotension (80/60 mm Hg). The patient's platelet count had dropped from $197 \times 10^9/L$ to $11 \times 10^9/L$ and his hemoglobin dropped from 132 to 98 g/L. The patient was intubated and diffuse exudation of blood from all pulmonary segments was discovered on fiberoptic bronchoscopy. Tirofiban was discontinued in addition to the patient's heparin and dual antiplatelet therapy. The patient expired within the next day.

A retrospective review conducted between March 2010 and January 2015 aimed to determine the safety and efficacy of tirofiban use for 40 patients undergoing stent-assisted coiling of intracranial aneurysms [54c]. Of the patients reviewed, two patients experienced intraprocedural aneurysmal rupture, two patients experienced cerebral infarction, and two patients experienced ventriculostomy-related hemorrhage. There were no cases of thrombocytopenia, retroperitoneal, gastrointestinal, or genitourinary bleeding reported.

P2Y12 RECEPTOR ANTAGONISTS
[SEDA-36, 533; SEDA-37, 427; SEDA-38, 373]

Cangrelor [SEDA-34, 427]

Hematologic

A total of 11 145 patients undergoing elective or urgent PCI were randomized to receive either cangrelor or clopidogrel therapy [55MC]. The primary safety end point was severe bleeding at 48 hours, defined used the GUSTO (global use of strategies to open occluded arteries) criteria. The odds of severe bleeding were similar in both women and men for both treatment groups. Cangrelor therapy increased the odds of moderate bleeding in women (0.9% vs 0.3%, $P = 0.02$), but not in men (0.2% vs 0.2%, $P = 0.68$).

Clopidogrel [SEDA-36, 533; SEDA-37, 427; SEDA-38, 373]

Hematologic

A subanalysis of a RCT evaluated the safety and efficacy of the combination of clopidogrel and aspirin administered within 12 hours for patients with minor stroke or transient ischemic attack (TIA) [56c]. The authors found that the combination of aspirin and clopidogrel was more effective than aspirin alone for the primary outcome of ischemic stroke risk within 90 days. Bleeding events occurred in 26/1293 patients for the clopidogrel-aspirin group and 18/1280 patients in the aspirin group (HR 1.31, 95% CI: 0.71–2.40, $P = 0.39$). There was no significant difference in severe, moderate, or mild bleeding for the two treatment groups.

A retrospective observational study conducted in Sweden investigated whether discontinuing clopidogrel or ticagrelor before surgery would increase the incidence of CABG-related major bleeding complications [57c]. Patients with acute coronary syndrome who underwent CABG and were on dual antiplatelet therapy with either ticagrelor ($n = 1266$) or clopidogrel ($n = 978$) were included in the study. It was determined that the incidence of major bleeding was 38% for ticagrelor and 31% for clopidogrel when the agent was discontinued less than 24 hours before surgery. For patients on ticagrelor therapy, there was no significant difference between discontinuation within 72–120 hours or >120 hours before surgery ($P=0.80$). However, patients treated with clopidogrel had a higher incidence of bleeding when the agent was discontinued 72–120 hours before surgery compared with patients who discontinued >120 hours before surgery ($P=0.033$).

A post-hoc analysis of the PLATO trial aimed to compare the treatment of 4949 patients with STEMI undergoing primary PCI who were treated with either ticagrelor or clopidogrel [58c]. The primary safety endpoint was major bleeding. A total of 6.7% of patients treated with ticagrelor experienced major bleeding compared with 6.8% of patients treated with clopidogrel ($P=0.79$).

A 67-year-old male developed thrombotic microangiopathy 3 months after clopidogrel administration, representing a much longer latent period than previously reported [59c]. The patient was prescribed clopidogrel 75 mg daily after a cerebral infarction. Three months later he experienced red urine, oliguria, and systemic edema and was admitted to the hospital. He was found to have renal failure (requiring dialysis), hemolytic anemia and thrombocytopenia. Clopidogrel was discontinued, and intravenous steroids were administered. The patient was eventually discharged 102 days after admission.

A meta-analysis was conducted to compare the safety and efficacy of prasugrel, ticagrelor, standard dose (75 mg/day) clopidogrel, and high dose (≥150 mg/day) clopidogrel [60M]. A total of 30 RCT were included. Primary safety outcomes included major bleeding (defined according to the thrombolysis in MI) and any bleeding (all bleeding incidents except nuance bleeding). Of the treatment arms, standard dose clopidogrel was found to have the lowest number of major bleeding events, followed by ticagrelor, and lastly prasugrel. For the outcome of any bleeding, both standard dose clopidogrel and ticagrelor were associated with the lowest incidence, followed by high-dose clopidogrel, and lastly prasugrel.

Drug–Drug Interactions

Patients treated with a combination of clopidogrel and aspirin post-PCI who were also taking sustained-release nitrates were assessed for potential drug interactions [61c]. A total of 266 patients were taking concomitant dual anti-platelet therapy and sustained-release nitrates vs 192 patients who were not taking nitrates. It was concluded that concomitant nitrate therapy significantly enhanced platelet inhibition after dual anti-platelet therapy ($P=0.008$). Comparatively, statins, calcium-channel blockers, beta blockers, angiotensin receptor blockers, ACE-inhibitors, diuretics, and anti-diabetic agents did not enhance platelet inhibition.

A report of a 60-year-old female with a suspected drug interaction with concomitant clopidogrel (dose unknown) and paclitaxel therapy was published [62A]. The patient eventually developed toxicity requiring discontinuation of paclitaxel. The authors propose the mechanism of interaction involves the inhibition of overall paclitaxel depletion and CYP2C8 inhibition by acyl-β-D-glucuronide, a metabolite of clopidogrel.

Prasugrel [SEDA-36, 535; SEDA-37, 429; SEDA-38, 374]

Hematologic

The safety of prasugrel in 1083 patients with STEMI was assessed in a prospective observational study [63c]. The primary outcome evaluated was the incidence of any major bleeding according to the Bleeding Academic Research Consortium (BARC) 3 or 5 definition, or minor bleeding according to the BARC 2 definition. The study found that patients treated with aspirin + prasugrel had fewer BARC 3 or 5 bleeding events compared with those treated with aspirin + clopidogrel ($P=0.04$) but more BARC 2 bleeding ($P<0.001$). However, the two treatment groups differed in baseline characteristics (prasugrel group was younger with less patients experiencing previous stroke), necessitating further research to make conclusions.

Drug–Drug Interactions

A double-blind, cross-over trial involving 12 patients assessed the potential drug–drug interaction between morphine and prasugrel [64c]. Patients received 60 mg prasugrel with either placebo or 5 mg morphine intravenously. Morphine did not diminish the total drug exposure, determined by liquid chromatography tandem mass spectrometry. However, morphine did reduce the maximal plasma concentrations of the prasugrel active metabolite by 31% ($P=0.019$).

Ticagrelor [SEDA-35, 617; SEDA-37, 429; SEDA-38, 374]

Cardiovascular

A 62-year-old male patient was administered ticagrelor after an angioplasty procedure [65A]. Seven hours after ticagrelor 180 mg loading dose, Mobitz type II atrioventricular block appeared on continuous ECG monitoring (heart rate of 40 beats/min). The patient remained in atrioventricular block for 7 days before ticagrelor was discontinued and prasugrel initiated. Three days after stopping ticagrelor, the patient was in normal sinus rhythm and first degree atrioventricular block. This is the first reported case of progressed asymptomatic atrioventricular block due to ticagrelor therapy.

Hematologic

A prospective trial followed 152 patients discharged on triple antithrombotic therapy after PCI for 12 months to determine if ticagrelor is safer compared with clopidogrel [66c]. The study compared BARC types 2, 3, or 5 bleeding. A total of 5/27 patients taking ticagrelor therapy experienced BARC 2, 3 or 5 bleeding (compared with 22/125 patients taking clopidogrel). There was no statistical difference in bleeding between the two groups. Low estimated glomerular filtration rate was an independent predictor of bleeding ($P = 0.03$).

A total of 13199 patients with non-severe ischemic stroke or high-risk TIA were randomly assigned to receive either ticagrelor or aspirin for 90 days to compare the occurrence of stroke, MI, or death [67C]. Safety endpoints included time to first major bleeding event, time to discontinuation of study treatment as a result of any bleeding event, incidence of intracranial hemorrhage, incidence of fatal bleeding, and incidence of serious and selected non-serious AE. Major bleeding occurred in 31 patients (0.5%) in the ticagrelor group and 38 patients (0.6%) in the aspirin group. There were no significant differences in the safety outcomes between the two treatment groups.

Respiratory

A report of a patient developing Cheyne-Stokes respiration with ticagrelor was published [68A]. The patient was prescribed aspirin and ticagrelor (doses not reported) after a non-ST-segment elevation MI. Within a few hours, the patient experienced dyspnea, particularly at night and in the supine position. However, arterial blood gas analysis and pulmonary function were both assessed and considered normal. After 1 month, the patient continued to have dyspnea and was further assessed with 24-hour cardiorespiratory monitoring which revealed Cheyne-Stokes respiration. Symptoms resolved after the patient discontinued ticagrelor and instead took clopidogrel.

HEMOSTATIC AGENTS [SEDA-36, 536; SEDA-37, 430; SEDA-38, 375]

Tranexamic Acid [SEDA-35, 625; SEDA-36, 536; SEDA-37, 430]

Hematologic

A series of small prospective RCT were performed to analyze TXA compared to placebo in reducing blood loss in total hip and knee replacement (THA/TKA) surgeries. The first trial ($n = 108$) concluded that a single preoperative dose of TXA or two infusions of lower dose TXA resulted in less blood loss during the first 2 days after THA and less need for blood transfusion [69C]. In the ROTEM analysis ($n = 55$), 10 mg/kg of tranexamic acid lead to less postoperative blood loss in patients undergoing THA [70c]. A third trial ($n = 100$) studied the efficacy of both intravenous (IV) and intra-articular (IA) TXA in reducing blood loss during TKA [71C]. The study found that both IV and IA TKA had comparable effect on perioperative blood loss. The authors concluded that IA TXA is a viable alternative to IV TXA.

A study examined 119 patients undergoing unilateral TKA who were given either IV TXA alone or IV TXA plus topical TXA solution before closure of arthrotomy [72C]. The combined TXA group had better results including lower mean calculated blood loss (590 mL vs 386 mL, $P < 0.001$), hemoglobin drop (1.82 vs 1.14, $P < 0.001$), and non-statistically significant blood transfusion rates (6.6% vs 1.6%, $P = 0.365$). The authors conclude that combined use of TXA topical and IV is safer and provides better results than with IV use alone.

A small cohort study compared 52 patients who received topical TXA during cardiac implantable electronic device (CIED) implantation against 83 patients assigned to the control group [73C]. The study found high risk bleeding patients to have reduced pocket hematoma and major bleeding complications with topical TXA vs the control group.

REVERSAL AGENTS

Idarucizumab [SEDA-38, 375]; Ciraparantag; Andexanet Alfa

℞ Special Review

Historically, a major limitation of the use of NOACs has been a lack of commercially available reversal agents and inability to stop major and life-threatening bleeding. Idarucizumab is the only true reversal agent currently available. Results of idarucizumab clinical trials were documented in SEDA-38. [74c]. This agent has been proven efficacious in reversing the direct thrombin inhibitor, dabigatran. Now, two new agents are undergoing phase III clinical trial investigations and are awaiting FDA approval for their use in reversing NOACs: ciraparantag and andexanet alfa [75R].

Ciraparantag is a small synthetic molecule that binds directly to direct factor Xa inhibitors, direct thrombin inhibitors, and unfractionated and low-molecular-weight heparin (LMWH). In a preliminary trial, single dose IV ciraparantag was administered after a 60-mg oral dose of edoxaban in 80 healthy individuals [76c]. Results showed that baseline hemostasis was restored from the anticoagulated state within 10–30 minutes after administration of 100–300 mg of ciraparantag and was sustained for 24 hours. Potential AEs related to the trial drug were mild perioral and facial flushing and dysgeusia, with one patient reporting moderate headache. Further phase III trials are currently being conducted.

Andexanet alfa is a recombinant and inactivated form of factor Xa engineered to be a universal antidote of the factor Xa inhibitors: apixaban, rivaroxaban, and edoxaban. Early results from the phase III ANNEXA trials have tested the safety and efficacy of andexanet alfa in healthy subjects anticoagulated with apixaban and rivaroxaban [77c]. When 24 patients were given a bolus of andexanet alfa for apixaban-mediated anticoagulation, anti-factor Xa activity decreased by 94% (P < 0.0001) and lasted for 1–2 hours. The clinical trials have not identified any AEs, but it is worth nothing that procoagulant AEs are possible due to andexanet alfa's binding of the tissue factor pathway inhibitor (TFPI).

Further phase III trial data are necessary before either medication can be deemed safe and effective; however, excitement builds for the possibility of new approved agents to reverse the potential life-threatening bleeding associated with NOACs.

Acknowledgement

Jennifer Helmen, Saint Joseph Health System, Mishawaka, IN, USA

References

[1] Chan PH, Hai JJ, Chan EW, et al. Use of the SAMe-TT₂R₂ score to predict good anticoagulation control with warfarin in Chinese patients with atrial fibrillation: relationship to ischemic stroke incidence. PLoS One. 2016;11(3)e0150674 [C].

[2] Kataoka T, Hoshi K, Ando T. Is the HAS-BLED score useful in predicting post-extraction bleeding in patients taking warfarin? A retrospective cohort study. BMJ Open. 2016;6:e010471 [C].

[3] Ng CY, Chieh ST, Chin CT, et al. Warfarin related nephropathy: a case report and review of the literature. BMC Nephrol. 2016;17:15 [A].

[4] Jones S, McLoughlin S, Piovesan D, et al. Safety and efficacy outcomes of a home and hospital warfarin management within a pediatric anticoagulation clinic. J Pediatr Hematol Oncol. 2016;38(3):216–20 [C].

[5] Lee S, Choi D, Jeong WK, et al. Frequency of hemorrhagic complications on abdominal CT in patients with warfarin therapy. Clin Imaging. 2016;40:435–9 [C].

[6] Lee M, Saver JL, Hong K, et al. Warfarin use and risk of stroke in patients with atrial fibrillation undergoing hemodialysis. Medicine. 2016;95(6)e2741 [M].

[7] Noseworthy PA, Yao X, Shah N, et al. Comparative effectiveness and safety of non-vitamin K antagonist oral anticoagulants versus warfarin in patients with atrial fibrillation and valvular heart disease. Int J Cardiol. 2016;209:181–3 [C].

[8] Han KH, O'Neill C. Increased peripheral arterial calcification in patients receiving warfarin. J Am Heart Assoc. 2016;5:e002665 [C].

[9] Al-ani M, Parperis K. Warfarin-induced calciphylaxis. BMJ Case Rep. 2016. http://dx.doi.org/10.1136/bcr-2015-214142 [A].

[10] Gouveia AI, Lopes L, Soares-Almeida L, et al. Bullous hemorrhagic dermatosis induced by enoxaparin. Cutan Ocul Toxicol. 2016;35(2):160–2 [A].

[11] Stephenson ML, Serra AE, Neeper JM, et al. A randomized controlled trial of differin doses of postcesarean enoxaparin thromboprophylaxis in obese women. J Perinatol. 2016;36:95–9 [c].

[12] Kikkert WJ, van Brussel PM, Damman P, et al. Influence of chronic kidney disease on anticoagulation levels and bleeding after primary percutaneous coronary intervention in patients treated with unfractionated heparin. J Thromb Thrombolysis. 2016;41:441–51 [C].

[13] Pinto DS, Kohli P, Fan W, et al. Bivalirudin is associated with improved clinical and economic outcomes in heart failure patients undergoing percutaneous coronary intervention: results from an observational database. Catheter Cardiovasc Interv. 2016;87:363–73 [C].

[14] Barria Perez AE, Rao SV, Jolly SJ, et al. Meta-analysis of effects of bivalirudin versus heparin on myocardial ischemic and bleeding outcomes after percutaneous coronary intervention. Am J Cardiol. 2016;117:1256–66 [M].

[15] Shah R, Rogers KC, Matin K, et al. An updated comprehensive meta-analysis of bivalirudin vs heparin use in primary percutaneous coronary intervention. Am Heart J. 2016;171:14–24 [M].

[16] Ng VG, Baumbach A, Grinfeld L, et al. Impact of bleeding and bivalirudin therapy on mortality risk in women undergoing percutaneous coronary intervention (from the REPLACE-2, ACUITY, and HORIZONS-AMI trials). Am J Cardiol. 2016;117:186–91 [R].

[17] Douketis JD, Healey JS, Brueckmann M, et al. Urgent surgery or procedures in patients taking dabigatran or warfarin: analysis of perioperative outcomes form the RE-LY trial. Thromb Res. 2016;139:77–81 [C].

[18] Nishtala PS, Gnjidic D, Jamieson HA, et al. 'Real-world' haemorrhagic rates for warfarin and dabigatran using population-level data in New Zealand. Int J Cardiol. 2016;203:746–52 [C].

[19] Avgil-Tsadok M, Jackevicius CA, Essebag V, et al. Dabigatran use in elderly patients with atrial fibrillation. Thromb Haemost. 2016;115:152–60 [C].

[20] Chan P, Huang D, Hai JJ, et al. Stroke prevention using dabigatran in elderly Chinese patients with atrial fibrillation. Heart Rhythm. 2016;13:366–73 [C].

[21] Darwiche W, Bejan-Angoulvant T, Dievart F, et al. Bleeding risk in patients treated with dabigatran or vitamin K antagonist for atrial fibrillation: a meta analysis of adjusted analysis in routine practice settings. Int J Cardiol. 2016;206:89–92 [M].

[22] Aslan O, Yaylali YT, Yildirim S, et al. Dabigatran versus warfarin in atrial fibrillation: multicenter experience in Turkey. Clin Appl Thromb Hemost. 2016;22(2):147–52 [C].

[23] Tziomalos K, Giampatzis V, Bouziana SD, et al. Acenocoumarol vs. low-dose dabigatran in real-world patients discharged after ischemic stroke. Blood Coagul Fibrinolysis. 2016;27:185–9 [c].

[24] Jones JM, Ryan HM, Tieszen M, et al. Successful hemostasis and reversal of highly elevated PT/INR after dabigatran etexilate use in a patient with acute kidney injury. Am J Emerg Med. 2016;34:758.e5–6 [A].

[25] Marchetti G, Giuliani E, Urbinati S, et al. Dabigatran anticoagulation and Stanford type A aortic dissection: not a lethal coincidence. Acta Anaesthesiol Scand. 2016;60:544 [A].

[26] Toya Y, Nakamura S, Tomita K, et al. Dabigatran-induced esophagitis: the prevalence and endoscopic characteristics. J Gastroenterol Hepatol. 2016;31:610–4 [c].

[27] Shibagaki K, Taniguchi H, Kobayashi K, et al. Dabigatran-induced asymptomatic esophageal mucosal injury. Gastrointest Endosc. 2016;83(2):472–3 [A].

[28] Wang K, Ehlers JP. Bilateral spontaneous hyphema, vitreous hemorrhage and choroidal detachment with concurrent dabigatran etexilate therapy. Ophthalmic Surg Lasers Imaging Retina. 2016;47(1):78–80 [A].

[29] Liu X, Thompson J, Phatak H, et al. Extended anticoagulation with apixaban reduces hospitalisations in patients with venous thromboembolism. An analysis of the AMPLIFY-EXT trial. Thromb Haemost. 2016;115(1):161–8 [R].

[30] Kearon C, Akl EA, Ornelas J, et al. Antithrombotic therapy for VTE disease: CHEST guideline and expert panel report. Chest. 2016;149(2):315–52.

[31] Ng KH, Shestavovska O, Connolly SJ, et al. Efficacy and safety of apixaban compared with aspirin in the elderly: a subgroup analysis from the AVERROES trial. Age Ageing. 2016;45(1):77–83 [R].

[32] Gard FJ, Chaudhary MR, Krishnamoorthy P, et al. Safety and efficacy of uninterrupted periprocedural apixaban in patients undergoing atrial fibrillation catheter ablation: a metaanalysis of 1,057 patients. J Atr Fibrillation. 2016;8(6):1368 [M].

[33] Lip GY, Mitchell SA, Liu X, et al. Relative efficacy and safety of non-Vitamin K oral anticoagulants for non-valvular atrial fibrillation: network meta-analysis comparing apixaban, dabigatran, rivaroxaban and edoxaban in three patient subgroups. Int J Cardiol. 2016;204:88–94 [M].

[34] Pollari F, Fischlein T, Fittkau M, et al. Anticoagulation with apixaban in a patient with a left ventricular assist device and gastrointestinal bleeding: a viable alternative to warfarin? J Thorac Cardiovasc Surg. 2016;151(4):e79–81 [A].

[35] Cordeanu M, Lambert A, Gaertner S, et al. Apixaban-induced hepatotoxicity. Int J Cardiol. 2016;204:4–5 [A].

[36] Goette A, Merino JL, Ezekowitz MD, et al. Edoxaban versus enoxaparin-warfarin in patients undergoing cardioversion of atrial fibrillation (ENSURE-AF): a randomised, open-label, phase 3b trial. Lancet. 2016;388(10055):1995–2003 [MC].

[37] Cappato R, Ezekowitz MD, Klein AL, et al. Rivaroxaban vs. vitamin K antagonists for cardioversion in atrial fibrillation. Eur Heart J. 2014;35(47):3346–55.

[38] Bohula EA, Giugliano RP, Ruff CT, et al. Impact of renal function on outcomes with edoxaban in the ENGAGE AF-TIMI 48 trial. Circulation. 2016;134(1):24–36 [R].

[39] Xu H, Ruff Ct, Giugliano RP, et al. Concomitant use of single antiplatelet therapy with edoxaban or warfarin in patients with atrial fibrillation: analysis from the ENGAGE AF-TIMI48 trial. J Am Heart Assoc. 2016;5(2):1–9 [R].

[40] Yamashita T, Korestune Y, Yang Y, et al. Edoxaban vs. warfarin in east Asian patients with atrial fibrillation—an ENGAGE AF-TIMI 48 subanalysis. Circ J. 2016;80(4):860–9 [R].

[41] Piccini JP, Hellkamp AS, Washam JB, et al. Polypharmacy and the efficacy and safety of rivaroxaban versus warfarin in the prevention of stroke in patients with nonvalvular atrial fibrillation. Circulation. 2016;133(4):352–60 [R].

[42] Fordyce CB, Hellkamp AS, Lokhnygina Y, et al. On-treatment outcomes in patients with worsening renal function with rivaroxaban compared with warfarin. Circulation. 2016;134:37–47 [C].

[43] Aslan AN, Sari C, Bastug S, et al. Severe jaundice due to intrahepatic cholestasis after initiating anticoagulation with rivaroxaban. Blood Coagul Fibrinolysis. 2016;27(2):226–7 [A].

[44] Radu C, Barnig C, de Blay F. Rivaroxaban-induced drug reaction with eosinophilia and systemic symptoms. J Investig Allergol Clin Immunol. 2016;26(2):124–6 [A].

[45] Hoeltzenbein M, Beck E, Meixner K, et al. Pregnancy outcome after exposure to the novel oral anticoagulant rivaroxaban in women at suspected risk for thromboembolic events: a case series from the German Embryotox Pharmacovigilance Centre. Clin Res Cardiol. 2016;105(2):117–26 [c].

[46] Kreutz R, Haas S, Holberg G, et al. Rivaroxaban compared with standard thromboprophylaxis after major orthopaedic surgery: co-medication interactions. Br J Clin Pharmacol. 2016;81(4):723–34 [MC].

[47] Tsuda K, Nishii T, Sakai T, et al. Thrombophylaxis with low-dose, short-term fondaparinux after elective hip surgery. J Thromb Thrombolysis. 2016;41:413–21 [C].

[48] Kolluri R, Plessa AL, Sanders MC, et al. A randomized study of the safety and efficacy of fondaparinux versus placebo in the prevention of venous thromboembolism after coronary artery bypass graft surgery. Am Heart J. 2016;171:1–6 [c].

[49] Kageyama T, Okanoue Y, Takai R, et al. Cardiovascular instability preceded by orolingual angioedema after alteplase treatment. Intern Med. 2016;55(4):409–12 [A].

[50] Osorio MJ, Ferrari L, Goette NP, et al. Long-term follow-up of essential thrombocythemia patients treated with anagrelide: subgroup analysis according to JAK2/CALR/MPL mutational status. Eur J Haematol. 2016;96(4):435–42 [c].

[51] Dezsi DA, Bokori G, Falukozy J, et al. Eptifibatide-induced thrombocytopenia leading to acute stent thrombosis. J Thromb Thrombolysis. 2016;41:522–4 [A].

[52] Pothineni NV, Watts TE, Ding Z, et al. Eptifibatide-induced thrombocytopenia when inhibitor turns killer. Am J Ther. 2016;23: e298–9 [A].

[53] Zhou X, Peng H, Yin Y, et al. Diffused alveolar hemorrhage: a rare and severe complication of tirofiban-induced thrombocytopenia. Int J Cardiol. 2016;206:93–4 [A].

[54] Kim S, Choi JH, Kang M, et al. Safety and efficacy of intravenous tirofiban as antiplatelet premedication for stent-assisted coiling in acutely ruptured intracranial aneurysms. Am J Neuroradiol. 2016;37:508–14 [c].

[55] O'Donoghue ML, Bhatt DL, Stone GW, et al. Efficacy and safety of cangrelor in women versus men during percutaneous coronary intervention. Circulation. 2016;133:248–55 [MC].

[56] Zixiao L, Wang Y, Zhao X, et al. Treatment effect of clopidogrel plus aspirin within 12 hours of acute minor stroke or transient ischemic attack. J Am Heart Assoc. 2016;5:e003038 [c].

[57] Hansson EC, Jideus L, Aberg B, et al. Coronary artery bypass grafting-related bleeding complications in patients treated with ticagrelor or clopidogrel: a nationwide study. Eur Heart J. 2016;37:189–97 [c].

[58] Velders MA, Abtan J, Angiolillo DJ, et al. Safety and efficacy of ticagrelor and clopidogrel in primary percutaneous coronary intervention. Heart. 2016;102:617–25 [c].

[59] Tada K, Ito K, Hamauchi A, et al. Clopidogrel-induced thrombotic microangiopathy in a patient with hypocomplementemia. Intern Med. 2016;55:969–73 [c].

[60] Singh S, Singh M, Grewal N, et al. Comparative efficacy and safety of prasugrel, ticagrelor, and standard-dose and high-dose clopidogrel in patients undergoing percutaneous coronary intervention: a network meta-analysis. Am J Ther. 2016;23: e52–62 [M].

[61] Lee DH, Kim MH, Guo LZ, et al. Concomitant nitrates enhance clopidogrel response during dual anti-platelet therapy. Int J Cardiol. 2016;203:877–81 [c].

[62] Bergmann TK, Filppula AM, Launiaien T, et al. Neurotoxicity and low paclitaxel clearance associated with concomitant clopidogrel therapy in a 60-year-old Caucasian woman with ovarian carcinoma. Br J Clin Pharmacol. 2015;81:313–5 [A].

[63] Bacquelin R, Oger E, Filippi E, et al. Safety of prasugrel in real-world patients with ST-segment elevation myocardial infarction: 1-year results form a prospective observational study. Arch Cardiovasc Dis. 2016;109:31–8 [c].

[64] Hobl E, Reiter B, Schoergenhofer C, et al. Morphine interaction with prasugrel: a double-blind, cross-over trial in healthy volunteers. Clin Res Cardiol. 2016;105:349–55 [c].

[65] Ozturk C, Unlu M, Yildirim AO, et al. The progressed atrioventricular block associated with ticagrelor therapy may not require permanent pacemaker after acute coronary syndrome; it may be reversible. Int J Cardiol. 2016;203:822–4 [A].

[66] Fu A, Singh K, Abunassar J, et al. Ticagrelor in triple antithrombotic therapy: predictors of ischemic and bleeding complications. Clin Cardiol. 2016;39:19–23 [A].

[67] Johnston SC, Amarenco P, Albers GW, et al. Ticagrelor versus aspirin in acute stroke or transient ischemic attack. N Engl J Med. 2016;375(1):35–43 [C].

[68] Giannoni A, Emdin M, Passino C. Cheyne-Stokes respiration, chemoreflex, and ticagrelor-related dyspnea. N Engl J Med. 2016;375(10):1004–6 [A].

[69] Barrachina B, Lopez-Picado A, Remon M, et al. Tranexamic acid compared with placebo for reducing total blood loss in hip replacement surgery: a randomized clinical trial. Anesth Analg. 2016;122(4):986–95 [C].

[70] Na HS, Shin HJ, Lee YJ, et al. The effect of tranexamic acid on blood coagulation in total hip replacement arthroplasty: rotational thromboelastographic (ROTEM®) analysis. Anaesthesia. 2016;71(1):67–75 [c].

[71] Chen JY, Chin PL, Moo IH, et al. Intravenous versus intra-articular tranexamic acid in total knee arthroplasty: a double-blinded randomised controlled noninferiority trial. Knee. 2016;23(1):152–6 [C].

[72] Jain NP, Nisthane PP, Shah NA. Combined administration of systemic and topical tranexamic acid for total knee arthroplasty: can it be a better regimen and yet safe? A randomized controlled trial. J Arthroplasty. 2016;31(2):542–7 [C].

[73] Beton O, Saricam E, Kaya H, et al. Bleeding complications during cardiac electronic device implantation in patients receiving antithrombotic therapy: is there any value of local tranexamic acid? BMC Cardiovasc Disord. 2016;16:73 [C].

[74] Pollack C, Reilly P, Eikelboom J. Idarucizumab for dabigatran reversal. N Engl J Med. 2015;373(6):511–20 [c].

[75] Hu TY, Vaidya VR, Asirvatham SJ. Reversing anticoagulant effects of novel oral anticoagulants: role of ciraparantag, andexanet alfa, and idarucizumab. Vasc Health Risk Manag. 2016;12:35–44 [R].

[76] Ansell JE, Bakhru SH, Laulicht BE, et al. Use of PER977 to reverse the anticoagulant effect of edoxaban. N Engl J Med. 2014;371(22):2141–2 [c].

[77] Crowther M, Levy G, Lu G, et al. ANNEXA-A: a phase 3 randomized, double-blind, placebo-controlled trial, demonstrating reversal of apixaban-induced anticoagulation in older subjects by andexanet alfa (PRT064445), a universal antidote for factor Xa (fXa) inhibitors. Circulation. 2014;130:2105–26 [c].

32

Gastrointestinal Drugs

Kirby Welston*, Dianne May†,1

*University of Georgia College of Pharmacy, Athens, GA, United States
†University of Georgia College of Pharmacy, Augusta, GA, United States
¹Corresponding author: dimay@augusta.edu

ACID-IMPACTING AGENTS

Antacids [SED-16; SEDA-36, 539; SEDA-37, 433]

Drug–Drug Interaction, Antiretrovirals

A systematic review assessed the presence of clinically meaningful drug interactions with dietary supplements and antiretrovirals [1R]. One pharmacokinetic study reviewed the effect of a single 1200 mg calcium carbonate dose on dolutegravir, an integrase inhibitor, in 24 healthy volunteers. Dolutegravir levels were significantly decreased when co-administered with calcium carbonate. Area under the curve (AUC) decreased by 39% (CI90%: 0.47–0.8), maximum concentration (C_{max}) decreased by 37% (CI90%: 0.5–0.81). The proposed mechanism was related to the ability of calcium carbonate to chelate with divalent or trivalent metal cation-containing medications.

Histamine-2 Receptor Antagonists (H2RAs) [SED-16, 751-753; SEDA-36, 545; SEDA-37, 433; SEDA-38, 379]

Ranitidine

NERVOUS SYSTEM

Case Report

A 42-year-old male hospitalized for alcoholic cirrhosis developed severe mania after 18 days of ranitidine 300 mg/day for gastroesophageal reflux (GERD) [2c, A]. Other medications included spironolactone, furosemide, and norfloxacin. Symptoms on Day 4 included disorganized speech and feeling persecuted. Severe psychomotor agitation, insomnia and obsessive-compulsive symptoms occurred on Day 7

and the patient left the hospital against medical advice. The patient was re-hospitalized on Day 18 with mania symptoms. On Day 20, ranitidine and norfloxacin were discontinued. Haloperidol was started for psychiatric symptoms and by Day 24, symptoms had improved. While considered a rare adverse effect, predisposing characteristics identified included older age, decreased renal or hepatic function, and polypharmacy. Alcohol may also be a contributing factor due to changes in blood–brain barrier and hepatic function.

AUTACOIDS

Out of 584 Korean patients identified as having a self-reported adverse effect to ranitidine, 99 patients (17%) reported anaphylaxis [3c]. Pharmacovigilance data from a medication safety database were retrospectively analyzed to characterize the incidence, clinical presentation and diagnosis of this ranitidine-induced anaphylaxis. Twenty-three patients with ranitidine-induced anaphylaxis went on to receive further testing with skin prick tests, oral provocation tests, and laboratory tests to further describe the ranitidine-induced anaphylaxis. Average age was 50 years old and 45% were male. Fifty-seven percent of the reactions were considered serious, although no deaths were reported. Intravenous (IV) ranitidine was four times more likely to be associated with anaphylaxis compared to oral ranitidine. The presence of ranitidine-specific immunoglobulin E (IgE) was not conclusive. After re-exposure to ranitidine, 42.9% had an anaphylactic recurrence.

Case Report

Perioperative anaphylaxis was reported in a 24-year-old male after receiving ranitidine 50 mg preoperatively for ureteroscopic lithotripsy with stent replacement [4A]. Tachycardia, bronchospasm, and hypotension were reported soon after induction. The surgery was cancelled and he was intubated and treated with epinephrine for anaphylaxis. Surgery was attempted using the same protocol 1 month later and anaphylaxis recurred. His profile revealed that he had experienced several previous reactions over a year ago to IV ranitidine including urticaria, flushing, and chest tightness that required treatment with IV steroids. Anaphylaxis with ranitidine may occur as the initial presentation or after minor reactions to previous exposures. Immunoglobulin E (IgE) concentrations were not assessed. Ranitidine avoidance was recommended to the patient.

Proton-Pump Inhibitors (PPIs) [SED-16, 1040-1045; SEDA-36, 535; SEDA-37, 435; SEDA-38, 379-385]

CARDIOLOGY

A meta-analysis assessed the association between cardiovascular risk and PPIs in GERD patients [5M]. Seventeen articles were included covering 7540 patients. Cardiovascular risk increased by 70% in PPI users vs non-PPI users (RR=1.7; CI95%: 1.13–2.56; $P=0.01$; $I^2=0\%$). Omeprazole demonstrated the highest risk for adverse cardiovascular events vs other PPIs (RR=3.17; CI95%: 1.43–7.03; $P=0.004$; $I^2=25\%$). Longer duration was also associated with increased risk of adverse cardiovascular events (RR=2.33; CI95%: 1.33–4.08; $P=0.003$; $I^2=0\%$).

A retrospective, population-based prospective cohort study was performed to evaluate the association between GERD and coronary heart disease [6MC]. GERD patients were identified from a Taiwanese insurance database ($n=12\,960$) and were matched with non-GERD patients ($n=51\,840$) for age, gender, and index year. GERD patients experienced a higher rate of coronary heart disease vs the control group (11.8 vs 6.5 per 1000 person-years). The rate was even higher in PPI use greater than 1 year (adjusted HR=1.67; CI95%: 1.34–2.08).

Case Report

A 40-year-old female taking omeprazole 20–40 mg daily for 13 years for GERD presented to the emergency department with worsening symptoms of fatigue, diarrhea, nausea, and palpitations [7A]. Symptoms started 1 week prior when she was unable to eat or drink as normal. Upon admission, her blood pressure was 103/80 mm Hg and heart rate was 125 beats per minute. Hemoglobin, white blood cell count, platelets, creatinine, sodium, troponin, and albumin were all elevated. Her EKG showed tachycardia and ST segment changes indicating cardiac arrest. She was

also diagnosed with acute renal failure secondary to dehydration and within 5 hours developed convulsions and lost consciousness. Torsades was identified and treated with IV magnesium. Serum magnesium level was <0.27 mmol/L. She was discharged on Day 14 with magnesium supplements but returned 3 months later, again with hypomagnesemia. At this time, the omeprazole was identified as the culprit and was discontinued. Impaired intestinal absorption of magnesium was proposed. Magnesium levels remained stable for the 5 months since omeprazole was discontinued.

NERVOUS SYSTEM

A prospective, multicenter observational study evaluated new-onset dementia in PPI users [8MC]. Data were collected from claims to a German health insurer database. Patients were at least 75 years old and were community dwellers without dementia at baseline. There were 2950 PPI users identified and matched with 70729 non-PPI users for age, sex, polypharmacy, stroke, ischemic heart disease, and diabetes. Dementia risk increased in PPI users (HR=1.44; [CI95%: 1.36–1.52]; $P<0.001$). Dementia was more common in males, those with depression, or previous stroke. Risk-benefit must be considered with PPI use in the elderly. Evaluation of cognitive changes may be warranted.

METAL METABOLISM

A prospective, cross-sectional study of 156 patients evaluated the effects of PPIs on magnesium levels in those newly started on PPIs, as well as those on chronic PPIs [9C]. PPI-naïve patients ($n=56$) were followed prospectively with magnesium levels obtained at 2, 4 and 8 months. For the remaining 100 chronic PPI users, magnesium levels were measured one time and the duration of therapy noted. Duration ranged from 1 to 5 years in the cross-sectional arm. No one in either group had clinically relevant hypomagnesemia while on PPIs regardless of duration. In PPI-naïve patients, there was a statistically significant decrease in magnesium level after starting a PPI. No relationship was found between the fractional excretion of magnesium in the urine and PPI duration; however, there was a significant increase in renal magnesium losses in those on concurrent diuretics. Magnesium conservation may be impaired with diuretic use and thus put the patient at greater risk for hypomagnesemia. While no clear guidance was given on how often magnesium levels should be monitored, targeting those at higher risk, such as those on concurrent diuretics and long-term PPI therapy, may be prudent.

A case-series described neurological symptoms associated with PPI-induced hypomagnesemia in hospitalized patients [10c]. Hypomagnesemia occurred in 14.1%

(85/604). Sixty-three patients with hypomagnesemia were on a PPI. Nine patients with hypomagnesemia developed neurological symptoms including confusion, delirium, depression, disorientation, and difficulty ambulating. Eight of the nine patients with neurological symptoms were PPI users. Elderly patients and duration greater than 1 year were common factors present in patients with neurological symptoms. Symptoms improved with PPI discontinuation.

A 91-year-old male was hospitalized for tetany. He experienced involuntary muscle twitching over the past several months [11c, R]. The twitching worsened and eventually affected his speech and use of his hands. He also experienced watery diarrhea for the past 3 weeks. Eighteen months prior to admission, pantoprazole was started secondary to nonsteroidal anti-inflammatory drug (NSAID) use. Upon admission, his magnesium and calcium levels were low. Symptoms resolved after electrolyte replacement and PPI discontinuation. Diarrhea was thought to be due to electrolyte derangement and improved once electrolytes replenished. Symptoms were possibly due to PPI-induced hypomagnesemia leading to hypocalcemia in patient who also had underlying hyperparathyroidism. Chronic renal failure and vitamin D deficiency were also present. The calcium may have further been affected by bisphosphonates and noncompliance with calcium carbonate and cholecalciferol.

A retrospective observational study assessed the prevalence of hypomagnesemia in patients on PPIs for at least 6 months (mean duration = 5.7 years) [12C]. Patients with hypomagnesemia were identified from a large health maintenance organization database. There were 414 PPI users and 57 (13.8%) had greater than one low serum magnesium level. All but eight of these had other causes for hypomagnesemia including diuretic use, chronic diarrhea, chronic kidney disease or malignancy. The hypomagnesemia in these remaining eight patients was considered mild. Results indicated that PPI-induced hypomagnesemia was uncommon without other known precipitating factors that put the patient at higher risk.

MOUTH AND TEETH

A retrospective cohort study evaluated the association between PPIs and risk of osseointegrated dental implant failure [13C]. A total of 1540 patients who received osseointegrated dental implants were included ($n = 799$ on PPI users; $n = 741$ non-PPI users). Patients did not have underlying disorders that would affect bone metabolism. PPI users were at higher risk for dental implant failure (6.8%) vs non-PPI users (3.2%) [HR = 2.73; CI95%: 1.1–6.78]. Most failures occurred between 10 and 20 months after implant. NSAIDs and smoking were also associated with more dental implant failures.

GASTROINTESTINAL

A systematic review with meta-analysis evaluated the risk of fundic gland polyps (FGP) in PPI users [14M]. Twenty articles were included representing 40218 patients. An increase in FGP was seen in PPI users vs controls (OR: 2.46; CI95%: 1.42–4.27; $P = 0.001$). Patients on PPIs for greater than 6 months were 4.71 times more likely to have FGP (OR: 4.71; CI95%: 2.22–9.99; $P < 0.001$). Durations greater than 12 months increased the risk for even further (OR: 5.32; CI95%: 2.58–10.99; $P < 0.001$).

An observational study compared the rate of gastric cancers, gastrointestinal cancers, and other cancers in patients receiving pantoprazole vs other shorter acting PPIs [15MC]. Potential confounders such as age, gender, cumulative PPI dose, total years of PPI treatment, *Helicobacter pylori* treatment, and index date were adjusted for using the Cox proportional hazards model. There were 34178 pantoprazole users and 27686 on other PPIs identified from a Kaiser Permanente database. Patients were followed for 27700 vs 272321 person-years, respectively. Pantoprazole did not increase risk of cancers compared to other PPIs [HR: 0.68; CI95%: 0.24–1.93].

A retrospective case–control study evaluated 138 geriatric patients (mean age = 83.7 ±4.8 years) [16r]. The first 46 patients admitted with their first episode of *Clostridium difficile* were matched 1:2 for age, gender, and antibiotic use with a control group without diarrhea. For the cases, PPI use was considered use prior to admission and continued in the hospital. For the matched controls it was considered PPI administration at least 3 days prior to the development of *C. difficile* infection while hospitalized. PPIs were not found to increase risk for nosocomial *C. difficile* infections in this geriatric population. Ninety percent of patients in the study received antibiotics that were considered high risk for developing *C. difficile* infection.

A retrospective case–control study evaluated the association between PPIs and NSAIDs and the risk of microscopic colitis [17MC]. A total of 1211 cases were identified using the British Clinical Practice Research Datalink and matched with 6041 controls. The mean age was 63.4 years and three-fourths of patients were female. Patients were categorized based on current PPI use (within 61–90 days of the index date), recent PPI use (within 91–150 days of the index day), past PPI use (greater than 150 days before the index date), or no use of PPIs. Current PPI use had a 3.37-fold increase in risk of microscopic colitis (adjusted OR = 3.37; CI95%: 2.77–4.09) compared to past use or no use. The risk increased by fivefold with concomitant PPI and NSAID use. Duration of therapy greater than 4–12 months increased the risk further.

Case Report

A case series reported on six Dutch infants who experienced discoloration of gastric juices after using esomeprazole or omeprazole used for GERD. A purple/red discoloration of regurgitated gastric juices was described [18r, c]. The dose of omeprazole was 10 mg daily. Two patients received tablets and two patients received capsules. Esomeprazole granule doses were 5 mg daily and 5 mg twice daily. The discoloration was attributed to the rapid degradation of omeprazole to a dark purple compound known to occur when the pH is less than 4. Dispersion in water or placement in the buccal space may contribute to the degradation of the enteric coating. While the discoloration was not harmful, it could be mistaken for blood and may lead to decreased bioavailability decreasing efficacy. Discoloration of gastric juices was not seen after PPI discontinuation.

URINARY TRACT

A retrospective observational study, using a large critical care research database, assessed the risk of acute kidney injury (AKI) during critical illness in PPI users [19MC]. A total of 15 063 critically ill patients were included and stratified according to prior use of PPIs, H2RAs, or neither. A total of 3725 (24.7%) were PPI users and AKI occurred in 747 (20%). This was compared to 18% and 16.2% of patients on an H2RA or no antisecretory therapy, respectively. When adjusted for demographics, cardiovascular comorbidities, indication, and severity of illness, PPIs did not increase risk for AKI (OR = 1.02; CI95%: 0.91–1.13; $P = 0.73$).

A prospective cohort observational study evaluated the association between PPI use and new onset chronic kidney disease (CKD) using a population-based database [20MC]. Patients had normal renal function at baseline and the mean age was 63 years. The study consisted of a population-based cohort ($n = 10482$) and a replication study ($n = 248751$). A total of 3.1% of patients in the cohort self-reported PPI use whereas 6.8% of patients in the replication study had actual prescriptions for PPIs. H2RAs or placebo were used as comparators. The cohort was followed for 13.9 years and the replication follow-up was approximately 6.2 years. The absolute risk of CKD was 3.3% for PPI users compared to non-PPI users in the cohort (HR = 1.5; CI95%: 1.14–1.96; $P = 0.003$). In the replication study, the hazard ratio was 1.17 (CI95%: 1.12–1.23; $P < 0.001$). The association still existed when baseline PPI use was directly compared to H2RA use (HR = 1.39; CI95%: 1.01–1.91; $P = 0.05$). Baseline PPI users had a 20%–50% higher risk of chronic kidney disease after adjusting for confounders.

A retrospective observational study assessed the risks and benefits of using PPIs prophylactically in 286 kidney transplant patients [21C]. All patients were within 5 days of transplant and were on tacrolimus and mycophenolate and were PPI-naïve prior to transplant. The duration of PPI use was greater than 30 days in the treatment group (mean duration 287 ± 120 days); $n = 171$. There were 115 patients in the control group. GI bleeding or ulceration was rare and thus the benefit of adding a PPI prophylactically was questionable. There were no differences seen in the risk of infectious or hematological adverse effects. However, biopsy-proven rejection was higher in PPI users compared to non-PPI users (9.4% vs 2.6%; $P = 0.03$).

A case–control study evaluated the association between end-stage renal disease (ESRD) and PPIs by analyzing data from the Taiwan National Health Insurance Research Database [22MC]. Patients with a diagnosis of GERD and ESRD were identified and all had received PPIs prior to study entry. Patients were matched using propensity scoring. Cases included those who went on to develop ESRD within the 6-year study period (mean age: 65.4 ± 13.1 years), whereas the controls did not go on to develop ESRD (mean age: 66.1 ± 13.8 years). PPIs were associated with a higher risk of developing ESRD vs control group (adjusted OR = 1.88; CI95%: 1.71–2.06).

SKIN

Case Report

Sticky palms was reported in two patients receiving PPIs [23r, A]. Both patients were in their 30s–40s and the PPI had been recently started within 2–3 weeks of the adverse effect occurring. One male patient was taking lansoprazole 30 mg and reported sticky palms in the third week of treatment. Symptoms improved 1 month after stopping lansoprazole. The other patient was taking esomeprazole 20 mg. She developed sticky palms within 2 weeks of starting treatment and symptoms resolved after 1 week of stopping esomeprazole.

MUSCULOSKELETAL

A prospective, open-label, comparative, parallel study evaluated 12-month changes in bone mineral density of the lumbar spine, femur neck, and total hip in 209 patients (age: 18–65 years old) [24C]. Patients on PPIs due to long-term NSAID therapy were compared to non-PPI users. Patients were stratified according to which PPI used and were matched for age, gender, body mass index, and baseline bone mineral density. Other medications that might affect bone mineral density were excluded. At 1 year, there were 42 patients in each group (e.g., control group, omeprazole group, esomeprazole group, lansoprazole group, and pantoprazole group) who were assessed for outcomes. PPI use was associated with lowering of femur neck and total hip bone mineral density T-scores. Only esomeprazole was independently associated with significant reduction of bone mineral density. These effects were seen soon after initiation of therapy, suggesting that bone mineral density screening early in the course of PPI therapy may be useful.

A cross-sectional study evaluated the effect of PPIs on bone mineral density in 80 patients aged 20–45 years old without a previous history of hip fracture [25c]. Forty patients were PPI users and 40 patients were non-PPI users and all were followed for up to at least 2 years. Patients were not at risk for osteoporosis at baseline. Multivariate linear regression analysis adjusted for age, gender, BMI, and serum vitamin D levels. There was an increased risk of developing osteoporosis and osteopenia in the femur bones in PPI users vs non-PPI users as shown by mean femoral T-scores (-0.44 ± 1.11 vs $+0.19 \pm 0.95$; $P = 0.007$). There was no association between PPI users vs non-PPI users in lumbar spine T-scores.

A case–control study evaluated time to first hip fracture in kidney transplant recipients receiving PPIs [26C]. Cases of first hip fracture in kidney transplant recipients ($n = 231$) were identified from the US Renal Data System and matched with controls ($n = 15\,575$) based on age, gender, race, and year of transplantation. A total of 65.4% of cases were on PPIs, while 57.4% of the control group was on PPIs within the year prior to the index date. About half of those patients had been on a PPI for greater than 80% of the year before the index date. PPI use increased the risk of hip fracture 1.39–1.41 times depending on PPI duration.

Case Report

A 45-year-old Korean male was seen in the Emergency Department for a 6-hour history of chest pain [27A]. Cardiac evaluation was unremarkable so he was given esomeprazole 40 mg IV. Twelve hours later, he developed severe right buttock pain with an area of muscle tenderness approximately 8 cm in diameter noted. Labs revealed a creatine kinase of 40 538 units/liter and a lactate dehydrogenase of 1326 units/liter which was consistent with rhabdomyolysis. He received a second dose of esomeprazole 40 mg IV the next day before it was determined as the culprit. Muscular symptoms and lab values improved with hydration and urine alkalinization with bicarbonate infusion and he was discharged on Day 12. At 6 months, there was no recurrence of rhabdomyolysis. Proposed mechanisms include higher peak concentrations achieved with IV administration, direct muscle toxicity, or a true idiosyncratic reaction.

IMMUNOLOGIC

A review article summarized the clinical presentation, diagnosis and treatment of immune-mediated hypersensitivity reactions related to PPIs [28R]. Lansoprazole, followed by omeprazole, pantoprazole, and esomeprazole were identified as the most likely PPIs to cause immediate

hypersensitivity reactions. The use of an immediate hypersensitivity skin test and oral provocation challenge test identified immediate hypersensitivity reactions to PPIs. Desensitization was suggested as a potential option when PPIs could not be avoided in allergic patients. Current literature regarding delayed cell-mediated dermatologic reactions, severe life-threatening delayed reactions, and subacute cutaneous lupus due to PPI use was also reviewed.

The US FDA Adverse Event Reporting System (FAERS) database was queried to determine the association between PPIs and subacute cutaneous lupus erythematosus (SCLE) [29C]. Of the 220 cases of drug-induced SCLE reported over the 2-year review period, 120 were thought to be due to PPIs. Symptoms improved upon PPI discontinuation and returned upon re-challenge. H2RAs also showed this association, although not as strong as with PPIs. Following this query, a search of the literature for case reports identifying PPI-induced SCLE was performed and 22 case reports were identified. The mean age was 58 years old and the majority were female. Educating high-risk patients (e.g., women of child-bearing age or going through hormonal changes, previous episode of SCLE, sun reactive skin, ultraviolet radiation exposure, previous drug allergies) to look for skin rashes and protect skin from sun exposure is important. If SCLE is suspected, discontinue the PPI.

A case series of 5 patients who developed anaphylaxis due to PPIs was reported. Anaphylaxis occurred within 5 minutes to 2.5 hours after administration [30r, c]. Reactions ranged from dyspnea, severe, angioedema of the face, lips or tongue, throat tightness to loss of consciousness. Two patients had taken pantoprazole, two patients had taken omeprazole, and one patient had taken esomeprazole. The patient taking esomeprazole had experienced generalized urticaria 1 year prior with omeprazole. All patients had a positive skin prick test or intradermal test confirming IgE-mediated hypersensitivity.

INFECTION RISK

A case–control study from Denmark evaluated the association of nonpregnancy-associated listeriosis in PPI users [31C]. A total of 721 patients (over 45 years old) identified as having nonpregnancy-related listeria from a population-based database served as the case group. A total of 34 800 patients served as the matched controls. Logistic regression was used to determine the association between PPIs, and other selected medications, use within 30 days (considered current use) and other time frames prior to the index date. PPI users were 2.81 times more likely to develop listeriosis (OR = 2.81; CI95%: 2.14–3.69). This remained significant up to 90 days before the index date. Age, comorbidities, and glucocorticoids increased the odds of PPI users developing listeriosis. There was no association seen with current H2RA use.

A prospective, observational study evaluated the association between PPIs and hospitalization due to infectious gastroenteritis in a population-based cohort [32MC]. Data were gathered from the Sax Institute's 45 and Up Study, an Australian national database. The median age was 69.7 years old and 57.3% were female. Patients were followed over 6 years. Infectious gastroenteritis hospitalizations were more common in PPI users compared to non-PPI users (adjusted HR=1.4 CI95%: 1.2–1.5). A dose–response relationship was noted ($P < 0.001$). Risk was not different based on which PPI used. No increase risk was noted in patients who had recently used H2RAs.

LONG-TERM EFFECTS

A nested case–control study examined the risk of periampullary adenocarcinoma in long-time PPI users [33MC]. Decreased enzymatic activity was thought to increase DNA damage and harmful cell mutation. Patients with periampullary cancers were identified from the Taiwan National Health Insurance Administration Database over a 10 year period ($n = 7681$ cases). Controls were matched for age, gender, and observation period ($n = 76762$). Mean follow-up was 6.6 ± 2 years. PPI exposure in patients with periampullary cancers was 1.35 times more likely than in the control group (OR: 1.35; CI95%: 1.16–1.57). Risk increased with increasing PPI dose.

Drug–Drug Interaction, Capecitabine

An ad hoc analysis of a phase III, randomized trial examined the effects of PPIs on the efficacy of capecitabine and oxaliplatin, with or without lapatinib, in 545 patients with ERBB2/HERS-positive metastatic gastroesophageal cancer [34C]. Median age was 60 years old and 74% were male. Median progression-free survival was decreased in PPI users (4.2 vs 5.7 months; HR=1.55; [CI95%: 1.29–1.81]; $P < 0.001$). Overall survival was also decreased in PPI users (9.2 vs 11.3 months; HR=1.34; [CI95%: 1.06–1.62]; $P = 0.04$). While PPI users also on lapatinib had less of a decrease in progression-free survival they actually had a significant difference in overall survival; HR=1.38; [CI95%: 1.06–1.66]; $P = 0.03$). Altered dissolution and absorption was due to the increase in pH decreased capecitabine efficacy. The effect of PPIs on lapatinib is unknown.

Drug–Drug Interaction, Clopidogrel

A meta-analysis examined the proposed drug interaction between clopidogrel and PPIs on adverse cardiovascular outcomes in patients undergoing high risk percutaneous coronary intervention (PCI) [35M]. All patients were followed for 6 months. Concomitant PPI therapy increased risk of composite MACE outcomes (HR=1.28; CI95%: 1.24–1.32). Individual outcomes that were also significantly increased included myocardial infarction (HR=1.51; CI95%: 1.4–1.62) and stroke (HR=1.46; CI95%: 1.15–1.86).

A double-blind, double-dummy, randomized study evaluated the drug interaction between clopidogrel with either ranitidine or omeprazole in stable coronary artery disease patients [36c]. Clopidogrel users were given either ranitidine ($n = 44$) or omeprazole ($n = 41$) after which the antiplatelet effect of clopidogrel was assessed. Antiplatelet effect was measured at baseline and after 1 week. The percent inhibition of platelets (IPA) was decreased significantly ($26.3\% \pm 32.9\%$ to $17.4\% \pm 33.1\%$; $P = 0.025$) with omeprazole but not with ranitidine.

A review article summarized the evidence regarding the drug interaction between clopidogrel and PPIs when used concomitantly in patients with coronary artery disease [37R]. While a potential pharmacodynamic interaction that may decrease clopidogrel's effectiveness was suggested, the data were conflicting and the risk of increased mortality was not substantiated. Continued monitoring is recommended and use of a PPI with the least cytochrome P450 2C19 inhibition is preferred.

Drug–Drug Interaction, Dasatinib
Case Report

A 16-year-old male with Philadelphia-positive acute lymphoblastic leukemia experienced a decrease in dasatinib absorption due to esomeprazole 40 mg/day daily [38A]. The C_{max} was 23.1 ng mL^{-1}. The esomeprazole was decreased to 20 mg/day then discontinued. The C_{max} of dasatinib 4 days after esomeprazole discontinuation increased from 23.1 to 52 ng mL^{-1}. The area under the curve also increased (89.6–130.6 ng mL^{-1}).

Drug–Drug Interaction, Melphalan

A retrospective observational study evaluated the impact of antisecretory medications (rabeprazole, famotidine) on the efficacy and toxicity of bortezomib plus melphalan plus prednisolone (VMP) in 10 multiple myeloma Japanese patients [39c]. Patients were divided into those taking an antisecretory medications ($n = 3$) and those not taking an antisecretory medications ($n = 7$). The level of M protein was significantly decreased in cycles 2 and 3 of chemotherapy in the control group vs those receiving antisecretory medications. A decrease in M protein is indicative of a more favorable clinical response. All control patients experienced a partial response whereas those in the antisecretory group were considered to have stable disease. Grade 1 gastrointestinal toxicities were lower in the antisecretory group vs the control group possibly related to the decreased solubility and absorption of melphalan with increasing gastric pH. Hematologic toxicities were comparable between the two groups. Avoid co-administration of antisecretory medications with oral melphalan.

Drug–Drug Interaction, Pemetrexed

PPIs, specifically lansoprazole, were shown to inhibit pemetrexed transport via human organic anion transporters (hOATs) [40C]. Inhibitors of hOAT3 may delay the elimination of pemetrexed leading to increased hematological toxicities. A study was undertaken to determine the effects of PPIs on hOAT3-expressing cultured cells in vitro, as well as a retrospective review of the incidence of hematologic toxicities in 108 patients with nonsquamous cell small-cell lung cancer who received pemetrexed and carboplatin concurrently with a PPI [40C]. In vitro, lansoprazole was found to inhibit hOAT3-mediated pemetrexed uptake more than other PPIs. When retrospectively reviewing the 108 cancer patients, concomitant use of lansoprazole with pemetrexed and carboplatin was an independent risk factor associated with hematologic toxicities (odds ratio: 10.004; $P = 0.005$). Forty-seven percent of lansoprazole users experienced a hematologic toxicity. This suggests that lansoprazole, but not other PPIs, should be avoided in patients receiving pemetrexed and carboplatin.

Drug–Drug Interaction, Voriconazole

A 44-year-old Caucasian male experienced fatigue, jaundice, and acute cholestatic hepatitis 5 days after starting lansoprazole [41c, R]. He was also on voriconazole which he had been taking for 1 year for pulmonary aspergillosis. Serum aspartate aminotransferase, alanine aminotransferase, alkaline phosphatase, total bilirubin level, and direct bilirubin were all elevated. All tests were normal 1 month prior to hospitalization. Liver function tests returned to normal within 4 weeks of voriconazole and lansoprazole discontinuation. Voriconazole was restarted after liver function tests normalized. Symptoms resolved after lansoprazole was discontinued. Voriconazole is metabolized by the cytochrome P450 enzyme, 2C19. This enzyme is inhibited by lansoprazole leading to decreased voriconazole metabolism and potential toxicity due to accumulation. PPIs should be used cautiously in patients receiving voriconazole.

Sucralfate [SED-16, 538-539]

Drug–Drug Interactions

A review summarized the drug interactions of sucralfate [42R]. Unabsorbed sucralfate within the

gastrointestinal tract can affect oral drug absorption and bioavailability of other medications by forming a barrier.

NSAIDs
- Single dose and multiple dose studies show decreased T_{max} of various NSAIDs. The C_{max} is reduced with this combination; however, not all analyses displayed significant differences. One proposed mechanism suggests sucralfate's antacid properties increase gastric emptying of NSAIDs.

Fluoroquinolones
- Concurrent administration of sucralfate with fluoroquinolones including ciprofloxacin, moxifloxacin, levofloxacin, gemifloxacin has shown bioavailability reductions of 29.6% and 8% with ciprofloxacin and levofloxacin, respectively. A stable chelation complex between the fluoroquinolone and aluminum within sucralfate is the most likely explanation. Administering the agents 2–4 hours apart may still impact the bioavailability of the fluoroquinolone, however, not as much as with concurrent administration.

Antifungals
- Concomitant administration of ketoconazole with sucralfate resulted in a 24% decreased bioavailability. Separation of doses by at least 2 hours is recommended.

ANTICONSTIPATION AND PROKINETIC

Domperidone [SED-16, 1067-1068; SEDA-36, 541, SEDA-37, 445, SEDA-38, 385]

QT Prolongation in Pediatric Patients

A review was performed to evaluate cardiovascular risks associated with domperidone, specifically QTc interval prolongation, ventricular arrhythmias, and sudden cardiac death in Canadian pediatric patients [43R]. Ventricular arrhythmias and sudden cardiac death have been reported with doses of 30 mg/day. Five trials were identified representing 137 patients that were included in the analysis. Patients ranged in age from 24 weeks gestational age to 9 months. No studies reported ventricular arrhythmias or sudden cardiac death. From the included trials, five patients had asymptomatic QTc interval increase >450 ms, while one patient had symptomatic increase. The patient experiencing symptomatic QTc interval increase was given 1.8 mg/kg/day divided three times daily. The QTc interval normalized after domperidone discontinuation. The randomized controlled trial evaluated low dose domperidone, 0.8 mg/kg/day. Difference in mean QTc interval from baseline and days 3 to 5 of therapy were not significant (404 ± 18 ms vs 402 ± 20 ms; $P = 0.758$). A prospective cohort of 45 preterm and term infants receiving 1.5–4 mg/kg/day domperidone observed QTc interval >460 ms in two patients. After domperidone discontinuation, the QTc interval returned to baseline. In the overall observed cohort, there was no difference in QTc interval after domperidone administration compared to baseline (389 ± 20 ms and 397 ± 31 ms; $P = 0.13$). This review of pediatric patients did not observe any serious cardiac adverse effects with domperidone; however, QTc interval prolongation was noted. It was often asymptomatic and returned to baseline with discontinuation.

Erythromycin [SED-16, 99-108; SEDA-38, 385]

Drug–Drug Interaction, Edoxaban

In a small, controlled trial, 33 healthy patients received erythromycin for 8 days with a single dose of edoxaban 60 mg, a factor Xa inhibitor, on Day 7 followed by an additional treatment sequence without erythromycin and a single dose of edoxaban 60 mg on Day 1 [44c]. Co-administration resulted a 68% and 85% increase in peak and total exposure of edoxaban, respectively. Change in prothrombin time (PT) from baseline was $44.9\% \pm 21.6\%$ with co-administration compared to $24.8\% \pm 9.2\%$ for edoxaban alone. Edoxaban is a substrate for CYP3A4 and transported via P-glycoprotein (P-gp) and combination with erythromycin, a CYP3A4 and P-gp inhibitor, likely resulted in the increased exposure. Co-administration of these medications could potentially increase bleeding risk.

Metoclopramide [SED-16, 976-980; SEDA-36, 542, SEDA-37, 446, SEDA-38, 385]

Drug–Drug Interaction, Olanzapine

Neuroleptic malignant syndrome (NMS) is a potential adverse effect with atypical antipsychotics but is most often seen with first generation antipsychotics [45A]. A 64-year-old male with a history of hypertension, diabetes, peripheral neuropathy, depression and recent diabetic foot infection (DFI) presented with edema in the lower extremities. Olanzapine/fluoxetine had been initiated 4 days prior for depression. Linezolid was started for his DFI which made him nauseous, resulting in the administration of metoclopramide IV 10 mg every 6 hours. On the Day 3 of hospitalization, after continuing to feel nauseous, he continued to desaturate, his blood pressure remained elevated at 160/90 mm Hg and he remained febrile. Right lower limb showed hyperreflexia with clonus and he was asymmetrically rigid in both upper and lower extremities. Creatine phosphokinase (CPK) value was elevated (1856 mcg/L). Recognition of NMS resulted in administration of dantrolene, carbidopa/levodopa, and baclofen. Rigidity improved after 12 hours and CPK level decreased by approximately 50%. The patient remained febrile, diaphoretic and hypertensive, leading physicians to believe this was a combination of NMS and serotonin syndrome due to the interaction between fluoxetine and linezolid. Although rare with atypical antipsychotics, NMS can result and be precipitated by co-administration with metoclopramide.

Methylnaltrexone [SED-16, 953]

A meta-analysis evaluated the safety and efficacy of methylnaltrexone in patients with opioid-induced constipation [46R]. Seven studies were included representing 1860 patients in a qualitative synthesis and 6 studies representing 1412 patients were included in the meta-analysis. Abdominal pain occurred more in patients receiving methylnaltrexone vs placebo (RR 2.38, CI95%: 1.75–3.23; $I^2 = 60\%$). Cancer patients (RR 2.42, CI95%: 1.62–3.61; $I^2 = 65\%$) and non-cancer patients (RR 2.34, CI95%: 1.46–3.75; $I^2 = 71\%$) experienced similar rates of abdominal pain. Methylnaltrexone users were not at a higher risk for nausea (RR 1.27, CI95%: 0.90–1.78, $I^2 = 12\%$) or diarrhea (RR 1.45, CI95%: 0.94–2.24, $I^2 = 45\%$) vs placebo.

A randomized, placebo controlled, open-label extension study evaluated the efficacy and safety of methylnaltrexone in chronic non-cancer pain patients [47C]. Patients were randomized to 12 mg methylnaltrexone once daily ($n = 150$), 12 mg methylnaltrexone every other day ($n = 148$) or placebo ($n = 134$) for 4 weeks. After 4 weeks, patients could enter an open-label extension study for 8 weeks using 12 mg methylnaltrexone as needed up to once daily. Adverse events were reported in 32.8% of the placebo group during the first 4 weeks of the trial vs 43.3% in the methylnaltrexone group. The most common adverse events were nausea (5.2% vs 6.7% in placebo), abdominal pain (9.7% vs 1.5% in placebo) and diarrhea (4.5% vs 3% in placebo) and were described as mild to moderate. Methylnaltrexone appears to be mostly well-tolerated with predictable adverse events and minimal serious adverse events.

Naloxegol

Common adverse events noted in a phase III randomized, open-label study with naloxegol vs usual care were abdominal pain (17.8% vs 3.3%), diarrhea (12.9% vs 5.9%), nausea (9.4% vs 4.1%), headache (9% vs 4.8%), flatulence (6.9% vs 1.1%) and upper abdominal pain

(5.1% vs 1.1%) [48r]. Adverse events were mild to moderate. Discontinuation due to adverse events occurred in 10.5% of patients. All adverse events resolved after naloxegol discontinuation.

Sodium Picosulfate and Magnesium Citrate [SEDA-16, 729-732]

Case Reports

A 69-year-old male scheduled for colonoscopy ingested sodium picosulfate/magnesium citrate powder without dissolving in water according to instructions [49A]. He presented with a 1 day history of epigastric pain. Esophagogastroduodenoscopy (EGD) 12 hours after ingestion showed longitudinal ulcers with hematin throughout the entire gastric body and antrum. After 6 weeks of lansoprazole, symptoms dissipated and repeat EGD showed a healing ulcer scar.

A 63-year-old female preparing for colonoscopy mixed sodium picosulfate/magnesium citrate powder with one spoonful of water instead of 200 mL [50A]. She described immediate burning in oropharynx. Computed tomographic (CT) scan revealed diffuse soft tissue edema and thickening in the neck and chest. Esophagography with gastrografin revealed diffuse esophageal wall edema. On Day 9 of hospitalization, EGD showed exudate covering esophagus and multiple ulcerative lesions. She was treated with parenteral nutrition and IV PPIs and discharged on Day 12.

Sorbitol
Case Reports

Sodium polystyrene sulfonate with sorbitol was administered to four males and two females between ages 48 and 75 years with chronic renal failure receiving dialysis for hyperkalemia [51A]. Within a week of the enema administration, all patients had developed symptoms including abdominal pain ($n=4$), bleeding per rectum ($n=1$) and sepsis in a renal transplant patient ($n=1$). Endoscopy revealed large ulcers with slough in the cecum, hepatic flexure and anorectal region. Biopsies revealed acute inflammatory exudate with underlying inflammatory granulation. It is unclear whether or not the sorbitol or sodium polystyrene sulfonate was responsible for the necrosis.

Teduglutide

A 12 week, open-label study including pediatric patients with short bowel syndrome evaluated the safety and efficacy of three doses of teduglutide, 0.0125 mg/kg/day ($n=8$), 0.025 mg/kg/day ($n=14$) and 0.05 mg/kg/day ($n=15$), vs standard of care [52c]. All patients were on parenteral nutrition (PN) and showed minimal or no advance in enteral nutrition (EN) feeds. At least one adverse event was reported in all patients. Most were reported as mild or moderate. More teduglutide users reported serious adverse events vs placebo (30% vs 20%). Vomiting was the most common adverse event reported and occurred more frequently in the 0.025 and 0.05 mg/kg/day doses (36% and 47%). Gastrointestinal adverse events were the most common and occurred in 67% of 0.05 mg/kg/day group, 71% of 0.025 mg/kg/day group, 50% of 0.0125 mg/kg/day group and 20% in standard of care group. No teduglutide discontinuations or death were reported. Serious adverse effects that have been observed in the adult population, including intestinal obstruction, fluid overload or gallbladder, biliary or pancreatic disease, were not observed in this pediatric population.

A review of studies examining the efficacy and safety of teduglutide in adult PN-dependent patients showed that 95.2% (79/83) reported at least one adverse event. The most common adverse events were abdominal pain, headache, and nausea [53r]. Another study reported an event rate of 96.2% (50/52) for any adverse event. Serious adverse events appeared similar with placebo, however, were more often present with teduglutide throughout the trials assessed. Patients receiving teduglutide 0.05 mg/kg/day were more likely to experience a serious adverse event (OR: 1.3 and OR: 1.44 for two individual trials) as well as for patients receiving 0.01 mg/kg/day (OR: 1.15). Serious adverse events related to treatment were small intestinal obstruction, fever, and catheter-related complications and infection.

ANTIDIARRHEAL AND ANTISPASMODIC AGENTS

Eluxadoline [SEDA-38, 386]

Pooled data from phase 2 and phase 3 trials included a safety assessment of patients who received at least one dose of eluxadoline [54R,55r,56R]. There were 1032, 807, and 974 patients in the eluxadoline 100 mg, eluxadoline 75 mg, and placebo groups, respectively. All were given twice daily. Duration was longer in the eluxadoline 75 mg group vs the 100 mg group (219.7 vs 192.4 days). More than 50% of patients reported at least one adverse event seen typically within the first 2 weeks. Pancreatitis was the most commonly reported serious adverse event (SAE); however, SAEs were low (4%–4.2% with eluxadoline vs 2.6% with placebo). Incidence of pancreatitis was 0.4% for both strengths of eluxadoline and not reported with placebo. Major cardiac adverse events were spread evenly throughout all three groups (0.2% in 100 mg; 0.1% in 75 mg; 0.3% in placebo), and were observed in patients ≥70 years with cardiovascular history or risk factors for cardiovascular disease. A 72-year-old female in the eluxadoline 100 mg group developed suspected colon ischemia 19 days after first administration [54R]. Less serious adverse events that occurred more commonly vs placebo in ≥2% of patients were constipation (7.4%), nausea (8.1%), abdominal pain (5.8%) [55r]. Adverse effects leading to eluxadoline discontinuation were higher than seen with placebo, but only ≤1.1% [54R,56R]. Antispasmodics can typically be used to treat abdominal pain associated with eluxadoline [56R].

Loperamide [SED-16, 668; SEDA-37, 450; SEDA-38, 386-387]

DEATHS

Loperamide is a P-glycoprotein (P-gp) substrate located, among other places, at the blood–brain barrier (BBB). The P-gp efflux pump is responsible for shuttling xenobiotics out of the brain. Saturating the P-gp efflux pump with supratherapeutic levels of loperamide can result in harmful substances reaching the brain. A North Carolina database identified 21 documented deaths related to or contributed by loperamide since 2012. Mean age of patients identified was 34 years (20–58 years) [57A]. Loperamide was attributed to 18/21 deaths as the primary or additive to cause of death. Mean plasma concentration of loperamide was 0.27 mg/L (range <0.01 to 0.89 mg/L), which is higher than that achieved with the maximum daily dose of 16 mg (0.0031 mg/L).

Case Report

A 45-year-old male with fatigue and loss of libido and history of ulcerative colitis was managing his symptoms with loperamide 40–50 mg/day [58A]. Testosterone level was low (2.9 nmol/L) and hypogonadism was confirmed. Hypothalamic–pituitary–adrenal (HPA) axis was evaluated due to fatigue. Plasma ACTH and gonadotropins were within normal limits inappropriately and peak cortisol level was low indicating pituitary dysfunction. Symptoms improved with hydrocortisone and testosterone therapy. Two years later, patient used loperamide 4–6 mg/day for 48 hours and after synacthen administration, cortisol level was appropriate at 833 nmol/L. When the patient began taking higher doses of loperamide (15–20 mg/day), cortisol level after synacthen administration was suboptimal at 483 nmol/L.

ANTIEMETIC AGENTS

Aprepitant and Fosaprepitant [SED-16, 657; SEDA-36, 544; SEDA-37, 450]

Drug–Drug Interaction, Anticoagulants

Aprepitant is a moderate inhibitor and inducer of CYP3A4 and inducer of CYP2C9. The more potent isomer of warfarin, S-warfarin, is primarily metabolized by CYP2C9, while R-warfarin is primarily metabolized through CYP3A4 and CYP1A2. A retrospective study was conducted of 14 Japanese hospitalized patients who were administered aprepitant and warfarin [59c]. Patients were included who had been administered warfarin for 10 days prior to receiving aprepitant and their prothrombin time–international normalized ratio (PT–INR) and warfarin dose changes were assessed 1 week before and 3 weeks after aprepitant administration. PT–INR mean values increased significantly after 1 week from 1.68 ± 0.44 to 2.3 ± 0.67 (P=0.0000149). PT–INR values decreased significantly 2 weeks after treatment to 1.35 ± 0.33 (P=0.00069). There was no change in mean warfarin dose. PT–INR should be monitored in patients receiving both aprepitant and warfarin for at least 2 weeks after aprepitant administration [59c].

Drug–Drug Interactions, Antineoplastic Agents

Aprepitant is approved for prevention of chemotherapy-induced nausea and vomiting (CINV); however, many antineoplastic medications are CYP3A4 substrates [60r]. Currently there have been case reports, pharmacokinetic, or theorized interactions reported with many medications including cyclophosphamide, doxorubicin, docetaxel, etoposide, ifosfamide, paclitaxel, and vinca alkaloids. When aprepitant is used concurrently with these medications, increased concentrations of the antineoplastic medications may result increasing risk for adverse events. Use caution when aprepitant is used in combination with these medications and monitor for adverse events.

Drug–Drug Interaction, Psychoactive Agents

A 44-year-old male received three doses of aprepitant, dexamethasone and ondansetron for prevention of CINV due to laryngeal carcinoma [60r]. The patient was given quetiapine, a CYP3A4 substrate, for relief of nightly anxiety and depression. An 11-fold increase in quetiapine plasma concentration was reported leading to deep somnolence. Quetiapine dose was reduced by 50% during the 3 day course of aprepitant and somnolence improved.

Ondansetron [SED-16, 343-347; SEDA-36, 544; SEDA-37, 453, SEDA-38, 388]

Case Report

A 45-year-old male with no significant history presented to hospital complaining of fever and nausea for 2 days [61A]. He was given ondansetron 8 mg IV and intramuscular paracetamol. Six hours later, he was unable to maintain standing position. Metabolic panel was unremarkable except for severely decreased potassium 2.36 mEq/L. Potassium level was repeated and found to be 1.87 mEq/L. U waves were seen on electrocardiogram (ECG). The patient was transferred to the ICU and administered potassium 10 mEq/hour IV. ECG and potassium levels recovered to normal. Prior to discharge, potassium level was 4.29 mEq/L. Hypokalemia with ondansetron is a rare occurrence, but potentially related to downregulation of the NKCC2 co-transporter, resulting in increased excretion of potassium.

ANTIINFLAMMATORY AGENTS

Aminosalicylates [SED-16, 242-254; SEDA-36, 555; SEDA-37, 454, SEDA-38, 389]

Nephrotoxicity

A registry study of patients receiving 5-aminosalicylate (5-ASA) was assessed for potential cases of nephrotoxicity [62c, H]. Patients were included if they had normal serum creatinine and estimated glomerular filtration rate (eGFR) prior to first administration of 5-ASA, ≥50% increase in serum creatinine after initiation, and/or serum creatinine that returned to normal after cessation. Researchers identified 146 cases of probable nephrotoxicity and 5 definite cases. Median duration prior to first observed rise in serum creatinine was 3 years (CI95%: 2.3–3.7). An abnormal serum creatinine was only reported in 13% of patients within the first year. Full recovery of renal function was seen by 30% of patients within the median follow-up period of 5.1 years (CI95%: 4.17–6.02). Patients taking 5-ASA for a shorter period were more likely to recover renal function before developing nephrotoxicity. An inverse correlation was observed with duration ($P=0.05$) and average dose ($P=0.03$), which suggested mechanisms related to cumulative toxicity. Genetic testing performed as part of the study indicated there was a potential link between a specific marker within the HLA region that could predispose patients to nephrotoxicity with 5-ASA.

Azathioprine [SED-16, 759-781; SEDA-36, 555; SEDA-38, 389-390]

Special Review

What Is the Risk of Acute Pancreatitis? Pancreatitis was first associated with azathioprine in the 1950s after an autopsy series revealed 53% of patients with ulcerative colitis had histological evidence of interstitial pancreatitis and there was definite pancreatic fibrosis or acinar atrophy observed in 12% of cases [63R]. Incidence of azathioprine-induced pancreatitis ranges from 0% to 5%, and if occurs, typically presents within the first 3 months of therapy [64C]. It is more often reported with Crohn's disease vs ulcerative colitis, however, reports have been published for both. During a 16-year period, a Danish study revealed Crohn's disease patients were four times more likely to experience acute pancreatitis with azathioprine and ulcerative colitis patients were twice as likely. Acute pancreatitis secondary to azathioprine can result in complications, not only in the pancreas, but also in the hepatobiliary system, resulting in cirrhosis and sclerosing cholangitis. It can also lead to portal and superior mesenteric vein thrombosis and portal hypertension [63R]. Risk factors include female gender, young age, smoking and presence of gallstones.

In a prospective, multicenter trial, patients with a first prescription for azathioprine for inflammatory bowel disease (IBD) were assessed for acute pancreatitis ($n=510$). Data was obtained from a German registry. In a larger percentage than expected, 7.25% of patients were diagnosed with azathioprine-induced acute pancreatitis after a median of 21 days [IQR 17; 34 days, range 7–63 days]. Sixty-five percent were female ($n=24$). The majority of patients had Crohn's disease (29/37) vs ulcerative colitis. Crohn's disease patients were more often smokers vs ulcerative colitis patients (31.6% vs 7.6% $P < 0.0001$). Smokers were more likely to experience azathioprine-induced acute pancreatitis vs non-smokers (OR 3.24, CI95%: 1.74–6.02). Laboratory and clinical criteria were fulfilled in all patients while imaging criteria was only confirmed in 3 cases. Lipase levels were almost 10 times higher than the upper limit of normal in the confirmed cases of acute pancreatitis [IQR 4.34; 23.44] and patients with higher lipase levels tended to be hospitalized more often, however, that was not statistically significant ($P=0.22$). Hospitalization occurred in 43% of patients. Not only are smoking and female gender considered risk factors, but those receiving oral budesonide were also at an increased risk. Nine patients (24.4%) who were diagnosed with acute pancreatitis received oral budesonide while 48 patients (10.1%) who were not diagnosed with acute pancreatitis were on oral budesonide at baseline.

Results from a recent prospective trial may reveal that azathioprine-induced pancreatitis is more common than previously noted. Smoking was identified as the most modifiable *contributing factor. Patient's should be educated regarding the signs and symptoms of pancreatitis and should be counseled on the benefits of smoking cessation.*

PURE RED CELL APLASIA

Case Report

Pure red cell aplasia (PRCA), a rare adverse event seen with azathioprine, is characterized by normocytic, normochromic anemia associated with reticulocytopenia, normal granulocyte and platelet counts, and isolated erythroblastopenia in bone marrow. A 14-year-old female on azathioprine 75 mg/day over 6 months for ileocolonic Crohn's disease developed progressive fever, headache, fatigue, sore throat and vomiting over a 3-week period [65A]. There were no signs of bleeding, however, her hemoglobin and hematocrit were low at 2.5 g/dL and 7.3%, respectively. Bone marrow aspirate displayed suppression of the erythroid series. Azathioprine was replaced with mesalamine and the patient received 2 units of packed red blood cells leading to anemia resolution. In a similar case, a 39-year-old male was initiated on azathioprine and gradually increased to 125 mg/day. After 5 months, he presented with increased fatigue for 1 week. The hemoglobin was low (6.8 g/dL), but other laboratory parameters were normal. Azathioprine discontinuation led to hemoglobin normalization over the following weeks.

Case Report

A 66-year-old male with past medical history of hypertension, diabetes, hyperlipidemia and biopsy-proven autoimmune hepatitis was initiated on azathioprine 75 mg/day [66A]. After 10 days, he presented with fever, lethargy, polyarticular arthralgia, and painful rash on lower and upper extremities. C-reactive protein level was elevated, indicating an acute inflammatory reaction. Rheumatoid factor was slightly elevated; however, all other lab results were normal. A delayed hypersensitivity reaction was expected leading to discontinuation of azathioprine. Complete resolution of symptoms occurred within 2 weeks.

Thiopurines [SED-16, 759-781; SEDA-37, 455; SEDA-38, 390]

Case Report

A 62-year-old male with left-sided ulcerative colitis developed acute myocarditis secondary to azathioprine [67A]. He presented with flu-like symptoms, elevated troponins, ejection fraction of 35% and cardiac magnetic resonance imaging (MRI) which revealed myocarditis. Previously, the patient had

similar results after taking 6-mercaptopurine, resulting in an ejection fraction of 20% and acute onset atrial fibrillation. Over the course of a few years, azathioprine was suspended and restarted as his symptoms were uncontrolled, leading to his most recent presentation of myocarditis. Azathioprine was discontinued and his repeated ejection fraction was 60%.

ANTICHOLINERGIC AGENTS

Glycopyrrolate [SED-16, 571; SEDA-38, 390]

Case Report

A 5-year-old male was admitted to the ICU with hypovolemic shock secondary to hematemesis [68A]. His history included cerebral palsy, congenital encephalopathy, microcephaly and visual and hearing impairment. He was intubated, mechanically ventilated, sedated and subsequently given fentanyl and antibiotics. Vital signs were stable on Day 10 but due to excessive salivation, he was given 0.1 mg of glycopyrrolate. He became agitated, developed apnea, and lost consciousness. Oxygen saturations decreased to 88%–92% despite mechanical ventilation and 100% oxygen. Symptoms were interpreted as central anticholinergic syndrome (CAS) and glycopyrrolate was discontinued. He died 2 days later due to acute respiratory distress syndrome after aspiration.

MISCELLANEOUS AGENTS

Misoprostol [SED-16, 1063-1068; SEDA-38, 391]

Safety of retrievable prostaglandin vaginal inserts for induction of labor was characterized in 678 patients receiving misoprostol and 680 patients receiving dinoprostone [69C]. Onset of active labor was the primary reason for removal occurring in 43.8% of misoprostol users and 34.1% of dinoprostone users. The most frequent intrapartum adverse events leading to removal occurred more with misoprostol. Median time of onset of adverse event was shorter with misoprostol (6 hours 45 minutes vs 9 hours 41 minutes, $P=0.002$). Time from insert retrieval to adverse event resolution was similar between the two groups, even though slightly longer for misoprostol (1 hour 39 minutes vs 47 minutes, $P=0.452$). No neonatal deaths were reported, however, 10.4% of neonates born misoprostol users were admitted to the intensive care unit vs 3.7% of neonates born to dinoprostone users ($P=0.44$).

Case Report

A 32-year-old female was admitted for medical abortion of monoamniotic twins without distinguished heartbeats [70A]. She was given 400 µg (2 tablets) sublingual and intravaginal misoprostol every 2 hours. She developed shivering, diarrhea and abdominal cramping 1 hour after the first sublingual placement. She required 22 tablets of misoprostol for confirmed abortion. One day following discharge she had several white bullae lesions in her buccal mucosa and hyperkeratotic lip plaques, as well as target lesions on dorsal aspect of left palm. She was diagnosed with erythema multiforme after exclusion of pemphigus and herpes simplex virus. Lesions subsided after 3-week treatment with triamcinolone oral paste.

Orlistat [SED-16, 392-394; SEDA-38, 391]

Drug–Drug Interaction, Cyclosporine

A 35-year-old male with Evan's syndrome secondary to antiphospholipid syndrome and restrictive lung disease presented with headache, shortness of breath on exertion and jaundice [71A]. He had been in remission for Evan's syndrome for 4 years after taking cyclosporine 200 mg daily. He was concerned about weight gain from steroids, so he started orlistat and took it at the same time as his cyclosporine. Two weeks later, he discontinued orlistat due to increasing jaundice and undetectable cyclosporine levels (1 month prior his level was 36 ng/mL). Platelets had fallen to 4×10^9/L, and INR was supratherapeutic at 3.4. He was started on prednisolone and platelets recovered over 4 months. Suspected mechanism was due to cyclosporine's lipid-soluble properties and primary absorption within the small intestine and as well as orlistat's effect's on lipid absorption.

BIOLOGICS

See Volume 36: 539–560 for further information.

STEROIDS

See Volume 38: 379–393 for further information.

References

[1] Jalloh MA, Gregory PJ, Hein D, et al. Dietary supplement interactions with antiretrovirals: a systematic review. Int J STD AIDS. 2017;28(1):4–15 [R].

[2] Mauran A, Goze T, Abadie D, et al. Mania associated with ranitidine: a case report and review of the literature. Fundam Clin Pharmacol. 2016;30(4):294–6 [c, A].

[3] Park KH, Pai J, Dong D-G, et al. Ranitidine-induced anaphylaxis: clinical features, cross-reactivity, and skin testing. Clin Exp Allergy. 2016;46:631–9 [c].

[4] Neema S, Sen S, Chatterjee M. Ranitidine-induced perioperative anaphylaxis: a rare occurrence and successful management. Indian J Pharmacol. 2016;48(2):221–2 [A].

[5] Sun S, Cui Z, Zhou M, et al. Proton pump inhibitor monotherapy and the risk of cardiovascular events in patients with gastro-esophageal reflux disease: a meta-analysis. Neurogastroenterol Motil. 2017;29:e12926; 1–10. http://dx.doi.org/10.1111/nmo.12926 [M].

[6] Chen CH, Lin CL, Kao CH. Association between gastroesophageal reflux disease and coronary heart disease. A nationwide population-based analysis. Medicine. 2016;95(27):e4089. http://dx.doi.org/10.1097/MD.0000000000004089 [MC].

[7] Hansen BA, Bruserud O. Hypomagnesemia as a potentially life-threatening adverse effect of omeprazole. Oxf Med Case Reports. 2016;7:147–9 [A].

[8] Gomm W, von Holt K, Thome F, et al. Association of proton pump inhibitors with risk of dementia. A pharmacoepidemiological claims data analysis. JAMA Neurol. 2016;73(4):410–6 [MC].

[9] Begley J, Smith T, Barnett K, et al. Proton pump inhibitor associated hypomagnesaemia—a cause for concern? Br J Clin Pharmacol. 2016;81(4):753–8 [C].

[10] Pasina L, Zanotta D, Puricelli S, et al. Acute neurological symptoms secondary to hypomagnesemia induced by proton pump inhibitors: a case series. Eur J Clin Pharmacol. 2016;72:641–3 [c].

[11] Sivakumar J. Proton pump inhibitor-induced hypomagnesaemia and hypocalcaemia: case review. Int J Physiol Pathophysiol Pharmacol. 2016;8(4):169–74 [c, R].

[12] Sharara A, Chalhoub JM, Hammound N, et al. Low prevalence of hypomagnesemia in long-term recipients of proton pump inhibitors in a managed care cohort. Clin Gastroenterol Hepatol. 2016;14(2):317–21 [C].

[13] Wu X, Al-Abedalla K, Abi-Nader S, et al. Proton pump inhibitors and the risk of osseointegrated dental implant failure: a cohort study. Clin Implant Dent Relat Res. 2017;19(2):222–32. http://dx.doi.org/10.1111/cid.12455 [C].

[14] Martin FC, Chenevix-Trench G, Yeomans ND. Systematic review with meta-analysis: fundic gland polyps and proton pump inhibitors. Aliment Pharmacol Ther. 2016;44:915–25 [M].

[15] Schneider JL, Kolitsopoulos F, Corley DA. Risk of gastric cancer, gastrointestinal cancers, and other cancers: a comparison of treatment with pantoprazole and other proton pump inhibitors. Aliment Pharmacol Ther. 2016;43:73–82 [MC].

[16] Depoorter L, Verhaegen J, Joosten E. Use of proton pump inhibitors and risk of nosocomial Clostridium Difficile infection in hospitalized elderly adults. J Am Geriatr Soc. 2016;64(3):667–9 [r].

[17] Verhaegh BPM, de Vries F, Masclee AAM, et al. High risk of drug induced microscopic colitis with concomitant use of NSAIDs and proton pump inhibitors. Aliment Pharmacol Ther. 2016;43:1004–13 [MC].

[18] Van Hunsel F, de Jong L, de Vries T. (Es)omeprazole and discoloration of regurgitated gastric contents in infants: worrying for care-takers and a sign of a reduced bioavailability. J Pediatr Pharmacol Ther. 2016;21(3):260–2 [r, c].

[19] Lee J, Mark RG, Celi LA, et al. Proton pump inhibitors are not associated with acute kidney injury in critical illness. J Clin Pharmacol. 2016;56(12):1500–6 [MC].

[20] Lazarus B, Chen Y, Wilson FP, et al. Proton pump inhibitor use and risk of chronic kidney disease. JAMA Intern Med. 2016;176(2):238–46 [MC].

[21] Courson AY, Lee JR, Aull MJ, et al. Routine prophylaxis with proton pump inhibitors and post-transplant complications in kidney transplant recipients undergoing early corticosteroid withdrawal. Clin Transplant. 2016;30:694–702. http://dx.doi.org/10.1111/ctr.12736 [C].

[22] Peng YC, Lin CL, Yeh HZ, et al. Association between the use of proton pump inhibitors and the risk of ESRD in renal diseases:

a population-based control study. Medicine. 2016;95(15):e3363. http://dx.doi.org/10.1097/MD.0000000000003363 [MC].

[23] Alkeraye S, Baclet Y, Delaporte E. Sticky palms following use of proton pump inhibitors. JAMA Dermatol. 2016;152(6):722–3 [r, A].

[24] Bahtiri E, Islami H, Hoxha R, et al. Esomeprazole use is independently associated with significant reduction of BMD: 1-year prospective comparative safety study of four proton pump inhibitors. J Bone Miner Metab. 2016;34:571–9 [C].

[25] Abbas ARJ, Mohsen RZ, Maryam Y, et al. Proton pump inhibitor use and change in bone mineral density. Int J Rheum Dis. 2016;19:864–8 [c].

[26] Lenihan CR, Sukumaran Nair S, Vangala C, et al. Proton pump inhibitor use and risk of hip fracture in kidney transplant recipients. Am J Kidney Dis. 2017;69(5):595–601. http://dx.doi.org/10.1053/j.ajkd.2016.09.019 [C].

[27] Jeon DH, Kim Y, Kim MJ, et al. Rhabdomyolysis associated with single-dose intravenous esomeprazole administration. Medicine. 2016;95(29):e4313. http://dx.doi.org/10.1097/MD.0000000000004313 [A].

[28] Otani IM, Banerji A. Immediate and delayed hypersensitivity reactions to proton pump inhibitors: evaluation and management. Curr Allergy Asthma Rep. 2016;16(17):1–7. http://dx.doi.org/10.1007/s11882-016-0595-8 [R].

[29] Aggarwal N. Drug-induced subacute cutaneous lupus erythematosus associated with proton pump inhibitors. Drugs Real World Outcomes. 2016;3:145–54 [C].

[30] Mota I, Gaspar A, Chambel M, et al. Anaphylaxis induced by proton pump inhibitors. J Allergy Clin Immunol Pract. 2016;4(3):535–6 [r, c].

[31] Jensen AK, Simonsen J, Ethelberg S. Use of proton pump inhibitors and the risk of listeriosis: a nationwide registry-based case-control study. Clin Infect Dis. 2017;64(7):845–51. http://dx.doi.org/10.1093/cid/ciw860 [C].

[32] Chen Y, Liu B, Glass K, et al. Use of proton pump inhibitors and the risk of hospitalization for infectious gastroenteritis. PLoS One. 2016;11(12):e0168618. http://dx.doi.org/10.1371/journal.prone.01688618 [MC].

[33] Chien LN, Huang YJ, Shao YHJ, et al. Proton pump inhibitors and risk of periampullary cancers—a nested case-control study. Int J Cancer. 2016;138:1401–9 [MC].

[34] Chu MP, Hecht R, Slamon D, et al. Association of proton pump inhibitors and capecitabine efficacy in advanced gastroesophageal cancer. Secondary analysis of the TRIO-013/LOGIC randomized clinical trial. JAMA Oncol. 2017;3(6):767–73. http://dx.doi.org/10.1001/jamaoncol.2016.3358 [C].

[35] Serbin MA, Guzauskas GF, Veenstra DL. Clopidogrel-proton pump inhibitor drug-drug interaction and risk of adverse clinical outcomes among PCI-treated ACS patients. A meta-analysis. J Manag Care Spec Pharm. 2016;22(8):939–47 [M].

[36] De Mendonca Furtado RH, Giugliano RP, Srunz CMC, et al. Drug interaction between clopidogrel and ranitidine or omeprazole in stable coronary artery disease: a double-blind, double dummy, randomized study. Am J Cardiovasc Drugs. 2016;16:275–84 [c].

[37] Nancy AM, Sandip KC, Sachin MM, et al. Risk of concomitant use of proton pump inhibitors and clopidogrel on clinical outcomes in patients with acute coronary syndrome—a review. World J Pharm Pharm Sci. 2016;5(7):723–9 [R].

[38] Pape E, Michel D, Scala-Bertola J, et al. Effect of esomeprazole on the oral absorption of dasatinib in a patient with Philadelphia-positive acute lymphoblastic leukemia. Br J Clin Pharmacol. 2016;81:1195–6 [A].

[39] Kitazawa F, Kado Y, Ueda K, et al. The interaction between melphalan and gastric antisecretory drugs: impact on clinical efficacy and toxicity. Mol Clin Oncol. 2016;4:293–7 [c].

[40] Ikemura K, Hamada Y, Kaya C, et al. Lansoprazole exacerbates pemetrexed-mediated hematologic toxicity by competitive inhibition of renal basolateral human organic anion transporter 3. Drug Metab Dispos. 2016;44:1543–9 [C].

[41] Lopez JL, Tayek JA. Voriconazole-induced hepatitis via simvastatin- and lansoprazole-mediated drug interactions: a case report and review of the literature. Drug Metab Dispos. 2016;44:124–6. http://dx.doi.org/10.1124/dmd.115.066878 [c, R].

[42] Sulochana SP, Syed M, Chandrasekar DV, et al. Clinical drug-drug pharmacokinetic interaction potential of sucralfate with other drugs: review and perspectives. Eur J Drug Metab Pharmacokinet. 2016;41:469–503 [R].

[43] Morris AD, Chen J, Lau E, et al. Domperidone-associated QT interval prolongation in non-oncologic pediatric patients: a review of the literature. Can J Hosp Pharm. 2016;69(3):224–30 [R].

[44] Parasrampuria DA, Mendell J, Shi M, et al. Edoxaban drug-drug interactions with ketoconazole, erythromycin and cyclosporine. Br J Clin Pharmacol. 2016;82:1591–600 [c].

[45] Mazhar F, Akram S, Haider N, et al. Overlapping of serotonin syndrome with neuroleptic malignant syndrome due to linezolid-fluoxetine and olanzapine-metoclopramide interactions: a case report of two serious adverse drug effects caused by medication reconciliation failure on hospital admission. Case Rep Med. 2016;2016:1–4 [A].

[46] Siemens W, Becker G. Methylnaltrexone for opioid-induced constipation: review and meta-analyses for objective plus subjective efficacy and safety outcomes. Ther Clin Risk Manag. 2016;12:401–12 [R].

[47] Viscusi ER, Barrett AC, Paterson C, et al. Efficacy and safety of methylnaltrexone for opioid-induced constipation in patients with chronic noncancer pain. Reg Anesth Pain Med. 2016;41:93–8 [C].

[48] Jones R, Prommer E, Backstedt D. Naloxegol: a novel therapy in the management of opioid-induced constipation. Am J Hosp Palliat Med. 2016;33(9):875–80 [r].

[49] Ze EY, Choi CH, Kim JW. Acute gastric injury caused by undissolved sodium picosulfate/magnesium citrate powder. Clin Endosc. 2017;50:87–90 [A].

[50] Yark SY. A case of upper airway and esophageal injury after ingestion of sodium picosulfate and magnesium citrate for colonoscopy. Toxicology. 2016;27(5):492–5 [A].

[51] Jacob SSK, Parameswaran A, Parameswaran SA, et al. Colitis induced by sodium polystyrene sulfonate in sorbitol: a report of 6 cases. Indian J Gastroenterol. 2016;35(2):139–42 [A].

[52] Carter BA, Cohran VC, Cole CR, et al. Outcomes from a 12-week, open-label, multicenter clinical trial of teduglutide in pediatric short bowel syndrome. J Pediatr. 2017;181:102–11 [c].

[53] Naberhuis JK, Tappenden KA. Teduglutide for safe reduction of parenteral nutrition and/or fluid requirements in adults: a systematic review. J Parenter Enteral Nutr. 2016;40(8):1096–105 [r].

[54] Cash BD, Lacy BE, Schoenfeld PS, et al. Safety of eluxadoline in patients with irritable bowel syndrome with diarrhea. Am J Gastroenterol. 2017;112:365–74 [R].

[55] Weber HC. New treatment options for irritable bowel syndrome with predominant diarrhea. Curr Opin Endocrinol Diabetes Obes. 2017;24:25–30 [r].

[56] Rivkin A, Rybalov S. Update on the management of diarrhea-predominant irritable bowel syndrome: focus on rifaximin and eluxadoline. Pharmacotherapy. 2016;36(3):300–16 [R].

[57] Bishop-Freeman SC, Feaster MS, Beal J, et al. Loperamide-related deaths in North Carolina. J Anal Toxicol. 2016;40:677–86 [A].

[58] Napier C, Gan EH, Pearce SHS. Loperamide-induced hypopituitarism. BMJ Case Rep. 2016;2016, 1–3. http://dx.doi.org/10.1136/bcr-2016-216384 [A].

[59] Takaki J, Ohno Y, Yamada M, et al. Assessment of drug-drug interaction between warfarin and aprepitant and its effects on PT-INR of patients receiving anticancer chemotherapy. Biol Pharm Bull. 2016;39:863–8 [c].

[60] Dushenkov A, Kalabalik J, Carbone A, et al. Drug interactions with aprepitant and fosaprepitant: review of literature and implications for clinical practice. J Oncol Pharm Pract. 2016;23:296–308 [r].

[61] Mathew SK, Kutty KK, Ramya I, et al. Ondansetron-induced life threatening hypokalemia. J Assoc Physicians India. 2016;64:81–2 [A].

[62] Heap GA, So K, Weedon M, et al. Clinical features and HLA association with 5-aminosalicylate (5-ASA)-induced nephrotoxicity in inflammatory bowel disease. J Crohns Colitis. 2016;10:149–58 [c, H].

[63] Jasdanwala S, Babyatsky M. Crohn's disease and acute pancreatitis. A review of literature. JOP. 2015;16(2):136–42 [R].

[64] Teich N, Mohl W, Bokemeyer B, et al. Azathioprine-induced acute pancreatitis in patients with inflammatory bowel disease—a prospective study on incidence and severity. J Crohns Colitis. 2016;10:61–8 [C].

[65] Kamath N, Pai CG, Deltombe T. Pure red cell aplasia due to azathioprine therapy for Crohn's disease. Indian J Pharmacol. 2016;48(1):86–7 [A].

[66] Ardalan ZS, Vasudevan A, Testro AG. Arthralgia and fevers in a patient with autoimmune hepatitis. JAMA. 2016;316(1):91–2 [A].

[67] Latushko A, Ghazi LJ. A case of thiopurine-induced acute myocarditis in a patient with ulcerative colitis. Dig Dis Sci. 2016;61:3633–4 [A].

[68] Toksvang LN, Plovsing RR. Symptoms of central anticholinergic syndrome after glycopyrrolate administration in a 5-year old child. A A Case Rep. 2016;6(2):22–4 [A].

[69] Rugarn O, Tipping D, Powers B, et al. Induction of labour with retrievable prostaglandin vaginal inserts: outcomes following retrieval due to an intrapartum adverse event. BJOG. 2017;124:796–803 [C].

[70] Sahraei Z, Mirabzadeh M, Eshraghi A. Erythema multiforme associated with misoprostol: a case report. Am J Ther. 2016;23(5): e1230–3 [A].

[71] Earnshaw I, Thachil J. Example of the drug interaction between ciclosporin and orlistat, resulting in relapse of Evan's syndrome. BMJ Case Rep. 2016;2016: [A].

33

Drugs That Act on the Immune System: Immunosuppressive and Immunostimulatory Drugs

Calvin J. Meaney[1], Mario V. Beccari

School of Pharmacy and Pharmaceutical Sciences, State University of New York at Buffalo, Buffalo, NY, United States

[1]Corresponding author: cjmeaney@buffalo.edu

IMMUNOSUPPRESSIVE DRUGS

Belatacept [SEDA-34, 609; SEDA-37, 471; SEDA-38, 407]

Multiple reviews have highlighted the lower risk of metabolic and cardiovascular adverse effects, similar risk of infections and post-transplant lymphoproliferative disorder (PTLD), and improved quality of life and renal function with belatacept use in renal transplant recipients when compared to calcineurin inhibitors (CNI) [1R,2R,3R,4R,5R,6R].

Observational Studies

A prospective study assessed the safety of belatacept after switching from a CNI or a mammalian target of rapamycin (mTOR) inhibitor in 79 renal transplant recipients with severely impaired renal function [7c]. Mean estimated glomerular filtration rate (eGFR) reached 34.0 ± 15.2 mL/min/1.73 m^2 by month 12 from a baseline value of 26.1 ± 15.0 mL/min/1.73 m^2 ($P < 0.001$). Mean proteinuria in patients previously on mTOR inhibitors ($n = 22$) decreased to 98 ± 28 mg/L by 12 months from a baseline of 331 ± 119 mg/L ($P < 0.05$). A total of 57 serious adverse events occurred with the most common being infection ($n = 19$). Therapy was discontinued in 7 patients due to an adverse event.

The safety of belatacept after switching from a CNI in 25 graft recipients who received kidneys from extended-criteria donors was assessed in a retrospective study [8c]. Patients experienced a significant increase in mean eGFR after 6 months. Nine patients developed an infection, and 2 were diagnosed with cancer.

A retrospective study examined the safety of belatacept in 8 lung transplant recipients with renal insufficiency [9c]. Patients experienced a mean decrease in serum creatinine and an increase in eGFR. Of the 3 patients on hemodialysis at baseline, 2 were able to discontinue renal replacement therapy between 6 and 13 days after belatacept initiation. De novo bacterial infection occurred in 2 patients, and 2 patients were diagnosed with seasonal influenza.

Comparative Studies

Two different 7-year, international, multicenter, prospective, randomized phase III clinical trials comparing belatacept to cyclosporine demonstrated an increase in mean eGFR from baseline in the belatacept groups and a decrease in the cyclosporine groups ($P < 0.001$ for each comparison) [10MC,11MC]. In both studies, the most common serious adverse event experienced was infection, which occurred at similar rates across the groups. In one study, 9 patients developed PTLD [10MC]. Of which, 8 were receiving belatacept and 5 were Epstein–Barr virus-seronegative.

A retrospective cohort study compared the clinical outcomes of belatacept, tacrolimus, and belatacept plus tacrolimus in 50 244 renal transplant recipients [12MC]. New-onset diabetes after transplantation (NODAT) occurred in 1.7% of patients on belatacept plus tacrolimus, 2.2% on belatacept alone, and 3.8% on tacrolimus alone ($P = 0.01$). The incidences of de novo PTLD and other malignancy were similar between the 3 groups.

The outcomes of de novo belatacept were compared to steroid-free tacrolimus in 59 renal transplant recipients from high risk donors [13c]. Mean eGFR was significantly higher in the belatacept group at months 2 ($P=0.0004$) and 3 ($P=0.007$) but not by month 6 ($P=0.73$). Compared to the tacrolimus group, patients on belatacept had a higher occurrence of viremia due to cytomegalovirus (11/24 vs 5/35; $P=0.008$) and polyomavirus (7/24 vs 3/35; $P=0.04$).

Skin

Two patients with a past medical history of psoriasis experienced recurrence of psoriatic plaques following initiation of belatacept [14A]. The plaques appeared after 15 days in 1 patient and after 15 months in the other. Both patients were successfully treated with corticosteroids.

Infection Risk

A 53-year-old female who underwent double lung transplantation developed invasive tracheobronchial aspergillosis 3 weeks after switching from cyclosporine to belatacept [15A]. Mycophenolate mofetil and prednisone were discontinued and she received multiple forms of treatment, but she was maintained on belatacept for unknown reasons. The patient improved after 6 weeks of therapy, but she subsequently developed worsening respiratory failure 2 weeks later. She was diagnosed with superficial bacterial colonization, disseminated adenovirus infection, ventilator-associated pneumonia, and septic shock. Her family withdrew care.

A 28-year-old female who underwent renal transplantation switched from tacrolimus to belatacept after 1 month of therapy and subsequently developed *Toxoplasma* chorioretinitis at month 6 post-transplant [16A]. The infection was believed to be opportunistic due to cumulative immunosuppression, since she was also receiving mycophenolate mofetil and prednisone.

CYCLOSPORINE (CICLOSPORIN) [SED-15, 743; SEDA-34, 609; SEDA-35, 699; SEDA-36, 591; SEDA-38, 407]

Systematic Reviews

The strategy to minimize or avoid calcineurin inhibitors (both cyclosporine and tacrolimus) in renal transplantation was evaluated in a meta-analysis of 88 randomized controlled trials [17M]. Renal function, assessed by estimated glomerular filtration rate, was improved with minimization (RR 0.32, 95% CI: 0.22–0.41) and avoidance (RR 0.49, 95% CI: 0.26–0.72) of calcineurin inhibitors. Incidence of cytomegalovirus infection was lower with a minimization strategy (RR 0.71, 95% CI: 0.55–0.92). Biopsy proven acute rejection and graft loss were less with minimization strategies but were increased when calcineurin inhibitors were withdrawn. This meta-analysis demonstrates that minimization of calcineurin inhibitors post-renal transplant can improve renal function, decrease CMV infections, and improve graft outcomes.

A meta-analysis of 10 randomized controlled trials evaluated calcineurin inhibitors for induction and maintenance of lupus nephritis [18M]. The risk of leukopenia was similar between the calcineurin inhibitors and mycophenolate mofetil but was lower with calcineurin inhibitors compared to azathioprine (RR 0.26, $P=0.0005$) and compared to cyclophosphamide (RR 0.37, $P=0.01$).

Comparative Studies

The side effect profile of cyclosporine was compared to prednisolone in 33 patients with erythema nodosum leprosum [19c]. Infection, acne, hypertricosis, gingival hyperplasia, and hypertension were reported with cyclosporine which is similar side effects observed with cyclosporine in other disease states.

Observational Studies

Thirty-five allogeneic hematopoietic stem cell transplant patients were reported to experience nephrotoxicity (20%), neurotoxicity (48.6%), hypertension (14.2%), hypercholesterolemia (68.5%), and hypertriglyceridemia (82.8%) while receiving cyclosporine for GVHD prophylaxis [20c].

Cardiovascular

The prevalence of cardiovascular risk factors was compared between cyclosporine, tacrolimus, and sirolimus in a retrospective study of 115 pediatric renal transplant recipients [21C]. Cyclosporine treated patient had increased LDL ($P<0.05$), increased serum phosphorus ($P<0.05$), and increased calcium-phosphorus product ($P<0.05$) compared to the other treatments.

Urinary Tract

A longitudinal cohort study of 1622 renal transplant biopsies in 200 patients evaluated the histopathologic nephrotoxicity of cyclosporine compared to tacrolimus [22C]. Cyclosporine was associated with more mild arteriolopathy, striped interstitial fibrosis, glomerular congestion, and tubular microcalcification compared to tacrolimus. The incidence of arteriolar hyalinosis was similar between treatments.

Teratogenicity

The teratogenic effects of cyclosporine and tacrolimus were investigated using an in vitro rat embryo culture

[23E]. Cyclosporine caused hematoma at 4 mcg/mL and an apoptotic effect at 40 mcg/mL. Tacrolimus caused an hematoma and an open neural tube at 20 mcg/mL and apoptotic effect at 15 mcg/mL.

Drug–Drug Interactions

The interaction between cyclosporine and imatinib was assessed in 16 hematopoietic stem cell transplant patients [24c]. After initiation of imatinib, the dose-corrected cyclosporine concentration increased by 94% ($P < 0.001$). The proposed mechanism of this interaction is competitive inhibition of p-glycoprotein and/or CYP3A4.

Co-administration of cyclosporine 500 mg and edoxaban 60 mg resulted in a 73% increase in total edoxaban exposure and a 74% increase in peak edoxaban concentrations among healthy subjects [25c]. Cyclosporine-mediated inhibition of CYP3A4, p-glycoprotein, and/or OATP1B1 was the proposed mechanism of this interaction.

Food–Drug Interactions

A systematic review and meta-analysis evaluated the interaction between citrus juices and cyclosporine in 7 studies [26M]. Grapefruit juice and pomelo juice were found to increase the total exposure of cyclosporine by 53% and 23%, respectively. Orange juice had no impact on cyclosporine pharmacokinetics.

EVEROLIMUS [SED-15, 1306; SEDA-34, 614; SEDA-35, 701; SEDA 36, 592; SEDA-37, 471; SEDA-38, 407]

Systematic Reviews

A meta-analysis of 7 randomized controlled trials evaluated the incidence of everolimus-induced stomatitis [27M]. Stomatitis occurred frequently: 67% in patients with solid tumors and 70% in patients with tuberous sclerosis complex. More than 90% of manifestations were grade 1 or 2 (mild-to-moderate) in severity. Initial occurrence of stomatitis was within 8 weeks of starting everolimus.

Observational Studies

A prospective pharmacokinetic and safety analysis of everolimus was conducted in 42 patients with advanced thyroid cancer [28c]. Dose reductions were necessary in 45% of the patients due to stomatitis (4), pneumonitis (4), fatigue (5), loss of appetite (1), diarrhea (1), edema (1), kidney toxicity (1), and liver toxicity (1). Everolimus

exposure was 52% higher in patients that required dose reductions compared to those that did not. The *ABCB1* TTT haplotype was associated with a 21% lower everolimus exposure.

A retrospective study examined everolimus toxicities in 181 patients with metastatic breast cancer [29C]. Adverse events were similar to those observed in other populations receiving everolimus and a majority were grade 1 or 2 (mild-to-moderate). Everolimus was discontinued or dose reduced in 6% and 27% of patients due to toxicity, respectively.

Safety of everolimus was assessed in 19 patients with renal angiomyolipomas due to tuberous sclerosis complex [30c]. Adverse effects were consistent with the known profile of everolimus and most often grade 1 or 2 in severity. However, 42.1% of patients required dose reductions as a result of adverse effects.

Everolimus was evaluated for epilepsy associated with tuberous sclerosis complex in 15 pediatric patients [31c]. Adverse effects were common with 93% of patients developing a grade 1 event. Four patients developed a grade 4 events (pneumonia in 3 and impetigo contagiosa in 1) that required temporary discontinuation of therapy. Overall, everolimus was viewed to be safe in this patient population but requires careful monitoring.

Respiratory

Everolimus-associated pneumonitis was evaluated in a retrospective study of 66 patients with neuroendocrine tumors [32c]. Pneumonitis occurred in 21% of the patients and was more common in non-smokers. Radiographic findings included cryptogenic organizing pneumonia and non-specific interstitial pneumonia. All patients had ground glass and reticular opacities.

The mechanism of everolimus associated lung toxicity was investigated in an in vitro/in vivo study including 13 everolimus treated patients and 13 tacrolimus treated patients [33c]. The in vitro analysis demonstrated an epithelial to mesenchymal transition in bronchial cell lines consistent with pulmonary fibrosis. This was corroborated by the in vivo experiment which showed higher pulmonary fibrosis index scores with everolimus compared to tacrolimus ($P = 0.03$) which correlated with trough everolimus concentrations.

Urinary Tract

Renal tubule epithelial injury and renal dysfunction were associated with everolimus in a 57-year-old female with breast cancer [34A]. Renal function improved after everolimus was discontinued, but recurred following a re-challenge of everolimus 6 months later.

Mouth and Teeth

Angioedema occurred in a 59-year-old female patient after starting everolimus which resolved after discontinuation of the drug [35A].

Skin

Hand-foot syndrome (palmar-plantar erythrodysethesia) was reported in a patient receiving everolimus for metastatic breast cancer [36A].

Stomatitis-cutaneous toxicity of everolimus was evaluated in 79 patients with metastatic renal cell carcinoma [37c]. Stomatitis-cutaneous toxicity occurred in 25% of patients and was associated with favorable disease response.

Everolimus associated stomatitis in a 48-year-old female renal transplant recipient was successfully managed with intralesional triamcinolone and topical clobetasol gel while continuing everolimus treatment [38A].

Symmetrical drug-related intertriginous and flexural exanthema (SDRIFE) was reported in a 76-year-old male receiving everolimus for lung adenocarcinoma [39A]. The eruption subsided with topical triamcinolone and continued everolimus therapy.

Infection Risk

Two cases of pneumonia caused by *Mycoplasma pneumonia* were reported in children treated with everolimus for tuberous sclerosis complex [40A].

FINGOLIMOD [SEDA-34, 616; SEDA-35, 703; SEDA-36, 593; SEDA-36, 591; SEDA-37, 471; SEDA-38, 407]

Systematic Reviews

A systematic review of fingolimod adverse effects included 30 clinical trials, 24 review articles and 15 case reports [41M]. Bradycardia occurred in 1.1%–26.4% of patients with heart block occurring in 0.2% of patients after the first dose. Common adverse effects were gastrointestinal upset, nasopharyngitis, upper respiratory infections, viral infections, lymphopenia, hypertension, fatigue, and abnormal liver function tests. Macular edema was reported in a small number of patients.

Observational Studies

A registry analysis in Sweden examined discontinuation rates for 876 courses of fingolimod in multiple sclerosis patients [42C]. Patients maintain on fingolimod for 1 year at rates of 83% (natalizumab naïve) and 76%

(prior natalizumab therapy). Discontinuation due to adverse effects was 9% (natalizumab naïve) and 12% (prior natalizumab therapy).

Another registry analysis of fingolimod was conducted in 684 multiple sclerosis patients in Denmark [43C]. Discontinuation due to side effects occurred in 44 (6.4%) patients. Reported adverse effects included pneumonia, urinary tract infections, hair loss, prurisit, hypertension, and macular edema. Among a subset of 204 patients who were intensely followed, 8 (3.9%) required prolonged cardiac monitoring with bradycardia, AV block, and sinus arrest occurring. Eleven of the 204 patients (5.4%) developed dyspnea. All of the cardiac adverse effects resolved spontaneously; 2 of the patients with dyspnea stopped therapy.

Cardiovascular

A prospective study evaluated the cardiac effects of fingolimod compared to natalizumab in 53 multiple sclerosis patients [44c]. Left ventricular ejection fraction decreased and end-diastolic volume increased at months 1 and 6 in patients receiving fingolimod but not natalizumab. The clinical consequences of this effect are unknown, but caution should be used in patients with pre-existing cardiovascular disorders.

Respiratory

Severe dyspnea with reduced pulmonary diffusion capacity was reported in two patients receiving fingolimod for multiple sclerosis [45A]. Both had resolution of dyspnea following drug discontinuation.

Sensory Systems

A review summarized the adverse ocular effects of fingolimod, including macular edema, retinal hemorrhage, and retinal vein occlusion [46r].

Mutagenicity

A 46-year-old male receiving fingolimod for multiple sclerosis developed Kaposi sarcoma [47A].

GLATIRAMER [SEDA-34, 617; SEDA-35, 703; SEDA-36; SEDA-37, 471; SEDA-38, 407]

Observational Study

The tolerability of glatiramer over 2 years was investigated in 754 patients with relapsing-remitting multiple sclerosis (RRMS) [48C]. Adverse effects were experienced by 19.1% of patients with the majority being injection-site reactions and mild or moderate in intensity. Serious adverse events occurred in 50 patients with 18 considered probably related to glatiramer use and 7 considered possibly related. Serious adverse effects occurring in more than 1 patient included dyspnea (3), swelling at the injection site (2), and drug hypersensitivity (2). Treatment was interrupted in 6 patients and discontinued in 64 patients due to adverse events.

Comparative Studies

A retrospective study assessed the incidence and severity of depression in 891 RRMS patients receiving either glatiramer or interferon beta [49C]. Depression was viewed as therapy-related in 21.9% of patients on glatiramer compared to 54.6% of interferon beta patients. One glatiramer patient experienced suicidal ideation, but it was not attributed to the medication.

A prospective cohort study compared pregnancy outcomes in women with RRMS exposed to glatiramer ($n = 151$) with women not on disease-modifying therapies (DMT) at pregnancy onset ($n = 95$) [50C]. In the glatiramer group, 3 infants were born with congenital anomalies compared to 6 infants in the unexposed group. Of the 3 infants, 1 had a patent foramen ovale, 1 had renal duplication, and 1 had pyloric stenosis. In all of these cases, glatiramer was discontinued in the first trimester.

Systematic Reviews

The number needed to harm (NNH) for DMT for RRMS was analyzed in a meta-analysis [51M]. For glatiramer, the NNH was 22 for a serious adverse event, 236 for discontinuation, 32 for chest pain, 9 for dyspnea, 9 for immediate post-injection reaction, and 4 for injection-site reaction.

A meta-analysis compared the incidences of injection-related adverse events (IRAE) and injection-site reactions (ISR) between glatiramer 40 mg/mL given three times per week, glatiramer 20 mg/mL given daily, and placebo [52M]. The incidences of mild IRAE and ISR were greater than two times higher in patients on 20 mg/mL of glatiramer when compared to those on 40 mg/mL. Additionally, moderate IRAE and ISR were experienced 5.7 and 4.4 times more, respectively, in glatiramer 20 mg/mL patients.

Liver

A 56-year-old female using glatiramer for just over 2 months for RRMS was found to have hepatic cytolysis and centro-lobular hepatocyte necrosis with inflammatory infiltrates comprised of eosinophils and lymphocytes, which was consistent with drug-induced toxic hepatitis [53A]. Glatiramer was determined to be the probable cause of the acute hepatitis based on the Naranjo adverse drug reaction probability scale.

Skin

A 43-year-old female receiving glatiramer for RRMS was diagnosed with stage IIIB melanoma, and she experienced a recurrence 7 months following resection and lymphadenectomy [54A]. Glatiramer was discontinued, and her disease was no longer radiographically or clinically detectable after 10 months.

Nicolau syndrome, injection-site reaction-associated panniculitis, and subcutaneous sclerosis were reported in a 51-year-old female with RRMS on glatiramer [55A].

A 37-year-old female with RRMS experienced lobular panniculitis with lymphocytic venulitis and eosinophilic infiltration in adjacent lobules following administration of the first dose of glatiramer [56A]. Her symptoms resolved following cessation of glatiramer and administration of oral antihistamines and topical corticosteroids for 1 month.

A review highlighted the injection-related adverse effects of glatiramer [57R].

Infection Risk

The relatively low risk of infections associated with glatiramer use in patients with multiple sclerosis was reviewed [58R].

Management of Adverse Drug Reactions

A review discussed mitigation strategies for the most common adverse events of glatiramer [59R].

LEFLUNOMIDE [SED-15, 2015; SEDA-34, 618; SEDA-35, 703; SEDA-36, 594; SEDA-37, 471; SEDA-38, 407]

Multiple reviews have highlighted the gastrointestinal, hepatic, hematologic, cardiovascular, infectious, and teratogenic effects of temsirolimus in rheumatoid arthritis patients [60M,61R,62R,63R,64R,65R,66R,67R].

Observational Studies

A multicenter, prospective, randomized controlled trial of 346 rheumatoid arthritis patients assessed the tolerability of leflunomide plus methotrexate and hydroxychloroquine [68C]. The prevalence of adverse events was 43.4% (150/346). The most common adverse effects were increased transaminase levels (14.2%) and upper abdominal complaints (13.0%). Discontinuation of treatment occurred in 24 patients due to toxicity and 8 required hospitalization.

Another multicenter, prospective, randomized controlled trial evaluated the safety of weekly leflunomide in 244 patients with early rheumatoid arthritis [69C]. A total of 33 adverse events occurred in 24 out of 126 patients receiving leflunomide 50 mg/week. Eight patients experienced an increase in transaminase levels, and 4 withdrew treatment due to an adverse event.

The safety of leflunomide in 15 patients with myasthenia gravis was investigated in open-label pilot study [70c]. Three patients experienced minor adverse events, which consisted of gastrointestinal disturbances, transient thrombocytopenia, thinning hair, and rash.

A prospective study evaluated the tolerability of anti-tumor necrosis factor drugs in 531 rheumatic patients [71C]. Concomitant DMARDs were utilized in 444 patients, with 160 of those specifically using leflunomide. Of these patients, 17.5% (28/160) discontinued treatment due to toxicity. Leflunomide-treated patients had a higher risk of therapy cessation compared to those not receiving it (OR=1.984; $P<0.05$).

A retrospective study assessed the safety of leflunomide plus methotrexate in 194 patients with refractory rheumatoid arthritis [72C]. Treatment was discontinued in 17 patients due to adverse events, and 2 patients died from lower respiratory tract infections. After 12 months, 10 patients developed new-onset hypertension.

The tolerability of leflunomide in 28 patients with BK viremia and nephropathy was assessed in a retrospective study [73c]. The most common adverse events were leukopenia (35.7%; 10/28), thrombocytopenia (10.7%; 3/28), and anemia (10.7%; 3/28).

A retrospective study assessed the safety of leflunomide in patients with BK virus-hemorrhagic cystitis [74c]. Of the 4 patients that received leflunomide, 3 experienced mild gastrointestinal effects, such as nausea and bloating.

Comparative Studies

A multicenter, prospective, randomized controlled trial of 399 patients with immunoglobulin A nephropathy assessed the safety of leflunomide plus telmisartan and clopidogrel in 4 different dosing regimens [75C]. Abnormal liver function was observed in 4 out of 199 patients receiving leflunomide 20 mg/day, and 2 of those required discontinuation of therapy. Skin purpura occurred in 1 patient at day 129.

A prospective, randomized trial compared the safety of leflunomide plus prednisone to cyclophosphamide plus prednisone in 52 patients with refractory nephrotic syndrome [76c]. Three patients in the leflunomide group experienced adverse events, such as increased alanine aminotransferase (ALT) level ($n=1$), fatigue ($n=2$), and poor appetite ($n=2$). Patients in the cyclophosphamide group experienced alopecia and irregular menstruation ($n=3$), leukopenia ($n=2$), and ALT elevation ($n=2$).

Systematic Reviews

Multiple systematic reviews and meta-analyses assessed the safety of leflunomide [77M,78M,79M, 80M,81M,82M]. Liu et al. found that 4.7% of patients (13/267) developed increased hepatic enzymes and 3.7% (10/267) had gastrointestinal symptoms [77M]. Conway et al. determined that treatment with leflunomide, when compared to other agents, was not associated with an increased risk of overall pulmonary adverse events (RR=0.99; 95% CI, 0.56–1.78; $I^2=88\%$) or infectious pulmonary events (RR=1.02; 95% CI, 0.58–1.82; $I^2=88\%$) [78M] Stine and Lewis discussed the risk of drug-induced liver injury with the use of leflunomide and its management with cholestyramine [79M]. Hazlewood et al. determined that leflunomide plus methotrexate resulted in a higher rate of ALT elevations compared to methotrexate alone (rate ratio=4.75; 95% CI, 1.16–20.70) [80M]. Feng et al. found a higher rate of abnormal hepatic function with leflunomide monotherapy compared to treatment with leflunomide plus total glucosides of peony (OR=0.32; 95% CI, 0.12–0.84; $P=0.02$) [81M]. Baldwin et al. discussed the teratogenic risk of leflunomide [82M]. Among 78 live births from pregnancies exposed to leflunomide, 7 infants had congenital abnormalities and 3 had functional abnormalities [82M].

Respiratory

A case series of 3 patients evaluated the use of leflunomide for recalcitrant cytomegalovirus infections [83A]. Although 2 patients did not experience any adverse events, pulmonary hypertension occurred in 1 patient after approximately 16 months of treatment.

Diffuse alveolar damage and leflunomide-related interstitial lung disease occurred in an 80-year-old female after receiving treatment for over 9 years [84A].

A review discussed the pulmonary effects of leflunomide [85R].

Metabolism

A retrospective study assessed the effects of disease-modifying antirheumatic drugs (DMARD) on body mass in 32 859 patients [86MC]. By 6 months, leflunomide demonstrated a greater risk of weight loss (OR=1.86; 95% CI, 1.71–1.97) and a larger body mass index loss (-0.47 kg/m^2; 95% CI, -0.42 to -0.53 kg/m^2) compared to methotrexate ($P<0.001$ for each comparisons).

Skin

The occurrence of Stevens-Johnson syndrome and toxic epidermal necrosis in association with drug-induced liver injury was evaluated [87c]. Of the 36 patients that met the criteria, 3 were receiving leflunomide, and all 3 did not survive the adverse event.

A 50-year-old female developed keratotic papules a few months after leflunomide initiation, but the medication was not discontinued [88A]. The papules recurred 2 years later, and the patient was diagnosed with eruptive keratoacanthomas. Her skin lesions completely resolved following leflunomide cessation and isotretinoin therapy for 3 months.

Leflunomide-induced subacute cutaneous lupus erythematosus following 3 years of treatment was reported in a 50-year-old female [89A]. The patient's symptoms improved following leflunomide cessation and utilization of methotrexate and corticosteroids.

Musculoskeletal

A review discussed the risk of articular disorders, tenosynovitis, and tendon rupture with the use of leflunomide [90R].

Genetic Factors

Pharmacogenetic factors that contribute to leflunomide cessation due to toxicity were evaluated in 105 rheumatoid arthritis patients [91C]. Carriers of the CYP1A2 C163A allele demonstrated a 2.29-fold (95% CI, 2.24–2.34) increase in cessation hazard compared to non-carriers ($P = 0.016$). Prior to day 365, leflunomide therapy was discontinued due to toxicity in 32.4% of patients (34/105).

Leflunomide demonstrated an increased risk of toxicity in patients with CYP1A2*1F CC genotype compared to those with the CYP1A2*1F A allele (OR = 9.708; 95% CI, 2.276–41.403; $P = 0.002$) [92R].

MYCOPHENOLIC ACID [SED-15, 2402; SEDA-34, 622; SEDA-35, 704; SEDA-36, 594]

Observational Studies

Monotherapy with mycophenolate mofetil was evaluated in 30 liver transplant patients [93c]. Side effects included diarrhea (10%) and anemia (3.3%) and were managed with dose reduction.

Respiratory infections, leukopenia, anemia, and gastrointestinal adverse effects occurred among 34 children receiving mycophenolate mofetil for nephrotic syndrome [94c]. There was no association between the adverse effects and mycophenolic acid exposure.

Mycophenolic acid trough concentration was a risk factor for adverse events (OR 2.28, 95% CI 1.25–4.16) among 54 renal transplant recipients [95c]. A trough concentration greater than 5.25 mg/L had 77.8% sensitivity and 86.7% specificity for adverse events.

Adverse events of mycophenolic acid in the treatment of Graves' orbitopathy were analyzed in a prospective longitudinal study of 50 patients [96c]. Overall, there were 88 adverse events reported in 36 (68%) patients. No patients discontinued therapy due to adverse events.

Cardiovascular

A retrospective study of 63 heart transplant recipients compared cardiac allograft vasculopathy between mycophenolate mofetil and everolimus [97c]. Intravascular ultrasound demonstrated the mycophenolate treatment was associated with an increased plaque volume ($P = 0.006$) and decreased lumen volume ($P < 0.001$) over a 1-year period compared to no change in these parameters for everolimus treatment. These results indicate that everolimus may be associated with less cardiac allograft vasculopathy compared to mycophenolate.

Psychological

Two cases of psychiatric side effects of mycophenolate mofetil (panic attacks with crying and moodiness with anhedonia) were reported in pediatric patients [98A]. Both had resolutions of symptoms within weeks of discontinuing mycophenolate therapy.

Gastrointestinal

A case report described mycophenolate mofetil induced colitis in a 31-year-old female with lupus nephritis [99A]. While this is a known side effect of mycophenolate, the novelty of this case was that colitis developed 10 years into therapy.

An infectious mechanism of mycophenolic acid induced diarrhea was investigated in retrospective study of 726 renal transplant recipients [100C]. There were 51 episodes of chronic diarrhea, with 38 (74.5%) attributed to infection. Resolution of diarrhea was 100% with mycophenolic acid discontinuation, 76.5% with a switch from mycophenolate mofetil to enteric-coated mycophenolate sodium and antibiotics, 22.7% with a dose reduction and antibiotics, and 19% with antibiotics alone.

Immunologic

A 46-year-old female with a history of hypersensitivity to mycophenolate mofetil was successfully desensitized in a 12 step procedure [101A].

SIROLIMUS (RAPAMYCIN) [SED-15, 3148; SEDA-34, 626; SEDA-35, 705; SEDA-36, 594]

Comparative Studies

Safety analysis of a prospective, open-label, randomized controlled trial compared adverse effects of tacrolimus to sirolimus in 119 renal transplant recipients [102C]. Cumulative incidence of all adverse effects and serious adverse effects were similar between treatments. Sirolimus was associated with more aphthous ulcers (28% vs 0%), sinusitis (10% vs 0%), dermatitis (15% vs 3%) and dyslipidemia (35% vs 14%) compared to tacrolimus.

Observational Studies

Sirolimus was evaluated in 61 patients with complicated vascular anomalies [103c]. Discontinuation due to adverse effects occurred in two patients because of hypertriglyceridemia and laryngospasm. Grade 3 or 4 toxicities included: hematologic (27%), gastrointestinal (3%), metabolic (3%), infection (2%), pulmonary (2%) and lymphatic (2%).

Cardiovascular

A pediatric heart transplant recipient developed abdominal pain, nausea, vomiting, and ventricular extrasystole attacks attributed to sirolimus [104A]. The symptoms improved following a decrease in sirolimus dose.

Immunologic

Successful oral desensitization to sirolimus was described in a patient with lymphangioleiomyomatosis using a 7-step procedure [105A].

TACROLIMUS [SED-15, 3279; SEDA-34, 629; SEDA-35, 705; SEDA-36, 596]

Observational Studies

The relationship of adverse effects to tacrolimus and tacrolimus metabolite (M-I and M-III) concentrations was evaluated in 81 renal transplant recipients [106c]. Estimated glomerular filtration rate and red blood cell count were inversely associated with M-III metabolite concentrations ($r = -0.244$, $P < 0.01$ and $r = -0.349$, $P < 0.05$, respectively). Patients with infections had higher tacrolimus and M-III concentrations compared to those without infections.

Cardiovascular

An open-label, multicenter, randomized trial compared the extent of left ventricular hypertrophy between tacrolimus and everolimus in 71 renal transplant recipients [107C]. There was no difference in left ventricular mass index between treatments after 24 months. Everolimus was associated with reduced concentric remodeling of the left ventricle, reduced procollagen type I N-terminal propeptide, and improved renal function.

Nervous System

Two cases of posterior reversible encephalopathy syndrome (PRES) were reported in renal transplant patients receiving tacrolimus [108A]. PRES resolved after switching tacrolimus to cyclosporine in one patient and after reducing the dose of tacrolimus in the other patient.

Factors associated with neurologic complications of tacrolimus were investigated in 90 pediatric liver transplant recipients [109c]. Twelve patients (13.3%) developed neurologic complications, predominately seizures. Total bilirubin concentrations greater than 4.3 mg/dL in the first week post-transplant were the only factor associated with neurologic complications (HR 1.588, 95% CI: 1.042–2.358).

Sensory Systems

A case report described a 42-year-old female that developed diplopia attributed to tacrolimus therapy [110A]. She was transitioned to cyclosporine with persistence of diplopia. After discontinuation of calcineurin inhibitor therapy, the diplopia resolved within 6 days.

Hematologic

A 61-year-old female liver transplant recipient developed severe thrombocytopenia attributed to tacrolimus [111A]. The nadir platelet count was 17 000. The thrombocytopenia resolved after conversion to cyclosporine.

Urinary Tract

Tacrolimus vascular toxicity was observed in a renal transplant biopsy of a 23-year-old male [112A]. Initial biopsy results found antibody mediated rejection, but further analysis suggested a toxic effect of tacrolimus as the culprit.

Genetic Factors

The impact of CYP3A5 expresser status (rs776746) on tacrolimus adverse effects was investigated in 29 ulcerative colitis patients [113c]. The CYP3A5 expressers had significantly higher tacrolimus concentration-to-dose ratio and experienced more adverse effects (62.5% had at least one adverse effect) compared to non-expressers (23.1% with at least one adverse effect; $P = 0.034$).

The association of pregnane X receptor (PXR) polymorphisms and tacrolimus adverse effects was studied in 336 renal transplant recipients [114C]. There were no adverse effect associations with the rs3842689, rs6785049, or rs1523127 polymorphisms. The rs3842689 homozygous wild-type (WW) genotype was associated with a 15.8-fold increased risk of gastrointestinal reactions compared to the homozygous mutant (MM) genotype.

Polymorphisms in FOXP3 and CCDC22 genes were evaluated in 114 Chinese renal transplant recipients [115C]. There was a 10-fold higher risk of tacrolimus nephrotoxicity with the FOXP3 rs3761548 AA and AC genotypes compared to the CC genotype. No other tested polymorphisms displayed associations with tacrolimus adverse effects.

Drug Formulations

Adverse effect profiles were similar between once-daily extended-release tacrolimus and conventional twice daily tacrolimus in a randomized controlled trial of 91 liver transplant recipients [116c].

Another comparison between formulations investigated the effect of converting from traditional twice daily tacrolimus to the once-daily extended release tacrolimus on diabetes mellitus measures [117c]. There was no improvement in beta cell function or insulin resistance in 28 renal transplant recipients who underwent conversion. There was an improvement in beta-cell function among 15 of the subjects who converted within 4 years of transplantation, suggesting a possible benefit if converted to the once-daily formulation earlier post-transplantation.

Drug–Drug Interactions

Renal toxicity attributed to elevated tacrolimus and sirolimus concentrations developed in a 65-year-old male hematopoietic stem cell transplant recipient following initiation of clotrimazole troches [118A]. Trough concentrations increased from 4.6 to 17.2 ng/mL for tacrolimus and 13.2 to >30.0 ng/mL for sirolimus. Clotrimazole is a known inhibitor of CYP3A4 which is the probable mechanism of this interaction. The patient's renal function improved to baseline after holding tacrolimus and sirolimus to allow the concentrations to decline into the target range.

An interaction between cobicistat and tacrolimus was described in a 50-year-old male renal transplant recipient [119A]. Following initiation of cobicistat, tacrolimus trough concentrations increased to 111.2 ng/mL (goal 4–6 ng/mL) with associated acute kidney injury. Both drugs were held and the patient's renal function returned to baseline.

A 67-year-old male developed tacrolimus toxicity after taking edible marijuana and testing positive for tetrahydrocannabinol (THC) [120A]. The patient was also receiving posaconazole which contributes to the interaction with tacrolimus, although therapeutic tacrolimus concentrations had been maintained on this combination prior to testing positive for THC.

TEMSIROLIMUS [SEDA-34, 632; SEDA-35, 707; SEDA-36, 597]

Two reviews discussed the risk of stomatitis, metabolic disturbances, non-infectious pneumonitis, and drug interactions with the use of temsirolimus [121R,122R].

Observational Studies

A multicenter, prospective, phase II trial explored the safety of temsirolimus in 22 ovarian cancer patients and 22 endometrial cancer patients [123c]. Overall, grade 3 adverse events were rare and grade 4 ileus occurred in 1 ovarian cancer patient. However, multiple grade 1 and 2 adverse effects, such as anemia, thrombocytopenia, edema, hypokalemia, and dyspnea, were considered probably attributed to temsirolimus.

Another multicenter, prospective, phase II trial assessed the toxicity of temsirolimus plus bevacizumab in 40 patients with metastatic renal cell carcinoma (mRCC) [124c]. Overall, 95% of patients experienced an adverse event with 70% being grade 3 or higher. The most common adverse effects were hypertriglyceridemia ($n = 6$), hypertension ($n = 5$), and proteinuria ($n = 4$). Unacceptable toxicity leads to discontinuation of therapy in 27.5% of patients.

The safety of temsirolimus in 37 patients with relapsed/refractory lymphoma was evaluated in a prospective phase II trial [125c]. The most common adverse events were hyperglycemia, infections, bone marrow suppression, and fatigue. Twenty-eight severe adverse effects occurred, and 5 patients died due to toxicity.

The tolerability of temsirolimus in 11 patients with endometrial carcinoma was assessed [126c]. Overall, 90.9% of patients (10/11) experienced an adverse event, and the most common was mucositis (63.6%; 7/11).

A prospective phase II pilot trial evaluated the toxicity of temsirolimus in 20 patients with myelodysplastic syndrome [127c]. The most common adverse events experienced were gastrointestinal disorders, infectious complications, and cytopenias. The trial was prematurely discontinued due to the occurrence of 13 serious adverse events that were related to temsirolimus use.

A phase I trial explored the safety of temsirolimus in combination with trebananib in 21 patients with advanced solid tumors [128c]. Of the 6 patients that received 25 mg of temsirolimus and 15 mg/kg of trebananib, 1 experienced grade 2 pneumonitis as a dose-limiting toxicity. In the temsirolimus 20 mg and trebananib 15 mg/kg group, a dose-limiting toxicity occurred in 2 out of 7 patients (grade 2 edema and grade 3 mucositis). Of the 8 patients in the temsirolimus 20 mg and trebananib 10 mg/kg group, grade 4 hypertriglyceridemia was observed in 1 and grade 5 multi-organ failure was observed in 1. Overall, the most common adverse events were fatigue (81%), edema (62%), and lymphopenia (57%).

Another phase I trial assessed the toxicity of temsirolimus plus pemetrexed in 8 patients with advanced non-small cell lung cancer [129c]. Of the 2 patients in the temsirolimus 15 mg and pemetrexed 500 mg/m^2 group, 1 experienced grade 4 thrombocytopenia, grade 3 leukopenia, and grade 3 neutropenia and the other experienced grade 3 leukopenia. However, in the temsirolimus 15 mg and pemetrexed 375 mg/m^2 group, no dose-limiting toxicities were observed.

The safety of the combination of temsirolimus, bevacizumab, and cetuximab in 21 patients with advanced malignancies was investigated in a phase I trial [130c]. In the temsirolimus 5 mg, bevacizumab 5 mg/kg, and cetuximab 100/75 mg/m^2 group, grade 3 or 4 toxicity was experienced by 1 out of 3 patients but was not dose limiting. In the temsirolimus 5 mg, bevacizumab 10 mg/kg, and cetuximab 100/75 mg/m^2 group ($n=16$), 11 grade 3 or 4 toxicities were observed and 3 were dose limiting. In the temsirolimus 12.5 mg, bevacizumab 2.5 mg/kg, and cetuximab 100/75 mg/m^2 group, the 2 patients experienced 5 grade 3 or 4 toxicities with 3 considered dose limiting. All 21 patients experienced at least 1 adverse event, and the most common was anemia (90.5%; 19/21).

The toxicity of temsirolimus plus metformin in 21 patients with advanced/refractory cancers was evaluated [131c]. The most common adverse effects experienced were fatigue, mucositis, and rash. Overall, 5 grade 2 or 3 toxicities occurred, and no grade 4 or 5 adverse events were noted. Two dose-limiting toxicities

were observed (grade 3 mucositis and grade 3 renal failure).

The toxicity of temsirolimus and everolimus in 18 patients with mRCC and renal insufficiency was studied [132c]. All of the adverse events experienced were considered grade 1 or 2 except for a single occurrence of grade 3 creatinine level elevation. Stomatitis occurred in 50% of patients (9/18). Two patients on temsirolimus required a dose reduction due to non-renal toxicity.

A retrospective study assessed the safety of targeted therapy plus radiotherapy in mRCC patients [133c]. Of the 136 treatment courses, 11 were associated with temsirolimus use. One case of mucositis occurred when temsirolimus was utilized as second-line therapy.

Comparative Studies

A prospective, randomized phase II trial compared temsirolimus plus radiotherapy to temozolomide plus radiochemotherapy in 111 patients with glioblastoma [134C]. In the temsirolimus arm, grade 3 neutropenia occurred in 1.8% (1/56) of patients, grade 3 lymphocytopenia in 16.1% (9/56), and grade 4 lymphocytopenia in 1.8% (1/56). In the temozolomide arm, grade 4 neutropenia was observed in 3.6% (2/55) of patients, grade 3 leukopenia in 3.6% (2/55), grade 3 lymphocytopenia in 25.5% (14/55), grade 4 lymphocytopenia in 3.6% (2/55), grade 3 thrombocytopenia in 1.8% (1/55), and grade 4 thrombocytopenia in 1.8% (1/55).

Systematic Reviews

Three systematic reviews and meta-analyses have assessed the safety of mTOR inhibitors, including temsirolimus [135M,136M,137M]. Chang et al. determined that temsirolimus plus bevacizumab was safer than interferon alpha plus bevacizumab (RR=1.19; 95% CI, 1.01–1.41; $P<0.05$), and temsirolimus was safer than interferon alpha (RR=0.42; 95% CI, 0.27–0.67; $P<0.05$) [135M]. Lew and Chamberlain found no difference in the RR of high-grade metabolic events between temsirolimus and everolimus ($P=0.835$) [136M]. Zhang et al. determined that the incidence of severe pneumonitis after temsirolimus use was 1.3% (95% CI, 0.5%–3.4%), and the OR was 7.02 (95% CI, 2.33–21.14; $P=0.001$) [137M]. However, there was no significant difference between temsirolimus and everolimus [137M].

Respiratory

The risk of interstitial lung disease with temsirolimus in cancer patients was reviewed [138R]. The incidence of interstitial lung disease at any grade was 14%–45%.

Mouth and Teeth

A retrospective study evaluated the occurrence of osteonecrosis of the jaw in the United States Food and Drug Administration's adverse event reporting system [139MC]. Of the 17119 cases of osteonecrosis of the jaw experienced, 28 were associated with the use of temsirolimus (OR = 3.1; 95% CI, 2.2–4.6; $P < 0.0001$).

A retrospective study assessed the safety of temsirolimus and everolimus in 4 mRCC patients undergoing hemodialysis [140c]. Of the 2 patients treated with temsirolimus, 1 experienced grade 2 mucositis.

The risk of stomatitis with mTOR inhibitors was highlighted in a review [141R]. The prevalence of oral mucosal lesions at any grade during temsirolimus treatment was 41%.

Liver

Lee and Chan reviewed the hepatic adverse events associated with the use of temsirolimus [142R]. The overall incidence of hepatotoxicity was 30%–70%. The incidence of grade 3 or 4 drug-induced liver injury was 2%–5%.

THIOPURINES [SED-15, 377; SEDA-34, 633; SEDA-35, 709; SEDA-36, 598]

Systematic Reviews

The safety of low dose azathioprine in the treatment of ulcerative colitis was evaluated in a meta-analysis of 6 studies including 211 patients [143M]. Adverse effects occurred in 25.0% (95% CI: 18.0%–31.0%) of patients. Leukopenia, abnormal liver function tests, gastrointestinal upset, and alopecia were the most common adverse effects.

Observational Studies

Toxicities of azathioprine were described in a cohort of 571 patients with myasthenia gravis [144C]. Myelosuppression occurred in 9.1% of patients at a median of 4 weeks after initiation and included normocytic anemia or pancytopenia. Hepatotoxicity occurred in 15.2% of patients at a median of 5 weeks after initiation with most developing GGT elevation.

Cardiovascular

A 62-year-old male developed myocarditis while on azathioprine for ulcerative colitis [145A]. The reaction resolved with azathioprine discontinued but did recur after re-challenge.

Endocrine

Incidence of and risk factors for pancreatitis was evaluated in 510 inflammatory bowel disease patients in a prospective registry study [146C]. Azathioprine-induced pancreatitis occurred in 37 patients, with smoking being the strongest risk factor for development of this adverse event.

Hematologic

Pure red cell aplasia occurred in two patients receiving azathioprine for Crohn's disease [147A]. Both patients recovered after discontinuation of azathioprine.

Skin

A 67-year-old male on azathioprine for inflammatory bowel disease developed eruptive lentiginosis which resolved after azathioprine discontinuation [148A].

Teratogenicity

The effect of paternal use of a thiopurine within 3 months of conception was evaluated in a Danish cohort study [149C]. Among 699 men, use of a thiopurine was not associated with congenital abnormalities, preterm birth, or small for gestation age compared to 1012624 controls.

Genetic Factors

The association between thiopurine toxicities and polymorphisms in thiopurine methyltransferase (TMPT), methylenetetrahydrofolate reductase (MTHFR), and glutathione S-transferase (GST) were investigated in 100 pediatric patients with acute lymphoblastic leukemia (ALL) [150C]. In combination with the presence of hepatitis C virus, hepatotoxicity was associated with the TMPT*3B G460A polymorphism ($P < 0.04$) and the MTHFR C677T polymorphism ($P < 0.001$). Myelotoxicity was not associated with any of the tested genetic polymorphisms.

Fifty-three patients with inflammatory bowel disease receiving a thiopurine were analyzed in a candidate gene study [151c]. TMPT loss-of-function mutation was associated with increased adverse effects (OR 3.64, 95% CI 0.55–24.23). Polymorphisms in inosine triphosphatase (ITPA) and GST were not associated with toxicities. Overall, 10 patients had to discontinue therapy due to adverse effects.

A retrospective study compared adverse effects between full dose and low dose thiopurine treatment in 134 patients with Crohn's disease and normal TMPT activity [152C]. Complications of thiopurine use occurred in 49% of the full dose and 49% of the reduced dose groups ($P=1$). Discontinuation due to adverse effects was 28% with full dose and 39% with reduced dose ($P=0.25$).

Thiopurine-induced leukopenia was investigated in a genome-wide association study [153C]. The variant p.A134T (rs79206939) in *FTO* was associated with leukopenia, a result that was validated in two separate cohorts.

A retrospective study of 305 pediatric ALL patients investigated the association between polymorphisms in *PACSIN2* and *ITPA* with thiopurine-induced toxicities [154C]. The *PACSIN2* rs2413739TT genotype was associated with increased hematologic toxicity among patients that were normal function TMPT.

Polymorphisms in *TMPT* and *ITPA* were associated with azathioprine toxicities in 82 inflammatory bowel disease patients [155c]. Myelotoxicity occurred in 11% of patients, of which 44.4% were heterozygous mutants in *TMPT* and 11.1% were compound heterozygous. There were no associations with *ITPA* polymorphisms and azathioprine toxicities.

The association of thiopurine metabolites and myelotoxicity was evaluated in 224 patients with inflammatory bowel disease [156C]. Concentrations of 6-thioguanine nucleotide (6-TGN) and 6-methylmercaptopurine ribonucleotide (6-MMPR) at 1 week were associated with leukopenia. Leukopenia was more pronounced with mercaptopurine compared to azathioprine treatment (OR 7.3, 95% CI: 3.1–17.0).

R. Pharmacogenetic Associations With Thiopurines: Focus on NUDT15 Gene

The nucleoside diphosphatase-linked moiety X-type motif 15 (NUDT15) gene is involved in the hydrolysis of nucleoside diphosphate derivatives which may have an impact on thiopurine pharmacokinetics and pharmacodynamics. Recent studies have identified polymorphisms in NUDT15 that are associated with toxicities of thiopurines.

Loss-of-function variants in NUDT15 (p.Arg139Cys, p.Arg139His, p.Val18Ile, and p.Val18_Val19insGlyVal) were evaluated in 270 pediatric ALL patients receiving thiopurine treatment [157C]. These variants were associated with a 74.4%–100% loss of function in nucleotide diphosphatase activity, which led to increased exposure of active thiopurine metabolites and increased in vitro cytotoxicity. NUDT15 loss-of-function diplotypes were associated with significantly lower tolerated 6-mercaptopurine dose. This seminal work provided the foundation for further investigation of NUDT15 genetic associations with thiopurine toxicity.

Myelosuppression and alopecia occurred in a 40-year Chinese male patient receiving azathioprine [158A]. The reaction was attributed to the presence of the NUDT15 c.415C>T polymorphism (rs116855232). TMPT activity was normal in this patient.

The association of the NUDT15 R139C mutation with thiopurine-induced myelosuppression and alopecia was examined in 142 Japanese patients with inflammatory bowel disease [159C]. Severe alopecia occurred in 5 patients that were all homozygous TT genotype. Dose reductions were more frequent with the CT genotype compared to CC ($P=0.0001$). The R139C mutation was also associated with early leukopenia ($P<0.001$) but not late leukopenia.

The effect of the NUDT15 c.415C>T polymorphism on azathioprine-induced leukopenia was evaluated in 81 Korean pediatric Crohn's disease patients [160c]. Early leukopenia occurred in 8 patients, of which 6 (75%) carried the variant NUDT15 c.415C>T allele. Three patients were homozygous variants, all of whom developed alopecia totalis and two experienced severe systemic infection.

The C415T polymorphism in NUDT15 was assessed in 69 Indian patients on thiopurine therapy [161c]. Nine patients had variant alleles, of which 6 developed leukopenia (66.7%). This was significantly increased compared to the homozygous wild-type patients, of which none (0/60) developed leukopenia ($P<0.001$ for comparison).

The c.415C>T polymorphism in NUDT15 was assessed in 121 pediatric ALL patients [162C]. NUDT15 heterozygotes were able to tolerate 33.3% of the planned mercaptopurine dose, compared to 76.0% tolerability in the homozygotes. Dose tolerability was determined by a protocol that maintained leukocyte count above 1500 cells per microliter.

Pharmacogenetic associations to leukopenia were evaluated in 253 Chinese patients with Crohn's disease receiving thiopurine treatment [163C]. Compared to wild-type, the NUDT15 R139C variant polymorphism was associated with leukopenia (OR 10.8, 95% CI: 5.9–19.8). Among the NUDT15 wild-type patients, 6TGN concentrations were significant higher in patients with leukopenia compared to those without ($P=0.006$).

Overall, polymorphisms in the NUDT15 gene are associated with thiopurine toxicity, namely leukopenia. The inclusion of this genetic test, in addition to TMPT activity, may provide value in personalization of thiopurine therapy.

IMMUNOENHANCING DRUGS

Levamisole [SED-15, 2028; SEDA-34, 638; SEDA-35, 710; SEDA-36, 460]

Observational Studies

A retrospective study assessed the safety of levamisole in 72 children with steroid-dependent or frequently relapsing nephrotic syndrome [164c]. Sixteen patients (22%) experienced reversible adverse events, such as allergic rash (13%), hypertransaminasemia (4%), abdominal pain (4%), arthralgia (3%), thrombocytopenia (1%), and leukopenia (1%).

A prospective study assessed the safety of levamisole over 5 years in 186 children with steroid-dependent nephrotic syndrome [165C]. Discontinuation of therapy was required in 3 patients due to a suspected vasculitic rash and in 2 patients due to gastrointestinal intolerance.

Cardiovascular

Multiple case reports and one case series have demonstrated the occurrence of erythematous cutaneous lesions and glomerulonephritis (GN) following exposure to levamisole-adulterated cocaine [166A,167,168A,169A]. Renal biopsy in a 50-year-old female revealed crescentic GN and accompanying membranous nephropathy, with the likely etiology being anti-neutrophil cytoplasmic antibody (ANCA)-associated vasculitis based on the presence of elevated myeloperoxidase antibody titers [166A]. A 49-year-old male also presenting with spontaneous weight loss (20 kg over 1 year) and arthralgia had a positive ANCA titer, leukocytoclastic vasculitis on skin biopsy, and pauci-immune crescentic GN on renal biopsy [167A]. Improvement of cutaneous lesions and renal function occurred after the use of corticosteroids and intravenous cyclophosphamide [167A]. A 48-year-old female also presenting with an unintentional 10-pound weight loss had a positive perinuclear-ANCA titer, leukocytoclastic vasculitis on skin biopsy, and pauci-immune necrotizing and crescentic GN [168A]. Her manifestations improved following treatment with corticosteroids alone [168A]. In a series of 11 cases of levamisole-induced vasculitis, necrosis of the ears occurred in 100% of patients, retiform purpura in 91%, positive ANCA in 91%, lymphopenia in 73%, and glomerulonephritis in 55% [169A]. Lesions resolved in all patients following treatment with prednisolone [169A].

Fluid Balance

An autopsy of a 26-year-old male revealed brain edema, pulmonary edema, and extensive hyperemia after a packet of cocaine ruptured within his digestive tract [170A].

Immunologic

An international, multicenter, prospective, randomized clinical trial assessed the safety of levamisole over 1 year in 99 children with steroid-sensitive idiopathic nephrotic syndrome [171C]. Asymptomatic moderate neutropenia (500–1000 cells/µL) occurred in 8% (4/50) of levamisole patients. This adverse event was determined to be potentially related to the drug and was reversible either spontaneously or following levamisole interruption. Additionally, ANCA-related arthritis was reported in 1 patient and was reversible with interruption of levamisole.

References

[1] Hardinger KL, Sunderland D, Wiederrich JA. Belatacept for the prophylaxis of organ rejection in kidney transplant patients: an evidence-based review of its place in therapy. Int J Nephrol Renovasc Dis. 2016;9:139–50 [R].

[2] Adams AB, Ford ML, Larsen CP. Costimulation blockade in autoimmunity and transplantation: the CD28 pathway. J Immunol. 2016;197(6):2045–50 [R].

[3] Bamgbola O. Metabolic consequences of modern immunosuppressive agents in solid organ transplantation. Ther Adv Endocrinol Metab. 2016;7(3):110–27 [R].

[4] Bamoulid J, Staeck O, Halleck F, et al. Immunosuppression and results in renal transplantation. Eur Urol Suppl. 2016;15(9):415–29 [R].

[5] Garcia VD, Meinerz G, Keitel E. A safety evaluation of belatacept for the treatment of kidney transplant. Expert Opin Drug Saf. 2016;15(8):1125–32 [R].

[6] Del Bello A, Marion O, Milongo D, et al. Belatacept prophylaxis against organ rejection in adult kidney-transplant recipients. Expert Rev Clin Pharmacol. 2016;9(2):215–27 [R].

[7] Brakemeier S, Kannenkeril D, Durr M, et al. Experience with belatacept rescue therapy in kidney transplant recipients. Transpl Int. 2016;29(11):1184–95 [c].

[8] Le Meur Y, Aulagnon F, Bertrand D, et al. Effect of an early switch to belatacept among calcineurin inhibitor intolerant graft recipients of kidneys from extended-criteria donors. Am J Transplant. 2016;16(7):2181–6 [c].

[9] Timofte I, Terrin M, Barr E, et al. Belatacept for renal rescue in lung transplant patients. Transpl Int. 2016;29(4):453–63 [c].

[10] Durrbach A, Pestana JM, Florman S, et al. Long-term outcomes in belatacept- versus cyclosporine-treated recipients of extended criteria donor kidneys: final results from BENEFIT-EXT, a phase III randomized study. Am J Transplant. 2016;16(11):3192–201 [MC].

[11] Vincenti F, Rostaing L, Grinyo J, et al. Belatacept and long-term outcomes in kidney transplantation. N Engl J Med. 2016;374(4):333–433 [MC].

[12] Wen X, Casey MJ, Santos AH, et al. Comparison of utilization and clinical outcomes for belatacept- and tacrolimus-based immunosuppression in renal transplant recipients. Am J Transplant. 2016;16(11):3202–11 [MC].

[13] Alameddine M, Gaynor J, Chen L, et al. Outcomes of de novo belatacept versus tacrolimus in kidney recipients of high risk donors. Transplantation. 2016;100(7):S82 [c].

[14] Cicora F, Roberti J. Recurrent psoriasis after introduction of belatacept in 2 kidney transplant recipients. Prog Transplant. 2016;26(2):109–11 [A].

[15] Haidar G, Crespo M, Maximous S, et al. Invasive tracheobronchial aspergillosis in a lung transplant recipient receiving belatacept as salvage maintenance immunosuppression: a case report. Transplant Proc. 2016;48(1):275–8 [A].

[16] Sharma R, Shah N, Claus J, et al. Toxoplasma chorioretinitis following renal transplantation. Kidney Int. 2016;89(3):724 [A].

[17] Sawinski D, Trofe-Clark J, Leas B, et al. Calcineurin inhibitor minimization, conversion, withdrawal, and avoidance strategies in renal transplantation: a systematic review and meta-analysis. Am J Transplant. 2016;16(7):2117–38 [M].

[18] Zhang X, Ji L, Yang L, et al. The effect of calcineurin inhibitors in the induction and maintenance treatment of lupus nephritis: a systematic review and meta-analysis. Int Urol Nephrol. 2016;48(5):731–43 [M].

[19] Lambert SM, Nigusse SD, Alembo DT, et al. Comparison of efficacy and safety of ciclosporin to prednisolone in the treatment of erythema nodosum leprosum: two randomised, double blind, controlled pilot studies in Ethiopia. PLoS Negl Trop Dis. 2016;10(2)e0004149 [c].

[20] Tavakoli Ardakani M, Tafazoli A, Mehdizadeh M, et al. A 16 month survey of cyclosporine utilization evaluation in allogeneic hematopoietic stem cell transplant recipients. Iran J Pharm Res. 2016;15(1):331–9 [c].

[21] Garcia-Bello JA, Romo-Del Rio EG, Mendoza-Gomez E, et al. Effect of immunosuppressive therapy on cardiovascular risk factor prevalence in kidney-transplanted children: comparative study. Transplant Proc. 2016;48(2):639–42 [C].

[22] Nankivell BJ, P'Ng CH, O'Connell PJ, et al. Calcineurin inhibitor nephrotoxicity through the lens of longitudinal histology: comparison of cyclosporine and tacrolimus eras. Transplantation. 2016;100(8):1723–31 [C].

[23] Unver Dogan N, Uysal II, Fazliogullari Z, et al. Investigation of developmental toxicity and teratogenicity of cyclosporine A, tacrolimus and their combinations with prednisolone. Regul Toxicol Pharmacol. 2016;77:213–22 [E].

[24] Atiq F, Broers AE, Andrews LM, et al. A clinically relevant pharmacokinetic interaction between cyclosporine and imatinib. Eur J Clin Pharmacol. 2016;72(6):719–23 [c].

[25] Parasrampuria DA, Mendell J, Shi M, et al. Edoxaban drug-drug interactions with ketoconazole, erythromycin, and cyclosporine. Br J Clin Pharmacol. 2016;82(6):1591–600 [c].

[26] Sridharan K, Sivaramakrishnan G. Interaction of citrus juices with cyclosporine: systematic review and meta-analysis. Eur J Drug Metab Pharmacokinet. 2016;41(6):665–73 [M].

[27] Rugo HS, Hortobagyi GN, Yao J, et al. Meta-analysis of stomatitis in clinical studies of everolimus: incidence and relationship with efficacy. Ann Oncol. 2016;27(3):519–25 [M].

[28] de Wit D, Schneider TC, Moes DJ, et al. Everolimus pharmacokinetics and its exposure-toxicity relationship in patients with thyroid cancer. Cancer Chemother Pharmacol. 2016;78(1):63–71 [c].

[29] Moscetti L, Vici P, Gamucci T, et al. Safety analysis, association with response and previous treatments of everolimus and exemestane in 181 metastatic breast cancer patients: a multicenter Italian experience. Breast. 2016;29:96–101 [C].

[30] Robles NR, Peces R, Gomez-Ferrer A, et al. Everolimus safety and efficacy for renal angiomyolipomas associated with tuberous sclerosis complex: a Spanish expanded access trial. Orphanet J Rare Dis. 2016;11(1):128 [c].

[31] Samueli S, Abraham K, Dressler A, et al. Efficacy and safety of Everolimus in children with TSC-associated epilepsy—pilot data from an open single-center prospective study. Orphanet J Rare Dis. 2016;11(1):145 [c].

[32] Nishino M, Brais LK, Brooks NV, et al. Drug-related pneumonitis during mammalian target of rapamycin inhibitor therapy in patients with neuroendocrine tumors: a radiographic pattern-based approach. Eur J Cancer. 2016;53:163–70 [c].

[33] Tomei P, Masola V, Granata S, et al. Everolimus-induced epithelial to mesenchymal transition (EMT) in bronchial/pulmonary cells: when the dosage does matter in transplantation. J Nephrol. 2016;29(6):881–91 [c].

[34] Chan S, Francis LP, Kark AL, et al. Everolimus-induced tubular toxicity in non-renal cancer. Intern Med J. 2016;46(12):1454–5 [A].

[35] Roe N, Twilla JD, Duhart B, et al. Breast cancer patient with everolimus-induced angioedema: a rare occurrence with potential for serious consequences. J Oncol Pharm Pract. 2017;23(4):318–20 [A].

[36] Arora S, Akhil R, Chacko RT, et al. Palmar-plantar erythrodysesthesia: an uncommon adverse effect of everolimus. Indian J Med Paediatr Oncol. 2016;37(2):116–8 [A].

[37] Conteduca V, Santoni M, Medri M, et al. Correlation of stomatitis and cutaneous toxicity with clinical outcome in patients with metastatic renal-cell carcinoma treated with everolimus. Clin Genitourin Cancer. 2016;14(5):426–31 [c].

[38] Ji YD, Aboalela A, Villa A. Everolimus-associated stomatitis in a patient who had renal transplant. BMJ Case Rep. 2016; 2016:1–4 [A].

[39] Kurtzman DJ, Oulton J, Erickson C, et al. Everolimus-induced symmetrical drug-related intertriginous and flexural exanthema (SDRIFE). Dermatitis. 2016;27(2):76–7 [A].

[40] Flores-Gonzalez JC, Estalella-Mendoza A, Lechuga-Sancho AM, et al. Severe pneumonia by Mycoplasma as an adverse event of everolimus therapy in patients with tuberous sclerosis complex. Eur J Paediatr Neurol. 2016;20(5):758–60 [A].

[41] Enjeti AK, D'Crus A, Melville K, et al. A systematic evaluation of the safety and toxicity of fingolimod for its potential use in the treatment of acute myeloid leukaemia. Anticancer Drugs. 2016;27(6):560–8 [M].

[42] Frisell T, Forsberg L, Nordin N, et al. Comparative analysis of first-year fingolimod and natalizumab drug discontinuation among Swedish patients with multiple sclerosis. Mult Scler. 2016;22(1):85–93 [C].

[43] Voldsgaard A, Koch-Henriksen N, Magyari M, et al. Early safety and efficacy of fingolimod treatment in Denmark. Acta Neurol Scand. 2017;135(1):129–33 [C].

[44] Racca V, Di Rienzo M, Cavarretta R, et al. Fingolimod effects on left ventricular function in multiple sclerosis. Mult Scler. 2016;22(2):201–11 [c].

[45] Bianco A, Patanella AK, Nociti V, et al. Severe dyspnoea with alteration of the diffusion capacity of the lung associated with fingolimod treatment. Mult Scler Relat Disord. 2016;9:11–3 [A].

[46] Mandal P, Gupta A, Fusi-Rubiano W, et al. Fingolimod: therapeutic mechanisms and ocular adverse effects. Eye (Lond). 2017;31(2):232–40 [r].

[47] Walker S, Brew B. Kaposi sarcoma in a fingolimod-treated patient with multiple sclerosis. J Clin Neurosci. 2016;31: 217–8 [A].

[48] Ziemssen T, Calabrese P, Penner IK, et al. QualiCOP: real-world effectiveness, tolerability, and quality of life in patients with relapsing-remitting multiple sclerosis treated with glatiramer acetate, treatment-naïve patients, and previously treated patients. J Neurol. 2016;263(4):784–91 [C].

[49] Schippling S, O'Connor P, Knappertz V, et al. Incidence and course of depression in multiple sclerosis in the multinational BEYOND trial. J Neurol. 2016;263(7):1418–26 [C].

[50] Herbstritt S, Langer-Gould A, Rockhoff M, et al. Glatiramer acetate during early pregnancy: a prospective cohort study. Mult Scler. 2016;22(6):810–6 [C].

[51] Mendes D, Alves C, Batel-Marques F. Benefit-risk of therapies for relapsing-remitting multiple sclerosis: testing the number needed to treat to benefit (NNTB), number needed to treat to harm (NNTH) and the likelihood to be helped or harmed (LHH): a systematic review and meta-analysis. CNS Drugs. 2016;30(10):909–29 [M].

[52] Zagmutt F, Wu Y, Grinspan A, et al. Is severity of adverse events affected by the dose and frequency of glatiramer acetate treatment of relapsing-remitting multiple sclerosis? Neurology. 2016;86(16):177 [M].

[53] Flaire A, Carra-Dalliere C, Ayrignac X, et al. Glatiramer acetate-induced hepatitis in a patient with multiple sclerosis. Acta Neurol Belg. 2016;116(1):99–100 [A].

[54] Walker J, Smylie A, Smylie M. An association between glatiramer acetate and malignant melanoma. J Immunother. 2016;39(7): 276–8 [A].

[55] Mott SE, Pena ZG, Spain RI, et al. Nicolau syndrome and localized panniculitis: a report of dual diagnoses with an emphasis on morphea profunda-like changes following injection with glatiramer acetate. J Cutan Pathol. 2016;43(11):1056–61 [A].

[56] Sánchez-González MJ, Barbarroja-Escudero J, Antolín-Amérigo D, et al. Flare-up reaction in the inoculation drug sites by

glatiramer acetate: first case described. Allergol Int. 2016;65(4):469–71 [A].

[57] Dubey D, Cano CA, Stüve O. Update on monitoring and adverse effects of first generation disease modifying therapies and their recently approved versions in relapsing forms of multiple sclerosis. Curr Opin Neurol. 2016;29(3):272–7 [R].

[58] Winkelmann A, Loebermann M, Reisinger EC, et al. Disease-modifying therapies and infectious risks in multiple sclerosis. Nat Rev Neurol. 2016;12(4):217–33 [R].

[59] Adis Medical Writers. Reduce the risk of adverse events associated with disease-modifying therapies for multiple sclerosis by following appropriate mitigation strategies. Drugs Ther Perspect. 2016;32(5):197–202 [R].

[60] Negrei C, Bojinca V, Balanescu A, et al. Management of rheumatoid arthritis: impact and risks of various therapeutic approaches (Review). Exp Ther Med. 2016;11(4):1177–83 [R].

[61] Hugle B, Horneff G. The role of synthetic drugs in the biologic era: therapeutic strategies for treating juvenile idiopathic arthritis. Expert Opin Pharmacother. 2016;17(5):703–14 [R].

[62] Bester FCJ, Bosch FJ, Van Rensburg BJJ. The specialist physician's approach to rheumatoid arthritis in South Africa. Korean J Intern Med. 2016;31(2):219–36 [R].

[63] Walker UA. Immunomodulation of rheumatologic disorders with non-biologic disease modifying antirheumatic drugs. Semin Hematol. 2016;53:S58–60 [R].

[64] Gerosa M, Schioppo T, Meroni PL. Challenges and treatment options for rheumatoid arthritis during pregnancy. Expert Opin Pharmacother. 2016;17(11):1539–47 [R].

[65] Ngian GS, Briggs AM, Ackerman IN, et al. Safety of anti-rheumatic drugs for rheumatoid arthritis in pregnancy and lactation. Int J Rheum Dis. 2016;19(9):834–43 [R].

[66] Cassina M, Cagnoli GA, Zuccarello D, et al. Human teratogens and genetic phenocopies. Understanding pathogenesis through human genes mutation. Eur J Med Genet. 2017;60:22–31 [R].

[67] Biehl AJ, Katz JD. Pharmacotherapy pearls for the geriatrician: focus on oral disease-modifying antirheumatic drugs including newer agents. Clin Geriatr Med. 2017;33(1):1–15 [R].

[68] Li R, Zhao JX, Su Y, et al. High remission and low relapse with prolonged intensive DMARD therapy in rheumatoid arthritis (PRINT): a multicenter randomized clinical trial. Medicine (Baltimore). 2016;95(28):e3968 [C].

[69] Ren LM, Li R, Chen LN, et al. Efficacy and safety of weekly leflunomide for the treatment of early rheumatoid arthritis: a randomized, multi-center study. Int J Rheum Dis. 2016;19(7):651–7 [C].

[70] Chen P, Feng H, Deng J, et al. Leflunomide treatment in corticosteroid-dependent myasthenia gravis: an open-label pilot study. J Neurol. 2016;263(1):83–8 [c].

[71] Varela H, Villamanan E, Plasencia C, et al. Safety of antitumour necrosis factor treatments in chronic rheumatic diseases: therapy discontinuations related to side effects. J Clin Pharm Ther. 2016;41(3):306–9 [C].

[72] Hodkinson B, Magomero KR, Tikly M. Combination leflunomide and methotrexate in refractory rheumatoid arthritis: a biologic sparing approach. Ther Adv Musculoskelet Dis. 2016;8(5):172–9 [C].

[73] Nesselhauf N, Strutt J, Bastani B. Evaluation of leflunomide for the treatment of BK viremia and biopsy proven BK nephropathy; a single center experience. J Nephropathol. 2016;5(1):34–7 [c].

[74] Park YH, Lim JH, Yi HG, et al. BK virus-hemorrhagic cystitis following allogeneic stem cell transplantation: clinical characteristics and utility of leflunomide treatment. Turk J Haematol. 2016. http://dx.doi.org/10.4274/Tjh.2015.0131 [Epub ahead of print] [c].

[75] Wu J, Duan SW, Sun XF, et al. Efficacy of leflunomide, telmisartan, and clopidogrel for immunoglobulin A nephropathy: a randomized controlled trial. Chin Med J (Engl). 2016;129(16):1894–903 [C].

[76] Liu Y, Qu X, Chen W, et al. Efficacy of leflunomide combined with prednisone in the treatment of refractory nephrotic syndrome. Ren Fail. 2016;38:1616–21 [c].

[77] Liu Y, Xiao J, Shi X, et al. Immunosuppressive agents versus steroids in the treatment of IgA nephropathy-induced proteinuria: a meta-analysis. Exp Ther Med. 2016;11(1):49–56 [M].

[78] Conway R, Low C, Coughlan RJ, et al. Leflunomide use and risk of lung disease in rheumatoid arthritis: a systematic literature review and metaanalysis of randomized controlled trials. J Rheumatol. 2016;43(5):855–60 [M].

[79] Stine JG, Lewis JH. Current and future directions in the treatment and prevention of drug-induced liver injury: a systematic review. Expert Rev Gastroenterol Hepatol. 2016;10(4):517–36 [M].

[80] Hazlewood GS, Barnabe C, Tomlinson G, et al. Methotrexate monotherapy and methotrexate combination therapy with traditional and biologic disease modifying anti-rheumatic drugs for rheumatoid arthritis: a network meta-analysis. Cochrane Database Syst Rev. 2016;29(8):CD010227, [M].

[81] Feng Z, Xu J, He G, et al. The efficacy and safety of the combination of total glucosides of peony and leflunomide for the treatment of rheumatoid arthritis: a systemic review and meta-analysis. Evid Based Complement Alternat Med. 2016;2016:9852793 [M].

[82] Baldwin C, Avina-Zubieta A, Rai SK, et al. Disease modifying anti-rheumatic drug use in pregnant women with rheumatic diseases: a systematic review of the risk of congenital malformations. Clin Exp Rheumatol. 2016;34(2):172–83 [M].

[83] El Chaer F, Mori N, Shah D, et al. Adjuvant and salvage therapy with leflunomide for recalcitrant cytomegalovirus infections in hematopoietic cell transplantation recipients: a case series. Antiviral Res. 2016;135:91–6 [A].

[84] Keng LT, Lin MW, Huang HN, et al. Diffuse alveolar damage in a patient with rheumatoid arthritis under prolonged leflunomide treatment. Medicine (Baltimore). 2016;95(26):e4044 [A].

[85] Papiris SA, Manali ED, Kolilekas L, et al. Acute respiratory events in connective tissue disorders. Respiration. 2016;91(3):181–201 [R].

[86] Baker JF, Sauer BC, Cannon GW, et al. Changes in body mass related to the initiation of disease-modifying therapies in rheumatoid arthritis. Arthritis Rheumatol. 2016;68(8): 1818–27 [MC].

[87] Devarbhavi H, Raj S, Aradya VH, et al. Drug-induced liver injury associated with Stevens-Johnson syndrome/toxic epidermal necrolysis: patient characteristics, causes, and outcome in 36 cases. Hepatology. 2016;63(3):993–9 [c].

[88] James Tidwell WA, Malone J, Callen JP. Eruptive keratoacanthomas associated with leflunomide. JAMA Dermatol. 2016;152(1):105–6 [A].

[89] Singh H, Sukhija G, Tanwar V, et al. Rare occurrence of drug induced subacute cutaneous lupus erythematosus with leflunomide therapy. J Clin Diagn Res. 2016;10(10):OD06–7 [A].

[90] Drug-induced tendon damage. Prescrire Int. 2016;25(174):212–3 [R].

[91] Hopkins AM, Wiese MD, Proudman SM, et al. Genetic polymorphism of CYP1A2 but not total or free teriflunomide concentrations is associated with leflunomide cessation in rheumatoid arthritis. Br J Clin Pharmacol. 2016;81(1):113–23 [C].

[92] Tarnowski M, Paradowska-Gorycka A, Dabrowska-Zamojcin E, et al. The effect of gene polymorphisms on patient responses to rheumatoid arthritis therapy. Expert Opin Drug Metab Toxicol. 2016;12(1):41–55 [R].

[93] Cruz CM, Pereira S, Gandara J, et al. Efficacy and safety of monotherapy with mycophenolate mofetil in liver transplantation patients with nephrotoxicity. Transplant Proc. 2016;48(7):2341–3 [c].

[94] Hackl A, Cseprekal O, Gessner M, et al. Mycophenolate mofetil therapy in children with idiopathic nephrotic syndrome: does therapeutic drug monitoring make a difference? Ther Drug Monit. 2016;38(2):274–9 [c].

[95] Ham JY, Jung HY, Choi JY, et al. Usefulness of mycophenolic acid monitoring with PETINIA for prediction of adverse events in kidney transplant recipients. Scand J Clin Lab Invest. 2016;76(4):296–303 [c].

[96] Riedl M, Kuhn A, Kramer I, et al. Prospective, systematically recorded mycophenolate safety data in Graves' orbitopathy. J Endocrinol Invest. 2016;39(6):687–94 [c].

[97] Watanabe T, Seguchi O, Nishimura K, et al. Suppressive effects of conversion from mycophenolate mofetil to everolimus for the development of cardiac allograft vasculopathy in maintenance of heart transplant recipients. Int J Cardiol. 2016;203:307–14 [c].

[98] Arkin L, Talasila S, Paller AS. Mycophenolate mofetil and mood changes in children with skin disorders. Pediatr Dermatol. 2016;33(3):e216–7 [A].

[99] Goyal A, Salahuddin M, Govil Y. A unique case of mycophenolate induced colitis after 10 years of use. Case Rep Gastrointest Med. 2016;2016:3058407 [A].

[100] von Moos S, Cippa PE, Wuthrich RP, et al. Intestinal infection at onset of mycophenolic acid-associated chronic diarrhea in kidney transplant recipients. Transpl Infect Dis. 2016;18(5):721–9 [C].

[101] Smith M, Gonzalez-Estrada A, Fernandez J, et al. Desensitization to Mycofenolate Mofetil: a novel 12 step protocol. Eur Ann Allergy Clin Immunol. 2016;48(4):147–8 [A].

[102] Felix MJ, Felipe CR, Tedesco-Silva H, et al. Time-dependent and immunosuppressive drug-associated adverse event profiles in de novo kidney transplant recipients converted from tacrolimus to sirolimus regimens. Pharmacotherapy. 2016;36(2):152–65 [C].

[103] Adams DM, Trenor 3rd CC, Hammill AM, et al. Efficacy and safety of sirolimus in the treatment of complicated vascular anomalies. Pediatrics. 2016;137(2):e20153257 [c].

[104] Karakas NM, Erdogan I, Ozdemir B, et al. Pain syndrome and ventricular arrhythmia induced by sirolimus and resolved by dosage adjustment in a child after heart transplant: a case report. Exp Clin Transplant. 2016. http://dx.doi.org/10.6002/ect.2015.0320 [Epub ahead of print] [A].

[105] Sebaaly J, Bowers L, Mazur J, et al. Rapid oral desensitization to sirolimus in a patient with lymphangioleiomyomatosis. J Allergy Clin Immunol Pract. 2016;4(2):352–3 [A].

[106] Zegarska J, Hryniewiecka E, Zochowska D, et al. Tacrolimus metabolite M-III may have nephrotoxic and myelotoxic effects and increase the incidence of infections in kidney transplant recipients. Transplant Proc. 2016;48(5):1539–42 [c].

[107] Cruzado JM, Pascual J, Sanchez-Fructuoso A, et al. Controlled randomized study comparing the cardiovascular profile of everolimus with tacrolimus in renal transplantation. Transpl Int. 2016;29(12):1317–28 [C].

[108] Song T, Rao Z, Tan Q, et al. Calcineurin inhibitors associated posterior reversible encephalopathy syndrome in solid organ transplantation: report of 2 cases and literature review. Medicine (Baltimore). 2016;95(14)e3173 [A].

[109] Sato K, Kobayashi Y, Nakamura A, et al. Early post-transplant hyperbilirubinemia is a possible predictive factor for developing neurological complications in pediatric living donor liver transplant patients receiving tacrolimus. Pediatr Transplant. 2017;21:e12843 [c].

[110] Gupta AK, Bahri N. Isolated diplopia associated with calcineurin inhibitor therapy in a patient with idiopathic membranous nephropathy: a case report. BMC Nephrol. 2016;17(1):116 [A].

[111] Arai K, Kuramitsu K, Fukumoto T, et al. A case report of drug-induced thrombocytopenia after living donor liver transplantation. Kobe J Med Sci. 2016;62(1):E9–E12 [A].

[112] Sugitani A, Takahashi C, Naka T, et al. Unusual case of tacrolimus vascular toxicity after deceased donor renal transplantation. Nephrology (Carlton). 2016;21(Suppl 1):60–2 [A].

[113] Asada A, Bamba S, Morita Y, et al. The effect of CYP3A5 genetic polymorphisms on adverse events in patients with ulcerative colitis treated with tacrolimus. Dig Liver Dis. 2017;49(1):24–8 [c].

[114] Wang ZP, Zhao M, Qu QS, et al. Effect of pregnane X receptor polymorphisms on tacrolimus blood concentrations and the resulting adverse reactions in kidney transplantation recipients. Genet Mol Res. 2016;15(3) gmr.15038464 [C].

[115] Wu Z, Xu Q, Qiu X, et al. FOXP3 rs3761548 polymorphism is associated with tacrolimus-induced acute nephrotoxicity in renal transplant patients. Eur J Clin Pharmacol. 2017;73(1):39–47 [C].

[116] Kim JM, Kwon CH, Joh JW, et al. Conversion of once-daily extended-release tacrolimus is safe in stable liver transplant recipients: a randomized prospective study. Liver Transpl. 2016;22(2):209–16 [c].

[117] Ruangkanchanasetr P, Sanohdontree N, Supaporn T, et al. Beta cell function and insulin resistance after conversion from Tacrolimus twice-daily to extended-release Tacrolimus once-daily in stable renal transplant recipients. Ann Transplant. 2016;21:765–74 [c].

[118] El-Asmar J, Gonzalez R, Bookout R, et al. Clotrimazole troches induce supratherapeutic blood levels of sirolimus and tacrolimus in an allogeneic hematopoietic cell-transplant recipient resulting in acute kidney injury. Hematol Oncol Stem Cell Ther. 2016;9(4):157–61 [A].

[119] Han Z, Kane BM, Petty LA, et al. Cobicistat significantly increases tacrolimus serum concentrations in a renal transplant recipient with human immunodeficiency virus infection. Pharmacotherapy. 2016;36(6):e50–3 [A].

[120] Hauser N, Sahai T, Richards R, et al. High on cannabis and calcineurin inhibitors: a word of warning in an era of legalized marijuana. Case Rep Transplant. 2016;2016:4028492 [A].

[121] Lin T, Leung C, Nguyen KT, et al. Mammalian target of rapamycin (mTOR) inhibitors in solid tumours. Clin Pharm. 2016;8(3). http://dx.doi.org/10.1211/CP.2016.20200813 [R].

[122] Studentova H, Vitaskova D, Melichar B. Safety of mTOR inhibitors in breast cancer. Expert Opin Drug Saf. 2016;15(8):1075–85 [R].

[123] Emons G, Kurzeder C, Schmalfeldt B, et al. Temsirolimus in women with platinum-refractory/resistant ovarian cancer or advanced/recurrent endometrial carcinoma. A phase II study of the AGO-study group (AGO-GYN8). Gynecol Oncol. 2016;140(3):450–6 [c].

[124] Mahoney KM, Jacobus S, Bhatt RS, et al. Phase 2 study of bevacizumab and temsirolimus after VEGFR TKI in metastatic renal cell carcinoma. Clin Genitourin Cancer. 2016;14(4):304–13. e6 [c].

[125] Korfel A, Schlegel U, Herrlinger U, et al. Phase II trial of temsirolimus for relapsed/refractory primary CNS lymphoma. J Clin Oncol. 2016;34(15):1757–63 [c].

[126] Santacana M, Coronado P, Matias-Guiu X, et al. Biological effects of temsirolimus on the mTOR pathway in endometrial carcinoma: a pharmacodynamic phase II study. Int J Gynecol Cancer. 2016. http://dx.doi.org/10.1097/IGC.0000000000000715 [Epub ahead of print] [c].

[127] Wermke M, Schuster C, Nolte F, et al. Mammalian-target of rapamycin inhibition with temsirolimus in myelodysplastic syndromes (MDS) patients is associated with considerable toxicity: results of the temsirolimus pilot trial by the German MDS Study Group (D-MDS). Br J Haematol. 2016;175(5):917–24 [c].

[128] Chiu JW, Hotte SJ, Kollmannsberger CK, et al. A phase I trial of ANG1/2-Tie2 inhibitor trebaninib (AMG386) and temsirolimus in advanced solid tumors (PJC008/NCImusical sharp9041). Invest New Drugs. 2016;34(1):104–11 [c].

[129] Waqar SN, Baggstrom MQ, Morgensztern D, et al. A phase I trial of temsirolimus and pemetrexed in patients with advanced non-small cell lung cancer. Chemotherapy. 2016;61(3):144–7 [c].

[130] Liu X, Kambrick S, Fu S, et al. Advanced malignancies treated with a combination of the VEGF inhibitor bevacizumab, anti-EGFR antibody cetuximab, and the mTOR inhibitor temsirolimus. Oncotarget. 2016;7(17):23227–38 [c].

[131] Khawaja MR, Nick AM, Madhusudanannair V, et al. Phase I dose escalation study of temsirolimus in combination with metformin in patients with advanced/refractory cancers. Cancer Chemother Pharmacol. 2016;77(5):973–7 [c].

[132] Kim KH, Kim JH, Lee JY, et al. Efficacy and toxicity of mammalian target rapamycin inhibitors in patients with metastatic renal cell carcinoma with renal insufficiency: the Korean cancer study group GU 14-08. Cancer Res Treat. 2016;48(4):1286–92 [c].

[133] Langrand-Escure J, Vallard A, Rivoirard R, et al. Safety assessment of molecular targeted therapies in association with radiotherapy in metastatic renal cell carcinoma: a real-life report. Anticancer Drugs. 2016;27(5):427–32 [c].

[134] Wick W, Gorlia T, Bady P, et al. Phase II study of radiotherapy and temsirolimus versus radiochemotherapy with temozolomide in patients with newly diagnosed glioblastoma without MGMT promoter hypermethylation (EORTC 26082). Clin Cancer Res. 2016;22(19):4797–806 [C].

[135] Chang X, Zhang F, Liu T, et al. Comparative efficacy and safety of first-line treatments in patients with metastatic renal cell cancer: a network meta-analysis based on phase 3 RCTs. Oncotarget. 2016;7(13):15801–10 [M].

[136] Lew S, Chamberlain RS. Risk of metabolic complications in patients with solid tumors treated with mTOR inhibitors: meta-analysis. Anticancer Res. 2016;36(4):1711–8 [M].

[137] Zhang X, Ran YG, Wang KJ. Risk of mTOR inhibitors induced severe pneumonitis in cancer patients: a meta-analysis of randomized controlled trials. Future Oncol. 2016;12(12):1529–39 [M].

[138] Willemsen AECAB, Grutters JC, Gerritsen WR, et al. MTOR inhibitor-induced interstitial lung disease in cancer patients: comprehensive review and a practical management algorithm. Int J Cancer. 2016;138(10):2312–21 [R].

[139] Zhang X, Hamadeh IS, Song S, et al. Osteonecrosis of the jaw in the United States food and drug administration's adverse event reporting system (FAERS). J Bone Miner Res. 2016;31(2):336–40 [MC].

[140] Omae K, Kondo T, Takagi T, et al. Use of mammalian target of rapamycin inhibitors after failure of tyrosine kinase inhibitors in patients with metastatic renal cell carcinoma undergoing hemodialysis: a single-center experience with four cases. Hemodial Int. 2016;20(3):E1–5 [c].

[141] Peterson DE, O'Shaughnessy JA, Rugo HS, et al. Oral mucosal injury caused by mammalian target of rapamycin inhibitors: emerging perspectives on pathobiology and impact on clinical practice. Cancer Med. 2016;5(8):1897–907 [R].

[142] Lee KWC, Chan SL. Hepatotoxicity of targeted therapy for cancer. Expert Opin Drug Metab Toxicol. 2016;12(7):789–802 [R].

[143] Luan ZJ, Li Y, Zhao XY, et al. Treatment efficacy and safety of low-dose azathioprine in chronic active ulcerative colitis patients: a meta-analysis and systemic review. J Dig Dis. 2016;17(10):652–9 [M].

[144] Jack KL, Koopman WJ, Hulley D, et al. A review of Azathioprine-associated hepatotoxicity and myelosuppression in Myasthenia Gravis. J Clin Neuromuscul Dis. 2016;18(1):12–20 [C].

[145] Latushko A, Ghazi LJ. A case of thiopurine-induced acute myocarditis in a patient with ulcerative colitis. Dig Dis Sci. 2016;61(12):3633–4 [A].

[146] Teich N, Mohl W, Bokemeyer B, et al. Azathioprine-induced acute pancreatitis in patients with inflammatory bowel diseases—a prospective study on incidence and severity. J Crohns Colitis. 2016;10(1):61–8 [C].

[147] Kamath N, Pai CG, Deltombe T. Pure red cell aplasia due to azathioprine therapy for Crohn's disease. Indian J Pharmacol. 2016;48(1):86–7 [A].

[148] Ramos-Rodriguez C, Murillo-Lazaro C, Mendoza-Chaparro C. "Eruptive Lentiginosis" in a patient with vitiligo and inflammatory bowel disease treated with azathioprine. Am J Dermatopathol. 2016;38(2):135–7 [A].

[149] Norgard BM, Magnussen B, Larsen MD, et al. Reassuring results on birth outcomes in children fathered by men treated with azathioprine/6-mercaptopurine within 3 months before conception: a nationwide cohort study. Gut. 2016. http://dx.doi.org/10.1136/gutjnl-2016-312123 [C].

[150] Abdelaziz DH, Elhosseiny NM, Khaleel SA, et al. Association between combined presence of hepatitis C virus and polymorphisms in different genes with toxicities of methotrexate and 6-mercaptopurine in children with acute lymphoblastic leukemia. Pediatr Blood Cancer. 2016;63(9):1539–45 [C].

[151] Al-Judaibi B, Schwarz UI, Huda N, et al. Genetic predictors of azathioprine toxicity and clinical response in patients with inflammatory bowel disease. J Popul Ther Clin Pharmacol. 2016;23(1):e26–36 [c].

[152] Benmassaoud A, Xie X, AlYafi M, et al. Thiopurines in the management of Crohn's disease: safety and efficacy profile in patients with normal TPMT activity-A retrospective study. Can J Gastroenterol Hepatol. 2016;2016:1034834 [C].

[153] Kim HS, Cheon JH, Jung ES, et al. A coding variant in FTO confers susceptibility to thiopurine-induced leukopenia in East Asian patients with IBD. Gut. 2016. http://dx.doi.org/10.1136/gutjnl-2016-311921 [C].

[154] Smid A, Karas-Kuzelicki N, Jazbec J, et al. PACSIN2 polymorphism is associated with thiopurine-induced hematological toxicity in children with acute lymphoblastic leukaemia undergoing maintenance therapy. Sci Rep. 2016;6:30244 [C].

[155] Steponaitiene R, Kupcinskas J, Survilaite S, et al. TPMT and ITPA genetic variants in Lithuanian inflammatory bowel disease patients: prevalence and azathioprine-related side effects. Adv Med Sci. 2016;61(1):135–40 [c].

[156] Wong DR, Coenen MJ, Vermeulen SH, et al. Early assessment of thiopurine metabolites identifies patients at risk of thiopurine-induced leukopenia in inflammatory bowel disease. J Crohns Colitis. 2016;11:175–84 [C].

[157] Moriyama T, Nishii R, Perez-Andreu V, et al. NUDT15 polymorphisms alter thiopurine metabolism and hematopoietic toxicity. Nat Genet. 2016;48(4):367–73 [C].

[158] Ailing Z, Jing Y, Jingli L, et al. Further evidence that a variant of the gene NUDT15 may be an important predictor of azathioprine-induced toxicity in Chinese subjects: a case report. J Clin Pharm Ther. 2016;41(5):572–4 [A].

[159] Kakuta Y, Naito T, Onodera M, et al. NUDT15 R139C causes thiopurine-induced early severe hair loss and leukopenia in Japanese patients with IBD. Pharmacogenomics J. 2016;16(3):280–5 [C].

[160] Lee YJ, Hwang EH, Park JH, et al. NUDT15 variant is the most common variant associated with thiopurine-induced early leukopenia and alopecia in Korean pediatric patients with Crohn's disease. Eur J Gastroenterol Hepatol. 2016;28(4):475–8 [c].

[161] Shah SA, Paradkar M, Desai D, et al. Nudt15 C415t variant as a predictor for thiopurine induced toxicity in Indian patients. J Gastroenterol Hepatol. 2017;32(3):620–4 [c].

[162] Zgheib NK, Akika R, Mahfouz R, et al. NUDT15 and TPMT genetic polymorphisms are related to 6-mercaptopurine intolerance in children treated for acute lymphoblastic leukemia at the Children's Cancer Center of Lebanon. Pediatr Blood Cancer. 2017;64(1):146–50 [C].

[163] Zhu X, Wang XD, Chao K, et al. NUDT15 polymorphisms are better than thiopurine S-methyltransferase as predictor of risk for

thiopurine-induced leukopenia in Chinese patients with Crohn's disease. Aliment Pharmacol Ther. 2016;44(9):967–75 [C].

[164] Kuzma-Mroczkowska E, Skrzypczyk P, Panczyk-Tomaszewska M. Levamisole therapy in children with frequently relapsing and steroid-dependent nephrotic syndrome: a single-center experience. Cent Eur J Immunol. 2016;41(3):243–7 [c].

[165] Abeyagunawardena A, Dharmawardena H, Jayaweera H, et al. Safety profile of long-termlevamisole therapy in maintaining remission in steroid dependent nephrotic syndrome. Pediatr Nephrol. 2016;31(10):1849 [C].

[166] Moinuddin I, Madhrira M, Bracamonte E, et al. Membranous nephropathy with crescents associated with levamisole-induced MPO-ANCA vasculitis. Pathol Res Pract. 2016;212(7):650–3 [A].

[167] Veronese FV, Dode RS, Friderichs M, et al. Cocaine/levamisole-induced systemic vasculitis with retiform purpura and pauci-immune glomerulonephritis. Braz J Med Biol Res. 2016;49(5): e5244 [A].

[168] Liu YW, Mutnuri S, Siddiqui SB, et al. Levamisole-adulterated cocaine nephrotoxicity: ultrastructural features. Am J Clin Pathol. 2016;145(5):720–6 [A].

[169] Munoz CH, Vanegas AL, Arbelaez A, et al. Cocaine-levamisole induced vasculitis: a series of 11 cases. Ann Rheum Dis. 2016;75:567 [A].

[170] Brajkovic G, Babic G, Stosic JJ, et al. Fatal cocaine intoxication in a body packer. Vojnosanit Pregl. 2016;73(2):198–201 [A].

[171] Gruppen M, Davin JC, Bouts A. Levamisole increases the time to relapse in children with steroid-sensitive idiopathic nephrotic syndrome: results of a multi-center, double-blind, placebo-controlled, randomized clinical trial. Pediatr Nephrol. 2016;31(10):1753 [C].

34

Corticotrophins, Corticosteroids, and Prostaglandins

Justin B. Kaplan*[†,1], Alison Brophy[‡]

*Rutgers, The State University of New Jersey, Piscataway, NJ, United States
[†]Hackensack University Medical Center, Hackensack, NJ, United States
[‡]Overlook Medical Center, Summit, NJ, United States
[1]Corresponding author: jbkaplan@pharmacy.rutgers.edu

CORTICOTROPHINS [SED-15, 906; SEDA-33, 841; SEDA-34, 653; SEDA-35, 719; SEDA-36, 603; SEDA-37,491; SEDA-38, 425]

Adrenocorticotropic hormone (ACTH) has been studied as a therapeutic option for treatment of infantile spasms in children, nephrotic syndrome, and several other rheumatic and dermatologic disorders [1M,2A,3c,4A].

Cardiovascular: A meta-analysis of 19 studies reviewing ACTH for the treatment of various glomerular diseases was performed. In the 12 studies that assessed tolerability, 7% of patients dropped out secondary to side effects. The most commonly reported adverse event was edema followed by insomnia, mood swings, and hyperglycemia [1M].

Nervous System: A 4-month-old infant girl diagnosed with infantile spasms was treated with vigabatrin for 1.5 months and then switched to intramuscular ACTH 3 IU/kg every other day. After 7 ACTH administrations, she developed dyskinetic movements such as arm elevations and tongue protrusion. There was no epileptic activity that correlated with the movements on video electroencephalography. The drug was immediately discontinued and symptoms abated over the next 2 months [2A].

Drug Tolerability: A randomized open-label crossover study of 18 healthy patients compared tolerability of porcine ACTH analogue 80 units subcutaneously daily to methylprednisolone 1000 mg IV daily for 5 days. After a 30-day washout period, the groups switched treatments. There were no major adverse events in the study. During ACTH administration, two patients reported a mild rash and one patient reported nausea. Rates of these adverse events were lower than the rates reported in the methylprednisolone group [3c]. In a different case report, a Japanese girl diagnosed with West Syndrome associated with tuberous sclerosis complex was treated with a course of ACTH 0.005 mg/kg IM daily for 2 weeks at 4 months and 8 months old. Epileptic spasms and hypsarrhythmia returned following the completion of each course. Due to the refractory nature, she was treated again at age 1 year with a third course of ACTH at a dose of 0.01 mg/kg IM daily for 2 weeks followed by weekly administration of the same dose through the age of 2 years and 10 months. Emergence of symptoms only occurred when the dose was reduced and therapy discontinued. No adverse events were associated with long-term weekly administration of ACTH [4A].

SYSTEMIC GLUCOCORTICOIDS [SED-15, 906; SEDA-33, 841; SEDA-34, 653; SEDA-35, 719; SEDA-36, 604; SEDA-37,492; SEDA-38, 425]

Systemic glucocorticoid therapy has been utilized for decades in the management of acute and chronic inflammatory and autoimmune conditions. The decision to prescribe corticosteroids must include a thorough evaluation of the associated risks. A recent editorial reviewing the use of systemic glucocorticoids for severe asthma highlighted common adverse effects including gastrointestinal disorders, hypertension, dyslipidemia, weight gain, hyperglycemia and diabetes mellitus, reduced bone density, as well as psychiatric and sleep disorders. The risk of developing adverse effects may depend on a host of different factors including dose, duration of therapy, age, and gender [5r]. While the risk is likely multifactorial, data suggest that even short courses of systemic glucocorticoid therapy such as 13-hour premedication regimens for patients with allergies to iodinated intravenous contrast media may be associated with increased risk of infection, longer hospital length of stay, and greater healthcare costs [6c]. For these reasons, a thorough risk-benefit analysis should be performed prior to initiating any systemic corticosteroid therapy.

Systematic Review: Six systematic reviews related to systemic corticosteroids were published by the Cochrane Library in 2016. Bell's Palsy patients treated with corticosteroids were less likely to have incomplete recovery of facial motor function 6 months or later compared to placebo (RR 0.63, 0.5–0.8, NNT = 10). There were no significant differences in rate of adverse effects [7M]. In two studies of 179 patients with leprosy-related nerve damage, prednisolone did not show a benefit compared to placebo in terms of improvement of nerve function at 12 months. There were no differences in reported adverse effects in those two studies. In a third study comparing different doses of prednisone, two major adverse effects were reported in the high-dose prednisone group with one patient who developed cataracts and another who had osteoporosis leading to collapse of the 10th dorsal vertebra [8M]. In a systematic review of nine studies that included 1337 patients with tuberculosis meningitis, addition of corticosteroids to standard anti-tuberculosis treatment was associated with reduced mortality compared to standard anti-tuberculosis treatment alone (RR 0.75, 0.65–0.87). There were no significant differences in incidence of adverse effects between patients who received steroids and those who did not [9M]. An analysis of several trials in Duchenne's muscular dystrophy patients suggested that prednisone or prednisolone 0.75 mg/kg/day for at least 3 months improved functional outcomes including timed walking test, stair climb, weight lifting strength, and others. Higher doses of steroids did not appear to provide incremental benefit. Adverse effects observed in the 12 studies of 667 patients included weight gain, Cushingoid appearance, hirsutism, and changes in behavior. The data suggest that hair growth and Cushingoid appearance may be dose-dependent and more common with a prednisone dose of 0.75 mg/kg/day compared to 0.3 mg/kg/day [10M]. A systematic review of 18 studies including 2438 adult and pediatric patients evaluated various oral corticosteroid regimens used for acute asthma exacerbations. Due to the heterogeneity in the patient population, drug, dosing regimen, and duration of treatment, the review was unable to identify a specific drug, dose, or duration that would optimize treatment efficacy and minimize

glucocorticoid-related adverse effects [11M]. A Cochrane review of eight trials (474 patients) assessed studies of chronic rhinosinusitis patients who received either 2 or 3 weeks of oral corticosteroids or placebo. Compared to placebo, patients who received glucocorticoids had improved health-related quality of life and disease severity. However, corticosteroids were associated with increased gastrointestinal adverse events (RR 3.45, 1.11–10.78) and insomnia (RR 3.63, 1.10–11.95) [12M].

Special Review: The Surviving Sepsis Campaign Guidelines for the Management of Severe Sepsis and Septic Shock suggest that hydrocortisone 200 mg/day be considered only for patients in septic shock who remain hemodynamically unstable despite adequate fluid resuscitation and vasopressor therapy [13R]. The role of corticosteroids in preventing the development of septic shock remains unknown. Published this year, the Hydrocortisone for Prevention of Septic Shock (HYPRESS) trial randomized 353 patients with severe sepsis to receive hydrocortisone 200 mg/day by continuous infusion or placebo. Hydrocortisone did not prevent the development of septic shock within 14 days (21.2% hydrocortisone vs 22.9% placebo, P = 0.7). There were no statistically significant differences in mortality at 28, 90, or 180 days. In the hydrocortisone group, there was more hyperglycemia compared to placebo (90.9% vs 81.5%, P = 0.009), although the difference in maximum glucose concentrations was likely not clinically significant. There were trends towards more secondary infections and muscle weakness with hydrocortisone, but these findings were not statistically significant [14C].

Cardiovascular: A study compared weight-based vs body surface area (BSA)-based prednisolone dosing in 100 children with idiopathic nephrotic syndrome. Patients in the BSA-based group received higher prednisolone doses and had a greater incidence of hypertension (P = 0.048) [15C]. A retrospective study of 220 consecutive patients who underwent transfemoral aortic valve implantation (TAVI) aimed to determine if steroids would influence the rate of vascular complications. After multivariate modelling, patients who were on steroids at the time of the TAVI procedure (n = 25) were more likely to have minor vascular complications based on VARC2 criteria (HR 2.65, 1.04–6.8, P = 0.042) including higher rates of femoral artery occlusion or stenosis and the need for more recanalization procedures [16c]. A study retrospectively analysed 200 patients undergoing a first-time elective CABG procedure who received a single dose of methylprednisolone 1 mg/kg intra-operatively or placebo. No serious steroid-related adverse events were reported and the risk of developing post-pericardiotomy syndrome was lower in the methylprednisolone group (OR 0.8, 0.25–0.91, P < 0.026) [17c]. A 39-year-old woman treated with corticosteroids for optic neuritis for 4 days (hydrocortisone 150 mg IV × 3 days, prednisone 60 mg orally × 1 day) experienced spontaneous coronary artery dissection (SCAD) of her left circumflex artery. The timing correlated with initiation of steroids. She had negative screening tests for antinuclear antibodies and genes associated with connective tissue disorders, and other common causes of SCAD were ruled out [18A].

Nervous System: Premature low birth-weight neonates receiving hydrocortisone within 36 hours of birth for 10 days to prevent bronchopulmonary dysplasia showed impaired neurodevelopment compared to infants receiving placebo. At pre-school age, the hydrocortisone group had lower performance IQ (88.3 vs 99.1, $P = 0.034$) and more children required physiotherapy (4 vs 0, $P = 0.034$) [19c]. A retrospective study revealed a higher rate of delayed CSF leak in pediatric patients in which Gelfoam soaked with 40 mg of triamcinolone acetonide injection was applied to the dura during lumbar decompression surgery (24% vs 0%, $P = 0.049$). In particular, 10/14 patients receiving triamcinolone for multilevel laminectomy developed CSF leaks compared to 0/10 who were not exposed to triamcinolone ($P < 0.001$) [20c].

Psychiatric: A prospective multicenter study of 685 patients with chronic rhinosinusitis (CRS) revealed that patients with CRS-related depression were more likely to have received oral corticosteroids within the past 90 days compared to patients without CRS-related depression [21c]. Children with idiopathic nephritis treated with oral prednisone 60 mg/m^2/day or 2 mg/kg/day for 6 weeks demonstrated significant behavioral changes based on the Child Behavior Checklist. Of 45 children (30 aged 2–5 years, 15 aged 6–14 years), 73% of the younger group and 60% of the older group demonstrated attention deficits and/or aggressive behavior which typically continued throughout the tapering period to 12 weeks [22c]. A review evaluating the link between different medication classes and suicide risk included two studies and one case series related to corticosteroids. The data were mixed and no definitive conclusion could be made regarding the use of corticosteroid and likelihood of attempting or committing suicide [23M].

Endocrine: A large multicenter trial randomized 2827 pregnant women at gestational age 34 to 36 weeks with a high likelihood to deliver in the late preterm period (up to 36 weeks and 6 days) to receive two doses of intramuscular betamethasone 12 mg or placebo at an interval of 24 hours apart. After birth, more neonates randomized to mothers who received betamethasone experienced hypoglycemia compared to those who received placebo (24% vs 15%, RR 1.60, 1.37–1.87, $P < 0.001$). Despite this finding, betamethasone was associated with a significant reduction in the primary composite outcome of early need for respiratory support within 72 hours of birth, stillbirth, or neonatal death within 72 hours. It also reduced the incidence of bronchopulmonary dysplasia, need for resuscitation at birth, and the need for surfactant administration. The authors concluded that the benefit of antenatal betamethasone in this population outweighed

the risks [24MC]. A prospective study of 16 healthy adult males demonstrated that dexamethasone administration at 2 mg/day for 2 days increased insulin resistance in hepatocytes and peripheral tissues and increased fat oxidation compared to placebo. When studied in combination with fish oil supplementation at 1.5 g by mouth daily for 3 weeks, it was found that fish oil augmented the effects of dexamethasone. Patients randomized to receive fish oil had further increases in insulin resistance, fat oxidation, and lipolysis. Authors hypothesized that worsening insulin sensitivity could be due to fish oil and dexamethasone additive effects on PI3K activity in the liver and muscle, but definite causality could not be determined [25c]. In a retrospective study of 118 patients treated for autoimmune hepatitis in Japan, a multivariate regression analysis showed that new onset diabetes was associated with corticosteroid use (OR 6.693, 1.391–32.210, $P = 0.049$). However, there was no difference in 10-year survival for patients who developed diabetes compared to those who did not [26c]. A prospective study of 58 children aged 2–20 years old who received ≥ 6 months of orally administered fluticasone propionate or budesonide for eosinophilic esophagitis revealed that despite low oral bioavailability, an abnormal ACTH stimulation test (peak cortisol ≤ 20 mcg/dL) occurred in 15% and biochemical adrenal insufficiency occurred in 10% of patients. All patients who had abnormal ACTH stimulation tests were receiving fluticasone propionate orally at doses greater than 440 mcg/day. No patients on oral budesonide had abnormal ACTH stimulation tests. Therefore the choice of glucocorticoid and dose used for eosinophilic esophagitis may both be factors in development of adrenal insufficiency [27c].

Metabolic: Ninety two patients with acute-stage allergic bronchopulmonary aspergillosis (ABPA) were randomized to receive medium-dose prednisolone (0.5 mg/kg/day for 2 weeks, then 0.5 mg/kg every other day for 8 weeks, then tapered to discontinuation by 3–5 months) or high-dose prednisolone (0.75 mg/kg/day for 6 weeks, then 0.5 mg/kg/day for 6 weeks, then tapered to discontinuation by 8–10 months). There were no differences in exacerbation rates or glucocorticoid-dependent ABPA, but patients in the high-dose prednisolone group experienced significantly more corticosteroid-related adverse effects including cushingoid habitus (79.6% vs 29.2%, $P = 0.0001$) and weight gain greater than 10% of baseline (54.6% vs 16.7%, $P = 0.0001$) [28c]. A prospective observational study of 15 patients with epileptic encephalopathy with continuous spike-and-wave during sleep patterns refractory to at least two antiepileptic drugs and prednisone were treated with dexamethasone 0.15 mg/kg/day for 4 weeks. The seven patients who were initial responders were continued and tapered for a total of 6–10 months of therapy. At 6 months, 7/7 had increased appetite and weight gain and 5/7 had Cushing syndrome.

Other adverse effects included behavioral changes, oral candidiasis, hypertension, and growth suppression [29c]. Similarly, a study of children with idiopathic nephrotic syndrome receiving 6 months of glucocorticoid therapy had a significant increase in BMI compared to healthy controls [30c].

Hematologic: A nested case–control study of adults with a primary diagnosis of pulmonary embolism (PE) who were prescribed vitamin K antagonists for treatment from 1998 to 2008 was performed. Three hundred eighty four patients with recurrent PE based on ICD-9 coding were matched to 1030 patients without recurrent PE. After logistic regression, oral corticosteroid use was associated with development of recurrent PE ($P = 0.02$). It was noted that current active use of corticosteroids increased the risk of recurrent PE (OR 3.74, 2.04–6.87) whereas previous corticosteroid use was actually associated with lower risk of PE (OR 0.46, 0.28–0.74). Causality could not be definitively determined due to the fact that underlying disease states necessitating the use of corticosteroids are often prothrombotic themselves and that flare-ups may lead to hospital admission and other risk factors for venous thromboembolism [31C].

Gastrointestinal: An open-label study analysed 113 patients with acute gouty arthritis randomized to receive either prednisolone 35 mg daily, etoricoxib 120 mg daily, or indomethacin 50 mg three times daily for 4 days. All three treatments yielded similar efficacy in reducing pain, tenderness, and increasing joint activity. Only 2/33 patients in the prednisolone group reported adverse effects, both of which were gastric or abdominal pain. The proportion of patients reporting adverse effects in the prednisolone group (6.1%) was similar to the etoricoxib group (6.8%) but significantly lower than the indomethacin group (30.6%) [32C]. A systematic review of short course ($\leq$14 days) oral corticosteroids in children aged 28 days to 18 years included 38 articles. The most common adverse effect was vomiting in 5.4% of patients followed by behavioral disturbances (4.7%), sleep disturbances (4.3%), nausea (1.9%), increased appetite (1.7%), and abdominal pain (1.3%) [33M]. A systematic review aimed at identifying predictors of acute diverticulitis found that corticosteroids were associated with more severe diverticular disease. However, causality cannot be assigned since this association may be attributed to the fact that patients with more severe disease were more likely to require steroids for management [34M]. In a meta-analysis of methylprednisolone for acute spinal cord injury, nine observational studies totalling 2857 patients identified a signal towards increased gastrointestinal bleeding (RR 2.18, 1.13–4.19, $P = 0.02$). However, there was concern about bias in the studies and data from the four included randomized trials did not support these findings [35M]. Similarly, a systematic review of corticosteroids for community acquired pneumonia found no

association between glucocorticoid therapy and gastrointestinal bleeding or any other significant increase in adverse effects [36M].

Liver: A 23-year-old woman with relapsing–remitting multiple sclerosis (MS) received methylprednisolone 1 g IV daily for 3 days for an MS relapse. At the time, her liver enzymes and bilirubin were normal. Three weeks later, she presented to a hepatology clinic with jaundice, abdominal pain, and elevated liver enzymes (AST 1515 U/L, ALT 2011 U/L, alkaline phosphatase 148 U/L, GGT 121 U/L, total bilirubin 117.1 micromoles/L). Viral and serological testing for other possible causes of liver injury were negative. Liver biopsy showed inflammation, hepatocyte congestion, and histology was consistent with drug-induced liver injury. The Roussel Uclaf causality assessment model was performed and suggested high probability of drug-induced liver injury. The hepatotoxicity resolved spontaneously with time. The patient had a similar event 9 months prior when she had received the same high-dose regimen of methylprednisolone for MS flare [37A].

Skin: A multicenter study of 376 patients presenting to the emergency department with acute gout randomized patients to receive either prednisolone (30 mg by mouth daily for 2 days, then 30 mg daily for 3 days) or indomethacin (50 mg by mouth three times daily for 2 days, then 25 mg three times daily for 3 days). In the first 2 hours of treatment, adverse effects were reported in 19% of patients in the indomethacin group and 6% in the prednisolone group ($P < 0.001$). Over the 14-day study period, patients in both groups reported a similar incidence of adverse events (37% vs 37%, $P = 1.0$). The only adverse effect that occurred more frequently in the prednisolone group was development of a skin rash (5.3% vs 1.0%, $P = 0.011$). No major adverse effects were reported in the study [38C]. A letter to the editor of British Journal of Dermatology reviewed the results of the Tight Control of Psoriatic Arthritis Trial. Given that corticosteroids are often used for psoriasis flares, the authors raised the point that intramuscular or intra-articular steroids may induce generalized pustular psoriasis or tapering of steroids may result in a rebound flare. In 101 patients who received 307 administrations of intra-articular or intramuscular steroid injections, there were no flares noted and no overall change in psoriasis severity after steroid use [39r].

Musculoskeletal: A prospective observational study of 200 patients with multifocal corticosteroid-related osteonecrosis followed patients annually for a minimum of 10 years. In total, 17.5% of patients developed new osteonecrotic lesions at the contralateral site and asymptomatic lesions became symptomatic requiring 258 total arthroplasty procedures by the end of the study. Continuation of peak doses of methylprednisolone >200 mg or equivalent steroid was associated with development of new lesions [40C]. In another study of patients over

40 years old, 516 patients who received prednisone ≥5 mg daily or equivalent for at least 3 months were matched to 1104 control subjects. Overall, no significant differences in areal bone mineral density (aBMD) were found between the groups, yet patients who received steroids scored lower on the Trabecular Bone Score (1.267 vs 1.298, $P < 0.001$). The authors concluded that these findings suggest that glucocorticoids impact bone microarchitecture and that aBMD may not be the best marker of fracture risk for patients taking corticosteroids [41C]. A study comparing data from 7195 patients in the Optimum Patient Care Research Database found that patients with severe asthma requiring ≥4 prescriptions for oral corticosteroids in 2 consecutive years had significantly more musculoskeletal complications compared to patients with mild-moderate asthma and non-asthmatics. The odds ratio for developing osteopenia in severe asthma patients requiring frequent steroids compared to mild-moderate asthma or non-asthmatics, respectively, was 5.26 (3.75–7.37, $P < 0.001$) and 6.68 (4.28–10.43, $P < 0.001$). Similarly, the odds ratio for osteoporosis was 5.23 (3.97–6.89, $P < 0.001$) and 6.53 (4.63–9.21, $P < 0.001$). Patients in the severe asthma group requiring frequent steroids had significantly more fractures compared to both control groups as well ($P < 0.001$) [42C]. A Japanese observational cohort study of 11 907 patients with rheumatoid arthritis revealed that the risk of proximal humerus fracture was related to the dose of prednisolone received. Authors suggested that steroid dosing should be judicious given that the hazard ratio per milligram of daily prednisolone was 1.07 (1.01–1.13, $P < 0.05$) [43C]. A 56-year-old woman who received an intraarticular injection of triamcinolone acetonide 40 mg (2 mL) and 1% lidocaine (2 mL) for osteoarthritis of the knee suffered severe pain and inflammation causing inability to walk 2 hours after injection. A synovial fluid sample yielded "butterscotch-colored" fluid containing 14 600 white blood cells/mL. Septic arthritis was ruled out with negative cultures and synovial fluid aspirate viewed with light microscopy revealed intracellular and extracellular crystals consistent with triamcinolone acetonide crystallization. The patient was discharged the following morning [44A].

Infection: A multicenter randomized controlled trial of 523 preterm infants born prior to 28 weeks gestation randomized patients to receive hydrocortisone (0.5 mg/kg IV twice daily × 7 days, then 0.5 mg/kg IV daily × 3 days) or placebo for the first 10 days after birth. Survival to week 36 without bronchopulmonary dysplasia favored administration of hydrocortisone (OR 1.48, 1.0–2.16, $P = 0.04$). The rate of sepsis prior to discharge was not significantly different between groups but was higher in hydrocortisone-treated infants in the subgroup born between 24 and 25 weeks gestational age (40% vs 23%, $P = 0.02$) [45C]. A study evaluated 1424 consecutive inpatients with reported iodinated contrast allergies who were premedicated with a 13-hour course of prednisone prior to CT scan. Compared to a matched control group, more patients who received the corticosteroid premedication regimen were diagnosed with a hospital-acquired infection during the admission (5.1% vs 3.1%, $P = 0.008$). Central line-associated bloodstream infections occurred in 1.3% of premedicated patients compared to 0.2% in the control group ($P < 0.001$) and *Clostridium difficile* infection occurred in 2.7% of premedicated patients compared to 1.6% of control patients ($P = 0.05$). There were no significant differences in surgical site infections or catheter-associated urinary tract infections [6c]. A prospective pilot of 33 Ethiopian patients with erythema nodosum leprosum (13 new ENL, 20 chronic ENL) were randomized to receive 16 weeks of tapering prednisolone therapy (prednisolone arm) or cyclosporine plus prednisolone (cyclosporine arm). In the cyclosporine arm, prednisolone was stopped after only 4 weeks and the cyclosporine dose was tapered through week 16. In the overall cohort, there were 23 infections attributed to prednisolone and 4 attributed to cyclosporine. There were 15 minor fungal infections attributed to prednisolone compared to two attributed to cyclosporine. Of the five serious adverse effects attributed to prednisolone, two patients were diagnosed with pulmonary tuberculosis and one patient died from sepsis after perforated peptic ulcer [46c]. In a prospective observational study after allogeneic hematopoietic stem cell transplant, 27 patients received a full methotrexate regimen (group 1) for prevention of acute graft-vs-host disease (GVHD), 38 patients did not finish the full course due to methotrexate tolerability issues and received no additional immunosuppression (group 2), and 12 patients did not finish the full methotrexate course but received methylprednisolone in its place (group 3). There was no significant difference in the development of acute GVHD in group 3 compared to group 1. However, the steroid group trended towards the lowest relapse-free survival at 2 years (46.3% in group 1, 49.3% in group 2, and 25% in group 3, $P = 0.329$). This trend towards poor outcome in the steroid group may be secondary to a higher infection rate (0% in group 1, 11.1% in group 2, 80% in group 3, $P = 0.002$) [47c]. A 75-year-old woman taking prednisone 7.5 mg daily for 7 years for rheumatoid arthritis developed pustules, nodules, and ulcers on her extremities and cavitary lesions were noted on chest CT scan. Diagnosis of disseminated infection with *Mycobacterium chelonae* was made via results from skin biopsy histology, polymerase chain reaction, and cultures. Skin lesions and pulmonary nodules improved after 1 month of clarithromycin, levofloxacin, and rifampicin. However, the patient died 6 months later from sudden respiratory failure [48A].

Death: A multicenter randomized controlled trial of 451 patients with HIV-associated cryptococcal meningitis treated with amphotericin B and fluconazole were randomized to receive 6 weeks of dexamethasone or placebo. Mortality at 10 weeks was 47% in the dexamethasone group and 41% in the placebo group ($P = 0.45$). The trend towards increased mortality may not have been statistically significant because the study was terminated early. Patients in the dexamethasone group were less likely to have a good outcome at 10 weeks (OR 0.42, 0.25–0.69, $P < 0.001$) or 6 months (OR 0.49, 0.31–0.77, $P = 0.002$) compared to placebo [49C]. A multicenter observational study of 601 critically ill patients with H1N1pdm09 influenza evaluated the impact of corticosteroid administration. In the 280 patients who received corticosteroids as part of their treatment regimen, the crude risk of mortality was higher compared to those who received no steroids (25.5% vs 16.4%, $P = 0.007$). After multivariate regression adjusting for baseline characteristics, the risk of death was still higher in patients who received steroids (OR 1.71, 1.05–2.78, $P = 0.03$). However, the results were no longer statistically significant after adjustment for time-dependent confounders [50C].

PROSTAGLANDINS AND ANALOGUES
[SED-15, 2955; SEDA-33, 846; SEDA-34, 660; SEDA-35, 000; SEDA-36, 604; SEDA-37,494; SEDA-38 428]

Systematic Reviews: Several reviews of therapy in pulmonary arterial hypertension (PAH) describe each of the prostacyclin medications, dosage forms, and adverse reactions. Authors for all articles highlighted the lack of studies comparing clinical efficacy and adverse events between prostacyclin therapies [51R,52R,53R].

Two published meta-analyses of prostacyclin therapies reviewed the class effects using the available literature. The first included 14 studies evaluating four prostacyclins in PAH; treprostinil, iloprost, beraprost, and epoprostenol. Epoprostenol was found to improve 6 minute walk test, exercise capacity, and fewer patients discontinued therapy compared to the other agents. The major limitation of this analysis is the lack of studies making direct comparisons between agents and the need for statistical inference [54M]. A second meta-analysis of therapy for PAH included 31 randomized controlled trials with 6565 patients. The risk ratio for improvement with prostacyclin therapy compared to placebo was 5.06 (2.32–11.04). There were no differences in mortality between therapies and placebo. Adverse events leading to discontinuation were the highest with prostacyclin therapy, RR 2.92 (1.68–5.06). Selexipag was also associated with increased risk of discontinuation due to

adverse events when compared to placebo, 2.06 (1.04–3.88) [55M].

Hemodynamics: A single center study evaluated prostacyclin therapy for PAH in patients with chronic obstructive pulmonary disease (COPD). This retrospective chart review of more than 500 right heart catheterization procedures evaluated patients over a 10 year period. A significant increase in cardiac index and decrease in pulmonary vascular resistance was demonstrated between baseline and follow-up procedures. This demonstrates improvement in cardiopulmonary functioning with prostacyclin therapy [56c].

Epoprostenol (PGI$_2$)

Cardiovascular: In a single center retrospective study comparing inhaled nitric oxide to inhaled epoprostonol for pulmonary hypertension following cardiac surgery, there was no difference in the rate of hypotension or bleeding complications. The study included a total of 98 patients and did find a significant cost savings using inhaled epoprostonol over inhaled nitric oxide ($363.53 vs $2562.50, $P < 0.01$) [57c].

Drug Formulations: Two formulations of inhaled epoprostonol are available; Flolan® is formulated with glycine and Veletri® is formulated with arginine. Veletri® (iVEL) is stable at room temperature for 24 hours and refrigerated for 7 days, while Flolan® (iFLO) is only stable for 8 hours at room temperature and 24 hours refrigerated. A single center retrospective chart review compared clinical outcomes of 52 patients receiving iFLO and iVEL after a formulary change. There was no difference in clinical outcomes of oxygenation, hospital length of stay, duration of inhaled therapy, or cost. Patients receiving iVEL had shorter duration of mechanical ventilation and ICU stay which the authors attributed to differences in baselines characteristics [58c].

Drug–Drug interactions: A study of 24 healthy male volunteers evaluated the effect of epoprostonol on platelet activity. In the presence of dual anti-platelet therapy with prasugrel and aspirin, epoprostonol reduced platelet aggregation from 75% to 19%, $P < 0.05$. This demonstrates the ability of epoprostonol to enhance the effects of P2Y12 inhibition [59E].

Iloprost (PGI$_2$ Analogue) [SED-15, 1716; SEDA-33, 847; SEDA-34, 660; SEDA-35, 726; SEDA-36, 604; SEDA-37, 495; SEDA-38, 428]

Systematic Review: A Cochrane review for treatment of Buerger's disease evaluated iloprost compared to both placebo and aspirin. The evaluation included 5 studies (602 subjects) for a variety of endpoints. Iloprost was found to improve pain at rest and healing of ischemic ulcers compared to aspirin. Treatment-related side effects including headache, flushing, and nausea were not associated with treatment interruptions [60R].

Ethnicity: A prospective open-label phase III study compared outcomes in Japanese patients to those of Western patients from the global phase III AIR study of inhaled iloprost. A total of 27 Japanese patients received iloprost and demonstrated improvement in pulmonary vascular resistance and 6 minute walk test at 12 weeks. Adverse effects reported included headache (37%), cough (15%), and one patient experienced hypotension. There was no difference in safety or efficacy of inhaled iloprost for pulmonary hypertension in Japanese patients compared to a subgroup of Western patients [61c].

Diagnostic Testing: Vasodilator testing in pulmonary hypertension including the use of iloprost was the subject of a brief review article. Authors highlighted benefits of inhaled iloprost for vasodilator challenge including improved tolerability compared to adenosine and the possibility of being more effective than inhaled nitric oxide in heart transplant patients. Side effects discussed included headache, flushing, jaw pain, dizziness, and systemic vasodilatation [62r].

Treprostinil

Drug Dosage Regimens: An observational study included 80 patients to evaluate high dose treprostinil safety and efficacy with pulmonary arterial hypertension. There was no comparator group. Patients receiving more than 9 puffs (54 mcg) of treprostinil were evaluated for a mean of 20.3 months. The dose was titrated up to 12 puffs (72 mcg) four times per day in 91% of patients. Side effects with initiation included cough (41%), headache (28%), and throat irritation (8%) which improved upon follow-up. Inhaled high dose treprostinil was discontinued in 25% of patients, but only 4 patients discontinued the medication for intolerable side effects [63c].

Misoprostol (PGE$_1$ Analogue) [SED-15, 2357; SEDA-33, 847; SEDA-34, 660; SEDA-35, 726; SEDA-36, 612; SEDA-37, 496; SEDA-38, 429]

Systematic Review: A systematic review of 32 trials evaluated misoprostol administration for cervical ripening before hysteroscopy. Misoprostol was effective in avoiding further cervical dilation, increasing cervical width, and time to dilatation. More adverse events were reported in patients treated with misoprostol than placebo, risk difference 0.07 (0.01–0.12). Side effects included abdominal cramping, diarrhea, vaginal bleeding, and fever [64M].

Nervous System: A reported side effect of misoprostol is shivering. In a non-inferiority study of misoprostol for primary vs secondary prevention of postpartum hemorrhage which included more than 2000 deliveries, shivering occurred at a greater rate in patients treated for primary prevention [65c]. In a randomized controlled trial of 1052 women, oxytocin and misoprostol were compared for prevention of postpartum hemorrhage. Chills were reported by 61.4% of patients treated with misoprostol compared to 5.2% treated with oxytocin ($P < 0.0001$) [66C].

Reproductive System: A multicenter retrospective cohort study evaluated women treated for spontaneous miscarriage with dilation and curettage (D&C) and misoprostol. In the 73 patient cohort, 41 patients had a D&C performed and 32 were given misoprostol. During subsequent in vitro fertilization (IVF) cycles, no difference was observed in baseline follicle-stimulating hormone levels, endometrial thickness, or other markers of ovarian response. Authors suggested that future IVF treatments were not affected after misoprostol was used for spontaneous miscarriage [67c]. After administration of an unknown dose of misoprostol for a missed abortion, a 25-year-old woman in Cameroon presented in hypovolemic shock. She was found to have uterine rupture requiring hysterectomy and transfusion of 1.5 L of whole blood during surgery. Her postoperative course was uneventful. Authors indicate use of misoprostol could have contributed to uterine rupture [68A].

Selexipag (Prostacyclin IP Receptor Agonist) [SEDA-38, 429]

Major Reviews: Two major reviews evaluated all of the available preclinical and clinical trial results for selexipag. Ghosh et al. highlighted the receptor selectivity of selexipag for the PGI$_2$ receptor as the reason for less dose-related nausea and vomiting. Additionally, a study in which selexipag demonstrated no effect on gastric emptying was reviewed. Other side effects included headache, jaw pain, myalgia, and nasopharyngitis [69R]. Similar side effects are highlighted in the review by Duggan et al. A notable additional side effect discussed by this review is hyperthyroidism, which occurred in 1.4% and 0% of patients treated with selexipag and placebo, respectively. Other additional adverse events highlighted include increased heart rate and transient hypotension [70R]. A small editorial review commented that the tolerability profile of selexipag is similar to other prostacyclin therapies [71r].

Pharmacokinetics: Two prospective open-label studies evaluated administration of selexipag and its active metabolite to healthy patients, those with severe renal impairment, and those with moderate or mild hepatic impairment. Despite increase in area under the concentration-time curve in patients with renal and hepatic dysfunction compared to healthy patients, authors concluded no dose adjustment would be necessary from the dose of 200 to 400 mcg. Caution with increasing dose titration was advised [72c].

Drug–Drug Interactions: In a double-blind, two-way crossover study of 18 healthy male subjects, selexipag was administered 400 mcg twice daily or placebo for 12 days and a single 20 mg warfarin dose was administered on day 8. There was found to be no difference in international normalized ratio between placebo and selexipag treatment and the area under the concentration-time curve for selexipag was not affected by the single warfarin dose. Authors concluded there was no significant drug–drug interaction between selexipag and warfarin [73c].

References

[1] Kittanamongkolchai W, Cheungpasitporn W, Zand L. Efficacy and safety of adrenocorticotropic hormone treatment in glomerular diseases: a systematic review and meta-analysis. Clin Kidney J. 2016;9(3):387–96 [M].

[2] Arita JH, Vale TC, Pedroso JL, et al. ACTH-induced dyskinesia in a child with West syndrome (infantile spasms). Parkinsonism Relat Disord. 2016;24:145–6 [A].

[3] Lal R, Bell S, Challenger R, et al. Pharmacodynamics and tolerability of repository corticotropin injection in healthy human subjects: a comparison with intravenous methylprednisolone. J Clin Pharmacol. 2016;56(2):195–202 [c].

[4] Nakata M, Kato T, Ide M, et al. Long-term weekly ACTH therapy for relapsed West syndrome in tuberous sclerosis complex: a case report. Brain Dev. 2016;38:431–4 [A].

[5] Choo XN, Pavord ID. Morbidity associated with oral corticosteroids in patients with severe asthma. Thorax. 2016;71(4):302–4 [r].

[6] Davenport MS, Mervak BM, Ellis JH, et al. Indirect cost and harm attributable to oral 13-hour inpatient corticosteroid prophylaxis before contrast-enhanced CT. Radiology. 2016;279(2):492–501 [c].

[7] Madhok VB, Gagyor I, Daly F, et al. Corticosteroids for Bell's Palsy (idiopathic facial paralysis). Cochrane Database Syst Rev. 2016;(7): Article No: CD001942 [M].

[8] Van Veen NHJ, Nicholls PG, Smith WCS, Richardus JH. Corticosteroids for treating nerve damage in leprosy. Cochrane Database Syst Rev. 2016;(5):Article No: CD005491. http://dx.doi.org/10.1002/14651858.CD005491.pub3 [M].

[9] Prasad K, Singh MB, Ryan H. Corticosteroids for managing tuberculosis meningitis. Cochrane Database Syst Rev. 2016;(4): Article No: CD002244 [M].

[10] Matthews E, Brassington R, Kuntzer T, et al. Corticosteroids for the treatment of Duchenne muscular dystrophy. Cochrane Database Syst Rev. 2016;(5):Article No: CD003725 [M].

[11] Normansell R, Kew KM, Mansour G. Different oral corticosteroid regimens for acute asthma. Cochrane Database Syst Rev. 2016;(5): Article No: CD011801 [M].

[12] Head K, Chong LY, Hopkins C, et al. Short-course oral steroids alone for chronic rhinosinusitis. Cochrane Database Syst Rev. 2016;(4):Article No: CD011991 [M].

[13] Rhodes A, Evans LE, Alhazzani W, et al. Surviving sepsis campaign: international guidelines for management of severe sepsis and septic shock: 2016. Crit Care Med. 2017;45(3):486–552 [R].

[14] Keh D, Trips E, Marx G, et al. Effect of hydrocortisone on development of shock among patients with severe sepsis: the HYPRESS randomized clinical trial. JAMA. 2016;316(17):1775–85 [C].

[15] Raman V, Krishnamurthy S, Harichandrakumar KT. Body weight-based prednisolone versus body surface area-based prednisolone regimen for induction of remission in children with nephrotic syndrome: a randomized, open-label, equivalence clinical trial. Pediatr Nephrol. 2016;31:595–604 [C].

[16] Fink N, Segev A, Barbash I, et al. Vascular complications in steroid treated patients undergoing transfemoral aortic valve implantation. Catheter Cardiovasc Interv. 2016;87:341–6 [c].

[17] Sevuk U, Baysal E, Altindag R, et al. Role of methylprednisolone in the prevention of postpericardiotomy syndrome after cardiac surgery. Eur Rev Med Pharmacol Sci. 2016;20:514–9 [c].

[18] Keir ML, Dehghani P. Corticosteroids and spontaneous coronary artery dissection: a new predisposing factor? Can J Cardiol. 2016; 32(3):395e7–8 [A].

[19] Peltoniemi OM, Lano A, Yliherva A, et al. Randomized trial of early neonatal hydrocortisone demonstrates potential undesired effects on neurodevelopment at preschool age. Acta Paediatr. 2016;105: 159–164 [c].

[20] Sellin JN, Vedantam A, Luerssen TG, et al. Safety of epidural triamcinolone acetonide use during lumbar decompression surgery in pediatric patients: an association with delayed pseudomeningocele formation. J Neurosurg Pediatr. 2016;17:667–71 [c].

[21] Schlosser RJ, Hyer JM, Smith TL, et al. Depression-specific outcomes after treatment of chronic rhinosinusitis. JAMA Otolaryngol Head Neck Surg. 2016;142(4):370–6 [c].

[22] Upadhyay A, Mishra OP, Prasad R, et al. Behavioural abnormalities in children with new-onset nephrotic syndrome receiving corticosteroid therapy: results of a prospective longitudinal study. Pediatr Nephrol. 2016;31:233–8 [c].

[23] Gorton HC, Webb RC, Kapur N, et al. Non-psychotropic medication and risk of suicide or attempted suicide: a systematic review. BMJ Open. 2016;6:e009074 [M].

[24] Gyamfi-Bannerman C, Thom EA, Blackwell SC, et al. Antenatal betamethasone for women at risk for late preterm delivery. N Engl J Med. 2016;374(14):1311–20 [MC].

[25] Delarue J, Allain-Jeannic G, Guillerm S, et al. Interaction of low dose of fish oil and glucocorticoids on insulin sensitivity and lipolysis in healthy humans: a randomized controlled study. Mol Nutr Food Res. 2016;60:886–96 [c].

[26] Matsumoto N, Ogawa M, Matsuoka S, et al. Prevalence and risk factors of diabetes mellitus in patients with autoimmune hepatitis. Intern Med. 2016;55:879–85 [c].

[27] Golekoh MC, Hornung LN, Mukkada VA, et al. Adrenal insufficiency after chronic swallowed glucocorticoid therapy for eosinophilic esophagitis. J Pediatr. 2016;170:240–5 [c].

[28] Agarwal R, Aggarwal A, Dhooria S, et al. A randomised trial of glucocorticoids in acute-stage allergic bronchopulmonary aspergillosis complicating asthma. Eur Respir J. 2016;47:490–8 [c].

[29] Chen J, Cai F, Jiang L, et al. A prospective study of dexamethasone therapy in refractory epileptic encephalopathy with continuous spike-and-wave during sleep. Epilepsy Behav. 2016;55:1–5 [c].

[30] Kuzma-Mroczkowska E, Panczyk-Tomaszewska M, Skrzypczyk P, et al. Body weight changes in children with idiopathic nephrotic syndrome. Dev Period Med. 2016;20(1):16–22 [c].

[31] Sneeboer MM, Hutten BA, Majoor CJ, et al. Oral and inhaled corticosteroid use and risk of recurrent pulmonary embolism. Thromb Res. 2016;140:46–50 [C].

[32] Xu L, Liu S, Guan M, et al. Comparison of prednisolone, etoricoxib, and indomethacin in treatment of acute gouty arthritis: an open-label, randomised, controlled trial. Med Sci Monit. 2016;22: 810–7 [C].

[33] Aljebab F, Choonara I, Conroy S. Systematic review of the toxicity of short-course oral corticosteroids in children. Arch Dis Child. 2016;101:365–70 [M].

[34] Tan JP, Barazanchi AW, Singh PP, et al. Predictors of acute diverticulitis severity: a systematic review. Int J Surg. 2016;26:43–52 [M].

[35] Evaniew N, Belley-Cote EP, Fallah N, et al. Methylprednisolone for the treatment of patients with acute spinal cord injuries: a systematic review and meta-analysis. J Neurotrauma. 2016;33:468–81 [M].

[36] Wan Y, Sun T, Liu Z, et al. Efficacy and safety of corticosteroids for community-acquired pneumonia. Chest. 2016;149(1):209–19 [M].

[37] Davidov Y, Ofir H, Pappo O, et al. Methylprednisolone-induced liver injury: case report and literature review. J Dig Dis. 2016;17:55–62 [A].

[38] Rainer TH, Cheng CH, Janssens HJ, et al. Oral prednisolone in the treatment of acute gout. Ann Intern Med. 2016;164(7):464–72 [C].

[39] Coates LC, Helliwell PS. Psoriasis flare with corticosteroid use in psoriatic arthritis. Br J Dermatol. 2016;174:219–21 [r].

[40] Flouzat-Lachaniette C, Roubineau F, Heyberger C, et al. Multifocal osteonecrosis related to corticosteroid: ten years later, risk of progression and observation of subsequent new osteonecrosis. Int Orthop. 2016;40:669–72 [C].

[41] Leib ES, Winzenrieth R. Bone status in glucocorticoid-treated men and women. Osteoporos Int. 2016;27:39–48 [C].

[42] Sweeney J, Patterson CC, Menzies-Gow A, et al. Comorbidity in severe asthma requiring systemic corticosteroid therapy: cross sectional data from the Optimum Patient Care Research Database and British Thoracic Difficult Asthma Registry. Thorax. 2016;71:339–46 [C].

[43] Ochi K, Furuya T, Ishibashi M, et al. Risk factors associated with the occurrence of proximal humerus fractures in patients with rheumatoid arthritis: a custom strategy for preventing proximal humerus fractures. Rheumatol Int. 2016;36:213–9 [C].

[44] Young P, Homlar KC. Extreme postinjection flare in response to intra-articular triamcinolone acetonide (Kenalog). Am J Orthop. 2016;45(3):E108–11 [A].

[45] Baud O, Maury L, Lebail F, et al. Effect of early low-dose hydrocortisone on survival without bronchopulmonary dysplasia in extremely preterm infants (PREMILOC): a double-blind, placebo-controlled, multicentre, randomised trial. Lancet. 2016;387:1827–36 [C].

[46] Lambert SM, Nigusse SD, Alembo DT, et al. Comparison of efficacy and safety of ciclosporin to prednisolone in the treatment of erythema nodosum leprosum: two randomised, double blind, controlled pilot studies in Ethiopia. PLoS Negl Trop Dis. 2016;10. http://dx.doi.org/10.1371/journal.pntd.0004149 [c].

[47] Kim S, Kim AR, Yoon SY, et al. Substitution of methotrexate with corticosteroid for acute graft-versus-host disease prevention in transplanted patients who develop methotrexate toxicity. Ann Hematol. 2016;95:483–91 [c].

[48] Tsutsumi R, Yamada N, Yoshida Y, et al. Disseminated *Mycobacterium chelonae* infection identified by repeated skin sampling and molecular methods in a patient with rheumatoid arthritis. Acta Derm Venereol. 2016;96:132–3 [A].

[49] Beardsley J, Wolbers M, Kibengo FM, et al. Adjunctive dexamethasone in HIV-associated cryptococcal meningitis. N Engl J Med. 2016;374(6):542–54 [C].

[50] Delaney JW, Pinto R, Long J, et al. The influence of corticosteroid treatment on the outcome of influenza A (H1N1pdm09)-related critical illness. Crit Care. 2016;20(75):1–11 [C].

[51] O'Connell C, Amar D, Boucly A, et al. Comparative safety and tolerability of prostacyclins in pulmonary hypertension. Drug Saf. 2016;39:287–94 [R].

[52] Velayati A, Valerio MG, Shen M, et al. Update on pulmonary arterial hypertenions pharmacotherapy. Postgrad Med. 2016;128(5):460–73 [R].

[53] Maccaulay TE, Covell MB, Pogue KT. An update on the management of pulmonary arterial hypertension and the pharmacist's role. J Pharm Pract. 2016;29(1):67–76 [R].

[54] Zhang H, Li X, Huang J, et al. Comparative efficacy and safety of prostacyclin analogs for pulmonary arterial hypertension. Medicine. 2016;95(4):e2575 [M].

[55] Jain S, Khere R, Girotra S, et al. Comparative effectiveness of pharmacologic interventions for pulmonary arterial hypertension. Chest. 2017;151(1):90–105 [M].

[56] Calcaianu G, Canuet M, Schuller Enache I, et al. Pulmonary arterial hypertension-specific drug therapy in COPD patients with severe pulmonary hypertension and mild-to-moderate airflow limitation. Respiration. 2016;91:9–17 [c].

[57] McGinn K, Reichert M. A comparison of inhaled nitric oxide versus inhale epoprostenol for acute pulmonary hypertension following cardiac surgery. Ann Pharmacother. 2016;50(1):22–6 [c].

[58] Torbic H, Szumita PM, Anger KE, et al. Clinical and economic impact of formulary conversion from inhaled Flolan to inhaled Veletri for refractory hypoxemia in critically ill patients. Ann Pharmacother. 2016;50(2):106–22 [c].

[59] Chan MV, Knowles RBM, Lundberg MH, et al. P2Y12 receptor blockade synergizes strongly with nitric oxide and prostacyclin to inhibit platelet activation. Br J Clin Pharmacol. 2016;81(4):621–33 [E].

[60] Cacione DG, Macedo CR, Baptista-Silva JCC. Pharmacological treatment for Buerger's disease. Cochrane Database Syst Rev. 2016;(3):Article No. CD011033 [R].

[61] Saji T, Myoshi M, Sugimura K, et al. Efficacy and safety of inhaled iloprost in Japanese patients with pulmonary arterial hypertension. Circ J. 2016;80:835–42 [c].

[62] Sharma A, Obiagwu C, Kenechukwu M, et al. Role of vasodilator testing in pulmonary hypertension. Prog Cardiovasc Dis. 2016;58:425–33 [r].

[63] Parolj KS, Rajagopal S, Fortin T, et al. Safety and tolerability of high-dose inhaled treprostinil in pulmonary hypertension. J Cardiovasc Pharmacol. 2016;67:322–32 [c].

[64] Zhuo Z, Yu H, Jiang X. A systematic review and meta-analysis of randomize controlled trials on the effectiveness of cervical ripening with misoprostol administration before hysteroscopy. Int J Gynaecol Obstet. 2016;132(3):272–7 [M].

[65] Raghavan S, Geller S, Miller S, et al. Misoprostol for primary versus secondary prevention of postpartum haemorrhage: a cluster-randomised non-inferioirty community trial. BJOG. 2016;123:120–7 [c].

[66] Diop A, Daff B, Saw M, et al. Oxutocin via Uniject versus oral misoprostol for prevention of postpartum hemorrhage at the community level: a cluster-randomized controlled trial. Lancet Glob Health. 2016;4:e37–44 [C].

[67] Tamir R, Allouche S, Weissman A, et al. The effect of medical versus surgical treatment of spontaneous miscarriage on subsequent in vitro fertilization cycles. Gynecol Endocrinol. 2016;32(3):231–3 [c].

[68] Egbe TO, Halle-Ekane GE, Tchente CH, et al. Management of uterine rupture: a case report and review of the literature. BMC Res Notes. 2016;9:492 [A].

[69] Ghosh RK, Ball S, Das A, et al. Selexipag in pulmonary arterial hypertension: most updated clinical evidence from recent preclinical and clinical studies. J Clin Pharmacol. 2017;57:547–57 [R].

[70] Duggan ST, Keam SJ, Burness CB. Selexipag: a review in pulmonary hypertension. Am J Cardiovasc Drugs. 2016;17(1):73–80 [R].

[71] Sharma K. Selexipag for the treatment of pulmonary arterial hypertension. Expert Rev Respir Med. 2016;10(1):1–3 [r].

[72] Kaufman P, Cruz HG, Krause A, et al. Pharmacokinetics of the novel oral prostacyclin receptor agonist selexipag in subjects with hepatic or renal impairment. Br J Clin Pharmacol. 2016;82(2):369–79 [c].

[73] Bruderer S, Okubo K, Mukai H, et al. Investigation of potential pharmacodynamic and pharmacokinetic interactions between selexipag and warfarin in healthy male subjects. Clin Ther. 2016;38(5):1228–36 [c].

35

Sex Hormones and Related Compounds, Including Hormonal Contraceptives

Sandra Hrometz[1], *Shaun P Say*

College of Pharmacy, Natural and Health Sciences, Manchester University, Fort Wayne, IN, United States
[1]Corresponding author: slhrometz@manchester.edu

ESTROGENS: [SED-15, 1253; SEDA-35, 731; SEDA-36, 615; SEDA-37, 499-500; SEDA-38, 433-439]

Diethylstilbestrol (DES) [SED-15, 1119; SEDA-35, 731; SEDA-36, 615; SEDA-37, 499-500; SEDA-38, 433-434]

Diethylstilbestrol (DES) is a nonsteroidal estrogen that was prescribed for decades to pregnant women in order to prevent miscarriage and premature delivery. It was banned in the United States in 1972 and in France in 1977. A retrospective, cohort study looked at the adverse health effects of the grandchildren (third-generation) of women who took DES during pregnancy. Questionnaires were completed by the women who were exposed to DES in utero (second-generation) about their own children (third-generation). In order to be included in the study, the women exposed to DES in utero had to be certain about their exposure via documentation or by providing consistent information. A total of 3436 women who were exposed to DES in utero reported on their 4409 children (50.5% female and 49.5% male). The control group was 3256 unexposed women who reported on their 6203 offspring (49.2% female and 50.8% male). Odds ratios (OR) with 95% confidence interval (CI) were used to compare the third-generation exposed and unexposed children as a whole and separately per gender. In order to compare observed cases with expected incidences in the general population, the standardized incidence rate (SIR) was also calculated. The offspring of the women exposed to DES in utero had a significant increase in global birth defects compared to the offspring of women who were not exposed to DES (OR, 2.29; 95% CI, 1.80–2.70,

$P < 0.001$) and with the general population (SIR, 2.39; 95% CI, 2.11–2.68).

Specific birth defects that were significantly increased in the third generation of DES-exposed subjects include esophageal anomalies (atresia/fistula), other digestive defects, urogenital tract defects in males (significant for both hypospadias and undescended testes), cleft lip and palate, musculoskeletal anomalies and congenital heart defects. There was a significant increase in cerebral palsy; potentially due to the substantial increase in pre-term births (24% in the DES-exposed group and 3.35% in the unexposed group). Since cerebral palsy is related to premature birth, it is not surprising that the exposed group had a significantly higher incidence (OR, 8.71; 95% CI, 7.4–10.1). There was not a significant increase in urogenital defects or reproductive cancers (breast, uterine, ovarian) in females; however, the author's point out that these types of cancers are usually diagnosed in women who are older than the study population (the average age of the daughters was 15.2 years with a range of 0–43 years) [1MC].

In another study, the daughters of women who took DES during pregnancy were studied to determine if the timing of in utero exposure and increasing age changed their risk of developing cancers of the lower genital tract. A total of 4062 DES-exposed and 1837 unexposed women were followed between 1982 and 2013. The cumulative incidence of cervical intraepithelial neoplasia grade ≥ 2 (CIN2+) was 5.3% in the DES group and 2.6% in the control group. The covariate adjusted hazard ratios (HR) for exposure to DES and diagnosis with CIN2+ was 2.10 (95% CI, 1.41–3.13). Women with in utero DES exposure at <8 weeks gestation had a higher risk of CIN2+ (HR, 2.64; 95% CI, 1.64–5.25) than those exposed ≥ 8 weeks gestation (HR, 1.41; 95% CI, 0.88–2.25). When looking at age brackets, only DES-exposed women ≤30 years of age had an increased risk of developing lower genital tract cancers with a HR of 2.66 (95% CI, 1.11–6.37). Although other age brackets show an increase in risk; the associated CI ranges were not statistically significant. Specifically the 50 participants ages 30–34 had a HR of 1.97 (95% CI, 0.94–4.15), the HR for the 30 participants ages 35–39 had a HR of 2.87 (95% CI, 0.98–8.42) and the HR for the 24 participants ages 40–44 was 3.11 (95% CI, 0.88–11.0). Once women reached age ≥45 ($n=27$), there is no increase in risk with a HR of 0.91 (95% CI, 0.39–2.10). The authors pooled the data and determined the HR for women up to age 44 to be significantly increased at 2.47 (95% CI, 1.55–3.94) [2MC].

Hormone Replacement Therapy (HRT): [SEDA-15, 1684, 1686, 1692; SEDA-35, 732; SEDA-36, 616; SEDA-37, 500-501; SEDA-38, 434-435]

Updated evidence-based clinical practice guidelines for the treatment of menopausal symptoms were published in November of 2015 by a task force appointed by the Endocrine Society. Updates and analysis of HRT for menopause has been widespread since the 2002 WHI report that HRT increased the risk of cardiovascular disease, deep vein thrombosis, stroke, breast cancer and all-cause mortality. Repeated analysis of WHI data and spin-off studies have continued to show that the benefits of HRT can outweight the risks for most women who are within 10 years of initial menopause symptoms, less than 60 years of age, and devoid of cardiovascular and breast cancer risk factors. The 2015 guidelines emphasize that HRT should be individualized based upon clinical factors and patient preference. Additionally, they recommend that women should be screened for cardiovascular and breast cancer risk before initiation of HRT as a way of choosing the most appropriate therapy that will yield the best risk-to-benefit ratio. It is also important to note that newest guidelines recommend that HRT be limited to the treatment of vasomotor and urogenital symptoms of climacteric [3S].

For clarification, HRT is hormone replacement and it can be a combination of estrogen and progestin therapy (EPT) or just estrogen alone, which is referred to as estrogen replacement therapy (ERT). Hormone replacement in women who still have a uterus should be combination EPT. If a women no longer has a uterus, hormone therapy can be limited to just ERT. Use of just ERT or unopposed estrogen in a woman with a uterus has been known to increase the incidence of endometrial cancer for decades. As such, EPT is the standard recommendation for women with a uterus, as the progestin helps to counteract the malignant effects of estrogen on endometrial tissue growth and hyperplasia.

Cancer

ENDOMETRIAL CANCER

A nationwide cohort study of Danish women aged 50–79 years were followed for an average of 9.8 years (from 1995 to 2009) to evaluate the risk of endometrial cancer with HRT. The investigators examined the types and routes of hormones use, the pattern of hormone use (cyclic combined vs continuous combined) and the duration of hormone use. A total of 914 595 women without previous cancer or hysterectomy were categorized as never users of HRT ($n=593 207$) and current/previous users of HRT ($n=321 388$). Exposure to HRT was obtained from the National Prescription Register while the incidence of endometrial cancers ($n=6202$) were identified from the National Cancer Registry. There were 4972 Type I endometrial tumors (which develop from abnormal tissue proliferation and are considered to be hormone-dependent) and 500 Type II tumors (which are atrophic and character and considered to be less hormone-dependent) identified.

The data were presented as incidence rate ratios (RRs) with 95% CIs and adjusted for confounders such as age, education and concomitant disease states. All HRT regimens were compared to women who never used HRT. The data revealed an increased risk of overall endometrial cancer in current users (RR, 2.03; 95% CI, 1.90–2.18), with a specific RR of 2.17 (95% CI, 2.02–2.34) for Type I endometrial cancer and 1.34 (95% CI, 1.03–1.74) for Type II cancer. When broken down by duration of use, the risk of type II tumors was no longer significant after 5–9 years of use (RR, 1.14; 95% CI, 0.73–1.78) and the risk decrease after 10+ years of use (RR, 0.12; 95% CI, 0.02–0.85). The RR was significantly increased for Type I tumors (RR, 1.55; 95% CI, 1.42–1.69), Type II tumors (RR, 1.31; 95% CI, 1.00–1.73) and overall endometrial cancer (RR, 1.54; 95% CI, 1.42–1.66) in previous users of HRT. The RR for Type II tumors was only significantly increased in those using for a duration of 2–4 years. When looking at the types of HRT, overall endometrial cancer, Type I and Type II tumors were significantly increased with the use of tibolone, oral cyclic combined HRT and vaginal ERT. Tibolone, a synthetic steroid with estrogen, progestin and androgen activity, was associated with the highest risk estimates of all therapies investigated, with a RR of 3.56 (95% CI, 2.94–4.32) for overall endometrial cancer, 3.80 (95% CI, 3.08–4.69) for Type I and 2.34 (95% CI, 1.04–5.25) for Type II tumors. With respect to the use of unopposed estrogen therapy, the vaginal preparations were found to have a significantly increased RR for endometrial cancer overall, Type I and Type II tumors, while the oral and transdermal estrogen was only significant for overall and Type I endometrial tumors.

The researchers also looked at the pattern of HRT use. A significantly increased RR was noted for endometrial tumors overall (RR, 2.06; 95% CI, 1.88–2.27), Type I and Type II tumors in those using cyclic combined HRT. With long-cycle combined HRT, RR was only significant for overall endometrial cancer (RR, 2.89; 95% CI, 2.27–3.67) and Type I tumors (RR, 3.25; 95% CI, 2.52–4.19) only. The authors speculate the reason to be the longer periods of unopposed estrogen with the long-cycle therapy. Women using continuous combined HRT actually experienced a decreased RR of Type II tumors (RR, 0.45; 95% CI, 0.20–1.01) and no increased risk of overall (RR, 1.02; 95% CI, 0.87–1.20) and Type I endometrial tumors (RR, 1.09; 95% CI, 0.92–1.30).

When looking at duration of HRT (data only reported for overall endometrial cancer), there was a significantly increased risk with ≥10 years of cyclic combined HRT (RR, 2.59; 95% CI, 2.01–3.33), long-cycle combined HRT (RR, 5.02; 95% CI, 2.84–8.86) and tibolone (RR, 3.80; 95% CI, 2.56–5.64) use. There was not a significant increased risk with continous combined HRT (RR, 0.8; 95% CI, 0.51–1.24) use ≥10 years [4MC].

OVARIAN CANCER

The association between ERT and ovarian cancer risk was investigated in a pooled analysis of 10 population-based case–control studies. A total of 906 women with primary ovarian cancer and 1220 controls (no ovarian cancer at time of the study) were in the analysis. Inclusion criteria were such that all participants had at least one ovary (thus had potential for developing ovarian cancer), had undergone a hysterectomy (which is why they would be on estrogen only therapy rather than combination EPT) and was ≥50 years of age when ERT was initiated (since 50 in the approximate age of menopausal symptom onset). Prior use of hormonal contraceptives was an adjusted variable. Both the duration and timing of estrogen therapy was characterized. Overall, 50.8% of the women with ovarian cancer and 43.5% of the control group reported use of ERT after age 50. Women using ERT at some point after the age of 50 (ever users) had a 30% increased risk of ovarian cancer (OR, 1.3; 95% CI, 1.06–1.59) compared to controls. When the women with a history of ever using ERT where further categorized as either current/recent users (those using within the last 5 years) or previous users (those using over 5 years ago) a significant increase in risk was only seen with the current/recent users (OR, 1.35; 95% CI, 1.09–1.67). When stratified for duration of ERT use, risk significantly

increased with ≥10 years of use (mean duration ~15 years) for both current/recent users (OR, 1.53; 95% CI, 1.17–2.02) and ever users (OR 1.54; 95% CI, 1.18–2.01). With respect to the types of ovarian tumors seen after ≥10 years of ERT use, only endometrioid (P < 0.001) and serous (P = 0.001) types were reported to be significantly increased. There was not an increase in mucinous, clear cell or "other" epithelial tumor types [5MC].

Hormonal Contraceptives SEDA-15, 1642, 1645, 2225; SEDA-35, 733; SEDA-36, 618, 622-623; SEDA-37, 501-504, 506; SEDA-38, 436-439]

Cardiovascular and Hemostatic Effects

The time for clotting factors to change with use of a combination oral contraceptives (COC) was studied in a single-arm, open-label pilot study of 17 subjects aged 18–35. Repeated blood samples were collected throughout the duration of a 21 day cycle of a COC containing 30 mcg EE and 150 mcg of levonorgestrel (LVNG). Levels of D-dimer more than doubled after 6 days of using the COC and remained elevated at day 21 (P = 0.012) compared to baseline. A significant increase in Factor VIII activity was seen after 2 days of using the COC, but was no longer significant by day 21. There was not a significant increase in Protein C with the first cycle of use of the COC [6c].

DROSPIRENONE [SEDA-35, 736; SEDA-36, 622; SEDA-37, 506; SEDA-38, 436-437]

A 20-year-old female suffered an acute inferior myocardial infarction (MI) 1 month after starting a COC containing 3 mg of the third-generation progestin drospirenone (DRSP) and 30 mcg EE. Her personal history did not revealed any cardiovascular risk factors (non-smoker, normal body weight, normal lipid profile, no family history of cardiovascular disease, no drug abuse). Since there were no identifiable risk factors and her biochemical and hematological labs were normal, the authors concluded that the acute inferior MI occurred secondary to the COC. Existing case reports of an MI with use of hormonal contraceptives tend to be in older women (≥39) and in those with other risk factors such as being a heavy smoker, use of the product for multiple years and/or having a positive family history of significant cardiovascular disease [7A].

Cervical Cancer

The impact on hormonal factors on the risk of developing cervical intraepithelial neoplasia grade 3 (CIN3)/carcinoma in situ (CIS) and invasive cervical cancer (ICC) was investigated in a cohort of 308036 female participants between the ages of 35 and 70 from the EPIC (European Prospective Investigation into Cancer and

Nutrition) Study. The authors set out to show that although the human papilloma virus (HPV) is a known cause of cervical cancer, hormonal factors (such as use of exogenous hormones, number of full-term pregnancies) may also have a relevant influence. After a 9-year median follow-up, 261 ICC and 804 CIN3/CIS cases were reported. Multivariate HR with a 95% CI were estimated to evaluate the risk of cervical cancer. In a nested case–control study, the sera from 609 cases and 1218 matched controls were tested for antibodies against specific HPV types associated with cervical cancer, Chlamydia trachomatis and Human herpesvirus 2. The data for the nested case–control study are presented as an OR with a 95% CI. The cohort analysis showed that full-term pregnancy was a factor that increased the risk of CIN3/CIS risk (HR, 1.5; 95% CI, 1.2–1.9), but not ICC of the cervix. The HR increases to 2.3 (95% CI 1.6–3.3) for ≥4 full-term pregnancies. In the nested case–control study, there is a significant increase in risk of CIN3/CIS, but not ICC with a history of full-term pregnancy. In the cohort study (but not the nested case–control study), having a history of induced abortion was associated with an increased risk of ICC (HR 1.9; 95% CI, 1.3–2.7), but not CIN3/CIS of the cervix. Use of an OC was compared to women who never used an OC in the cohort study (reported as HR) and the nested case–control study (reported as OR). Current use of an oral contraceptive (OC) was shown to be a risk for CIN3/CIS (HR, 1.8; 95% CI, 1.4–2.4) and CIS (HR 2.2; 95% CI, 1.3–4.0). In the cohort study, ever and past use of an OC was associated with an increase risk in CIS, but not CIN3/CIS of the cervix. There was not a significant increase in either tumor type with use of OC in the nested case–control study. When OC use was stratified into duration of use, a clearer picture emerged. Use of an OC for 5 to 9 years increased the risk of ICC (HR 2.0; 95% CI, 1.3–3.0). It took 10 to 14 years of OC use (no data after this time point) to increase the risk of CIN3/CIS in the nested case–control study (OR, 1.6; 95% CI, 1.0–2.5). The risk of both CIN3/CIS and ICC (HR, 1.6; 95% CI, 1.2–2.2 and HR, 1.8; 95% CI, 1.1–2.9, respectively) significantly increased after ≥15 years of OC use. There was not an increased risk of CIN3/CIS cervical cancer noted in the cohort or nested case-controlled studies. However, use of menopausal HRT (currently and ever) was associated with a reduced risk of ICC in the cohort (HR, 0.5; 95% CI, 0.3–0.8 and HR, 0.5; 95% CI 0.4–0.8, respectively) and nested case-control studies (OR for current use is 0.2 with 95% CI, 0.1–0.5 and OR forever use is 0.3 with 98% CI, 0.1–0.7). Based upon these significant associations between the development of cervical cancer and hormone exposure (via OC, menopausal HRT and parity), the authors interject their opinion of the importance of following cervical cancer screening guidelines [8MC].

Bone Mineral Density

MEDROXYPROGESTERONE [SEDA-15, 225; SEDA-35, 737; SEDA-36, 623; SEDA-37, 506; SEDA-38, 437-438]

A longitudinal cohort study analyzed the effects of depot medroxyprogesterone acetate (DMPA) on bone mineral density (BMD) in physically active female cadets at West Point Military Academy (New York, USA). The mean age of participants at the time of enrollment was 18.4 ± 0.8 years. Ninety one cadets (75 Caucasians, 9 Asians, and 7 African Americans) remained in the study over the course of 4 years. All participants had very active lifestyles, which included daily marching, 3 hours of physical education weekly, participation in NCAA, club or company level sports and an average of at least 14 hours per week at sports practices. Contraception use was distinguished as either use of an OC or DMPA, and was included in analysis if the participant utilized the contraceptive for ≥3 months per year or >12 months over the 4-year study period. Participants were categorized as DMPA users ($n=19$) or non-DMPA users ($n=72$). No details were provided on dosage or composition of the OCs in the non-DMPA users. Least square means regression was applied to account for covariates including race, weight change, an eating disorder index and baseline BMD and served as a statistical test for assessing the difference between BMD loss and DMPA. The results demonstrated significant bone loss at the spine and hip with the use of DMPA in all races (Spine: $P < 0.01$; Hip: $P < 0.01$). DMPA users had bone loss at the spine, hip and calcaneus while those who never used DMPA maintained or gained bone at these three sites ($P < 0.05$). Thus the researchers suggested that it would be advisable to follow the boxed warning (do not use for greater than 2 years and unless other birth control methods are considered inadequate) for DMPA since bone loss was still likely to occur even with a high level of exercise in healthy young physically active women [9C].

Ophthalmic

DROSPIRENONE [SEDA-35, 736; SEDA-36, 622; SEDA-37, 506; SEDA-38, 436-437]

The impact of COC use on corneal connective tissue (CCT) was assessed in an observational study. The study had a total of 90 participants, with 50 women taking a COC containing 3 mg DRSP and 30 mcg EE, for a minimum of 3 months prior to the study (mean age of 32.8 ± 5.8 years) and a control group of 40 women who never used a COC (mean age of 31.3 ± 6.9 years). Exclusions for the study included women outside a BMI range of 19–24.8 kg/m^2, were pregnant or lactating, had various ophthalmic disorders or irregularities, or a previous history of dry eye, glaucoma, keratitis, uveitis, ocular surgery or trauma. Women were also excluded if they wore contact lenses or were using corticosteroids (systemic or topical) or other topical ocular medications. Each subject underwent a full ophthalmologic exam, and all CCT and intraocular pressure (IOP) readings were performed by the same physician at the same period of the day during the luteal phase of each woman's menstrual cycle, as determined by date of last menses and gynecological exam. Women using the COC had a significantly higher mean CCT compared to those not taking a COC (530.9 ± 30.4 and 519.6 ± 35.6 μm, $P = 0.003$). The findings suggest that ophthalmologist should be cognizant of patients using COC due to potentially elevated CCT values, which may lead to inaccurate IOP values [10c].

Sexual Function

DROSPIRENONE [SEDA-35, 736; SEDA-36, 622; SEDA-37, 506; SEDA-38, 436-437]

A small prospective, randomized study investigated the effect of a COC containing 30 mcg EE and 3 mg DRSP on female sexual function. DRSP is a third-generation progestin with anti-androgen and anti-aldosterone properties. A Female Sexual Function Index (FSFI) exam was administered before beginning the COC and after 3 months of COC use. FSFI is a validated questionnaire that assesses different domains of sexual function (desire, arousal, lubrication, orgasm, satisfaction and pain) in addition to providing an overall score regarding sexual function. Possible FSFI total score ranges from 2.0 to 36.0. A score ≤26.55 categorizes one as being at risk of female sexual dysfunction. The study had 40 participants in the COC and the comparable control group. All participants were considered healthy, reported to be sexually active in monogamous relationships, with a mean age of approximately 25. The control group utilized non-hormonal contraceptive methods (barrier methods, natural family planning, etc.). The two study groups had similar baseline qualities (age, BMI, marital status, education level, number of pregnancies, number of children and baseline FSFI scores ≤26.55), with the exception of smoking status. Forty percent of the COC group were smokers compared to 20% of the non-hormonal group ($P = 0.04$). The main outcome of interest was change in sexual function from baseline in the two groups. The COC group reported a significant decrease in desire ($P = 0.04$), arousal ($P = 0.03$) and total FSFI score ($P < 0.0001$) at their 3 month follow-up. Alternatively, the control group (non-hormonal contraceptive users) showed a significant increase in sexual desire ($P = 0.05$), arousal ($P = 0.005$), orgasm ($P = 0.0004$), satisfaction ($P = 0.02$) and total FSFI score ($P = 0.02$) at their 3 month follow-up from baseline. Additionally, after 3 months, there were significantly more women ($P = 0.0001$) with an FSFI score ≤26.55 in the COC group ($n = 26$) compared to the control group ($n = 10$). When comparing the amount of change in sexual function after 3 months between the two groups, the

hormonally treated women has significantly lower scores for desire ($P = 0.01$), arousal ($P = 0.002$) and total FSFI score ($P < 0.001$) compared to the non-hormonal contraception control group. Adjustment for smoking status did not alter the statistically significant findings. The risk of deterioration in sexual function associated with use of the DRSP-containing COC was 2.01 times higher than in those using non-hormonal contraception ($P < 0.001$) [11c].

A cross-sectional analysis of 1938 women examined the effect of different types of hormonal contraceptives on sexual desire. The participants came from a pool of 9256 women who were enrolled in the prospective, cohort contraceptive CHOICE Project. A predominant goal of the CHOICE Project was to remove barriers to all contraceptive methods and promote the use of reversible, long-acting contraceptive methods. This study offers interesting results concerning not only changes in sexual desire with the use of contraceptives, but also with participant demographics.

Inclusion criteria included age 14 to 45, no desire for pregnancy for at least 12 months, willingness to switch to or initiate a new contraceptive method, and being sexually active with a male partner or anticipating sexual activity in the next 6 months. Women with tubal ligation or hysterectomy were excluded. The participant demographics are as follows: mean age of 25, 50% black, 59% single or never married, 51% nulliparous, 36% received public assistance, 68% ranked their health as very good or excellent and the average BMI was 27.7.

The 1938 participants completed a baseline and 6-month telephone survey regarding their level of interest in having sex. Women were scored as lacking interest in sex if they answered "yes" when asked "During the past 6 months, has there even been a time of several months or more when you lacked interest in having sex?" The control group were women using a non-hormonal, copper intrauterine device (IUD; $n = 262$). After 6 months, the change in sexual desire from baseline for the control group (18.3% reported a lack of interest in sex) was compared to the change reported in women using different types of hormonal contraceptives. When compared to the control group, a significant lack of interest in sex was reported in women using DMPA, the implant and the contraceptive ring, but not in any of the other hormonal contraceptive products.

The largest effect occurred in the DMPA group ($n = 110$), where 37.3% reported lacking sexual interest at 6 months (adjusted OR, 2.61; 95% CI, 1.47–4.61). In women using the contraceptive vaginal ring ($n = 98$), 27.6% (adjusted OR, 2.53; 95% CI, 1.37–4.69) experienced a lack of interest in sex; while 25.6% of those using the contraceptive implant ($n = 454$) were found to have a lack of interest in sex over the study period (adjusted OR, 1.60; 95% CI, 1.03–2.49). Compared to controls, there was not a significant lack of interest in sex for those using the hormonal IUD (838), oral contraceptive pills ($n = 133$), and the contraceptive patch ($n = 43$). The women who experienced a decrease in sexual desire were more likely to be young (younger than 18 years: adjusted OR, 2.04), black (adjusted OR, 1.78), and married or living with a partner (adjusted OR, 1.82).

Confounding variables associated with a lack of interest in sex included age, in that younger women (<18 age group and 18–20 age group) were more likely to report a lack of interest in sex at 6 months compared to those in the 21–25 year age group. Black women were more likely to experience a lack of interest in sex than white women (adjusted OR, 1.78; 95% CI, 1.33–2.40) and women who were married or living with a partner were more likely to experience a loss of desire compared to single women (adjusted OR, 1.82; 95% CI, 1.38–2.40). The multivariable analysis did not find a significant association between lack of interest in sex and parity, depression, use of public assistance, level of self-reported general health, BMI or history of sexually transmitted infection [12MC].

Psychological: Depression

A nationwide prospective cohort study with >1 million subjects utilizing 2 national registries (Denmark) investigated the association of hormonal contraceptive use with depression. Data were collected on all women aged 15–34 from 1985 through 2013. Exclusion criteria included women with a history of psychiatric diagnosis, use of anti-depressants, use of infertility medications and contraindications to hormonal contraceptive use (cancer, venous thrombosis). Depression was determined by either the first fill of a prescription for an antidepressant or a first discharge diagnosis of depression from the Psychiatric Central Research Register database. All forms of hormonal contraceptives (oral, non-oral, progestin only) were included. The participants were categorized into two groups: current and recent users (cessations within the previous 6 months) or never and former (last use a minimum of 6 months ago) users of hormonal contraceptives. To ensure that subjects who discontinued a hormonal contraceptive due to depression but before they initiated treatment for depression were still considered to have been exposed to hormonal contraceptives, recent users were put in the same category as current users. A total of 1 061 997 women, with a mean age of 24.4 (±0.001) years were followed for a mean of 6.4 (±0.004) years. During follow-up, 55.5% of the participants were current or recent users of some form of hormonal contraceptive. Compared with nonusers, users of hormonal contraceptives had an increased RR of first use of an antidepressant. The RR for the following contraceptives (from lowest to highest) are as follows: COC, 1.23 (95% CI, 1.22–1.25); progestin-only pills, 1.34 (95% CI, 1.27–1.40); LVNG IUD, 1.4 (95% CI, 1.31–1.42);

contraceptive vaginal ring, 1.6 (95% CI, 1.55–1.69); contraceptive patch, 2.0 (95% CI, 1.76–2.18); contraceptive implant, 2.1 (95% CI, 2.01–2.24); and DMPA, 2.71 (95% CI, 2.45–2.87). For depression diagnoses, similar or slightly lower estimates were found. Age stratified analysis found adolescents (15–19 years) had a higher RR of a first use of an antidepressant while using a COC (RR, 1.8; 95% CI, 1.75–1.84) and progestin-only pills (RR, 2.2; 95% CI, 1.99–2.52) compared to other age groups. The RR of antidepressant use peaked at 6 months after initiation at 1.4 (95% CI, 1.34–1.46) [13MC].

In Vitro Fertilization

Ophthalmic

The exact cause of keratoconus, which is forward bulging (ectasia) and thinning of the cornea, is unknown, but considered to have genetic and environmental influences (hormonal changes, microtraumas). Microtraumas, such as chronic eye rubbing, chronic eye irritation and oxidative stress have been the most frequently associated causes. Corneal changes and progression of keratoconus has been reported to occur during pregnancy, presumably due to elevated estrogen levels. A retrospective review of medical records of patients with keratoconus produced three patients who underwent *in vitro fertilization* (IVF) therapy. The mean and maximum keratometry values increased and corrected distance visual acuity decreased in all 6 eyes after an average of 2.3 IVF treatments. This is the first report of keratoconus progression associated with IVF therapy. None of the women were pregnant before or after the IVF treatments. All 3 patients complained of decreased vision 1 or 2 months after the second or third treatment IVF treatment cycle. The IVF therapies were slightly different for the three women, but all three received human chorionic gonadotropin and intravaginal progesterone in addition to either a gonadotropin-releasing hormone (GnRH) agonist, clomiphene and/or recombinant DNA follicle-stimulating hormone. During follow-up, corneal cross-linking treatment was performed to harden the cornea and halt or delay disease progression in 4 eyes of the 3 patients. The authors offer that corneal cross-linking could be offered before IVF procedures as a way to minimize the risk of keratoconus progression [14c].

Selective Progesterone Receptor Modulator [SEDA-35, 738; SEDA-36, 625; SEDA-37, 506-507; SEDA-38, 439]

Ulipristal Acetate [SEDA-36, 626; SEDA-37, 504, 507]

Ulipristal acetate (UPA) is a selective progesterone receptor modulator approved for use as an emergency contraceptive in the United States and Europe and for preoperative treatment of uterine myomas in Europe (used "off-label" in the United States). Generally, UPA is administered for 3 months, which not only decreases myoma size before surgery, but also decreases symptoms such as abnormal uterine bleeding, dysmenorrhea and pelvic pain. Surgical removal of myomas can occur via hysterectomy or myomectomy, if wishing to preserve fertility. Three cases of myoma migration were recently reported to occur 1 month after completion of the standard pre-surgical 3 month regimen of UPA. The myomas were all noted to be submucosal. The first case was a nulliparous women, 31 years of age who was planning on a hysteroscopic myomectomy after UPA. At the time of the surgery, the 70% decrease in size and migration of the myoma resulted in changing the surgical approach to a less invasive laparoscopy of the entire myoma without opening the endometrial cavity. The second case was a 28-year-old multiparous woman who was scheduled to undergo a hysteroscopic myoma resection after the course of UPA. The ultrasound right before surgery showed a 55% reduction in myoma size and the myoma was no longer impacting the mucosa. The surgery was cancelled since this patient was not planning on having additional children. The third case was a 26-year-old multiparous woman, who opted for a laparoscopic myomectomy (she was still a virgin and did not want a vaginal procedure). However, after treatment with UPA, it was noted that the myoma had decreased in size by 27%, had separated from the submucosa and was being expelled through the cervix. The surgery was switched from laparoscopic to a vaginal myomectomy. The authors note that myoma migration has been reported to occur after other pre-surgical myoma therapies (uterine artery embolization and GnRH agonists); however, there has only been one other report of myoma migration following pre-operative treatment with UPA. The authors warn that a pre-operative ultrasound should be performed to confirm myoma location and surgical approach after treatment with UPA [15A].

Gonadotropin-Releasing Hormone Agonist—Triptorelin Acetate [SEDA-36, 631; SEDA-37, 509-510]

Pseudotumor cerebri is a known adverse effect to GnRH analogs in adults. A 9-year-old girl receiving depot triptorelin acetate (3.75 mg/month) for precocious puberty developed a headache and elevated blood pressure after the fourth dose. Further analysis led to the diagnosis of pseudotumor cerebri. Triptorelin was discontinued and she was treated with acetazolamide until cerebrospinal fluid pressure, funduscopic examinations and blood pressure returned to normal. This is the first case of pseudotumor cerebri development after use of a GnRH analog in a child [16A].

Aromatase Inhibitor—Anastrozole [SEDA-35, 735; SEDA-36, 619; SEDA-37, 504]

The characteristics and risk factors for the development of carpal tunnel syndrome (CTS) in women using anastrozole was explored via analysis of participants in the International Breast Cancer Intervention Study II (IBIS-II). Anastrozole is an aromatase inhibitor and functions to reduce estrogen levels by blocking the peripheral conversion of androgens into estrogen. Participants in IBIS-II (double-blinded, randomized clinical trial) were women at increased risk of breast cancer who were randomly assigned to treatment with anastrozole ($n=1920$) or placebo ($n=1944$). A total of 96 participants with CTS were identified. The anastrozole group had a significantly higher OR than placebo ($P < 0.001$). Sixty-five (3.4%) participants in the anastrozole group and 31 (1.6%) in the placebo group (OR, 2016; 95% CI, 1.40–3.33) developed CTS. With respect to risk factors for the development of CTS, those with a BMI between 25 and 30 kg/m^2 and a BMI >30 mg/m^2 had a significantly higher risk ($P = 0.02$) than those with a BMI of ≤25 kg/m^2 (OR, 1.78; 95% CI 1.07–2.96). Age, smoking and prior history of menopausal HRT were not found to be risk factors for developing CTS [17MC].

ANABOLICS, ANDROGENS AND RELATED COMPOUNDS [SEDA-35, 738; SEDA-36, 627; SEDA-37, 507-508; SEDA-38, 439-441]

Testosterone [SEDA-36, 631; SEDA-37, 509; SEDA-38, 439-440]

Venous Thromboembolism (VTE)

A large, population-based case–control study investigated the VTE risk with testosterone utilizing the United Kingdom Clinical Practice Research Datalink (CPRD) database. A total of 19 215 men (over the age of 18) with confirmed VTE (includes deep venous thrombosis and pulmonary embolism) were compared with 909 530 age-matched controls (who did not have a confirmed VTE) using records between January 1, 2001 and May 31, 2013. The researchers reported on current and recent testosterone use, the duration of therapy in current users, the presence or absence of VTE risk factors and whether testosterone was being used to treat hypogonadism. The overall incident rate of VTE was determined to be 15.8 (95% CI 15.6–16.0) per 10 000 years based upon the 19 215 cases of VTE out of the 2.92 million men in the database population. At the time of first occurrence of VTE (the index date), testosterone use was measured. Men were categorized as current users within their first

6 months of initiating therapy, current users with >6 months of use and recent users (not current users but had used within the previous 2 years).

All RRs reported were adjusted for age, history of hypogonadism and other risk factors for VTE. When compared to controls, only current users within the first 6 months of initiating therapy had a significantly higher risk of VTE (RR, 1.63; CI, 1.12–2.37). The risk was not increased for current users collectively, current users beyond 6 months or initiating testosterone and recent users. The author's report that the risk of VTE peaks at about 3 months into therapy and then decreases back towards pretreatment baseline. Although the increased risk is transient in those within 6 months of initiating treatment, this corresponds to an additional 10.0 VTE cases per 10,000 person years.

In men with a diagnosis of hypogonadism, there was never an increase in risk of VTE for current (collectiviely, within and beyond 6 months of therapy initiation) or recent testosterone users. In men who did not have a diagnosis of hypogoandism, the adjusted RR of VTE in current testosterone users collectively was significantly increased compared to controls (RR, 1.69; 95% CI, 1.09–2.63). Current user subgroup analysis revealed an increased risk in those within the first 6 months of initiating testosterone (RR, 1.88; 95% CI, 1.02–3.45), but not in those who had been using for more than 6 months [18MC].

The presence or absence of risk factors for VTE was also explored. In men who were not known to have any VTE risk factors, the risk was increased in current testosterone users collectively (RR, 1.57; 95% CI, 1.06–2.32) and in those within the first 6 months of starting therapy (RR, 1.91; 95% CI, 1.13–3.23). There was not a significant risk in those who had been using beyond 6 months.

Anabolic Steroids [SEDA-35, 738; SEDA-36, 627; SEDA-37, 507-508; SEDA-38, 440-441]

Anabolic androgens consist of testosterone and synthetic derivatives that have been modified to enhance anabolic over androgenic effects. Coveted anabolic effects include muscle growth, erythropoiesis, reduced body fat, faster recover from muscle strain/injury and increased athletic training intensity and ability.

A 13-year-old boy suffered from massive cardiomegaly and eventually death secondary to anabolic steroid use. He went into ventricular fibrillation during physical exertion. Although defibrillation resuscitated him, severe neurological damage had already occur and life-support was withdrawn the following week. His heart weighed 465 g compared to an expected weight of 175 g. On the basis of previous health records and physical changes (adrenal atrophy, mature genitalia with reduced gonadal size, muscular development, skin striae at biceps and thighs and cardiovascular changes) at the time of cardiac arrest, it was estimated that steroid use was likely initiated when he was 11 years of age. Evaluation by his primary physician revealed a considerable increase in muscle mass and precocious development of secondary sex characteristics since his last exam, but his health status was otherwise excellent. His personal and family history was negative for hypertrophic cardiomyopathy, arrhythmias or sudden death. All first-degree relatives actually underwent EKG and echocardiogram screens, which were all found to be normal [19A].

Androgen Deprivation Therapy (ADT) [SEDA-35, 740; SEDA-36, 628; SEDA-37, 508-509]

Dementia

Electronic medical records from Stanford University (1994–2013) and Mt. Sinai (2000–2013) health systems were utilized in a retrospective cohort study of 16 888 men with prostate cancer. All participants had prostate cancer and were studied throughout their treatment to determine if there is an association between ADT and Alzheimer's disease risk. The 14.2% of men receiving ADT (n = 2397) were followed for a mean of 2.7 years. The follow-up period ended with the last available record or time of Alzheimer's disease diagnosis. For inclusion, subjects must have data for the propensity scoring covariates and follow-up data for at least 180 days after prostate cancer diagnosis. The 180 day deferral period was a way of ruling out those with pre-existing Alzheimer's disease. Subjects were excluded if they had any characteristics that were associated with increased risk for cognitive decline or Alzheimer's disease (history of chemotherapy use, dementia or stroke). The follow-up period was defined as either the time of starting ADT and at least 180 days after cancer diagnosis, or for non-ADT users, 180 days after prostate cancer diagnosis plus the median time to ADT use in the study.

The participant groups were men with prostate cancer receiving ADT and men with prostate cancer not receiving ADT. Before propensity scoring (to account for differences in demographics), men receiving ADT were significantly older and more likely to be Caucasian have a positive history for smoking, cardiovascular disease or diabetes (P < 0.001 for all variables). Those receiving ADT were also more likely to be current users of antiplatelet, anticoagulant and antihypertensive medications (P < 0.001 for all variables). Propensity score matching analysis unveiled a statistically significant association between ADT use and Alzheimer's disease risk P = 0.021). Propensity score-matched Cox regression analysis revealed a statistically significant association between ADT use and Alzheimer's disease risk (P = 0.031). Lastly, a statistically significant increased risk of Alzheimer's disease was noted in those using ADT ≥12 months compared to those using ADT for <12 months (P = 0.016) [20MC].

This same research group published a second observational cohort study an association between androgen deprivation therapy (ADT) and risk of dementia. This time, they only utilized the electronic medical record data from Stanford University (1994–2013) health systems. After excluding for age <18 at time of prostate cancer diagnosis and history of dementia, a total of 9272 men were followed for a median of 3.4 years. The follow-up period was defined as either the time of starting ADT or for non-ADT users, the time of prostate cancer diagnosis plus the median time to ADT use in the study. The follow-up period ended with the last available record or time of diagnosis of dementia. Their statistical analysis was based on HRs calculated using propensity score-matched and traditional multivariable adjusted Cox proportional hazards regression.

Before propensity scoring, men receiving ADT were significantly older and more likely to be Caucasian have a positive history for smoking, cardiovascular disease, diabetes or prior malignant disease ($P < 0.001$ for all variables). Those receiving ADT were also and more likely to be current users of antiplatelet and antihypertensive medications ($P < 0.001$ for all variables). The 1826 men who used ADT (19.7% of the participants) had a significantly increased risk of dementia ($P < 0.001$). In sensitivity analysis, the results were still significant when excluding those receiving chemotherapy ($P < 0.001$), excluding those diagnosed with dementia within the first 2 years of eligible follow-up as to avoid the bias of a pre-existing condition ($P < 0.001$), and excluding those with Alzheimer's disease ($P < 0.001$). During the study, there were 314 new cases of dementia. The mean time to dementia diagnosis was 4.0 years. The absolute increased risk of developing dementia in those on ADT was 4.4% at 5 years, which represents 7.9% in ADT users and 4.4% in controls. The results showed a positive correlation between use of ADT and development of dementia using the propensity score-matched ($P < 0.001$) and Cox proportional hazards regression ($P < 0.001$) analyses.

The cumulative probability of developing dementia was calculated for 4 groups of men based upon age and whether they were treated with ADT. The cumulative probability of developing dementia at 5 years was 13.7% in men ≥70 years receiving ADT, 6.6% in men ≥70 years who did not receive ADT, 2.3% in men <70 years receiving ADT and 1% in men <70 years who did not receive ADT. Each value is significantly different from the other three groups ($P < 0.05$) [21MC].

Enzalutamide [SEDA-35, 740; SEDA-36, 629; SEDA-37, 508-509]

Acute generalized exanthematous pustulosis (AGEP) was reported in a 62-year-old man receiving enzalutamide for metastatic prostate cancer. Enzalutamide, a competitive antagonist at the androgen receptor, is second-line therapy when androgen suppression (degarelix and bicalutamide in his case) and first-line chemotherapy (docetaxel) fail. The subject was started on oral prednisone 40 mg/day, oral enzalutamide 160 mg/day, and a subcutaneous GnRH analog implant providing 10.8 mg of goserelin over 12 weeks. Ten days after starting enzalutamide and 4 days after introduction of the first goserelin implant, he experienced an acute skin reaction consisting of large areas of edematous and erythematous plaques on his chest, back and upper extremities. The plaques were covered with millimeter non-follicular pustules on groin, trunk and axilla. The eruption evolved to diffuse desquamation after 4 days, with slightly painful multiple erythematous targetoid papular lesions on his inferior members. He did not have any mucosal lesions or a fever. Blood work revealed a moderate inflammatory syndrome with peripheral leukocytosis with neutrophilia and elevated C-reactive protein (53 mg/L, normal range <5 mg/dL). Cholestasis was also diagnosed with gamma-glutamyl transferase and alkaline phosphatase levels three to seven times higher than the normal values. A skin biopsy gave further evidence of AGEP. Enzalutamide treatment was stopped, but the goserelin implant could not be removed and continued to deliver stable plasma levels over the next 12 weeks. Supportive treatment included continuation of the oral steroid, addition of topic betamethasone, wet dressings and oral anti-histamines. Complete resolution of the skin lesions occurred within 4 weeks of discontinuing enzalutamide. The prednisolone and goserelin (since it was an implant that could not be removed) were continued as the AGEP cleared up. The slow resolution of symptoms (4 weeks) is speculated to be due to the long half-life (5.8 days) of enzalutamide an accumulation of at least 10 doses before the medication was discontinued [22A].

References

[1] Tournaire M, Epelboin S, Devouche E, et al. Adverse health effects in children of women exposed in utero to diethylstilbestrol (DES). Therapie. 2016;71(4):395–404. ISBN or ISSN: 00405957 [MC].

[2] Troisi R, Hatch EE, Palmer JR, et al. Prenatal diethylstilbestrol exposure and high-grade squamous cell neoplasia of the lower genital tract. Am J Obstet Gynecol. 2016;215:322.e1–8 [MC].

[3] Stuenkel CA, Davis SR, Gompel A, et al. Treatment of symptoms of the menopause: an endocrine society clinical practice guideline. J Clin Endocrinol Metab. 2015;100(11):3975–4011 [R].

[4] Mørch LS, Kjær SK, Keiding N, et al. The influence of hormone therapies on type I and II endometrial cancer: a nationwide cohort study. Int J Cancer. 2016;138(6):1506–15 [MC].

[5] Lee AW, Ness RB, Roman LD, et al. Association between menopausal estrogen-only therapy and ovarian carcinoma risk. Obstet Gynecol. 2016;127(5):828–36 [MC].

[6] Westhoff CL, Eisenberger A, Tang R, et al. Clotting factor changes during the first cycle of oral contraceptive use. Contraception. 2016;93:70–6 [c].

[7] Aslan AN, Süygün H, Sivri S, et al. Low-dose oral contraceptive-induced acute myocardial infarction. Eur J Contracept Reprod Health Care. 2016;21(6):499–501 [A].

[8] Roura E, Travier N, Waterboer T, et al. The influence of hormonal factors on the risk of developing cervical cancer and pre-cancer: results from the EPIC Cohort. PLoS One. 2016;11(1):1–17 [MC].

[9] Nieves JW, Ruffing JA, Zion M, et al. Eating disorders, menstrual dysfunction, weight change and DMPA use predict bone density change in college-aged women. Bone. 2016;84:113–9 [C].

[10] Kurtul BE, Inal B, Ozer PA, et al. Impact of oral contraceptive pills on central corneal thickness in young women. Indian J Pharmacol. 2016;48:665–8 [c].

[11] Čiaplinskienė L, Žilaitienė B, Verkauskienė R, et al. The effect of a drospirenone-containing combined oral contraceptive on female sexual function: a prospective randomised study. Eur J Contracept Reprod Health Care. 2016;1362-5187. 21(5):395–400. http://dx.doi.org/10.1080/13625187.2016.1217324 [c].

[12] Boozalis A, Tutlam NT, Robbins CC, et al. Sexual desire and hormonal contraception. Obstet Gynecol. 2016;127(3):563–72 [MC].

[13] Scovund CW, March LS, Kessing LV, et al. Association of hormonal contraception with depression. JAMA Psychiat. 2016;73(11):1154–62 [MC].

[14] Yuksel E, Yalinbas D, Aydin B, et al. Keratoconus progression induced by in vitro fertilization treatment. J Refract Surg. 2016;32(1):60–3 [c].

[15] Willame A, Marci R, Petignat P, et al. Myoma migration: an unexpected "effect" with ulipristal acetate treatment. Eur Rev Med Pharmacol Sci. 2016;20:1439–44 [A].

[16] Gül U, Bayram AK, Kendirci M, et al. Pseudotumour cerebri presentation in a child under the gonadotropin-releasing hormone agonist treatment. J Clin Res Pediatr Endocrinol. 2016;8(3):365–7 [A].

[17] Spagnolo F, Sestak I, Howell A, et al. Anastrozole-induced carpal tunnel syndrome: results from the International Breast Cancer Intervention Study II prevention trial. J Clin Oncol. 2016;34(2):139–44 [MC].

[18] Martinez C, Suissa S, Rietbrock S, et al. Testosterone treatment and risk of venous thromboembolism: population based case-control study. BMJ. 2016;355:i5968 [MC].

[19] Lichtenfeld J, Deal BJ, Crawford S. Sudden cardiac arrest following ventricular fibrillation attributed to anabolic steroid use in an adolescent. Cardiol Young. 2016;26:996–8 [A].

[20] Nead KT, Gaskin G, Chester C, et al. Androgen deprivation therapy and future Alzheimer's disease risk. J Clin Oncol. 2016;34(6):566–71 [MC].

[21] Nead KT, Gaskin G, Chester C, et al. Association between androgen deprivation therapy and risk of dementia. JAMA Oncol. 2017;3(1):49–55 [MC].

[22] Alberto C, Konstantinou MP, Martinage C, et al. Enzalutamide induced acute generalized exanthematous pustulosis. J Dermatol Case Rep. 2016;2:35–8 [A].

36

Thyroid Hormones, Iodine and Iodides, and Antithyroid Drugs

Haley Ethredge, Irandokht K. Najafabadi*, Rahul Deshmukh†,*
Ajay Singh‡, Vicky Mody,1*

*PCOM School of Pharmacy, Suwanee, GA, United States
†College of Pharmacy, Rosalind Franklin University of Medicine and Science, North Chicago, IL, United States
‡South University School of Pharmacy, Savannah, GA, United States
1Corresponding author: vickymo@pcom.edu

THYROID HORMONES [SED-15, 3409; SEDA-31, 687; SEDA-32, 763; SEDA-33, 881; SEDA-34, 679; SEDA-35,747; SEDA-36, 635; SEDA-37, 513]

Agents which mimic the activity of thryroid hormones such as eprotirome, levothyroxine (T4), and triiodothyronine (liothyronine, T3) are used in the treatment of hypothyroidism. Hypothryodisim can be of two types, overt and subclinical, and both of them are presented with elevated TSH levels. Clinically, overt hypothyroidism is further defined by low levels of free triiodothyronine (fT3) and free levothyroxine (fT4). Patients presenting with overt or subclinical hypothyroidism are at increased risk of developing various metabolic disorder which can lead to cardiovascular disease hence care has to be sought as soon as discovered.

Eprotirome

Eprotirome, a thyroid mimitic hormone, has shown to lower serum low-density lipoprotein (LDL) cholesterol concentrations in patients with dyslipidemia. Mechanistically it acts on the hepatic β receptor. Abnormal lipid levels put patients at risk for cardiovascular disease, which is sometimes becomes difficult to reverse with stand-alone statin therapy [1R]. The use of thyroid hormone mimetics in these patients can help lower levels of LDL cholesterol. Various adverse events have been reported during the use of eprotirome. All of them have been listed below.

Cardiovascular Disorders

A low-density lipoprotein (LDL) has been correlated with the increased cardiovascular disease (CVD) risk in various populations, such as postmenopausal women. Anagnostis et al. published a systematic review to evaluate the effect of various drugs including eprotirome on patients cardiovascular function. Eprotirome is a liver-selective thyroid hormone receptor agonist on LDL receptors [2R]. Authors found that eprotirome causes upregulation of LDL receptors at a maximum dose of 200 mcg/day [2R].

Cartilage Defect in Dogs

It was found by Anderson et al. that a 12- to 15-month eprotirome treatments in dog lead to cartilage defects in them. This was unexpected as there is no evidence of defect in cartilage occurring in humans [3M].

Levothyroxine

Levothyroxine is one of the most important medications which are used to treat hypothyroidism. However, there is no recourse from this agent, and it becomes a life-long companion of patient. Hence, it is also associated with various adverse effects from quality of life, to neurological developmental issues on fetus to its effects on bone. These effects have to be carefully reviewed and monitored over the period of time so as soon as patient becomes symptomatic needful action is taken.

ISSN: 0378-6080
http://dx.doi.org/10.1016/bs.seda.2017.06.017

Neurodevelopmental Issues

Korevaar et al. conducted a population-based prospective cohort study on pregnant women in the Netherlands [4M]. They followed women requiring thyroid therapies during pregnancy until their children were 6 years old. They found that there was an association between high maternal-free thyroxin and IQ level of the child [4M]. In fact they showed a reduction in child's average IQ of 1.4–3.8 as compared to the control. Authors concluded that the thyroid hormone is involved in brain development and levothyroxine therapy during pregnancy might put unborn child at the risk of neurodevelopment issues.

Quality of Life

Quality of life (QOL) can be effected by primary hypothyroidism. The association between QOL and various parameters in hypothyroid patients who were taking levothyroxine was studied by Kelderman-Bolk et al. [5R]. The authors evaluated the QOL for 90 patients (20 males and 70 females) who were treated for primary hypothyroidism. The evaluation was done using Short-Form 36, Hospital Anxiety and Depression Scale, and MFI20. Authors found an inverse relationship between QOL and BMI. Similarly, an inverse relationship was found between QOL and hypothyroid patients who were on thyroxine treatment. Authors concluded that the weight gain might be responsible for the lower QOL of the patients who were on levothyroxine therapy.

Rheumatoid Arthritis (RA)

Patients taking levothyroxine over the period of time have shown to increase the risk of developing rheumatoid arthritis in patients with autoimmune disorders [6R]. In this study, authors compared 1998 patients using levothyroxine along with 2252 controls for incident RA cases. They found that patients on levothyroxine were at twofold risk for RA [6R].

Vitamin D Deficiency

The effect on levothyroxine for vitamin D deficiency was evaluated by comparing the levels of 25-hydroxyvitamin D and parathyroid hormone (PTH) on 59 non-lactating women [7C]. Patients were divided into four groups, A, B, C, and D. Group A and B, both consisted of 14 hypothyroid and euthyroid females with post-partum thyroiditis, respectively. Group C included 16 females with non-autoimmune hypothyroidism, whereas group D was a control which included 15 healthy euthyroid females. The patients in both groups A and C were treated with L-thyroxine for 6 months. After 6 months, it was found that the serum levels of 25-hydroxyvitamin D were lowered in group A than in group B, as well as in group C in comparison with group D. Hence, the authors concluded that there is an association of vitamin D status with post-partum thyroiditis and levothyroxine treatment.

Multiple Subungual Pyogenic Granulomas

A case study was reported for a 54-year-old woman on levothyroxine for 3 months presented with rapidly growing lesions in her nail beds [8R]. During examination it was found that red nodules had invaded patients nail plates. A wide excision was performed but the symptoms relapsed as noted during the 3-month follow-up period. During this time levothyroxine treatment was stopped, and the symptoms did not recur [8R].

Bone Loss

Kim et al. examined the effect of levothyroxine (LT4) on bone losses in 93 patients after initiating levothyroxine therapy [9C]. Authors found that there was a mean bone losses in the lumbar spine, femoral neck, and total hip. Additionally, the bone loss was more prominent in postmenopausal women. It was found that postmenopausal women who received supplementation of calcium/vitamin D showed less bone loss as compared to others who did not. Thus, the authors concluded that levothyroxine therapy can accelerate bone loss predominantly in postmenopausal women who are not taking calcium/vitamin D supplement. These losses can be reduced by adding calcium/vitamin D to the therapy.

Nyandege and coworkers suggested that the concomitant use of bisphosphonates and other medications can stimulate bone metabolism. For example, acid-suppressive therapy, levothyroxine, thiazolidinediones (TZDs), and selective serotonin reuptake inhibitors (SSRIs) can increase the risk of fracture [10R]. Authors found that the concomitant use of acid suppressive agents with bisphosphonate can precipitate the risk of fracture. However, they suggested that TZDs, SSRIs, and levothyroxine can have similar implications based on their pharmacological action. Hence, precaution should to be taken while using bisphosphonates along with these other medications.

Cardiovascular Disorders

Bakiner et al. conducted a prospective, controlled, single-blind study to determine plasma Fetuin A levels in hypothyroid patients ($n = 39$) before and after levothyroxine treatment [11C]. Authors found that there was no correlation between Fetuin A levels and cardiovascular risk factors; however, the mean HDL cholesterol levels decreased in those patients from 49.3 (23–83.9) to 44 (28.3–69.0) [11C].

Drug Overdose

Toxic effects of high doses of levothyroxine on cardiac cells were reported by Stuijver et al. [12A]. Authors reported a case of 23-year-old woman who attempted suicide by ingesting 25 mg of levothyroxine. Patient experienced hypercoagulation and a hypofibrinolytic effect, reflecting an increased risk of venous thrombosis [12A]. Similarly, a 61-year-old patient who accidentally ingested 1000 times excess of levothyroxine rather than the actual dose of 50 mg exhibited altered mental consciousness, acute respiratory failure, and atrial fibrillation [13A].

Drug–Drug Interaction

Levothyroxine can interact with various other drugs. In an observational study carried out by Irving and coworkers, authors evaluated the effect of drugs co-administered with thyroxine [14C]. In this study, authors evaluated 10 999 patients (mean age 58 years, 82% female) who were prescribed levothyroxine on at least three occasions within a 6-month period, prior to the start of a study. They found that both iron and calcium supplements, proton pump inhibitors, and oestrogen were responsible for the increase in serum TSH concentration (7.5%, 4.4%, 5.6%, and 4.3%), respectively. However, there was a decrease in the TSH concentration (0.17 mU/L) for those patients on statins. Hence, authors concluded that there is a significant interaction between levothyroxine and iron, calcium, proton pump inhibitors, statins and oestrogens. Co-administration of these drugs with levothyroxine may reduce the effectiveness of levothyroxine therapy, and hence the TSH concentrations in those patients should be carefully monitored.

The amount of levothyroxine absorbed can also be affected by the co-administration of other drugs such as ciprofloxacin or rifampin [15A]. In a randomized, double-blind, placebo-controlled study on 8 healthy volunteers who received either 1000 μg of levothyroxine and placebo, or 1000 μg of levothyroxine and 750 mg ciprofloxacin, or 1000 μg of levothyroxine and 600 mg rifampin authors found that the co-administration of ciprofloxacin significantly decreased the area T4 levels by ~39% ($P=0.035$)], whereas rifampin co-administration significantly increased T4 by 25% ($P=0.003$)].

Octreotide

The use of preoperative administration of octreotide in cohort of patients with TSH secreting pituitary adenomas (TSHoma) was evaluated by Fukuhara et al. [16C]. Authors discovered that of 81 patients who underwent surgery for TSHoma at Toranomon Hospital between January 2001 and May 2013, 44 received preoperative short-term octreotide. Further, among these 44 patients 19 received octreotide as a subcutaneous injection, and 24 patients received octreotide as a long-acting release (LAR) injection, and one of them was excluded due to side effects. It was found that the use of short-term preoperative octreotide administration was highly effective in suppressing TSHoma shrinkage. Some common side effects such as mild diarrhea (5 patients), constipation (1 patient), nausea and elevation of bilirubin (1 patient) were observed. Hence, the authors concluded that preoperative octeroide is effective in suppressing TSHoma and should be recommended to patients to avoid problems with hyperthyroidism.

IODINE AND IODIDES [SED-15, 1896; SEDA-32, 764; SEDA-33, 883; SEDA-34, 680; SEDA-35,752; SEDA-36; SEDA-37, 514]

Dietary Iodine

Dietary iodine is essential for thyroid hormone production and regulation of many important biochemical processes in the body. Iodine deficiency can have multiple adverse effects on growth and development, and it also can critically jeopardize children's mental health and often their very survival. Iodine deficiency disorders (IDD) in pregnant women can result in stillbirth, spontaneous abortion, and congenital abnormalities such as cretinism, a grave, irreversible form of mental retardation. The World Health Organization (WHO) recommends that iodine deficiency in patients should be corrected through intake of iodized salt. Significant progress has been made to eliminate iodine deficiencies worldwide since WHO's initiation in 1990 [17R]. Moreover, iodine deficiency and its side effects routinely reported worldwide [18R,19C,20M,21C], particularly from the underdeveloped countries of Africa and Asia [22R].

In a case of a 27-year-old gravid 1 at 27 weeks 6 days with a history of hypothyroidism had an ultrasound that demonstrated a 3.9 × 3.2 × 3.3-cm well-circumscribed anterior neck mass, an extended fetal head, and polyhydramnios. Further characterization by MRI showed a fetal goiter. Patient revealed she was taking nutritional iodine supplements for treatment of her hypothyroidism which might be an underlying cause of the fetal goiter. Patient was ingesting 62.5 times the recommended amount of daily iodine in pregnancy. The excessive iodine consumption caused the fetal hypothyroidism and goiter formation. After the iodine supplement was discontinued, the fetal goiter decreased in size. At delivery, the airway was not compromised. The infant was found to have reversible hypothyroidism and bilateral hearing loss postnatally [23A].

In a data analysis of large-scale cross-country (46 countries) studies (89 national surveys between 1994 and 2012), a general association between the household unavailability of iodized salt and child growth was determined [24R]. Data consisted of 390 328 children for the stunting analysis, 397 080 children for the underweight analysis, 384 163 children for the wasting analysis, and 187 744 children for the low-birth-weight analysis. The unavailability of iodized salt was associated with 3% higher odds of being stunted (95% CI of ORs: 1.00, 1.06; $P=0.04$), 5% higher odds of being underweight (95% CI: 1.02, 1.09; $P<0.01$), and 9% higher odds of low birth weight (95% CI: 1.02, 1.17; $P=0.01$).

Iodine-Containing Solutions

Excessive iodine intake due to a long-term topical exposure like iodine solution dressings or by intravenous administration of iodine-containing agents can lead to hyperthyroidism [25R]. Excessive iodine intake can also lead to hypothyroidism.

A unique case of a 3-day-old neonate born with a giant omphalocele, who was being treated with topical povidone-iodine dressings to promote escharification was presented with a suppressed thyroid stimulating hormone of 0.59 μIU/mL, elevated free thyroxine of 5.63 ng/dL, and frank cardiovascular manifestations of thyrotoxicosis. After replacement of the topical iodine dressings with iodine-free silver sulfadiazine, the thyroid status gradually improved with complete resolution of hyperthyroidism by 17th DOL [26A].

ANTITHYROID DRUGS [SEDA-32, 765; SEDA-33, 884; SEDA-34, 681; SEDA-35, 754; SEDA-36, 638; SEDA-37, 518]

Thionamides, a class of antithyroid drugs (ATDs), are compounds that are known to inhibit thyroid hormone synthesis. Iodine is incorporated into thyroglobulin for the production of thyroid hormone, which is achieved after the oxidation of iodide by peroxide. Thioamides inhibit organification of iodine to tyrosine residues in thyroglobulin and the subsequent coupling of iodotyrosines [27R]. The commonly available thionamides are propylthiouracil (PTU) and methimazole (MMI). Compared to propylthiouracil, MMI exhibits longer half-life of the drug. This pharmacokinetic advantage allows for once daily dosing and better patient compliance. The safety profile of MMI is also significantly better compared to PTU, with less hepatotoxicity observed with MMI. Carbimazole (CBZ) an another agent available as an ATD is a prodrug of methimazole and is currently not available in the United States.

Common Side Effects

Some of the common side effects associated with PTU and MMI include pruritus, rash, urticaria, arthralgias, arthritis, fever, abnormal taste sensation, nausea, and vomiting. These adverse effects were observed in 13% of patients ($n=389$) taking thionamide drugs in one study [28C].

Agranulocytosis

Agranulocytosis, although not common, is a serious complication of thionamide therapy. A prevalence of as high as 0.5% has been observed within the first 2 months of treatment with thionamide drugs [29R].

A 6-year-old girl was reported to develop agranulocytosis after about 18 months on MMI therapy. In most instances, this condition develops within few months of therapy. A late onset though not common is still observed in about 4% of children [30A]. A study aimed to estimate the incidence, mortality, and risk of the drugs associated with agranulocytosis in Chinese patients was carried out using clinical data analysis and monitoring system, between January 2004 and December 2013. The study concluded that carbimazole had the highest risk of agranulocytosis (adjusted OR 416.7, 95% confidence interval 51.5–3372.9) with an incidence of 9.2 (95% confidence interval 6.9–12.1) per 10 000 users and 3.6 (95% confidence interval 2.7–4.8) per 10 000 user-years [31c].

A study aimed to identify genetic variants associated with antithyroid drug-induced agranulocytosis in a white European population using Genome-wide association studies concluded that drug-induced agranulocytosis was associated with HLA-B*27:05 and with other SNPs on chromosome 6. The study further concluded that to avoid one case of agranulocytosis, based on the possible risk reduction roughly 238 patients would need to be genotyped for all the three SNPs identified [32C].

ANCA-Positive Vasculitis

Propylthiouracil (PTU)-associated vasculitis is normally associated with tetrad of fever, sore throat, arthralgia, and skin lesions but may also involve multiple systems. Recently a perinuclear antineutrophil cytoplasmic antibody-associated vasculitis developed during treatment with PTU for Grave's disease was reported [33R]. Also a case reported the challenges and complication associated with management of hyperthyroidism has been reported. A patient suffering from hyperthyroidism exhibited propylthiouracyl-induced vasculitis with renal involvement. The vasculitis reversed completely after cessation of PTU therapy. This was followed by treatment with thiamazole that caused agranulocytosis with fever. After transient lithium carbonate therapy a successful thyroidectomy was performed. This case highlights some of the challenges and complications encountered in the management of hyperthyroidism [34A].

A 60-year-old woman was admitted because of hyperthyroidism and leukopenia. A terminal diagnosis of PTU-induced AAV was made. After PTU withdrawal and use of steroid, the patient recovered well and then accepted RAI therapy [35A]. Another fatal case of 41-year-old woman was attributed to extreme PTU-associated vasculitis, and skin necrosis that eventually led to death due to septic shock and multisystem organ failure. The patient tested positive for p-ANCA, MPO-ANCA and proteinase 3-ANCA. The skin lesions caused infection requiring debridement and leg amputation but also led to septic shock [36A]. In another case study, a 27-year-old woman presenting with refractory hypoxaemic respiratory failure, haemoptysis, and thyrotoxicosis was attributed by the authors as a rare manifestation of propylthiouracil therapy resulting from the development of c-ANCA [37A]. A 34-year-old female was being treated for autoimmune hyperthyroidism; six weeks later she developed purpuric plaques with central necrosis on the gluteal areas [38A]. Laboratory results showed the presence of cryoglobulin, cryofibrinogen, and c-ANCA. PTU is considered to be the most common inducer of ANCA-associated microscopic polyangiitis [39R]. When PTU was stopped and replacing it with MMI, the skin lesions improved within a week, but the cryoglobulins, cryofibrinogens, c-ANCA and anti-SSA remained positive even after 5 months.

Hepatotoxicity

DILI (drug-induced liver injury) is a major problem for pharmaceutical industry and drug development. Although MMI has been associated with liver disease, it is typically due to cholestatic dysfunction, not hepatocellular inflammation [40R]. Due to the idiosyncratic nature of the injury, the understanding of the mechanism of these toxicities is limited. It appears that reactive metabolite formation and immune-mediated toxicity may play a role in antithyroids liver toxicity, especially those caused by MMI, though other mechanism including reactive metabolites formation, oxidative stress induction, intracellular targets dysfunction may be possible [41H]. A recent report presents two women with cholestatic jaundice due to methimazole treatment. Before initiating therapy, both women had normal liver function and complete blood counts. DILI was inferred based on the relationship between methimazole therapy initiation and cholestasis onset. After methimazole was discontinued, the symptoms gradually resolved. DILI is a rare condition that is more likely to occur in females and has dose dependent relationship [42A].

Pancreatitis

Pancreatitis has very rarely been reported in association with MMI treatment [43A]. A population-based case–control study analyzing the database of the Taiwan National Health Insurance Program involving 5764 individuals aged 20–84 years with a first attack of acute pancreatitis from 1998 to 2011 was evaluated to estimate the relative risk of acute pancreatitis associated with the use of MMI. The study did not detect a substantial association between the use of MMI and risk of acute pancreatitis [44A]. Recently, a sixth case of MMI-induced pancreatitis (according to the authors), in a patient with toxic multinodular goiter, was reported. The authors suggest exploring the possibility of pancreatitis in subjects treated with MMI in the presence of suggestive symptoms. Discontinuation of the drug is recommended if the diagnosis is confirmed by elevated pancreatic enzymes [45A].

Miscellaneous Side Effects

For the first time a case of an erythema annulare mimicking a figurate inflammatory dermatosis of infancy has been reported in a 11-year-old female with GD on MMI treatment. Fifteen days after MMI administration, generalized itching erythematous rash developed all over the body. Erythema disappeared slowly after MMI withdrawal. The clinicians suspect the rash to be due to methimazole use. Recently a case of Insulin-induced Autoimmune Syndrome (IAS) has been reported. A 76-year-old female with history of hyperthyroidism also exhibited hypotension and low blood glucose which was attributed to use of MMI. Though this condition is rare, patients exhibiting hypoglycemia with autoimmune patients, prior use of MMI is these patient should be evaluated. Once discontinuing her methimazole and treating with dextrose and octreotide, the hypoglycemic episodes resolved [46A]. In another first report methimazole-induced chronic cutaneous lupus erythematosus (CCLE) was documented in literature. A 30-year-old female with autoimmune thyroid disease developed an erythematous patch on her nasal pyramid. The patch appeared after 1 month on methimazole therapy and worsened on sun exposure. After discontinuing MMI therapy, the symptoms gradually resolved [47A].

References

[1] France M, Schofield J, Kwok S, et al. Treatment of homozygous familial hypercholesterolemia. Clin Lipidol. 2014;9(1):101–18. http://dx.doi.org/10.2217/clp.13.79 [R].

[2] Anagnostis P, Karras S, Lambrinoudaki I, et al. Lipoprotein(a) in postmenopausal women: assessment of cardiovascular risk and therapeutic options. Int J Clin Pract. 2016;70(12):967–77. http://dx.doi.org/10.1111/ijcp.12903 [R].

[3] Andersen SL, Olsen J, Wu CS, et al. Birth defects after early pregnancy use of antithyroid drugs: a Danish nationwide study. J Clin Endocrinol Metab. 2013;98(11):4373–81. http://dx.doi.org/10.1210/jc.2013-2831. Epub 2013/10/24. PubMed PMID: 24151287 [M].

[4] Korevaar TIM, Muetzel R, Medici M, et al. Association of maternal thyroid function during early pregnancy with offspring IQ and brain morphology in childhood: a population-based prospective cohort study. Lancet Diabetes Endocrinol. 2016;4(1):35–43. http://dx.doi.org/10.1016/S2213-8587(15)00327-7 [M].

[5] Kelderman-Bolk N, Visser TJ, Tijssen JP, et al. Quality of life in patients with primary hypothyroidism related to BMI. Eur J Endocrinol. 2015;173(4):507–15. http://dx.doi.org/10.1530/eje-15-0395. Epub 2015/07/15. PubMed PMID: 26169304 [R].

[6] Bengtsson C, Padyukov L, Källberg H, et al. Thyroxin substitution and the risk of developing rheumatoid arthritis; results from the Swedish population-based EIRA study. Ann Rheum Dis. 2014;73(6):1096–100. http://dx.doi.org/10.1136/annrheumdis-2013-203354 [R].

[7] Krysiak R, Kowalska B, Okopien B. Serum 25-hydroxyvitamin D and parathyroid hormone levels in non-lactating women with post-partum thyroiditis: the effect of L-thyroxine treatment. Basic Clin Pharmacol Toxicol. 2015;116(6):503–7. http://dx.doi.org/10.1111/bcpt.12349. Epub 2014/11/15. PubMed PMID: 25395280 [C].

[8] Keles MK, Yosma E, Aydogdu IO, et al. Multiple subungual pyogenic granulomas following levothyroxine treatment. J Craniofac Surg. 2015;26(6):e476–7. http://dx.doi.org/10.1097/scs.0000000000001922. Epub 2015/09/12. PubMed PMID: 26355986 [R].

[9] Kim MK, Yun KJ, Kim MH, et al. The effects of thyrotropin-suppressing therapy on bone metabolism in patients with well-differentiated thyroid carcinoma. Bone. 2015;71:101–5. http://dx.doi.org/10.1016/j.bone.2014.10.009. Epub 2014/12/03. PubMed PMID: 25445448 [C].

[10] Nyandege AN, Slattum PW, Harpe SE. Risk of fracture and the concomitant use of bisphosphonates with osteoporosis-inducing medications. Ann Pharmacother. 2015;49(4):437–47. http://dx.doi.org/10.1177/1060028015569594. Epub 2015/02/11. PubMed PMID: 25667198 [R].

[11] Bakiner O, Bozkirli E, Ertugrul D, et al. Plasma fetuin-A levels are reduced in patients with hypothyroidism. Eur J Endocrinol. 2014;170(3):411–8. http://dx.doi.org/10.1530/EJE-13-0831. PubMed PMID: 24366942 [C].

[12] Stuijver DJ, van Zaane B, Squizzato A, et al. The effects of an extremely high dose of levothyroxine on coagulation and fibrinolysis. J Thromb Haemost. 2010;8(6):1427–8. http://dx.doi.org/10.1111/j.1538-7836.2010.03854.x. PubMed PMID: 20345725 [A].

[13] Kreisner E, Lutzky M, Gross JL. Charcoal hemoperfusion in the treatment of levothyroxine intoxication. Thyroid. 2010;20(2):209–12. http://dx.doi.org/10.1089/thy.2009.0054. PubMed PMID: 20151829 [A].

[14] Irving SA, Vadiveloo T, Leese GP. Drugs that interact with levothyroxine: an observational study from the Thyroid Epidemiology, Audit and Research Study (TEARS). Clin Endocrinol (Oxf). 2015;82(1):136–41. http://dx.doi.org/10.1111/cen.12559. Epub 2014/07/22. PubMed PMID: 25040647 [C].

[15] Goldberg AS, Tirona RG, Asher LJ, et al. Ciprofloxacin and rifampin have opposite effects on levothyroxine absorption. Thyroid. 2013;23(11):1374–8. http://dx.doi.org/10.1089/thy.2013.0014. Epub 2013/05/08. PubMed PMID: 23647409 [A].

[16] Fukuhara N, Horiguchi K, Nishioka H, et al. Short-term preoperative octreotide treatment for TSH-secreting pituitary adenoma. Endocr J. 2015;62(1):21–7. http://dx.doi.org/10.1507/endocrj.EJ14-0118. Epub 2014/10/03. PubMed PMID: 25273395 [C].

[17] Pearce EN, Andersson M, Zimmermann MB. Global iodine nutrition: where do we stand in 2013? Thyroid. 2013;23(5):523–8. http://dx.doi.org/10.1089/thy.2013.0128. Epub 2013/03/12. PubMed PMID: 23472655 [R].

[18] Laillou A, Sophonneary P, Kuong K, et al. Low urinary iodine concentration among mothers and children in Cambodia. Nutrients. 2016;8(4):172. http://dx.doi.org/10.3390/nu8040172. Epub 2016/04/09. PubMed PMID: 27058551; PMCID: Pmc4848647 [R].

[19] Mizehoun-Adissoda C, Desport JC, Houinato D, et al. Evaluation of iodine intake and status using inductively coupled plasma mass spectrometry in urban and rural areas in Benin, West Africa. Nutrition. 2016;32(5):560–5. http://dx.doi.org/10.1016/j.nut.2015.11.007. Epub 2016/01/23. PubMed PMID: 26796150 [C].

[20] Yang J, Zhu L, Li X, et al. Iodine status of vulnerable populations in henan province of China 2013–2014 after the implementation of the new iodized salt standard. Biol Trace Elem Res. 2016;173(1):7–13. http://dx.doi.org/10.1007/s12011-016-0619-1. Epub 2016/01/19. PubMed PMID: 26779621 [M].

[21] Edmonds JC, McLean RM, Williams SM, et al. Urinary iodine concentration of New Zealand adults improves with mandatory fortification of bread with iodised salt but not to predicted levels. Eur J Nutr. 2016;55(3):1201–12. http://dx.doi.org/10.1007/s00394-015-0933-y. Epub 2015/05/29. PubMed PMID: 26018655 [C].

[22] Gernand AD, Schulze KJ, Stewart CP, et al. Micronutrient deficiencies in pregnancy worldwide: health effects and prevention. Nat Rev Endocrinol. 2016;12(5):274–89. http://dx.doi.org/10.1038/nrendo.2016.37. PubMed PMID: PMC4927329 [R].

[23] Overcash RT, Marc-Aurele KL, Hull AD, et al. Maternal iodine exposure: a case of fetal goiter and neonatal hearing loss. Pediatrics. 2016;137(4) [A].

[24] Krämer M, Kupka R, Subramanian S, et al. Association between household unavailability of iodized salt and child growth: evidence from 89 demographic and health surveys. Am J Clin Nutr. 2016;104(4):1093–100. http://dx.doi.org/10.3945/ajcn.115.124719 [R].

[25] Deshmukh R, Singh AN, Martinez M, et al. Thyroid hormones, iodine and iodides, and antithyroid drugs. In: Sidhartha DR, editor. Side effects of drugs annual. United States: Elsevier; 2016. p. 443–52 [chapter 39] [R].

[26] Malhotra S, Kumta S, Bhutada A, et al. Topical iodine-induced thyrotoxicosis in a newborn with a giant omphalocele. AJP Rep. 2016;06(02):e243–5. http://dx.doi.org/10.1055/s-0036-1584879 [A].

[27] Cooper DS. Antithyroid drugs. N Engl J Med. 2005;352(9):905–17. http://dx.doi.org/10.1056/NEJMra042972. PubMed PMID: 15745981 [R].

[28] Werner MC, Romaldini JH, Bromberg N, et al. Adverse effects related to thionamide drugs and their dose regimen. Am J Med Sci. 1989;297(4):216–9. PubMed PMID: 2523194 [C].

[29] Watanabe N, Narimatsu H, Noh JY, et al. Antithyroid drug-induced hematopoietic damage: a retrospective cohort study of agranulocytosis and pancytopenia involving 50,385 patients with Graves' disease. J Clin Endocrinol Metab. 2012;97(1):E49–53. http://dx.doi.org/10.1210/jc.2011-2221. PubMed PMID: 22049174 [R].

[30] Arrigo T, Cutroneo PM, Vaccaro M, et al. Lateralized exanthem mimicking figurate inflammatory dermatosis of infancy after methimazole therapy. Int J Immunopathol Pharmacol. 2016;29(4):707–11. http://dx.doi.org/10.1177/0394632016652412. PubMed PMID: 27272160 [A].

[31] Sing CW, Wong IC, Cheung BM, et al. Incidence and risk estimate of drug-induced agranulocytosis in Hong Kong Chinese. a population-based case-control study. Pharmacoepidemiol Drug Saf. 2017;26:248–55. http://dx.doi.org/10.1002/pds.4156. PubMed PMID: 28083886 [c].

[32] Hallberg P, Eriksson N, Ibañez L, et al. Genetic variants associated with antithyroid drug-induced agranulocytosis: a genome-wide association study in a European population. Lancet Diabetes Endocrinol. 2016;4(6):507–16. http://dx.doi.org/10.1016/S2213-8587(16)00113-3 [C].

[33] Criado PR, Grizzo Peres Martins AC, Gaviolli CF, et al. Propylthiouracil-induced vasculitis with antineutrophil cytoplasmic antibody. Int J Low Extrem Wounds.

2015;14(2):187–91. http://dx.doi.org/10.1177/1534734614549418. PubMed PMID: 25256279 [R].

[34] Sohar G, Kovacs M, Gyorkos A, et al. Rare side effects in management of hyperthyroidism. Case report. Orv Hetil. 2016;157(22):869–72. http://dx.doi.org/10.1556/650.2016.30465. PubMed PMID: 27211356 [A].

[35] Yi X-Y, Wang Y, Li Q-F, et al. Possibly propylthiouracil-induced antineutrophilic cytoplasmic antibody-associated vasculitis manifested as blood coagulation disorders: a case report. Medicine. 2016;95(41):e5068. http://dx.doi.org/10.1097/MD.0000000000005068. PubMed PMID: PMC5072949 [A].

[36] Wall AE, Weaver SM, Litt JS, et al. Propylthiouracil-associated leukocytoclastic necrotizing cutaneous vasculitis: a case report and review of the literature. J Burn Care Res. 2017;38:e678–85. http://dx.doi.org/10.1097/bcr.0000000000000464. Publish Ahead of Print. PubMed PMID: 01253092-900000000-98491 [A].

[37] Ortiz-Diaz EO. A 27-year-old woman presenting with refractory hypoxaemic respiratory failure, haemoptysis and thyrotoxicosis: a rare manifestation of propylthiouracil therapy. BMJ Case Rep. 2014;2014:1. http://dx.doi.org/10.1136/bcr-2014-204915. Epub 2014/08/26. PubMed PMID: 25150234 [A].

[38] Akkurt ZM, Ucmak D, Acar G, et al. Cryoglobulin and antineutrophil cytoplasmic antibody positive cutaneous vasculitis due to propylthiouracil. Indian J Dermatol Venereol Leprol. 2014;80(3):262–4. http://dx.doi.org/10.4103/0378-6323.132261. Epub 2014/05/16. PubMed PMID: 24823411 [A].

[39] Bonaci-Nikolic B, Nikolic MM, Andrejevic S, et al. Antineutrophil cytoplasmic antibody (ANCA)-associated autoimmune diseases induced by antithyroid drugs: comparison with idiopathic ANCA vasculitides. Arthritis Res Ther. 2005;7(5):R1072–81. http://dx.doi.org/10.1186/ar1789. PubMed PMID: 16207324; PMCID: 1257438 [R].

[40] Arab DM, Malatjalian DA, Rittmaster RS. Severe cholestatic jaundice in uncomplicated hyperthyroidism treated with methimazole. J Clin Endocrinol Metab. 1995;80(4):1083–5. http://dx.doi.org/10.1210/jcem.80.4.7714072. PubMed PMID: 7714072 [R].

[41] Heidari R, Niknahad H, Jamshidzadeh A, et al. An overview on the proposed mechanisms of antithyroid drugs-induced liver injury. Adv Pharm Bull. 2015;5(1):1–11. http://dx.doi.org/10.5681/apb.2015.001. PubMed PMID: 25789213; PMCID: PMC4352210 [H].

[42] Zou H, Jin L, Wang LR, et al. Methimazole-induced cholestatic hepatitis: two cases report and literature review. Oncotarget. 2016;7(4):5088–91. http://dx.doi.org/10.18632/oncotarget.6144. PubMed PMID: 26498145; PMCID: PMC4826268 [A].

[43] Yang M, Qu H, Deng HC. Acute pancreatitis induced by methimazole in a patient with Graves' disease. Thyroid. 2012;22(1):94–96. http://dx.doi.org/10.1089/thy.2011.0210. PubMed PMID: 22136208 [A].

[44] Lai S-W, Lin C-L, Liao K-F. Use of methimazole and risk of acute pancreatitis: a case–control study in Taiwan. Indian J Pharmacol. 2016;48(2):192–5 [A].

[45] Agito K, Manni A. Acute pancreatitis induced by methimazole in a patient with subclinical hyperthyroidism. J Investig Med High Impact Case Rep. 2015;3(2):1–4. http://dx.doi.org/10.1177/2324709615592229. 2324709615592229. PubMed PMID: 26425645; PMCID: PMC4557366 [A].

[46] Jain N, Savani M, Agarwal M, et al. Methimazole-induced insulin autoimmune syndrome. Ther Adv Endocrinol Metab. 2016;7(4):178–81. http://dx.doi.org/10.1177/2042018816658396. PubMed PMID: 27540463; PMCID: PMC4973408 [A].

[47] Venturi M, Ferreli C, Pinna AL, et al. Methimazole-induced chronic cutaneous lupus erythematosus. J Eur Acad Dermatol Venereol. 2017;31(2):e116–7. http://dx.doi.org/10.1111/jdv.13857. PubMed PMID: 27519167 [A].

37

Insulin and Other Hypoglycemic Drugs

Jasmine M. Pittman*, *Laura A. Schalliol*[†,1], *Sidhartha D. Ray*[‡]

*Parkwest Medical Center, Knoxville, TN, United States
[†]South College School of Pharmacy, Knoxville, TN, United States
[‡]Manchester University College of Pharmacy, Natural & Health Sciences, Fort Wayne, IN, United States
[1]Corresponding author: lschalliol@southcollegetn.edu

ALPHA-GLUCOSIDASE INHIBITORS
[SEDA-31, 691; SEDA-32, 772; SEDA-33, 893; SEDA-36, 647; SEDA-37, 523]

Acarbose

Cardiovascular

Acarbose was associated with a reduced risk of recurrent major adverse cardiovascular events (MACE) in patients recently diagnosed with impaired glucose tolerance (IGT) and acute coronary syndrome (ACS). In this randomized controlled trial (RCT), 135 patients newly diagnosed with IGT and hospitalized with ACS were randomized to the acarbose 150 mg/day group ($n = 67$) or the control group (no acarbose, $n = 68$). After a mean follow-up of 2.3 years, there was a significant reduction in the risk of recurrent MACE in the acarbose group (26.67% vs 46.88% in the control group, $P < 0.05$). Thickening of carotid intima-media thickness was also significantly slower in the acarbose group [1.28 ± 0.42 vs 1.51 ± 0.64 mm in the control group, $P < 0.05$] [1C].

AMYLIN ANALOGS

Pramlintide

Cardiovascular

Cardiovascular (CV) safety was reviewed from five randomized controlled phase III and IV trials in adults with type 2 diabetes mellitus (T2DM). The duration of these trials ranged from 16 to 52 weeks. Four studies compared pramlintide with placebo, and one study compared pramlintide with a mealtime rapid-acting insulin analog. No differences were seen in the number of investigator-reported MACE between pramlintide (4.7%) and comparator (4.5%) groups with a risk ratio (RR) of 1.034 (95% CI 0.694–1.540) [2M].

BIGUANIDES [SEDA-33, 893; SEDA-34, 687; SEDA-36, 647; SEDA-37, 523-526; SEDA-38, 459-461]

Metformin

Metabolism

A meta-analysis including six RCTs was conducted of 301 adolescents with type 1 diabetes mellitus (T1DM) receiving metformin in addition to insulin. Patients had an average diabetes duration of five to ten years, were an average age of less than 20 years, and were taking metformin for an average of three to nine months. Metformin doses ranged from 1000 to 2000 mg per day. Metformin use significantly decreased both body mass index (BMI) [standardized mean difference (SMD) −0.36, 95% CI −0.59 to −0.14] and body weight [mean difference (MD) −1.93, 95% CI −2.58 to −1.27] in participants, especially in those who were overweight or obese [3M].

Acid–Base Balance

Metformin-associated lactic acidosis (MALA) was reported in a 52-year-old female with a past medical history of hypertension, alcohol dependence, and T2DM. The patient presented with altered mental status, hypoglycemia, and shock. Her metformin concentration was 51 µg/mL (therapeutic range 1–2 µg/mL), making MALA probable. The patient ultimately recovered after prolonged critical illness [4A].

A study with a duration of 12 weeks assessed glycemic control in 240 patients with T2DM. Patients received delayed-release metformin, extended-release metformin, or placebo. A patient in the extended-release metformin 2000 mg group experienced an increase in blood lactate levels for 16 days (up to 5.9 mmol/L). The patient experienced no other adverse effects, and the treatment regimen was not changed [5c].

Skin

A 41-year-old female developed a fixed-drug eruption (FDE) demonstrated by erythematic pustular lesions on the soles of the feet and the palms of the hands. The reaction occurred after using immediate release metformin 1000 mg twice daily (BID). The dose of metformin was reduced to 500 mg BID, and some improvement was seen. Symptoms fully resolved after total discontinuation of metformin. The patient tried metformin nine months later, and the reaction returned. Once again symptoms resolved after discontinuation of metformin [6A].

Musculoskeletal

In a retrospective analysis of patients undergoing surgical repair of femoral or tibial fractures, those with diabetes were compared to matched controls without diabetes. The control group was composed of 166 patients (138 males), and the treatment group included 36 patients (25 males). This study found that medications used for the treatment of diabetes, including biguanides used as monotherapy or in combination with a sulfonylurea (SU) or a dipeptidyl peptidase 4 inhibitor (DPP4I), impair the healing process through slowing the formation of callus ($P < 0.001$) or bridging ($P = 0.014$). Additionally, non-union of the bones was more likely in those patients on one of the studied medications ($P = 0.006$) in comparison to those without antidiabetic medications [7c]. Of note, the retrospective study design of this trial prevents determining causality. With data showing diabetes can impair healing time, the result shown in this study may be due to the disease state itself rather than the medications associated with its treatment. A more ideal control would have been to include those with diabetes controlled without medications in order to identify if it is the disease state or the medications themselves that may be associated with impaired fracture healing. Additional studies determining the effects of these medications on bone healing may be warranted.

DIPEPTIDYL PEPTIDASE-4 INHIBITORS (DPP4Is) [SEDA-33, 894; SEDA-34, 688; SEDA-36, 648; SEDA-37, 526-528; SEDA-38, 454-457]

Cardiovascular

In a large analysis investigating the association between DPP4Is and heart failure (HF) hospitalizations, patients with diabetes on a DPP4I were identified in the National Health Insurance Claims database of Taiwan. This was a large study including a total of 239 669 patients (sitagliptin $n = 159\,330$; saxagliptin $n = 38\,561$; and vildagliptin $n = 41\,778$). The primary outcome was first hospitalization for heart failure (HHF). Follow-up ranged from 269 to 313 days. The crude incidence rate of HF was 1.91, 2.63, and 2.77 per 100 person-years for vildagliptin, saxagliptin, and sitagliptin, respectively. Saxagliptin showed similar risk as sitagliptin, with a hazard ratio (HR) of 0.98 (95% CI 0.91–1.06). Of note, vildagliptin displayed a lower risk of HF (HR 0.85, 95% CI 0.78–0.93) [8MC].

Use of DPP4Is was associated with an increased risk of HF (RR 1.13, 95% CI 1.01–1.26) in a systematic review which included 35 RCTs published before May 2015 and the Trial Evaluating Cardiovascular Outcomes with Sitagliptin (TECOS). This review included data from 54 664 patients [9M].

An evaluation of the FDA Adverse Event Reporting System (FAERS) data from 2006 to 2013 was undertaken to investigate the incidence of HF with DPP4I use from 2006 through 2013. HF during DPP4I use was recorded in 390 reports (4.4% of total reports). Statistically significant reporting odds ratios (RORs) emerged for DPP4Is as a class (ROR 1.17, 95% CI 1.05–1.29) and for individual agents within the class. Associations were found with saxagliptin (ROR 1.68, 95% CI 1.29–2.17) and vildagliptin (ROR 2.39, 95% CI 1.38–4.14). In consolidated analyses the RORs for saxagliptin (2.60, 95% CI 1.92–3.50) and vildagliptin (4.07, 95% CI 2.28–7.27) increased, and the ROR for sitagliptin became significant (1.61, 95% CI 1.40–1.86). Concomitant medications that increase the risk of developing HF were reported in more than 50% of cases; when adjusted, the RORs of saxagliptin (2.30, 95% CI 1.70–3.10), vildagliptin (3.15, 95% CI 1.76–5.63), and sitagliptin (1.48, 95% CI 1.28–1.71) all remained significant. The FAERS data are consistent with other clinical studies that have found saxagliptin to have a possible association with HF [10C].

A meta-analysis of 43 trials ($n = 68\,775$) and 12 observational studies ($n = 1\,777\,358$) found low-quality evidence for no increased risk of HF associated with DPP4I use in comparison to the control. Five trials reporting HF admission provided moderate-quality evidence for an increased risk in patients treated with DPP4I vs control.

The pooling of adjusted estimates from observational studies similarly suggests a possible increased risk of HHF although the quality of that evidence is considered very low-quality [11M].

Respiratory

Acute respiratory failure (ARF) was reported in a 38-year-old Japanese female with newly diagnosed DM. The patient developed ARF one day after administration of vildagliptin 100 mg daily. The patient was admitted in a comatose state after several hours of dyspnea and hyperpnea. The patient was diagnosed with acute kidney failure and diabetic ketoacidosis (DKA) and received insulin and intravenous saline. Nonsegmental ground-glass opacities in the lower lobes of both lungs were seen on chest computed tomography (CT), which was initially treated with empiric antibiotic therapy and oxygen. Pulmonary problems resolved within weeks. The patient fully recovered after discontinuation of vildagliptin. Of note, due to the development of DKA and insulin-deficient hyperglycemia, the patient met the diagnostic criteria for acute-onset T1DM [12A].

Pancreas

DPP4Is were associated with a significantly increased risk of acute pancreatitis (RR 1.57, 95% CI 1.03–2.39) in a systematic review of 36 double-blind RCTs that included data for 54 664 patients [9M].

In a case–control review of the FAERS database from November 1968 to December 2013, there was an increased risk of pancreatic cancer associated with all of the DPP4Is, with the exception of alogliptin. A reported EB_{05} of ≥ 2 was associated with an increased risk of pancreatic cancer. The study found an EB_{05} of <2 for alogliptin, 4.9 for linagliptin, 7.1 for saxagliptin, and 10.3 for sitagliptin [13M].

Musculoskeletal

In a retrospective analysis of patients undergoing surgical repair of femoral or tibial fractures, those with diabetes were compared to matched controls without diabetes. The control group was composed of 166 patients (138 males), and the treatment group included 36 patients (25 males). This study found that diabetic medications, including biguanides used as monotherapy or in combination with a SU or a DPP4I, impair the healing process through slowing the formation of callus ($P < 0.001$) or bridging ($P = 0.014$). Additionally, nonunion of the bones was more likely in those patients on one of the studied diabetic medications ($P = 0.006$) in comparison to those without diabetic medications [7c]. As discussed earlier in the chapter, the retrospective study design of this trial prevents determining causality. Also a more ideal control would have been to include those with diabetes controlled without medications to identify if it is the disease state or the medications themselves that may be associated with impaired fracture healing.

In a meta-analysis including 51 RCTs published between 2006 and 2014, there was no association found between DPP4I use and fracture risk. The individual studies included varied populations with nine RCTs being multi-site trials and 39 being multi-country studies. The meta-analysis included two RCTs investigating vildagliptin, three with linagliptin, five with alogliptin, 12 with saxagliptin, and 29 with sitagliptin [14M].

Saxagliptin

Cardiovascular

In a meta-analysis of 100 RCTs involving 54 758 incretin-based therapy users and 48 175 controls, saxagliptin was associated with an increased risk of HF [odds ratio (OR) 1.23, 95% CI 1.03–1.46). These results are primarily driven by SAVOR-TIMI-53, and when that trial was excluded, the difference in risk was not present [15M].

In a study using data from the FDA Mini-Sentinel program including information from 178 million persons and 358 million person-years from 2000 to 2014, saxagliptin was found to be significantly less associated with HHF than insulin (adjusted HR 0.66, 95% CI 0.51–0.85) and pioglitazone (adjusted HR 0.58, 95% CI 0.41–0.83). It is worth noting that in those with a high risk of developing HF, the difference between treatment groups was not found to be significant between any groups assessed [16MC].

Pancreas

Acute pancreatitis was reported in a 33-year-old male with a five-year history of T2DM. Saxagliptin 5 mg daily was initiated, and the patient was assessed in an outpatient clinic a few months later. During the outpatient visit, treatment was changed to glimepiride and saxagliptin/metformin 5 mg/1000 mg daily. A few months later, the patient was hospitalized with complaints of breathlessness, dizziness, nausea, vomiting, and palpitations. The patient was initially thought to have DKA, but acute pancreatitis was considered due to the presence of abdominal pain, nausea, and vomiting. An abdominal ultrasound revealed irregular, turbid fluid around the pancreas. Abdominal CT scan with contrast revealed edema, evidence of necrotic changes in the tail of the pancreas, and signs of acute pancreatitis. Upon resolution of the acute condition, the patient was eventually discharged on extended-release metformin and premixed insulin [17A].

Musculoskeletal

A case of arthralgia was reported in a 55-year-old female patient with T2DM taking saxagliptin 5 mg daily and metformin, which she had been on for the previous two years. Two months after starting saxagliptin, the patient reported bilateral knee pain. Saxagliptin was discontinued, and the knee pain resolved completely after one month without saxagliptin therapy [18A].

Sitagliptin

Cardiovascular

Patients with end-stage renal disease (ESRD) on dialysis and T2DM who were treated with sitagliptin between 2009 and 2011 ($n=870$) were matched to a control cohort ($n=3480$). The majority of patients were ≥65-years-old, male, receiving hemodialysis, and had diabetes for roughly nine years. The mean follow-up was one year. HHF was more likely in the sitagliptin cohort than in the control cohort (1130 vs 754 per 10000 person-years, adjusted HR 1.52, 95% CI 1.21–1.90). Additionally, increased sitagliptin doses were significantly associated with increased HHF risk. Those at greater risk of HHF after taking sitagliptin were those without severe hypoglycemia, without treatment with angiotensin-converting enzyme (ACE) inhibitors, with a history of HF, or on hemodialysis [19C].

A study from Taiwan's National Health Insurance database evaluated the risk of HHF in a sample of sitagliptin ever-users ($n=85859$) and never-users ($n=85859$). Groups were followed for the first event of HHF. Incidence of HHF was 1020.16 and 832.54 per 100000 person-years for ever- and never-users, respectively, with an overall HR of 1.262 (95% CI 1.167–1.364). Additional risk factors for HHF in sitagliptin users were older age, longer duration of diabetes, male gender, and use of insulin, SUs, calcium channel blockers (CCBs), aspirin, ticlopidine, clopidogrel, and dipyridamole [20MC].

In a study using data from the FDA Mini-Sentinel program, including information from 178 million persons and 358 million person-years from 2000 to 2014, sitagliptin was found to be significantly less associated with HHF than insulin (adjusted HR 0.71, 95% CI 0.63–0.81), pioglitazone (adjusted HR 0.68, 95% CI 0.58–0.81), and SUs (0.83, 95% CI 0.73–0.93). Of note, in those with a high risk of developing HF, the difference between treatment groups was not found to be significant between any groups assessed [16MC].

Endocrine

A study of Taiwanese patients with newly diagnosed T2DM evaluated the risk of cancer in those who were newly treated with sitagliptin ($n=58238$ ever-users) or other antidiabetic agents ($n=312853$ never-users).

Thyroid cancer developed in 28 ever-users and 172 never-users, with a respective incidence of 29.34 and 22.13 per 100000 person-years and an overall HR of 1.516 (95% CI 1.011–2.271), suggesting a significantly higher risk associated with sitagliptin [21MC].

Pancreas

A retrospective analysis of Taiwan's National Health Insurance database included data from 1999 to 2010. Participants were at least 25-years-old with newly diagnosed T2DM. The incidence of pancreatic cancer was followed for ever-users of sitagliptin ($n=71137$) and never-users ($n=933046$) until December 31, 2011. Eighty-three ever-users and 3658 never-users developed pancreatic cancer, with an incidence of 73.6 and 55.0 per 100000 person-years and an overall HR of 1.40 (95% CI 1.13–1.75) [22MC].

Urinary Tract

A 56-year-old male patient with a history of T2DM and stage 2 chronic kidney disease (CKD) secondary to diabetic nephropathy presented with an acute decline of kidney function and complaints of nausea, fatigue, and vomiting. He reported starting sitagliptin 50 mg daily two weeks prior. Non-invasive work-up did not divulge the cause of acute kidney failure. An ultrasound revealed normal kidney size. Kidney biopsy revealed acute tubulointerstitial nephritis (ATIN), which was attributed to sitagliptin use. Sitagliptin was discontinued and replaced with an insulin regimen. The patient was treated with prednisone 20 mg PO daily for six weeks. Creatinine levels trended downwards after three to six weeks. Prednisone was then tapered over a period of six weeks. The patient's kidney function returned to baseline [23A].

Musculoskeletal

A 60-year-old female was hospitalized due to complaints of generalized weakness, muscle aches, and atypical chest pain for one week after starting sitagliptin. The patient also reported taking atorvastatin during this time frame, but she correlated her symptoms with initiating sitagliptin. The patient's creatinine phosphokinase (CPK) was elevated at 13456 U/L. Sitagliptin and atorvastatin were discontinued as the case authors felt the rhabdomyolysis was due to a potential interaction between the medications through their metabolism as CYP3A4 substrates, and the CPK dropped to 1220 U/L at discharge [24A].

Linagliptin

Urinary Tract

Linagliptin-associated acute kidney injury (AKI) was reported in a 54-year-old African-American male with preexisting CKD. His kidney function was stable with a baseline SCr of 4.3 mg/dL, estimated glomerular filtration rate (GFR) of 18 mL/min/1.73 m^2, and a BUN of 64 mg/dL. Potassium level was 6.4 mmol/L. The patient's hyperkalemia was attributed to orange juice that patient was ingesting daily for the prevention and treatment of recurrent hypoglycemic episodes during the prior week. Due to hypoglycemic risk, the patient's glimepiride was discontinued, and linagliptin 5 mg once daily was started. One week later, SCr and BUN increased to 7.0 and 101 mg/dL, and hyperkalemia continued. The patient was admitted for evaluation of AKI. Linagliptin was discontinued as the onset of AKI corresponded with its initiation. Oral kayexalate was administered along with intravenous normal saline over 24 hours. SCr and potassium levels improved to 5.7 mg/dL and 5.1 mmol/L, respectively. The patient refused further treatment and was discharged. The patient's lisinopril and linagliptin was not restarted, and his SCr improved to 3.4 mg/dL in 10 days, remaining stable for the next two months. The authors concluded the patient's AKI was caused by renal hypoperfusion due to concomitant lisinopril with linagliptin-induced natriuresis [25A].

GLUCAGON-LIKE PEPTIDE-1 (GLP-1) RECEPTOR AGONISTS [SEDA-33, 896; SEDA-34, 690; SEDA-36, 650; SEDA-37, 528-530; SEDA-38, 457-458]

Exenatide

Cardiovascular

In a subgroup analysis of a larger study, 114 Latin Americans with T2DM currently on insulin glargine and metformin were randomized to receive either exenatide twice daily or insulin lispro three times daily. Three patients in the exenatide group experienced serious adverse events, including osteomyelitis (resolved), congestive heart failure (CHF) (resolved), and hemorrhagic stroke resulting in death, but study investigators determined this side effect was unrelated to study treatment [26c].

An increased risk of arrhythmia was associated with exenatide use (OR 2.83; 95% CI, 1.06–7.57) in a meta-analysis of 100 RCTs involving 54 758 incretin-based therapy users and 48 175 controls [20M].

INSULINS [SEDA-15, 1761; SEDA-34, 685; SEDA-36, 645-647; SEDA-37, 521-523, SEDA-38, 453-454]

Cardiovascular

There was a case report regarding a subdural hematoma in a male patient with a 40-year history of T1DM.

The patient was on both insulin aspart and insulin detemir, and he had been injecting those doses into the same part of his abdomen for years, causing lipohypertrophy. Injecting into an area of lipophyertrophy causes delayed absorption of the insulin, increasing the risk of hypoglycemia. The patient experienced a hypoglycemia-induced fall that caused the subdural hematoma. The authors recommend monitoring all patients on long-term insulin for areas of lipohypertrophy through palpation of the injections site(s); they recommend monitoring at least once a year and any time a patient presents with recurrent hypoglycemia [27A].

In a meta-analysis comparing metformin to insulin for the treatment of gestational diabetes, the investigators found less incidence of pregnancy-induced hypertension in those on metformin in comparison to insulin therapy (RR 0.54, 95% CI 0.31–0.91, $P = 0.02$), with no significant differences in other outcomes including large for gestational age infants, neonatal hypoglycemia, phototherapy use, respiratory distress syndrome, and perinatal death [28M].

In an observational study focused on initiating basal insulins in an insured population of adults with T2DM, there was a 27% increased risk of acute MI in those randomized to premixed insulins when compared to long-acting insulin analogs (HR 1.27, 95% CI 1.02–1.58, $P < 0.001$); this risk was not shown when comparing insulin NPH to the long-acting insulin analogs (HR 0.94, 95% CI 0.74–1.19, $P = 0.594$). Other risk factors associated with an increased risk of acute MI include previous MI (HR 1.78, 95% CI 1.41–2.24, $P < 0.001$), CHF (HR 1.28, 95% CI 1.03–1.59, $P = 0.029$), hyperlipidemia (HR 1.26, 95% CI 1.03–1.53, $P = 0.023$), diabetic retinopathy (1.27, 95% CI 1.03–1.57, $P = 0.025$), use of a CCB (HR 1.32, 95% CI 1.08–1.60, $P = 0.006$), and use of a nitrate (HR 1.71, 95% CI 1.36–2.16, $P < 0.001$) [29c].

In a study using data from the FDA Mini-Sentinel program, including information from 178 million persons and 358 million person-years from 2000 to 2014, both saxagliptin and sitagliptin were found to be significantly less associated with HHF than insulin (adjusted HR 0.66, 95% CI 0.51–0.85, and adjusted HR 0.71, 95% CI 0.63–0.81, respectively). As stated earlier in the chapter, the difference between treatment groups was not found to be significant between any groups determined to have a high risk of developing HF [16MC].

Endocrine

A meta-analysis using 301 RCTs that involved a total of 118 094 participants investigated CV mortality associated with medications for the management of diabetes. When comparing basal insulin as monotherapy against other antihyperglycemic agents, the risk of hypoglycemia, a secondary safety outcome, was much greater with basal insulin (odds ratio (OR) 17.9, 95% CI 1.97–162) [30M].

In a trial involving hospitalized patients with T2DM treated with diet, oral agents, and/or insulin, starting the patient on a regimen of 70% insulin aspart protamine/30% insulin aspart was compared to a basal-bolus regimen with insulin glargine and insulin glulisine. Hypoglycemia was more likely to occur in the premixed insulin (64.1% vs 24.2%, $P = 0.001$) [31c].

In a phase IV, randomized, open-label trial comparing basal-bolus insulin (using insulin glargine U-100 and once daily insulin glulisine) to premixed insulin (70% insulin aspart protamine/30% insulin aspart twice daily) in adults with T2DM, there was more nocturnal hypoglycemia associated with the premixed dosing [rate ratio (RR) 1.57, 95% CI 1.08–2.29, $P = 0.019$], although there was no difference in overall hypoglycemia (RR 0.84, 95% CI 0.64–1.11, $P = 0.22$) [32C].

When premixed insulin degludec and insulin aspart BID was compared to premixed insulin aspart protamine and insulin aspart BID in insulin-naïve patients with T2DM, there was less incidence of hypoglycemia, RR of 0.46, 95% CI 0.35–0.61, $P < 0.001$ and nocturnal hypoglycemia (RR 0.25, 95% CI 0.16–0.38, $P < 0.001$) with the degludec combination over the course of 24 weeks [33C].

In a 26-week-long open-label trial comparing insulin degludec to detemir, there were no differences in confirmed or severe hypoglycemia. Of note, there was less nocturnal hypoglycemia with insulin degludec (RR 0.67, 95% CI 0.51–0.88, $P < 0.05$) [34C].

In a meta-analysis comparing insulin glargine U-300 to other basal insulins, nocturnal hypoglycemia was less likely with insulin glargine U-300 than premixed insulin (risk ratio 0.36, 95% CI 0.14–0.94) and insulin NPH (risk ratio 0.18, 95% CI 0.05–0.55). There was no difference in nocturnal hypoglycemia between insulin glargine U-300 and insulin degludec or insulin detemir. No P-values were reported for these comparisons [35M].

An open-label RCT investigated the use of insulin glargine U-300 as basal insulin in adults with T2DM in comparison to insulin glargine U-100. There was less incidence of the composite of severe hypoglycemia and nocturnal hypoglycemia with insulin glargine U-300 [rate ratio (RR) 0.63, 95% CI 0.42–0.96, $P = 0.0308$]. Additionally, there was less incidence of nocturnal hypoglycemia (RR 0.61, 95% CI 0.41–0.92) [36C].

In a randomized, open-label, parallel group trial including participants from 12 countries that compared insulin glargine U-300 to insulin glargine U-100 for the treatment of T1DM in adults stable on their current insulin regimen, there was less incidence of documented symptomatic hypoglycemia defined as a BG <70 mg/dL, [rate ratio (RR) 0.62, 95% CI 0.44–0.86, P-value not reported] and severe hypoglycemia, defined as a BG

<54 mg/dL, (RR 0.63, 95% CI 0.41–0.98, P-value not reported), during the first eight weeks of treatment. There was no difference noticed after that point for the six-month duration of the trial [38C].

In an open-label, treat-to-target trial involving insulin-naïve adults with T2DM started on basal insulin with insulin degludec in comparison to insulin glargine, there was no difference between hypoglycemia rates between the two groups. The rate ratio (RR) for confirmed hypoglycemia was 0.87 (95% CI 0.51–1.48), and the RR for nocturnal hypoglycemia was 0.50 (95% CI 0.19–1.32) with no reported P-values [38C].

Metabolism

A case report of a 60-year-old female with a 25-year history of T2DM revealed her developing interscapular lipoatrophy while receiving a total daily dose of 50 units SubQ of premixed 70% insulin NPH/30% insulin R into her anterior abdomen. This patient was also on 2 g of metformin per day. Upon changing her injection site to the anteriolateral aspects of her thighs, the lipoatrophy was partially reversed two months later [39A].

An open-label RCT investigated the use of insulin glargine U-300 as basal insulin in adults with T2DM, in comparison to insulin glargine U-100. There was significantly less incidence of weight gain with insulin glargine U-300 in comparison to the U-100 formulation (−0.7 kg, 95% CI −1.3 to 0.2 kg, $P = 0.009$) [36C].

When comparing insulin glargine U-300 to insulin glargine U-100 for the treatment of T1DM in adults stable on their current insulin regimen over a treatment duration of six months, there was less incidence of weight gain (−0.06 kg, 95% CI −1.1 to −0.03 kg, $P = 0.037$) [37C].

In adults with T2DM started on basal insulin with insulin degludec in comparison to insulin glargine, there was no significant difference between the two groups in terms of body weight (weight −0.17 kg, 95% CI −0.59 to 0.26, $P = 0.44$) [38C].

In a meta-analysis comparing insulin glargine U-300 to other basal insulins in adults with T2DM, insulin glargine U-300 was associated with significantly less weight gain than premixed insulin (−1.83 kg, 95% CI −2.85 to −0.75 kg). No P-value was reported for this association [35M].

In a study that compared premixed insulin (insulin degludec/insulin aspart) administered BID to basal-bolus insulin (once daily insulin degludec and insulin aspart injected two to four times daily) in adult patients with T2DM, the weight gain over 26 weeks was significantly less with premixed insulin (−1.04 kg, 95% −1.99 to −0.10, $P < 0.05$) [40C]. This benefit may have been associated with the opportunity for more frequent administration of rapid-acting insulin with the basal-bolus regimen in comparison to the premixed formulation.

Musculoskeletal

In a retrospective analysis of patients undergoing surgical repair of femoral or tibial fractures, those with diabetes were compared to matched controls without diabetes. The control group included 166 patients (138 males), and the treatment group included 36 patients (25 males). This study found that diabetic medications, including biguanides used as monotherapy or in combination with a SU or a DPP4I, impair the healing process through slowing the formation of callus ($P < 0.001$) or bridging ($P = 0.014$). Additionally, non-union of the bones was more likely in those patients on one of the studied medications ($P = 0.006$) in comparison to those without antidiabetic medications [7c]. Of note, the retrospective study design of this trial prevents determining causality. With data showing diabetes can impair healing time, the result shown in this study may be due to the disease state itself rather than the medications associated with its treatment. A more ideal control would have been to include those with diabetes controlled without medications to identify if it is the disease state or the medications themselves that may be associated with impaired fracture healing. Additional studies determining the effects of these medications on bone healing may be warranted.

Breasts

In a retrospective review of the Taiwanese National Health Insurance database from 1996 to 2009 comparing patients on human insulin (ever-users) to those who have not used human insulin (never-users), those on human insulin for a longer duration of time (≥ 21.8 months) or received more doses ($\geq 39\,000$ units) were at a higher risk of developing breast cancer in comparison to never-users (HR 1.257, 95% CI 1.094–1.446, P-value 0.0013 and HR 1.260, 95% CI 1.096–1.450, P-value 0.0012, respectively). It is worth noting that there were significant differences between the groups at baseline, with ever-users of human insulin being older, more obese, and having a longer duration of diabetes [41MC].

Immunologic

An allergy to insulin aspart, insulin R and all long-acting insulin analogs was reported in a 36-year-old female patient with T2DM. This allergy presented at the age of 32 years when the patient tried an insulin pump for glycemic control. The symptoms of this allergy were managed with topical betamethasone valerate and oral cetirizine. When the patient tried insulin degludec, however, allergic symptoms were alleviated. The patient was then managed on insulin degludec and liraglutide. It was hypothesized by the authors that the insulin degludec's crystallized structure masked the allergen, preventing the allergic reaction she had experienced with other long-acting insulin analogues [42A].

SODIUM-GLUCOSE COTRANSPORTER 2 (SGLT2) INHIBITORS [SEDA-33, 898; SEDA-34, 695; SEDA-36, 652; SEDA-37, 530-531; SEDA-38, 458-459]

Canagliflozin

Acid–Base Balance

DKA associated with canagliflozin use was reported in a 62-year-old woman with T2DM. The patient recovered after five days in the intensive care unit. She was discharged on insulin, and canagliflozin was not restarted [43A].

A case of euglycemic metabolic acidosis was reported in a 52-year-old male with T2DM who was taking canagliflozin [44A]. Another report of euglycemic metabolic acidosis was reported in a 54-year-old Middle Eastern male with T1DM who had been taking canagliflozin for three years, in addition to insulin glargine. Acidosis resolved 72 hours after discontinuing canagliflozin [45A]. Another case of euglycemic metabolic acidosis was reported in a 42-year-old woman with a past medical history of T2DM who was taking canagliflozin in addition to metformin and basal-bolus insulin [46A].

Gastrointestinal

A case of non-occlusive mesenteric ischemia (NOMI) was diagnosed in a 60-year-old male patient who was taking insulin aspart with meals, insulin glargine daily, metformin 1000 mg daily, and canagliflozin 300 mg daily (initiated two weeks prior). The patient had originally been diagnosed with T2DM at the age of 42 but during his hospitalization for NOMI was subsequently diagnosed with slowly progressive T1DM, based on high titers of glutamic acid decarboxylase antibody and insulinoma-associated protein 2 antibodies in combination with a maintained depletion of insulin secretion [47A].

Musculoskeletal

The potential association between canagliflozin use and fracture risk was investigated in a trial that included data from nine placebo- and active-controlled studies ($n = 10194$), a single trial of patients high-risk patients [defined as those with risk factors for or a prior history of CV disease; The CANagliflozin cardioVascular Assessment Study (CANVAS); $n = 4327$] and a pooled population of eight non-CANVAS studies ($n = 5867$). Fracture risk was increased with canagliflozin, driven by CANVAS patients who were older, had a prior history or risk of CV disease, had higher baseline diuretic use, and had a lower baseline estimated GFR [48MC].

Dapagliflozin

Cardiovascular

A meta-analysis of 81 trials, including 37195 patients with T2DM, showed potential harm with dapagliflozin with regards to CV mortality (OR 2.15, 95% CI 0.92–5.04, $P=0.08$) [49M].

Acid–Base Balance

DKA was reported in a 44-year-old obese male patient with poorly controlled T2DM. The patient was admitted with DKA five days after initiating dapagliflozin. The patient was treated with insulin, glucose, and saline and was discharged home on insulin therapy after 72 hours. After one month, dapagliflozin was added to insulin therapy with no recurrence of DKA [50A]. Another case of DKA was reported in a 48-year-old female with a 16-year history of T2DM who had been taking dapagliflozin for ten months [51A].

A 56-year-old female patient with T2DM treated with insulin and dapagliflozin was diagnosed with acute kidney injury and DKA precipitated by gastroenteritis and SGLT2 inhibitors after six months of dapagliflozin use [52A].

Urinary Tract

Acute renal failure was reported in a 75-year-old female with a 15-year history of T2DM. The patient presented with nausea, vomiting, and weakness. The patient reported dapagliflozin was started one week prior. The patient was admitted with a diagnosis of acute renal failure secondary to tubulointerstitial nephritis. After hydration urine output increased and BUN, creatinine levels, and clinical status returned to normal [53A].

Empagliflozin

Acid–Base Balance

A 61-year-old female with T2DM presented with abdominal pain. The patient reported taking only one medication, empagliflozin. Abdominal ultrasound revealed evidence of acute, calculous cholecystitis. She was admitted for laparoscopic cholecystectomy and was given intravenous fluids with normal saline. Lab results revealed ketoacidosis with normal serum glucose, which was attributed to empagliflozin use. A dextrose-containing intravenous solution and insulin were started. Her status improved in the next 48 hours, and she was able to proceed with the cholecystectomy [54A].

A case report of euglycemic DKA was reported in a 57-year-old male patient with a past medical history of T2DM for ten years who had been taking empagliflozin for 189 days [55A]. Euglycemic DKA was also reported in a 64-year-old female patient who had T2DM for the past 15 years and had been taking empagliflozin for five days [56A]. Another case of euglycemic DKA occurred in a 42-year-old male patient who had T2DM for seven years and had been taking empagliflozin for four days [57A].

SULFONYLUREAS (SUs) [SEDA-33, 898; SEDA-34, 695; SEDA-36, 652; SEDA-37, 531-532; SEDA-38, 461]

Cardiovascular

In a case–control study investigating CV risk associated with medications for the management of diabetes, patients currently using SUs had a higher risk of MI (OR 1.67, 95% CI 1.10–2.55) but not an increased risk of stroke. Prior use of SUs was not associated with an increased risk of CV disease [58C].

In a systematic review of observational studies that report MI and stroke, SUs were associated with an increased risk of CV disease when compared to metformin (summary relative risk 1.24, 95% CI 1.14–1.34) [59M].

In a study using data from the FDA Mini-Sentinel program including information from 178 million persons and 358 million person-years from 2000 to 2014, sitagliptin users were less likely to experience HHF than those on SUs (0.83, 95% CI 0.73–0.93). Notably, the difference between treatment groups was not found to be significant in those with a high risk of developing HF [16MC].

Endocrine

In a meta-analysis comparing SUs to other antidiabetic agents, there was a significantly increased risk of hypoglycemia with SU monotherapy (OR 3.13, 95% CI 2.39–4.12). The combination of SU and metformin was the most associated with hypoglycemia [30M].

In regards to identifying risk factors of developing hypoglycemia on SU treatment, a recent study found that some anti-hyperlipidemic agents were more associated with SU-associated hypoglycemia. Using propensity-score adjusted HRs for the first 181 days of cohort entry, concomitant use of fenofibrate or gemfibrozil was more associated with severe hypoglycemia than pravastatin, the comparator. For fenofibrate, concomitant use with glyburide was associated with a HR of 1.69 (95% CI 1.02–2.82), and a HR of 1.75 (95% CI 1.05–2.89) was associated with glimepiride use. Using fenofibrate with glipizide did not significantly increase the risk of hypoglycemia (HR 0.69, 95% CI 0.35–1.35). When gemfibrozil was used concomitantly with glyburide (HR 1.52, 95% CI 1.01–2.29) or glipizide (HR 1.63, 95% CI 1.08–2.47), there was a significant increase in hypoglycemia risk. Use of gemfibrozil with glimepiride was not associated with a significant increase in the risk of hypoglycemia (HR 1.58, 95% CI 0.89–2.80). No P-values were reported for these comparisons [60MC].

Metabolism

In a meta-analysis comparing SUs to other antidiabetic agents, the combination of a SU and metformin was the combination most associated with weight gain [30M].

Musculoskeletal

In a retrospective analysis of patients undergoing surgical repair of femoral or tibial fractures, those with diabetes were compared to matched controls without diabetes. The control group included 166 patients (138 males), and the treatment group included 36 patients (25 males). This study found that antidiabetic medications including biguanides used as monotherapy or in combination with a SU or a DPP4I impair the healing process through slowing the formation of callus ($P < 0.001$) or bridging ($P = 0.014$). Additionally, non-union of the bones was more likely in those patients on one of the studied antidiabetic medications ($P = 0.006$) in comparison to those without antidiabetic medications [7c]. There are limitations to this study. The retrospective study design of this trial prevents determining causality. With data showing diabetes can impair healing time, the result shown in this study may be due to the disease state rather than the medications used in treatment. An ideal control would have been to include those with diabetes controlled without medications to identify if it is the disease state or the medications themselves that may be associated with impaired fracture healing.

Glimepiride

Cardiovascular

In a case report involving a 40-year-old male with an eight-year history of diabetes due to partial pancreas removal, the patient experienced myocardial injury due to an overdose of zolpidem and glimepiride, as evidenced by elevations in CK, CK-MB, and troponin I. There were no changes on the electrocardiogram. The total dose of zolpidem was 50 mg, and the total dose of glimepiride was 42 mg. With supportive care the patient made a full recovery [61A].

Glyburide

Cancer

When glyburide was compared to other second-generation SUs in a UK population, there was an association between the duration of glyburide use and total dosage and cancer risk. When glyburide was used for >36 months, there was a significantly increased risk of developing cancer (HR 1.21, 95% CI 1.03–1.42). Use of

more than 1096 defined daily doses was also significantly associated with the development of cancer (HR 1.27, 95% CI 1.06–1.51). Of note, there was less incidence of lung cancer associated with glyburide use (HR 0.93, 95% CI 0.88–0.99) [62MC].

THIAZOLIDINEDIONES (TZDs) [SEDA-32, 779; SEDA-33, 899; SEDA-34, 696; SEDA-36, 653; SEDA-37, 532-534]

Musculoskeletal

In a retrospective analysis of the ACCORD trial, TZDs were associated with an increased risk of bone fracture development. For women who were on TZDs currently, the risk trended to increase with an increased duration of treatment with an overall P-value <0.01. Those who were on TZDs for ≤one year had a HR of 1.84 (95% CI 1.17–2.89) which increased to a HR of 2.32 (95% CI 1.49–3.62) in those on TZDs for one to two years. In women on TZD therapy for >two years, bone fracture HR was 2.01 (95% CI 1.35–2.98). For those who had stopped TZDs, the risk of developing bone fractures was significantly reduced after one to two years of treatment cessation, in comparison to those who were continued on TZD therapy with a HR of 0.57 (95% CI 0.35–0.92). The risk further decreased after TZD treatment had been stopped for >two years, with a HR of 0.42 (95% CI 0.24–0.74) [63MC].

Pioglitazone

Cardiovascular

In a systematic review of observational studies that report MI and stroke, pioglitazone was associated with an increased risk of acute MI in comparison to metformin [summary relative risk (sRR) 1.02, 95% CI 0.75–1.38], which was not statistically significant [59M].

A study comparing pioglitazone to placebo in adults with insulin resistance and previous ischemic stroke or TIA found that there was significantly less risk of the composite of stroke and MI with pioglitazone (HR 0.76, 95% CI 0.62–0.93, $P = 0.007$) [64MC].

In a study using data from the FDA Mini-Sentinel program, which includes information from 178 million persons and 358 million person-years from 2000 to 2014, both saxagliptin and sitagliptin were found to be significantly less associated with HHF than pioglitazone (adjusted HR 0.58, 95% CI 0.41–0.83 and adjusted HR 0.68, 95% CI 0.58–0.81, respectively). It is worth noting that in those with a high risk of developing HF, the difference between treatment groups was not found to be significant between any groups assessed [16MC].

Endocrine

In a study comparing pioglitazone to placebo in adults with insulin resistance and previous ischemic stroke or TIA, there was significantly less risk of diabetes development with pioglitazone use (HR 0.48, 95% CI 0.33–0.69, $P < 0.001$) [64MC].

Urinary Tract

In a population-based observational study looking at adult, treatment-naïve T2DM patients, pioglitazone was associated with an increased risk of bladder cancer (HR 1.63, 95% CI 1.22–2.19) when compared to those who never received a TZD, with the risk of cancer significantly increasing after two years of therapy (HR 1.78, 95% CI 1.21–2.64, $P < 0.01$). Higher cumulative doses were also associated with an increased risk of bladder cancer with cumulative doses >28 000 mg associated with a HR of 1.70 (95% CI 1.04–2.78) [65MC].

A nested case–control study of South Korean patients with T2DM investigated the incidence of bladder cancer associated with TZD use and included 85 patients with bladder cancer and 850 control patients. No significant association was found with pioglitazone use and bladder cancer (adjusted OR 0.95, 95% CI 0.34–2.68), adding to this debate [66MC].

Rosiglitazone

Cardiovascular

In a systematic review of observational studies that report MI and stroke, rosiglitazone was associated with an increased risk of acute MI, in comparison to metformin (sRR 1.42, 95% CI 1.03–1.98) and pioglitazone (sRR 1.13, 95% CI 1.04–1.24). In comparison to pioglitazone, rosiglitazone was associated with an increased risk of stroke (sRR 1.18, 95% CI 1.02–1.36) [59M].

In a meta-analysis investigating the CV safety of the TZDs, rosiglitazone had an increased risk of stroke and MI. The NNH for MI with rosiglitazone use in comparison to non-TZDs was 51 (95% CI 32–131), with a NNH of 69 (95% CI 32–379) when compared to pioglitazone. The NNH for stroke with rosiglitazone use compared to non-TZDs was 28 (95% CI 15–225) with a NNH of 36 (95% CI 20–225) in comparison to pioglitazone [67M].

An evaluation of the FAERS data from 2006 to 2013 showed an association between rosiglitazone and the incidence of HF, with a statistically significant ROR of 13.98 (95% CI 13.30–14.70) [10C].

Urinary Tract

A nested case–control study of South Korean patients with T2DM investigated the incidence of bladder cancer associated with TZD use and included 85 patients with bladder cancer and 850 control patients. Rosiglitazone use was associated with an increased risk of bladder cancer (adjusted OR 3.07, 95% CI 1.48–6.37) [66MC].

References

[1] Yun P, Du AM, Chen XJ, et al. Effect of acarbose on long-term prognosis in acute coronary syndromes patients with newly diagnosed impaired glucose tolerance. J Diabetes Res. 2016;2016:1602083 [C].

[2] Herrmann K, Zhou M, Wang A, et al. Cardiovascular safety assessment of pramlintide in type 2 diabetes: results from a pooled analysis of five clinical trials. Clin Diabetes Endocrinol. 2016;1(2):1–8 [M].

[3] Liu W, Yang XJ. The effect of metformin on adolescents with type 1 diabetes: a systematic review and meta-analysis of randomized controlled trials. Int J Endocrinol. 2016;2016:3854071 [M].

[4] White S, Driver B, Cole J. Metformin-associated lactic acidosis presenting as acute ST-elevation myocardial infarction. J Emerg Med. 2016;50(1):32–6 [A].

[5] Buse JB, DeFronzo RA, Rosenstock J, et al. The primary glucose-lowering effect of metformin resides in the gut, not the circulation: results from short-term pharmacokinetic and 12-week dose-ranging studies. Diabetes Care. 2016;39(2):198–205 [c].

[6] Steber C, Perkins S, Harris K. Metformin-induced fixed-drug eruption confirmed by multiple exposures. Am J Case Rep. 2016;17:231–4 [A].

[7] Simpson C, Jayaramaraju D, Agraharam D, et al. The effects of diabetes medications on post-operative long bone fracture healing. Eur J Orthop Surg Traumatol. 2015;25(8):1239–43 [c].

[8] Chang C, Chang Y, Lin J, et al. No increased risk of hospitalization for heart failure for patients treated with dipeptidyl peptidase-4 inhibitors. Int J Cardiol. 2016;220:14–20 [MC].

[9] Rehman MB, Tudrej BV, Soustre J, et al. Efficacy and safety of DPP-4 inhibitors in patients with type 2 diabetes: meta-analysis of placebo-controlled randomized clinical trials. Diabetes Metab. 2017;43:48–58 [M].

[10] Raschi E, Poluzzi E, Koci A, et al. Dipeptidyl peptidase-4 inhibitors and heart failure: analysis of spontaneous reports submitted to the FDA adverse event reporting system. Nutr Metab Cardiovasc Dis. 2016;26(5):380–6 [C].

[11] Li L, Li S, Deng K, et al. Dipeptidyl peptidase-4 inhibitors and risk of heart failure in type 2 diabetes: systematic review and meta-analysis of randomised and observational studies. BMJ. 2016;352: i610 [M].

[12] Ohara N, Kaneko M, Sato K, et al. Vildagliptin-induced acute lung injury: a case report. J Med Case Rep. 2016;10(1):225 [A].

[13] Nagel AK, Ahmed-Sarwar N, Werner PM, et al. Dipeptidyl peptidase-4 inhibitor-associated pancreatic carcinoma: a review of the FAERS database. Ann Pharmacother. 2016;50(1):27–31 [M].

[14] Mamza J, Marlin C, Wang C, et al. DPP-4 inhibitor therapy and bone fractures in people with Type 2 diabetes—a systematic review and meta-analysis. Diabetes Res Clin Pract. 2016;116: 288–98 [M].

[15] Wang T, Wang F, Zhou J, et al. Adverse effects of incretin-based therapies on major cardiovascular and arrhythmia events: meta-analysis of randomized trials. Diabetes Metab Res Rev. 2016;32(8):843–57 [M].

[16] Toh S, Hampp C, Reichman ME, et al. Risk for hospitalized heart failure among new users of saxagliptin, sitagliptin, and other antihyperglycemic agents. Ann Intern Med. 2016;164:705–14 [MC].

[17] Alajaj A, Elrishi M. Acute pancreatitis associated with saxagliptin treatment presented by metabolic acidosis. Pract Diabetes. 2016;33(5) 158–158a [A].

[18] Dahiwele A, Kansal D, Sood A, et al. Saxagliptin induced bilateral knee arthralgia: a rare case report. Int J Basic Clin Pharmacol. 2016;5(5):2283–5 [A].

[19] Hung Y-C, Lin C-C, Huang W-L, et al. Sitagliptin and risk of heart failure hospitalization in patients with type 2 diabetes on dialysis: a population-based cohort study. Sci Rep. 2016;6:30499 [C].

[20] Tseng C. Sitagliptin and heart failure hospitalization in patients with type 2 diabetes. Oncotarget. 2016;7(38):62687–96 [MC].

[21] Tseng C. Sitagliptin use and thyroid cancer risk in patients with type 2 diabetes. Oncotarget. 2016;7(17):24871–9 [MC].

[22] Tseng CH. Sitagliptin and pancreatic cancer risk in patients with type 2 diabetes. Eur J Clin Invest. 2016;46(1):70–9 [MC].

[23] Alsaad AA, Dhannoon S, Pantin S-A, et al. Rare allergic reaction of the kidney: sitagliptin-induced acute tubulointerstitial nephritis. BMJ Case Rep. 2016; http://dx.doi.org/10.1136/bcr-2016-216297 [A].

[24] Khan MW, Kurian S, Bishnoi R. Acute-onset rhabdomyolysis secondary to sitagliptin and atorvastatin interaction. Int J Gen Med. 2016;9:103–6 [A].

[25] Nandikanti DK, Gosmanova EO, Gosmanov AR. Acute kidney injury associated with linagliptin. Case Rep Endocrinol. 2016;2016:5695641 [A].

[26] de Lapertosa SB, Frechtel G, Hardy E, et al. The effects of exenatide twice daily compared to insulin lispro added to basal insulin in Latin American patients with type 2 diabetes: a retrospective analysis of the 4B trial. Diabetes Res Clin Pract. 2016;122:38–45 [c].

[27] Boon IS, Saeed MA. Cautionary tale: subdural haematoma following frequent hypoglycaemia from insulin-induced lipohypertrophy. BMJ Case Rep. 2015;2015:26628309 [A].

[28] Zhao LP, Sheng XY, Zhou S, et al. Metformin versus insulin for gestational diabetes mellitus: a meta-analysis. Br J Clin Pharmacol. 2015;80(5):1224–34 [M].

[29] Kollhorst B, Behr S, Enders D, et al. Comparison of basal insulin therapies with regard to the risk of acute myocardial infarction in patients with type 2 diabetes: an observational cohort study. Diabetes Obes Metab. 2015;17(12):1158–65 [c].

[30] Palmer SC, Mavridis D, Nicolucci A, et al. Comparison of clinical outcomes and adverse events associated with glucose-lowering drugs in patients with type 2 diabetes: a meta-analysis. JAMA. 2016;316(3):313–24 [M].

[31] Bellido V, Suarez L, Rodriguez MG, et al. Comparison of basal-bolus and premixed insulin regimens in hospitalized patients with type 2 diabetes. Diabetes Care. 2015;38(12):2211–6 [c].

[32] Vora J, Cohen N, Evans M, et al. Intensifying insulin regimen after basal insulin optimization in adults with type 2 diabetes: a 24-week, randomized, open-label trial comparing insulin glargine plus insulin glulisine with biphasic insulin aspart (LanScape). Diabetes Obes Metab. 2015;17(12):1133–41 [C].

[33] Franek E, Haluzik M, Canecki VS, et al. Twice-daily insulin degludec/insulin aspart provides superior fasting plasma glucose control and a reduced rate of hypoglycaemia compared with biphasic insulin aspart 30 in insulin-naive adults with type 2 diabetes. Diabet Med. 2016;33(4):497–505 [C].

[34] Davies M, Sasaki T, Gross JL, et al. Comparison of insulin degludec with insulin detemir in type 1 diabetes: a 1-year treat-to-target trial. Diabetes Obes Metab. 2016;18(1):96–9 [C].

[35] Freemantle N, Chou E, Frois C, et al. Safety and efficacy of insulin glargine 300 U/mL compared with other basal insulin therapies in patients with type 2 diabetes mellitus: a network meta-analysis. BMJ Open. 2016;6(2)e009421 [M].

[36] Yki-Jarvinen H, Bergenstal RM, Bolli GB, et al. Glycaemic control and hypoglycaemia with new insulin glargine 300 U/mL versus insulin glargine 100 U/mL in people with type 2 diabetes using basal insulin and oral antihyperglycaemic drugs: the EDITION 2 randomized 12-month trial including 6-month extension. Diabetes Obes Metab. 2015;17(12):1142–9 [C].

[37] Home PD, Bergenstal RM, Bolli GB, et al. New insulin glargine 300 units/mL versus glargine 100 units/mL in people with type 1 diabetes: a randomized phase 3a, open-label clinical trial (EDITION 4). Diabetes Care. 2015;38(12):2217–25 [C].

[38] Osonoi T, Onishi Y, Nishida T, et al. Insulin degludec versus insulin glargine, both once daily as add-on to existing orally administered antidiabetic drugs in insulin-naive Japanese patients with uncontrolled type 2 diabetes: subgroup analysis of a pan-Asian, treat-to-target phase 3 trial. Diabetol Int. 2016;7(2):141–7 [C].

[39] Chakraborty PP, Biswas SN. Distant lipoatrophy: a rare complication of subcutaneous insulin therapy. Postgrad Med J. 2016;92(1083):57–8 [A].

[40] Rodbard HW, Cariou B, Pieber TR, et al. Treatment intensification with an insulin degludec (IDeg)/insulin aspart (IAsp) co-formulation twice daily compared with basal IDeg and prandial IAsp in type 2 diabetes: a randomized, controlled phase III trial. Diabetes Obes Metab. 2016;18(3):274–80 [C].

[41] Tseng CH. Prolonged use of human insulin increases breast cancer risk in Taiwanese women with type 2 diabetes. BMC Cancer. 2015;15:846 [MC].

[42] Fujishiro M, Izumida Y, Takemiya S, et al. A case of insulin allergy successfully managed using multihexamer-forming insulin degludec combined with liraglutide. Diabet Med. 2016;33(11): e26–9 [A].

[43] Turner J, Begum T, Smalligan RD. Canagliflozin-induced diabetic ketoacidosis case report and review of the literature. J Investig Med High Impact Case Rep. 2016;4(3) 2324709616663231 [A].

[44] Danford C, Chan P, Magill S. 'Euglycemic' ketoacidosis in a patient with type 2 diabetes being treated With canagliflozin. WMJ. 2016;115(4):206–9 [A].

[45] Gelaye A, Haidar A, Kassab C, et al. Severe ketoacidosis associated with canagliflozin (Invokana): a safety concern. Case Rep Crit Care. 2016;2016:1656182 [A].

[46] Clement M, Senior P. Euglycemic diabetic ketoacidosis with canagliflozin: not-so-sweet but avoidable complication of sodium-glucose cotransporter-2 inhibitor use. Can Fam Physician. 2016;62(9):725–8 [A].

[47] Gocho N, Aoki E, Okada C, et al. Non-occlusive mesenteric ischemia with diabetic ketoacidosis and lactic acidosis following the administration of a sodium glucose co-transporter 2 inhibitor. Intern Med. 2016;55(13):1755–60 [A].

[48] Watts NB, Bilezikian JP, Usiskin K, et al. Effects of canagliflozin on fracture risk in patients with type 2 diabetes Mellitus. J Clin Endocrinol Metab. 2016;101(1):157–66 [MC].

[49] Saad M, Mahmoud AN, Elgendy IY, et al. Cardiovascular outcomes with sodium-glucose cotransporter-2 inhibitors in patients with type II diabetes mellitus: a meta-analysis of placebo-controlled randomized trials. Int J Cardiol. 2016;228:352–8 [M].

[50] Storgaard H, Bagger JI, Knop FK, et al. Diabetic ketoacidosis in a patient with type 2 diabetes after initiation of sodium-glucose cotransporter 2 inhibitor treatment. Basic Clin Pharmacol Toxicol. 2016;118(2):168–70 [A].

[51] West K, et al. Possible risk factors for the development of sodium-glucose cotransporter 2 inhibitor-associated diabetic ketoacidosis in type 2 diabetes. Br J Diabet. 2016;16(2):78–81 [A].

[52] Kalidindi S, et al. A case of diabetic ketoacidosis (DKA) precipitated by sodium glucose cotransporter 2 inhibitor (SGLT2) in a patient with Type 2 diabetes. Diabet Med. 2016;33(Suppl S1): 103. abstr. P231 [A].

[53] Akın A, Keşkek ŞÖ, Özdemir E, et al. Acute renal failure after dapagliflozin treatment: a case report. Int J Intern Med Papers. 2016;1(1):1–4 [A].

[54] Candelario N, Wykretowicz J. The DKA that wasn't: a case of euglycemic diabetic ketoacidosis due to empagliflozin. Oxf Med Case Reports. 2016;2016(7):144–6 [A].

[55] Farjo PD, Kidd KM, Reece JL. A case of euglycemic diabetic ketoacidosis following long-term empagliflozin therapy. Diabetes Care. 2016;39(10):e165–6 [A].

[56] Roach P, Skierczynski P. Euglycemic diabetic ketoacidosis in a patient with type 2 diabetes after treatment with empagliflozin. Diabetes Care. 2016;39(1):e3 [A].

[57] Rashid O, et al. Euglycaemic diabetic ketoacidosis in a patient with type 2 diabetes started on empagliflozin. BMJ Case Rep. 2016; [A].

[58] Floyd J, Wiggins K, Christiansen M, et al. Case-control study of oral glucose-lowering drugs in combination with long-acting insulin and the risks of incident myocardial infarction and incident stroke. Pharmacoepidemiol Drug Saf. 2016;25(2):151–60 [C].

[59] Pladevall M, Riera-Guardia N, Marqulis A, et al. Cardiovascular risk associated with the use of glitazones, metformin and sufonylureas: meta-analysis of published observational studies. BMC Cardiovasc Discord. 2016;16:14 [M].

[60] Leonard CE, Bilker WB, Brensinger CM, et al. Severe hypoglycemia in users of sulfonylurea antidiabetic agents and severe antihyperlipidemics. Clin Pharmacol Ther. 2016;99(5):538–47 [MC].

[61] Chou S, Ayabe S, Sekine N. Myocardial injury without electrocardiographic changes after a suicide attempt by an overdose of glimepiride and zolpidem: a case report and literature review. Intern Med. 2015;54(21):2727–33 [A].

[62] Tuccori M, Wu JW, Yin H, et al. The use of glyburide compared with other sulfonylureas and the risk of cancer in patients with type 2 diabetes. Diabetes Care. 2015;38(11):2083–9 [MC].

[63] Schwartz AV, Chen H, Ambrosius WT, et al. Effects of TZD use and discontinuation on fracture rates in ACCORD bone study. J Clin Endocrinol Metab. 2015;100(11):4059–66 [MC].

[64] Kernan WN, Viscoli CM, Furie KL, et al. Pioglitazone after ischemic stroke or transient ischemic attack. N Engl J Med. 2016;371(14):1321–31 [MC].

[65] Tuccori M, Filion KB, Yin H, et al. Pioglitazone use and risk of bladder cancer: population based cohort study. BMJ. 2016;352:i1541 [MC].

[66] Han E, Jang SY, Kim G, et al. Rosiglitazone use and the risk of bladder cancer in patients with type 2 diabetes. Medicine (Baltimore). 2016;95(6)e2786 [MC].

[67] Mendes D, Alves C, Batel-Marques F. Number needed to harm in the post-marketing safety evaluation: results for rosiglitazone and pioglitazone. Pharmacoepidemiol Drug Saf. 2015;24(12):1259–70 [M].

38

Miscellaneous Hormones

Renee McCafferty[1], *Rozette Fawzy*

Manchester University College of Pharmacy, Natural and Health Sciences, Fort Wayne, IN, United States
[1]Corresponding author: rmccafferty@manchester.edu

CALCITONIN [SEDA-35, 789; SEDA-36, 659; SEDA-37, 539; SEDA-38, 463]

Seizure

A 29-year-old male had a tonic-clonic seizure immediately after his first dose of 50 mg calcitonin. He lost consciousness for 5 minutes but regained consciousness without residual symptoms. He had received 7.5 mg metopimazine 30 minutes prior to his calcitonin dose. On the day of the seizure, he was found to have normal chemistries, TSH, liver enzymes, creatine phosphokinase, and coagulation studies. Serum calcium was normal and protein was 84 g/L (normal values: 64–82 g/L). Alcohol was negative and lactic acid was 5.8 mmol/L (normal values: 0.4–2 mmol/L). Electroencephalogram performed the next day found no focal epileptogenic focus. Encephalic MRI performed 11 days after the seizure found a dilation of the spaces of Virchow Robin on the left without visible anomalies or atrophy. Authors conclude that although no relationship between calcitonin and the seizure can be established, a possible link may exist, but that metopimazine injection prior to calcitonin must be taken into account [1A].

GONADOTROPINS (GONADORELIN, GnRH AND ANALOGUES) [SEDA-36, 660; SEDA-37, 539; SEDA-38, 463]

Thyroid Function

Oral dosing regimens of MK-8389, an oral low molecular weight follicle-stimulating hormone (FSH) agonist, were tested in healthy, young female volunteers. Safety, pharmacokinetics and pharmacodynamics were tested at 5–40 mg once daily for up to 14 days. Daily doses of 10 mg were found to result in dose-dependent decreases in TSH levels. Free T3 and T4 correspondingly decreased. Daily doses of 30 mg and 40 mg suppressed TSH to below reference range of 0.3 mIU/L. Thyroid function test values returned to baseline within 6 days after last dose of MK-8389. Authors state that clinical symptoms of hyperthyroidism did not occur, including heart rate changes. They theorize that since FSH treatment is usually brief, such changes in TSH may not be clinically relevant. Since FSH and TSH receptors are similar, cross-reactivity may occur when an FSH agonist lacks specificity. In vitro studies, however, showed 100-fold less MK-8389 activity at TSH receptors compared to FSH receptors. Since this 100-fold window of difference in FSH to TSH activation was not observed in vivo, authors were forced to hypothesize. They offer that this variance may be due to different concentrations of MK-8389 being present at TSH vs FSH receptors, or that pharmacokinetic differences could exist between species (monkeys, dogs, humans). Developments of MK-8389 were ceased since thyroid function parameters were adversely affected at doses insufficient to aid fertility. This unexpected finding can help guide future investigations and raise questions regarding plan differences between species in such agents [2C].

Recombinant Human FSH Tolerability

Ovaleap® was compared to Gonal-f® for safety and efficacy for ovarian stimulation in an open-label study of up to 3 cycles while undergoing assisted reproductive technology. Both are recombinant follitropin alfa products. No hypersensitizing reactions occurred and local tolerability was mostly rated "very good" or "good" by patients in both groups. In cycle 3, mild, moderate and severe injection site reactions were reported but frequencies were comparable between groups. Authors conclude that these findings support continued use of Ovaleap® for multiple cycles or substituting Ovaleap® if Gonal-f® does not initially result in pregnancy [3C].

Lipodystrophy

Leuprolide administration resulted in lipohypertrophy in a 70-year-old man during the 2-month period after his first leuprolide acetate 22.5 mg injection. The patient had a prior history of heavy alcohol intake and CT evidence of cirrhosis. The patient's first symptom was swelling over his deltoids that interfered with his clothing fitting. This swelling interfered with activities of daily living, including inability to abduct and forward flex his shoulder joints, making reaching objects in cupboards difficult. These raised, soft tissue masses measured 10 cm in diameter when leuprolide injections were stopped. Thorax CT established the masses to be adipose tissue. Liposuction was performed with good effect. Authors postulate that an androgen surge occurred after leuprorelin administration which was converted to estrogen due to increased aromatase activity from cirrhosis in this patient. Authors suggest watching for signs and symptoms of lipodystrophy when using leuprolide, especially in patients with cirrhosis. [4A].

SOMATROPIN (HUMAN GROWTH HORMONE, hGH) [SEDA-36, 661; SEDA-37, 542; SEDA-38, 463]

Clinical Report: Brain Tumors in Noonan Syndrome

Caution is suggested in the use of growth hormone therapy in children due to occurrences of dysembryoplastic neuroepithelial tumor (DNET) and other brain tumors in Noonan syndrome. Noonan syndrome (NS) is an autosomal dominant developmental disorder caused by mutations in the RAS-MAPK signaling pathway that is well known for its relationship with oncogenesis. Noonan syndrome has been associated with an increased risk in cancer of 8.1-fold. A total of 22 NS patients are known to have brain tumors. It is unknown whether the development or progression of tumors is augmented by GH therapy; however, there is concern based on epidemiological, animal and in vitro studies. There is not enough data available to assess the safety of GH therapy in children with neoplasia-predisposition syndromes. Authors recommended that GH use in children with such disorders, including NS, be undertaken with appropriate surveillance for malignancies [5r].

Creutzfeldt Jakob Disease

Cadaver-sourced growth hormone has not been available for use in the United Kingdom for more than 30 years but patients with Creutzfeldt Jakob disease (CJD) from its exposure are still being identified. In this study, cases of CJD presenting between 2000 and 2014 that were determined to be iatrogenic from cadaver-sourced pituitary growth hormone. These diagnoses are estimated to occur 0–6 times annually. It is estimated that the incubation period after exposure to this growth hormone product is 18–40 years. Authors discussed prion protein genotype, PrP^{sc} type by Western blot, related to incubation periods. Neuropathology and disease course was also described. Since cadaver-sourced growth hormone was available until 1985 and the incubation period is now understood to be up to 40 years, new CJD diagnoses from this source may still occur [6c].

Cochlear Implant Performance Decrease

Two pediatric patients had decreased cochlear transplant performance after receiving hGH for treatment of short stature. Patient 1 had a cochlear implant placed in the right ear at 10 months of age and the left ear at 4 years 3 months for bilateral labyrinthine dysplasia. After 4 months of hGH when he was 8 years of age, word recognition scores decreased from 90% to 72% in the right ear and were stable at 40% on the left. Additional decreases were found down to 52% in the right ear and 28% in the left. Word recognition scores improved to 74% (right) and 68% (left) 1 month before hGH was discontinued. Patient 2 had a left cochlear implant placed at 7 years 10 months of age for severe to progressive bilateral sensorineural hearing loss. Word recognition scores decreased from 92% to 82% after 2 months of hGH treatment which had been started around age 11. Treatment with hGH was discontinued after being given for 10 months. Two months later, word recognition increased to 86%. Authors concluded that speech perception decreases after treatment with hGH in pediatric patients with cochlear implants is reversible after discontinuation of hGH treatment. They stress the importance of inquiring whether patients receiving cochlear implants are taking, or plan to take hGH so they can be appropriately monitored [7A].

Case Report: Lichen planus-like drug reaction associated with RHGH

Turner syndrome (TS) is a genetic disease with phenotypic abnormalities that are related to monosomy of the X-chromosome. The feature of short stature is almost always present in patients with TS. Recombinant Human Growth Hormone (RHGH) is usually given for the treatment of short stature in girls with TS in childhood. A 9-year-old girl who had been receiving RHGH for 2 months after being diagnosed as having monosomy of the X-chromosome, experienced burning of the mouth to the point at which she was unable to eat. Numerous interlacing white keratotic lines were noted involving labial and buccal mucosa. Scaly papules on the palms and soles were found 1 month after starting RHGH treatment. Biopsy was conducted and histological findings reported lichen planus-like drug reaction. Treatment with topical clobetasol propionate 0.05% cream was initiated to the palmoplantar lesions which completely resolved after 1 month of treatment. Dexamethasone 0.5 mg elixir was prescribed as mouthwash thrice daily for oral lesions. Unfortunately, oral lesions remained present and did not resolve until RHGH was discontinued [8A]. Another case was described in a 9-year-old boy with dwarfism who presented with skin-colored discrete pinpoint papules in the skin and violaceous, polygonal plaque on the glans penis during RHGH treatment. His condition was diagnosed as lichen planus and it remained resistant to treatment during RHGH therapy [9A]. In conclusion, there was no causal relationship established between RHGH and the lichenoid reaction in the girl with TS but it appears to be likely [8A].

MELATONIN AND ANALOGUES
[SEDA-35, 792; SEDA-36, 664; SEDA-37, 545; SEDA-38, 464]

Reviews

A review examining melatonin, its receptors and drugs discussed that melatonin agonists are contraindicated in patients with liver failure, renal failure, alcohol addiction and high lipid levels. Most common side effects related to melatonin agonists have been reported as headache, somnolence, palpitations and abdominal pain. The adverse events of melatonin agonists are as follows: nausea, headache and elevations in some liver parameters, rebound insomnia, withdrawal symptoms when used for 6 to 12 month or addiction. In experimental animal studies, melatonin was found to be carcinogenic at very high doses. Melatonin has been developed into a controlled-release dosage form despite the fact that it has been most commonly used for reduction of sleep latency (at 0.1–0.3 mg/day) and has a desired short action for that purpose. Melatonin up to 2 mg/day is now approved by the European Medicines Agency for insomnia. Doses as high as 300 mg/day for up to 2 years have been found to be safe when used in amyotrophic lateral sclerosis patients. Agomelatine is a melatonin receptor agonist and serotonergic agonist with anxiolytic and antidepressant effects. It is discussed here as being very effective in small doses without affecting sleep, which is a benefit as many antidepressants affect sleep quality [10R].

Melatonin and related agonists were reviewed for the treatment of circadian rhythm sleep-wake disorders (CRSWDs). Misalignment between the body's circadian timing of functions and a person's external environment can cause general decrease in work or health quality and may predispose to adverse consequences such as metabolic, cardiovascular, psychiatric or oncologic disease. CRSWDs are subdivided as exogenous (e.g., jet lag disorder, shift work disorder) or endogenous in which genetic or biological disruptions occur to system, behavioral or environmental factors (e.g., maladaptive exposure to light cues). Only one melatonin receptor agonist, tasimelteon, has been approved in the US for CRSWD although melatonin has long been used for this purpose as a natural augmentation to sleep cycle regulation. Agomelatine and ramelteon have also been investigated for use in CRSWD. This review cites the American Academy of Sleep Medicine's guidelines which state concerns regarding potency, purity, dissolvability, and safety between lots and brands of dietary supplements containing melatonin. Common adverse events when 2 mg prolonged-release melatonin was taken 1–2 hours prior to bed and after food were headache, nasopharyngitis, back pain, and arthralgia. Ramelteon 8 mg daily taken within 30 minutes of bed time and without food reports an adverse event rates of ≥3% with somnolence, dizziness, fatigue, nausea, and exacerbated insomnia. Tasimelteon 20 mg daily taken just prior to bed time and without food reported ≥5% adverse event rates (at least twice as high as placebo) with headache, increased ALT level, nightmares or unusual dreams, upper respiratory infection, urinary tract infection. Agomelatine is the most different listing adverse event incidence rates of ≥1% to ≤10% as nausea, dizziness, headache, somnolence, insomnia, migraine, diarrhea, constipation, abdominal pain, vomiting, hyperhidrosis, back pain, fatigue, anxiety, increases in AST and ALT level. Authors conclude that tremendous opportunity exists for additional research to explore the diverse properties of melatonergic compounds for the estimated millions of patients suffering with CRSWDs worldwide [11R].

Management of sleep disturbances in Alzheimer's disease (AD) patients was reviewed. Authors explain that sleep and circadian disorders are more frequent in AD than in the general population and they begin early after the onset of AD. Many approaches are used for these sleep disturbances but there is scarce evidence of efficacy or comparison between treatments. Authors conclude that behavioral light therapy (BLT) and melatonin are the only treatments with substantial evidence to support use. This review included 8 randomized placebo-controlled studies of melatonin in the treatment of Alzheimer's disease. Authors stated that no relevant side effects to melatonin had been reported in these 8 studies. However, one of them, a multicenter double-blind study found that melatonin improved sleep onset latency and total sleep time but it had adverse effects on mood and aggravated withdrawn behavior in patients with AD. These researchers additionally reported that the combination of BLT with the melatonin allows avoidance of these adverse effects. It is therefore suggested to accompany melatonin therapy for sleep disturbances in AD with BLT. Authors of the review express a need for effective BLT protocols to be established [12R].

Agomelatine

A retrospective pooled analysis was performed on 7605 patients who had taken either 25 mg or 50 mg agomelatine daily in phase II or phase III trials looking at hepatic safety. The analysis was restricted to patients who had at least one post-baseline transaminase value. Patients without transaminase levels during the studied period were excluded. Each case of transaminase increase was evaluated by a liver safety committee, composed of 4 hepatologists and one internist. This panel classified each case as probably, possibly, unlikely, or not related to the agomelatine treatment based on evidence and confounding factors. "The pooled incidence of increased serum transaminases to >3× ULN in the 9234 patients analyzed was 1.3% and 2.5% in patients treated with 25 mg and 50 mg/day of agomelatine, respectively (agomelatine 25 mg/day vs 50 mg/day, $P < 0.001$) compared with 0.5% in placebo-treated patients (agomelatine 25 or 50 mg/day vs placebo, $P < 0.001$) [13M]. No fatalities or liver failures were reported. None even had severe liver injury but 20 had transaminase increases >10× ULN. One had elevated bilirubin but this was determined to be due to concomitant itraconazole. When transaminase increase >3× ULN was determined to be "possibly" of "probably" related to agomelatine, it occurred with the first 12 weeks of treatment in 64% of patients. Many of these transaminase increases resolved during continued treatment with agomelatine. This phenomenon is described by the authors as adaptation. It is not known whether this adaptation will normally occur in all patients during the first 12 weeks of agomelatine treatment or if there may be some who will progress to liver injury or failure if they are unable to "adapt." The European Medicines Agency (EMA) approved agomelatine for the treatment of major depressive episodes in adults in 2009. EMA and the marketing authorization holder (MAH) recommended careful consideration before use in several patient types that maybe at increased hepatic risk. This analysis found that female sex and older age were not associated with risk of increased transaminase levels. Those factors associated with transaminase increase were baseline elevations of AST, ALT, GGT, triglyceride, or presence of metabolic syndrome. Authors conclude that baseline and regular transaminase testing should be done for agomelatine therapy. They do not suggest adjustments in current treatment or monitoring recommendations, despite safety findings [13M].

OXYTOCIN AND ANALOGUES [SEDA-36, 665; SEDA-37, 546; SEDA-38, 465]

Oxytocin Adverse Reaction Mimicking Allergy

A retrospective study of patients reported to have had an allergic reaction to oxytocin who were subsequently referred for allergy testing was performed to determine whether these reactions were more consistent with allergy or adverse effect. A total of 409 patients were investigated by the Danish Anaesthesia Allergy Centre, 30 of which had been exposed to oxytocin so they were tested. Most of these 30 women had received oxytocin doses of at least 10 IU. Authors assessed that of 30 women tested for oxytocin allergy over the 10-year period, none were allergic to oxytocin as all 30 women had negative skin tests to it. Authors discuss that side effects of oxytocin are related to dose and rate of administration. They surmise these side effects (e.g., flushing, tachycardia, hypotension) mimicked an allergic reaction but could have been avoided if the oxytocin dose given was more appropriately lower. They discuss the lowering of recommended oxytocin doses in many countries over recent years and state that a dose of 0.5–3 IU at elective caesarean sections reduces maternal side effects and is usually sufficient. Authors stress that new recommendations should be reported widely and identically by all national societies. Further, they recommend obstetricians and anesthesiologists both be knowledgeable and in agreement on oxytocin dosing [14c].

Intranasal Oxytocin & Vasopressin Have Different Effects in Men vs Women

A double-blind, placebo-controlled trial comparing male and female responses to intranasal oxytocin and vasopressin was conducted in 153 men and 151 women, all between 18 and 22 years of age. Test subjects were imaged with fMRI as they participated in social interaction testing with same-sex human and computer partners. Pretreatment with oxytocin attenuated negative social interaction in men. In women, oxytocin attenuated the amygdala and anterior insula responses to interactions with computer but not human partners, in contrast to the effect in men. This is hypothesized to be related to women having higher endogenous oxytocin levels. Discussion includes a previous work that showed oxytocin had been found to increase women's amygdala response to fearful faces and negative scenes. While authors conclude that oxytocin may reduce stress of negative social interactions among men and support continued research into oxytocin use in treatment for anxiety disorders, they note that responses in men and women can be different so studies should be structured to reveal this inconsistency before clinical treatments can be designed [15C].

Case Report: Ventricular tachycardia

A 32-year-old female weighing 56 kg was ordered to receive 5 units of oxytocin mixed in 500 mL of crystalloid solution to be delivered intravenously over 30 minutes along with 0.2 mg of methylergometrine maleate to be injected intravenously over 10 minutes as uterotonic after a repeat cesarean section birth. She had been found to have no signs or symptoms of cardiovascular disease prior to surgery. At 8 minutes after the start of spinal anesthesia, her blood pressure dropped to 85/30 which was corrected with 8 mg ephedrine. At 17 minutes after the start of anesthesia, the child was born so oxytocin and methylergometrine were started. Sixteen minutes after the start of oxytocin and methylergometrine, ventricular tachycardia appeared. Only 2.5 mg of oxytocin had infused at this time and it was stopped. Upon cessation of oxytocin infusion, the arrhythmia disappeared. During the arrhythmia, blood pressure was approximately 110/50 mmHg. Oxytocin administration is known to possibly induce arrhythmias. Methylergometrine was not ruled out as a causative factor but its relationship to arrhythmia onset was less clear. Naranjo's adverse drug reaction scale was used by the authors to rate oxytocin as a score of 4 and ergometrine as a score of 2. Authors state that autonomic nervous imbalance after surgical anesthesia along with ephedrine which preceded the oxytocin and methylergometrine administration could have contributed to the arrhythmia in this case [16A].

Case Report: Iatrogenic water intoxication

A gravida-3, para-2 woman of 31 years of age presented to a hospital obstetric department in labor with irregular labor pain and spontaneous vaginal discharge at 38 + weeks gestation. Her medical history and current pregnancy had no remarkable problems. On examination, all labs and vital signs were within normal limits except for a slightly low hemoglobin level of 10.6 g/dL. Serum sodium was 137 mEq/L and potassium 3.85 mEq/L at that time. Normal vaginal delivery was planned. Oxytocin was prepared in 5% dextrose at a concentration of 10 mU/mL to be given by continuous infusion to help improve her weak uterine contractions. It was first administered at a rate of 7 mU/min and increased by 0.3 mU/min every 30 minutes to reach a uterine contraction rate of 3–4/10 minutes with a duration of about 30–40 seconds. Oxytocin infusion was discontinued 30 minutes postpartum. She received a total of 9 units

of oxytocin and 2270 mL of 5% aqueous dextrose solution. Soon after oxytocin discontinuation, the patient became unresponsive and started having tonic-clonic convulsions, clenching strongly on her teeth while bleeding from the mouth. Diazepam 5 mg was immediately administered intravenously. She was resuscitated and intubated. Eclampsia was considered a possible cause of convulsions so magnesium sulfate 4 g was loaded intravenously, followed by continuous infusion at 1 g/hour. A dentoalveolar fracture carrying all mandibular incisors associated with muco-gingival laceration was found and repaired in surgery. Lab results were then found to be sodium level of 118 mEq/L, potassium of 3.1 mEq/L, blood sugar of 279 mg/dL, normal kidney and liver function tests, hemoglobin of 10.6 g/dL, and white cell count of 22 600 mL. Authors discuss that because of its structural similarity to antidiuretic hormone, oxytocin exerts an antidiuretic activity, which can cause water retention during labor. The risk of hyponatremia in association with oxytocin administration is increased when oxytocin is diluted in 5% dextrose water, which is hypotonic and deficient in necessary electrolytes, most importantly sodium. During labor, the body does not have normal tolerance to fluids; therefore, administration of hypotonic fluid should be avoided. Convulsions in the peri-partum period can be precipitated by multiple causes, underlying convulsive disorder, eclampsia, stressful physiological changes, labor complications, co-existing diseases, and iatrogenic mishaps. The mouth bleeding in this case was observed prior to the patient's intubation and was found to originate from the dentoalveolar trauma during seizure. Authors caution against administration of hypotonic fluid during labor because hyponatremia may occur [17A].

SOMATOSTATIN (GROWTH HORMONE RELEASE-INHIBITING HORMONE) AND ANALOGUES [SEDA-35, 794; SEDA-36, 666; SEDA-37, 549; SEDA-38, 466]

Lanreotide

Lanreotide is a somatostatin analog that has undergone several studies for inhibiting tumor growth and controlling hormonal symptoms in gastroenteropancreatic neuroendocrine tumors (GEP-NETs). This review was written to summarize literature to date on lanreotide for GEP-NETs. Lanreotide has low oral bioavailability and short half-life so it is given in a sustained-release depot formulation. In the CLARINET core study intent-to-treat population, 101 patients received lanreotide and 103 patients received placebo. Lanreotide depot was well tolerated in general as 88% of patients had any adverse events compared with placebo at 90%. Most adverse events were mild (17%) or moderate (44%) in both lanreotide and placebo groups. The most common adverse event was diarrhea at 26% in the lanreotide group, 9% with placebo. Abdominal pain was recorded in 14% of patients taking lanreotide but only occurred in 2% of patients taking placebo. Cholelithiasis occurred in 10% of patients but only in 3% in the placebo group. Hyperglycemia occurred in 5% of lanreotide patients but was not observed in those receiving placebo [18R].

A placebo-controlled phase 3 trial studied lanreotide 120 mg depot auto gel efficacy and safety for 16 weeks in 115 patients with carcinoid syndrome. Adverse event data were collected by patient diaries and at each post-screening visit. Patients in the lanreotide and placebo groups reported the same rates and types of adverse events. Authors conclude a favorable tolerability profile [19C].

A CLARINET open-label extension was conducted including 88 patients enrolled within 4 weeks of their last core CLARINET study visit. Adverse event data were collected at monthly treatment visits. Of the 88 patients, 47 had been on placebo during the core CLARINET study, 41 had been on lanreotide. Now all were on open-label lanreotide. The only adverse event the authors noted in discussion was transient diarrhea which was more common in the group new to lanreotide (31.9% vs 9.8%). They explain that diarrhea is a common transient side effect when somatostatin analogue therapy is initiated. A median progression free survival of 32.8 months was reached in the lanreotide group with no new safety concerns. This review and its corollary studies provide encouraging information regarding sustained-release lanreotide for GEP-NETs [20c].

Octreotide

Nine children were given long-acting octreotide for intractable chronic gastrointestinal bleeding from 2000 until 2009. The dose ranged from 2.5 to 20 mg monthly and patients were studied for a median of 62 months (12–111 months). One patient developed diarrhea and abdominal bleeding with subcutaneous octreotide which resolved after the long-acting octreotide was started. He was also found to have growth hormone deficiency during treatment with subcutaneous octreotide. Authors speculate that the patient may not have experienced these adverse events if the long-acting octreotide had been used from the start of therapy. No adverse events were attributed to use of long-acting octreotide in this group of children [21c].

Octreotide was observed in 16 children determined to be dependent on intravenous total parenteral nutrition due to chronic intestinal pseudo-obstruction (CIPO). Median age was 5 years (age range 1–18 years). The majority (69%, 11/16) of patients had what researchers considered a beneficial enteral feeding increase. Octreotide was dosed at 0.2–1 mcg/kg/day divided as two doses daily. The four patients experiencing adverse events were all taking 0.5 mcg/kg/day. One of these had a rash which resolved upon discontinuation of octreotide. Desensitization of octreotide was attempted but failed. One patient had hyperglycemia while on octreotide and could not advance enteral feeding until octreotide was discontinued. Another patient of the 16 developed hypertension but could continue octreotide when its dose was decreased. The fourth adverse event was cholecystitis with gallstones then pancreatitis. In this patient, octreotide was stopped but successfully restarted after cholecystectomy. Although this study was small, retrospective and open-label, authors note that the patient population has limited options and is difficult to sustain with adequate nutrition. They consider these results to show octreotide to be a safe option in children with CIPA [22c].

Case Report: Pituitary apoplexy

Pituitary apoplexy was reported in an 18-year-old boy with pituitary adenoma that had presented as acromegaly. Octreotide 100 mcg thrice daily had been given along with levothyroxine and prednisolone. The patient had improvement of headache and blurred vision within 1 week. He went on to receive 3 months of octreotide long-acting release (LAR) depot injections.

He was then found to have complete resolution of soft tissue and visual changes. MRI of his brain showed tumor resolution but also hemorrhagic and cystic areas of the pituitary gland. This was diagnosed as subclinical pituitary apoplexy and the octreotide LAR was discontinued. Within 6 months, the patient achieved biochemical remission consisting of insulin-like growth factor-1 and GH being 140 ng/mL and 0.06 ng/mL after glucose load, respectively. At 2-year follow-up, the patient still takes prednisone 5 mg and levothyroxine 75 mcg once daily and is symptom-free [23A].

Pasireotide

Complete control of acromegaly is not always achieved with octreotide or lanreotide, but pasireotide, a newer somatostatin analogue, has shown some increased efficacy [24C]. Its glucose homeostasis-related safety when compared to the first-generation somatostatin analogues was explored in the extended analysis of the PAOLA study. Glucose and HbA1C levels remained similar in octreotide and lanreotide patients.

These levels increased rapidly in the pasireotide long-acting release (LAR) patients, plateaued, then remained stable the remaining 24 weeks. Authors report this is consistent with other study observations in which glucose elevations associated with pasireotide usually plateaued after 2–3 months when treating patients with acromegaly and Cushing's disease with pasireotide. Patients' baseline glucose control was found to have predictive value for the development of hyperglycemia during pasireotide treatment [25C]. An editorial article remarks that long-acting pasireotide "could be seen as a trigger in diabetes-prone subjects" as he refers to the statistic that 52% and 71% of patients receiving pasireotide LAR 40 mg and 60 mg, respectively, that already had BG >101 at study entry developed hyperglycemia during the 24 weeks of the study [26r].

VASOPRESSIN RECEPTOR ANTAGONISTS [SEDA-35, 797; SEDA-36, 668; SEDA-37, 552; SEDA-38, 466]

Conivaptan

When conivaptan was tested against hypertonic saline (HS) for the treatment of hyponatremia due to syndrome of inappropriate antidiuretic hormone, thrombophlebitis was the only adverse event seen in each group of 40 patients it occurred much more often (75% of patients) in the HS group than the conivaptan group (10% of patients). Three patients died in each group, all with similar treatments and severities. APACHE II score was 17.05 and 17.1 in the HS and conivaptan groups, respectively, and predicted mortality was 26% in both groups [27c].

Tolvaptan

Tolvaptan 7.5 mg or 15 mg was given enterally to 38 patients during admission in an intensive care unit for refractory hyponatremia. This case series was conducted in a university hospital in Italy, from January 2012 to January 2014. Patient age was 53 ± 15 years. Admission types were 26 (68.4%) medical, 12 (31.6%) unscheduled surgical. No relevant difference was found between 7.5 mg and 15 mg tolvaptan dose response. Successful primary outcome was achieved in 31 (81.6%) of patients as defined by serum sodium increase ≥ 4 mmol/L 24 hours after tolvaptan administration. Rapid correction of hyponatremia was experienced in 4 (10.5%) patients. All patients increased their serum sodium by 14 mEq/L. One patient developed mild hypernatremia (Na 147 mEq/L). No symptoms or other adverse events were documented. Authors acknowledge limitations of this study being a small, heterogeneous population not adequately powered to draw conclusions

about adverse events. The lack of significant adverse events encourages future study [28c].

Short- and long-term tolvaptan use was evaluated in a retrospective study of 371 elderly Japanese patients receiving tolvaptan between January 2013 and December 2015. Heart failure was the primary target disease for tolvaptan treatment (91.1% of subjects), the other was liver cirrhosis (8.9% of subjects). Duration of treatment was divided into 7 days for 138 patients, 8–30 days for 110 patients and 1 month for 123 patients. Prescriptions were written for up to 3 month's duration. Hypernatremia occurred in 95 patients (25.6%), 71 of these within the first 7 days. Over the next month, the other 24 hypernatremia cases occurred. Stepwise logistic regression analysis determined risk factors for early onset (≤ 7 days) of hypernatremia to be baseline serum sodium ≥ 140 mEq/L, initial tolvaptan dosage >7.5 mg daily, and a BUN/creatinine ratio ≥ 20. Authors suggest that while elderly patients may be considered for long-term tolvaptan treatment, they have a higher risk of hypernatremia [29c].

VASOPRESSIN AND ANALOGUES [SEDA-34, 714; SEDA-35, 798; SEDA-36, 669; SEDA-37, 552; SEDA-38, 466]

Terlipressin

A case of torsade de pointes (TdP) developed in a 67-year-old man and was only temporarily responsive to the suggested treatment modalities, according to the authors. Transcutaneous pacing and external defibrillation were not effective treatments. It was not until terlipressin was discontinued and transvenous overdrive pacing begun that ventricular arrhythmias ceased. The onset of TdP in this patient was confounded by the fact that the patient had a highly complicated, multifactorial case leading up to the receipt of terlipressin. Authors of this case report assess that only one other known case of terlipressin-induced ventricular arrhythmia has occurred and it was in a patient with temporary risk factors. They suggest terlipressin be avoided in patients with QT prolongation and that QT-interval be evaluated prior to terlipressin use [30A].

DESMOPRESSIN (N-DEAMINO-8-D-ARGININE VASOPRESSIN, DDAVP) [SEDA-35, 798; SEDA-36, 669; SEDA-37, 552; SEDA-38, 467]

Occurrence of hyponatremia was compared in 136 elderly men with ($n=81$) and without ($n=55$) nocturnal polyuria. This retrospective cohort study included men who were ≥65 years of age and had lower urinary tract symptoms (LUTS) consistent with benign prostate hyperplasia (BPH) enrolled and prospectively followed from January 2006 to June 2010. Patients were excluded for urolithiasis, previous prostate surgery, or active urinary tract infection. Standard medications were allowed such as alpha blockers, 5 alpha-reductase inhibitors, antimuscarinics, and imipramine. Desmopressin was only added in patients with refractory nocturia. Duration of desmopressin therapy was 22.28 ± 13.42 months and 23.95 ± 14.80 months in the without nocturnal polyuria (non-NP) group and with nocturnal polyuria (NP) group, respectively. Most patients in both groups started with 0.05 mg daily. In the non-NP group, 7/55 men stayed at that dose, 44/55 increased to 0.1 mg daily, 1/55 to 0.15 mg daily, and 3/55 increased to 0.2 mg daily. In the NP group, 10/81 patients continued taking the 0.05 mg daily, 62/81 increased to 0.1 mg daily, 2/81 to 0.15 mg daily, and 7/81 increase to 0.2 mg desmopressin daily. There was one case of hyponatremia in each group (Na <125 mmol/L) but neither had symptoms and both continued desmopressin treatment. When the dose was decreased to 0.05 mg, adverse event rates were low and similar between the groups. In those with non-NP, 1 had dizziness, 1 had nausea, 1 had diarrhea, 1 had oliguria, and 1 reported incontinence for a total of 9 ADRs in the study (6.61%). Authors conclude that long-term treatment with low-dose desmopressin is safe and effective for nocturia in elderly men but stress that patients should be educated about their disease and monitored closely [31c].

A retrospective analysis of children with mild bleeding disorders prescribed subcutaneous DDAVP between January 2008 and December 2013 were identified through records in an Australian hospital. Authors note that there was no standard guideline of fluid restriction to prevent pediatric hyponatremia so their institution developed and was testing a protocol of two-thirds maintenance fluid restriction. Data were collected on 69 children aged 2–18 years of age. If multiple doses of desmopressin were given, sodium was checked prior to each dose. Seven cases of hyponatremia (Na 129–133 mmol/L) occurred, all asymptomatic. Transient facial flushing was documented after receiving desmopressin in 28% of patients. Two children had headache and one had transient, asymptomatic hypotension. The fact that this study is retrospective and performed at a single site does limit its applicability but the age and case range of patients does enhance the encouragement that no symptomatic hyponatremia occurred over their 5-year period of observation. Authors conclude that subcutaneous DDAVP was well tolerated and no serious side effects were observed. They state that a two-thirds maintenance fluid regimen for these patients is now standard protocol in their institution [32c].

Case Report: Severe hyponatremia

A 68-year-old woman was given 20 mcg IV DDAVP for bleeding prophylaxis for von Willebrand disease (vWD). She also took valsartan and hydrochlorothiazide for HTN. She was drinking 3 L of water daily for a healthy lifestyle. She presented to the emergency department 5 days after receiving the DDAVP injection reporting 3 days of nausea, vomiting and fatigue. Sodium level was 116, uric acid 2 mg/dL, serum osmolality 250 mOsm/kg, urine osmolality 398 mOsm/kg, urine Na 38 mEq/L. Hyponatremia from water intoxication was diagnosed and necessitated discontinuation of hydrochlorothiazide. She was treated with hypertonic saline and discharged with fluid restriction. Patients on DDAVP should avoid concomitant thiazide diuretics if possible and follow fluid restriction instructions. Practitioners are advised to check sodium before, and regularly after starting DDAVP therapy [33A].

HUMAN CHORIONIC GONADOTROPIN (HCG)

Gonadotropin-releasing hormone agonist (GnRHa) was tested against human chorionic gonadoptropin (hCG) in 227 patients with polycystic ovary syndrome (PCOS) undergoing IVF to determine relative safety and efficacy. Ovarian hyperstimulation syndrome (OHSS) is an iatrogenic complication of fertility treatments. OHSS can manifest as mild, moderate and severe degrees, with severe being possibly life-threatening. Participating patients were instructed to seek medical care for early symptoms of OHSS (abdominal distension or pain, nausea, vomiting, diarrhea). OHSS occurred in 53 patients in the hCG group vs only 2 patients in the GnRHa group (P<0.001). Efficacy was also better in the GnRHa group. Age, BMI, parity, seminal parameters, and causes/duration of infertility were similar in both groups. Authors explain that hCG, endogenous or exogenous, is often the trigger for OHSS. Both agents tested here were useful as trigger therapy during IVF in PCOS but GnRHa is associated with a much lower incidence of OHSS when compared to hCG [34C].

References

[1] Maison O, Pierre S, Charpiat B, et al. Convulsion apres administration de calcitonine de saumon: a propose d'un cas. Therapie. 2016;71:529–31 [A].
[2] Gerrits MGF, Kramer H, el Galta R, et al. Oral follicle-stimulating hormone agonist tested in healthy young women of reproductive age failed to demonstrate effect on follicular development but affected thyroid function. Fertil Steril. 2016;105(4):1056–62 [C].
[3] Strowitzki T, Kuczynski W, Mueller A, et al. Safety and efficacy of Ovaleap® (recombinant human follicle-stimulating hormone) for

up to 3 cycles in infertile women using assisted reproductive technology: a phase 3 open-label follow-up to main study. Reprod Biol Endocrinol. 2016;14:31 [C].

[4] Chang J, Bucci J. Unusual side effect from a luteinizing hormone-releasing hormone agonist, leuprorelin, in the treatment of prostate cancer: a case report. J Med Case Reports. 2016;10:323 [A].

[5] McWilliams GD, SantaCruz K, Hart B, et al. Occurrence of DNET and other brain tumors in Noonan syndrome warrants caution with growth hormone therapy. Am J Med Genet A. 2016;170(1):195–201 [r].

[6] Rudge P, Jaunmuktane Z, Adlard P, et al. Iatrogenic CJD due to pituitary-derived growth hormone with genetically determined incubation times of up to 40 years. Brain. 2015;138(11):3386–99 [c].

[7] Lafer MP, Green JE, Heman-Ackah SE, et al. Reduced cochlear implant performance after the use of growth hormone with regain of function after cessation of growth hormone therapy. Otol Neurotol. 2015;36(6):1006–9 [A].

[8] Soares MQS, Mendonca EF. Lichen planus-like drug reaction associated with recombinant human growth hormone therapy in a child patient with Turner syndrome. Dermatol Online J. 2016;22(3): pii: 13030/qt4k61f5jn, [A].

[9] Oono T, Arata J. Childhood lichen planus in a patient receiving growth hormone for dwarfism. Dermatology. 1996;192:87–8 [A].

[10] Emet M, Ozcan H, Ozel L, et al. A review of melatonin, its receptors and drugs. Eurasian J Med. 2016;48:135–41 [R].

[11] Williams WP, McLin DE, Dressman MA, et al. Comparative review of approved melatonin agonists for the treatment of circadian rhythm sleep-wake disorders. Pharmacotherapy. 2016;36(9):1028–41 [R].

[12] Urrestarazu E, Iriarte J. Clinical management of sleep disturbances in Alzheimer's disease: current and emerging strategies. Nat Sci Sleep. 2016;8:21–3 [R].

[13] Perlemuter G, Cacoub P, Valla D, et al. Characterisation of agomelatine-induced increase in liver enzymes: frequency and risk factors determined from a pooled analysis of 7605 treated patients. CNS Drugs. 2016;30:877–88 [M].

[14] Kjær BN, Krøigaard M, Garvey LH. Oxytocin use during caesarean sections in Denmark—are we getting the dose right? Acta Anaesthesiol Scand. 2016;60(1):18–25 [c].

[15] Chen X, Hackett PD, DeMarco AC, et al. Effects of oxytocin and vasopressin on the neural response to unreciprocated cooperation within brain regions involved in stress and anxiety in men and women. Brain Imaging Behav. 2016;10(2):581–93 [C].

[16] Nakanishi M, Masumo K, Oota T, et al. Ventricular tachycardia observed during cesarean section in a patient without structural cardiac disease. JA Clin Rep. 2015;1:23 [A].

[17] Abu Halaweh SA, Aloweidi AS, Qudaisat IY, et al. Iatrogenic water intoxication in healthy parturient causing convulsions and fractured mandible. Saudi Med J. 2014;35(2):192–4 [A].

[18] Wolin EM, Manon A, Chassaing C, et al. Lanreotide depot: an antineoplastic treatment of carcinoid or neuroendocrine tumors. J Gastrointest Cancer. 2016;47:366–74 [R].

[19] Vinik AI, Wolin EM, Liyanage N, et al. Evaluation of lanreotide depot/autogel efficacy and safety as a carcinoid syndrome treatment (ELECT): a randomized, double-blind, placebo-controlled trial. Endocr Pract. 2016;22(9):1068 [C].

[20] Caplin ME, Pavel M, Cwikta JB, et al. Anti-tumor effects of lanreotide for pancreatic and intestinal neuroendocrine tumours: the CLARINET open-label extension study. Endocr Relat Cancer. 2016;23(3):191–9 [c].

[21] O'Meara M, Cicalese MP, Bordugo A, et al. Successful use of long-acting octreotide for intractable chronic gastrointestinal bleeding in children. JPGN. 2015;60(1):48–53 [c].

[22] Ambartsumyan L, Flores A, Nurko S, et al. Utility of octreotide in advancing enteral feeds in children with chronic intestinal pseudo-obstruction. Paediatr Drugs. 2016;18:387–92 [c].

[23] Kumar S, Sharma S. Pituitary apoplexy causing spontaneous remission of acromegaly following long-acting octreotide therapy: a rare drug side effect or just a coincidence. Oxf Med Case Reports. 2016;4:81–3 [A].

[24] Gadelha MR, Bronstein MD, Brue T, et al. Pasireotide versus continued treatment with octreotide or lanreotide in patients with inadequately controlled acromegaly (PAOLA): a randomised, phase 3 trial. Lancet Diabetes Endocrinol. 2014;2(11):875–84 [C].

[25] Schmid HA, Brue T, Colao A, et al. Effect of pasireotide on glucose- and growth hormone-related biomarkers in patients with inadequately controlled acromegaly. Endocrine. 2016;53:210–9 [C].

[26] Luger A. Hyperglycemia in pasireotide-treated patients with acromegaly and its treatment. Endocrine. 2016;54:1–2 [r].

[27] Reddy SNV, Rangappa P, Jacob I, et al. Efficacy of conivaptan and hypertonic (3%) saline in treating hyponatremia due to syndrome of inappropriate antidiuretic hormone in a tertiary intensive care unit. Indian J Crit Care Med. 2016;20(12):714–8 [c].

[28] Umbrello M, Mantovani ES, Formenti P, et al. Tolvaptan for hyponatremia with preserved sodium pool in critically ill patients. Ann Intensive Care. 2016;6:1 [c].

[29] Hirai K, Shimomura T, Moriwaki H, et al. Risk factors for hypernatremia in patients with short- and long-term tolvaptan treatment. Eur J Clin Pharmacol. 2016;72:1177–83 [c].

[30] Jao YTFN. Refractory torsade de pointes induced by terlipressin (Glypressin). Int J Cardiol. 2016;222:135–40 [A].

[31] Chen SL, Huang YH, Hung TW, et al. Comparison of nocturia response to desmopressin treatment in elderly men with and without nocturnal polyuria in real-life practice. Int J Clin Pract. 2016;70(5):372–9 [c].

[32] Mason JA, Robertson JD, McCosker J, et al. Assessment and validation of a defined fluid restriction protocol in the use of subcutaneous desmopressin for children with inherited bleeding disorders. Haemophilia. 2016;22:700–5 [c].

[33] Yalcin A, Silay K, Yilmaz T, et al. Severe hyponatremia after desmopressin diacetate arginine vasopressin infusion in an older woman. J Am Geriatr Soc. 2016;64(5):1532–5415 [A].

[34] Krishna D, Dhoble S, Praneesh G, et al. Gonadotropin—releasing hormone agonist trigger is a better alternative than human chorionic gonadotropin in PCOS undergoing IVF cycles for an OHSS free clinic: a randomized control trial. J Hum Reprod Sci. 2016;9(3):164 [C].

39

Drugs That Affect Lipid Metabolism

Asima N. Ali*,†,1, Jennifer J. Kim‡,§, Mary E. Pisano¶, Nathan T. Goad†

*Campbell University College of Pharmacy and Health Sciences, Buies Creek, NC, United States
†Wake Forest Baptist Health, Internal Medicine Clinic, Winston-Salem, NC, United States
‡Greensboro Area Health Education Center, Greensboro, NC, United States
§University of North Carolina Eshelman School of Pharmacy, Chapel Hill, NC, United States
¶Novant Health, Winston Salem, NC, United States
¹Corresponding author: ali@campbell.edu; asima.nuz.ali@gmail.com

BILE ACID SEQUESTRANTS [SED-15, 1902; SEDA-36, 676; SEDA-37, 559; SEDA-38, 469]

Cholestyramine, Colesevelam and Colestipol

No relevant publications from the review period were identified.

CHOLESTEROL ABSORPTION INHIBITOR [SEDA-35, 810; SEDA-36, 677; SEDA-37, 560; SEDA-38, 469]

Ezetimibe

A few case reports have demonstrated hepatotoxicity with ezetimibe [1R]. Studies have shown that ezetimibe, when added to statin therapy, confers no increased risk of adverse events compared to statin monotherapy. Adverse events evaluated in these studies included cancer, gallbladder-related or musculoskeletal-related events, creatinine kinase or liver injury test changes, renal failure or progression of chronic kidney disease, treatment-related drug discontinuation, and, more recently, diabetes.

The risk for new-onset diabetes with ezetimibe was initially disproven by a subgroup analysis of the Improved Reduction of Outcomes: Vytorin Efficacy International (IMPROVE-IT) Trial [2r], and was further dispelled by a recent observational study [3C]. This recent retrospective cohort included 877 patients treated for dyslipidemia in a lipid clinic in Greece (median age of 55 years, 44% males). Results showed that the addition of ezetimibe to statin treatment did not increase the risk of incident diabetes in normoglycemic (adjusted odds ratio, 1.05 [95% CI, 0.34–3.23]) or prediabetic patients (adjusted odds ratio, 0.89 [95% CI, 0.36–2.22]).

The presence of NPC1L1 in the liver raises questions regarding the impact of ezetimibe at this site of action such as the potential benefits or harms in liver disease [1R]. A recent study examined the effects of ezetimibe in patients with hepatobiliary disease [4c]. Eleven patients (six males, mean age 58.5 years) with dyslipidemia were treated for 12 months with ezetimibe. Eight patients had gallstones; three patients had fatty liver disease; four patients had previously undergone laparoscopic cholecystectomy. Baseline lipid-lowering agents were continued (eight patients on ursodeoxycholic acid (UDCA), two patients on statins, one patient on bezafibrate). Results showed that the lithogenic index was unchanged overall, indicating that ezetimibe did not worsen biliary lithogenicity or pathophysiology.

NICOTINIC ACID DERIVATIVE [SED-15, 2512; SEDA-36, 679; SEDA-37, 560; SEDA-38, 470]

Niacin

In a recent review article on use of lipid-lowering medications in pediatrics, authors noted niacin lacks FDA approval for pediatric patients and is an unlikely therapeutic option due multiple known adverse effects [5R].

A recent dose-finding study in nondiabetic obese children ages 6–12 years evaluated the dose of niacin required to reduce free fatty acid (FFA) concentrations and increase growth hormone (GH) concentrations [6c]. Twelve patients were enrolled with a mean age of 9.7 ± 1.8 years and BMI of 26.4 ± 3.1 kg/m^2. Using three different dosing regimens, 250 mg every 2 hours for three doses ($n = 2$), 500 mg every 2 hours for three doses ($n = 5$), or 500 mg every hour for four doses ($n = 5$), the investigators measured serum FFA, GH, blood glucose, and insulin concentrations every 30 minutes through an intravenous catheter. Adverse effects were assessed hourly through structured interviews. After the first dose of niacin, 100% of patients experienced flushing and/or warmth, 60% experienced tingling, up to 40% had GI complaints (nausea, abdominal discomfort), and 20% experienced emesis when given the highest dosing regimen. No serious adverse effects were reported and tachyphylaxis developed to all adverse effects. This is the first study to investigate FFA and GH concentrations in obese children in response to niacin administration and provides information concerning the adverse effect profile of niacin in children, an area where there is minimal data. Though limited by its size, design as a dose-finding trial, and lack of randomization or comparison to placebo, this study provides an early look at the safety, tolerability, and potential therapeutic use of niacin in pediatric patients.

Endocrine

A recent prespecified secondary intention to treat (ITT) analysis of the 2011 AIM-HIGH trial sought to elucidate the effect of extended release niacin (Niaspan) on fasting glucose (FG) and insulin levels in statin-treated nondiabetic patients with a history of cardiovascular disease [7MC]. Patients included in this trial were 45 years or older had established cardiovascular disease, low HDL-C, triglycerides 100–400 mg/dL, and LDL-C <180 mg/dL. After an open-label run-in phase, patients who tolerated 1500 mg or more of Extended-release niacin (ERN) were randomized to ERN plus simvastatin/ezetimibe combination or placebo (immediate release niacin 50 mg) plus simvastatin/ezetimibe. When compared to placebo, patients who received ERN had significantly increased FG by 7.9 ± 15.8 vs 4.3 ± 10.3 ($P < 0.001$) at year 1 and 8.5 ± 13.6 vs 5.7 ± 12.3 ($P = 0.002$) at year 2 in patients with NFG at baseline. In patients with impaired fasting glucose (IFG) at baseline compared to placebo, FG increased by 4.1 ± 18.7 vs 1.4 ± 14.9 ($P = 0.02$) at year 1 and 5.0 ± 19.6 vs 1.7 ± 14.8 ($P = 0.007$) at year 2. More patients with normal fasting glucose (NFG) at baseline randomized to placebo maintained NFG at year 3 compared to those in the ERN group (34.2% vs 52.9%, $P < 0.001$; NNH = 5), and more patients randomized to ERN developed IFG at year 3 (27.4% vs 16.8%,

$P = 0.002$; NNH = 9). Development of new-onset diabetes was not significantly different between treatment arms. In those with IFG at baseline, more patients randomized to placebo exhibited NFG (10.0% vs 5.0%, $P = 0.016$; NNH = 20). Measures of insulin resistance, such as the homeostatic model assessment for insulin resistance (HOMA-IR), were statistically worse in those randomized to ERN in patients with NFG, IFG, and diabetes at baseline. HOMA-IR was significantly increased in patients randomized to ERN treatment who had NFG at baseline at years 1 and 3 ($P < 0.001$), IFG at baseline at year 1 ($P < 0.001$), and diabetes at baseline at year 1 ($P = 0.007$). These significant differences in HOMA-IR values were accompanied by statistically significant increases in insulin concentrations between ERN and placebo groups in the respective year and baseline FG category.

A recent meta-analysis sought to confirm an association between niacin and new-onset diabetes [8M]. In 11 trials ($n = 26\,340$) designed primarily to assess niacin's effects on cardiovascular endpoints, niacin at doses of 1–4 g daily was associated with a RR of 1.34 for new onset diabetes compared to placebo over a median follow-up of 3.6 years (5.53% vs 4.89%; [95% CI, 1.21–1.49]). In sensitivity analyses these results were consistent across prespecified subgroups showing a significant association regardless of statin therapy or combination with laropiprant (P values for interaction 0.88 and 0.52, respectively). This meta-analysis showed limited heterogeneity between studies with an I^2 statistic of 0.0% ($P = 0.87$). Findings remained consistent after removal of the heaviest weighted trial for new-onset diabetes (RR 1.38, [95% CI, 1.16–1.65]), which persisted regardless of fixed-effects or random effects modeling.

Hematologic

A nonrandomized observational study ($n = 46$) analyzed the hemorheological effects of nicotinic acid/laropiprant in patients with elevated Lp(a) levels (≥500 mg/L) and a prior arterial thrombotic event [9c]. This study found that despite the ability of niacin to improve lipid profiles of included patients, several rheologic and vascular endpoints worsened when patients received doses of 1 g/20 mg for 1 month followed by 2 g/40 mg to complete 12 months. A significant worsening of endothelial function was noted as peripheral arterial tonometry (PAT) values significantly decreased from baseline ($P = 0.001$). More patients had a reactive hyperemia index (RHI) <1.5 after treatment (39.1% vs 17.4%). Lastly, erythrocyte deformability was impaired after treatment compared to baseline ($P < 0.0001$). Whole blood viscosity, plasma viscosity, and red cell aggregation were no different from baseline. While statistically significant differences in surrogate markers were found, the clinical significance is unclear.

Neomycin

No relevant publications from the review period were identified.

Probucol

No relevant publications from the review period were identified.

FIBRIC ACID DERIVATIVES [SED-15, 1358; SEDA-35, 812; SEDA-37, 561; SEDA-38, 471]

A Cochrane review and meta-analysis evaluated benefits and harms of fibrates versus placebo or usual care, as well as fibrates plus other lipid-modifying drugs vs other lipid-modifying drug monotherapy for primary prevention of cardiovascular disease events [10M]. Six trials were included with a total of 16 135 patients. Mean age ranged of 47.3–62.3 years, and mean treatment duration was 4.8 years. Overall, the risk ratio (RR) for therapy discontinuation due to adverse effects was 1.38 [95% CI, 0.71–2.68]; participants = 4805; studies = 3; $I^2 = 74\%$; very low-quality of evidence), suggesting that fibrates do not increase risk for adverse effects. Serum creatinine levels were increased with fibrate compared with placebo (RR, 1.88 [95% CI, 1.65–2.15]; participants = 4173; studies = 3; $I^2 = 0\%$), whereas other adverse effects were not significantly increased [serum transaminases (RR, 2.94 [95% CI, 0.47–18.21]), pancreatitis (RR, 2.74 [95% CI, 0.11–66.88]), venous thrombotic events (RR, 1.46 [95% CI, 0.24–8.78]), gallbladder disease (RR, 1.33 [95% CI, 0.68–2.62]), and therapy discontinuation due to unspecified adverse effects (RR, 1.38 [95% CI, 0.71–2.68]).

Fenofibrate

A retrospective cohort study examined the effects of fenofibrate in combination with ursodeoxycholic acid (UDCA) for primary biliary cholangitis (PBC) patients with incomplete response to 12 months of UDCA [11c]. The study was conducted in a PBC specialist center in the United Kingdom and included 23 female patients with a median age of 56 years. Fenofibrate was discontinued in 4 patients (17.3%) due to intolerance (nausea, vomiting, abdominal pain, bloating), and 2 patients (8.7%) due to fenofibrate-induced liver injury (ALT peaks of about 4–5 × ULN without liver failure which subsided after fenofibrate discontinuation). Two patients (8%) developed self-limiting nausea and dizziness during the first week of therapy. No significant adverse effects were reported for patients taking fenofibrate for 12 months or longer.

A case–control study of the Action to Control Cardiovascular Risk in Diabetes evaluated risk factors for hypoalphalipoproteinemia, a paradoxical reduction in HDL-C and apolipoprotein A-I from the combination of fenofibrate with rosiglitazone [12c]. A total of 60 patients were included, with a mean age of 62 years, and 85% were male. The study found that an imbalance in HDL proteins, namely, paraoxonase/arylesterase 1 and apolipoprotein Cs, may be unique to diabetes patients and predispose to hypoalphalipoproteinemia from fenofibrate-rosiglitazone combination.

Gemfibrozil

A recent review article described the effects of gemfibrozil as an inhibitor of CYP2C8 and membrane transporters [13R]. Although in vitro data are lacking, caution is recommended when gemfibrozil is given concomitantly with a CYP2C8 substrate (e.g. dasabuvir, repaglinide, montelukast, thiazolidinediones, statins, paclitaxel, enzalutamide, imatinib) due to its potential to boost substrate drug pharmacokinetics and risk for adverse effects.

HMG-CoA REDUCTASE INHIBITORS [SED-15, 1632; SEDA-35, 812; SEDA-37, 562; SEDA-38, 472]

Cognition

In a review of randomized controlled trials regarding statin safety and efficacy, authors suggested deletion of labeling indicating adverse effects of statins on cognition or memory [14R]. Further studies provide positive evidence regarding statin use and impact on cognition.

A cross-sectional analysis including 120 patients (ages 50–75 years) assessed whether low LDL levels (<1.5 mmol/L) were associated with poor cognition in statin users with coronary artery disease [15C]. After controlling for covariates no association was found between lower LDL concentration and global cognition impairment using Montreal Cognitive Assessment (OR 0.56; 95% CI 0.24–1.32, $P = 0.19$). An association was found between high-dose statin and lower risk of impairment on visuospatial memory (OR, 0.12 [95% CI, 0.02–0.66, $P = 0.01$) and executive functioning (OR, 0.25 [95% CI, 0.06–0.99]; $P = 0.05$). The authors concluded statins may be used safely in CAD patients without concern for adverse impact on cognition. Due to various limitations including observational methodology, it is difficult to determine causality.

A prospective, randomized, double-blind, placebo-controlled study evaluated a 14-week trial of lovastatin for neurobehavioral function in Neurofibromatosis Type I patients ($n = 44$) [16c]. Lovastatin was tolerated with no serious adverse effects, and a positive effect on working memory using an MRI paradigm was found (effect size $f^2 = 0.70$, $P < 0.01$) with doses ranging from 40 to 80 mg daily. Authors concluded preliminary results suggest beneficial effects of lovastatin on learning and memory function. Due to small sample and inherent limitations of mouse modeling, clinical trial results are not generalizable and causality is not proven. Further studies are needed to demonstrate true impact.

Cataracts

Adding to inconsistencies previously reported in the literature on the role of statins impacting cataract progression, a multicenter, prospective study analysis including 2771 participants demonstrated a negative association [17C]. Researchers found statin users had an increased risk of cataract surgery (HR, 1.9 [95% CI, 1.17–3.10]), cortical lens opacity progression (HR, 1.52 [95% CI, 1.08–2.12]), and posterior subcapsular (PSC) lens opacity progression (HR, 1.84 [95% CI, 1.25–2.71]). Females were at increased risk of cataract progression (HR, 1.67 [95% CI, 1.03–2.71]) and cataract surgery (HR, 2.46 [95% CI, 1.25–4.85]). Individuals less than 75 years were at increased risk of PSC lens opacity progression (HR, 2.11 [95% CI, 1.22–3.65]) and cataract surgery (HR, 2.52 [95% CI, 1.20–5.33]). Strengths of the study include a large sample size, longitudinal design and 5-year median follow-up. Results based on self-reported statin use in patients with intermediate to late acute macular degeneration limit external validity; therefore, evidence should be reviewed in context of previously published literature.

Diabetes

Previous evidence supported an increased risk of new onset diabetes (NODM) with statins (atorvastatin, rosuvastatin, and simvastatin) was dose dependent. There is an increasing body of evidence indicating that the cardiovascular benefits of statins highly likely outweigh any increase in diabetes related morbidity, particularly in higher risk patients [14R, 18C]. Newer data suggest potential genetic associations [19M] while others consider pitavastatin as the safest choice [20C, 21r].

In a review article, multiple randomized trial data and genetic polymorphism data were combined and analyzed [19M]. Two polymorphisms of the Hydroxymethylglutaryl-CoA reductase (HMGCR) gene (rs12916 and rs17238484 alleles) were associated with higher weight, waist circumference, glucose, and diabetes risk. The authors conclude that genetic studies suggest that the increased diabetes risk with statins is likely to be a true on target effect of statins and further data are necessary for identifying additional LDL pathways.

A Delphi study in Spain evaluated the consensus rate of 497 experts (58.4% primary care physicians, 13.7% endocrinologists, 13.9% internal medicine, 7.0% cardiologists, and 7.0% nephrologists) on aspects of diabetogenicity of statins and found influential factors on statin selection in this regard [20C]. Using a 9 point Likert scale consensus was deemed "reached" when a questions obtained 80% responses grouped in scores 1–3 (consensus in disagreement) or scores 7–9 (consensus in agreement). Experts agreed that the most diabetogenic statin was atorvastatin (60.6% $P < 0.0001$) and the least was pitavastatin (4.4%, $P = 0.15$). Authors concluded that regardless of LDL lowering ability, the effect of statins on other metabolic effects, patient characteristics, and diabetogenicity need to be considered during statin selection. A major limitation of this study includes those inherent to survey research as it is more descriptive in nature and likely hypothesis generating.

Pancreatitis

A population-based case–control study in Taiwan aimed to explore the relationship between pancreatitis and atorvastatin [22C]. Authors identified 5810 cases of patients with first time diagnosis of acute pancreatitis. Subsequent logisitic regression analysis found an increased association of acute pancreatitis with atorvastatin use (OR, 1.67 [95% CI, 1.18–2.38]). It is unclear if risk is dose related, however authors did find that late atorvastatin users (last dose noted greater than 7 days prior to diagnosis) demonstrated a nonstatistically significantly decrease in acute pancreatitis risk (OR, 1.1 [95% CI, 0.87–2.38]). Authors concluded that atorvastatin is associated with diagnosis of acute pancreatitis independent of other comorbidities and that clinicians should consider this as a possibility.

Intracerebral Hemorrhage

Low serum cholesterol concentrations have been associated with increased risk of intracerebral hemorrhage (ICH), though results of major studies investigating the relationship between statin use and ICH have yielded inconsistent results [23M]. Meta-analyses of recently published studies are also not consistent in their findings on the risk of statin use and ICH incidence [24M]. Pandit et al. conducted a meta-analysis of randomized control trials that focused specifically on high-dose statins and ICH risk in a population of patients with cardiovascular disease. Seven studies were included in the analysis and involved 31 099 high-dose statin users and 31 105 placebo users in total. Results point to an increase risk of ICH with the use of high dose statins (RR, 1.53 [95%, CI, 1.16–2.01]) but no increase in all-cause mortality (RR, 0.95 [95% CI, 0.86–1.06]). This study was not able to account for the reason for the increased ICH risk, while others have suggested that patients with low total cholesterol and LDL-C and who are at high risk of ICH should exercise caution in statin use [24M].

℞ Special Review

Acute Kidney Injury

Evidence from previous randomized controlled trials does not support the negative association of statins on kidney outcomes except potentially in perioperative settings [14a, 25MC]. Caution is warranted particularly if statin therapy is continued in the setting of statin induced myopathy as this may lead to kidney failure [14R].

A retrospective cohort study in a military health care system was conducted to investigate the association of statin use and risk of chronic kidney disease (CKD) with a median duration of follow-up of 6.5 years [26MC]. Two cohorts were included: an overall cohort of all patients (statin and nonstatin users), and a healthy cohort. Propensity score matches were created for each group with 6342 pairs of statin users and nonusers in the overall cohort and 3351 pairs in the healthy cohort. In the overall cohort, statin users were at increased risk for acute kidney injury (AKI) (OR, 1.30 [95% CI, 1.14–1.48]), CKD (OR, 1.36 [95% CI, 1.22–1.52]), and nephritis/nephrosis/renal sclerosis (OR 1.35, [95% CI, 1.05–1.73]). In the healthy cohort statin use was associated with increased risk of CKD, but not the other renal-related conditions seen in the overall cohort. Secondary sensitivity analyses found that high-intensity statin users in the overall cohort had a higher incidence of aforementioned negative renal outcomes compared to low-to-moderate intensity statin users. Authors conclude that long-term statin use is associated with increased risk of AKI and CKD with differing effects seen in shorter term statin trials. Given the observational nature of the study results do not prove causality and are hypothesis generating.

When presented in context of previous literature, aforementioned evidence may be cautionary, indicating a need for renal function monitoring in users. While in the setting of secondary prevention, cardiovascular benefit of statin use may outweigh potential negative renal risk [14R], further studies are needed in the setting of primary prevention as well as in the elderly and populations in which there is an inherent deterioration of renal function or increased risk of renal injury.

Musculoskeletal

Muscle-related issues such as myalgia and myopathy are well documented in the literature [14R,27R,28R]. Statins have been reported to induce tendinopathy and tendon rupture; however, the molecular mechanism for this simvastatin mediated rupture has not been described until recently [29E]. An in vitro study was conducted to explore this mechanism by adding mevalonate, farnesyl pyrophosphate (FPP) or Geranylgeranyl pyrophosphate (GGPP) to simvastatin treated tendon cells. GGPP inhibited the effect of simvastatin on tendon cells leading authors to conclude that GGPP prevents the adverse effect of simvastatin in tendon cells. Further studies need to be conducted to better determine clinical implications.

Cancer

A retrospective epidemiological study evaluating the association between statin use and breast cancer incidence was conducted [30C]. The study included 79 518 participants without history of cancer and over 823 086 person-years follow-up; 3055 cases of breast cancer occurred with similar rates found between former (HR 0.96; 95% CI: 0.82–1.1) and current statin users (HR 1.1, 95% CI: 0.92–1.3), although not statistically significant. Authors concluded that statin use was not associated with risk of invasive breast cancer despite subtype or estrogen receptor status.

Drug–Drug Interactions

In a case report, a 60-year-old female with hyperlipidemia, diabetes, and coronary artery disease presented to the emergency department with chest pain, generalized weakness, myalgias, subjective fever, and chills [31A]. Due to these symptoms and persistent elevated CPK levels, potential causes for rhabdomyolysis were evaluated. Resolution of CPK and considerable reduction in muscle aches and chest pain occurred after discontinuation of sitagliptin and atorvastatin. After ruling other causes, authors concluded that the drug interaction between atorvastatin 40 mg and recently added sitagliptin 100 mg daily (started a week prior to presentation) was the culprit. Although causality is unproven and confounding factors exist, this evidence encourages close monitoring for signs and symptoms of rhabdomyolysis with concomitant use of atorvastatin and sitagliptin.

PROPROTEIN CONVERTASE SUBTILISIN/ KEXIN TYPE 9 (PCSK9) INHIBITORS [SEDA-38, 474]

Alirocumab

A pooled analysis reviewed 10 ODYSSEY Phase 3 randomized double-blind, controlled trials with subcutaneous alirocumab every 2 weeks for 6–18 months [32C]. Patients were randomized to either alirocumab, placebo, or ezetimibe, and only those with pre-diabetes ($n=1969$) or normoglycemia ($n=1479$) were evaluated. Overall, the HR was not significant for an increased incidence of diabetes in the alirocumab group compared with placebo controls (0.64 [95% CI, 0.36–1.14]) or ezetimibe controls (0.55, 0.22–1.41). There was no increase in progression to new-onset diabetes in the alirocumab group as compared to placebo or ezetimibe (0.90 [95% CI, 0.63–1.29] and 1.10 [95% CI, 0.57–2.12], respectively). Likewise, in the normoglycemic group there was not increase in progression to prediabetes for alirocumab group compared to placebo or ezetimibe (1.20, [95% CI, 0.96–1.49] and 0.88 [95% CI, 0.59–1.32], respectively).

The ODYSSEY OPTIONS II trial randomized 305 patients on rosuvastatin 10 mg ($n=145$) or 20 mg ($n=160$) daily to either add-on alirocumab 75 mg every 2 weeks, add-on ezetimibe 10 mg daily, or double-dose rosuvastatin [33C]. Patients either had cardiovascular disease (CVD) with LDL $\geq$70 mg/dL or CVD risk factors with LDL $\geq$100 mg/dL. Although P values were not provided for adverse events, incidence was similar across groups (56.3% in the alirocumab add-on, 53.5% in the ezetimibe add-on, and 67.3% in the double-dose rosuvastatin). General allergic events occurred with 9% of alirocumab patients compared to 2% of ezetimibe and 7% of double-dose rosuvastatin patients. To detect immunogenicity, patients were tested for development of anti-drug antibodies (ADA). Two (2.5%) alirocumab add-on patients who were negative at baseline resulted positive after receiving alirocumab, and both patients appeared to demonstrate a treatment-emergent ADA response.

A recent case report described vocal fold lesions in a 68-year-old female temporally associated with alirocumab therapy [34c]. Altered voice quality and episodic aphonia presented the day after receiving alirocumab 75 mg and worsened by about 1 week later to include flu-like symptoms, nonproductive cough, and dryness of the throat and nose. The patient eventually recovered after prednisone treatment. Authors hypothesize that alirocumab may stimulate immunogenicity contributing to inflammation leading to vocal fold lesions.

Evolocumab

Patients with elevated LDL-C levels who were intolerant to effective doses of statins due to muscle-related adverse effects were enrolled in the GAUSS 3 trial [35C]. This was a two-phase randomized clinical trial, with phase A being a 24-week crossover procedure of patients on either atorvastatin or placebo to identify those with intolerance only on atorvastatin. Phase B patients ($n=208$) were randomized to ezetimibe or evolocumab for 24 weeks. Overall there were approximately equal numbers of men and women, with a mean age of approximately 60 years. Muscle symptoms were reported in 28.8% of ezetimibe-treated patients and 20.7% of evolocumab-treated patients (HR, 0.68 [95% CI, 0.39–1.19]). Any investigator-reported increase in CK level occurred in 1.4% of ezetimibe patients and 2.8% of evolocumab patients. Injection site reaction occurred in 2.7% of placebo and 4.8% of evolocumab patients. One patient developed evolocumab-binding antibodies.

A post hoc analysis of phase two and phase three randomized trials reviewed evolocumab in patients with mixed hyperlipidemia [36C]. The safety analysis included 2246 patients from phase two and three studies and 1698 patients from their open-label extension studies. Overall, adverse events were similar among evolocumab, ezetimibe, and placebo. Inferential statistics were not performed.

Aside from their efficacy for LDL-C lowering, the overall safety and tolerability of ezetimibe, bile acid sequestrants, and PCSK-9 inhibitors have contributed to their inclusion in the 2016 American College of Cardiology (ACC) recommendations for use of nonstatin therapy to reduce atherosclerotic cardiovascular disease risk.

References

[1] Kei AA, Filippatos TD, Elisaf MS. The safety of ezetimibe and simvastatin combination for the treatment of hypercholesterolemia. Expert Opin Drug Saf. 2016;15(4):559–69 [R].

[2] Qamar A, Alexander KM. Incidence of new-onset diabetes in the IMPROVE-IT Trial: does adding ezetimibe to simvastatin increase risk compared to simvastatin alone?, 2015. Available at: http://www.acc.org/latest-in-cardiology/articles/2015/11/20/14/20/incidence-of-new-onset-diabetes-in-the-improve-it-trial [r].

[3] Barkas F, Elisaf M, Liberopoulos E, et al. Statin therapy with or without ezetimibe and the progression to diabetes. J Clin Lipidol. 2016;10:306–13 [C].

[4] Kishikawa N, Kanno K, Sugiyama A, et al. Long-term administration of a Niemann-Pick C1-like 1 inhibitor, ezetimibe, does not worsen bile lithogenicity in dyslipidemic patients with hepatobiliary diseases. J Hepatobiliary Pancreat Sci. 2016;232(2):125–31 [c].

[5] Miller ML, Wright CC. Use of lipid lowering medications in youth [Updated 2016 Jun 5]. In: De Groot LJ, Chrousos G, Dungan K, et al., editors. Endotext. South Dartmouth (MA): MDText.com, Inc.; 2000. Available from: https://www.ncbi.nlm.nih.gov/books/NBK395575/ [R].

[6] Galescu OA, Crocker MK, Altschul AM, et al. A pilot study of the effects of niacin administration on free fatty acid and growth hormone concentrations in children with obesity. Pediatr Obes. 2016;1–8 [c].

[7] Goldberg RB, Bittner VA, Dunbar RL, et al. Effects of extended-release niacin added to simvastatin/ezetimibe on glucose and

insulin values in AIM-HIGH. Am J Med. 2016;129(7):753. e13–22 [MC].

[8] Goldie C, Taylor AJ, Nguyen P, et al. Niacin therapy and the risk of new-onset diabetes: a meta-analysis of randomised controlled trials. Heart. 2016;102(3):198–203 [M].

[9] Cioni G, Mannini L, Liotta AA, et al. Detrimental effects of niacin/laropiprant on microvascular reactivity and red cell deformability in patients with elevated lipoprotein(a) levels. J Thromb Thrombolysis. 2016;41(3):433–5 [c].

[10] Jakob T, Nordmann AJ, Schandelmaier S, et al. Fibrates for primary prevention of cardiovascular disease events. Cochrane Database Syst Rev. 2016;11:CD009753 [M].

[11] Hegade VS, Khanna A, Walker LJ, et al. Long-term fenofibrate treatment in primary biliary cholangitis improves biochemistry but not the UK-PBC risk score. Dig Dis Sci. 2016;61(10):3037–44 [c].

[12] Ronsein GE, Reyes-Soffer G, He Y, et al. Targeted proteomics identifies paraoxonase/arylesterase 1 (PON1) and apolipoprotein Cs as potential risk factors for hypoalphalipoproteinemia in diabetic subjects treated with fenofibrate and rosiglitazone. Mol Cell Proteomics. 2016;15(3):1083–93 [c].

[13] Tornio A, Neuvonen PJ, Niemi M, et al. Role of gemfibrozil as an inhibitor of CYP2C8 and membrane transporters. Expert Opin Drug Metab Toxicol. 2017;13(1):83–95 [R].

[14] Collins R, Reith C, Emberson J, et al. Interpretation for the efficacy and safety of statin therapy. Lancet. 2016;388:2532–61 [R].

[15] Rej S, Saleem M, Herrman N, et al. Serum low-density lipoprotein levels, statin use and cognition in patients with coronary artery disease. Neuropsychiatr Dis Treat. 2016;12:2913–20 [C].

[16] Bearden CE, Hellemann GS, Rosser T, et al. A randomized placebo-controlled lovastatin trial for neurobehavioral function in neurofibromatosis I. Ann Clin Transl Neurol. 2016;3(4):266–79 [c].

[17] Al-Holou SH, Tucker WR, Agron W, et al. The association of statin use with cataract progression and cataract surgery: the AREDS2 report number 8. Ophthalmology. 2016;123(4):916–7 [C].

[18] Duvnjak L, Blaslov K. Statin treatment is associated with insulin sensitivity decrease in type 1 diabetes mellitus: a prospective, observational 56 month follow-up study. J Clin Lipidol. 2016;10(4):1004–10 [C].

[19] Preiss D, Swerdlow DI. Genetic insights into statin-associated diabetes risk. Curr Opin Lipidol. 2016;27(2):125–30 [M].

[20] Nunez-Cortes JM, Amenos AC, Ascaso Gimilio JF, et al. Consensus on the statin of choice in patients with impaired glucose metabolism: results of the DIANA study. Am J Cardiovasc Drugs. 2017;2:135–42 [C].

[21] Barrios V, Escobar C. Clinical benefits of pitavastatin: focus on patients with diabetes or at risk of developing diabetes [abstract]. Future Cardiol. 2016;12(4):449–66 [r].

[22] Lai SW, Lin CL, Liao KF. Atorvastatin use associated with acute pancreatitis: a case-control study in Taiwan. Medicine. 2016;95(7):1–5 [C].

[23] Ma Y, Li Z, Li X. Blood lipid levels, statin therapy and the risk of intracerebral hemorrhage. Lipids Health Dis. 2016;15(43):1–9 [M].

[24] Pandit AK, Kumar P, Kumar A, et al. High-dose statin therapy and risk of intracerebral hemorrhage: a meta-analysis. Acta Neurol Scand. 2016;134(1):22–8 [M].

[25] Zheng Z, Jayaram R, Jiang L, et al. Perioperative rosuvastatin in cardiac surgery. N Engl J Med. 2016;374:1744–53.

[26] Acharya T, Huang J, Tringali S, et al. Statin use and the risk of kidney disease with long term follow up (8.4 year study). Am J Cardiol. 2016;117:647–55 [M,C].

[27] Thompson PD, Panza G, Zleski A, et al. Statin associated side effects. J Am Coll Cardiol. 2016;67(20):2395–410 [R].

[28] Ramkumar S, Raghunath A, Ragunath S. Statin therapy: a review of safety and potential side effects. Acta Cardiol Sin. 2016;32:631–9 [R].

[29] Tsai WC, Yu TY, Lin LP, et al. Prevention of simvastatin-induced inhibition of tendon cell proliferation and cell cycle progression by geranylgeranyl pyrophosphate. Toxicol Sci. 2016;149(2):326–34 [E].

[30] Borgquist S, Tamimi RM, Chen WY, et al. Statin use and breast cancer risk in the Nurses's health study. Cancer Epidemiol Biomarkers Prev. 2016;251(1):201–6 [C].

[31] Khan M, Kurian S, Bishnoi R, et al. Acute-onset rhabdomyolysis secondary to sitagliptin and atorvastatin interaction. Int J Gen Med. 2016;29(9):103–6 [A].

[32] Colhoun HM, Ginsberg HN, Robinson JG, et al. No effect of PCSK9 inhibitor alirocumab on the incidence of diabetes in a pooled analysis from 10 ODYSSEY Phase 3 studies. Eur Heart J. 2016;37(39):2981–9 [C].

[33] Farnier M, Jones P, Severance R, et al. Efficacy and safety of adding alirocumab to rosuvastatin versus adding ezetimibe or doubling the rosuvastatin dose in high cardiovascular-risk patients: the ODYSSEY OPTIONS II randomized trial. Atherosclerosis. 2016;244:138–46 [C].

[34] Benedict PA, Abdou RM, Dion GR, et al. Association of alirocumab therapy with inflammatory lesions of the vocal folds: a case report. Laryngoscope. 2016;127(7):1652–4. http://dx.doi.org/10.1002/lary.26426 [Epub ahead of print] [c].

[35] Nissen SE, Stroes E, Dent-Acosta RE, et al. Efficacy and tolerability of evolocumab vs ezetimibe in patients with muscle-related statin intolerance. JAMA. 2016;315(15):1580–90 [C].

[36] Rosenson RS, Jacobson TA, Preiss D, et al. Efficacy and safety of the PCSK9 inhibitor evolocumab in patients with mixed hyperlipidemia. Cardiovasc Drugs Ther. 2016;30:305–13 [C].

40

Cytostatic Agents: Monoclonal Antibodies Utilized in the Treatment of Solid Malignancies

David Reeves[1]

College of Pharmacy and Health Sciences, Butler University, Indianapolis, IN, United States

St. Vincent Indianapolis Hospital, Indianapolis, IN, United States

[1]Corresponding author: dreeves@butler.edu

INTRODUCTION

The discovery of pathways driving cancer cell growth, proliferation, and survival has revolutionized the treatment of malignancies. Many agents now exist which target these different pathways either by inhibiting signaling intracellularly or by binding to cell receptors and blocking ligand binding or by binding ligand to inhibit its interaction with the cell receptors. One method of interrupting these pathways is to utilize monoclonal antibodies directed at the specific receptors or ligands implicated in cancer cell signaling. In addition to simple blockade of ligand binding and subsequent signal interruption, monoclonal antibodies may also be used to deliver chemotherapy molecules to malignant cells via drug conjugates or to affect the host's immune response to the cancers cells. Monoclonal antibodies have led to multiple improvements in patient outcomes and have been incorporated into the mainstay of treatment for multiple malignancies including, breast cancer, colon cancer, and lung cancer, to name a few. Due to their unique mechanisms of action, distinct from traditional chemotherapeutic agents, adverse effects differ greatly and are largely predicted by the pathways they target. Monoclonal antibodies are more targeted in their effects on cells than traditional chemotherapy agents; however, they can have unique adverse effects, which may be serious. Given their frequent use in the management of solid malignancies and ever increasing role in cancer treatment, it is important to be able to recognize adverse effects of these commonly utilized anticancer medications.

Though other methods of targeting cancer cell signaling exist (i.e., tyrosine kinase inhibitors—see *SEDA* 38:479–492), this chapter will focus on the monoclonal antibodies utilized for the treatment of solid tumors. This review will include inhibitors of the vascular endothelial growth factor (VEGF), epidermal growth factor receptor (EGFR), and platelet-derived growth factor receptor (PDGFR) pathways, as well as, immune checkpoint inhibitors [cytotoxic T-lymphocyte-associated antigen 4 (CTLA-4), program cell death-1 (PD-1), and programmed cell death ligand-1 (PD-L1)-directed therapies]. This chapter will focus on developments related to the tolerability of these medications published in the literature between January 1, 2016 and December 31, 2016.

VASCULAR ENDOTHELIAL GROWTH FACTOR (VEGF) PATHWAY INHIBITORS

Currently, two monoclonal antibodies targeting the VEGF pathway are approved by the FDA. Bevacizumab binds the ligand VEGF, preventing its interaction with VEGF receptors while ramucirumab binds the VEGF receptor, preventing its ability to bind VEGF ligand. The hallmark of both of the medications is the ability to inhibit angiogenesis, a critical process for cancer cell growth and survival. Three recent phase three trials (2 with bevacizumab and 1 with ramucirumab) have demonstrated that the most common adverse effects continue to be increased risk of hemorrhages, arterial and venous thrombosis, proteinuria, and hypertension [1C,2C,3C].

Patients receiving bevacizumab for the treatment ovarian cancer were analyzed in two meta-analyses [4M,5M]. The first meta-analysis included 4994 patients with newly diagnosed or recurrent ovarian cancer from 5 randomized controlled trials and demonstrated that grade 3 or higher hypertension (RR 21.27, 95% CI: 9.42–48.02), proteinuria (RR 4.77, 95% CI: 2.15–10.61), wound healing disruption (RR 3.55, 95% CI: 1.09–11.59), and bleeding (RR 3.16, 95% CI 1.59–5.03) were more common in those receiving bevacizumab in addition to chemotherapy [4M]. Any grade gastrointestinal perforation (RR 2.76, 95% CI: 1.51–5.03), arterial thrombosis (RR 2.39, 95% CI: 1.39–4.10), and venous thrombosis (RR 1.43, 95% CI: 1.04–1.96) were also increased in the bevacizumab group. Another meta-analysis of 3 phase three trials of bevacizumab for recurrent ovarian cancer demonstrated similar results with increased incidence of grade 3 or higher hypertension (RR 19.02, 95% CI: 7.77–46.55), proteinuria (RR 17.31, 95% CI: 5.42–55.25), arterial thrombosis (RR 4.99, 95% CI: 1.29–19.27), and bleeding (RR 3.14, 95% CI: 1.35–7.32) [5M]. Bevacizumab increased the risk of similar adverse effects in meta-analyses of non-small-cell lung cancer (NSCLC), colorectal cancer, and glioblastoma [6M,7M,8M]. Patients included in the glioblastoma meta-analysis were also at an increased risk for fatigue (OR 1.72, 95% CI: 1.0–2.96) which was not described in the previously mentioned meta-analyses [8M]. In the meta-analysis of patients with NSCLC, bevacizumab plus chemotherapy or erlotinib (a tyrosine kinase inhibitor targeted at the EGFR) was compared chemotherapy or erlotinib [6M]. This analysis of 3745 patients from nine clinical trials demonstrated similar increases in hypertension, proteinuria, and hemorrhagic events. Interestingly, there was no difference in grade 5 (fatal) adverse effects between groups (RR 1.21, 95% CI: 0.85–1.73).

In the older population, unfit for aggressive therapy, bevacizumab with a fluoropyrimide was compared to fluoropyrimide monotherapy alone [9M]. Toxicities of any grade occurring most frequently in the bevacizumab group included hand-foot syndrome (57.4%), diarrhea (42.1%), and hypertension (27.1%). Common grade 3 or higher toxicities included hand-foot syndrome (16.3%), diarrhea (15.7%), venous thrombosis (7.4%), and hypertension (6.9%). Those occurring more frequently in the bevacizumab arm included hypertension (27% vs 5%), bleeding (24% vs 6%), thromboembolic events (10% vs 5%), and proteinuria (26% vs 8%). This analysis demonstrated that bevacizumab likely has a manageable toxicity profile in an older, unfit population.

In the final meta-analysis of bevacizumab use published in 2016, neoadjuvant bevacizumab plus chemotherapy was compared to chemotherapy for the treatment of non-metastatic breast cancer [10M]. This analysis demonstrated a slightly different adverse effect profile, compared to the above analyses. Bevacizumab increased the risk for grade 3 or higher neutropenia (OR 1.18, 95% CI: 1.03–1.36), hand-foot syndrome (OR

1.63, 95% CI 1.21–2.20), and fatigue (OR 1.46, 95% CI: 1.01–2.11). Likewise, there was an increased risk for any grade febrile neutropenia (OR 1.99, 95% CI: 1.52–2.6) and surgical complications (OR 2.38, 95% CI 1.04–5.47). Overall, this analysis demonstrated an increased risk for myelosuppression not otherwise described in the other analyses. An increased risk for myelosuppression was also demonstrated in a study of ramucirumab plus paclitaxel vs paclitaxel monotherapy in patients with gastric or gastroesophageal junction adenocarcinoma [3C]. This study was a subgroup analysis of the East Asian population enrolled in the phase three Rainbow trial. East Asians developed grade 3 or higher neutropenia more frequently in the ramucirumab group (60% vs 28%, respectively). A similar increase in leukopenia was also present in this population (34% vs 13%, respectively). Among those of non-East Asian descent, neutropenia occurred less frequently than in the East Asian population; however, the rate was still increased compared to chemotherapy alone (31% vs 14%, respectively). Interestingly, neuropathy was also increased among those of non-East Asian decent receiving bevacizumab (10% vs 5%, respectively). In concordance with prior reports, bleeding/hemorrhage and hypertension occurred more frequently in those receiving ramucirumab in both the East Asian and non-East Asian populations.

Despite these adverse effects, patients receiving ramucirumab may have better quality of life outcomes than those not receiving this medication. In a quality of life analysis of a phase three trial of 665 patients with previously treated gastric or gastroesophageal junction adenocarcinoma receiving paclitaxel with or without ramucirumab, time to deterioration was significantly better with ramucirumab compared to placebo [11C]. Additionally, nausea/vomiting (HR 0.746, 95% CI: 0.574–0.969) and emotional functioning (HR: 0.642, 95% CI 0.491–0.840) significantly favored the ramucirumab arm. The only symptom more common in those receiving ramucirumab was diarrhea (HR 1.333, 95% CI: 1.007–1.764). Similar results for the phase three REVEL trial were also published in which patients with advanced or metastatic NSCLC receiving docetaxel with or without ramucirumab after progression on platinum-based chemotherapy resulted in no impairment in quality of life, symptoms, or functioning with the addition of ramucirumab [12C].

Cardiovascular Adverse Effects

Cardiovascular effects of inhibitors of the VEGF pathway are a significant concern for those utilizing these agents. In the phase three trials of bevacizumab during the past year, cardiovascular adverse effects comprised the majority of the most common adverse effects [1C,2C]. In a phase three trial of cisplatin and pemetrexed with or without bevacizumab for the treatment of mesothelioma, any grade and grade 3 or higher hypertension occurred in 56.3% receiving bevacizumab vs 1.3% not receiving bevacizumab and 23% receiving bevacizumab vs 0% not receiving bevacizumab, respectively [1C]. Likewise, the risk of any grade and grade 3 or higher arterial and venous thromboembolic events was higher with bevacizumab (any grade: 7.2% and 1.3%, respectively; grade 3 or higher: 5.8% and 0.9%, respectively). Risk of any grade hemorrhages was elevated in the bevacizumab group (37.4% vs 6.3%, respectively); however, the majority of these were grade 1 or 2 epistaxis. One grade 5 (fatal) brain hemorrhage occurred in the bevacizumab group. Lastly, proteinuria was increased in those receiving bevacizumab compared to control (all grades: 16.7% vs 0.4%, respectively; grade 3 or higher: 3.2% vs 0%, respectively). Similar results were demonstrated in the phase three trial of maintenance pemetrexed with or without bevacizumab in patients with non-squamous NSCLC [2C]. A significant increase compared to control any grade nasal hemorrhage (20% vs 2.9%, respectively), grade 3 or higher hypertension (15.6% vs 0%, respectively), and any grade proteinuria (44.4% vs 14.3%, respectively) were noted. The cardiovascular side effects noted in these phase three trials are comparable to those noted in the aforementioned meta-analyses.

A meta-analysis specifically describing the risk of cardiovascular adverse effects associated with ramucirumab use in 5694 patients with solid tumors demonstrated a significant increase in risk for all grade hypertension (RR 2.83, 95% CI: 2.43–3.29) and all grade bleeding (RR 1.98, 95% CI: 1.77–2.21) [13M]. Interestingly there was no increase in risk for any grade arterial or venous thromboembolic events, any grade congestive heart failure, or high-grade bleeding. There was an increased risk for high-grade hypertension with ramucirumab (RR 3.73, 95% CI: 2.82–4.93).

Hypertension was specifically analyzed in a meta-analysis of 2649 patients receiving ramucirumab or standard therapy for the treatment of cancer [14M]. All grade hypertension occurred in 16.4% of the patients receiving ramucirumab (RR 2.29, 95% CI: 1.61–3.24) with the highest incidence in those with advanced hepatocellular carcinoma and the lowest incidence in those with NSCLC. High-grade hypertension occurred in 9.8% of those patients receiving ramucirumab (RR 3.59, 95% CI: 2.32–5.54) with the highest incidence in the colorectal cancer population and the lowest incidence in occurring in the breast cancer population.

The risk of hemorrhage was specifically assessed in two meta-analyses, one with ramucirumab and one with bevacizumab [15M,16M]. In the meta-analysis of hemorrhagic events of 4963 patients, the overall incidence of all

grade hemorrhagic events in those receiving ramucirumab was significantly higher than control at 27.6% (RR 2.06, 95% CI: 1.85–2.29), while the incidence of high-grade events was not significantly elevated, occurring in 2.3% (RR 1.19, 95% CI: 0.80–1.76) [15M]. Overall the risk of low-grade hemorrhage was comparable between the different tumor types included (gastric cancer, gastroesophageal junction cancer, NSCLC, and metastatic breast cancer). High-grade hemorrhage did appear to be more common in the ramucirumab group among those with gastric cancer and gastroesophageal junction cancer. The drug dosing schedule did not appear to play any role in the incidence of low-grade thromboembolic events; however, there was an increase in the risk of high-grade hemorrhage in those receiving 8 mg/kg every 2 weeks compared to 10 mg/kg every 3 weeks. In the bevacizumab meta-analysis of 10 030 colorectal patients, the overall incidence of all grade hemorrhage was 5.8% (RR 1.96, 95% CI: 1.27–3.02) [16M]. The relative risk of high-grade hemorrhage was also increased with bevacizumab (RR 1.41, 95% CI 1.01–1.97). A significant difference was apparent between the group receiving 2.5 mg/kg/week and those receiving 5 mg/kg/week (RR 1.73 vs 4.67, respectively, $P = 0.001$). A difference was also present between those receiving bevacizumab for greater than 6 months or less than 6 months (RR 1.43 vs 4.13, respectively, $P = 0.001$). This indicates that like ramucirumab, increasing dose intensity may increase the risk for hemorrhagic events. Furthermore, this data with bevacizumab may signify that the majority of hemorrhagic events occur within the first 6 months of therapy.

The risk of thromboembolism associated with bevacizumab was also investigated in a meta-analysis of 13 185 patients with colorectal cancer [17M]. Thromboembolic events occurred in 9.9% of those receiving bevacizumab which corresponded with a significant increase in risk compared to control (RR 1.334, 95% CI: 1.191–1.494). This translated to an increased risk for both venous thromboembolism (incidence 8% with bevacizumab; RR 1.224, 95% CI: 1.091–1.415) and arterial thromboembolism (incidence 2.3% with bevacizumab; RR 1.627, 95% CI: 1.162–2.279).

In addition to the meta-analyses describing cardiovascular adverse effects, two case reports describing cardiac failure and cardiomyopathy were published [18A,19A]. In one case report, a 66-year-old male receiving cisplatin, gemcitabine, and bevacizumab for advanced urothelial carcinoma was admitted to the hospital for epigastric pain, nausea, intermittent diarrhea, and lightheadedness. The patient received their first cycle dose of bevacizumab 15 mg/kg 2 weeks prior to admission and developed chest pain that was accompanied with tachycardia, ST elevation, and conduction abnormalities. Troponin 1 levels were elevated, and the patient developed hypoxemia and metabolic acidosis; echocardiogram showed a reduced ejection fraction of 10%–20%. Ultimately the patient died 48 hours after admission and post mortem examination of the heart showed borderline cardiomegaly, diffuse microvasculopathy and changes due to global hypoperfusion. In the second case, a 70-year-old female with metastatic colon cancer was admitted to the hospital comatose within 4 days of receiving bevacizumab [19A]. The patient was experiencing lower limb spasticity and hypertension. An extensive workup was negative and the patient regained consciousness without any treatment other than nicardipine and urapidil. The patient had imaging consistent with posterior reversible encephalopathy syndrome that also involved the frontal lobes and echocardiographic changes. Both cardiac and neurologic symptoms improved with 10 days.

Wound Healing Complications

Wound healing complications have been described in multiple studies with VEGF-directed therapy and are likely due to disruption of angiogenesis in the wound healing process. In a meta-analysis of 5147 patients, those receiving bevacizumab had an increased risk for wound healing complications (OR 2.32, 95% CI: 1.43–3.75) [20M]. Patients with colon cancer appeared to be at highest risk (OR 5.81, 95% CI 2.0–16.85) as there was no difference between bevacizumab and control in those with breast cancer, NSCLC, renal cell carcinoma, or gastroesophageal adenocarcinoma. Operative patients were also at an increased risk (OR 2.68, 95% CI: 1.55–4.62), while non-operative patients did not demonstrate any significant increase in risk. Interestingly, ovarian cancer patients were not included in this analysis; however, in the meta-analysis of patients receiving bevacizumab and chemotherapy for ovarian cancer described previously, there was an increase in the risk of grade 3 or higher wound healing disruption (RR 3.35, 95% CI: 1.09–11.59) [4M]. In another meta-analysis of colorectal patients receiving bevacizumab prior to resection of liver metastases, wound healing complications were increased (OR 1.81, 95% CI: 1.12–2.91) [21M]. The impact of bevacizumab on wound healing was greater in those receiving more than 6 cycles preoperatively.

Gastrointestinal Adverse Effects

VEGF pathway-directed monoclonal antibodies have been implicated as a causative agent in various adverse gastrointestinal effects such as diarrhea; however, the most worrisome gastrointestinal adverse effect is likely the potential for gastrointestinal perforation. Though the risk is low, there appears to be a significant increase in the risk of perforation in those receiving bevacizumab. In the meta-analysis of bevacizumab use in ovarian cancer, the risk of grade 3 or higher gastrointestinal perforation was significantly greater than control (RR 2.76, 95% CI: 1.51–5.03) [4M]. Another meta-analysis of patients receiving bevacizumab for the treatment of advanced or metastatic colorectal cancer demonstrated a similar increase in risk of grade 3 or greater perforation (RR 3.63, 95% CI: 1.31–10.09) [7M]. In a meta-analysis of 26 833 patients with cancer specifically investigating this risk, all grade gastrointestinal perforation risk was significantly elevated in those receiving bevacizumab (RR 3.35, 95% CI: 2.35–4.79) [22M]. The risk of fatal perforations was also elevated (RR 3.08, 95% CI: 1.04–9.08). Overall, there was no difference in risk based on bevacizumab dose or schedule, treatment line, or patient age. In a meta-analysis of 4579 patients receiving ramucirumab, the incidence of gastrointestinal perforations was 1.5% (RR 2.56, 95% CI 1.29–5.09) with a mortality rate of 29.8% in those developing a perforation [23M].

In addition to these meta-analyses, 4 case reports were also recently published [24A,25A,26A]. The first report described a 56-year-old male presenting 5 days after receiving bevacizumab, procarbazine, lomustine, and vincristine for glioblastoma [24A]. He was diagnosed with a sigmoid perforation and underwent a sigmoid resection with colostomy. Pathologic review of the removed tissue revealed inflammation near the perforation area. The authors concluded that the inflammation observed supports the hypothesis that perforations may be caused by decreased wound healing of ulcerative lesions within the gastrointestinal tract. The second case described a male patient with rectal cancer receiving chemotherapy (modified FOLFOX6) and bevacizumab [25A]. Thirteen days after receiving bevacizumab, the man presented with a perforation and underwent surgery. The third case was another patient with rectal cancer who developed a perforation of the transverse colon while receiving capecitabine, oxaliplatin, and bevacizumab. The patient was treated surgically and required peritoneal drainage for approximately 1 month postoperatively. Lastly, a 54-year-old man receiving bevacizumab and chemotherapy for the treatment of lung cancer was admitted with lower abdominal pain [26A]. Opioid pain medication doses were increased, and within 6 days, the abdominal pain intensified. The patient was diagnosed with multiple perforations on the transverse and descending colon.

Another adverse gastrointestinal effect reported with bevacizumab is the formation of fistulas. In a case report of a 53-year-old woman with a history of ovarian and uterine cancer, a sigmoid-vaginal fistula developed after 15 cycles of bevacizumab [27A]. This was managed by performing a colostomy and continuing chemotherapy without bevacizumab.

Neurologic Adverse Events

Two cases describing neurologic adverse events attributed to the use of bevacizumab have recently been reported [19A,28A]. The first case was described earlier as the patient also developed cardiomyopathy [19A]. This patient was a 70-year-old female with colon cancer presenting to the intensive care unit with coma and lower limb spasticity 4 days after receiving bevacizumab and chemotherapy. The patient was found to have posterior reversible encephalopathy syndrome upon magnetic resonance imaging and improved completely without any treatment. The second case is a 67-year-old female receiving bevacizumab and chemotherapy for recurrent ovarian cancer that developed altered mental status, dizziness, double vision, difficulty focusing, imbalance, nausea and vomiting 2 days after her first cycle [28A]. An extensive neurologic workup was negative besides the presence of cranial sixth nerve palsy. The patient's mental status improved within 1 week and she was discharged, and the sixth nerve palsy resolved over the next 3 months.

Pulmonary Adverse Effects

Pulmonary adverse effects, outside of pulmonary embolism, were described in one case report of a 61-year-old woman receiving bevacizumab and chemotherapy for breast cancer [29A]. After three cycles the patient developed respiratory failure with bilateral pulmonary infiltrates which responded to steroid therapy. An infectious workup was negative, and the patient was determined to have an acute drug-induced lung injury.

EPIDERMAL GROWTH FACTOR PATHWAY INHIBITORS

Three monoclonal antibodies target the epidermal growth factor pathway, all of which are targeted at the epidermal growth factor receptor (EGFR). Signaling via the EGFR is often increased in malignancies and blocking the binding of EGFR ligands to the receptor with a monoclonal antibody inhibits this signaling thereby decreasing cell growth and inducing apoptosis, among other effects. The most recent Food and Drug Administration (FDA) approved EGFR monoclonal antibody, necitumumab, had two studies published recently which demonstrated a similar adverse effect profile to the other EGFR antibodies (cetuximab and panitumumab), including skin rash and electrolyte abnormalities among the most commonly reported [30C,31C]. Despite an increase in adverse effects with necitumumab, the two groups had similar qualities of life, and those receiving necitumumab

actually experienced a delayed time to deterioration of their appetite (HR 0.47, 95% CI: 0.23–0.95).

In a meta-analysis of 1338 patients describing the use of panitumumab in combination with irinotecan-based chemotherapy for the treatment of metastatic colorectal cancer, the overall incidence of adverse events was 56% [32M]. Grade 3 or higher skin toxicity, diarrhea, fatigue, vomiting, neutropenia, stomatitis, dehydration, hypomagnesemia, mucositis, and asthenia all occurred more frequently in those receiving the EGFR-targeted monoclonal antibody. In a meta-analysis of 4212 patients with head and neck squamous cell carcinoma that compared cisplatin to cetuximab with radiation, there was no difference in total toxicity (HR 0.34, 95% CI: −0.72 to 0.04) [33M]. However, there was an increase in the incidence of acneiform rash in those receiving cetuximab (HR 3.49, 95% CI: 1.23–5.74).

Cardiovascular Adverse Effects

Compared to therapies targeted at the VEGF pathway, cardiovascular adverse effects are less common among those agents targeted at the EGFR. Thromboembolism has been attributed to patients receiving EGFR monoclonal antibodies and was investigated in a meta-analysis of 12 870 patients with various cancers who were enrolled in studies investigating cetuximab or panitumumab [34M]. The overall incidence of venous thromboembolism was 7.8% in those receiving an EGFR monoclonal antibody compared to 4.6% in the control group (RR 1.27, 95% CI: 1.27–1.69). The incidence of pulmonary embolism was also increased 3.8% vs 2.7%, respectively (RR 1.55, 95% CI: 1.2–2.0). The relative risk increase for venous thromboembolism and pulmonary embolism was similar among those receiving cetuximab and panitumumab (cetuximab: venous thromboembolism RR 1.46, 95% CI: 1.2–1.79; pulmonary embolism RR 1.6, 95% CI: 1.08–2.37 vs panitumumab: venous thromboembolism RR 1.46, 95% CI: 1.18–1.80; pulmonary embolism RR 1.51, 95% CI 1.08–2.13). In addition to thromboembolism being described with cetuximab and panitumumab, a subgroup analysis of Germans from the phase three necitumumab trial also demonstrated an increased risk compared to control of grade 3 or higher venous thromboembolism (16.7% vs 5.6%, respectively) and arterial thromboembolism (4.8% vs 1.9%, respectively) [31C].

Dermatologic Adverse Events

Skin reactions are a well-known adverse effect of EGFR-targeted therapies and the monoclonal antibodies are no exception, as described in the phase three trials and meta-analyses discussed earlier. In an update to Italian recommendations for the management of skin reactions during cetuximab, the guideline panel recommended multiple prophylactic strategies in attempt to lessen the impact of EGFR-targeted therapy skin reactions [35R]. These included avoidance of the following: tight footwear and clothing, direct sunlight in the absence of protection, aggravators of dry skin including alcohol-based cosmetics and aftershave, excessive beard growth, depilatory wax and plucking, and incorrect nail cutting. Furthermore, they encourage the use of the following: sunscreen, additive-free and alcohol-free creams and bath oils, minimal make-up, and cleansing milk/lukewarm water to remove any make-up. General treatment strategies recommended involved supportive care such as topical antibiotics and steroids, systemic tetracycline, and potential dose modifications and/or systemic steroids for severe reactions.

Electrolyte Abnormalities

Similar to skin reactions, electrolyte abnormalities have been recognized as a common adverse effect with EGFR inhibitors. The mechanism by which this occurs is believed to be either via inhibition of transient receptor potential channel 6 (TRPM6) within the nephron that leads to magnesium wasting or indirect tubular nephrotoxicity [36c]. In the analysis of tolerability of the phase three trial of necitumumab (SQUIRE trial), grade 3 or higher hypomagnesemia occurred in 8.9% of those receiving necitumumab [30C]. This risk was also demonstrated in the panitumumab meta-analysis described earlier in which there was a significant increase in the risk of hypomagnesemia with panitumumab ($P < 0.001$) [32M]. In a retrospective analysis of hypomagnesemia in 27 metastatic colorectal patients receiving cetuximab either as monotherapy (14.8%) or with chemotherapy (85.2%), the incidence of hypomagnesemia was 29.6%. The majority were grade 1 in severity (22.2%) while only one patient each had grade 2 or 3 toxicity [36c].

Pulmonary Adverse Events

Besides pulmonary embolism, EGFR monoclonal antibodies have been associated with the rare development of interstitial lung disease. Of note, none of the recently published meta-analyses or the phase three trials included above described the presence of interstitial lung disease [30C,31C,32M,33M]. A case report describing a separate potential pulmonary toxicity was published recently. This case involved a 64-year-old male who developed pneumocystis pneumonia after receiving cetuximab and radiation for laryngeal cancer [37A]. The patient improved with treatment directed at pneumocystis (trimethoprim/sulfamethoxazole).

Miscellaneous Adverse Effects

Two additional case reports were recently published describing potential adverse effects in patients receiving EGFR-targeted monoclonal antibodies [38A,39A]. The first case described a 71-year-old male receiving chemotherapy with panitumumab for the treatment of rectal cancer who developed thrombocytopenia requiring plate transfusion [38A]. The patient progressed to develop jaundice and hematuria with elevated lactate dehydrogenase levels and anti-ADAMS13 antibodies as well as the presence of schistocytes on peripheral blood smear. The patient was diagnosed with thrombotic thrombocytopenic purpura and died 1 day after initiating plasma exchange.

The second case published described a 50-year-old male with pyriform sinus squamous cell cancer who developed a hypersensitivity reaction to cetuximab within 15 minutes of starting the first infusion [39A]. Subsequently, the patient had a negative skin prick test and a positive intradermal test with cetuximab, and he was diagnosed with IgE-mediated hypersensitivity to cetuximab. Hypersensitivity has been reported in the past due to IgG antibodies to galactose-alpha-1,3-galactose present on the Fab portion of the cetuximab heavy chain. This patient underwent a successful desensitization protocol that included 10 steps of increasingly concentrated cetuximab at increasing rates which lasted over approximately 225 minutes. The patient received 9 weekly desensitization protocols and tolerated all without any hypotension or any other symptoms. Based on this report, desensitization appears to be an option for patients experiencing immediate hypersensitivity to cetuximab.

HER2/*neu* PATHWAY INHIBITORS

HER2/*neu* is a member of the EGFR family; however, adverse effects associated with anti-HER2 therapies tend to differ slightly from the EGFR-targeted monoclonal antibodies described earlier. Currently there are three therapies directed at HER2: trastuzumab, panitumumab, and ado-trastuzumab emtansine. Ado-trastuzumab emtansine is an antibody–drug conjugate that includes an antimicrotubule agent (emtansine) linked to trastuzumab. In a subgroup of patients receiving trastuzumab monotherapy from a phase three trial of patients receiving adjuvant trastuzumab with or without lapatinib (an anti-HER2 tyrosine kinase inhibitor), grade 3 or higher toxicities occurred in 25% with 8% withdrawing from the study due to toxicity [40C]. A meta-analysis of 14 546 patients enrolled in trastuzumab trials demonstrated an increased risk in the following serious adverse effects among those receiving trastuzumab in the adjuvant setting: neutropenia (69.1% trastuzumab vs 54.2%

control, $P < 0.0001$), leukopenia (57.1% vs 48.8% respectively, $P < 0.0001$), diarrhea (2.9% vs 1.6% respectively, $P = 0.002$), LVEF reduction (8.6% vs 4.4% respectively, $P = 0.007$), congestive heart failure (2.4% vs 0.4% respectively, $P < 0.0001$), and skin/nail changes (3.2% vs 2.0% respectively, $P = 0.02$) [41M]. In the neoadjuvant setting, no differences were observed in neutropenia, febrile neutropenia, stomatitis, or LVEF reduction between the trastuzumab and control groups.

Incorporation of emtansine with trastuzumab does alter the adverse effect profile. In a meta-analysis of 2050 patients receiving ado-trastuzumab or control, the most common adverse effects were anemia, fatigue, transaminase elevations, nausea, thrombocytopenia, arthralgia and headache [42M]. Grade 3 or higher adverse effects were relatively rare, with severe thrombocytopenia occurring in 10.7% of those receiving ado-trastuzumab emtansine. Among the studies that included control arms, there was a significant increase in transaminase elevations (OR 4.04, 95% CI 1.429–11.427), thrombocytopenia (OR 8.50, 95% CI: 3.964–18.226), and fatigue (OR 1.288, 95% CI: 1.041–1.593) in those receiving ado-trastuzumab emtansine. Likewise, there was a significant increase in the risk for grade 3 or higher thrombocytopenia with ado-trastuzumab emtansine (OR 7.271, 95% CI: 1.098–48.133).

Cardiovascular Adverse Effects

HER2-directed therapies are well known for their adverse cardiac effects. The most common malignancy for which these medications are used, breast cancer, is particularly challenging in relation to the adverse cardiovascular risk due to the common use of anthracyclines in this population which also carry a potential for cardiac toxicity. This increase in risk was investigated in the meta-analysis of trastuzumab mentioned earlier [41M]. In this analysis, those receiving both concurrent and sequential anthracyclines had an increased risk for both LVEF reductions (concurrent anthracycline use RR 1.54, 95% CI: 1.27–1.86; sequential anthracycline use RR 4.66, 95% CI 2.89–7.53) and congestive heart failure (concurrent anthracycline use RR 4.79, 95% CI: 2.80–8.17; sequential anthracycline use RR 12.63, 95% CI: 3.90–40.92). This analysis also investigated the impact of schedule (weekly vs every 3-week administration) and determined that there as an increase in the risk of both LVEF reduction and congestive heart failure in those receiving the every 3-week regimen (LVEF reduction RR 4.62, 95% CI: 2.88–7.41; congestive heart failure RR 11.2, 95% CI: 3.76–33.35). Cardiac adverse effect risk was further investigated in an analysis of a phase three trial of trastuzumab in the adjuvant therapy of breast cancer [43MC]. The overall incidence in cardiac events after 6 years was 2.8% in those receiving paclitaxel and trastuzumab sequentially and 3.4% in those receiving paclitaxel and trastuzumab simultaneously. Risk factors for cardiac events were age greater than 60 years, reduced baseline LVEF and the use of antihypertensive medications.

In addition to the analyses above, meta-analyses specifically investigating the cardiotoxic effects of anti-HER2 monoclonal antibodies have recently been published in attempt to further describe this adverse event [44M,45M,46M]. In a meta-analysis of 6527 patients, the risk factors for trastuzumab-induced cardiotoxicity in patients with breast cancer were elucidated [44M]. Death due to cardiac complications occurred in 0.09%. Risk factors for the development of cardiotoxicity included: hypertension (OR 1.61, 95% CI: 1.14–2.26), diabetes mellitus (OR 1.62, 95% CI: 1.10–2.38), prior anthracycline use (OR 2.14, 95% CI: 1.17–3.92), increased age ($P = 0.013$), and family history of cardiac disease ($P < 0.001$). Another meta-analysis of 29 598 patients with breast cancer attempted to determine the risk for severe cardiotoxicity with trastuzumab [45M]. The overall incidence of severe cardiotoxicity was 3.0% with 2.62% of those with early breast cancer and 3.14% of those with metastatic breast cancer experiencing severe cardiotoxicity. Lastly, another meta-analysis of congestive heart failure in 18 111 patients receiving adjuvant trastuzumab for the treatment of early breast cancer described the risk for high-grade congestive heart failure [46M]. The incidence of high-grade congestive heart failure was 1.44% (RR 3.04, 95% CI 1.12–7.85). A higher incidence occurred in those receiving an 8 mg/kg loading dose (1.64%, RR 6.79, 95% CI: 2.03–22.73) compared to those receiving a 4 mg/kg loading dose (0.95%, RR 2.64, 1.62–4.33). Likewise higher risks were associated with 1 year and 2 years of therapy compared to receiving only 9 weeks of therapy (1 year 1.45%, RR 3.30, 95% CI: 2.07–5.25; 2 years 1.09%, RR 9.54, 95% CI: 2.20–41.44; 9 weeks 0.94%, RR 0.50, 95% CI: 0.05–5.49).

A phase two trial was recently published describing the risk of cardiac events with pertuzumab in 69 patients with metastatic breast cancer [47M]. Asymptomatic reductions in LVEF were noted in 3%, while none of the patients experienced symptomatic heart failure. Global longitudinal strain was noted to be stable throughout (19% at baseline, 19% at 6 months, 19% at 12 months). Detectable troponin-1 was observed in 4.3% and 3% developed an elevated brain natriuretic peptide.

Ocular Adverse Effects

HER2 is expressed by corneal, limbal and conjunctival epithelial tissue and ocular adverse effects have been reported with the use of HER2-directed monoclonal antibodies. Usually these effects are mild with approximately 2.5% of those receiving trastuzumab experiencing conjunctivitis [48A]. A more serious effect, corneal ulceration, was described in a case report of a 49-year-old female receiving adjuvant trastuzumab for early stage breast cancer [48A]. Ten days after the 12th dose, the patient experienced burning, water eyes, and impaired vision. The patient developed conjunctival congestion with perikeratic hyperemia and light perilimbal conjunctival edema with corneal marginal infiltrates. Topical steroids and antibiotics were administered leading to improvement. After the 13th dose of trastuzumab, the patient's symptoms worsened. The patient received autologous serum drops and after 7 days, experienced epithelial healing and disappearance of marginal infiltrates. Trastuzumab was restarted without any further worsening of symptoms.

Miscellaneous Adverse Effects

Radiation recall is a rarely reported adverse effect of multiple anticancer medications and has been reported previously with trastuzumab. In a case report of a 55-year-old receiving trastuzumab, the patient developed dermatitis in the area of previously irradiated skin 9 days after the fifth dose [49A]. The boarders were well demarcated and consistent with the radiated area. The recall reaction resolved within 1 week without steroids or antihistamines, and the patient continued trastuzumab without any further issues.

A case of thrombocytopenia was also recently published describing a 70-year-old patient with breast cancer receiving trastuzumab [50A]. The patient received trastuzumab with docetaxel for three cycles, and for the fourth cycle, only trastuzumab was administered. After the fourth cycle of trastuzumab, the platelet count dropped to 39 k/mm^3. Bone marrow biopsy demonstrated abundant megakaryocytes, moderate erythrocytic and granulocytic dysplasia series and a lack of iron, normal cytogenetics, no myelodysplasia and no tumor infiltration. Additional causes of thrombocytopenia were ruled out. The patient received prednisone 1 mg/kg for 4 weeks and was not re-challenged with trastuzumab.

Another adverse event described in a case report involved an anaphylactic reaction to pertuzumab in a 38-year-old woman within minutes of starting her second infusion of pertuzumab for the treatment of breast cancer [51A]. Skin prick and intradermal tests were negative at both 2 and 8 weeks after this hypersensitivity; however, a basophil activation test was positive. The patient proceeded to receive a 16-step desensitization. The patient tolerated the desensitization without any further reactions and proceeded to receive 3 additional doses without any complications.

PLATELET-DERIVED GROWTH FACTOR PATHWAY INHIBITORS

Olaratumab was recently approved by the FDA for the treatment of soft tissue sarcoma. It is a monoclonal antibody that binds platelet-derived growth factor receptor α (PDGFRα). A recent open-label phase 1b/randomized phase two trial of doxorubicin with or without olaratumab was recently published [52C]. This study enrolled 133 patients with locally advanced or metastatic soft tissue sarcoma in the phase two portion of the trial. Grade 3 or higher adverse effects occurred in 80% receiving olaratumab and doxorubicin compared to 69% of those receiving doxorubicin monotherapy. Adverse effects resulted in treatment discontinuation in 13% of those patients receiving olaratumab and doxorubicin compared to 18% of those receiving doxorubicin monotherapy. The most common adverse effects of any grade occurring in the combination group were nausea (73%, grade 3 or higher: 2%), fatigue (69%, grade 3 or higher: 9%), neutropenia (58%, grade 3 or higher: 53%), and mucositis (53%, grade 3 or higher: 3%). Infusion reactions occurred in 13% of those receiving olaratumab. The incidence of grade 3 or higher fatigue, neutropenia, and febrile neutropenia was similar among both groups.

IMMUNE CHECKPOINT INHIBITORS

Monoclonal antibodies serving as immune checkpoint inhibitors have multiple therapeutic targets. Currently, four agents are available in the United States with three distinct mechanism of action. Ipilimumab binds to and inhibits CTLA4. CTLA4 serves as an inhibitory receptor on T-cells which is subsequently inhibited by ipilimumab leading to increased immune destruction of tumors. Similarly, nivolumab and pembrolizumab bind to PD-1 which inhibits the inhibitory signal of PD-1 on the T-cells leading to increased immune destruction of tumors. Atezolizumab, the final drug in this class, inhibits PD-L1 by binding to the ligand for PD-1 on tumor cells, preventing activation of the inhibitory signal. Due to increased immune system activity, immune-mediated effects dominate the adverse effect profile of these medications.

In a phase three trial of adjuvant ipilimumab for the treatment of melanoma, grade 3 or higher immune-related adverse effects occurred in 41.6% of those receiving ipilimumab compared to 2.7% of those receiving placebo [53C]. The most common sites of grade 3 or higher autoimmune adverse effects were the gastrointestinal track (16.1%), liver (10.8%), and endocrine system (7.9%). The average time to onset of the immune mediate adverse effects was 4 weeks for dermatologic adverse effects and 13.1 weeks for neurologic adverse effects. Overall, 82%–97% of grade 2–4 adverse effects resolved within 4–8 weeks and 1.1% died.

In two trials of pembrolizumab, similar adverse effects were noted [54C,55C]. In one trial, immune-mediated adverse effects occurred in 29.2% of those receiving pembrolizumab compared to 4.7% of those receiving chemotherapy with the most common of any grade being diarrhea (14.3%) [54C]. Grade 3 or higher adverse immune-mediated adverse effects occurred in 9.7% vs 0.7%, respectively with the most common being diarrhea (3.9%) and pneumonitis (2.6%). In the other trial, immune-mediated adverse effects occurred in 20% of those receiving 2 mg/kg and 19% of those receiving 10 mg/kg [55C]. The most common immune mediate adverse effects were hypothyroidism, hyperthyroidism, and pneumonitis. Similarly, two trials of atezolizumab demonstrated a significant risk of adverse effects, the most common being fatigue, nausea, anorexia, pruritus [56C,57C]. The most common immune-related adverse effects included pneumonitis, elevated liver function tests, colitis, and hepatitis.

Meta-analyses confirmed trends observed in clinical trials. In a meta-analysis of 9 trials of nivolumab, any grade adverse effects occurred in 63%, with fatigue (28%), decreased appetite (13%), nausea (12%), and asthenia (10%) being the most common [58M]. Despite the common occurrence of adverse effects, when compared to chemotherapy, nivolumab led to a decreased risk of any grade adverse effect (RR 0.65 [95% CI: 0.55–0.76]) and grade 3 or higher adverse effects (RR 0.12 [95% CI: 0.09–0.15]) [59M]. Overall, there was a significantly decreased risk of anemia, anorexia, asthenia, febrile neutropenia, neutropenia, vomiting, alopecia, leukopenia, myalgia, and pruritus compared to control. Similar outcomes were demonstrated in another meta-analysis of nivolumab use in melanoma [60M]. Compared to decarbonize, nivolumab had a lower risk of grade 3 or higher fatigue (RR 0.23, 95% CI: 0.05–1.01) and all grade vomiting (RR 0.27, 95% CI 0.17–0.43). A higher risk of all grade pruritus was associated with nivolumab (4.96, 95% CI: 1.47–16.72). In this same analysis, the combination of nivolumab and ipilimumab when compared to ipilimumab monotherapy led to increased risk of grade 3 or higher rash (RR 2.7, 95% CI: 1.11–6.75), fatigue (RR 4.51, 95% CI: 1.44–14.15), and vomiting (RR 5.41, 95% CI: 1.03–28.34). The risk of all grade diarrhea (RR 1.32, 95% CI: 1.1–1.59), rash (RR 1.28, 95% CI: 1.05–1.56), and vomiting (RR 1.91, 95% CI: 1.25–2.92) was also increased with the combination.

Finally, the dose effect relationship for adverse effects was explored in a systematic review of pembrolizumab for the treatment of NSCLC [61M]. In this analysis of 2 mg/kg vs 10 mg/kg, there was no increased risk of rash, vitiligo, diarrhea, pneumonitis, hypothyroidism, hepatitis, or nephritis with the higher dose.

Cardiovascular Adverse Effects

Cardiovascular adverse effects have been rarely associated with immune checkpoint inhibitors. In an analysis of 146 patient receiving nivolumab for renal cell carcinoma, there was no clinically meaningful effect on QTc observed at doses up to 10 mg/kg [62C]. In addition to this report, a multi-center, retrospective review of patients receiving pembrolizumab or nivolumab for metastatic melanoma demonstrated 8 cardiac disorders in 5 patients (atrial flutter, left ventricular systolic dysfunction, myocarditis with cardiomyopathy, sinus tachycardia, hypertension, stable angina pectoris, ventricular arrhythmia, and asystole) [63c].

Two case reports were also published describing cardiovascular adverse effects. In the first case, a 65-year-old receiving ipilimumab for four doses developed a moderate pleural effusion and large pericardial effusion 6 months after completing therapy [64A]. The patient received pericardiocentesis, a subxiphoid pericardial window, and aggressive IV fluid resuscitation. Pathology demonstrated lymphocytic pericarditis and intravenous methylprednisolone was started. Improvement was noted over 24 hours, and steroids were tapered over 6 weeks. The second case involved a 60-year-old male receiving ipilimumab for metastatic melanoma who developed left ventricular dysfunction after the second dose with an asymptomatic reduction in his ejection fraction from 55%–60% to 40%–50% [65A]. Five months after discontinuation of ipilimumab and initiation of lisinopril and carvedilol, the patient's ejection fraction returned to baseline.

SPECIAL REVIEW

Gastrointestinal Adverse Effects

Immune-mediated gastrointestinal adverse effects have been described in many patients receiving immune checkpoint inhibitors and generally manifest as colitis or hepatitis. In the multicenter, retrospective analysis of nivolumab and pembrolizumab described earlier, gastrointestinal adverse effects (diarrhea, colitis, abdominal pain, coprostasis, xerostomia, and esophagitis) occurred in 4.2% of the 496 patients [66c]. Hepatitis occurred in 2.2% of patients in this report. Supporting this risk for hepatitis is a meta-analysis of 9 trials of nivolumab (with or without ipilimumab) or pembrolizumab which demonstrated PD-1 inhibitors were associated with an increased risk for all grade ALT elevations (RR 2.09, 95% 1.1–3.95) and AST elevations (RR 2.02, 95% CI: 1.01–4.03) [67M]. There was no increase in the risk for high-grade elevations in AST or ALT. In those receiving the combination of nivolumab and ipilimumab, there was an increase in risk compared to ipilimumab monotherapy for both all grade and high-grade elevations of

ALT (RR 2.09, 95% CI: 2.66–8.09 and RR 5.55, 95% CI: 2.27–13.57, respectively) and AST (RR 4.43, 95% CI: 2.48–7.90 and RR 8.98, 95% CI: 2.47–32.65, respectively). However, when comparing nivolumab and pembrolizumab, there was no difference in risk for hepatic toxicity between these agents.

Multiple reports of colitis have been published in 2016. In the largest report, 83 patients receiving ipilimumab for melanoma were described [68c]. Diarrheal illness occurred in 19.3% of the patients (5 developed after cycle 1, 6 after cycle 2, 4 after cycle 3, and 1 after cycle 4). Overall, 2 resolved spontaneously, while 9 patients with grade 2 or higher diarrhea received steroids or infliximab (8 received steroids and 4 of those received infliximab; one patient with grade 3 diarrhea received infliximab without steroids). The infliximab dose utilized was 5 mg/kg (3 received one dose and 2 received 2 doses). Symptoms resolved in all patients receiving infliximab and antidiarrheal medications alone led to resolution in all patients with grade 1 diarrhea. In a case series of patients receiving ipilimumab, the outcomes of 13 patients receiving infliximab for severe, steroid refractory colitis were described [69A]. Infliximab alone managed 62% of the patients while 33% required surgical intervention and one expired due to bowel perforation. Overall, 4 patients had resolution 1 month after infliximab administration.

A case report of a 51-year-old female, who received ipilimumab for metastatic melanoma, also described the use of infliximab for colitis [70A]. The patient experienced grade 4 diarrhea and hypovolemic shock after two doses of ipilimumab. No response was observed with intravenous methylprednisolone; therefore, infliximab 5 mg/kg was initiated, and improvement was noted within 7 days. Two weeks after hospital discharge, colitis symptoms recurred, and the patient was restarted on methylprednisolone. Clostridium difficile toxin was present, and the patient was treated with oral vancomycin. A colonoscopy and biopsy demonstrated ipilimumab-mediated colitis with numerous infiltrating T-cells. The patient received a second dose of infliximab after clearance of the toxin. Infliximab was also utilized in a case of 83-year-old male experiencing enteritis after receiving ipilimumab for melanoma [71A]. One month after starting ipilimumab, grade 3 diarrhea occurred with electrolyte disturbances and acute kidney injury. Steroids were initiated and a colonoscopy demonstrated a normal mucosa. Steroids were weaned; however, symptoms occurred. On endoscopy, duodenal inflammation was observed, and the patient was restarted on steroids. After tapering of steroids, the patient developed bloody diarrhea and a sigmoidoscopy with biopsy demonstrated ipilimumab-associated colitis for which steroids were restarted, and one dose of infliximab was administered. In the last case report describing colitis to be published in 2016, a 63-year-old patient with metastatic melanoma developed diarrhea after the second dose of ipilimumab [72A]. Upon admission to the hospital, the patient was determined to have a perforated colon and underwent a subtotal colectomy. Pathology revealed intestinal necrosis with increased lymphocyte infiltration. High dose steroids were started; however, 8 weeks later, the patient experienced another colon perforation and palliative care was initiated.

Due to the seriousness of colitis and the success of infliximab in the treatment of these gastrointestinal toxicities, a case series describing 3 cases of colitis proposed a treatment algorithm for colitis management [73A]. Based on the cases presented, the authors proposed an algorithm in which they suggested patients with grade 1 and 2 diarrhea be managed by holding ipilimumab along with symptom management. If symptoms resolved within 1 week, ipilimumab may be restarted, if not, steroids may be initiated. In those with grade 3 or higher diarrhea, ipilimumab should be discontinued permanently and high dose intravenous steroids should be administered with an oral taper over 6–8 weeks. If the patient does not improve after 3 days, infliximab may be administered, and a second dose may be considered after 2 weeks if no response is observed.

Dermatologic Adverse Effects

In the phase three trials and meta-analyses described earlier, immune checkpoint inhibitors caused rash in 4%–13% [56C,58M,59M]. In addition to this, the multicenter, retrospective analysis of nivolumab and pembrolizumab described earlier demonstrated dermatologic (pruritus, rash, eczema, vitiligo, alopecia) side effects in 8.7% of the 496 patients included [66c]. In addition to these analyses, dermatologic adverse effects were reported in multiple case reports and a case series over the past year.

Toxic epidermal necrolysis (TEN) was demonstrated in a 64-year-old female receiving nivolumab for ipilimumab refractory melanoma [74A]. The patient developed a grade 1 maculopapular rash after 2 doses of nivolumab and was started on oral prednisone. The rash increased to grade 2 within 1 week, and the patient was started on methylprednisolone for 4 days followed by prednisone with some response. After another week, the patient developed wide spread maculopapular rash with bullae on the trunk and extremities. Methylprednisolone and intravenous immunoglobulin was initiated and a biopsy demonstrated interface dermatitis with lymphocyte infiltrate and apoptotic keratinocytes present along with some necrosis of the dermis. Cyclosporine was added, and the patient had a gradual improvement. Another case described a Grover's like drug eruption in a 73-year-male receiving ipilimumab for metastatic melanoma [75A]. Five weeks after starting ipilimumab, the patient developed a wide spread grade 2 polymorphic papulovesicular dermatosis on the trunk and extremities with pruritus. Biopsy demonstrated acantholytic dyskeratosis with interface dermatitis. Topical steroids led to resolution of the symptoms and ipilimumab was continued. Similar to these cases, a case series described 6 patients with bullous skin eruptions during treatment with nivolumab or pembrolizumab [76A]. The patients ranged in age from 59 to 75. Symptoms developed 21–112 days after starting therapy and involved the extremities and trunk. All patients had a partial or complete response with systemic corticosteroids and discontinuation of the immune checkpoint inhibitor.

Due to the upregulation of the immune system, patients with autoimmune disorders, such as psoriasis are at risk for exacerbation of their disease. A case report of an 87-year-old male receiving nivolumab for the treatment of metastatic melanoma described a psoriasis flare with pulmonary involvement [77A]. After the second infusion of nivolumab, the patient developed a pulmonary infiltrate, and CT demonstrated ground glass opacities and consolidation of the lungs which did not respond to treatment with ampicillin/sulbactam. Prednisolone was initiated with improvement in the lung and psoriatic lesions.

In yet another case published in 2016, a patient receiving pembrolizumab for metastatic melanoma experienced pembrolizumab-induced radiosensitization [78A]. The patient was a 30-year-old male with metastatic melanoma who received radiation to sites of metastases in the elbow and knee. He was started on pembrolizumab 3 days after finishing radiation and developed a well-defined inflammatory erythematous eruption of the left elbow, confided to the irradiated area. Topical steroids led to regression over 3 weeks and the patient received additional cycles of pembrolizumab without further issues.

Sarcoid-Like Adverse Effects

Sarcoid-like reactions, many involving the skin have been reported. In 2016, 4 case reports and a case series were published describing sarcoid-like reactions associated with immune checkpoint inhibitors. In the first case, a 60-year-old female receiving ipilimumab plus nivolumab experienced a rash consisting of pink firm papules, some coalescing into annular papules, after three doses of ipilimumab and 10 doses of nivolumab [79A]. A skin biopsy was consistent with sarcoidosis and topical steroids led to some improvement. A case report of a 46-year-old female with metastatic melanoma who developed sarcoid-like reaction while receiving ipilimumab was also published [80A]. The patient developed generalized pruritus and cutaneous lesions on her lower extremities which were shown to be consistent with sarcoidosis on biopsy. Again, topical steroids demonstrated improvement; however, this patient developed progressive dyspnea 1 month after stopping ipilimumab that improved within a few days of starting oral steroids. In a case of nivolumab treatment for unresectable

melanoma, a 57-year-old male developed lymphadenopathy with hypermetabolism of the upper lip, appendectomy scars, and hilar/mediastinal lymph nodes on PET scan [81A]. Biopsy of a subcutaneous nodule of the appendectomy scar was consistent with a sarcoid-like reaction. No treatment was necessary and lesions regressed over the following year. In the final case report published in 2016, a 56-year-old male receiving nivolumab for metastatic melanoma developed pulmonary symptoms, dry eyes, and bilateral swelling of the parotid glands [82A]. Bronchial biopsy demonstrated sarcoidosis, and oral steroids led to a quick resolution within 4 weeks. In the published case series, 3 patients with melanoma, who were receiving ipilimumab or pembrolizumab for melanoma, developed symptoms after the second, third, and sixth cycles of therapy. Symptoms resolved without steroids and one patient required opioids and non-steroidal anti-inflammatory drugs to control pain [83A].

Endocrine Adverse Effects

In the phase three trial of adjuvant ipilimumab described earlier, grade 3 or higher endocrinopathies occurred in 7.9% of those receiving ipilimumab [53C]. Those with grade 2–4 adverse effects resolved in 51.5% with a median of 54.3 weeks to resolution. In the multicenter, retrospective analysis of patients receiving nivolumab or pembrolizumab described earlier, 6% developed endocrinopathies (hypothyroidism, hyperthyroidism, hypophysitis, adrenal insufficiency, Hashimoto's disease, and diabetes) [66c]. In a meta-analysis of 10 trials of patients receiving ipilimumab or nivolumab, the risk for all grade hypothyroidism (RR 8.26, 95% CI: 4.67–14.62), hyperthyroidism (RR 5.48, 95% CI: 1.33–22.53), hypophysitis (RR 22.03, 95% CI: 8.52–56.94), and adrenal insufficiency (RR 3.87, 95% CI: 1.12–13.41) was all increased [84M]. In addition to these, thyroid effects were described in a two case reports. The first one involved nivolumab-induced transient hyperthyroidism associated with thyroiditis in a patient with no history of a thyroid disorder [85A]. The second report was another case of hyperthyroidism after two doses of ipilimumab for metastatic melanoma [86A]. Ipilimumab was held and methimazole was administered. Once under control, ipilimumab was restarted without further exacerbation.

Case reports have also been published describing hypophysitis. In 50-year-old with unresectable melanoma who was receiving nivolumab, the patient developed fatigue, appetite loss, and weakness after the sixth dose [87A]. The patient was diagnosed with nivolumab-induced hypophysitis and hydrocortisone was initiated. Improvement occurred over the next few days, and nivolumab was re-administered with steroid supplementation without exacerbating the condition. A similar case report was also published describing a 67-year-old female with metastatic melanoma who developed fatigue, nausea, and headaches after their third dose of ipilimumab [88A]. The patient was diagnosed with autoimmune hypophysitis and started on a glucocorticoid which led to normalization of pituitary size and resolution of symptoms. In addition to developing endocrinopathies during therapy with immune checkpoint inhibitors, a unique case of a late onset endocrinopathy in a patient receiving ipilimumab for metastatic melanoma was published [89A]. Nine months after completing four doses of ipilimumab, the patient was diagnosed with panhypopituitarism. They also showed a reduction in the size of the pituitary gland which was postulated to be due to a late atrophic phase of autoimmune hypophysitis. Treatment with oral cortisone, levothyroxine, and intramuscular testosterone were initiated with resolution of symptoms.

As demonstrated in the multi-center retrospective analysis of adverse effects associated with pembrolizumab and nivolumab described earlier, diabetes may develop while receiving these medications [66c]. In a case report of a 76-year-old male with metastatic NSCLC receiving pembrolizumab, carboplatin, and nab-paclitaxel, the patient developed a blood glucose level of 616 mg/dL during the second cycle [90A]. Prior to pembrolizumab, the patients glucose ranged 120–140 mg/dL with a hemoglobin AIC of 6.3%. Long-acting and short-acting insulin were started and the patient's glycemic control improved. Pembrolizumab was re-initiated with good glucose level control with insulin.

The last case report of an endocrinopathy associated with immune checkpoint inhibitors involved a 43-year-old patient receiving nivolumab for metastatic melanoma [91A]. After four cycles, the patient's sodium level began to decrease, and by the end of the fifth cycle, it was 127 mmol/L. The patient was determined to be cortisol deficient, and hydrocortisone was initiated with improvement in fatigue, anorexia, and weight loss. Sodium levels remained at 127 mm/L and fludrocortisone was added. Sodium returned to normal, and the patient went on to receive 1 year of nivolumab with a normal sodium levels.

Neurologic Adverse Effects

Neurologic adverse effects were not commonly reported in phase three trials of immune checkpoint inhibitors. In studies of nivolumab, asthenia occurred in 3%–10.4% of the population; however, there was no distinction whether or not this was neurologic in origin [56C,59M]. Despite this, multiple case reports have been published describing neurologic effects associated with these medications. Likewise, in the multi-center, retrospective review of nivolumab and pembrolizumab described earlier, neurologic effects (paresthesia, paresis, polyneuropathy, seizures, Guillain-Barré syndrome, mining-radiculitis, aphasia, bradykinesia, parkinsonian syndrome) were reported in 1.4% of the population [63c].

Three case reports have been published describing demyelination [92A,93A]. The first report included a 45-year old receiving pembrolizumab for unresectable melanoma who developed motor weakness in the legs, areflexia, and peripheral facial paralysis after the second dose [92A]. The patient received intravenous immunoglobulin and symptoms resolved over the next 2 weeks. In the second case, an 85 year old with metastatic melanoma receiving pembrolizumab developed painful paresthesia, motor weakness, and areflexia after the sixth pembrolizumab dose [92A]. The patient did not improve despite treatment with oral and intravenous steroids and plasma exchange. The last case involved a 60-year-old male with metastatic melanoma receiving nivolumab who developed confusion, apathy, a fixed gaze, and psychomotor slowing [93A]. MRI demonstrated tumefactive demyelination, and the patient received high dose intravenous methylprednisolone and intravenous immunoglobulin that resulted in improvement.

In addition to the above case reports, 6 additional case reports describing neurologic effects were published in 2016. In an 81-year-old female receiving nivolumab for metastatic melanoma, symptoms of proximal limb weakness, dyspnea, bilateral ptosis, diplopia, and muscle weakness developed [94A]. Lab tests for AChR-binding antibody were elevated; however, the patient declined ventilator assistance and died. A 46-year-old female receiving ipilimumab for metastatic melanoma developed bilateral hearing loss with asthenia and severe ataxia after her fourth dose [95A]. The patient was diagnosed with cerebellar syndrome without vestibular defect that improved on steroids. In a 51-year-old female receiving pembrolizumab for metastatic melanoma, acute confusion and weakness occurred 18 months after starting therapy [96A]. This was thought to be intracranial vasculitis which resolved after starting aspirin. A 56-year-old male with metastatic melanoma developed meningoencephalitis 6 weeks after their last dose of ipilimumab [97A]. Eventually a trial of steroids was initiated for non-infectious, non-neoplastic meningoencephalitis. Improvement occurred over 48 hours and within 6 months was back to baseline. In a 53-year old with recurrent melanoma, visions changes developed 5 months after starting ipilimumab [98A]. He was determined to have possible inflammatory optic neuropathy and aseptic meningitis that improved with methylprednisolone. Due to the inability to wean steroids without recurrence of symptoms, mycophenolate mofetil was added to therapy. Lastly, a patient receiving pembrolizumab for melanoma developed progressive cognitive decline 1 year after starting therapy [99A]. Cerebral spinal fluid analysis demonstrated an elevated white blood cell count and protein and an MRI demonstrated signal changes within the limbic structure which was treated with steroids.

Pulmonary Adverse Effects

Pulmonary adverse effects, such as pneumonitis, have been described in patients receiving immune checkpoint inhibitors. In fact, a meta-analysis of 11 trials with pembrolizumab, nivolumab, and ipilimumab that included 6671 patients demonstrated an increased risk for all grade pneumonitis with these medications (OR 3.96, 95% CI: 2.02–7.79) [100A]. The overall incidence for all grade pneumonitis was 1.3%–11% and 0.3%–2% developed high-grade pneumonitis. There was no increase in the risk of high-grade pneumonitis. Compared to ipilimumab monotherapy, patients receiving nivolumab in combination with ipilimumab demonstrated an increased risk for all grade pneumonitis (RR 3.68, 95% CI: 1.59–8.50) without a significant increase in high-grade pneumonitis. Likewise, the multi-center, randomized analysis of nivolumab and pembrolizumab, described earlier, demonstrated an incidence of 1.6% for autoimmune-related pneumonitis [63c].

In addition to this, case reports of pulmonary sarcoidosis (see above) have been published along with two case reports demonstrating the ability of these medications to cause pulmonary adverse effects. The first involved a 70-year-old female with metastatic melanoma who developed a drop in oxygen saturation and bilateral basal fine crackles 28 days after her third dose of nivolumab [101A]. Bronchoscopy results were suggestive of organizing pneumonia. Dexamethasone was started and the patient improved over the next 3 months. In the second case, a 77-year old with metastatic melanoma developed fever, cough, and dyspnea during treatment with ipilimumab and was diagnosed with bronchiolitis obliterans organizing pneumonia [102A]. Clarithromycin was initiated, taking advantage of its anti-inflammatory effects, and the patient responded.

Ocular Adverse Effects

In the multi-center, randomized analysis of nivolumab and pembrolizumab, described earlier, ocular side effects occurred in 1.6% of the population and included iritis, uveitis, conjunctivitis, dry eyes and blurry vision [63c]. In another retrospective review, within a single institution, 4 patients developed orbital inflammation (treated with systemic corticosteroids), 2 developed uveitis (treated with topical and systemic corticosteroids), and one developed peripheral ulcerative keratitis (treated with topical corticosteroids) [103A]. Overall, 4 presented after the second dose, 2 after the third dose, and one after the first dose.

In addition to these studies, 8 cases of ocular adverse effects were reported in the literature in 2016. Two patients developed dry eye with nivolumab and were treated with lubricating ointment, artificial tears and topical cyclosporine drops [104A]. One of the patients developed a corneal perforation that was managed with topical loteprednol, autologous serum tears, oral doxycycline, and vitamin C in addition to topical cyclosporine. Both patients were able to restart nivolumab with this eye care regimen. Five cases of uveitis with pembrolizumab were reported and all resolved with steroid treatment (three received topical and oral steroids and two received topical steroids alone) [105A,106A,107A,108A]. One patient also required topical mydriatic agents, a topical non-steroidal anti-inflammatory drug, a topical beta-blocker, and carbonic anhydrase inhibitor [105A]. Another of these patients developed cataracts and developed crystoid macular edema 1 month postoperatively that was treated with topical steroids and intravitreal triamcinolone [106A]. The last case report included a 44-year-old male receiving ipilimumab for metastatic melanoma who developed bilateral ocular inflammation and was found to have anterior chamber inflammation and bilateral optic nerve edema [109A]. Topical prednisolone, brimonidine tartrate, timolol maleate, and oral prednisone were administered. Due to the continued presence of optic nerve edema and macular edema, the oral prednisone was increased and the patient responded. The patient self-discontinued steroids and developed a flare of anterior uveitis that responded to topical difluprednate. After 2 months, the patient's vision improved and the anterior chamber reaction stabilized.

Renal Adverse Effects

Renal adverse effects, though rare, have been described with immune checkpoint inhibitors. In the multi-center, retrospective analysis of patients receiving nivolumab or pembrolizumab described earlier, renal failure and nephritis occurred in two patients [66c]. In addition to this, a case report and a case series were published in 2016. The first case report was of a 75-year-old patient receiving nivolumab and ipilimumab for melanoma [110A]. The patient developed rash and severe acute tubulointerstitial nephritis after two doses. Serum creatinine increased to 3.96 mg/dL and the patient also developed 2+ proteinuria. Intravenous methylprednisolone was administered for 3 days followed by a steroid taper. One week later the patient was readmitted with a serum creatinine of 4.64 mg/dL and a worsening rash. Treatment with methylprednisolone and mycophenolate mofetil was initiated. The serum creatinine peaked at 7.31 mg/dL and decreased to 3.37 mg/dL over 10 days. In the case series, 6 patients developed acute kidney injury with interstitial nephritis on biopsy while receiving anti-PD-1 monoclonal antibodies [111A]. The patients were all receiving other medications associated with acute interstitial nephritis but had been tolerating them prior to initiating therapy with immune checkpoint inhibitors. The authors postulated that anti-PD-1 therapies may decrease renal tolerance for drugs associated with nephritis.

Hematologic Adverse Effects

In 2016, six cases of hematologic toxicity were reported. Two patients experienced autoimmune hemolytic anemia during treatment with pembrolizumab (one after two doses, the other after 3 doses); one responding to prednisone and the other requiring additional therapy [112A,113A]. In the first case, nivolumab was reintroduced for the treatment of the patients recurrent, refractory Hodgkin's lymphoma without recurrence of hemolysis [112A]. In the second case, the patient had an initial response to glucocorticoids; however, upon tapering of the dose, the pure red-cell aplasia flared [113A]. The patient responded to a dose of intravenous immune globulin and steroids was able to be tapered without any further recurrence.

In another case, a patient receiving ipilimumab for the adjuvant treatment of melanoma developed neutropenia [114A]. Based on a bone marrow biopsy, the neutropenia was determined to be due to an ipilimumab-induced immune assault on the myeloid precursors. Prednisone was administered without response followed by cyclosporine, immunoglobulin, and filgrastim without response. After not responding, therapy was changed to rabbit anti-thymocyte globulin, cyclosporine, prednisone, and filgrastim which led to improvement in the neutrophil count. Steroids were tapered over 5 months after finishing anti-thymocyte globulin and the neutrophil count remained stable within normal limits.

Three cases of idiopathic thrombocytopenic purpura were reported, one with nivolumab and two with pembrolizumab [115A,116A]. The patient receiving nivolumab responded to prednisolone, intravenous immunoglobulin, romiplostim, and platelet transfusion [115A]. In the patients receiving pembrolizumab, both patients responded quickly, one with steroids alone and one with steroids and intravenous immunoglobulin [116A].

Miscellaneous Effects

In addition to the adverse events described earlier, there were multiple additional reports of adverse effects associated with immune checkpoint inhibitors. A meta-analysis of 17 trials with ipilimumab, nivolumab, pembrolizumab, and tremelimumab investigated their association with fatigue [117M]. Overall, there was an increase in the risk with ipilimumab and tremelimumab for both all grade fatigue (OR 1.23, 95% CI: 1.07–1.41) and high-grade fatigue (OR 1.72, 95% CI: 1.26–2.33). Conversely, nivolumab and pembrolizumab led to a decreased risk for both all grade fatigue (RR 0.72, 95% CI: 0.62–0.84) and high-grade fatigue (RR 0.36, 95% CI: 0.23–0.56). This demonstrates that the PD-1 inhibitors may be more tolerable, in terms of fatigue. Four case reports were also published describing additional adverse effects.

Multiple case reports describing miscellaneous adverse effects were also published. Tumor lysis syndrome was reported in a 73-year old with metastatic melanoma 6 days after receiving ipilimumab [118A]. The patient experienced hyperkalemia, hypocalcemia, hyperuricemia, cardiac arrhythmia and renal failure. Another case involved an 82-year-old male with metastatic melanoma who experienced autoimmune inner ear disease after two doses of pembrolizumab [119A]. The patient experienced bilateral sensorineural hearing loss that recovered after intratympanic dexamethasone injections. Ipilimumab was also associated with the development of an anorectal fistula 1 month after starting treatment [120A]. The patient was a 74-year-old woman with metastatic melanoma who initially experienced ipilimumab-induced colitis that partially responded to steroids, but the patient subsequently developed anal pain and was found to have an anorectal fistula that was treated with a deroofing fistulectomy. Due to delayed healing, two doses of infliximab were administered; however, the patient passed away a few months later due to their malignancy. The last case report involved a 52-year-old male receiving ipilimumab for the treatment of metastatic melanoma who experienced osteonecrosis of the jaw [121A]. Six days after this second dose of ipilimumab, the patient developed gingival swelling that progressed over 1 month to a necrotic area of bone measuring 2×2 mm and further increased in size to 10×5 mm. The patient was receiving chlorhexidine all along and over the next 2 months fully resolved.

CONCLUSION

Monoclonal antibodies have become a mainstay of therapy for many malignancies. Although they lack traditional adverse effects observed with cytotoxic chemotherapeutic agents, toxicity can be severe with these medications. Many of these adverse effects may be predicted based on the target of the monoclonal antibody. Due to the frequency of adverse effects with these medications, patients need to be followed closely and educated regarding potential side effects prior to starting therapy.

References

[1] Zalcman G, Mazieres J, Margery J, et al. Bevacizumab for newly diagnosed pleural mesothelioma in the Mesothelioma Avastin Cisplatin Pemetrexed Study (MAPS): a randomized, controlled, open-label, phase 3 trial. Lancet. 2016;387:1405–14 [C].

[2] Karayama M, Inui N, Fujisawa T, et al. Maintenance therapy with pemetrexed and bevacizumab versus pemetrexed monotherapy after induction therapy with carboplatin, pemetrexed, and bevacizumab in patients with advanced non-squamous non-small cell lung cancer. Eur J Cancer. 2016;58:20–37 [C].

[3] Muro K, Cheul Oh S, Shimada Y, et al. Subgroup analysis of East Asians in RAINBOW: a phase 3 trial of ramucirumab plus paclitaxel for advanced gastric cancer. J Gastroenterol Hepatol. 2016;31:581–9 [C].

[4] Wu YS, Shiu L, Shen D, et al. Bevacizumab combined with chemotherapy for ovarian cancer: an updated systemic review and meta-analysis of randomized controlled trials. Oncotarget. 2017;8:10703–13 [M].

[5] Marchetti C, De Felice F, Palaia I, et al. Efficacy and toxicity of bevacizumab in recurrent ovarian disease: an update meta-analysis on phase III trials. Oncotarget. 2015;7:13221–7 [M].

[6] Lai X, Xu R, Li Y, et al. Risk of adverse events with bevacizumab addition to therapy in advanced non-small-cell cancer: a meta-analysis of randomized controlled trials. Onco Targets Ther. 2016;9:2421–8 [M].

[7] Botrel TE, Clark LG, Paladini L, et al. Efficacy and safety of bevacizumab plus chemotherapy compared to chemotherapy alone in previously untreated advanced or metastatic colorectal cancer: a systematic review and meta-analysis. BMC Cancer. 2016;16:1677 [M].

[8] Li Y, Hou M, Lu G, et al. The prognosis of anti-angiogenesis treatments combined with standard therapy for newly diagnosed glioblastoma: a meta-analysis of randomized controlled trials. PLoS One. 2016;11:e0168264 [M].

[9] Pinto C, Antonuzzi L, Porcu L, et al. Efficacy and safety of bevacizumab combined with fluoropyrimidine monotherapy for unfit or older patients with metastatic colorectal cancer: a systematic review and meta-analysis. Clin Colorectal Cancer. 2017;16:e61–72. epub ahead of print Aug 31 [M].

[10] Cao L, Yao G, Liu M, et al. Neoadjuvant bevacizumab plus chemotherapy versus chemotherapy alone to treat non-metastatic breast cancer: a meta-analysis of randomized controlled trials. PLoS One. 2015;10:e0145442 [M].

[11] Al-Batran SE, Van Cutsem E, Oh SC, et al. Quality-of-life and performance status results from the phase III RAINBOW study of ramucirumab plus paclitaxel versus placebo plus paclitaxel in patients with previously treated gastric or gastroesophageal junction adenocarcinoma. Ann Oncol. 2016;27:673–9 [C].

[12] Perol M, Ciuleanu TE, Arrieta O, et al. Quality of life results from the phase 3 REVEL randomized clinical trial of ramucirumab-plus-docetaxel versus placebo-plus-docetaxel in advanced/metastatic non-small cell lung cancer patients with progression after platinum-based chemotherapy. Lung Cancer. 2016;93:95–103 [C].

[13] Abdel-Rahman O, ElHalawani H. Risk of cardiovascular adverse events in patients with solid tumors treated with ramucirumab: a meta analysis and summary of other VEGF targeted agents. Crit Rev Oncol Hematol. 2016;102:89–100 [M].

[14] Qi WX, Fu S, Zhang Q, et al. Incidence and risk of hypertension associated with ramucirumab in cancer patients: a systematic review and meta-analysis. J Cancer Res Ther. 2016;12:775–81 [M].

[15] Tian R, Yan H, Zhang F, et al. Incidence and relative risk of hemorrhagic events associated with ramucirumab in cancer patients: a systematic review and meta-analysis. Oncotarget. 2016;7:66182–91 [M].

[16] Zhu X, Tian X, Yu C, et al. Increased risk of hemorrhage in metastatic colorectal cancer patients treated with bevacizumab: an updated meta-analysis of 12 randomized controlled trials. Medicine. 2016;95:e4232 [M].

[17] Alahmari A, Almalki Z, Alahmari A, et al. Thromboembolic events associated with bevacizumab plus chemotherapy for patients with colorectal cancer: a meta-analysis of randomized controlled trials. Am Health Drug Benefits. 2016;9:221–32 [M].

[18] Gruenberg J, Manivel J, Gupta P, et al. Fatal acute cardiac vasculopathy during cisplatin-gemcitabine-bevacizumab (GCB) chemotherapy for advanced urothelial carcinoma. J Infect Chemother. 2016;22:112–6 [A].

[19] Frantzen L, Rondeau-Lutz M, Mosquera F, et al. Reversible posterior encephalopathy syndrome and cardiomyopathy after bevacizumab therapy. Rev Med Interne. 2016;1:50–2 [A].

[20] Zhang H, Huang Z, Zou X, et al. Bevacizumab and wound-healing complications: a systematic review and meta-analysis of randomized controlled trials. Oncotarget. 2016;7: 82473–81 [M].

[21] Volk AM, Fritzmann J, Reissfelder C, et al. Impact of bevacizumab on parenchymal damage and functional recovery of the liver in patients with colorectal liver metastases. BMC Cancer. 2016;16:84 [M].

[22] Qi WX, Shen Z, Tang L, et al. Bevacizumab increases the risk of gastrointestinal perforation in cancer patients: a meta-analysis with a focus on different subgroups. Eur J Clin Pharmacol. 2014;70:893–906 [M].

[23] Wang Z, Zhang J, Zhang L, et al. Risk of gastrointestinal perforation in cancer patients receiving ramucirumab: a meta-analysis of randomized controlled trial. J Chemother. 2016;28:328–34 [M].

[24] Ozturk MA, Erdik B, Eren OO. Sigmoid colon perforation related to bevacizumab in a patient with glioblastoma. Am J Ther. 2016;23:e241–2 [A].

[25] Miyake Y, Ikeda K, Murakami M, et al. Two cases of bowel perforation during chemotherapy with bevacizumab to metastatic rectal cancer. Gan To Kagaku Ryoho. 2015;42:75–8 [A].

[26] Kurata T, Makita N, Hagino S, et al. A case of multiple bevacizumab-related colonic perforations during opioid use. Gan To Kagaku Ryoho. 2016;42:95–7 [A].

[27] Hayashi C, Takada S, Kasuga A, et al. Sigmoid-vaginal fistula during bevacizumab treatment diagnosed by fistulography. J Clin Pharm Ther. 2016;41:725–6 [A].

[28] Momeni M, Veras L, Zakashamansky K. Bevacizumab-induced transient sixth nerve palsy in ovarian cancer: a case report. Asia Pac J Clin Oncol. 2016;12:e196–8 [A].

[29] Yamaguchi Y, Tada Y, Takaya S, et al. A case of drug-induced lung injury associated with paclitaxel plus bevacizumab therapy. Gan To Kagaku Ryoho. 2016;43:781–4 [A].

[30] Reck M, Socinski MA, Luft A, et al. The effect of necitumumab in combination with gemcitabine plus cisplatin on tolerability and on quality of life: results from the phase 3 SQUIRE trial. J Thorac Oncol. 2016;11:808–18 [C].

[31] Reck M, Thomas M, Kropf-Sanchen, et al. Necitumumab plus gemcitabine and cisplatin as first-line therapy in patients with stage IV EGFR-expressing squamous non-small-cell lung cancer: German subgroup data from an open-label, randomized controlled phase 3 study (SQUIRE). Oncol Res Treat. 2016;39:539–47 [C].

[32] Chen Q, Cheng M, Wang Z, et al. The efficacy and safety of panitumumab plus irinotecan-based chemotherapy in the treatment of metastatic colorectal cancer: a meta-analysis. Medicine. 2016;95(50)e5284 [M].

[33] Huang J, Zhang J, Shi C, et al. Survival, recurrence and toxicity of HNSCC in comparison of a radiotherapy combination with

cisplatin versus cetuximab: a meta-analysis. BMC Cancer. 2016;16:689 [M].

[34] Miroddi M, Sterrantino C, Simmonds M, et al. Systematic review and meta-analysis of the risk of severe and life-threatening thromboembolism in cancer patients receiving anti-EGFR monoclonal antibodies (cetuximab or panitumumab). Int J Cancer. 2016;139:2370–80 [M].

[35] Pinto C, Barone C, Girolomoni G, et al. Management of skin reactions during cetuximab treatment in association with chemotherapy or radiotherapy. Am J Clin Oncol. 2016;39:407–15 [R].

[36] Streb J, Puskulluoglu M, Glanowska I, et al. Assessment of frequency and severity of hypomagnesemia in patients with metastatic colorectal cancer treated with cetuximab. Oncol Lett. 2015;10:3749–55 [c].

[37] Shinohara A, Kogo R, Uryu H, et al. A case of pneumocystis pneumonia after cetuximab-based bioradiotherapy. Nihon Jibiinkoka Gakkai Kaiho. 2016;119:204–9 [A].

[38] Kato K, Michishita Y, Oyama K, et al. A case of thrombotic thrombocytopenic purpura in a patient undergoing FOLFOX6 plus panitumumab therapy for unresectable recurrent rectal cancer with a rapidly progressive course. Gan To Kagaku Ryoho. 2016;43:133–6 [A].

[39] Garcia-Menaya JM, Cordobes-Duran C, Gomez-Ulla J, et al. Successful desensitization to cetuximab in a patient with a positive skin test to cetuximab and specific IgE to alpha-gal. J Investig Allergol Clin Immunol. 2016;26:111–43 [A].

[40] Piccart-Gebhart M, Holmes E, Baselga J, et al. Adjuvant lapatinib and trastuzumab for early human epidermal growth factor receptor 2-positive breast cancer: results from the randomized phase III adjuvant lapatinib and/or trastuzumab treatment optimization trial. J Clin Oncol. 2016;34:1034–42 [C].

[41] Chen Y, Want L, Chen F, et al. Efficacy, safety and administration timing of trastuzumab in human epidermal growth factor receptor 2 positive breast cancer patients: a meta-analysis. Exp Ther Med. 2016;11:1721–33 [M].

[42] Shen K, Ma X, Zhu C, et al. Safety and efficacy of trastuzumab emtansine in advanced human epidermal growth factor receptor 2-positive breast cancer: a meta-analysis. Sci Rep. 2016;6:23262 [M].

[43] Krug D. Cardiac toxicity of trastuzumab in adjuvant therapy of breast cancer patients: results of the NCCTG-N9831study. Rayenther Onkol. 2016;192:193 [MC].

[44] Jawa Z, Perez RM, Garlie L, et al. Risk factors of trastuzumab-induced cardiotoxicity in breast cancer: a meta-analysis. Medicine. 2016;95(44):e5195 [M].

[45] Mantarro S, Rossi M, Bonifazi M, et al. Risk of severe cardiotoxicity following treatment with trastuzumab: a meta-analysis of randomized and cohort studies of 29,000 women with breast cancer. Intern Emerg Med. 2016;11:123–40 [M].

[46] Long H, Lin Y, Zhang J, et al. Risk of congestive heart failure in early breast cancer patients undergoing adjuvant treatment with trastuzumab: a meta-analysis. Oncologist. 2016;21:547–54 [M].

[47] Yu AF, Manrique C, Pun S, et al. Cardiac safety of paclitaxel plus trastuzumab and pertuzumab in patients with HER2-positive metastatic breast cancer. Oncologist. 2016;21:418–24 [M].

[48] Orlandi A, Fasciani R, Cassano A, et al. Trastuzumab-induced corneal ulceration: successful no-drug treatment of a "blind" side effect in a case report. BMC Cancer. 2015;15:973 [A].

[49] Moon D, Koo JS, Suh C, et al. Radiation recall dermatitis induced by trastuzumab. Breast Cancer. 2016;23:159–63 [A].

[50] Miarons M, Velasco M, Campins L, et al. Gradual thrombocytopenia induced by long-term trastuzumab exposure. J Clin Pharm Ther. 2016;41:563–5 [A].

[51] Gonzalez-de-Olano D, Juarez-Guerrero R, Sanchez-Munoz L, et al. Positive basophil activation test following anaphylaxis to pertuzumab and successful treatment with rapid desensitization. J Allergy Clin Immunol Pract. 2016;4:338–40 [A].

[52] Tap WD, Jones RL, Van Tine BA, et al. Olaratumab and doxorubicin versus doxorubicin alone for treatment of soft-tissue sarcoma: an open-label phase 1b and randomized phase 2 trial. Lancet. 2016;338:488–97 [C].

[53] Eggermont AMM, Chiarion-Sileni V, Grob JJ, et al. Prolonged survival in stage III melanoma with ipilimumab adjuvant therapy. N Engl J Med. 2016;375:1845–55 [C].

[54] Reck M, Rodriguez-Abreu D, Robinson AG, et al. Pembrolizumab versus chemotherapy for PD-L1-positive non-small-cell lung cancer. N Engl J Med. 2016;375:1823–33 [C].

[55] Herbst RS, Baas P, Kim D, et al. Pembrolizumab versus docetaxel for previously treated, PD-L1-positive, advanced non-small-cell lung cancer (KEYNOTE-010): a randomized controlled trial. Lancet. 2016;387:1540–50 [C].

[56] Rosenberg JE, Hoffman-CenSits J, Powles T, et al. Atezolizumab in patients with locally advanced and metastatic urothelial carcinoma who have progressed following treatment with platinum-based chemotherapy: a single-arm, multicenter, phase2 trial. Lancet. 2016;387:1909–20 [C].

[57] Fehrenbacher L, Spira A, Ballinger M, et al. Atezolizumab versus docetaxel for patients with previously treated non-small-cell lung cancer (POPLAR): a multicenter, open-label, phase 2 randomised controlled trial. Lancet. 2016;387:1837–46 [C].

[58] Huang J, Zhang Y, Sheng J, et al. The efficacy and safety of nivolumab in previously treated advanced non-small-cell lung cancer: a meta-analysis of prospective clinical trials. Onco Targets Ther. 2016;9:5867–74 [M].

[59] Tie Y, Ma X, Zhu C, et al. Safety and efficacy of nivolumab in the treatment of cancers: a meta-analysis of 27 prospective clinical trials. Int J Cancer. 2017;140:948–58 [M].

[60] Jin C, Zhang X, Zhao K, et al. The efficacy and safety of nivolumab in the treatment of advanced melanoma: a meta-analysis of clinical trials. Onco Targets Ther. 2016;9:1571–8 [M].

[61] Abdel-Rahman O. Evaluation and safety of different pembrolizumab dose/schedules in treatment of non-small-cell lung cancer and melanoma: a systematic review. Immunotherapy. 2016;8:1383–91 [M].

[62] Agrawal S, Waxman I, Lanbert A, et al. Evaluation of the potential for QTc prolongation in patients with solid tumors receiving nivolumab. Cancer Chemother Pharmacol. 2016;77:635–41 [C].

[63] Zimmer L, Goldinger SM, Hofman L, et al. Neurological, respiratory, musculoskeletal, cardiac and ocular side-effects of anti-PD-1 therapy. Eur J Cancer. 2016;60:210–25 [c].

[64] Dasanu CA, Jen T, Skulski R, et al. Late-onset pericardial tamponade, bilateral pleural effusions and recurrent immune monoarthritis induced by ipilimumab use for metastatic melanoma. J Oncol Pharm Pract. 2017;23:231–4. Epub ahead of print Mar 4 2016 [A].

[65] Roth ME, Muluneh B, Jensen BC, et al. Left ventricular dysfunction after treatment with ipilimumab for metastatic melanoma. Am J Ther. 2016;23:e1925–8 [A].

[66] Hofmann L, Forschner A, Loquai C, et al. Cutaneous, gastrointestinal, hepatic, endocrine, and renal side-effects of anti-PD-1 therapy. Eur J Cancer. 2016;60:190–209 [c].

[67] Zhang X, Ran Y, Wang K, et al. Incidence and risk of hepatic toxicities with PD-1 inhibitors in cancer patients: a meta-analysis. Drug Des Devel Ther. 2016;10:3153–61 [M].

[68] O'Connor A, Marples M, Mulatero C, et al. Ipilimumab-induced colitis: experience from a tertiary referral center. Therap Adv Gastroenterol. 2016;9:457–62 [c].

[69] Hillock NT, Heard S, Kichenadasse G, et al. Infliximab for ipilimumab-induced colitis: a series of 13 patients. Asia Pac J Clin Oncol. 2016. Epub ahead of print Dec 16 2016 [A].

[70] Aya F, Gaba L, Victoria I, et al. Life-threatening colitis and complete response with ipilimumab in a patient with metastatic BRAF-mutant melanoma and rheumatoid arthritis. ESMO Open. 2016;1:e000032 [A].

[71] Messmer M, Upreti S, Tarabishy Y, et al. Ipilimumab-induced enteritis without colitis: a new challenge. Case Rep Oncol. 2016;9:705–13 [A].

[72] Gonzalez-cao M, Boada A, Teixido C, et al. Fatal gastrointestinal toxicity with ipilimumab after BRAF/MEK inhibitor combination in a melanoma patient achieving pathological complete response. Oncotarget. 2016;7:56619–27 [A].

[73] Klair JS, Girotra M, Hutchins LF, et al. Ipilimumab-induced gastrointestinal toxicities: a management algorithm. Dig Dis Sci. 2016;61:2132–9 [A].

[74] Nayar N, Briscoe K, Penas PF. Toxic epidermal necrolysis-like reaction with severe satellite cell necrosis associated with nivolumab in a patient with ipilimumab refractory metastatic melanoma. J Immunother. 2016;39:149–52 [A].

[75] Koelzer VH, Buser T, Willi N, et al. Grover's-like drug eruption in a patient with metastatic melanoma under ipilimumab therapy. J Immunother Cancer. 2016;4:47 [A].

[76] Jour G, Glitza IC, Ellis RM, et al. Autoimmune dermatologic toxicities from immune checkpoint blockade with anti-PD-1 antibody therapy: a report on bullous skin reactions. J Cutan Pathol. 2016;43:688–96 [A].

[77] Matsumura N, Ohtsuka M, Kikuchi N, et al. Exacerbation of psoriasis during nivolumab therapy for metastatic melanoma. Acta Derm Venereol. 2016;96:259–60 [A].

[78] Sibaud V, David I, Lamant L, et al. Acute skin reaction suggestive of pembrolizumab-induced radiosensitization. Melanoma Res. 2015;25:555–8 [A].

[79] Suozzi KC, Stahl M, Ko CJ, et al. Immune-related sarcoidosis observed in combination ipilimumab and nivolumab therapy. JAAD Case Rep. 2016;2:264–8 [A].

[80] Leborans LM, Martinez AE, Martinez AMV, et al. Cutaneous sarcoidosis in a melanoma patient under ipilimumab therapy. Dermatol Ther. 2016;29:306–8 [A].

[81] Danlos FX, Pages C, Baroudjian B, et al. Nivolumab-induced sarcoid-like granulomatous reaction in a patient with advanced melanoma. Chest. 2016;149:e133–6 [A].

[82] Montaudie H, Pradelli J, Passeron T, et al. Pulmonary sarcoid-like granulomatosis induced by nivolumab. Br J Dermatol. 2017;176:1060–3. Epub ahead of print Jun 13 2016 [A].

[83] Firwana B, Ravilla R, Raval M, et al. Sarcoidosis-like syndrome and lymphadenopathy due to checkpoint inhibitors. J Oncol Pharm Pract. 2016. Epub ahead of print Sep 2 2016 [A].

[84] Abdel-Raham O, ElHalawani H, Fouad M. Risk of endocrine complications in cancer patients treated with immune check point inhibitors: a meta-analysis. Future Oncol. 2016;12:413–25 [M].

[85] Verma I, Modi A, Tripathi H, et al. Nivolumab causing painless thyroiditis in a patient with adenocarcinoma of the lung. BMJ Case Rep. 2016; [A].

[86] Azmat U, Liebner D, Joehlin-Price A, et al. Treatment of ipilimumab induced Graves' disease in a patient with metastatic melanoma. Case Rep Endocrinol. 2016;2016:2087525 [A].

[87] Okana Y, Satoh T, Horiguchi K, et al. Nivolumab-induced hypophysitis in a patient with advanced malignant melanoma. Endocr J. 2016;63:905–12 [A].

[88] Marques P, Grossman A. Ipilimumab-induced autoimmune hypophysitis: diagnostic and management challenges illustrated by a clinical case. Acta Med Port. 2015;28:775–9 [A].

[89] Vancieri G, Bellia A, Lauro D. Late-onset panhypopituitarism in a 72-year-old male patient treated with ipilimumab for metastatic melanoma: a case report. J Endocrinol Invest. 2016;39:805–6 [A].

[90] Chae YK, Chiec L, Mohindra N, et al. A case of pembrolizumab-induced type-1 diabetes mellitus and discussion of immune checkpoint inhibitor-induced type 1 diabetes. Cancer Immunol Immunother. 2017;66:25–32 [A].

[91] Trainer H, Hulse P, Higham CE, et al. Hyponatremia secondary to nivolumab-induced primary adrenal failure. Endocrinol Diabetes Metab Case Rep. 2016. Epub ahead of print [A].

[92] De Maleissye MF, Nicolas G, Saiag P. Pembrolizumab-induced demyelinating polyradiculoneuropathy. N Engl J Med. 2016;375:296–7 [A].

[93] Maurice C, Schneider R, Kiehl TR, et al. Subacute CNS demyelination after treatment with nivolumab for melanoma. Cancer Immunol Res. 2015;3:1299–302 [A].

[94] Shirai T, Sano T, Kamijo F, et al. Acetylcholine receptor binding antibody-associated myasthenia gravis and rhabdomyolysis induced by nivolumab in a patient with melanoma. Jpn J Clin Oncol. 2016;46:86–8 [A].

[95] Koessler T, Oliver T, Fertani S, et al. Ipilimumab-related hypophysitis may precede severe CNS immune attack. Ann Oncol. 2016;27:1975–6 [A].

[96] Khoja L, Maurice C, Chapell M, et al. Eosinophilic fasciitis and acute encephalopathy toxicity from pembrolizumab treatment of a patient with metastatic melanoma. Cancer Immunol Res. 2016;4:175–8 [A].

[97] Stein MK, Summers BB, Wong CA, et al. Meningoencephalitis following ipilimumab administration in metastatic melanoma. Am J Med Sci. 2015;350:512–3 [A].

[98] Wilson MA, Guld K, Galetta S, et al. Acute visual loss after ipilimumab treatment for metastatic melanoma. J Immunother Cancer. 2016;18:66 [A].

[99] Salam S, Lavin T, Turan A. Limbic encephalitis following immunotherapy against metastatic malignant melanoma. BMJ Case Rep. 2016;23: bcr2016215012. [A].

[100] Abdel-Rahman O, Fouad M. Risk of pneumonitis in cancer patients treated with immune checkpoint inhibitors: a meta-analysis. Ther Adv Respir Dis. 2016;10:183–93 [M].

[101] Sano T, Uhara H, Mikoshiba Y, et al. Nivolumab-induced organizing pneumonia in a melanoma patient. Jpn J Clin Oncol. 2016;46:270–2 [A].

[102] Mailleux M, Cornelis F, Colin GC, et al. Unusual pulmonary toxicity of ipilimumab treated by marcolides. Acta Clin Belg. 2015;70:442–4 [A].

[103] Papavasileiou E, Prasad S, Freitag SK, et al. Ipilimumab-induced ocular and orbital inflammation—a case series and review of the literature. Ocul Immunol Inflamm. 2016;24:140–6 [A].

[104] Nguyen AT, Elia M, Materin MA, et al. Cyclosporine for dry eye associated with nivolumab: a case progressing to corneal perforation. Cornea. 2016;35:399–401 [A].

[105] Diem S, Keller F, Ruesch R, et al. Pembrolizumab-triggered uveitis: an additional surrogate marker for responders in melanoma immunotherapy. J Immunother. 2016;39:379–82 [A].

[106] Basiliou A. Posterior subcapsular cataracts and hypotony secondary to severe pembrolizumab induced uveitis: case report. Can J Ophthalmol. 2016;51:e4–6 [A].

[107] Samra KA, Valdes-Navarro M, Lee S, et al. A case of bilateral uveitis and papillitis in a patient treated with pembrolizumab. Eur J Ophthalmol. 2016;26:e46–8 [A].

[108] Hanna KS. A rare case of pembrolizumab-induced uveitis in a patient with metastatic melanoma. Pharmacotherapy. 2016;36:e183–8 [A].

[109] Hahn L, Pepple KL. Bilateral neuroretinitis and anterior uveitis following ipilimumab treatment for metastatic melanoma. J Ophthalmic Inflamm Infect. 2016;6:14 [A].

[110] Murakami N, Borges TJ, Yamashita M, et al. Severe acute interstitial nephritis after combination immune-checkpoint inhibitor therapy for metastatic melanoma. Clin Kidney J. 2016;9:411–7 [A].

[111] Shirali AC, Perazella MA, Gettinger S. Association of acute interstitial nephritis with programmed cell death 1 inhibitor therapy in lung cancer patients. Am J Kidney Dis. 2016;68:287–91 [A].

[112] Tardy MP, Gastaud L, Boscagli A, et al. Autoimmune hemolytic anemia after nivolumab treatment in Hodgkin lymphoma responsive to immunosuppressive treatment: a case report. Hematol Oncol. 2016. Epub ahead of print Aug 19 2016 [A].

[113] Nair R, Gheith S, Nair SG. Immunotherapy-associated hemolytic anemia with pure red-cell aplasia. N Engl J Med. 2016;374:11096–7 [A].

[114] Ban-Hoefen M, Burack R, Sievert L, et al. Ipilimumab-induced neutropenia in melanoma. J Investig Med High Impact Case Rep. 2016;9:1–5 [A].

[115] Kanameishi S, Otsuka A, Nonomura Y, et al. Idiopathic thrombocytopenic purpura induced by nivolumab in a metastatic melanoma patient with elevated PD-1 expression on B cells. Ann Oncol. 2016;27:546 [A].

[116] Le Roy A, Kempf E, Ackermann F, et al. Two cases of immune thrombocytopenia associated with pembrolizumab. Eur J Cancer. 2016;54:172–4 [A].

[117] Abdel-Rahman O, Helbling D, Schmidt J, et al. Treatment-associated fatigue in cancer patients treated with immune checkpoint inhibitors; a systematic review and meta-analysis. Clin Oncol. 2016;28:e127–38 [M].

[118] Masson Regnault M, Ofaiche J, Boulinguez S, et al. Tumour lysis syndrome: an unexpected adverse event associated with ipilimumab. J Eur Acad Dermatol Venereol. 2017;31: e73–4 [A].

[119] Zibelman M, Pollak N, Olszanski AJ. Autoimmune inner ear disease in a melanoma patient treated with pembrolizumab. J Immunother Cancer. 2016;4:8 [A].

[120] Balaphas A, Restellini S, Robert-Yap J, et al. A case of ipilimumab-induced anorectal fistula. J Crohns Colitis. 2016;10:501–2 [A].

[121] Owosho AA, Scordo M, Yom SK, et al. Osteonecrosis of the jaw a new complication related to ipilimumab. Oral Oncol. 2015;51: e100–1 [A].

41

Radiological Contrast Agents

Makoto Hasegawa[1], Tatsya Gomi

Ohashi Medical Center, Toho University, Tokyo, Japan

[1]Corresponding author: makoto.hasegawa@med.toho-u.ac.jp

INTRODUCTION

Contrast agents are substances, which are widely used to improve diagnostic performance of medical imaging. Various types of these agent exist depending on the imaging modality; iodinated contrast agents which absorb more X-rays than human tissue are used for radiographic examinations such as computed tomography (CT), gadolinium-based agents which have T1 relaxation time shortening effects are used for magnetic resonance imaging (MRI), and microbubbles which have a higher echogenicity compared to human tissue are used for ultrasound (US). Most of these agents are known to be stable. Although these agents are indispensable in medical imaging, they are not risk free.

Adverse reactions to contrast agents can be classified as acute, late and very late by the timing of the reaction after administration of the agent. Acute reactions can be categorized as allergic-like or physiological by the type of reaction, and mild, moderate, or severe by the severity. Adverse reactions may affect various organ systems. Recent publications which cover various aspects of adverse reactions to contrast agents will be discussed in this chapter, including the recently reported gadolinium accumulation.

Water-Soluble Intravascular Iodinated Contrast Agents [SEDA-33, 963; SEDA-34, 749; SEDA-35, 863; SEDA-36, 695; SEDA-37, 583; SEDA-38, 493]

Intravascular iodinated contrast agents can be classified into four types according to their physicochemical properties (Table 1). Most of these agents are used intravascularly, but they can also be injected into body cavities, particularly the low-osmolar contrast agents. Some are also used for oral or rectal administration, and the high-osmolar water-soluble contrast agent diatrizoate is suitable only for these purposes. Low-osmolar and iso-osmolar iodinated contrast media have almost completely replaced high-osmolar agents for intravascular use and administration into body cavities.

Drug Interactions

Metformin, a biguanide oral antihyperglycaemic agent, is used to treat patients with noninsulin-dependent

TABLE 1 List of Few Iodinated Water-Soluble Contrast Media

Properties	Examples (INNs)	Brand names
High-osmolar ionic monomers	Diatrizoate	Angiografin, Hypaque, Gastrografin, Renografin, Urografin
	Iotalamic acid	Conray
	Ioxitalamic acid	Telebrix
	Metrizoate	Isopaque, Triosil
Low-osmolar ionic dimers	Ioxaglic acid	Hexabrix
Low-osmolar non-ionic monomers	Iobitridol	Xenetrix
	Iohexol	Omnipaque
	Iomeprol	Iomeron
	Iopamidol	Isovue, Niopam, Solutrast
	Iopentol	Imagopaque
	Iopromide	Ultravist
	Ioversol	Optiray
	Metrizamide	Amipaque
Iso-osmolar non-ionic dimmers	Iodixanol	Visipaque
	Iosimenol	Iosmin
	Iotrolan	Isovist

diabetes mellitus. Metformin is thought to act by decreasing hepatic glucose production and enhancing peripheral glucose uptake as a result of increased sensitivity of peripheral tissues to insulin. The most significant adverse effect of metformin therapy is the potential for the development of metformin-associated lactic acidosis in susceptible patients. Metformin is excreted by the kidneys, therefore patients with renal insufficiency are at risk for this condition. Iodinated contrast is not an independent risk factor for patients taking metformin, but is a concern in the presence of underlying conditions of delayed renal excretion of metformin, decreased metabolism of lactic acid, or increased anaerobic metabolism. In patients with normal renal functions and no known comorbidities, there is no need of discontinuation of metformin prior to intravenous administration of iodinated contrast media. However, patients with comorbidities, it should be withheld for 48 hours and administration can resume after reassessment of renal function [1M,2M]

Types of Reactions

Adverse reactions that occur after contrast media injection typically occur within 20 minutes of the injection. An acute adverse reaction is an adverse reaction that occurs within 1 hour of injection. Acute reactions are classified as being of mild, moderate, and severe intensity. Types of reactions include mild symptoms such as nausea and itching and severe reactions such as hypotensive shock and convulsions. Most of these reactions resolve spontaneously. A late adverse reaction to contrast medium is defined as a reaction that occurs at 1 hour to 1 week after injection. Maculopapular rashes, erythema, and pruritus are the most common types of late reactions. A very late adverse reaction is a reaction that occurs more than 1week after contrast injection; this includes reactions such as thyrotoxicosis [3R].

A study retrospectively evaluated the incidence of acute adverse reactions of two iodinated contrast agents, Ultravist-370 and Isovue-370. The study included 137 473 patients. Four hundred and twenty-eight (0.31%) patients experienced acute adverse reactions, which included 330 (0.24%) patients with mild acute adverse reactions, 82 (0.06%) patients with moderate acute adverse reactions, and 16 (0.01%) patients with severe acute adverse reactions (including 3 cases of cardiac arrest and 1 case of death). The incidence of acute adverse reactions was higher with Ultravist-370 than with Isovue-370 (0.38% vs 0.24%, $P < 0.001$), but only for mild acute adverse reactions (0.32% vs 0.16%, $P < 0.001$). Cutaneous manifestations (50.52%) were the most frequent mild acute adverse reactions [4C].

Endocrine

Thyroid dysfunction may occur due to the effect of excess iodine within the contrast medium. This may either cause hypo or hyperthyroidism. Thyrotoxicosis is a type of very late adverse reaction seen after iodine-based contrast media. Untreated Graves' disease and multinodular goiter and thyroid autonomy are risks for this adverse reaction. Patients with hyperthyroidism are usually advised not to have iodinated contrast media injection. Patients with normal thyroid function are thought to be at low risk for this condition [1M]. However, a study investigating the effect of contrast media injection in children found that the incidence of incident hypothyroidism was significantly higher in patients who received intravenous contrast medium (odds ratio 2.60; 95% confidence interval, 1.43–4.72; $P < 0.01$). The authors suggest monitoring of thyroid dysfunction in children undergoing iodinated contrast medium administration [5c].

Another study investigated the incidence of thyroid dysfunction in euthyroid nodular goiter patients. The study compared 334 patients with euthyroid nodular goiter, and 2672 matched patients without thyroid nodule as controls. The study found that patients with euthyroid nodular goiter had a higher risk of thyroid dysfunction (hazard ratio 5.43, confidence interval (CI) 3.01–9.80) compared with controls after iodinated contrast media exposure. Risks of hyperthyroidism and hypothyroidism were both increased in these cases compared with controls. Half of the euthyroid nodular goiter cases developed thyroid dysfunction within 1 year after iodinated contrast media exposure. These data suggest that the risk of thyroid dysfunction may be higher in euthyroid patients in the presence of nodular goiter [6c].

SALIVARY GLANDS

Iodide mumps is a rare adverse reaction after administration of iodinated contrast agents. Painless bilateral enlargements of the salivary glands are seen after administration of contrast agents. It is speculated to be due to accumulation of high concentration of iodine in the ductal system, which induces inflammation. Prognosis is reported to be good with conservative treatment alone [7c,8c].

RADIATION

Radiation dose increase in iodine-charged tissue has been previously been reported in in vitro and in vivo experiments [9r,10R]. This may result in induction of DNA double-strand break induction [11E]. This was demonstrated in vitro and in vivo in patients undergoing paediatric cardiac catheterization [12c].

Iodinated Radiocontrast-Induced Nephropathy

Contrast-induced nephropathy is defined as renal hypofunction with an increase in the serum creatinine concentration of 25% or more or by 44 μmol/L (0.5 mg/dL) or more, developing within 3 days after injection of an intravascular contrast medium in the absence of other causes [1M]. The incidence of CIN is thought to be less common than previously believed. In patients with a stable baseline eGFR $\geq$45 mL/min/1.73 m^2, IV iodinated contrast media are not an independent nephrotoxic risk factor, and in patients with a stable baseline eGFR 30–44 mL/min/1.73 m^2, IV iodinated contrast media are rarely nephrotoxic [2M].

Some studies have reported no differences in the rates of CIN following administration of iodixanol compared to iohexol. However, iodixanol tends to be used in patients with an estimated glomerular filtration rate (eGFR) between 45.0 and 59.9 mL/min. Also, it is known that iodixanol is more expensive. The study included patients with a glomerular filtration rate (GFR) of 45.0 to 59.9 mL/min/1.73 m^2 which was obtained within 48–96 hours of their scheduled outpatient CT examination. Patients were randomized to receive 100 mL of iohexol ($n = 47$) or iodixanol ($n = 55$). CIN rate for iohexol was 2% compared to 9% for iodixanol. These results do not suggest a benefit of iodixanol over iohexol in the study population [13c].

Another study investigated the incidence of CIN in adult patients ($\geq$18 years) with active cancer who underwent CE-CT had a baseline creatinine level of 1.5 mg/dL or less. The incidence of CIN in this series was 8.0% (66/820 patients). CECT examinations, hypotension before the CT scan, liver cirrhosis, dehydration, and peritoneal carcinomatosis seem to predispose patients to CIN [14c]. Another study included 860 patients who underwent coronary intervention. 40 patients developed CIN. SCr levels significantly increased from a baseline of 1.55 ± 1.08 to 1.79 ± 1.26 mg/dL on the following day in patients with CIN ($P < 0.0001$). eGFR significantly decreased from a baseline of 47.3 ± 28.3 to 40.6 ± 26.7 mL/min/1.73 m^2 on the following day in patients with CIN ($P < 0.0001$). Receiver operating characteristic curve analysis indicated that SCr change $\geq$0.1 mg/dL and eGFR change $\leq$−1.1 mL/min/1.73 m^2 were the best cut-off values for predicting CIN [15c].

Susceptibility Factors, Diagnosis and Prevention of Adverse Reaction

In patients who are at risk for an adverse reaction (patients who previously had moderate or severe acute reaction to an iodine-based contrast agent, patients with asthma or any allergy requiring medical treatment), premedication should be considered. In patients who have previously reacted to iodinated contrast media, European Society of Urogenital Radiology guidelines on contrast media suggest the use of a different agent. Although clinical evidence of premedication is limited, the use of prednisolone 30 mg or methylprednisolone 32 mg orally 12 and 2 hours before the contrast agent should be considered for patients at risk [1M].

771 patients undergoing contrast enhanced CT with previous adverse reactions was assessed to compare the protective effect of changing the contrast media and premedications. The study found that although premedications for patients with previous adverse reactions to contrast media was effective, changing the contrast media was more effective [16c].

Currently, predicting adverse reactions to iodinated contrast agents is not possible. Skin tests are known to have a limited sensitivity and high specificity for patients with hypersensitivity. However, preliminary intradermal skin testing with contrast agents is not predictive of adverse reactions, and testing itself be dangerous, and is not recommended [17C]. They may have a modest utility in retrospectively evaluating severe adverse reactions. In vitro tests such as basophil activation test, lymphocyte transformation test, and lymphocyte activation test have been reported to be useful in previous reactors. However, the sensitivity and specificity of these tests have not been firmly established.

Thirty-five patients who experienced at least one breakthrough reaction who underwent contrast enhanced CT with iodinated contrast media were retrospectively reviewed to evaluate the efficacy of skin prick test, intradermal test, and patch test. 29% (10/35) of patients with prior breakthrough reactions resulted positive to STs compared to 57% (16/28) of the control group ($P < 0.05$). These results suggest that patients with breakthrough reaction have a low incidence of positive skin tests, which may suggest that many of these reactions may be nonallergic hypersensitivity reactions [18c].

A prospective randomized study investigated the protective effect of oral hydration for the prevention of adverse reactions. The study included 2244 patients who were given oral rehydration and 3715 patients as controls who were not given oral rehydration. The overall incidence of an acute adverse reaction was 4.3%. The study found that there was no significant difference between the rehydration group and adjusted control group in the overall incidence of adverse reactions (99/2244 [4.4%] vs 100/2244 [4.5%], respectively). This study suggests that dehydration and oral hydration does not affect the incidence of acute adverse reactions [19C].

MRI CONTRAST MEDIA

Gadolinium Salts [SEDA-33, 968; SEDA-34, 754; SEDA-35, 866; SEDA-36, 701; SEDA-37, 588; SEDA-38, 497]

Contrast enhancement is obtained by the T1 relaxation time shortening characteristics of gadolinium (Gd). From the type of use, these agents can be categorized into extracellular fluid agents, blood pool agents, and organ

TABLE 2 Some Gadolinium Salts That Have Been Used as Contrast Media in Magnetic Resonance Imaging

Name (INN)	Brand name	Charge	Structure
Gadobenic acid	Multihance	Ionic	Linear
Gadobutrol	Gadovist	Non-ionic	Macrocyclic
Gadocoletic acid			
Gadodenterate			
Gadodiamide	Omniscan	Non-ionic	Linear
Gadofosveset	Ablavar	Ionic	Linear
Gadomelitol	Vistarem		
Gadopenamide			
Gadopentetic acid	Magnevist	Ionic	Linear
Gadoteric acid	Dotarem	Ionic	Macrocyclic
Gadoteridol	Prohance	Non-ionic	Macrocyclic
Gadoversetamide	OptiMARK	Ionic	Linear
Gadoxetic acid	Eovist, Primovist	Ionic	Ionic

specific agents. Extracellular gadolinium-based contrast agents can be categorized as non-ionic and ionic from their charge, and linear or macrocyclic by structure (Table 2). Blood pool agents can be categorized into albumin-binding gadolinium complexes such as gadofosveset and gadocoletic acid, and polymeric gadolinium complexes such as gadomelitol.

Gadolinium agents are considered to have little nephrotoxicity at approved dosages for MRI. However, renal insufficiency is a risk factor for gadolinium deposition and nephrogenic systemic fibrosis. Therefore, gadolinium contrast agents should be used with caution in these patients.

Observational Studies

The incidence of acute adverse reactions to gadolinium-based contrast agents has been reported to be low (less than 2.4%) [20R].

Five different gadolinium-based contrast agents, Gd-BOPTA (MultiHance), Gd-DTPA (Magnevist), Gd-EOBDTPA (Primovist), Gd-DOTA (Dotarem), and Gd-BTDO3A (Gadovist) in 10608 MRI examinations were retrospectively evaluated for acute adverse reactions. The study found 32 acute adverse reactions, accounting for 0.3% of all administrations. Twelve reactions were associated with Gd-DOTA injection (0.11%), 9 with Gd-BOPTA injection (0.08%), 6 with Gd-BTDO3A (0.056%), 3 with Gd-EOB-DTPA (0.028%), and 2 with Gd-DTPA (0.018%). Twenty-four reactions (75.0%) were mild, four (12.5%) moderate, and four (12.5%) severe. The most severe

reactions were seen associated with use of Gd-BOPTA, with 3 severe reactions in 32 total reactions [21C]. Another report retrospectively investigated the incidence of acute adverse side effects of three gadolinium contrast agents; MultiHance((R)) (Bracco Diagnostics Inc., Princeton, NJ), Magnevist((R)) (Bayer Healthcare Pharmaceuticals, Wayne, NJ) or Gadavist((R)) (Bayer HealthCare Pharmaceuticals)] in 2393 paediatric patients. 40 of the 2393 patients who received gadolinium contrast agents experienced acute side effects, representing an incidence of 1.7%. The majority of the acute side effects (in 30 patients) were nausea and vomiting. The incidence of both nausea and vomiting was significantly higher in children receiving MultiHance, with a 4.48% incidence of nausea when compared with Magnevist (0.33%, $P < 0.0001$) and Gadavist (0.28%, $P < 0.0001$) and a 2.36% incidence of vomiting compared with those for Magnevist (0.50%, $P = 0.0054$) and Gadavist (0.28%, $P = 0.014$), whereas no difference was observed between Magnevist and Gadavist [22C].

Immunologic

Anaphylactic reactions to contrast media in most cases are not IgE-mediated (in other words they are what used to be called "anaphylactoid", now called non-IgE-mediated anaphylactic reactions), and may occur without previous sensitization. Nor do they occur consistently in patients who have had previous reactions to contrast media.

An anaphylactic reaction to a gadolinium contrast agent presenting with severe abdominal pain has been reported. 48-year-old woman with a history of chronic abdominal pain and Raynaud disease was injected with a gadolinium contrast agent. The patient developed severe diffuse abdominal pain and diaphoresis, and en route to the emergency department, decreased blood pressure and diffuse maculopapular rash. After receiving an intramuscular injection of epinephrine 0.5 mg twice, and methylprednisolone 125 mg, diphenhydramine 50 mg, famotidine 20 mg intravenously, her symptoms improved [23c].

Multiorgan Damage

Nephrogenic systemic fibrosis (NSF) is a multisystem disease in patients with renal insufficiency. Administration of gadolinium-based contrast agents, especially linear-structured agents has been associated with the development of NSF (Table 3). After the restriction of gadolinium-based agents in high risk patients in guidelines, the number of new cases has decreased sharply. *Yet, clinicians should continue to be cautious when administering gadolinium-based contrast agents; renal insufficiency should be screened for patients prior to administration* [24r,25R,26C,27R].

TABLE 3 Risks of Systemic Fibrosis From Gadolinium-Containing Salts

Name (INN)	Chelate	Charge	Structure	Risk
Gadodiamide	DTPA-BMA	Non-ionic	Linear	High (3%–7%)
Gadopentetic acid	DTPA	Ionic	Linear	High (0.1%–1%)
Gadoversetamide	DTPA-BMEA	Non-ionic	Linear	High
Gadobenic acid	BOPTA	Ionic	Linear	Intermediate
Gadofosveset	DTPA-DPCP	Ionic	Linear	Intermediate
Gadoxetic acid	EOB-DTPA	Ionic	Linear	Intermediate
Gadobutrol	BT-DO3A	Non-ionic	Cyclic	Low
Gadoteric acid	DOTA	Ionic	Cyclic	Low
Gadoteridol	HP-DO3A	Non-ionic	Cyclic	Low

BMA, 5,8-bis(carboxymethyl)-11-[2-(methylamino)-2-oxoethyl]-3-oxo-2,5,8,11-tetra-azatridecan-13-oic acid; BMEA, N,N'-bis[methoxyethylamide); BOPTA, benzyloxypropionic tetra-acetic-acid; BT-DO3A, 10-[2,3-dihydroxy-1-hydroxymethylpropyl]-1,4,7,10-tetra-azacyclododecane-1,4,7-triacetic acid; DOTA, 1,4,7,10-tetra-azacyclododecane-N,N',N'',N''''-tetra-acetic acid; DPCP, N,N'-bis[pyridoxal-5-phosphate)-trans-1,2-cyclohexyldiamine-N,N'-diacetic acid; DTPA, diethylene triamine penta-acetic acid; EOB-DTPA, ethoxybenzyldiethylene triamine penta-acetic acid; HP-DO3A, 10-[2-hydroxypropyl)-1,4,7-tetra-azacyclododecane-1,4,7-triacetic acid.

There is no specific treatment for NSF. Improvement of skin lesions after recovery of renal function [28c], and response to therapeutic plasma exchange have previously been reported [29c].

℞ Special Review

Gadolinium Accumulation

Free gadolinium ions are toxic in tissues. Gd3+ ions have the same diameter as Ca2+ ions and can act as an inorganic blocker of voltage-gated calcium channels [30R]. Cell membrane modification has also been reported in an in vitro study [31E]. Gadolinium contrast agents also target iron-recycling CD163- and ferroportin-expressing macrophages to release labile iron that may mediate gadolinium toxicity and NSF [32R].

The chemical stability of gadolinium contrast agents are different according to their structure, with macrocyclic chelates being the most stable, and non-ionic linear chelates the least stable. Ionic agents are more stable than non-ionic agents. Evidence of stability have been demonstrated in in vivo experiments which found evidence that more gadolinium retention are found in animals administered with non-ionic linear agent gadodiamide than ionic linear agent gadopentetate diglumine. Very small amounts of gadolinium were retained after macrocyclic agent administration [33R]. In vivo the presence of metal ions that compete with gadolinium for chelation such as Na+, K+, Ca2+, Fe3+ could result in transmetallation, which results in free gadolinium ions [34].

In 2014, Kanda et al. described increased T1WI hyperintensity in the globus palidus in patients who underwent contrast enhanced MRI using gadolinium contrast agents, which

suggested gadolinium deposition in these areas [35C]. This has been confirmed in various studies, even in the pediatric brain [36c,37c,38c,39c,40c]. A study which observed the increased T1WI hyperintensity of the dentate nucleus intraindividually found that administration of a linear gadolinium contrast agent gadopentetate dimeglumine was associated with an increased signal intensity while subsequent applications of the macrocyclic gadolinium contrast agents gadobutrol or gadoterate meglumine in the same patients were not. Also, a decrease in preexisting hyperintensities over time when linear agents were changed to macrocyclic agents suggested a washout effect or precipitation of gadolinium [41c]. However, another study investigated the effect of cumulative dose of gadobutrol, a macrocyclic agent, in patients with relapsing-remitting multiple sclerosis, found that administration of the same total amount of gadobutrol over a shorter period caused greater signal intensity increase within dentate nucleus and globus pallidus on unenhanced T1-weighted images. The study suggests that macrocyclic agents may cause gadolinium deposition, with a cumulative effect [42c]. Increased T1WI signal has also been reported in a study which investigated patients who underwent intrathecal administration of gadolinium contrast agents, which may suggest a glymphatic pathway [43c].

Gadolinium deposition itself has been confirmed by studies using inductively coupled mass spectrometry, and deposition seems to occur even in patients with normal renal function [44c,45c]. Accumulation in the dentate nucleus seems to be lower for macrocyclic agents [46r,47R]. Gadolinium accumulation has also been confirmed in bone in autopsy cases [48c], in liver tissue in patients who underwent allogenic hematopoietic stem cell transplantation [49c], and skin in patients without renal impairment nor evidence of NSF [50c].

There is lack of knowledge of the long-term effects of gadolinium retention as well as adverse health effects. Yet, clinician should be aware of the accumulation, and caution may be necessary when using linear agents as well as macrocylic agents.

Superparamagnetic Iron Oxide (SPIO) MRI Contrast Agents [SEDA-33, 970; SEDA-34, 757]

Iron oxide-containing contrast agents consist of suspended colloids of iron oxide nanoparticles, which reduce T2 MRI signals. They are taken up by the reticuloendothelial system. Superparamagnetic iron oxide (SPIO) contrast agents are taken up by the liver and spleen. The ultra-small superparamagnetic iron oxide (USPIO) contrast agents have a longer plasma circulation time and have greater uptake into marrow and lymph nodes. They also have a greater T1 shortening effect than SPIO contrast agents. For these characteristics, they have been investigated for liver imaging, macrophage imaging or blood pool agents.

References

[1] European Society of Urogenital Radiology. ESUR guidelines on contrasts media 9.0. Vienna, Austria: European Society of Urogenital Radiology; 2014. Available from: http://www.esur-cm.org/index.php/en/ [M].

[2] American College of Radiology. ACR manual on contrast media, Version 10.2. Reston, VA: American College of Radiology; 2016 [M].

[3] Morcos SK, Thomsen HS. Adverse reactions to iodinated contrast media. Eur Radiol. 2001;11(7):1267–75 [R].

[4] Zhang B, Dong Y, Liang L, et al. The incidence, classification, and management of acute adverse reactions to the low-osmolar iodinated contrast media isovue and ultravist in contrast-enhanced computed tomography scanning. Medicine (Baltimore). 2016;95(12)e3170 [C].

[5] Barr ML, Chiu HK, Li N, et al. Thyroid dysfunction in children exposed to iodinated contrast media. J Clin Endocrinol Metab. 2016;101(6):2366–70 [c].

[6] Kornelius E, Chiou JY, Yang YS, et al. Iodinated contrast media-induced thyroid dysfunction in euthyroid nodular goiter patients. Thyroid. 2016;26(8):1030–8 [c].

[7] Ghosh RK, Somasundaram M, Ravakhah K. Iodide mumps following fistulogram in a haemodialysis patient. BMJ Case Rep. 2016;2016, https://dx.doi.org/10.1136/bcr-2015-214037 [c].

[8] Elder AM, Ng MK. Iodide mumps complicating coronary and carotid angiography. Heart Lung Circ. 2017;26(2):e14–5 [c].

[9] Riley P. Does iodinated contrast medium amplify DNA damage during exposure to radiation. Br J Radiol. 2015;88(1055): 20150474 [r].

[10] Hasegawa M, Gomi T. Chapter 44—Radiological contrast agents and radiopharmaceuticals. In: Sidhartha DR, editor. Side effects of drugs annual. Amsterdam, The Netherlands: Elsevier; 2016. p. 493–501 [R].

[11] Deinzer CK, Danova D, Kleb B, et al. Influence of different iodinated contrast media on the induction of DNA double-strand breaks after in vitro X-ray irradiation. Contrast Media Mol Imaging. 2014;9(4):259–67 [E].

[12] Gould R, McFadden SL, Horn S, et al. Assessment of DNA double-strand breaks induced by intravascular iodinated contrast media following in vitro irradiation and in vivo, during paediatric cardiac catheterization. Contrast Media Mol Imaging. 2016;11(2):122–9 [c].

[13] Cernigliaro JG, Haley WE, Adolphson DP, et al. Contrast-induced nephropathy in outpatients with preexisting renal impairment: a comparison between intravenous iohexol and iodixanol. Clin Imaging. 2016;40(5):902–6 [c].

[14] Hong SI, Ahn S, Lee YS, et al. Contrast-induced nephropathy in patients with active cancer undergoing contrast-enhanced computed tomography. Support Care Cancer. 2016;24(3):1011–7 [c].

[15] Watanabe M, Saito Y, Aonuma K, et al. Prediction of contrast-induced nephropathy by the serum creatinine level on the day following cardiac catheterization. J Cardiol. 2016;68(5):412–8 [c].

[16] Abe S, Fukuda H, Tobe K, et al. Protective effect against repeat adverse reactions to iodinated contrast medium: premedication vs. changing the contrast medium. Eur Radiol. 2016;26(7):2148–54 [c].

[17] Yamaguchi K, Katayama H, Takashima T, et al. Prediction of severe adverse reactions to ionic and nonionic contrast media in Japan: evaluation of pretesting. A report from the Japanese Committee on the Safety of Contrast Media. Radiology. 1991;178(2):363–7 [C].

[18] Berti A, Della-Torre E, Yacoub M, et al. Patients with breakthrough reactions to iodinated contrast media have low incidence of positive skin tests. Eur Ann Allergy Clin Immunol. 2016;48(4):137–44 [c].

[19] Motosugi U, Ichikawa T, Sano K, et al. Acute adverse reactions to nonionic iodinated contrast media for CT: prospective randomized evaluation of the effects of dehydration, oral rehydration, and patient risk factors. AJR Am J Roentgenol. 2016;207(5):931–8 [C].

[20] Kanal E. Gadolinium-based contrast agents (GBCA): safety overview after 3 decades of clinical experience. Magn Reson Imaging. 2016;34(10):1341–5 [R].

[21] Granata V, Cascella M, Fusco R, et al. Immediate adverse reactions to gadolinium-based MR contrast media: a retrospective analysis on 10,608 examinations. Biomed Res Int. 2016;2016:3918292 [C].

[22] Neeley C, Moritz M, Brown JJ, et al. Acute side effects of three commonly used gadolinium contrast agents in the paediatric population. Br J Radiol. 2016;89(1063):20160027 [C].

[23] Pourmand A, Guida K, Abdallah A, et al. Gadolinium-based contrast agent anaphylaxis, a unique presentation of acute abdominal pain. Am J Emerg Med. 2016;34(8). 1737.e1–2 [c].

[24] Weller A, Barber JL, Olsen OE. Gadolinium and nephrogenic systemic fibrosis: an update. Pediatr Nephrol. 2014;29:1927–37 [r].

[25] Thomsen HS, Morcos SK, Almen T, et al. Nephrogenic systemic fibrosis and gadolinium-based contrast media: updated ESUR Contrast Medium Safety Committee guidelines. Eur Radiol. 2013;23(2):307–18 [R].

[26] Edwards BJ, Laumann AE, Nardone B, et al. Advancing pharmacovigilance through academic-legal collaboration: the case of gadolinium-based contrast agents and nephrogenic systemic fibrosis—a Research on Adverse Drug Events and Reports (RADAR) report. Br J Radiol. 2014;87(1042):20140307 [C].

[27] Canga A, Kislikova M, Martinez-Galvez M, et al. Renal function, nephrogenic systemic fibrosis and other adverse reactions associated with gadolinium-based contrast media. Nefrologia. 2014;34(4):428–38 [R].

[28] Schad SG, Heitland P, Kuhn-Velten WN, et al. Time-dependent decrement of dermal gadolinium deposits and significant improvement of skin symptoms in a patient with nephrogenic systemic fibrosis after temporary renal failure. J Cutan Pathol. 2013;40(11):935–44 [c].

[29] Poisson JL, Low A, Park YA. The treatment of nephrogenic systemic fibrosis with therapeutic plasma exchange. J Clin Apher. 2013;28(4):317–20 [c].

[30] Idee JM, Fretellier N, Robic C, et al. The role of gadolinium chelates in the mechanism of nephrogenic systemic fibrosis: a critical update. Crit Rev Toxicol. 2014;44(10):895–913 [R].

[31] Gianulis EC, Pakhomov AG. Gadolinium modifies the cell membrane to inhibit permeabilization by nanosecond electric pulses. Arch Biochem Biophys. 2015;570:1–7 [E].

[32] Swaminathan S. Gadolinium toxicity: iron and ferroportin as central targets. Magn Reson Imaging. 2016;34:1373–6 [R].

[33] Thomsen HS, Morcos SK, Almen T, et al. Nephrogenic systemic fibrosis and gadolinium-based contrast media: updated ESUR Contrast Medium Safety Committee guidelines. Eur Radiol. 2013;23(2):307–18 [R].

[34] Kanda T, Nakai Y, Oba H, et al. Gadolinium deposition in the brain. Magn Reson Imaging. 2016;34:1346–50 [r].

[35] Kanda T, Ishii K, Kawaguchi H, et al. High signal intensity in the dentate nucleus and globus pallidus on unenhanced T1-weighted MR images: relationship with increasing cumulative dose of a gadolinium-based contrast material. Radiology. 2014;270(3):834–41 [C].

[36] Flood TF, Stence NV, Maloney JA, et al. Pediatric brain: repeated exposure to linear gadolinium-based contrast material is associated with increased signal intensity at unenhanced T1-weighted MR imaging. Radiology. 2016;28:160356 [c].

[37] Hinoda T, Fushimi Y, Okada T, et al. Quantitative assessment of gadolinium deposition in dentate nucleus using quantitative susceptibility mapping. J Magn Reson Imaging. 2017;45:1352–8 [c].

[38] Hu HH, Pokorney A, Towbin RB, et al. Increased signal intensities in the dentate nucleus and globus pallidus on unenhanced T1-weighted images: evidence in children undergoing multiple gadolinium MRI exams. Pediatr Radiol. 2016;46(11):1590–8 [c].

[39] Roberts DR, Holden KR. Progressive increase of T1 signal intensity in the dentate nucleus and globus pallidus on unenhanced T1-weighted MR images in the pediatric brain exposed to multiple doses of gadolinium contrast. Brain Dev. 2016;38(3):331–6 [c].

[40] Zhang Y, Cao Y, Shih GL, et al. Extent of signal hyperintensity on unenhanced T1-weighted brain MR images after more than 35 administrations of linear gadolinium-based contrast agents. Radiology. 2016;11:152864 [c].

[41] Radbruch A, Weberling LD, Kieslich PJ, et al. Intraindividual analysis of signal intensity changes in the dentate nucleus after consecutive serial applications of linear and macrocyclic gadolinium-based contrast agents. Invest Radiol. 2016;51(11):683–90 [c].

[42] Stojanov DA, Aracki-Trenkic A, Vojinovic S, et al. Increasing signal intensity within the dentate nucleus and globus pallidus on unenhanced T1W magnetic resonance images in patients with relapsing-remitting multiple sclerosis: correlation with cumulative dose of a macrocyclic gadolinium-based contrast agent, gadobutrol. Eur Radiol. 2016;26(3):807–15 [c].

[43] Oner AY, Barutcu B, Aykol S, et al. Intrathecal contrast-enhanced magnetic resonance imaging-related brain signal changes: residual gadolinium deposition? Invest Radiol. 2017;52:195–7 [c].

[44] McDonald RJ, McDonald JS, Kallmes DF, et al. Intracranial gadolinium deposition after contrast-enhanced MR imaging. Radiology. 2015;275(3):772–82 [c].

[45] Kanda T, Fukusato T, Matsuda M, et al. Gadolinium-based contrast agent accumulates in the brain even in subjects without severe renal dysfunction: evaluation of autopsy brain specimens with inductively coupled plasma mass spectroscopy. Radiology. 2015;276(1):228–32 [c].

[46] Kanda T, Oba H, Toyoda K, et al. Macrocyclic gadolinium-based contrast agents do not cause hyperintensity in the dentate nucleus. AJNR Am J Neuroradiol. 2016;37(5)E41 [r].

[47] Radbruch A. Are some agents less likely to deposit gadolinium in the brain? Magn Reson Imaging. 2016;34:1351–4 [R].

[48] Murata N, Gonzalez-Cuyar LF, Murata K, et al. Macrocyclic and other non-group 1 gadolinium contrast agents deposit low levels of gadolinium in brain and bone tissue: preliminary results from 9 patients with normal renal function. Invest Radiol. 2016;51(7):447–53 [c].

[49] Maximova N, Gregori M, Zennaro F, et al. Hepatic gadolinium deposition and reversibility after contrast agent-enhanced MR imaging of pediatric hematopoietic stem cell transplant recipients. Radiology. 2016;281(2):418–26 [c].

[50] Roberts DR, Lindhorst SM, Welsh CT, et al. High levels of gadolinium deposition in the skin of a patient with normal renal function. Invest Radiol. 2016;51(5):280–9 [c].

42

Drugs Used in Ocular Treatment

Lisa V. Stottlemyer[*],[†],[1],[2]

*Pennsylvania College of Optometry, Elkins Park, PA, United States
†Wilmington VA Medical Center, Wilmington, DE, United States
[2]Corresponding author: Lisa.stottlemyer@VA.GOV

INTRODUCTION

Many different classes of drugs are utilized for the treatment of ocular disease and all pose risk of side effects, some severe. Ocular medications can be administered topically, orally or injected into the eye, and each route allows for potential of local and systemic side effects. For example, the most common side effects of any topically applied eye drops are burning upon installation and conjunctival hyperemia, which may be related to either the therapeutic agent or preservatives [1M], while medication injected into the vitreous cavity often leaves the patient reporting floaters or a spot in their vision as they can appreciate the shadow of the depot of drug [2A].

By far, topical application is the most common route of administration of medications used for the treatment of ocular disease and some conditions, such as glaucoma, require frequent, chronic dosing. Often the preservatives therein contribute ocular surface disease [1M]. Symptoms such as redness, stinging, burning and foreign body sensation are reported to be present in up to 60% of patients using topical anti-glaucoma medications [3A].

There are several classic side effects for each class of medications that are so prevalent, we almost expect them. For example, beta blockers classically cause bradycardia even when topically applied, and steroids are well known to cause increased IOP and posterior sub-capsular cataracts. Systemic side effects of topically applied ocular medications have been attributed to the "first pass" effect that up to 80% of topically applied medication drains through the nasolacrimal system and is absorbed into the bloodstream through the nasal mucosa. By this route,

organ systems are exposed to concentration of drug prior to the drugs first pass through the liver where many are metabolized [4A,5A]. Infants and children may be more at risk for serious systemic side effects due to the fact that there is often no weight adjusted dose available and struggling with an uncooperative child may lead to a greater number of drops instilled [5A]. This chapter is meant to serve as a review of both the common and lesser occurring side effects of ocular medications reported in the literature.

ANTI-VASCULAR ENDOTHELIAL GROWTH FACTOR (VEGF) MEDICATIONS

Pegaptanib, Bevacizumab, Aflibercept, Ranibizumab

General

Anti-VEGF medications are injected into the vitreous cavity through the pars plana and are used for the treatment of many conditions including age-related macular degeneration (AMD), central retinal vein occlusion, diabetic macular edema and proliferative diabetic retinopathy, and retinopathy of prematurity (ROP). Reported adverse events following anti-VEGF injections include vitreous hemorrhage, retinal tear, retinal detachment, macular hole formation, endophthalmitis, intraocular inflammation, increased intraocular pressure, and retinal vascular occlusions [6R] as well as systemic events such as blood pressure elevation, myocardial infarction, stroke and death. Dedania and Bakri suggest that a risk factor for stroke with anti-VEGF treatment may be a prior history of stroke and therefore recommend exerting caution when treating patients that have had a history of a stroke within the preceding 3 months [7R].

---

[1] Board Certified: American Board of Certification in Medical Optometry.

Corneal complications of anti-VEGF injections include corneal edema, delayed healing and limbal insufficiency [8A].

A comparison of age-related treatment trials (CATT) reported incidence of endophthalmitis after intravitreal injection of anti-VEGF to be 0.085% [9M]. Sterile intraocular inflammation has been reported with all intravitreal anti-VEGF medications injected intravitreally. A review of the literature of a large-scale clinical trials showed that enrolled patients that were treated with ranibizumab experienced inflammation rates of 1.4%–2.9%. Lower rates of inflammation, 0.09%–1.3%, were reported for those treated with bevacizumab [6R].

The overall risk of rhegmatogenous retinal detachment is low. Meyer et al. reviewed 35942 injections of either 0.05 mL of ranibizumab, 0.05–0.1 mL of bevacizumab or 0.05 bevacizumab rtPA combined with 0.2 mL SF6 gas. 5 retinal detachments occurred between day 2 and day 6 post injection (4 of the 5 occurring in myopic eyes) yielding an overall incidence of 0.013% per injection [10c]. Zhang et al. suggest the risk of retinal adverse effects after intravitreal injections is greater in myopic eyes where degenerative changes already exist [11R].

The Pan-American Collaborative Retina Study Group (PACORES) conducted a retrospective multicenter, interventional case series ($n=81$) and reported an incidence of 5.2% of eyes with proliferative diabetic retinopathy treated with bevacizumab developed a tractional retinal detachment, thought to result from contraction of fibrovascular tissue following a brisk halt to proliferating neovascular vessels, that required vitrectomy [12c].

Elevated intraocular pressure (IOP) is an important risk factor for the development of glaucoma. Increased post-injection IOP is common and has been reported with all anti-VEGF drugs; however, it is generally a transient rise in IOP that resolves within several hours without treatment [13M]. Possible risk factors for sustained increase in IOP, and therefore increased risk of developing glaucoma, are the following: increased number of injections, pre-existing glaucoma, male gender and frequency of repeat injection within 8 weeks or less [14C]. It has been theorized that the recurrent stress to the endothelium of Schlemm's canal from the repeated injections causes the IOP to rise [15R].

Bevacizumab

Significantly higher serum levels have been detected following intravitreal injection with bevacizumab as compared to similar injections with pegaptanib and ranibizumab [16M]. Frequently reported systemic adverse events with bevacizumab include blood pressure increases, deep vein thrombosis, transient ischemic attack, congestive heart failure and myocardial infarction [15R]. Mickacic and Bosnar performed a systematic review the literature and report a high level of

uncertainty related to cardiovascular risk in patients treated with IV bevacizumab, stating that the low number of randomized controlled trials with low numbers of enrolled patients, short follow-up and an overall low overall incidence of cardiovascular disease and cerebrovascular accidents in the study populations yield very little confidence in an assessment of associated risk [17R].

In recent years, bevacizumab has been investigated for the treatment of ROP, and although treatment responses are promising, there is some concern for the effects of systemically absorbed drug on developing preterm infants. VEGF plays an important role in blood vessel and organ development, suppression of which can cause developmental compromise. In a prospective cohort study ($n=10$), serum VEGF levels were suppressed for 2 months after treatment with intravitreal bevacizumab, longer and to a greater degree than with intravitreal ranibizumab [18c].

Morin et al. performed a retrospective analysis of data (gathered prospectively as part of an observational cohort study) comparing neurodevelopment at 18 months corrected age of pre-term infants that were treated with either bevacizumab or laser ablation. They reported significantly increased risk of severe neurodevelopmental disorders in patients treated with bevacizumab when compared to conventional laser treated group (51.9% vs 28.6%) [19c]. The investigators did note that the database did not contain decision making details for anti-VEGF treatment vs laser and therefore concede that it is possible that sicker infants, and therefore infants that are more likely to develop neurodevelopmental defects were selected to receive anti-VEGF treatment. Large-scale studies of this emerging ROP treatment are needed to evaluate systemic toxicity given this developmentally fragile patient base; two trials are presently underway, one of which the Pediatric Eye Disease Investigative Group (PEDIG) is assessing some safety outcomes with bevacizumab [20R].

A case of choroidal ischemia resulting in hypotony and exudative retinal detachment occurred in a 6-week-old preterm infant hours after injection of bevacizumab for the treatment of severe retinopathy of prematurity [21A].

Intravitreal use of bevacizumab (1.25 mg/0.05 mL) in the pediatric population (average age 8.7 years) for the treatment of retinal and choroidal conditions (with the exclusion of ROP) was investigated with a recent multi-center, retrospective, consecutive case series ($n=95$ eyes) and reported 8 eyes developing increased IOP that required treatment, 3 patients with rapid progression of tractional retinal detachment and a statistically significant increase in diastolic blood pressure [22c].

A retrospective cohort study of 174 patients (201 eyes) reported a sustained rise in IOP occurred in 11% of patients treated with bevacizumab. It is postulated that the rise in IOP is related to mechanical obstruction of aqueous outflow due to the repackaging of bevacizumab in plastic syringes and that these syringes may cause contamination with materials such as silicone oil [14C]. Repackaging also increases the risk of microbial contamination and incidence of endophthalmitis [11R].

Onoda et al. reported 2 cases of severe gastrointestinal effects post intravitreal injection of bevacizumab (1.25 mg/0.05 mL). The first, a 78-year-old woman with a distant history of colon cancer and post-operative ischemic colitis suffered a recurrence of ischemic colitis 1 day after injection. The second, a 64-year-old man experienced abdominal pain 2 days after injection. 9 days later he was given a second injection after vitrectomy surgery and the following day developed paralytic ileus with symptoms of vomiting and severe abdominal pain and distention. The authors hypothesized that systemically absorbed drug reduced nitric oxide production which resulted in vasoconstriction and ultimately decreased gastrointestinal blood flow. Both patients were admitted to the hospital for treatment and symptoms improved without surgery [23A].

Ranibizumab

Although the most common side effect of ranibizumab is uveitis [24R], other drug-induced effects may occur.

Bosanquet et al. reported a case of acute generalized exanthematous pustulosis, a cutaneous drug reaction, occurring in a 90-year-old female. Four days after receiving an intravitreal injection of ranibizumab, she developed malaise and a progressive erythematous rash involving the torso and limbs. Early in the course, the rash spread despite treatment with topical and oral corticosteroid before finally resolving spontaneously 6 weeks after the initial appearance [25A].

A case of marginal keratitis developed in a 56-year-old man being treated with ranibizumab for diabetic macular edema. One day after injection, he presented with pain, redness and pain in the injected eye. Multiple peripheral subepithelial infiltrates and a mild anterior chamber reaction were present. This case of marginal keratitis is thought to be related to a hypersensitivity reaction to reflux of ranibizumab onto the ocular surface. The patient was treated with topical moxifloxacin and dexamethasone eye drops and condition resolved over the course of a week [8A].

Ueta et al. conducted a meta-analysis of existing trials which looked at treatment of AMD with intravitreal ranibizumab reported a statistically significant increase of CVAs, non-ocular hemorrhage, and arterial thromboembolic events (ATE) in those treated with 0.5 mg ranibizumab when compared to 0.3 mg ranibizumab and no ranibizumab-treated groups [26R].

Aflibercept

A prospective, open-label, non-randomized clinical trial of 49 patients treated with aflibercept (2 mg) reported the occurrence of cataract progression (4 patients), atrial fibrillation (2 patients), syncope (2 patients) and sub-macular hemorrhage (2 patients) as well as an average IOP rise of 1.45 ± 0.95 mmHg over the 12-month study duration, but this minor increase was not considered to be clinically significant [27c].

Medications Used to Treat Glaucoma

Topical therapy is the mainstay of glaucoma management. Life-threatening adverse events including central nervous system depression and cardiogenic shock are described in 2 infants treated with topical antiglaucoma medications (brimonidine and timolol) [5A]. These cases highlight the fact that systemic absorption and lack of weight adjusted dosages likely subject infants to greater risk of systemic side effects.

PROSTAGLANDIN (PGF$_{2\alpha}$) ANALOGUES

Latanoprost, Bimatoprost, Travoprost

General

Prostaglandin analogue side effects are local and involve hyperemia, increased lash growth, periocular skin pigmentation and increased iris pigmentation [28c]. Hamroush and Cheung report an interesting case of an 84-year-old man treated for glaucoma in the left eye only whose unilateral prostaglandin-induced hypertrichosis partially masked lash loss from a malignant lid lesion [29A]. A small ($n = 69$) prospective observational case study reported statistically significant increase of periocular skin hyperpigmentation in patients treated with bimatoprost and latanoprost after 3 months of treatment, occurring more frequently and to a greater degree with the bimatoprost-treated group [30c]. Deepening of the superior lid sulcus [28c] and sunken eye appearance [31A] has also been described. No systemic adverse events have been attributed to prostaglandin therapy [32C].

Prostaglandin analogues have also been reported to cause nongranulomatous, and to a far lesser extent granulomatous, anterior uveitis presumably because the prostaglandin activity causes a pro-inflammatory state [33A]. Latanoprost's pro-inflammatory properties were further implicated in the development of a choroidal detachment with inflammatory membranes in the suprachoroidal space (noted on Bscan) which occurred in a 64-year-old man 7 weeks after cataract surgery [34A]. The authors speculate that the post-operative topical steroid masked the inflammation explaining the late development of the choroidal effusion after the topical steroids were discontinued.

Parchand et al. report a case of a serous macular detachment occurring 7 days after routine cataract surgery in a 66-year-old man treated with bimatoprost for primary open-angle glaucoma; the authors suggest the use of prostaglandin was directly related [35A].

Benzalkonium chloride (BAK) is the most commonly use preservative for ocular medications and is associated with conjunctival inflammation and corneal compromise [32C]. BAK interferes with the lipid component of the tear film which results in a more rapid tear breakup time (TBUT) [36c] and therefore frequent dosing of BAK containing glaucoma medications are well known to increase the symptoms of dry eye disease. A prospective, open-label, single-arm, multicenter, 8 weeks study evaluated the effect of switching patients actively taking BAK-containing latanoprost ophthalmic solution 0.005% to BAK-free latanoprost ophthalmic solution 0.005% and reported significant improvements in inferior corneal staining, ocular surface disease index (OSDI) scores and TBUT. Conjunctival hyperemia was also notably decreased with BAK-free regimen; however, this finding was not clinically significant [36c].

Latanoprost is a highly selective agonist of the prostaglandin F2a receptor (PTGFR) [37c]. Evidence that specific genetic variants can impact drug responses is provided by a recent prospective study ($n = 89$) that identified a single-nucleotide polymorphism (SNP) of the PTGFR gene (rs3766355) and a SNP of the solute carrier organic anion transporter family 2A1 (SLCO2A1) gene (rs4241366) that were associated with treatment response of latanoprost in Han Chinese patients with glaucoma [37c].

Beta Blockers

While localized side effects of beta blockers are in keeping with the other classes of glaucoma medications (predominantly burning upon installation of drops and conjunctival hyperemia), the prevalence of systemic effects is a frequent limitation of these agents [1M]. Beta blockers effect on heart rate and respiration is widely reported and includes bradycardia, blood pressure decreases, worsening of asthma attacks and chronic obstructive pulmonary disease (COPD). Rana et al. highlight serious systemic effects in a case report of an 84-year-old male with hypertension diabetes and hypercholesterolemia and open-angle glaucoma developed a bradycardia arrhythmia, confusion and hypoglycemia that required ICU admission while being treated with topical beta blocker (timolol) for the treatment of open-angle glaucoma [38A].

Timolol

A self-controlled case series study reported an increased risk of hospitalization due to bradycardia in the second to sixth month after initiation of medication [39A]. One recent case report details a 68-year old who experienced 2 episodes of syncope with sinus bradycardia occurring shortly after initiating topical timolol [40A].

Levobunolol

A case recently reported an 88-year-old man developed symptomatic bradycardia after instillation of drops, which resolved with discontinuation of drug, highlights the potential cardiac side effects of topical beta blockers [41A].

Carbonic Anhydrase Inhibitors (CAI)

A single dose of acetazolamide is frequently prescribed by cataract surgeons and to prevent an acute rise of IOP postoperatively. Zimmerman et al. report a case of a 76-year-old male who collapsed 30 minutes after ingestion of 250 mg acetazolamide, prescribed by his cataract surgeon [42A]. He developed nausea, progressive dyspnea, shock and pulmonary edema which, after detailed history of a similar event occurring immediately after ingestion of acetazolamide prescribed after his had cataract surgery 2 months prior, suggests the acetazolamide is the most likely trigger for this event. Zimmerman et al. make note of the fact that pulmonary edema is not a recognized pharmacogenic side effect of acetazolamide but argues that this patient's lack of prior exposure to a related sulfonamide make an anaphylactic mechanism less likely.

Sympathetic Alpha2-Receptor Antagonists

Local ocular side effects of sympathomimetic agents include conjunctival hyperemia, irritation, pupil dilation and allergic conjunctivitis [1M].

More serious systemic side effects can result from systemic absorption of the topically applied formulations and can be severe in pediatric patients. A small case series reports four children who experienced somnolence minutes after topical administration of brimonidine. The central nervous system depression is speculated to be the result of poor ability to metabolize the systemically absorbed drug and/or an immature blood–brain barrier [43A].

Fixed Combinations (FC)

The treatment of glaucoma often requires 2 or more medications for adequate IOP control and therefore fixed combinations are an increasingly favorable option because they limit the inconvenience of dosing with multiple bottles while also limiting exposure to preservatives contained in each single agent.

An open-label retrospective review of patients treated with FC dorzolamide/timolol that were switched to FC brinzolamide/brimonidine, reported significantly less redness and ocular stinging after the switch; however, two treatment-related adverse events were reported (one increased hyperemia and one episode of allergic conjunctivitis) but resolved promptly upon discontinuation of the FC brinzolamide–brimonidine suspension [44c].

While the most common reported effect of tafluprost/timolol (a preservative-free FC manufactured in unit dose pipettes) is ocular hyperemia, there is theoretical concern for corneal injury associated with improper handling of the dose dispensers and therefore Hollo and Katsanos advocate for careful assessment of manual dexterity of patients prior to prescribing this novel therapy presentation [45R].

A patient developed a hemorrhagic choroidal detachment and severely reduced visual acuity 1 day after initiation of treatment with fixed combination 0.5% timolol maleate/0.004% travoprost. This effect was attributed to the sudden decrease in intraocular pressure [46A]. Treatment was immediately discontinued; full resolution and visual recovery occurred within the following 4 months.

A 12-week prospective, interventional, single-arm study ($n = 47$) evaluating the efficacy and safety of adding fixed combination brinzolamide/timolol to existing prostaglandin therapy reported the most common side effect was headache. Other noteworthy side effects reported were allergic conjunctivitis, burning, eyelid swelling, blur, conjunctival discomfort, metallic taste, ocular foreign body sensation and one serious side effect of pseudostenocardia which required patient to be removed from the study [47c].

ANTIMICROBIALS

Sulfonamides

High dose sulfadiazine may crystalize in the urine, but resultant obstructive nephropathy is rare [New #13]. Kabha et al. report a case of a 31-year-old female treated for acute ocular toxoplasmosis for 2 weeks with sulfadiazine (a sulfonamide), pyrimethamine and steroid who developed severe flank pain and left hydronephrosis with urine extravasation at the uretero-pelvic junction. Management consisted of IV hydration, placement of an internal ureteral stent and change of medications from sulfadiazine–pyrimethamine to trimethoprim–sulfamethoxazole. The stent was removed 4 weeks later and a follow-up CT confirmed resolution of the condition. As dehydration increases the risk of crystal deposition, educating patients on the importance of significantly increasing their fluid intake while on this medication is of paramount importance [48A].

Sulfacetamide: A 15-year-old boy was hospitalized with Toxic Epidermal Necrolysis (TEN) 3 days after using sulfacetamide eye drops for conjunctivitis. He presented with a fever, widespread blistering rash and severe ocular inflammation with cicatricial lid changes, symblepharon and reduced vision. Over the next few days, the rash spread to involve greater than 30% of his body with erosions on all mucosal membranes. The exact pathogenesis is unknown, although most patients with TEN are noted to have abnormal metabolism of the drug. It is unusual for topical medications to incite TEN. This case highlights the importance of a strong history given that this medication was acquired over-the-counter [49A].

Aminoglycosides

Gentamicin is the most toxic antibiotic used in ophthalmology, and toxicity can mimic a retinal vaso-occlusive event involving macular infarction and optic atrophy [50A,51A]. One such case was presented by Lartey et al. wherein total loss of vision occurred after a routine cataract surgery utilizing the use of a sub-conjunctival gentamicin injection (20 mg in 0.5 mL) for endophthalmitis prophylaxis. The vision loss was the result of macular infarction noted on postoperative day 1, followed by notable optic atrophy 2 months later [50A]. This effect may occur if gentamicin, when injected sub-conjunctivally, enters the interior of the eye through the corneal scleral wound [52A]. A similar case of suspected aminoglycoside toxicity occurred in a 52-year-old male who developed severe vision loss after sutureless vitrectomy with sub-conjunctival injection of 0.5 mL of 0.4 mg/mL gentamicin [53A]. Fundus examination revealed extensive retinal hemorrhages, retinal edema and micro-infarcts and fluorescein angiography demonstrated capillary non-perfusion, mostly in the posterior pole, consistent with this patient's dense central scotoma and poor visual acuity. The authors believe that this clinical presentation resulted from toxicity to the gentamicin which gained access to eye through the sutureless sclerotomies [53A].

Additionally, two patients developed toxic anterior segment syndrome (TASS) within 2 weeks after a single sub-conjunctival injection of gentamicin (20 mg in 0.5 mL) used during routine cataract surgery. The associated effects were corneal edema, dilated pupil, cystoid macular edema and uveitis [54A]. The corneal edema, macular edema (present in only one of the two reported cases) and uveitis resolved slowly in the following months; in both cases, however, the pupil dilation was permanent.

Topical gentamicin has been implicated in the development of acute renal failure in a 67-year-old woman being treated for endophthalmitis. Once topical gentamicin and fortified vancomycin were discontinued, the patient experienced a dramatic improvement in renal status prompting her physicians to suspect toxicity. Serum gentamicin levels were 0.34 mg/L 2 days after discontinuation of the drug, the first ever report of measurable serum gentamicin resulting from topical administration. Acute renal failure completely resolved after her eye drops were stopped [55A].

Fluoroquinolones

General

Corneal precipitates with topical fluoroquinolone use are widely reported, occurring in approximately 15% of patients treated with ciprofloxacin but also with ofloxacin, norfloxacin and gatifloxacin [56A]. Precipitates appear to occur with greater frequency in older patients, and while they do not slow the rate of infection resolution, they may result in a delay of re-epithelialization [56A,57r].

Ciprofloxacin

While oral and IV administrations of ciprofloxacin have been noted to decrease serum levels of phenytoin and decrease seizure threshold, Malladi et al. report a case of topical fluroquinolone administration where use of 0.3% ciprofloxacin eye drops four times a day for 2 weeks led to reduced serum phenytoin levels and increased seizure activity [58A]; serum levels rose steadily upon discontinuation of the eye drops and were back to therapeutic levels within a week.

Levofloxacin

Contact urticaria syndrome characterized by conjunctival hyperemia, nasal discharge, sneezing, facial edema, pruritic rash, and mild dyspnea was reported with topical administration of 0.5% levofloxacin hydrate eye drops for bacterial conjunctivitis [59A]. Symptoms of conjunctival hyperemia, nasal discharge and sneezing developed immediately, followed by the other symptoms.

Vancomycin

A retrospective case series reviewed cases of postoperative hemorrhagic occlusive retinal vasculitis (HORV) after cataract surgery and reported that all (11/11 eyes) were treated with intercameral vancomycin for endophthalmitis prophylaxis. All patients experienced painless vision loss, uveitis, vasculitis and extensive retinal hemorrhages between postoperative day 1 and 14. Authors speculate that HORV represents a type III hypersensitivity reaction to vancomycin [60c].

Lenci et al. report a case of a 65-year-old woman that was given an injection of intracameral vancomycin as routine endophthalmitis prophylaxis after cataract surgery in the right eye (OD). Her vision was 20/20 on post-op day 1 but decreased to 20/400 post-op day 3. At that time, she presented with an afferent pupillary defect (APD) OD and a relatively quiet anterior segment (mild conjunctival injection, trace corneal edema, few cells in anterior chamber), but dilated fundus exam revealed attenuated retinal vessels and scattered dot-blot hemorrhages in the periphery [61A]. A fluorescein angiogram showed delayed retinal and choroidal filling, multiple peripheral branch artery occlusions and vessel wall hyperfluorescence consistent with retinal ischemic vasculitis which prompted an inflammatory work-up. Vision gradually improved over the course of the following week without treatment (other than the previously prescribed post-operative regimen of ofloxacin and prednisolone acetate drops) and returned to 20/20 with complete resolution of the APD at her 2-month follow-up. As the laboratory work-up was negative and no other sign/symptoms of uveitis were present, the authors believe this case to represent a rapidly normalizing event related to vancomycin toxicity [61A].

AMIKACIN

Lodhi et al. report a case of last-onset endophthalmitis, occurring 45 days after cataract surgery, in a 50-year-old female treated with intravitreal amikacin (200 μg/0.1 mL) that developed a macular infarction suspected to be amikacin induced [62A].

Mydriatics/Cycloplegics

Mydriatics and cycloplegics cause pupillary dilation and congestion of the anterior chamber angle yielding increased risk for acute angle closure in at risk patients. Additional side effects include potential central nervous system toxicity which can induce seizures, coma and death [63A].

Atropine/Homatropine

A small case series report reminds clinicians that children are particularly at risk for systemic side effects. A 6-month-old boy was admitted to the ER with acute urinary retention for greater than 36 hours. Symptoms began 3 hours after instillation of 2 drops homatropine 1%, and a 2-year-old boy was admitted for drowsiness, thirst and dry mouth which occurred after being given 3 drops of atropine 1% [64A]. Maximum concentration of 0.3% atropine is recommended for infants to reduce risk of systemic side effects.

Delirium, a feature of anti-cholinergic syndrome, was reported in a 55-year-old male. Onset of delirium occurred 30 minutes after 0.6-mg injection of atropine given as a pre-anesthetic medication prior to bronchoscopy. Patient was treated immediately with psychiatric medications and symptoms resolved. One day later, the patient was given a single drop of atropine 1% in each eye for fundus evaluation and again developed delirium [65A]. The delirium resolved promptly after 8 mg of midazolam was given intravenously [65A].

A lethal dose of atropine is between 100 and 200 mg. Atropine eye drops are up to 10 times more concentrated than oral and injectable formulations, and a massive oral dose of eye drops has been cited in an intentional case of homicide by poisoning. Based on toxicological analysis of the disease dense peripheral blood, urine and tissue samples, the administered dose was estimated to be the equivalent of 200–500 milligrams of atropine. A 172-mg dose is the equivalent of ingesting two 10-mL bottles of atropine eye drops; evidence in the case revealed those charged with the crime purchased three 10-mL bottles of atropine 1% 1 month before the crime [66A].

Cyclopentolate

A recent prospective observational cohort study ($n = 912$) investigated the use of 2 drops of cyclopentolate 1% in both eyes (C+C) or one drop of cyclopentolate followed by one drop of 1% tropicamide (C+T) and reported the presence and nature of adverse reactions occurring with the use of these two regimens used to elicit cycloplegia among a pediatric population. Adverse reactions were reported in 10.3% of patients on the C+C regimen (95.2% of which were central nervous system (CNS) effects) compared to 4.8% of participants on the C+T regimen (91.7% of which were CNS effects). The most common reported effect was drowsiness which was twice as likely in the C+C group when compared to the C+T group (7.8% vs 3.7%) and more commonly occurring in younger patients with lower BMIs [67c].

In a recent survey of pediatric ophthalmologists, Wygnanski-Jaffe et al. report 5 cases of epileptic seizures resulting from administration of 1.0% cyclopentolate eye drops. Seizures occurred within the first hour of dosing in all 5 cases. The median age of patients was 5 years, and patients had no prior history of seizure activity. Lower body weight and immaturity of the central nervous system in children is thought to predispose patients to the toxic effects of cycloplegic agents [63A]. The susceptibility of children to central nervous system effects of cyclopentolate was further evidenced in a case where a 4-year-old boy experienced the inability to walk, disequilibrium, dysarthria and disorientation 3 hours after the instillation of 6 drops of 1% cyclopentolate in both eyes [68A].

Anti-cholinergic addiction has been reported with cyclopentolate eye drops [69A]. The eye drops were initially prescribed for the treatment of uveitis; however,

the patient enjoyed the "tingling" feeling and "felt high" when he used them. He gradually increased the dose over a period of 10 years, ultimately using 300–400 drops per day to achieve the desired high. He was unable to go more than a few hours without the drops because he would experience withdrawal symptoms of anxiety, sweating and nausea. He was admitted to an alcohol and drug treatment center to address the addiction [69A].

Recently, a case of fatal necrotizing enterocolitis was reported in a preterm infant dilated with 0.5% cyclopentolate and 1.25% phenylephrine. While necrotizing enteral colitis is commonly feared in preterm infants, it is thought that cyclopentolate-induced parasympatholytic effect on the gut and the phenylephrine-induced vasoconstriction are important risk factors for this condition [70A].

Cyclomidril (0.2% Cyclopentolate and 1% Phenylephrine Combination)

Cardiopulmonary arrest was reported in a pre-term infant after topical administration of cyclomidril to effect dilation for a ROP screening [4A]. Three sets of eye drops were administered at 15-minute intervals. Fifteen minutes after the third set, the baby became unresponsive. The baby was resuscitated but experienced a second event 3 hours later. Follow-up ROP screenings with 1.0% tropicamide and 2.5% phenylephrine (instead of cyclomydril) were uneventful [4A].

Phenylephrine

Topical phenylephrine is widely reported to cause a transient rise in blood pressure and bradycardia; however, a systematic review and meta-analysis including 8 randomized clinical trials with a total of 918 patients concluded that phenylephrine 2.5% leads to no clinically relevant rise in blood pressure, and the elevation associated with 10% phenylephrine is short-lived [71M].

Anti-Inflammatory Agents

CORTICOSTEROIDS

It is widely known that topical corticosteroids frequently cause elevated intraocular pressure, decreased corneal healing and posterior sub-capsular cataracts. Elevated intraocular pressure usually occurs within the first 4 weeks of treatment; however, delayed onset has been reported with difluprednate 0.05% emulsion dosed two to four times daily for 1 year prior to the significant IOP rise [72A].

Fluorometholone (FML) has recently been noted to have caused a manic episode in a 76-year-old man, marking the first report of psychiatric side effects of topical administration [73A], and growth suppression was observed in a small case series of children, aged 6–10, treated with one drop FML in each eye three times daily for allergic conjunctivitis [74A].

Dexamethosone A 35-year-old man developed central serous chorioretinopathy days after using dexamethasone 0.1% eye drops intranasally for the treatment of rhinitis. The conditions spontaneously resolved but recurred several times over the course of the year, each time occurring 5–7 days after intranasal use of dexamethasone eye drops [75A].

Intravitreal injections and implants offer high potency and sustained dose of corticosteroid and major concerns with use are elevated intraocular pressure and cataract formation, although more severe side effects are reported. Of note, one case of scleral melt over the site of the fluocinolone implant is reported. This effect occurred in a 42-year-old female 18 months after the placement of the implant and required treatment with a scleral graft [76A]. Furthermore, local intraocular immune suppression is suggested as causative for reactivation of viral eye disease. A case of cytomegalovirus endotheliitis after *fluocinolone acetonide* implant was inserted into the eye of a 40-year-old immunocompetent patient [77A], acute retinal necrosis developed in a 52-year-old woman 1 month after intravitreal *dexamethasone* implantation [78A] and CMV retinitis developed in a 54-year-old male 3 months after intravitreal dexamethasone implantation [79A].

A retrospective chart review ($n=234$) comparing patients treated with anti-VEGF (bevacizumab or ranibizumab) injections given alone ($n=150$) vs in combination with 2 mg IVT ($n=42$) for the treatment of diabetic macular edema reported greater likelihood of a significant increase in IOP (>10 mmHg) in adjunct IVT-treated group (21% vs 3.3%) as well as increased risk of cataract progression warranting cataract surgery (36.3% vs 4.7%) [80c].

Lifitegrast A multicenter, randomized, double-masked, placebo-controlled phase 3 study ($n=331$) evaluating the safety of lifitegrast ophthalmic solution for the treatment of dry eye disease reported the most common non-ocular effect was dysgeusia (change in taste) occurring in 16.4% of patients in the lifitegrast group and 1.8% of the placebo group [81C].

Tacrolimus Tacrolimus 0.1%, a potent immunosuppressive agent used for the treatment of allergic ocular diseases can potentially increase risk of infection. An open cohort study ($n=791$) reported the risk of infection (Staphylococcus, Streptococcus, pseudomonas aeruginosa, adenovirus, herpes simplex virus) in patients treated with 0.1% tacrolimus eye drops was increased in patients with giant papillae at baseline [82C]. Hazarika and Singh and Barot et al. report the most commonly observed side effects in patients treated with 0.03% tacrolimus eye ointment were transient foreign-body sensation, burning and transient blurring of vision in their prospective observational studies ($n=41$ and $n=36$, respectively) [83c,84c].

Ocriplasmin

Ocriplasmin, a recombinant protease with activity against fibronectin and laminin, is used for the treatment of vitreomacular adhesion. Laminin is present not only in the vitreous but also throughout retina, leading to potential retinal toxicity [85A]. Barteselli et al. report a case of a 69-year-old woman who developed decreased vision (20/50) and dyschromatopsia 1 day after intravitreal ocriplasmin injection (0.125 mg/0.1 mL) that was associated with transient retinal structural abnormalities noted on both fundus autofluorescence (FAF) and spectral domain optical coherence tomography (OCT). Vision improved to 20/40 1 week later; FAF and OCT changes resolved 4 months post-injection [85A].

Han and Scott report a case of a 67-year-old woman that developed decreased vision, pain and photophobia, 2 hours after an intravitreal injection of ocriplasmin (0.125 mg/0.1 mL), symptoms that are a common post-injection response [86A]. However, vision further decreased to counting fingers over 24 hours as was associated with conjunctival hyperemia and severe anterior chamber inflammation with layered pseudohypopyon which resolved with topical intensive steroid treatment and cycloplegia [86A].

Special Review on Drug Delivery

Drug delivery to the intended site of action can be a challenge because pharmacologic agents must overcome anatomic and physiologic barriers that serve to protect the eye [87R,88R]. The viscosity, concentration, chemical structure of a compound and frequency of application all impact the bioavailability of a topically applied ophthalmic medication. For example, more viscous formulations of eye drops are less affected by tear dilution which allows for longer ocular contact time to maximize absorption. Similarly, the multiple layers of the cornea form a natural barrier that is more easily breached by the lipid solubility of prednisolone acetate then prednisolone phosphate, which is more hydrophilic [89c]. The presence of the blood ocular barrier, comprised of blood-aqueous and blood-retinal barriers, poses another challenge to drug delivery, accounting for the reason that systemic and IV medications are infrequently employed for the treatment of eye disease. Improvements in the use of biomaterials and nanotechnology as non-invasive drug distribution techniques offer major advancements in ocular delivery systems [88R]. Significant advances in the use of polymeric and lipid nanoparticles in topical ophthalmic formulations have allowed for increased corneal contact time and ocular penetration of topically applied medications [90R].

Conditions that require frequent topical dosing constitute a significant treatment burden for patients, which often lead to poor patient adherence to prescribed regimens. Non-compliance rates are reported to be as high as 59% in glaucoma patients [91c] and are therefore a significant risk factor for progression of disease. Novel controlled release delivery systems are being studied as a means to offers sustained IOP control without requiring patients to instill eye drops at all. One such delivery system, the travoprost punctum plug (OTX-TP), utilizes encapsulated travoprost microspheres embedded in a punctal plug to be inserted into the inferior canaliculus. The microspheres slowly released travoprost over a period of 30 days. A prospective, single-arm feasibility study ($n=17$) evaluated the effectiveness and safety of the OTX-TP and reported a 24% reduction in IOP from baseline at day 10 which lessened to a 15.6% decrease in IOP by day 30. Reported effects were foreign body sensation (38.5%), itchiness (15.4%), epiphora (3.8%) and ocular pain (3.8%) [91c]. 100% of the plugs were retained and visible in the puncta at day 10 but decreased to 42% at day 30 which likely contributed to the reduced effect on IOP over time [New #33]. Overall the authors report the OTX-TP to be a feasible option for IOP management and noncompliant patients. Another option being explored entails the use of brimonidine-loaded microspheres deposited into the supraciliary space, adjacent to the ciliary body, via a microneedle is showing promise in early animal studies [92E].

Presently intravitreal injections offer the most efficient drug delivery to the posterior segment and intravitreal injection of anti-VEGF agents have become the mainstay of treatment for age-related macular degeneration. High clearance rates, unfortunately, require frequent injections which expose patients repeatedly to potential adverse effects. Drug delivery systems that reduce the frequency of injection are presently being explored. A capsule drug ring (CDR) has been developed which researchers suggest may extend the duration of action of anti-VEGF agents to 90 days [93R]. Additionally, nanosystems that utilize polymers to release drug in response to a stimulus, such as ultrasound application or oxidative stress, are being developed and offer a novel way to trigger drug released the posterior segment [New #35]. Finally, evolving cell-based therapy such as stem cell transplantation and encapsulated cell technologies (ECT) offer exciting potential to preserve and restore visual function [93R].

References

[1] Inoue K. Managing adverse effects of glaucoma medications. Clin Ophthalmol. 2014;8:903–13 [M].

[2] Charalampidou S, Nolan J, Ormonde GO, et al. Visual perceptions induced by intravitreous injections of therapeutic agents. Eye. 2011;25(4):494–501 [A].

[3] Shah A, Modi Y, Wellik S, et al. Brimonidine allergy presenting as vernal-like keratoconjunctivitis. J Glaucoma. 2015;24(1):89–91 [A].

[4] Lee J, Kodsi S, Gaffar M, et al. Cardiopulmonary arrest following administration of cyclomydril eyedrops for outpatient retinopathy of prematurity screening. J AAPOS. 2014;18(2):183–4 [A].

[5] Kiryazov K, Stefova M, Iotova V. Can ophthalmic drops cause central nervous system depression and cardiogenic shock in infants? Pediatr Emerg Care. 2013;29(11):1207–9 [A].

[6] Pozarowska D, Pozarowski P. The era of anti-vascular endothelial growth factor (VEGF) drugs in ophthalmology, VEGF and anti-VEGF therapy. Cent Eur J Immunol. 2016;41(3):311–6 [R].

[7] Dedania V, Bakri S. Systemic safety of intravitreal anti-vascular endothelial growth factor agents in age-related macular degeneration. Curr Opin Ophthalmol. 2016;27(3):224–43 [R].

[8] Bayhan S, Bayhan H, Adam M, et al. Marginal keratitis after intravitreal injection of ranibizumab. Cornea. 2014;33(11): 1238–9 [A].

[9] Haddock L, Ramsey D, Young L. Complications of subspecialty ophthalmic care: endophthalmitis after intra-vitreal injections of anti-vascular endothelial growth factor medications. Semin Ophthalmol. 2014;29(5–6):257–62 [M].

[10] Meyer CH, Michels S, Rodrigues EB, et al. Incidence of rhegmatogenous retinal detachments after intravitreal avascular endothelial factor injections. Acta Ophthalmol. 2011;89:70–5 [c].

[11] Zhang Y, Han Q, Ru Y, et al. Anti-VEGF treatment for myopic choroidal neovascularization: from molecular characterization to update on clinical application. Drug Des Devel Ther. 2015;9:3413–21 [R].

[12] Arevalo J, Lasave A, Wu L, et al. Intravitreal bevacizumab for proliferative diabetic retinopathy: results from the Pan-American Collaborative Retina Study Group (PACORES) at 24 months of follow-up. Retina. 2017;37(2):334–43 [c].

[13] Gismondi M, Salati C, Salvetat ML, et al. Short-term effect of intravitreal ranibizumab on intraocular pressure. J Glaucoma. 2009;18(9):658–61 [M].

[14] Mathalone N, Arodi-Golan A, Sar A, et al. Sustained elevation of intraocular pressure after intravitreal injections of bevacizumab in eyes with neovascular age-related macular degeneration. Graefes Arch Clin Exp Ophthalmol. 2012;250:1435–40 [C].

[15] Ziemssen F, Sobolewska B, Deissler H, et al. Safety of monoclonal antibodies and related therapeutic proteins for the treatment of neovascular macular degeneration: addressing outstanding issues. Expert Opin Drug Saf. 2015;15(1):1–13 [R].

[16] Hard A, Hellstrom A. On safety, pharmacokinetics and dosage of bevacizumab in ROP treatment—a review. Acta Paediatr. 2011;100:1523–7 [M].

[17] Mikacic I, Bosnar D. Intravitreal bevacizumab and cardiovascular risk in patients with age-related macular degeneration: systematic review and meta-analysis of randomized controlled trials and observational studies. Drug Saf. 2016;39:517–41 [R].

[18] Wu W, Shih C, Lien R, et al. Serum vascular endothelial growth factor after bevacizumab or ranibizumab treatment for retinopathy of prematurity. Retina. 2017;37(4):694–701 [c].

[19] Morin J, et al. Neurodevelopmental outcomes following bevacizumab injections for retinopathy of prematurity. Pediatrics. 2016;137(4) [2016 Apr, Epub 2016 Mar 17]. pii: e20153218. http://dx.doi.org/10.1542/peds.2015-3218 [c].

[20] Hartnett M. Role of cytokines and treatment algorithms and retinopathy of prematurity. Curr Opin Ophthalmol. 2017;28:282–8 [epub ahead of print]. [R].

[21] Chhablani J, Rani PK, Balakrishnan D, et al. Unusual adverse choroidal reaction to intravitreal bevacizumab in aggressive posterior retinopathy of prematurity: the Indian Twin Cities ROP screening (ITCROPS) Data Base Report #7. Semin Ophthalmol. 2014;29(4):222–5 [A].

[22] Henry C, et al. Long-term follow-up of intravitreal bevacizumab for the treatment of pediatric retinal and choroidal diseases. J AAPOS. 2015;19(6):541–8 [c].

[23] Onoda Y, Shiba T, Hori Y, et al. Two cases of acute abdomen after intravitreal injection of bevacizumab. Case Rep Ophthalmol. 2015;6:110–4 [A].

[24] Tolentino M. Systemic and ocular safety of intravitreal anti-vegF therapies for ocular neovascular disease. Surv Ophthalmol. 2011;56(2):95–113 [R].

[25] Bosanquet DC, Davies WL, May K, et al. Acute generalized exanthematous pustulosis following intravitreal ranibizumab. Int Wound J. 2011;8:317–9 [A].

[26] Ueta T, Noda Y, Toyama T, et al. Systemic vascular safety of ranibizumab for age-related macular degeneration. Ophthalmology. 2014;121(11):2193–203 [R].

[27] Chang A, Broadhead G, Hong T, et al. Intravitreal aflibercept for treatment-resistant neovascular age related macular degeneration: 12-month safety and efficacy outcomes. Ophthalmic Res. 2016;55:84–90 [c].

[28] Nakakura A, Tabuchi H, Kiuchi Y. Latanoprost therapy after sunken eyes caused by travoprost or bimatoprost. Optom Vis Sci. 2011;88(9):1140–4 [c].

[29] Hamroush A, Cheung D. Irregularly luscious lashes: difficult to say but a sinister sign to miss. BJM Case Rep. 2016;2016. pii: bcr2016215590. http://dx.doi.org/10.1136/bcr-2016-215590 [A].

[30] Karslioglu MZ, Hosal MB, Tekeli O. Periocular changes in topical bimatoprost and latanoprost use. Turk J Med Sci. 2015;45(4):925–30 [c].

[31] Ung T, Currie Z. Periocular changes following long-term administration of latanoprost 0.005%. Ophthal Plast Reconstr Surg. 2012;28(2):e42–4 [A].

[32] Peace J, Ahlberg P, Wagner M, et al. Polyquaternium-1-preserved travoprost 0.003% or benzalkonium chloride-preserved travoprost 0.004% for glaucoma and ocular hypertension. Am J Ophthalmol. 2015;60(2):266–74 [C].

[33] Chiam P. Travoprost induced granulomatous anterior uveitis. Case Rep Ophthalmol Med. 2011;2011:507073 2 p. [A].

[34] Krishnamurthy R, Senthil S, Garudadri C. Late postoperative choroidal detachment following an uneventful cataract surgery in a patient on topical latanoprost. BMJ Case Rep. 2015;2015 [2015 Jul 14]. pii: bcr2015211408. http://dx.doi.org/10.1136/bcr-2015-211408 [A].

[35] Parchand A, Kaliaperumal S, Deb A, et al. Bimatoprost-induced serous macular detachment after cataract surgery. Case Rep Ophthalmol Med. 2016;2016:7260603 3 p. [A].

[36] Walimbe T, Chelerkar V, Bhagat P, et al. Effect of benzalkonium chloride free latanoprost ophthalmic solution on ocular surface in patients with glaucoma. Clin Ophthalmol. 2016;10:821–7 [c].

[37] Zhang P, Jiang B, Xie L, et al. PTGFR and SLCO2A1 gene polymorphisms determine intraocular pressure response to latanoprost in Han Chinese patients with glaucoma. Curr Eye Res. 2016;41(12):1561–5 [c].

[38] Rana MA, Mady AF, Rehman BA, et al. From eyedrops to ICU, a case report of 3 side effects of ophthalmic timolol maleate in the same patient. Case Rep Crit Care. 2015;2015:714919 4 p. [A].

[39] Pratt N, Ramsay E, Ellett L, et al. Association between ophthalmic timolol and hospitalization for bradycardia. J Ophthalmol. 2015;2015:567387 6 p. [A].

[40] Eyal A, Braun E, Naffaa ME. Syncope caused by intraocular atenolol. Harefuah. 2015;154(11):701–2. 742. [A].

[41] Lin L, Wang Y, Chen Y, et al. Bradyarrhythmias secondary to topical levobunolol hydrochloride solution. Clin Interv Aging. 2014;9:1741–5 [A].

[42] Zimmerman S, et al. Recurrent shock and pulmonary edema due to acetazolamide medication after cataract surgery. Heart Lung. 2014;43:124–6 [A].

[43] Levy Y, Zadok D. Systemic side effects of ophthalmic drops. Clin Pediatr. 2004;43(1):99–101 [A].

[44] Lo J, Pang P, Lo S. Efficacy and tolerability of brinzolamide/brimonidine suspension and prostaglandin analogues in patients previously treated with dorzolamide/timolol solution and prostaglandin analogues. Clin Ophthalmol. 2016;10:583–6 [c].

[45] Hollo G, Katsanos A. Safety and tolerability of the tafluprost/timolol fixed combination for the treatment of glaucoma. Expert Opin Drug Saf. 2015;14(4):609–17 [R].

[46] Coban DT, Erol MK, Yucel O. Hemorrhagic choroidal detachment after use of anti-glaucomatous eyedrops: case report. Arq Bras Oftalmol. 2013;76(5):309–10 [A].

[47] Hommer A, Hubatsch DA, Cano-Parra J. Safety and efficacy of adding fixed-combination brinzolamide/timolol maleate to prostaglandin therapy for treatment of ocular hypertension or glaucoma. J Ophthalmol. 2015;2015:131970 7 p. [c].

[48] Kabha M, Dekalo S, Barnes S, et al. Sulfadiazine-induced obstructive nephropathy presenting with upper urinary tract extravasation. J Endourol Case Rep. 2016;2(1):159–61 [A].

[49] Byrom L, Zappala T, Muir J. Toxic epidermal necrolysis caused by over the counter eye drops. Aust J Dermatol. 2013;54:144–6 [A].

[50] Lartey S, Armah P, Ampong A. A sudden total loss of vision after routine cataract surgery. Ghana Med J. 2013;47(2):96–9 [A].

[51] Kuo H, Lee J. Macular infarction after 23-gauge trans-conjunctival sutureless vitrectomy and sub-conjunctival gentamicin for macular pucker: a case report. Can J Ophthalmol. 2009;44(6):720–1 [A].

[52] Salati C, Migliorati G, Brusin P. Sclero-retinal necrosis after a sub-conjunctival injection of gentamicin in a patient with surgically repaired episcleral retinal detachment. Eur J Ophthalmol. 2004;14(6):575–7 [A].

[53] Brouzas D, Moschos M, Koutsandrea C, et al. Gentamicin-induced macular toxicity in 25-gauge sutureless vitrectomy. Cutan Ocul Toxicol. 2013;32(3):258–9 [A].

[54] Litwin A. Toxic anterior segment syndrome after cataract surgery secondary to sub-conjunctival gentamicin. J Cataract Refract Surg. 2012;38:2196–7 [A].

[55] Tang R, Tse R. Acute renal failure after topical fortified gentamicin and vancomycin eyedrops. J Ocul Pharmacol Ther. 2011;27(4):411–3 [A].

[56] Wilhelmus K, Abshire R. Corneal ciprofloxacin precipitation during bacterial keratitis. Am J Ophthalmol. 2003;136(6):1032–7 [A].

[57] Patwardhan A, Khan M. Topical ciprofloxacin can delay recovery from viral ocular surface infection. J R Soc Med. 2005;98:274–5 [r].

[58] Malladi A, Liew E, Ng X, et al. Ciprofloxacin eyedrops-induced subtherapeutic serum phenytoin levels resulting in breakthrough seizures. Singapore Med J. 2014;55(7):e114–5 [A].

[59] Saito M, Nakada T. Contact urticaria syndrome from eyedrops: levofloxacin hydrate ophthalmic solution. J Dermatol. 2013;40(2):130–1 [A].

[60] Witkin AJ, Shah AR, Engstrom RE, et al. Postoperative hemorrhagic occlusive retinal vasculitis. Expanding the clinical spectrum and possible association with vancomycin. Ophthalmology. 2015;122:1438–51 [c].

[61] Lenci L, Chin E, Carter C, et al. Ischemic retinal vasculitis associated with cataract surgery and intracameral vancomycin. Case Rep Ophthalmol Med. 2015;2015:683194 4 p. [A].

[62] Lodhi S, Reddy G, Sunder C. Post-operative nocardia endophthalmitis and the challenge of managing with intravitreal amikacin. Case Rep Ophthalmol Med. 2016;2016:2365945 6 p. [A].

[63] Wygnanski-Jaffe T, Nucci P, Goldchmit M, et al. Epileptic seizures induced by cycloplegic eyedrops. Cutan Ocul Toxicol. 2014;33(2):103–8 [A].

[64] Princelle A, Hue V, Pruvost I, et al. Systemic adverse effects of topical ocular instillation of atropine in 2 children. Arch Pediatr. 2013;20:391–4 [A].

[65] Panchasara A, Mandavia D, Anovadiya A, et al. Central anti-cholinergic syndrome induced by single therapeutic dose of atropine. Curr Drug Saf. 2012;7:35–6 [A].

[66] Carlier J, Escard E, Peoch M, et al. Atropine eyedrops: an unusual homicidal poisoning. J Forensic Sci. 2014;59(3):859–64 [A].

[67] Van Minderhout HM, Joosse MV, Grootendorst DC, et al. Adverse reactions following routine anticholinergic eye drops in a paediatric population: an observational cohort study. BMJ Open. 2015;5(12): e008798. http://dx.doi.org/10.1136/bmjopen-2015-008798 [c].

[68] Derinoz O, Anil E. Inability to walk, disequilibrium, incoherent speech, disorientation following the instillation of 1% cyclopentolate eyedrops: case report. Pediatr Emerg Care. 2012;28(1):59–60 [A].

[69] Darcin A, Dilbaz N, Yilmaz S, et al. Cyclopentolate hydrochloride eyedrops addiction: a case report. J Addict Med. 2011;5(1):84–5 [A].

[70] Ozgun U, Demet T, Ozge A, et al. Fatal necrotizing enterocolitis due to mydriatic eyedrops. J Coll Physicians Surg Pak. 2014;24(Special Suppl 2):S147–9 [A].

[71] Stavert B, McGuinness M, Harper A, et al. Cardiovascular adverse effects of phenylephrine eyedrops. A systematic review and meta-analysis. JAMA Ophthalmol. 2015;133(6):647–52 [M].

[72] Kurz P, Chheda L, Kurz D. Effects of twice daily topical difluprednate 0.05% emulsion in a child with pars planitis. Ocul Immunol Inflamm. 2011;19(1):84–5 [A].

[73] Kumagi R, Ichimiya Y. Manic episode induced by steroid (fluorometholone) eye drops in an elderly patient. Psychiatry Clin Neurosci. 2014;68:652–3 [A].

[74] Wolthers O. Growth suppression caused by corticosteroid eyedrops. J Pediatr Endocrinol Metab. 2011;24(5–6):393–4 [A].

[75] Prakash G, Shephali J, Tirupati N, et al. Recurrent central serous chorioretinopathy with dexamethasone eyedrops used nasally for rhinitis. Middle East Afr J Ophthalmol. 2013;20(4):363–5 [A].

[76] Georgalas I, Koutsandrea C, Papaconstantinou D, et al. Scleral melt following Retisert intravitreal fluocinolone implant. Drug Des Devel Ther. 2014;8:2373–5 [A].

[77] Park U, Kim S, Yu H. Cytomegalovirus endotheliitis after fluocinolone acetonide (Retisert) implant in a patient with Behçet uveitis. Ocul Immunol Inflamm. 2011;19(4):282–3 [A].

[78] Kucukevcilioglu M, Eren M, Sobaci G. Acute retinal necrosis following intravitreal dexamethasone implant. Arq Bras Oftalmol. 2015;78(2):118–9 [A].

[79] Vannozzi L, Bacherini A, Beccastrini E, et al. Cytomegalovirus retinitis following intravitreal dexamethasone implant in a patient with central retinal vein occlusion. Acta Ophthalmol. 2016;94(2): e158–60 [A].

[80] Garoon R, Coffee R, Lai Jiang L, et al. Adjunct intravitreous triamcinolone acetonide in the treatment of diabetic macular edema with anti-VEGF agents. J Ophthalmol. 2016;2016:5282470 6 p. [c].

[81] Donnenfeld E, Karpecki P, Majmudar P, et al. Safety of lymphocytic graft ophthalmic solution 5.0% in patients with dry eye disease: a 1 year, multicenter, randomized, placebo controlled study. Cornea. 2016;35(6):741–8 [C].

[82] Miyazaki D, Fukashima A, Ohashi Y, et al. Steroid sparing effect of 0.1% tacrolimus eyedrop for treatment of shield ulcer in corneal epitheliopathy in refractory allergic ocular diseases. Ophthalmology. 2016;124(3):287–94. pii: S0161-6420(16) 31135-6. [C].

[83] Barot R, Shitole S, Bhaghat N, et al. Therapeutic effects of 0.1% tacrolimus eye ointment in allergic ocular diseases. J Clin Diagn Res. 2016;10(6):NC05–9 [c].

[84] Hazarika A, Singh K. Efficacy of topical application of 0.03% tacrolimus eye ointment in the management of allergic conjunctivitis. J Nat Sci Biol Med. 2015;6(Suppl 1): S10–2 [c].

[85] Barteselli G, Carinia E, Invernizzi A, et al. Early panretinal abnormalities on fundus autofluorescence and spectral domain optical coherence tomography after intravitreal ocriplasmin. Acta Ophthalmol. 2016;94(2):e160–2 [A].

[86] Han I, Scott A. Sterile endophthalmitis after intravitreal ocriplasmin injection: report of a single case. Retin Cases Brief Rep. 2015;9(3):242–4 [A].

[87] Fraunfelder FT, Fraunfelder FW, Chambers WA. Drug-induced ocular side effects: clinical ocular toxicology. 7th ed. Philadelphia: Elsevier; 2015 [R].

[88] Gaudana R, Ananthula HK, Parenky A, et al. Ocular drug delivery. AAPS J. 2010;12(3):348–60. http://dx.doi.org/10.1208/s12248-010-9183-3 [R].

[89] Stringer W, Bryant R. Dose uniformity of topical corticosteroid preparations: difluprednate ophthalmic emulsion 0.05% versus branded and generic prednisolone acetate ophthalmic suspension 1%. Clin Ophthalmol. 2010;4:1119–24. http://dx.doi.org/10.2147/OPTH.S12441 [c].

[90] Almeida H, Amaral MH, Lobao P, et al. Nanoparticles in ocular drug delivery systems for topical administration: promises and challenges. Curr Pharm Des. 2015;21(36):5212–24 [R].

[91] Perera S, Ting D, Nongpiur M, et al. Feasibility study of sustained released travoprost punctum plug for intraocular pressure reduction in Asian population. Clin Ophthalmol. 2016;10:757–64 [c].

[92] Chiang B, Kim YC, Doty AC, et al. Sustained reduction of intraocular pressure by supraciliary delivery of brimonidine-loaded poly (lactic acid) microspheres for the treatment of glaucoma. J Control Release. 2016;228:48–57 [E].

[93] Vibhuti A, Agrahari V, Mandal A, et al. How are we improving the delivery to back of the eye? Advances and challenges of novel therapeutic approaches. Expert Opin Drug Deliv. 2016;28:1–17 [R].

43

Safety of Complementary and Alternative Medicine (CAM) Treatments and Practices

Renee A. Bellanger[1], Christina M. Seeger, Helen E. Smith

Feik School of Pharmacy, University of the Incarnate Word, San Antonio, TX, United States

[1]Corresponding author: bellange@uiwtx.edu

INTRODUCTION

Spending on herbal dietary supplements in the United States totaled $6.92 Billion in 2015. This represents a 7.5% increase from the previous year, and an "all-time high," according to the American Botanical Council, which also reports 12 years of consecutive growth, despite media attention on the possibility of contamination, adulteration and safety concerns [1H,2R]. The global acceptance and use of herbal medicines and natural products continue to experience exponential growth, and likewise issues relating to safety and adverse reactions are becoming more prominent as evidence compounds to show that "natural" and "safe" are not synonymous, as is often misconceived [3R,4R]. However, with the increasing uses of these products, the pharmacovigilance of herbal medicines and natural products is becoming more pressing, and it continues to be important to monitor their safety. The methods of pharmacovigilance, the science and activities related to the detection, assessment, understanding and prevention of adverse effects or any other drug-related problem [5S], were developed for monitoring the safety of pharmaceuticals, but can and should be used to monitor herbal products "aiming to increase their safety profile" [6H]. While this is not a new concept, Naranjo et al. offered a systematic method of monitoring adverse drug reactions (ADRs) and determining the probability of a causal relationship between a substance and the suspected ADR that remains the gold standard [7c]. The study of causality of natural and herbal products in ADRs has progressed with the increase in use of these products worldwide, especially in countries that generally practice Western-style medicine. The Naranjo nomogram is utilized to detect the potential for safety concerns from herbal and natural supplements.

There is a lack of quality publication on the clinical efficacy of natural products, and due to the variability in preparation and composition of herbal products, studies may not be comparable [4R]. The efficacy of non-patentable herbs is not a research priority in the same way new prescription medications are, and in fact, the research can be financially unfeasible. Some of the issues with herbal products, hindering comparison, include unknown composition or pharmaceutical form of the herbal preparation, lack of standardization in dosing and active components, inappropriate or improper dosing or labeling, contamination and herb–drug interactions [8r]. The majority of evidence is found in case reports, which are often of poor quality, and the best level of evidence, systematic reviews, "strongly rely on the quality and quantity of primary data (clinical trials), which is low in the field of herbal medicine" [4R], making it difficult to incorporate herbal products into the evidence-based medicine criteria for clinical use [8r]. In addition, the majority of systematic reviews of adverse effects do not include unpublished data, which introduces a publication bias as well as an omission bias that could be a serious threat to the validity of systematic reviews on adverse effects, further complicating the availability of evidence for clinical decision making [9R].

Herbal and dietary supplements are related to an increase in hepatotoxicity reports in the United States and elsewhere, increasing the urgency to identify a means of diagnosing and predicting toxicity, adverse effects and interactions of herbal and natural products [10R]. Databases of spontaneous reporting of potential ADRs allow for timely diagnosis and treatment, as well as possible prevention, and serve as a major function in worldwide safety surveillance and detection. One such attempt is the World Health Organization Global Individual Case Safety Report database (VigiBase®), the largest international pharmacovigilance database of spontaneous ADR reports of reactions to medicines, including herbal based and other natural supplements, and vaccines [11C].

A study across the Italian Surveillance System of Natural Products, which collects reports of suspected adverse effects occurring following the use of dietary supplements, herbal preparations, natural non-plant preparations and homeopathic products, and utilizes data from VigiBase®. A report from this surveillance system on the adverse events reported from a single dietary supplement highlighted two potential safety issues. The authors called for continued pharmacovigilance and reporting of suspect reports, as well as appropriate education for clinicians and consumers on the safety risks and reporting mechanisms for suspected adverse effects [12C].

METHODS

A literature search of PubMed, Google Scholar, NIH, CINAHL, Science Direct, Cochrane, and WHO databases for meta-analyses, case studies, and case reports published in English from January 1, 2016 through January 1, 2017 included the terms: CAM therapies, herbal therapies, mind–body therapy, yoga, tai chi, chiropractic, manipulative therapy, acupuncture, traditional Chinese medicine, and adverse effects (psychiatric, cardiac, endocrine, gastrointestinal, pulmonary, neurotoxic, nephrotoxicity, hepatotoxicity), side effects, adverse reactions, contaminants. Specific products searched include: soybean, *Camellia sinensis*, *Gingko biloba*, *Citrus aurantium* (bitter orange), *Cinnamomum verum* (cinnamon), *Cimcifuga racemosa* (black cohosh), *Echinacea purpurea*, *Vitex agnus castus* (chaste tree), *Hypericum perforatum* (St. John's wort), *Panax ginseng*, *Panax* species, *Valeriana officinalis*, *Serenoa repens* (Saw palmetto), *Silybum marianum* (Milk thistle), *Amorphophallus konjac*, *Paullinia cupana* (Guarana), Primrose, Acai, *Garcinia cambogia*, *Cascara sagrada*, Turmeric (curcumin), *Zingiber officinale* (ginger), *Glycyrrhiza glabra* (licorice), and energy drinks are included in this document by body system.

DIETARY AND HERBAL SUPPLEMENTS

Adverse Effects: Central Nervous System

The potential effects of herbals and herbal medications on central nervous system function are of great concern.

Few reviews, case reports, or studies of the neurotoxicity of these compounds were published in the English language literature within the last year.

In a post-hoc review of a Phase 1 study of St. John's wort (SJW) drug interactions with rifampicin revealed dose-dependent adverse effects on only the female participants. Paresthesia and phototoxic erythrodermia occurred in 5 of 6 of the female participants of the study at the dose of 1800 mg SJW per day within 6 days of a 3-week period, symptoms worsened on exposure to sun light. The symptoms did not occur at lower doses given prior to this point. Rifampicin was not being administered when the symptoms appeared. The subjects developed phototoxic skin reactions and became sensitive to cold temperature, developed allodynia and intermittent or persistent paresthesia and dysaesthesia. The neurologic symptoms were limited to the areas of skin changes. When the SJW was discontinued, symptoms disappeared within 12–16 days. There were no sequelae noted. None of the male participants in the study had these manifestations [13c].

A double-blind, placebo-controlled crossover design compared the effects on cognition with six different tests on a laptop computer and cardiac parameters, blood pressure and heart rate, of *P. ginseng* or *G. biloba* on 28 female and 20 male young adult volunteers. Each participant was randomized to either ginkgo or ginseng and then they attended a practice day and three test days with a placebo, and two different doses, medium or high, of the chosen supplement with wash out periods of 48 hours between each supplement level or placebo day. Difference was seen in the *G. biloba* group on cognitive performance measured by the Berg card sorting test, including, the total number of errors in females ($P < 0.011$) and the perseverative errors both in males and females ($P = 0.004$). No differences between ginkgo and ginseng groups of either gender in the other cognitive tasks. Females in the high dose *G. biloba* after the BERG test had reduced diastolic blood pressure readings compared to placebo ($P = 0.005$). There were no other blood pressure or heart rate reading effects on any of the cognitive tests in either supplement group or by gender [14c].

A case of tumefactive demyelination in a 32-year-old man presenting with facial drooping and dysarthria was linked to a multiple ingredient homeopathic supplement for restless leg syndrome. The patient had experienced mild symptoms of an upper respiratory infection a week prior to developing the neurologic symptoms. He had taken the homeopathic supplement which contained arsenic, zinc, lycopodium, pulsatilla, and *Rhus toxicodendron* among other ingredients. The authors consider the homeopathic product possibly contributed to a proinflammatory response to a viral illness leading to the demyelination [15A].

Adverse Effects: Cardiac, Pulmonary, and Hematologic Systems

Some recent investigations of the risk of developing adverse effects or toxicity on the heart, lungs or blood/coagulation systems with the use of some herbal medications are described. A few case reports of ill effects on these body systems associated with the use of herbal dietary supplements in the past year were published.

Healthy active duty military volunteers (20 men and 6 women) were enrolled in a randomized controlled study to assess the effects of energy drinks on blood pressure and cardiac parameters. The subjects were given a standardized caffeinated energy shot drink or placebo in a crossover design twice daily for 7 days. After the first energy shot, systolic BP was elevated at 3 and 5 hours with energy drink consumption compared with placebo ($P = 0.050$ and $P = 0.038$, respectively), and diastolic BP was elevated at 1 and 5 hours with energy drink consumption ($P = 0.019$ and $P = 0.043$, respectively). Heart rate and ECG parameters were not significantly different at any point in the evaluation. The effects on blood pressure were similar to baseline after 7 days of consistent energy shot ingestion [16c].

In another study, otherwise healthy patients, aged 15–39 years, that presented to an emergency department with complaint of "heart palpitations" were surveyed by questionnaire. The questionnaire assessed energy drink consumption and any pre-existing or family history of cardiac disease. Baseline characteristics and vital signs were obtained, as well as an electrocardiogram. Of the 60 participants, 42 (70%) had consumed an energy drink at some time in their life. Among these "consumers," 15 (25%) had consumed energy drinks withing the past 24 hours. Of these 15, 8 had consumed 5 or more drinks and 1 had consumed 12 energy drinks with alcohol. The survey participants that drank at least 2 energy drinks regularly were considered high volume consumers and had a significant increase in the frequency of palpitations experienced within 24 hours of consumption. There was no association with chest pain or shortness of breath with any energy drink consumption. Co-ingestion of alcoholic beverages and energy drinks increased the findings of palpitations. The ECGs from the participants did not show differences between consumers and non-consumers of energy drinks [17c].

Caffeinated products, such as coffee, tea or chocolate, may affect cardiac rate and rhythm. A group of participants from the Cardiovascular Health Study of the National Heart, Lung, and Blood Institute underwent 24-hour ambulatory electrocardiography monitoring during their study assessment period. During this time, they also provided a baseline food frequency questionnaire with a validated visual component, including information about caffeinated beverages or food items. Patients ($n = 1388$) without persistent atrial fibrillation and who completed the food frequency questionnaire were included in this evaluation. Chronic consumption of caffeinated items was considered the average frequency over the past 12 months from never to almost every day. Those who consumed at least one serving of a caffeinated product per day were women, but no other differences in this group vs those who did not. There were no associations between groups, including those with underlying disease states, diabetes, hypertension, congestive heart failure, coronary artery disease, or atrial fibrillation, with caffeinated product consumption and additional cardiac episodes, including Premature Atrial Contractions, Premature Ventricular Contractions, Supraventricular Tachycardia or Ventricular Tachycardia, as seen on the monitor [18C].

A case report linked bidirectional ventricular tachycardia and a traditional Chinese medicine product Fu Zi (aconite, *Radix Aconiti praeparata*) in a middle-aged woman experiencing syncope [19A]. The product is used for anti-inflammatory effects [19A] and as a cardiotonic (20R). The patient recovered after 2 hours on discontinuance of the product. The patient received amiodarone, metoprolol, potassium, and lidocaine with no change in cardiac symptoms. Fu Zi's effects on cardiac rhythm and rate vary due to product dose, origin, processing method, composition of extract used and individual patient variation [20R]. The risk of cardiac toxicity depends on which dose and variation is used [19A].

Horse chestnut (*Aesculus hippocastanum* L.) paste ingested over a 6-week period was implicated in a case involving a 32-year-old man who developed an acute pericardial effusion, an exudative pleural effusion and cardiac decomposition. This patient was previously healthy. His admission laboratory included a C-reactive protein (CRP) level of 124.3 mg/dL and alanine transaminase (ALT) of 245 U/L. All other causes, infectious, oncologic, and rheumatic, were ruled out. The patient required steroid injections and a surgical procedure to mitigate the acute effects of the horse chestnut paste. The patient required administration of a long-term steroid taper over 2 months with ibuprofen and colchicine therapy for 3 months. The patient was advised to not take the supplement. At 90 days post the acute event the patient was symptom free and the effusion had resolved. The authors calculated the Naranjo Probability scale of 6 points to suggest a causal relationship of the adverse events with the horse chestnut paste [21A].

Caffeine intoxication, including agitation, palpitations, shortness of breath and chest pain, from ingesting a large volume of a cola beverage in an otherwise healthy 27-year-old woman was reported from Israel.

The woman ingested approximately 400 mg of caffeine over a 2-hour period. The patient presented with tachycardia (160 bpm) and an elevated leukocytosis. She had worsening lactic acidosis, hypokalemia and hyperglycemia. She was admitted to the intensive care unit on broad spectrum antibiotics with the suspicion of diabetic ketoacidosis and sepsis. An electrocardiogram (ECG) revealed sinus tachycardia but no underlying cardiac damage. The patient's hypotension, acidosis and hypokalemia were resistant to treatment with fluid and electrolyte therapy in the acute phase. All symptoms and laboratory values resolved within 24 hours of admission without further treatment and the patient was discharged the following day [22A].

Adverse Effects: Renal

The potential nephrotoxic effects of herbals and herbal medications are of concern. However, very few reviews, case reports, or studies of the nephrotoxicity of these compounds were published in the English language literature within the last year.

Nauffal and Gabardi [23R] published a review of reported cases of apparent nephrotoxicity associated with ingestion of natural products. Cases were identified using a key word search in Medline and were defined as significant reduction in glomerular filtration rate (GFR). The authors categorized the reviewed cases into the following nephrotoxic mechanisms of action: direct nephrotoxicity, immune-mediated responses, nephrolithiasis, rhabdomyolysis, and hepatorenal syndrome. They also included a category for nephrotoxicity caused by contaminants in the natural products. Twenty-three different natural products were reported to have caused cases of nephrotoxicity reported in the literature. The doses of the natural products patients ingested were not always available, and the causality of the natural product related to the various types of nephrotoxicity cannot be determined.

A review of studies investigating the nephrotoxicity of ingredients of some traditional Chinese medicine preparations (TCM) in animal models was published in the last 20 years. Based on their literature search, the authors found that the administration of TCM products made from plants containing aristolochic acids (AAs), alkaloids, and several anthraquinones, flavonoids, and glycosides resulted in nephrotoxicity in the studied animals. AAs detected in TCM products usually are made from plants of the Aristolochiaceae family. Alkaloids and the other less common nephrotoxic compounds come from a wide variety of plants used in TCM for a variety of uses. Both acute and chronic renal effects have been observed with the administration of these nephrotoxic ingredients [24R].

Adverse Effects: Hepatic

There have been recent investigations of the risk of developing hepatotoxicity with the use of some herbal medications, case reports, and reviews of hepatotoxicity associated with the use of herbal dietary supplements in the last year.

A randomized controlled clinical trial was conducted to evaluate the efficacy of S. marianum as a protectant against drug-induced liver injury caused by medications used to treat tuberculosis [25C]. S. marianum is often used in China to prevent hepatotoxicity when treating tuberculosis (TB). Three hundred seventy TB patients were enrolled in the study. 183 subjects were randomized to the experimental group received standard TB treatment with S. marianum 200 mg orally in capsules twice daily as a hepatoprotectant. 187 subjects were randomized to the control group receiving standard TB treatment with vitamin C. Probable and possible anti-tuberculosis drug-induced liver were the primary outcomes evaluated. Probable drug-induced liver injury was defined as serum ALT or AST values three times and a total bilirubin (TBiL) twice the upper limit of normal in asymptomatic patients or those with hepatitis symptoms. Possible drug-induced liver injury was defined by elevated AST, ALT, and TBiL elevated by twice the upper limits of normal. The study found that S. marianum was not significantly protective of drug-induced liver injury caused by TB treating medications for either the probable or possible liver injury category. There was some indication that S. marianum itself caused some hepatotoxicity.

An investigation of reports of herb-induced hepatotoxicity using data from the Berlin Case–control Surveillance Study was published by Douros [26C]. In this study, 10 cases associated with herbs were identified from the one hundred ninety-eight cases of liver injury reported at all the hospitals in Berlin from October 2002 through December 2011. Cases of liver injury caused by herbal use were determined by using the Council for International Organizations of Medical Sciences (CIOMS) scale. Cases were identified if they had elevated ALT or AST three times the upper limit of normal or total bilirubin >2 mg/dL and did not have underlying hepatic disease. Several herbals were determined to be associated with liver injury. An Ayurvedic herbal tea was considered the probable cause of one patient's liver toxicity. Valeriana, Mentha piperita, Pelargonium sidoides, H. perforatum, and Eucalyptus globulus were the possible cause of other patients' liver injuries.

Kombucha tea is a drink made from steeping black tea with a combination of yeast and bacterial cultures. It is sometimes called mushroom tea, although mushrooms are not used to make it. It is also known as Manchurian or Kargasok tea. It has a reputation of having a wide variety of health benefits, although these have not been proven. Gedela et al. [27A] reported in January of 2016 a case of cholestatic hepatitis associated with Kombucha tea ingestion. A 58-year-old woman was admitted to the hospital with epi-gastric pain, clay-colored bowel movement that resolved before admittance, dark urine, pruritus and jaundice after consuming Kombucha tea for a month. She showed the signs of cholestatic liver injury due to a high alkaline phosphatase to aminotransferase ratio, and bilirubinemia. Other factors likely to cause signs and symptoms of cholestasis were ruled out. A liver biopsy and the temporal relationship between tea ingestion and symptoms suggested drug-induced hepatotoxicity. No details were reported by these authors regarding the amount of tea consumed, beyond the statement that "the patient had been consuming a significant amount of Kombucha tea for 1 month prior to her admission." The mechanism for the drug-induced liver injury by this drink is not known.

Papafragkakis reported a recent case of acute hepatitis resulting from consumption of Chinese skullcap and black catechu by a 54-year-old woman treating arthralgia [28A]. Chinese skullcap, or *Scutellaria baicalensis*, is used for a wide variety of medical purposes. There have been some reports of adverse effects with its use, including acute thromobocytopenic purpura, pneumonitis, and hepatotoxicity with pulmonary infiltrates. Black catechu is used for its blood stabilization, liver protecting, antifungal, antibacterial, anti-inflammatory, antioxidant, and antidiarrheal properties. There have been a few reports of hepatotoxicity reported with the use of Chinese skullcap and black catechu combinations. In this case report, the patient was admitted to the hospital complaining of pruritus, diarrhea, weakness, jaundice, dark colored urine, and a four-pound weight loss over the 2 weeks these symptoms had been occurring. Blood work found elevated levels of aspartate aminotransferase (AST), alanine aminotransferase (ALT), alkaline phosphatase (ALP), TbiL, and lipase with an elevated partial thromboplastin time. All stool and serological evaluations for infectious agents were negative. Imaging studies revealed dilated intrahepatic biliary ducts. Based on all diagnostic results and the resolution of her symptoms in relation to the time of consumption of the Chinese skullcap and black catechu, no other cause was found for the hepatitis besides ingestion of these herbals. Using the Roussel Uclaf Causality Assessment Method (RUCAM) for determining causality of hepatotoxicity from Chinese herbal medicines, the authors stated that the patient's ingestion of Chinese skullcap and black catechu was the probable cause of the patient's hepatitis.

G. cambogia is a herbal supplement often used to for weight loss. Corey [29A] recently published a case report of a 52-year-old woman who developed liver failure after taking *G. cambogia* for weight loss. This patient ingested two 1000-mg capsules twice a day for about 25 days until she began to suffer from decreased appetite, fatigue, and confusion. She was found to have elevated total bilirubin, AST, ALT, INR and platelet count, and mild jaundice. Severe acute hepatitis was diagnosed with a liver biopsy. The patient underwent liver transplantation about 50 days after presenting with symptoms. Using the CIOMS scale to determine the association between ingested substances and liver failure, the authors determined that the patient's ingestion of *G. cambogia* was the probable cause of her liver failure.

A case of hepatotoxicity after the use of a home-made flower pollen preparation was reported by Rollason [30A]. The 43-year-old female patient presented to her provider complaining of fatigue, nausea, vomiting and jaundice for 10 days prior to being seen. It was determined the patient ingested a home-made flower pollen preparation harvested from local fields for fatigue, consuming one tablespoon daily for up to 4 weeks. She had also taken five 500-mg paracetamol tablets for 3 days prior to seeking medical care for a headache, but had not taken any other medications or supplements. The flower pollen was analyzed and was found to contain significant levels of a pyrrolizidine alkaloid that is metabolized to a hepatotoxic metabolite via the activity of CYP2B6 and CYP3A4. The patient was found to have elevated AST, ALT, gamma-glutamyltransferase (GGT), and serum bilirubin. A liver biopsy diagnosed mostly lobular hepatocellular necrosis, portal inflammation and cholestasis. The patient's CYP3A4 phenotype was determined using a marker substrate, revealing she had high CYP3A4 activity. Using the RUCAM scoring, the authors concluded that the flower pollen exposure in conjunction with the patient's ability to metabolize the pyrrolizidine alkaloid to a hepatotoxic product was the probable cause of the patient's hepatotoxicity.

Several reviews herb-induced liver injury (HILI) have been published in the last year. One by Valdivia-Correa et al. [31R] was a review of HILI. The authors state that the use of herbal medicines and herbal supplements is high in Mexico, but there is limited information in the literature about level of knowledge and use of medicinal plants in Mexico. There is also limited information regarding which herbal medicines or supplements are causally associated with HILI in that country. Efforts are being made to catalog the plants used medicinally and their associated HILI. The authors of this review cited the Digital Library of Traditional Mexican Medicine as a source of information on Mexican herbal medicines, their use, and their known hepatotoxicity. Seven herbal medicines associated with hepatotoxicity were listed in the Digital Library. These were *Scoparia dulcis* (maidenhair), *C. aurantium* (citrus orange), *Prunus persica* (peach), *Rosmarinus officinalis* (rosemary), *Equisetum hyemale* (horse tail), *Tilia mexicana* (tilia), and *Morus alba* (white mulberry). In the Valdivia-Correa review itself, the authors provided a list of herbs commonly used in Mexico with known hepatotoxicity.

Bedi et al. published a review of hepatoprotective and hepatotoxic herbal drugs in 2016 [32R]. The authors of this review published a list of herbal medications available in India. A second review published in 2016 was authored by Garcia-Cortes and includes a comprehensive discussion of the hepatotoxicity of herbal dietary supplements [33R]. These authors defined herbal dietary supplements to be herbal products that are used for weight loss, constipation, or to improve nutrition. Herbal dietary supplements made of single ingredients as well as those with multiple ingredients are discussed in this chapter. Single-ingredient herbal dietary supplements that have been associated with significant hepatotoxicity included in the chapter were green tea extract, linoleic acid, usnic acid, 1.3-dimethylamylamin, vitamin A, *G. cambogia*, and ma huang. Multiple-ingredient dietary supplement products whose consumption has resulted in known hepatotoxicity include Herbalife™ products, Hydroxycut™, LipoKinetix™, UCP-1 and OxyELITE™. Anabolic androgenic steroids were also included in this chapter as products that pose a risk of hepatotoxicity. The severity of the liver toxicity associated with the use of these products was included in this review.

Frenzel and Teschke also published a systematic review of HILI cases reported in the medical literature from 1990 to 2016 [34R]. The pathogenesis and clinical picture of HILI by a variety of herbs and herbal medications, as well as common contaminants of these herbal products were presented. The authors also discussed the difficulties in determining causality in HILI, suggesting that standardization of determining causality may be reached if cases are assessed using a method such as the RUCAM tool.

An important addition to the literature on HILI is an update to the Roussel Uclaf Causality Assessment Method (RUCAM). RUCAM is a tool used to determine the causality between both drug-induced liver injury (DILI) and herb-induced liver injury (HILI). This update was published by Danan and Teschke [35S]. The update allows for the differentiation between hepatocellular injury compared to cholestatic and mixed liver injury. A checklist to use when considering differential diagnoses of DILI and HILI compared to other causes of liver injury was added to the update, as well as information on how to evaluate the results of re-exposure. The updated RUCAM was intentionally developed for use in prospective analysis, an approach that makes it easier to gather complete data for evaluating causality. The authors of this RUCAM update encourage the use of the term RUCAM for this assessment tool rather than its previous name Council for International Organizations of Medical Sciences (CIOMS) as a way of harmonizing the efforts at determining HILI and DILI.

Adverse Effects: Endocrine

The documentation of adverse effects of herbals and herbal medications on endocrine function is lacking. No reviews were found from the past year. One case report and a limited study of the neurotoxicity of herbals and herbal medications were published in the English language literature within the last year.

A prospective study of St. John's wort (SJW) reported that it caused elevated glucose tolerance in 10 healthy men. An oral glucose tolerance test (OGTT) was administered at baseline, the morning after completion of 21 days of SJW capsules, and at least 6 weeks after the last SJW dose was ingested. Each SJW capsule contained 240–294 mg of dry extract which was standardized to 900 micrograms of hypericin and given orally twice daily. The men were 18–40 years of age with a body mass index (BMI) less than 30 kg/m^2 and laboratory values of serum glucose and hemoglobin A1C levels within normal limits. Fasting laboratory values of glucose, serum insulin and C-peptide did not differ between the phases. After the 75 g glucose challenge, the 2-hour glucose ($P = 0.003$), and the total ($P < 0.001$) and incremental glucose ($P < 0.001$) area under the curve (AUC) at the 21st day and 6-week values after SJW ingestion varied from baseline. At the 6-week laboratory assessments, the glucose AUC had continued to increase from the 21-day point without additional SJW ingestion. No differences were seen in the serum insulin or C-peptide values. Insulin response ($P = 0.003$) and insulin response adjusted for insulin sensitivity ($P = 0.01$) were also shown to be different from baseline in 9 subjects evaluated for these parameters [36c].

Licorice-containing cough lozenges were associated with a new diagnosis hypertension and hypokalemia in a 66-year-old man. The patient's blood pressure was 152/80 mmHg. His laboratory findings were within normal limits except for his serum potassium at 2.5 mmol/L (normal range of 3.5–5.3 mmol/L) and with a metabolic alkalosis, serum bicarbonate 34.6 mmol/L (normal range of 24–31 mmol/L). He did not meet laboratory or steroid suppression criteria for Cushing's syndrome. On further questioning, the patient admitted to ingesting up to 160 licorice containing cough lozenges (approximately 288 mg of glycyrrhizin) per day as a distraction from neuropathic pain. The patient was told to discontinue the lozenge intake. On follow-up 6 weeks later he admitted to continuing the lozenges but at half of his previous intake per day. His serum potassium at this time was within normal parameters but he was still hypertensive. His 24-hour urinary-free cortisol level was elevated at

133 mg. Seven weeks after completely discontinuing the lozenges, all parameters normalized [37A].

Adverse Effects: Dermatology

In a recent correspondence, researchers support the relationship of dietary psoralens/furocoumarins from citrus with melanoma. The contention is that skin cell changes can occur with consistent but not intermittent exposure to ultraviolet light in the presence of these chemicals. The authors assert that ingestion of furocoumarins may enhance development of both melanoma and non-melanoma skin cancer [38r].

Ranunculus arvensis has been shown to cause chemical burns despite the fact that this product is generally used topically to treat joint and muscle pain, burns and inflammatory conditions such as hemorrhoids. Fresh plant preparations seem to cause more adverse effects than dried or boiled preparations. Although the primary toxic substance, protoanemonin, has been reported to be absent in dried or boiled plants, cases of skin burns have been reported with the boiled plant in Turkey [39r].

CONCERNS WITH HERBAL PRODUCT CONTAMINATION

Contamination of herbal products is of concern as the consumer is exposed to ingredients they did not intend to ingest. These contaminants can cause adverse effects. Cross contamination of herbal plants with plants containing pyrrolizidine alkaloids (PAs) has been documented. Nowak [40E] investigated whether horizontal transfer of PAs into herbal plants could occur. Horizontal contamination may occur if the growing herbal plants are mulched with PA containing plants, and the PAs are subsequently taken up from the soil into the growing herb. Nowak conducted a study to evaluate the extent of PA uptake into plants cultivated in pots and mulched with ragwort (*Senecio jacobaea*). The following herbals were cultivated: *Melissa officinalis* (lemon balm), *M. piperita* (peppermint), *Matricaria chamomilla* (chamomile) and *Petroselinum crispum* (parsley). The ragwort was dried in the laboratory and milled into mulch that was applied only to the soil of the growing herbs. The mulch was dampened before application and covered with filter paper through which the plants were watered to prevent dust getting onto the growing herbs. 2 g of mulch was applied to the lemon balm while 1 g of mulch was applied to the other herbs. A second mulching occurred for a subset of the plants 7 days after the first mulching. The herbs were harvested in two groups, at either 7 or 14 days after mulching. The authors of this experiment found that the PAs from the ragwort were taken up into all four of the cultivated herbs. The quantity of PAs taken up into the herbs differed across the species, as well as the types of PAs found in the herbal species. This study proved that PAs, are a source of herbal contamination and can cause adverse effects when ingested, can indeed be absorbed from the soil into herbs when PA containing plants contaminate the soil in which the herbs are grown.

The contamination of herbal products with heavy metals is also of concern as heavy metals can have significant toxicity. They may contaminate herbal products both during growth of the herb and during the production process of the herbal product. Lemus-Olalde published a systematic review of herbal supplement contamination by heavy metals [41M]. This review evaluated the levels of metals contaminating herbal supplements and assessed the risks associated with ingesting herbal supplements contaminated with heavy metals. These authors noted the following heavy metals were found in herbal supplements: aluminum, arsenic, barium, cadmium, cobalt, chromium, copper, iron, lanthanum, lead, lithium, manganese, mercury, methyl mercury, molybdenum, nickel, selenium, strontium, vanadium, and zinc. Some of these metals were present in high enough concentrations in various herbal supplements that consumption of the herbal product would expose the consumer to levels of the heavy metal greater than what is considered safe.

Shaban et al. also published a review in 2016 on the contamination of heavy metals and pesticides in herbal products [42R]. Medical herbal products have been found to be contaminated with heavy metals and pesticides. Heavy metal contamination of herbal products has been reported when treated or untreated water is used to irrigate the plants, when they grow near highly used roads, and when grown on old landfills. Pesticides contaminate herbal products when sprayed on the growing plants or when harvested plants are fumigated during storage.

It has been reported that many herbal products used as sexual enhancers and weight loss products are contaminated. The extensive use of these products puts many people at risk of exposure to heavy metals and synthetic medications that have been detected in these herbal products. Skalicka-Woźniak published a review in 2016 of the heavy metal and synthetic compound contamination of herbal sexual enhancers and weight loss products [43R]. Herbal sexual enhancers were found to often be contaminated with sildenafil, vardenafil, and tadalafil, erectile dysfunction prescription medications, as well as some analogs of those medications that are not approved for use. Herbal dietary products were found to be contaminated with sibutramine, sibutramine analogs, thyroid hormones, appetite suppressants, diuretics, stimulants, and laxatives, all products used in weight loss programs. These prescription medications are not listed on the label of the herbal products which is against FDA rules.

Yang published a review analyzing the patterns of contamination of herbs and dietary supplements in Taiwan [44R]. The authors queried from the Taiwanese FDA's analysis of Chinese herbal medicines (CHMs) and dietary supplements for adulterants between 2005 and 2014. CHMs used for health promotion or as aphrodisiacs or analgesics were the most adulterated herbal products. CHMs taken without a prescription were the most likely to be contaminated compared to those administered by prescription. Some prescription medications were commonly found as contaminants, including sildenafil, caffeine, hydrochlorothiazide and some analgesics. Dietary supplements used as aphrodisiacs or weight loss agents were most highly contaminated with sildenafil, sibutramine, phenolphthalein, caffeine, or tadalafil. The authors found that the measured levels of contamination in dietary supplements decreased over the time of the study.

A study was conducted at the German Hospital of Traditional Chinese Medicine to screen TCMs for possible contaminants. TCMs used in the hospital from the beginning of September 2012 until the end of 2013 were evaluated for the presence of contaminating microbes, aflatoxin, pesticides, and heavy metals. Twenty-three TCMs were tested. Five were found to be contaminated with microbes, pesticides, and heavy metals. Dicofol, an organochlorine miticide related to DDT, and fenpropathrin, a pyrethroid insecticide, were the most common pesticides detected. Lead was detected in these samples as well. Any sample found to be contaminated was removed from the hospital's inventory and was not administered to patients [45E].

Calahan et al. also published a review of contaminants in herbal products in 2016 [46R]. This review provided a compilation of cases of toxicity reported between 1990 and 2015 due to adulteration of herbal medicines. Their review also discussed the various analytical methods used to detect the contaminants. The authors did not include cases of toxicity from herbal medical products that had been contaminated with pesticides or heavy metals. The authors listed the following chemicals as common adulterants in herbal medicinal products: sildenafil, famotidine, ibuprofen, promethazine, diazepam, nifedipine, captopril, amoxicillin, and dextromethorphan. The authors list many other medications that are thought to be intentional adulterants of herbal medical products. Herbal medications used for sleep, weight loss, and bodybuilding were reported to be commonly adulterated. These products are contaminated with clonazepam, sibutramine or fenfluramine, and steroids, respectively. The contamination of these commonly used herbal medications with these prescription drugs poses a great deal of risk to patients consuming the herbal product, as the patient is exposed to a medication they did not intend to ingest.

HOMEOPATHY

Homeopathic intervention is an alternative medicine system which includes components of lifestyle consultation and use of extremely diluted medicinal remedies. Many health care providers and consumers consider these products safe because of the negligible amounts of active agent. To test this supposition, a recent systematic review and meta-analysis of the potential adverse effects/aggravations caused by homeopathic remedies that are reported in the literature was conducted using the PICO (population, intervention, comparison, outcome) format [47H]. A potential for adverse events from the use of homeopathic interventions was found, 68% ($n = 488$) mild/grade 1 decreasing to 0.2% ($n = 2$) severe/grade 5. Homeopathic aggravations, cases of an increase in the symptoms being treated with homeopathic agents, were reported in 12% of the RCTs studied, for a total of 158 events overall, 91 in treatment groups and 67 in controls. The meta-analysis showed no differences in adverse effects data from 39 RCTs with 5902 subjects between homeopathy and control or placebo or conventional or herbal medicine comparators. Bias in results may be due to lack of standard reporting procedures or differences in risk terminology used in the reviewed studies [48M].

MIND–BODY THERAPIES

The potential ill effects of mind–body therapies on various body system functions are not well defined or reported. These few reviews, case reports, or studies were published in the English language literature within the last year.

Adverse Effects: Manipulative Therapy, Chiropractic Therapy

A patient with lower back pain undergoing long-term chiropractic care is described as developing "ponytail" syndrome where compression of the roots at the level of the lumbar vertebral canal radiculopathies occurs. The patient recovered after surgical intervention and bladder rehabilitation [49A].

Adverse Effects: Acupuncture

Bee venom, either by bee sting or as diluted venom, is used as part of acupuncture therapy in Asia and other parts of the world. A case of immune thrombocytopenia, including ecchymosis and gum bleeding, is described in an obese 61-year-old woman having bee venom injections weekly to relieve back pain secondary to lumbar disc prolapse. She presented with a large ecchymosis (5 cm) on her abdomen and one on her right forearm (2 cm). Her presenting laboratory values was remarkable for a low platelet count (9×10^9/L) which compared unfavorably to her normal platelet count taken just prior to bee venom treatment (240×10^9/L). Her other laboratory values were not suggestive of any underlying hematologic disorder. Other reports of platelet aggregation inhibition from the venom of bees and wasps led the authors to suspect adverse effect was due to the bee venom therapy [50A].

Adverse Effects: Yoga

Falls resulting from yoga or meditation practices were analyzed in a sub-study analysis of survey data obtained from women aged 59 through 64 years that participated in the Australian Longitudinal Study on Women's Health (ALSWH). Of the entire cohort of 10011 women completing the survey questionnaire, 4413 (44.1%) had slipped, tripped or stumbled, 2770 (27.7%) women had a fall to the ground, 1398 (14.0%) women had been injured as a result of a fall, and 901 (9.0%) women had sought medical attention for an injury from a fall, within the previous 12 months. Also, yoga or meditation was practiced often by 746 (7.5%) women. Of these reported falls, only four were associated with women who practiced yoga or meditation. A comparison of women who practiced yoga and meditation with those who did not and the fall or injury rate did not show a difference. There was a slight non-statistical advantage of practicing yoga or meditation on reduction of slips, trips or stumbles (OR = 0.92; 95% CI: 0.79–1.08) and the number of times medical attention was sought for injury secondary to a fall (OR = 0.93; 95% CI: 0.70–1.22) during the past 12 months [51M].

Cardiac arrest secondary to heat exhaustion from participating in a "hot" yoga class occurred in a previously healthy 35-year-old woman who was 12 weeks postpartum. CPR was begun promptly at the site. She was placed on vasopressor support. She developed disseminated intravascular coagulation but not hemolysis. Trans-esophageal echocardiogram revealed a mild systolic dysfunction with an ejection fraction of 45%–50% and reduced apical myocardium function. The patient received an implantable cardioverter defibrillator [52r].

CONCLUSIONS

The continuous exponential growth in the global acceptance and use of herbal medicines and natural products raises the question of the need for increased pharmacovigilance and better regulation of the industry. Safety concerns of improper use and unforeseen adverse reactions from these products are being reported from many different areas of medicine, including emergency rooms and other "Western" or alternative healthcare practitioners. The literature regarding natural dietary supplements and herbal therapies, though not robust, is increasing in both strength and depth. Standardization of the methods of data gathering and analysis is beginning in several countries around the globe [5S]. Manufacturers should be held to higher standards worldwide to reduce contamination, adulteration, misidentification and substitution of plant materials. Strict enforcement of labeling and content verification may lead to fewer adverse effects [11C].

References

[1] Herbal dietary supplement sales in US increased by 7.5% in 2015 [homepage on the Internet], 2016, Austin, TX: American Botanical Council; 2016. [H]. Available from: http://cms.herbalgram.org/press/2016/Herbal_Dietary_Supplement_Sales_in_US_Increased.html?ts=1485712018&signature=7eea853e4b1228fe75503baa215b228f.

[2] Smith T, Kawa K, Eckl V, et al. Sales of herbal dietary supplements in US increased 7.5% in 2015 consumers spent $6.92 billion on herbal supplements in 2015, marking the 12th consecutive year of growth, HerbalGram. Fall 2016;(111):67–73. [R]. Available from: http://cms.herbalgram.org/herbalgram/issue111/hg111-mktrpt.html.

[3] Ekor M. The growing use of herbal medicines: issues relating to adverse reactions and challenges in monitoring safety. Front Pharmacol. 2014;4:177 [R].

[4] Izzo AA, Hoon-Kim S, Radhakrishnan R, et al. A critical approach to evaluating clinical efficacy, adverse events and drug interactions of herbal remedies. Phytother Res. 2016;30(5):691–700 [R].

[5] World Health Organization. The importance of pharmacovigilance-safety monitoring of medicinal products. Geneva: WHO; 2002 [S].

[6] Hassan MAG. Need to incorporate pharmacovigilance of herbal medicine to the curriculum. Natl J Physiol Pharm Pharmacol. 2014;4(2):99–100 [H].

[7] Naranjo CA, Busto U, Sellers EM, et al. A method for estimating the probability of adverse drug reactions. Clin Pharmacol Ther. 1981;30(2):239–45 [c].

[8] Toklu HZ. Pharmacovigilance of herbal medicine: herbavigilance. Adv Pharmacoepidemiol Drug Saf. 2016;5:208. 21671052 [r].

[9] Golder S, Loke YK, Wright K, et al. Most systematic reviews of adverse effects did not include unpublished data. J Clin Epidemiol. 2016;77:125–33 [R].

[10] Sarges P, Steinberg JM, Lewis JH. Drug-induced liver injury: highlights from a review of the 2015 literature. Drug Saf. 2016;39(9):801–21 [R].

[11] Pokladnikova J, Meyboom RH, Meincke R, et al. Allergy-like immediate reactions with herbal medicines: a retrospective study using data from VigiBase(R). Drug Saf. 2016;39(5):455–64 [C].

[12] Mazzanti G, Moro P, Raschi E, et al. Adverse reactions to dietary supplements containing red yeast rice: assessment of cases from the Italian surveillance system. Br J Clin Pharmacol. 2016;83(4):894–908 [C].

[13] Hohmann N, Maus A, Carls A, et al. St. John's wort treatment in women bears risks beyond pharmacokinetic drug interactions. Arch Toxicol. 2016;90(4):1013–5 [c].

[14] Teik DOL, Lee XS, Lim CJ, et al. Ginseng and Ginkgo biloba effects on cognition as modulated by cardiovascular reactivity: a randomised trial. PLoS One. 2016;11(3):1–20 [c].

[15] Dubey D, Golden E, Suss A, et al. Tumefactive demyelination following herbal supplement use: cause or coincidence? J Postgrad Med. 2016;62(2):136–7 [A].

[16] Shah SA, Dargush AE, Potts V, et al. Effects of single and multiple energy shots on blood pressure and electrocardiographic parameters. Am J Cardiol. 2016;117(3):465–8 [c].

[17] Busuttil M, Willoughby S. A survey of energy drink consumption among young patients presenting to the emergency department with the symptom of palpitations. Int J Cardiol. 2016;204:55–6 [c].

[18] Dixit S, Stein PK, Dewland TA, et al. Consumption of caffeinated products and cardiac ectopy. J Am Heart Assoc. 2016;5(1)e002503 [C].

[19] Zhao Y, Wang L, Yi Z. An unusual etiology for bidirectional ventricular tachycardia. Can J Cardiol. 2016;32(3):395.e5–6 [A].

[20] Zhao D, Wang J, Cui Y, et al. Pharmacological effects of Chinese herb aconite (Fuzi) on cardiovascular system. J Tradit Chin Med. 2012;32(3):308–13 [R].

[21] Edem E, Kahyaoglu B, Cakar MA. Acute effusive pericarditis due to horse chestnut consumption. Am J Case Rep. 2016;17: 305-8 [A].

[22] Love IY, Perl S, Rapoport MJ. A rare case of caffeine storm due to excessive coca-cola consumption. Isr Med Assoc J. 2016;18(6):366–7 [A].

[23] Nauffal M, Gabardi S. Nephrotoxicity of natural products. Blood Purif. 2016;41(1–3):123–9 [R].

[24] Xu XL, Yang LJ, Jiang JG. Renal toxic ingredients and their toxicology from traditional Chinese medicine. Expert Opin Drug Metab Toxicol. 2016;12(2):149–59 [R].

[25] Zhang S, Pan H, Peng X, et al. Preventive use of a hepatoprotectant against anti-tuberculosis drug-induced liver injury: a randomized controlled trial. J Gastroenterol Hepatol. 2016;31(2):409–16 [C].

[26] Douros A, Bronder E, Andersohn F, et al. Herb-induced liver injury in the Berlin case–control surveillance study. Int J Mol Sci. 2016;17(1):10 [C].

[27] Gedela M, Potu KC, Gali VL, et al. A case of hepatotoxicity related to kombucha tea consumption. S D Med. 2016;69(1):26–8 [A].

[28] Papafragkakis C, Ona MA, Reddy M, et al. Acute hepatitis after ingestion of a preparation of Chinese skullcap and black catechu for joint pain, Case Reports Hepatol. 2016;2016:3, Article ID 4356749. http://dx.doi.org/10.1155/2016/4356749 [A].

[29] Corey R, Werner KT, Singer A, et al. Acute liver failure associated with garcinia cambogia use. Ann Hepatol. 2016;15(1):123–6 [A].

[30] Rollason V, Spahr L, Escher M. Severe liver injury due to a homemade flower pollen preparation in a patient with high CYP3A enzyme activity: a case report. Eur J Clin Pharmacol. 2016;72(4):507–8 [A].

[31] Valdivia-Correa B, Gómez-Gutiérrez C, Uribe M, et al. Herbal medicine in Mexico: a cause of hepatotoxicity. A critical review. Int J Mol Sci. 2016;17(2):235 [R].

[32] Bedi O, Bijjem KRV, Kumar P, et al. Herbal induced hepatoprotection and hepatotoxicity: a critical review. Indian J Physiol Pharmacol. 2016;60(1):6–21 [R].

[33] Garcia-Cortes M, Robles-Diaz M, Ortega-Alonso A, et al. Hepatotoxicity by dietary supplements: a tabular listing and clinical characteristics. Int J Mol Sci. 2016;17(4):537 [R].

[34] Frenzel C, Teschke R. Herbal hepatotoxicity: clinical characteristics and listing compilation. Int J Mol Sci. 2016;17(5):588 [R].

[35] Danan G, Teschke R. RUCAM in drug and herb induced liver injury: the update. Int J Mol Sci. 2016;17(1):14 [S].

[36] Stage TB, Damkier P, Christensen MMH, et al. Impaired glucose tolerance in healthy men treated with St. John's wort. Basic Clin Pharmacol Toxicol. 2016;118(3):219–24 [c].

[37] Dai DW, Singh I, Hershman JM. Lozenge-induced hypermineralcorticoid state—a unique case of licorice lozenges resulting in hypertension and hypokalemia. J Clin Hypertens (Greenwich). 2016;18(2):159–60 [A].

[38] Dowdy JC, Sayre RM. Melanoma risk from dietary furocoumarins: how much more evidence is required? J Clin Oncol. 2016;34(6):636–7 [r].

[39] Kocak AO, Saritemur M, Atac K, et al. A rare chemical burn due to Ranunculus arvensis: three case reports. Ann Saudi Med. 2016;36(1):89–91 [r].

[40] Nowak M, Wittke C, Lederer I, et al. Interspecific transfer of pyrrolizidine alkaloids: an unconsidered source of contaminations of phytopharmaceuticals and plant derived commodities. Food Chem. 2016;213:163–8 [E].

[41] Lemus-Olalde R. A review of heavy metal levels in herbal supplements. Toxicol Lett. 2016;259(Suppl):S57 [M].

[42] Shaban NS, Abdou KA, Hassan NEY. Impact of toxic heavy metals and pesticide residues in herbal products. Beni-Suef Univ J Basic Appl Sci. 2016;5(1):102–6 [R].

[43] Skalicka-Woźniak K, Georgiev MI, Orhan IE. Adulteration of herbal sexual enhancers and slimmers: the wish for better sexual well-being and perfect body can be risky. Food Chem Toxicol. 2016: in press. http://dx.doi.org/10.101?/j.fct.2016. 06.018 [R].

[44] Yang CC. Pattern and trend of pharmaceutical adulteration of Chinese herbs and dietary supplements in Taiwan: roles of the Taiwan FDA. Toxicol Lett. 2016;259(Suppl):S57 [R].

[45] Melchart D, Hager S, Dai J, et al. Quality control and complication screening programme of Chinese medicinal drugs at the first German hospital of traditional Chinese medicine—a retrospective analysis. Forsch Komplementmed. 2016;23(Suppl 2):21–8 [E].

[46] Calahan J, Howard D, Almalki AJ, et al. Chemical adulterants in herbal medicinal products: a review. Planta Med. 2016;82(6):505–15 [R].

[47] Asking a good question (PICO) [homepage on the Internet]. Los Angeles, CA, USA: University of Southern California; 2017. [cited 2/8/2017]. Available from: https://www.usc.edu/hsc/ebnet/ ebframe/PICO.htm [H].

[48] Stub T, Musial F, Kristoffersen AA, et al. Adverse effects of homeopathy, what do we know? A systematic review and meta-analysis of randomized controlled trials. Complement Ther Med. 2016;26:146–63 [M].

[49] Undabeitia J, Samprón N, Úrculo E. Síndrome de cola de caballo tras tratamiento quiropráctico. Neurocirugia. 2016;27(3):151–3 [A].

[50] Abdulsalam MA, Ebrahim BE, Abdulsalam AJ. Immune thrombocytopenia after bee venom therapy: a case report. BMC Complement Altern Med. 2016;16:107 [A].

[51] Cramer H, Sibbritt D, Adams J, et al. The association between regular yoga and meditation practice and falls and injuries: results of a national cross-sectional survey among Australian women. Maturitas. 2016;84:38–41 [M].

[52] Boddu P, Patel S, Shahrrava A. Sudden cardiac arrest from heat stroke: hidden dangers of hot yoga. Am J Med. 2016;129(8): e129–30 [R].

Reviewers

Reviewer 1st Name	Surname	Affiliation
Adrienne	Black, PhD, DABT	Senior Regulatory Authoring Analyst- 3E Company, and, Adjunct Faculty at the Institute of Public Health of New York Medical College, Valhalla, NY, 7173 North Crest Court Warrenton, VA 20187
Alison	Brophy, Pharm D, BCPS	Critical Care Pharmacist, Saint Barnabas Medical Center, Clinical Assistant Professor, Ernest Mario School of Pharmacy, Rutgers, The State University of New Jersey, USA
Dana R.	Fasanella, PharmD, CDE, BCACP	Assistant Professor and Vice Chair of Education, Department of Pharmacy Practice and Administration, School of Pharmacy and Health Professions, University of Maryland Eastern Shore, 212 Somerset Hall, Princess Anne, MD 21853, USA
Joshua P.	Gray, Ph.D.	Associate Professor of Chemistry & Biochemistry, United States Coast Guard Academy, Department of Science, 27 Mohegan Ave, New London, CT 06320, USA
Herb	Halley, PharmD, BCPS	Director Experiential Education (Rtd), Manchester University College of Pharmacy, 10627 Diebold Road, Fort Wayne, IN 46845
Sandy	Hrometz, PharmD, PhD	Professor of Pharmaceutical Sciences, Manchester University College of Pharmacy, Natural & Health Sciences, 10627 Diebold Rd, Fort Wayne, IN 46845, USA
Jason	Isch, PharmD.	Ambulatory Care Pharmacy Resident Saint Joseph Regional Medical Center 611 E Douglas Rd. #412 Mishawaka, IN 46545
Cassandra	Maynard, PharmD, BCPS	Clinical Pharmacy Specialist - IM/Cardiology, St. Mary's Health Center, Clinical Associate Professor, SIUE - School of Pharmacy, Edwardsville, IL

Reviewer 1st Name	Surname	Affiliation
Dayna	Mcmannus, PharmD, BCPS, AQ-ID	Infectious Diseases Senior Clinical Pharmacy Specialist, Department of Pharmacy Services, Yale-New Haven Hospital, 20 York Street, New Haven, CT 06510
Vaibhab	Mundra, BPharm, MPharm, PhD	Assistant Professor of Pharmaceutical Sciences, Manchester University, College of Pharmacy, Natural and Health Sciences, 10627 Diebold Road, Fort Wayne, IN 46845
Toshio	Nakaki, MD, PhD	Professor & Chair, Department of Pharmacology, Teikyo University School of Medicine, Tokyo, Japan
Yekaterina	Opsha, PharmD., BCPS-AQ Cardiology	Clinical Assistant Professor, Ernest Mario School of Pharmacy Rutgers, The State University of NJ, Clinical Specialist-Cardiovascular Medicine, Saint Barnabas Medical Center, Livingstone, NJ, USA
Sreekumar	Othumpangat, PhD	Sr. Scientist, Allergy and Clinical Immunology Branch, HELD/NIOSH/CDC, 1095 Willowdale Road, Morgantown, WV 26505, USA
Mayur	Parmar, Bpharm, MS, PhD	Center of Translational Research in Neurodegenerative Disease Department of Neurology University of Florida, Gainsville, FL 32610
Hanna	Raber, PharmD, BCPS	Assistant Professor/ Dept of Clinical Sciences, University of Utah School of Medicine, Pharmacotherapy Specialist, Salt Lake City, UT 84112, USA
Sidhartha	D. Ray, PhD.	Professor, Department of Pharmaceutical Scs, College of Pharmacy, Manchester University, USA
Brian	Skinner, PharmD, BCPS	Assistant Professor of Pharmacy Practice Manchester University, Clinical Pharmacy Specialist – Internal Medicine, St. Vincent Hospital, 10627 Diebold Road, Fort Wayne, IN 46845

Reviewer 1st Name	Surname	Affiliation	Reviewer 1st Name	Surname	Affiliation
Thomas	Smith, PharmD	Assistant Professor of Pharmacy Practice, Manchester University College of Pharmacy, 10627 Diebold Road Fort Wayne, IN 46845, USA	Sidney	Stohs, RPh, MS, PhD, ATS, BABT, FACN	Dean Emeritus, Gilbert H. Taffe Endowed Chair & Professor, Department of Pharmacy Sciences, Creighton University School of Allied Health Professions, Omaha, NE 68178
Brian	Spoelhoff, PharmD., BCPS	Neurocritical Care and Neurosciences, Johns Hopkins Bayview Medical Center, Department of Pharmacy, 4940 Eastern Ave, Baltimore, MD 21224	Kelsi	Wurm, PharmD.	Pharmacy Resident, PARKVIEW REGIONAL MEDICAL CENTER 11109 Parkview Plaza Drive Fort Wayne, Indiana 46845

Index of Drugs

For drug–drug interactions see the separate index. In pages 523–524

Index of Drug-Drug Interactions

Index of Adverse Effects and Adverse Reactions

CPI Antony Rowe

Chippenham, UK

2017-10-23 11:40